2003/04

Twelfth Edition

The Complete Directory for People with Disabilities

A Comprehensive Source Book for Individuals and Professionals

A SEDGWICK PRESS Book

Grey House Publishing

PUBLISHER: Leslie Mackenzie

EDITORIAL DIRECTOR: Laura Mars-Proietti
EDITORIAL ASSISTANT: Pamela Michaud

PRODUCTION MANAGER: Karen Stevens
ASST. TO PRODUCTION MANAGER: Cecilia Fletcher
PRODUCTION ASSISTANTS: Debra Giordano, Gail Kusek, Megan McClune, Caitlin Stupak

MARKETING DIRECTOR: Jessica Moody

A Sedgwick Press Book
Grey House Publishing, Inc.
185 Millerton Road
Millerton, NY 12546
518.789.8700
FAX 518.789.0545
www.greyhouse.com
e-mail: books @greyhouse.com

First edition published 1991
Twelfth edition published 2003

The complete directory for people with disabilities : products, resources, books, services. -- 1992-2003.
1022p. ; 29 cm.

Other title: Directory for people with disabilities
Title varies.
Annual.

ISSN: 1063-0023

1. People with disabilities--Services for--United States--Directories. 2. People with disabilities--Services for--United States--Periodicals. 3. Disabled Persons--United States--Bibliography. 4. Disabled Persons--United States--Directory. 5. Information Services--United States--Bibliography. 6. Information Services--United States--Directory. 7. Mental Retardation--Rehabilitation--United States--Bibliography. 8. Mental Retardation--Rehabilitation--United States--Directory. 9. Rehabilitation--United States--Bibliography. 10. Rehabilitation--United States--Directory. I. Title: Directory for people with disabilities.
HV1553 .C58
362.4/048/02573 92-658843
Printed in the USA
ISBN 1-59237-007-1 softcover

TABLE OF CONTENTS

INTRODUCTION

Welcome to the 12th and most comprehensive edition of *The Complete Directory for People with Disabilities (CDD)*. Like its previous award-winning editions, this directory contains thousands of resources, products and services for people with disabilities. Coverage extends from associations that provide important support for families, individuals and professionals, to products that enable and enhance lifestyle of people with disabilities. *CDD* includes summer camps, living facilities, print and electronic resources and so much more. Be sure to use the Table of Contents as your guide through the 27 chapters and more than 100 subchapters contained in this rich resource.

Our update efforts for this 12th edition were especially successful. In addition to several fax campaigns, we mailed out thousands of questionnaires that resulted in a terrific response. We also reached out individually to all associations for updated information. As a result, the information in *CDD* is not only more accurate, but there is more of it. You will find 9,924 listings, with descriptions and key contacts, 8,775 fax numbers, 5,293 e-mail addresses and 6,019 web sites.

The careful research and compilation of the best data available is a year–long effort. As the reputation of *The Complete Directory for People with Disabilities* among educators, librarians and the disability community continues to grow, professionals and organizations in the field send us new and updated information, as well as editorial feedback. Their cooperation and support are, in large part, responsible for the strength of this directory.

We are confident that this resource will save hours of research time. Even if you search the web, it can often take hours to find the wide range of comparative health care resources on the Internet, and these resources are often scattered and unedited. *CDD* provides comprehensive, critical and immediate information in just one source that can be accessed in minutes.

In addition to the nearly 10,000 listings in *The Complete Directory for People with Disabilities*, there are three indexes to help you access the data through a variety of ways:

Disability & Subject Index: Organized alphabetically by hundreds of topics relevant to people with disabilities, this index groups together all listings on a particular subject (i.e., autism or language disorders), regardless of type.

Entry Index: This alphabetical list of all listings saves time searching for a listing that may be located in one of several different chapters.

Geographic Index: Organizes listings alphabetically by state.

The Complete Directory for People with Disabilities is also available via subscription on the Internet, as well as in a customized database. As always, we welcome your comments and suggestions, and look forward to another year of serving the disability community.

User Guide

Descriptive listings in *The Complete Directory for People with Disabilities* (*CDD*) are organized into 27 chapters, by resource type. You will find the following types of listings throughout the book:

- National Agencies & Associations
- State Agencies & Associations
- Camps & Exchanges Programs
- Manufacturers of Assistive Devices, Clothing, Computer Equipment & Supplies
- Print & Electronic Media
- Living Centers & Facilities
- Libraries & Research Centers
- Conferences & Trade Shows

Below is a sample listing illustrating the kind of information that is or might be included in an Association entry. Each numbered item of information is described in the paragraphs on the following page.

---

1 → **1234**
2 → **Advocacy Center for Seniors with Disabilities**
3 → 1762 South Major Drive
New Orleans, LA 98087

4 → 800-000-0000
5 → 058-884-0709
6 → Fax: 058-884-0568
7 → TDD: 800-000-0001
8 → e-mail: info@sadvoc.com
9 → www.sadvoc.com

10 → Barbara Pierce, Executive Director
Diane Watkins, Marketing Director
Robert Goldfarb, Administrative Assistant

11 → The mission of the Center is to advance the dignity, equality, self-determination and choices of senior citizens with disabilities. It provides referrals, publishes information, including a monthly newsletter, offers workshops and consultation on legal, social, travel, and medical issues. The Center works with various local organizations to help seniors with disabilities stay active in their community.

12 → Founded 1964

13 → 18 pages

14 → Monthly

User Key

1 → **Record Number:** Entries are listed alphabetically within each category and numbered sequentially. Entry numbers, rather than page numbers, are used in the indexes to refer to listings.

2 → **Organization Name:** Formal name of company or organization. Where organization names are completely capitalized, the listing will appear at the beginning of the alphabetized section. In the case of publications, the title of the publication will appear first, followed by the publisher.

3 → **Address:** Location or permanent address of the organization.

4 → **Toll Free Number:** This is listed when provided by the organization.

5 → **Phone Number:** The listed phone number is usually for the main office of the organization, but may also be for the sales, marketing, or public relations office as provided by the organization.

6 → **Fax Number:** This is listed when provided by the organization.

7 → **TDD Number:** This is listed when provided. It refers to Telephone Device for the Deaf.

8 → **E-Mail:** This is listed when provided by the organization and is generally the main office e-mail.

9 → **Web Site:** This is also referred to as an URL address. These web sites are accessed through the Internet by typing *http://* before the URL address.

10 → **Key Personnel:** Names and titles of department heads of the organization.

11 → **Organization Description:** This paragraph contains a brief description of the organization and their services.

12 → **Year Founded:** The year in which the organization was established or founded. If the organization has changed its name, the founding date is usually for the earliest name under which it was known.

13 → **Number of Pages:** Number of pages if the listing is a publication.

14 → **Frequency:** The frequency of the listing if it is a publication.

Resources for the Disabled

1 **Accentuate the Positive: Expressive Arts for Children with Disabilities**

MMB Music
3526 Washington Avenue
Saint Louis, MO 63103
314-531-9635
800-543-3771
FAX: 314-531-8384
e-mail: info@mmbmusic.com
www.mmbmusic.com

Designed to promote awareness of learning potential in creative abilities for young children who have moderate to severe disabilities. *$20.00*

2 **American Art Therapy Association (AATA)**

1202 Allanson Road
Mundelein, IL 60060
847-837-1190
FAX: 847-566-4580
www.arttherapy.org

Organization of professionals who believe the art process is a beneficial and healing process.

3 **American Dance Therapy Association (ADTA)**

2000 Century Plaza
Suite 930
Columbia, MD 21044
410-997-4040
FAX: 410-997-4048
www.adta.org

Dance-movement therapy is a psychotherapeutic use of movement as a process which furthers the emotional, cognitive and physical integration of the individual.

4 **American Music Therapy Association (AMTA)**

8455 Colesville Road
Suite 1000
Silver Spring, MD 20910
301-589-3300
FAX: 301-589-5175
e-mail: info@musictherapy.org
www.musictherapy.org

Andrea H Farbman, Executive Director
Judy Simpson, Director of Government Relations

AMTA's purpose is the progressive development of the therapeutic use of music in rehabilitation, special education and community settings. Predecessors to the American Music Therapy Association included the National Association for Music Therapy founded in 1950 and the American Association for Music Therapy founded in 1971. AMTA is committed to the advancement of education, training, professional standards, credentials and research in support of the music therapy profession.

5 **Arena Stage**

1101 6th Street SW
Washington, DC 20024
202-488-3300
FAX: 202-488-4056
e-mail: jbarasch@arenastage.org
www.arenastage.org

Jody Taylor Barasch, Access Ability Director

A pioneer in providing access to theater for people with disabilities and the birthplace of Audio Description. Offers infrared assistive listening devices (both loop and headset), program books in Braille, large print and wheelchair accessible seating with adjacent companion seating. Audio cassette format available upon request. Sign Interpretation and Audio Description are offered at selected performances. Cafe menus and shop lists in Braille. Wheelchair-accessible with lifts and ramps.

6 **Art and Disabilities**

Brookline Books
PO Box 97
Newton Upper Falls, MA 02464
617-558-8010
800-666-2665
FAX: 617-558-8011
e-mail: brbooks@yahoo.com
www.brooklinebooks.com

Florence Ludins-Katz, Author
Elias Katz, Author

A step-by-step guide to establishing creative arts centers for people with disabilities. Includes philosophy and making creative arts centers happen.

7 **Art for All the Children: Approaches to Art Therapy for Children with Disabilities**

2600 S First Street
Springfield, IL 62704
217-789-8980
800-258-8980
FAX: 217-789-9130
e-mail: books@ccthomas.com
www.ccthomas.com

This second edition is for art therapists in training and for in-service professionals in art therapy, art education and special education who have children with disabilities as a part of their case/class load. Cloth cover edition available for $72.95 (ISBN# 0-398-05797-4) *$72.95*

398 pages Paperback
ISBN 0-398060-60-7

8 **Association for Theatre and Accessibility**

300 UCLA Medical Plaza
Suite 3330
Los Angeles, CA 90095
310-794-1141
e-mail: oraynor@mednet.ucla.edu
www.npi.ucla.edu/ata

Dr. Olivia Raynor, Executive Director
Beth Sotffmacher, Technical Coordinator
John Clare, President

A nonprofit with the purpose of fostering the full participation and involvement of individuals with all types of disabilities in drama and theater. Newsletters and annual conferences.

9 **Deaf Artists of America**

87 N Clinton Avenue
Suite 408
Rochester, NY 14604
585-244-3460
FAX: 585-325-2413
TTY:716-325-2400

10 **Disability and Social Performance: Using Drama to Achieve Successful Acts**

Brookline Books
PO Box 1046
Cambridge, MA 02238
617-868-0360
800-666-2665
FAX: 617-868-1772
e-mail: brooklinebks@delphi.com
www.brooklinebooks.com

This book makes a major contribution to the understanding of disability, people with disabilities and the creative power they possess which can be unleashed through performance. *$17.95*

11 **Freedom to Create**

National Institute of Art and Disabilities
551 23rd Street
Richmond, CA 94804
510-620-0290
FAX: 510-620-0326
e-mail: reddot@niadart.org
www.niadart.org

Elias Katz, Author

Presents philosophy and practical experiences enabling teachers to stimulate creativity in the visual arts for students with and without disabilities.

12 **Friends-In-Art**

American Council of the Blind
1155 15th Street NW
Suite 1004
Washington, DC 20005
202-467-5081
800-424-8666
FAX: 202-467-5085
e-mail: info@acb.org
www.acb.org

Aims to enlarge the art experience of blind people, encourages blind people to visit museums, galleries, concerts, the theater and other enjoyable public places, offers consultation to program planners in establishing accessible art and museum exhibits and presents Performing Arts Showcases at the American Council of the Blinds' national convention.

13 **Institute for Therapy Throughout the Arts**

7 Happ Road
Suite A
Northfield, IL 60093
847-635-1654
FAX: 847-446-8458

Ted Rubenstein, Managing Director
Victoria Storm, Associate Director

In its twentieth year of service, ITA provides creative arts therapies for adults and children with special needs through the use of music, art, drama and or dance. Services include: assessment, treatment planning, one-to-one services and group therapy. ITA also offers adaptive lessons to students with special needs and workshops on topics related to the expressive arts therapies.

14 **Manual of Sequential Art Activities for Classified Children and Adolescents**

Charles C Thomas
2600 S First Street
Springfield, IL 62704
217-789-8980
800-258-8980
FAX: 217-789-9130
e-mail: books@ccthomas.com
www.ccthomas.com

Offers information to the special education professional on art therapy and management. *$41.95*

246 pages Softcover
ISBN 0-39805 -85-6

15 **National Arts and Disability Center (NADC)**

300 UCLA Medical Plaza
Suite 3330
Los Angeles, CA 90095
e-mail: oraynor@npimain.medsch.ucla.edu
www.dcp.ucla.edu/nadc

Dr. Olivia Raynor, Executive Director

NADC has a database and website which deals with access to and participation in the arts by people with disabilities.

16 **National Association for Drama Therapy**

5505 Connecticut Avenue NW
Suite 280
Washington, DC 20015
FAX: 301-990-9771
e-mail: nadt@mgmtsol.com

17 **National Theatre Workshop of the Handicapped (NTWH)**

535 Greenwich Street
New York, NY 10013
212-206-7789
FAX: 212-206-0200
e-mail: admissions@ntwh.org
www.ntwh.org

18 **Non-Traditional Casting Project**

1560 Broadway
Suite 1600
New York, NY 10036
212-730-4750
FAX: 212-730-4820
e-mail: info@ntcp.org
www.ntcp.org

Sharon Jensen, Executive Director

19 **VSA Arts**

JFK Center for the Performing Arts
1300 Connecticut Avenue NW
Suite 700
Washington, DC 20036
202-628-2800
800-933-8721
FAX: 202-737-0725
TTY:202-737-0645
e-mail: info@vsarts.com
www.vsarts.org

Doris Dixon, CEO

International coordinating agency for quality arts programs for disabled individuals from 68 countries. Purpose is to assure that disabled individuals have year-round opportunities to participate in educational programs demonstrating the value of the arts and to provide experiences to help them become active participants in mainstream society.

Automobile

20 **Ability Center**
Contact Technologies
11600 Western Avenue
Stanton, CA 90680
714-890-8262
FAX: 714-901-1492
e-mail: terry@abilitycenter.com

Terry Barton, Manager

Offers rear or side entry designed with painstaking craftsmanship using steel and lead.

21 **Acc-u-trol**
Ahnafield Corporation
3219 W Washington Street
Indianapolis, IN 46222
317-636-8061
800-636-8060
FAX: 317-636-8098

Bruce Ahnafield, President
Jeff Ahnafield, Sales Manager

Computer-controlled device that operates all secondary accessory functions. These functions may include ignition, lift and door operation, windows, wipers, lights and flashers.

22 **Adaptive Vans for the Physically Challenged**
Mobility Works
810 Moe Drive
Akron, OH 44310
800-638-8267
FAX: 330-633-0330
e-mail: bkoeblitz@mobility-works.com
www.mobility-works.com

Bill Koeblitz, President
Taylor F Clark, VP/General Manager

Mobility Works builds adaptive vans for the disabled and their special needs. Adaptations include lowered floors, raised roofs, wheelchair lifts, custom interiors, custom exteriors, driving systems, power transfer seats, wheelchair tie downs, wheelchair ramps, remote entry systems and rooftop wheelchair carriers for cars.

23 **Adaptive Vans for the Physically Challenge d**
Mobility Works
1965 E Avis
Madison Heights, MI 48071
800-638-8267
FAX: 248-616-3055
e-mail: bkoeblitz@mobility-works.com
www.mobility-works.com

Steve Young
Jan Hart

Mobility Works builds adaptive vans for the disabled and their special needs. Adaptations include lowered floors, raised roofs, wheelchair lifts, custom interiors, custom exteriors, driving systems, power transfer seats, wheelchair tie downs, wheelchair ramps, remote entry systems and rooftop wheelchair carriers for cars.

24 **Aeroquip Wheelchair Securement System**
Aeroquip Corporation
300 S E Avenue
Jackson, MI 49203
517-789-4144
FAX: 517-789-4716

Wheelchair users can have adaptable, safe, easily attached securement during transportation.

25 **Arcola Mobility**
51 Kero Road
Carlstadt, NJ 07072
201-507-8500
800-ARC-OLA1
FAX: 201-507-5372
www.arcolasales.com

Micheal Kohler, Vehicles Sales Representative
Brian Pruiksma, Lifts/Ramps/Etc Sales Rep

Arcola sells new and used accessible vehicles and adaptive driving equipment including hand controls, wheelchair lifts and securement systems. Daily, weekly and monthly vehicle rentals available. Stairway lift, porch elevators and ramps for the home sold and rented.

26 **Automobile Lifts for Scooters, Wheelchairs and Powerchairs**
Bruno Independent Living Aids
1780 Executive Drive
PO Box 84
Oconomowoc, WI 53066
262-567-4990
800-882-8183
FAX: 262-953-5501
e-mail: webmaster@bruno.com
www.bruno.com

Patrick Foy, National Sales Manager
Karla Branham Shaw, Marketing

Over 18 different styles of automobile lifts for scooters, wheelchairs and powerchairs for nearly any car, van, truck or sport utility vehicle that can raise most scooters or wheelchiars under 200 pounds and powerchairs up to 300 pounds. All Bruno lifts are eligible for reimbursement of up to $1000.00 from GM, Saturn, Ford, and Chrysler under the terms of their Mobility Programs.

27 **Ball Bearing Spinner**
Kroepke Kontrols
104 Hawkins Street
Bronx, NY 10464
718-885-1100
FAX: 212-885-1110

One lever fingertip control which is custom designed for each car but does not interfere with normal operation of your car and ball joints for perfect alignment. *$44.00*

28 **Blinker Buddy II Electronic Turn Signal**
HARC Mercantile
1111 W Centre Avenue
Portage, MI 49024
269-324-1615
800-445-9968
FAX: 269-324-2387
e-mail: home@harcmercantile.com
www.harcmercantile.com

Ronald Slager, President

Sounds a loud tone and flashes a light when the turn signal is on. *$79.95*

29 **Braun Corporation**
631 W 11th Street
Winamac, IN 46996
800-843-5438
FAX: 574-946-4670
www.braunlift.com

Jeff Ruff, Executive Vice President Sales

Manufactures wheelchair lifts and lowered floor minivans as well as many other mobility products.

30 Chevy Lowered Floor

Ahnafield Corporation
3219 W Washington Street
Indianapolis, IN 46222
317-631-8061
800-636-8060
FAX: 317-636-8098

Jeff Ahnafield, Sales Manager
Bruce Ahanfield, President

Full size Chevy van lowered floor from 4 to 12 depths.

31 Classic

Ricon
7900 Nelson Road
Panorama City, CA 91402
800-322-2884
FAX: 818-267-3001
e-mail: sales@riconcorp.com
www.riconcorp.com

Deluxe van conversion with equipment and accessories to offer freedom to the physically challenged.

32 Classic Coach Interiors

Classic Coach Interiors
1935 Burlington Avenue
Kewanee, IL 61443
309-852-4656
800-209-7225
FAX: 309-852-3463

George Giesenhagen, Manager

Offers van conversions with state-of-the-art equipment for the physically challenged.

33 DW Auto & Home Mobility Specialties

1208 N Garth Avenue
Columbia, MO 65203
573-449-3859
800-568-2271
FAX: 573-449-4187
e-mail: info@dwauto.com
www.dwauto.com

Sheila Lynch, Business Manager
Shawn Bright, Owner

Paratransit conversions and personalized conversions for the physically challenged. Home elevators and lifts.

34 Dodge Lowered Floor

Ahnafield Corporation
3219 W Washington Street
Indianapolis, IN 46222
317-631-8061
800-636-8060
FAX: 317-636-8098

Jeff Ahnafield, Sales Manager
Bruce Ahanfield, President

Full size Dodge van lowered floor from 4 to 12 depths.

35 Drive Master Company

9 Spielman Road
Fairfield, NJ 07004
973-808-9709
FAX: 973-808-9713
e-mail: sales@drivemaster.net
www.drivemaster.net

Peter B Ruprecht, President
Tina Knapik, VP Operations Manager
Shelby , Sales

Full service mobility center, raised tops/doors, drop floors, custom driving equipment, distributor of name brand devices and systems for full sized and mini vans. Sister company Van Master rents mobility equipped vans.

36 Dual Brake Control

Kroepke Kontrols
104 Hawkins Street
Bronx, NY 10464
718-885-1100
FAX: 212-885-1110

One lever fingertip brake controls, precision machines of the finest quality steel, are inconspicuous and do not take up lots of leg room. *$105.00*

37 Entervan

Braun Corporation
1014 S Monticello
PO Box 310
Winamac, IN 46996
800-THE-LIFT
www.entervan.com

The Entervan accessible features are designed to blend seamlessly into the original design of the Chrysler minivan. In fact, you'll find the Entervan to be virtually indistinguishable from other minivans on the road, with the only differences being the easily accessible qualities of the van.

38 Escort II XL

Worldwide Mobility Products
720 N Golden Street
Suite B6
Gilbert, AZ 85233
480-497-4692
800-848-3433
FAX: 480-497-3834
www.worldwide-mobility.com

Automatically lifts and secures for transportation a fully assembled three wheel electric scooter. *$1625.00*

39 Foot Steering

Drive Master Company
9 Spielman Road
Fairfield, NJ 07004
973-808-9709
FAX: 973-808-9713
e-mail: drivemstr1@aol.com

Custom installed system to steer a vehicle with your foot.

40 Foot Steering System

Ahnafield Corporation
3219 W Washington Street
Indianapolis, IN 46222
317-631-8061
800-636-8060
FAX: 317-636-8098

Jeff Ahnafield, Sales Manager
Bruce Ahnafield, President

41 Ford Lowered Floor

Ahnafield Corporation
3219 W Washington Street
Indianapolis, IN 46222
317-631-8061
800-636-8060
FAX: 317-636-8098

Jeff Ahnafield, Sales Manager
Bruce Ahanfield, President

Full size Ford van lowered floor from 4 to 12 depths.

42 Gresham Driving Aids

30800 Wixon Road
PO Box 930334
Wixom, MI 48096
248-624-1533
800-521-8930
FAX: 248-624-6358

Larry Pratt, Sales Manager

Offers a full-service package to physically challenged individuals including lowered floors, raised roofs and doors and high-quad driver control systems. Dealer for Braun, Ricoh, Crow River and Bruno wheelchair lifts.

43 **Hand Brake Control Only**

Kroepke Kontrols
104 Hawkins Street
Bronx, NY 10464
718-885-1100
FAX: 212-885-1110

One lever fingertip brake controls that are custom designed to fit each car, completely adjustable and offer positioning operation at your fingertips. *$130.00*

44 **Hand Control Systems**

Wright-Way
PO Box 460907
Garland, TX 75046
972-240-8839
800-241-8839
FAX: 972-240-0412
e-mail: mobility@wrightwayinc
www.wrightwayinc.com

Various automobile control systems that use hand, foot and steering aids for the disabled, including complete vehicle modifications.

45 **Hand Dimmer Switch**

Gresham Driving Aids
PO Box 930334
Wixom, MI 48393
248-624-1533
800-521-8930
FAX: 248-624-6358

This switch is recommended for left leg handicaps or when a right leg handicap uses a left foot throttle. *$36.25*

46 **Hand Dimmer Switch with Horn Button**

Gresham Driving Aids
PO Box 930334
Wixom, MI 48393
248-624-1533
800-521-8930
FAX: 248-624-6358

Attaches to the handle of control with a chrome plated steel insulated switch box, giving an instant warning without removing your hand from the steering wheel. *$28.75*

47 **Hand Gas & Brake Control**

Kroepke Kontrols
104 Hawkins Street
Bronx, NY 10464
718-885-1100
FAX: 212-885-1110

Driving controls that are attached by a control level right on to the gas and brake pedals for easy maneuvering and convenience. *$220.00*

48 **Hand Operated Parking Brake**

Gresham Driving Aids
PO Box 930334
Wixom, MI 48393
248-624-1533
800-521-8930
FAX: 248-624-6358

Converts foot parking brake to a hand operation for easy access and maneuverability. *$30.20*

49 **Hand Parking Brake**

Kroepke Kontrols
104 Hawkins Street
Bronx, NY 10464
718-885-1100
FAX: 212-885-1110

One lever fingertip brake controls for your car that offer easy installment, complete adjustability, complete independence and more. *$25.00*

50 **Handicapped Driving Aids**

Handicapped Driving Aids of Michigan
4020 2nd Street
Suite 30
Wayne, MI 48184
734-595-4400
FAX: 734-595-4520

Automobiles and vans customized, modified and equipped with industry approved handicapped equipment for ease of operation.

51 **Headlight Dimmer Switch**

Kroepke Kontrols
104 Hawkins Street
Bronx, NY 10464
718-885-1100
FAX: 212-885-1110

One lever fingertip controls for the disabled driver. *$23.00*

52 **Health & Mobility Systems**

9151 Hampton Overlook
Capitol Heights, MD 20743
301-499-1000
800-835-2002
FAX: 301-324-0121

Denise Terribile, Sales

Mobility needs, van conversions, ramps and lifts, retail products, healthcare equipment and medical supplies, orthodontics and prosthetics, seating systems, augmentative communications, assistive technology, rehab and technical support services.

53 **Horizontal Steering**

Drive Master Company
9 Spielman Road
Fairfield, NJ 07004
973-808-9709
FAX: 973-808-9713
e-mail: drivemaster@drivemaster.net
www.drivemaster.net

Peter Ruprecht, President
Christina Ruprecht, VP
Shelby Wells, Sales Manager

Horizontal steering system is customized to meet the needs of the high-level spinally injured and all others who experience limited arm strength and range of motion.

54 **Horn Control Switch**

Kroepke Kontrols
104 Hawkins Street
Bronx, NY 10464
718-885-1100
FAX: 212-885-1110

One lever fingertip controls that do not interfere with the normal operation of your car. *$23.00*

55 **Institute for Driver Rehabilitation**

156 E Commodore Boulevard
Jackson, NJ 08527
609-734-8000
800-866-1529
FAX: 732-928-2449

Debra Jackrel, President
Ted Jackrel, Program Director

Driver evaluation training for the physically/mentally challenged offering state certified driving instructors. Door-to-door pickup at home, work or rehab centers.

56 **Joystick Driving Control**

Ahnafield Corporation
3219 W Washington Street
Indianapolis, IN 46222
317-631-8061
800-636-8060
FAX: 317-636-8098

Jeff Ahnafield, Sales Manager
Bruce Ahnafield, President

Single lever, two axis remote control system for steering, brakes, and accelerator.

57 **Key Holders, Ignition & Door Keys**

Gresham Driving Aids
PO Box 930334
Wixom, MI 48393
248-624-1533
800-521-8930
FAX: 248-624-6358

Easy for arthritic hands to handle. Easily installed. *$18.70*

58 **Kneelkar Mednet**

Kneelkar Mednet
555 Industrial Park Drive
Battle Creek, MI 49015
269-964-7920
FAX: 269-962-8841

Offers the ultimate van conversions with equipment that is easily installed and accessible for the physically challenged.

59 **Latchloc Automatic Wheelchair Tiedown**

Ahnafield Corporation
3219 W Washington Street
Indianapolis, IN 46222
317-631-8061
800-636-8060
FAX: 317-636-8098

Jeff Ahnafield, Sales Manager
Bruce Ahanfield, President

An independent wheelchair tiedown system utilized primarily by individuals who drive from their wheelchairs.

60 **Lazy Days RV Center**

Lazy Days RV Center
6130 Lazy Days Boulevard
Seffner, FL 33584
813-246-4777
800-626-7800
FAX: 813-246-4408
www.lazydays.com

Jack Graham

Customized recreational vehicles for people with disabilities. Specializing in wheelchair accessible bathrooms.

61 **Left Foot Accelerator**

Gresham Driving Aids
PO Box 930334
Wixom, MI 48393
248-624-1533
800-521-8930
FAX: 248-624-6358

A custom pedal designed for left-foot usage. Stainless steel cross bar attaches above the throttle pedal and leaves right pedal free for right foot use. *$80.50*

62 **Left Foot Gas Pedal**

Kroepke Kontrols
104 Hawkins Street
Bronx, NY 10464
718-885-1100
FAX: 212-885-1110

One lever fingertip controls that offer custom design, easy installment and complete freedom for the disabled driver. *$90.00*

63 **Left Hand Shift Lever**

Gresham Driving Aids
PO Box 930334
Wixom, MI 48393
248-624-1533
800-521-8930
FAX: 248-624-6358

Converts steering wheel lever or automatic transmission selector lever to left hand usage for right arm handicaps. *$34.50*

64 **Low Effort and No Effort Steering**

Drive Master Company
9 Spielman Road
Fairfield, NJ 07004
973-808-9709
FAX: 973-808-9713
e-mail: drivemstr1@aol.com

Peter B Ruprecht, President
Christina M Ruprecht, General Manager
J Shelby Wells, Sales Manager

Reduced effort steering modifications available for nearly all vehicles. Additional products are pedal extensions which are 1 inch to 4 inch clamp-on aluminum blocks and 6 inch to 12 inch adjustable fold-down pedals.

65 **Mini-Bus and Mini-Vans**

Arcola Bus Sales
51 Kero Road
Carlstadt, NJ 07072
201-507-8500
800-ARC-OLA1
FAX: 201-507-5372
e-mail: tonyp@arcolamobility.com
www.arcolamobility.com

Tony Perez, Mobility Sales Representative
Brian Pruiksma, Sales Representative

Offers a virtually unlimited choice of chassis size, body style, floor plan and optional features. We provide transporters for almost every use, including school buses, vans, mini-coaches, medium-duty buses and personalized vans for the disabled.

66 **Mini-Rider**

Ricon
12450 Montague Street
Pacoima, CA 91331
818-899-7588
800-322-2884
FAX: 818-890-3354

Deluxe van conversions.

67 **Mobility Vehicle Stairlifts and Ramps**

Arcola Bus Sales
51 Kero Road
Carlstadt, NJ 07072
201-507-8500
800-ARC-OLA1
FAX: 201-507-5372
e-mail: tonyp@arcolamobility.com
www.arcolamobility.com

Tony Perez, Mobility Sales Representative
Brian Pruiksma, Accessibility Products

Arcola Mobility is a leading dealer of personal Accessible mini and full size vans with custom conversions and modifications available. We offer a complete line of adaptive driving equipment, including wheelchair lifts, ramps, hand controls, steering devices, scooter lifters, car top wheelchair carriers and power transfer seats. In addition to new custom vehicles, we also have an extensive selection of used vehicles for the physically challenged.

68 **Monarch Mark 1-A**

Manufacturing & Product Services
7948 Ronson Road
San Diego, CA 92111
619-292-1423

System of hand controls which incorporates a popular method of operation by pushing the control handles directly toward the brakes.

69 **Monmouth Vans, Access and Mobility**

5105 Routes 33/34
Farmingdale, NJ 07727
732-919-1444
800-221-0034
FAX: 732-919-0256
e-mail: info@monmouthvans.com
www.monmouthvans.com

Eugene Morton, President
Raymond Morton, VP
Arthur Smith, Sales Manager

Full vehicle modifications for driving and for transport of people with disabilities. Access equipment for buildings, e.g. ramps, stair lifts, pool lifts, automatic door openers and patient transfer lifts, pride jazzy portable and modular wheelchairs and scooters. Large selection of modified vans in stock.

70 **New Quad Grip**

Gresham Driving Aids
PO Box 930334
Wixom, MI 48393
248-624-1533
800-521-8930
FAX: 248-624-6358

Automobile aids for the disabled. *$40.25*

71 **PAC Unit**

Ahnafield Corporation
3219 W Washington Street
Indianapolis, IN 46222
317-631-8061
800-636-8060
FAX: 317-636-8098

Jeff Ahnafield, Sales Manager
Bruce Ahnafield, President

Low effort accelerator and brake remote serves hand control.

72 **Pedal Ease**

Ahnafield Corporation
3219 W Washington Street
Indianapolis, IN 46222
317-631-8061
800-636-8060
FAX: 317-636-8098

Jeff Ahnafield, Sales Manager
Bruce Ahnafield, President

Low effort accelerator and brake remote serves foot control.

73 **Portable Hand Controls**

Ahnafield Corporation
3219 W Washington Street
Indianapolis, IN 46222
317-631-8061
800-636-8060
FAX: 317-636-8098

Jeff Ahnafield, Sales Manager
Bruce Ahanfield, President

74 **Portable Vehicle Controls**

Contact Technologies
1033 Business Center Court
Newbury Park, CA 91320
805-498-8157
FAX: 805-498-2747

Fully portable integrated automotive hand control unit.

75 **Power Seat Base (6-Way)**

Ricon
12450 Montague Street
Pacoima, CA 91331
818-899-7588
800-322-2884
FAX: 818-890-3354

Facilitates a driver's self-transfer from a wheelchair to the driving seat and allows optimal driving positioning.

76 **Quad Grip with Pin**

Gresham Driving Aids
PO Box 930334
Wixom, MI 48393
248-624-1533
800-521-8930
FAX: 248-624-6358

Automobile aids for the disabled. *$40.25*

77 **Rampvan**

Independent Mobility Systems
4100 W Piedras Street
Farmington, NM 87401
505-326-4538
800-467-8267
FAX: 505-326-4846
e-mail: info@imsvans.com
www.ims-vans.com

Fully accessible minivan conversions with automatic doors and ramps, manufactured by Toyota, Chrysler, Dodge and Ford minivans.

78 **Reduced Effort Steering**

Ahnafield Corporation
3219 W Washington Street
Indianapolis, IN 46222
317-631-8061
800-636-8060
FAX: 317-636-8098

Jeff Ahnafield, Sales Manager
Bruce Ahanfield, President

79 **Right Hand Turn Signal Switch Lever**

Gresham Driving Aids
PO Box 930334
Wixom, MI 48393
248-624-1533
800-521-8930
FAX: 248-624-6358

Converts signal switch to right hand usage for left arm handicaps. *$34.50*

80 **Slim Line Brake Only**

Gresham Driving Aids
PO Box 930334
Wixom, MI 48393
248-624-1533
800-521-8930
FAX: 248-624-6358

A chrome plated steel handle, contour shaped, with a left hand or right hand unit available. *$155.25*

81 **Slim Line Control**

Gresham Driving Aids
PO Box 930334
Wixom, MI 48393
248-624-1533
800-521-8930
FAX: 248-624-6358

A plated, strong, compact unit designed to be easily transferred from car to car. Built of heavy steel tubing, welded and chrome plated and contour-shaped for maximum driving room. *$201.25*

82 **Slim Line Control: Brake and Throttle**

Gresham Driving Aids
PO Box 930334
Wixom, MI 48393
248-624-1533
800-521-8930
FAX: 248-624-6358

Brake is actuated by pushing the control lever directly towards the brake. Throttle is actuated by moving the lever at right angles to the brake movement, toward the seat. The weight of the operator's hand is sufficient to hold the throttle at any designed speed. *$300.00*

83 **Steering Backup System**

Ahnafield Corporation
3219 W Washington Street
Indianapolis, IN 46222
317-631-8061
800-636-8060
FAX: 317-636-8098

Jeff Ahnafield, Sales Manager
Bruce Ahanfield, President

84 **Superarm Lift**

Handicaps
4335 S Santa Fe Drive
Englewood, CO 80110
303-781-2062
800-782-4335
FAX: 303-761-6811
e-mail: Forest77@earthlink.com
www.handicapsinc.com

Made for vans and motorhomes. No platform is necessary and no doorways are blocked by lift that is simple and safe to use.

85 **Tim's Trim**

25 Bermar Park
Rochester, NY 14624
585-429-6270
888-468-6784
FAX: 585-429-6355
e-mail: timstrim@aol.com
www.theoptionstore.com

Timothy A Miller, President

Offers vehicle modifications, drop floors, raised tops/doors, driving equipment, touch pads and lifts.

86 **Transportation Equipment for People with Disabilities**

Drive Master Company
9 Spielman Road
Fairfield, NJ 07004
973-808-9709
877-282-8267
FAX: 973-808-9713
e-mail: drivemstr1@aol.com

Wheelchair lifts and ramps, hand and foot controls, steering and braking modifications, complete van conversions, home modifications, wheelchairs and scooters and wheelchair accessible van rentals.

87 **Tri-Post Steering Wheel Spinner**

Gresham Driving Aids
PO Box 930334
Wixom, MI 48393
248-624-1533
800-521-8930
FAX: 248-624-6358

Three nylon posts, adjustable for proper fit to drivers hand, to control the wheel, for use by persons with weak or limp wrists. *$40.25*

88 **Trunk Lift**

Fortress
PO Box 489
Clovis, CA 93613
559-322-5437
FAX: 559-323-0299

Scooters trunk lifts.

89 **Ultra-Lite XL Hand Control**

Drive Master Company
9 Spielman Road
Fairfield, NJ 07004
973-808-9709
FAX: 973-808-9713
e-mail: drivemstr1@aol.com

Allows the driver to operate gas and brake by hand— push for brake— pull for gas. Can be installed in nearly every vehicle.

90 **Vantage Mini-Vans**

Vantage Mini-Vans
5202 S 28th Place
Tempe, AZ 85040
602-243-2700
FAX: 602-304-2804
www.vantagemobility.com

Personalized vehicles with lowered floors and swing-away ramps.

91 **Voice Choice**

Ahnafield Corporation
3219 W Washington Street
Indianapolis, IN 46222
317-631-8061
800-636-8060
FAX: 317-636-8098

Jeff Ahnafield, Sales Manager
Bruce Ahnafield, President

Voice recognition system for accessories.

92 **Voice Scan**

Ahnafield Corporation
3219 W Washington Street
Indianapolis, IN 46222
317-631-8061
800-636-8060
FAX: 317-636-8098

Jeff Ahnafield, Sales Manager
Bruce Ahnafield, President

Voice feedback control for accessories.

93 **Warp Drive**

Ahnafield Corporation
3219 W Washington Street
Indianapolis, IN 46222
317-631-8061
800-636-8060
FAX: 317-636-8098

Jeff Ahnafield, Sales Manager
Bruce Ahnafield, President

Low effort steering wheel attachment accelerator and brake hand control serves system.

94 **XL Steering**

Ahnafield Corporation
3219 W Washington Street
Indianapolis, IN 46222
317-631-8061
800-636-8060
FAX: 317-636-8098

Jeff Ahnafield, Sales Manager
Bruce Ahnafield, President

Extra light, small diameter, remote steering system.

Bath

95 **ARJO**

50 N Gary Avenue
Roselle, IL 60172
630-307-2756
800-323-1245
FAX: 888-594-2756
e-mail: lchevrie@arjousa.com
www.arjo.com

Lorena Chevrie, Marketing Communications

Concerto shower and procedure trolley allows patients to be cleansed and changed while laying in a supine position.

96 **Adaptive Design Shop**

12847 Point Pleasant Drive
Fairfax, VA 22033
703-631-1585
800-351-2327
FAX: 775-256-2556
e-mail: rickerso@email.com
www.adaptivedesignshop.com

Joe Rickerson, Marketing Director

Offers various adjustable models of bath and shower chairs, as well as adjustable toilet and commode supports for toddlers through adults. Call for a free brochure. Prices range from $200 to $800.

97 **Adjustable Bath Seat**

Arista Surgical Supply Company
67 Lexington Avenue
New York, NY 10010
212-679-3694
800-223-1984
FAX: 212-696-9046
e-mail: aristasurgical@juno.com
www.aristasurgical.com

Bath seat that fits easily in any size tub. Easily adjustable to any height for easier maneuverability. *$44.00*

98 **Adjustable Raised Toilet Seat & Guard**

Frohock-Stewart
39400 Taylor Parkway
N Ridgeville, OH 44035
440-329-6000
FAX: 440-365-4558

The seat features an exclusive pivot locking system so it won't slip or tip and the adjustable guard rail fits all toilets.

99 **AirLift Toileting System from Mobility**

5726 La Jolla Boulevard #104
La Jolla, CA 92037
858-456-8121
866-456-8121
FAX: 858-456-8139
e-mail: info@mobilityinc.net
www.mobilityinc.net

Steve Winston, VP Sales
Eric Proffitt, VP Marketing

The Mobility AirLift toileting system makes it easy and painless to get on and off the toilet with or without an assistant. The AirLift absorbs the user's weight, providing gentle lowering to a sitting position and smooth lifting to a standing position.

100 **BIT Talking Scale Bathroom Scale**

Sense-Sations
919 Walnut Street
Philadelphia, PA 19107
215-627-0600
FAX: 215-922-0692

Push the on button and the scale will invite you to jump on and discover how much weight you have lost or gained. *$91.50*

101 **Bath Products**

Snug Seat
PO Box 1739
Matthews, NC 28106
704-882-0668
800-336-7684
FAX: 704-882-0751
e-mail: sales@snugseat.com
www.snugseat.com

Steve Scribner, National Sales Manager
Kirk MacKenzie, President

Offers a wide range of products to meet the transportation, mobility, seating and bath aid needs for people of all ages. From car seats and standers for children with special needs to versatile wheelchairs that offer adults customized options and the freedom to go anywhere with confidence.

102 **Bath Shower & Commode Chair**

Clarke Health Care Products
1003 International Drive
Oakdale, PA 15071
724-695-2122
888-347-4537
FAX: 724-695-2922
e-mail: info@clarkehealthcare.com
www.clarkehealthcare.com

Posterior and anterior tilt, fits over most toilets. Includes soft seat, collection pan, adjustable footrest and headrest.

103 **BathEase**

3815 Darston Street
Palm Harbor, FL 34685
727-786-2604
888-747-7845
FAX: 727-786-2604
e-mail: bathease@aol.com
www.bathease.com

Tom FitzGerald, President
Terry Stickler, Director R&D
Gerry Grondin, Production Manager

BathEase is the original standard size, residential style, acrylic bathtub with a door. Ideal for use in private homes by all who are ambulatory, the award winning design was specially created as an aid to daily living for the elderly and physically challenged. BathEase also features the first shower stall that may be converted to a bathtub with a door. *$1897.00*

104 **Bathtub Safety Rail**

Arista Surgical Supply Company
67 Lexington Avenue
New York, NY 10010
212-679-3694
800-223-1984
FAX: 212-696-9046
e-mail: aristasurgical@juno.com
www.aristasurgical.com

Made of stainless steel, this safety rail fits in any size bathtub and offers safety and independence at bathing time. *$55.00*

105 **Braun Corporation**

Braun Corporation
1014 S Monticello Street
Suite 310
Winamac, IN 46996
574-946-6153
800-843-5438
FAX: 574-946-4670

Carolyn Watts, Public Affairs Contact

Offers a variety of assistive devices for the bath and surrounding environment.

106 **Columbia Medical Manufacturing**

PO Box 633
Pacific Palisades, CA 90272
310-454-6612
800-454-6612
FAX: 310-305-1718
e-mail: cmedonline@aol.com
www.columbiamedical.com

Offers a full line of toilet supports, positioning commodes, wrap-around bath supports, reclining chairs and car seats for children from 20 to 102 pounds.

107 **Commode**

Maxi Aids
42 Executive Boulevard
Suite 3209
Farmingdale, NY 11735
631-752-0521
800-522-6294
FAX: 631-752-0689
e-mail: sales@maxiaids.com
www.maxiaids.com

Adjustable seat height for patient comfort. *$65.95*

108 **Crane Plumbing/Fiat Products**

1235 Hartrey Avenue
Evanston, IL 60202
847-864-7600
FAX: 847-864-7652
www.craneplumbing.com

Manufacturers plumbing fixtures for the disabled. Products include toilets, lavatories, showers and tub/shower units.

109 **DSI**

16141 Runnymede Street
Van Nuys, CA 91406
818-782-6793
FAX: 818-782-6485
e-mail: info@wavegrip.com
www.wavegrip.com

Greg Paquin, Marketing Manager

Designer grab bars with ergonomic grip. Available in colors and custom shapes. New fold down shower seat. Support grips extend out from the wall 24 or 30. Concealed fastener and modular components for many design possibilities. Price ranges from $30.00 to $280.00.

110 **Deluxe Bath Bench with Adjustable Legs**

Maxi Aids
42 Executive Boulevard
Suite 3209
Farmingdale, NY 11735
631-752-0521
800-522-6294
FAX: 631-752-0689
e-mail: sales@maxiaids.com
www.maxiaids.com

Bath bench with back support and adjustable legs. *$ 49.95*

111 **Electric Leg Bag Emptier and Tub Slide Shower Chair**

RD Equipment
230 Percival Drive
W Barnstable, MA 02668
508-362-7498
FAX: 508-362-7498
e-mail: info@rdequipment.com
www.rdequipment.com

Richard J Dagostino, Inventor/President
Diana M Pontieri, Sales Manager

Designed for independence, this small, lightweight battery-operated valve attaches to the bottom of the leg bag. A simple flip of the switch empties the leg bag, allowing the user to take in unlimited amounts of fluids. Tub Slide Shower Chair is a complete bathroom care system, with no need of costly renovations. Eliminates all transfers in the bathroom. *$200.00*

112 **Great Big Safety Tub Mat**

Maxi Aids
42 Executive Boulevard
Suite 3209
Farmingdale, NY 11735
631-752-0521
800-522-6294
FAX: 631-752-0689
e-mail: sales@maxiaids.com
www.maxiaids.com

Tub mat provides security against falls in the bath and shower. *$16.95*

113 **Long Handled Bath Sponges**

Therapro
225 Arlington Street
Framingham, MA 01702
508-872-9494
800-257-5376
FAX: 508-875-2062
e-mail: info@theraproducts.com
www.theraproducts.com

Plastic-handled, 18-inch bath sponge. Handle may be heated and bent for easy reach. *$2.50*

114 **Modular Wall Grab Bars**

Frohock-Stewart
39400 Taylor Parkway
N Ridgeville, OH 44035
440-329-6000
FAX: 440-365-7483

Engineered for strength and beauty, these bars can be assembled in various combinations to fit any bath or shower.

115 **Pik Stik**

Mobilelectrics Company
4014 Bardstown Road
Louisville, KY 40218
800-URM-OVIN
FAX: 502-495-2476

Provides reaching and grasping power with accuracy and ease.

116 **Portable Shampoo Bowl**

Ambulatory Cosmetology Technicians
12762 Brookhurst
Suite 532
Garden Grove, CA 92640
949-833-1432

Shirley D Smith

A bowl designed to allow a person who is in a wheelchair or sitting on a regular chair to shampoo hair.

117 **Prelude**

Arjo
50 N Gary Avenue
Roselle, IL 60172
630-307-2756
800-323-1245
FAX: 888-594-2756
e-mail: lchevrie@arjousa.com
www.arjo.com

Lorena Chevrie, Marketing Communications

Prelude shower cabinet allows patients to be showered in comfort and privacy, at the same time as protecting staff from excessive splashing.

118 **SLIDER**

Assistive Technology
530 S Whittaker Street
#240
New Buffalo, MI 49117
574-522-7201
800-478-2363
FAX: 574-293-0202
e-mail: info@pvcdme.com
www.pvcdme.com

The SLIDER bathing system eliminates costly roll-in shower renovations, bathroom transfers and other family members don't lost access to a bathtub. The SLIDER works with any standard built-in tub and rolls directly over any commode. The SLIDER utilizes 5 inch lock casters and has two swing-away arm rests for lateral transfers. Sliding sear functions in either direction. The SLIDER bathing system...a cost effective alternative to bathroom renovation.

119 **Suregrip Bathtub Rail**

Frohock-Stewart
39400 Taylor Parkway
N Ridgeville, OH 44035
440-329-6000
FAX: 440-365-7483

Compact and versatile, the bars have a soft-touch, contoured, white vinyl gripping area for added safety.

120 **Talking Bathroom Scale**

Independent Living Aids
200 Robbins Lane
Jericho, NY 11753
516-937-1848
800-537-2118
FAX: 516-937-3906
e-mail: can-do@independentliving.com
www.independentliving.com

Marvin Sandler, President

Talking scale. *$59.95*

121 **Terry-Wash Mitt: Medium Size**

Therapro
225 Arlington Street
Framingham, MA 01702
508-872-9494
800-257-5376
FAX: 508-875-2062
e-mail: info@theraproducts.com
www.theraproducts.com

Includes a thumb socket and a palm pocket to hold a bar of soap. *$8.00*

122 **Toilet Guard Rail**

Maxi Aids
42 Executive Boulevard
Suite 3209
Farmingdale, NY 11735
631-752-0521
800-522-6294
FAX: 631-752-0689
e-mail: sales@maxiaids.com
www.maxiaids.com

Made of chrome-plated, heavy gauge steel. Fits securely to the toilet for maximum sturdiness. *$43.95*

123 **Transfer Tub Bench**

Arista Surgical Supply Company
67 Lexington Avenue
New York, NY 10010
212-679-3694
800-223-1984
FAX: 212-696-9046
e-mail: aristasurgical@juno.com
www.aristasurgical.com

Curved padded backrest for comfortable support. Backrest also assists patient during lateral transfer. *$64.00*

124 **Tri-Grip Bathtub Rail**

Maxi Aids
42 Executive Boulevard
Suite 3209
Farmingdale, NY 11735
631-752-0521
800-522-6294
FAX: 631-752-0689
e-mail: sales@maxiaids.com
www.maxiaids.com

Two gripping heights for easy bathtub entrance or exit. *$36.95*

125 **Tub Slide Shower Chair**

RD Equipment
230 Percival Drive
W Barnstable, MA 02668
508-362-7498
FAX: 508-362-7498
e-mail: info@rdequipment.com
www.rdequipment.com

Richard J Dagostino, Proprietor/Inventor
Diana M Pontieri, Sales Manager

The tub slide shower chair was designed for the elderly and disabled to make any bathroom (at home or when travelling) accessible with little or no renovations. Go from the bed, to the commode and over to the bathtub for a shower using one product. No transfers in the bathroom whatsoever. *$2000.00*

Bed

126 **Adjustable Bed**

Golden Technologies
401 Bridge Street
Old Forge, PA 18518
570-451-7477
800-624-6374
FAX: 570-451-7494
e-mail: info@goldentech.com
www.goldentech.com

Rich Golden, CEO
Fred Kiwax, VP
Bob Smith, Sales VP

Trouble-free gear motor, safety features, dual massage variable speed timer and more, for the ultimate sleep experience.

127 **Bed Shaker**

Assistive Devices Network
5975 W Western Way
Tucson, AZ 85713
866-674-3549
FAX: 520-883-3172
e-mail: info@assistivedevices.net
www.assistivedevices.net/alarm-clocks-for-hea

Sells hearing, visual and mobility aid devices. *$39.00*

128 **Bye-Bye Decubiti Air Mattress Overlay**

Ken McRight Supplies
7456 S Oswego Avenue
Tulsa, OK 74136
918-492-9657
FAX: 918-492-9694

Ken McRight, President

Originally designed for hospital beds, converts any bed into an exceptionally therapeutic flotation unit when used between the conventional mattress and pad. The complete overlay is comprised of five individually inflatable, 100 percent natural rubber, ventilated sections enclosed within separate pockets of a soft fleece cover. Conforms to any configuration of electric or manual beds. *$731.50*

129 **Cervical Support Pillow**

Wise Enterprises
5017 El Don Drive
Rocklin, CA 95677
916-624-3848
888-947-3368
FAX: 916-624-3848
e-mail: wisent@pacbell.net
www.wisent.com/pillows.htm

Tom Wise, Owner

These hypoallergenic, antimicrobial fiber pillows support the neck in a natural position. Standard, midsize and petite pillows support the neck while sleeping on the back or side. The compact travel pillow offers support while sitting or lying down. The cervical roll has a gentle center and firm ends to ensure maximum comfort and proper support. Position the roll under the neck, back or knees. Standard and midsize fits adults, petite fits children and small adults.

130 **Foam Decubitus Bed Pads**

Profex/Professional
PO Box 16043
Saint Louis, MO 63105
314-727-2996

Convoluted foam provides extra back support and comfort for wheelchair users.

131 **Hard Manufacturing Company**

230 Grider Street
Buffalo, NY 14215
716-893-1800
800-873-4273
FAX: 716-896-2579
e-mail: currier@hardmfg.com
www.hardmfg.com

Kevin Currier, Corporate Sales

Manufacturer of pediatric cribs and age appropriate youth beds. Free catalog.

132 **Helping Handle**

Access with Ease
PO Box 1150
Chino Valley, AZ 86323
928-636-9469
800-531-9479
FAX: 928-636-0292
e-mail: KMJC@northlink.com

Gives you a hand getting out of bed. Fits any standard mattress and can be relocated up or down alongside the bed.
$44.95

133 **Jackson Cervipillo**

Wise Enterprises
5017 El Don Drive
Rocklin, CA 95677
916-624-3848
888-947-3368
FAX: 916-624-3848
e-mail: wisent@pacbell.net
www.wisent.com/ordering_lifestyle_products

Tom Wise, Owner

The Jackson Cervipillo confortably supports the neck vertebrae when sleeping on the side or on the back. Pillow measures 7 in diameter and is 17 long. A machine-washable cover is available separately.

134 **NeckEase**

Wise Enterprises
5017 El Don Drive
Rocklin, CA 95677
916-624-3848
888-947-3368
FAX: 916-624-3848
e-mail: wisent@pacbell.net
www.wisent.com/ordering_lifestyle_products

Tom Wise, Owner

Microwave NeckEase for penetrating heat that sooths stiff necks and shoulders, easing tension. NeckEase features a unique filling of organic, long grain rice and aromatic herbs and spices. When heated, this filling provides soothing, moist aromatherapy. Heat lasts about 30-45 minutes. Available in two sizes: small fits snugly around the neck, applying gentle pressure at the base of the skull; Large may be worn for a snug fit, or loosely for application on the shoulder and upper back.

135 **Permaflex Home Care Mattress**

BG Industries
8550 Balboa Boulevard
Suite 214
Northridge, CA 91325
630-257-1077
800-822-8288
www.bgind.com

Mattress with flame retardant upholstery material, water-repellant, anti-microbial and tear-resistant cover, for extra comfort.

136 **Priva**

PO Box 448
Champlain, NY 12919
514-356-8881
800-761-8881
FAX: 514-356-0055
e-mail: piv@priva-inc.com
www.priva-inc.com

David Horowitz, President
Natasha Pietramala, Director, HHC Division

Reusable incontinence care products including briefs, liners, inserts and sheet protectors. Manufacturers of Quorum Zip & Block anti-allergen bedding.

137 **SleepSafe Beds**

English Avenue Industries
3635 English Avenue
Morrisville, NY 13408
315-684-7976
866-852-2337
www.sleepsafebed.com

Perfect for adult home or home care use. Offering twin or full size bed frames in classic style, these beds offer an attractive alternative to a hospital bed. Keeps the user safe during rest and electrically adjusts smoothly for user comfort and caregiver ease of use.

138 **SleepSafe Plus**

English Avenue Industries
3635 English Avenue
Morrisville, NY 13408
315-684-7976
866-852-2337
www.sleepsafebed.com

Perfect for adult home or home care use. Offering twin or full size bed frames in classic style, these beds offer an attractive alternative to a hospital bed. Keeps the user safe during rest and electrically adjusts smoothly for user comfort and caregiver ease of use. Adaptive partial length side safety rails combine the strength of solid wood with clear, acrylic panels and exceed bed safety standards.

139 **Sonic Alert Bed Shaker**

Assistive Devices Network
2241 S Triangle X Lane
Tucson, AZ 85713
866-674-6549
www.assistivedevices.net/about.htm

$49.00

140 **Vibes Bed Shaker**

Assistive Devices Network
2241 S Triangle X Lane
Tucson, AZ 85713
866-674-3549
FAX: 520-883-3172
e-mail: info@assistivedevices.net
www.assistivedevices.net/about.htm

141 **Vibration Watch/Countdown Timer**

Global Assistive Devices
4950 N Dixie Highway
Fort Lauderdale, FL 33334
954-784-0035
888-778-4237
FAX: 954-784-0047
e-mail: info@globalassistive.com
www.globalassistive.com

Peggy Hewitt, Marketing Manager

This useful innovation reminds you and alerts you. Use for medical conditions. It can even be used as a travel alarm. Unique Auto Repeat Countdown Timer resets itself each time it reaches zero.

142 **Waterproof Sheet-Topper Mattress and Chair Pad**

Pillow Talk
348 Pond Road
Freehold, NJ 07728
732-780-9483
FAX: 732-708-0279
e-mail: pillowtalkusa2@aol.com
www.pillowtalkusa.com

Jack Fajerman, President

This soft pad lies on the top sheet, absorbing accidents from incontinence, pregnancy or medical problems. Waterproof barrier locks out moisture, soiling and stains and eliminates midnight linen changes and the resulting laundry. Available in bed sizes W/4 Anchor; twin; full; queen; king; and crib.

Communication

143 **ACS Wireless: Advanced Cyber Solutions**

3744 Civic Center Drive
North Las Vegas, NV 89030
702-364-1114
FAX: 702-364-1718
e-mail: info@advancedcyber.com
www.advancedcyber.com

This company makes a telephone headset.

144 **ADA Hotel Built-In Alerting System**

HARC Mercantile
PO Box 3055
Kalamazoo, MI 49003
269-324-1615
800-445-9968
FAX: 269-324-2387
e-mail: home@harcmercantile.com
www.harcmercantile.com

Ronald Slager, President
Ronald Damstra, Technical Sales Manager

Visual alerting system for ADA compliance for multi housing/rooms facilities, like hospitals, dorms, senior housing for persons who are hard of hearing or deaf. Alerts to five conditions: smoke, door bell, telephone ring, wake up and House central alarm.

145 **Able-Phone 110**

DQP
14167 Meadow Drive
Grass Valley, CA 95945
800-456-4979
FAX: 530-477-7122

Cordless headset telephone with keypad.

146 **Able-Phone 2500**

DQP
14167 Meadow Drive
Grass Valley, CA 95945
800-456-4979
FAX: 530-477-7122

Remote control emergency message telephone.

147 **Able-Switch 300**

DQP
14167 Meadow Drive
Grass Valley, CA 95945
800-456-4979
FAX: 530-477-7122

Wireless remote control.

148 **Able-Switch 500**

DQP
14167 Meadow Drive
Grass Valley, CA 95945
800-456-4979
FAX: 530-477-7122

Wireless remote receiver/controller.

149 **Able-Switch SW-1**

DQP
14167 Meadow Drive
Grass Valley, CA 95945
800-456-4979
FAX: 530-477-7122

Touch switch.

150 **Adaptek Systems**

2320 Brighton-Henrietta Town Line
Rochester, NY 14623
800-685-4566
FAX: 585-475-9889

Developers of a voice output module designed to work with the Kurzweil voice-recognition system. The device provides voice output of what the computer hears for persons with visual impairments.

151 **Akron Resources**

20 La Porte Street
Arcadia, CA 91006
626-254-9005
FAX: 626-254-9266
www.akron.com

Lisa Avalos, Operations Manager

Manufacturers of infrared amplification systems for televisions or stereos. $29-$69.00.

152 **Ameriphone**

12082 Western Avenue
Garden Grove, CA 92841
800-874-3005
FAX: 714-897-4703
e-mail: ameriphone@ameriphone.com
www.ameriphone.com

Lisa DeLeuil, Sales Manager
Michael Hartberger, President
John Koste, Product Manager

The Ameriphone Dialogue RC is a remote controlled speakerphone that can be activated up to 40 feet away. It features up to 20 memory buttons that you scan and select by gently pressing the remote control or blowing in the optional Airswitch or squeezing the optional pillow switch. Features voice activated answering for complete independence and access to telephone company services such as call waiting. Phones $299.00-$399.00. Accessories $39-$99.

153 **Ameriphone Hearing Assistance Telephone**

12082 Western Avenue
Garden Grove, CA 92841
800-874-3005
FAX: 714-897-4703
e-mail: ameriphone@ameriphone.com
www.ameriphone.com

Lisa DeLeuil, Sales Manager
Michael Hartberger, President
John Koste, Product Manager

A communication enhanced telephone with a large button and contrasting graphics for optimum visibility and dialing ease. Amplifies incoming voice by 30 db gain and has a frequency screening feature that permits user to identify sound frequencies. *$119.95*

154 Amplified Handsets

HARC Mercantile
PO Box 3055
Kalamazoo, MI 49003
269-324-1615
800-445-9968
FAX: 269-324-2387
e-mail: home@harcmercantile.com
www.harcmercantile.com

Ronald Slager, President

Choices of touch activated electronic control, rotary (thumb wheel) volume control, that can directly replace old handset, stocked in round and square styles. This also includes an electric transmitter with variable settings. *$39.95*

155 Amplified Phones

HARC Mercantile
PO Box 3055
Kalamazoo, MI 49003
269-324-1615
800-445-9968
FAX: 269-324-2387
e-mail: home@harcmercantile.com
www.harcmercantile.com

Ronald Slager, President

Low frequency ringer, indicator light, enhances or amplifies sound, some that automatically return to normal dial tone when phone receiver is hung up, lighted easy to read dial pad and volume control boosts incoming sound. *$95.00*

156 Amplified Portable Phone

HARC Mercantile
PO Box 3055
Kalamazoo, MI 49003
269-324-1615
800-445-9968
FAX: 269-324-2387
e-mail: home@harcmercantile.com
www.harcmercantile.com

Ronald Slager, President

Portable amplified phones. *$199.00*

157 Answerall 100

DQP
14167 Meadow Drive
Grass Valley, CA 95945
800-456-4979
FAX: 530-477-7122

Answering machine for TDD and voice.

158 Artificial Larynx

HARC Mercantile
PO Box 3055
Kalamazoo, MI 49003
269-324-1615
800-445-9968
FAX: 269-324-2387
e-mail: home@harcmercantile.com
www.harcmercantile.com

Ronald Slager, President

For people unable to use their larynx, a hand held speaking aid that simulates the natural vibrations of voice. *$220.00*

159 Assistive Technology

7 Wells Avenue
Newton, MA 02459
617-641-9000
800-793-9227
FAX: 617-641-9191
e-mail: customercare@assistivetech.com
www.assistivetech.com

Jane Oles, Customer Service Manager
Roxanne Varteressian, Marketing Specialist

A premiere developer of innovative technology solutions for people with physical and learning disabilities. Breakthrough products enable people of all ages and abilities to live and learn independently. Supportive material for teachers, clinicians and those with disabilities.

160 BESTspeech

Berkeley Speech Technologies
2409 Telegraph Avenue
Berkeley, CA 94704
510-843-1852
FAX: 415-841-5083

This text-to-speech facility is useful to persons who are blind or vision impaired and may be used by those with speech, hearing and learning difficulties.

161 Circline Illuminated Magnifer

Dazor Manufacturing Corporation
4483 Duncan Avenue
Saint Louis, MO 63110
314-652-2400
800-345-9103
FAX: 314-652-2069
e-mail: info@dazor.com
www.dazor.com

Kirk Cressey, Marketing Director
Bob Smith, National Sales Manager

Provides even, shadow free light under the magnifying lens with a 22-watt circline fluorescent. The magnifier is mounted on a floating arm that allows you to position the light source and lens with the touch of a finger.

162 Cornell Communications

7915 N 81st Street
Milwaukee, WI 53223
414-351-4660
800-558-8957
FAX: 414-351-4657
e-mail: sales@cornell.com
www.cornell.com

David D Thompson, Account Executive
Pauline Haack, Customer Service
Randy Stell, Account Executive

Cornell's Rescue Assistance Systems allow personnel to request emergency assistance. Applications include handicapped evacuations, parking garages and elevators. Voice, intercom and visual only signaling systems are available.

163 Davis Center for Hearing, Speech, Learning and Well-Being

98 Route 46 W
Budd Lake, NJ 07828
973-347-7662
FAX: 973-691-0611
e-mail: info@daviscenter.net
www.thedaviscenter.com

Dorinne S Davis, President

Sound-based therapies that help hearing, learning, speech and well-being. Complete hearing, speech and CAP testing.

164 Environment Control System: NHX Nurse Call System

Aiphone Corporation
1700 130th Avenue NE
Bellevue, WA 98005
800-692-0200
FAX: 425-455-0071
e-mail: info@aiphone.com
www.aiphone.com

Chuck Watkins, VP National Accounts
Nancy McAlister, VP National Accounts
Roy Paeth, VP National Accounts

AIPHONE manufactures audio and video intercom systems for home or business to help the physically disabled answer doors and communicate through physical barriers; also ADA-compliant emergency call intercom stations for use in public facilities and an Environmental Control System for persons with limited mobility.

165 Flashing Lamp Telephone Ring Alerter

Independent Living Aids
200 Robbins Lane
Jericho, NY 11753
516-937-1848
800-537-2118
FAX: 516-937-3906
e-mail: can-do@independentliving.com
www.independentliving.com

Once your phone is plugged into the Telephone Ring Alerter, the lamp light will flash with each ring, alerting you that there is a phone call. *$62.00*

166 Gabbi Talk Phone

Sense-Sations
919 Walnut Street
Philadelphia, PA 19107
215-627-0600
FAX: 215-922-0692

The talking telephone for mistake-free dialing lets the individual know what numbers they have dialed. *$28.50*

167 Genesis One

2827B Cleveland Road
Wooster, OH 44691
330-263-0015
888-221-5032
FAX: 775-252-4834
e-mail: info@apt-technology.com
www.apt-technology.com

Larry Shirer, President

Dedicated to sales and manufacturing of user friendly, and reliable assistive technology products and systems. These products are designed to increase independence and improve the quality of life for persons with disabilities.

c pages

168 Headmaster Plus

Prentke Romich Company
1022 Heyl Road
Wooster, OH 44691
330-262-1984
800-262-1984
FAX: 330-263-4829
e-mail: info@prentrom.com
www.prentrom.com

A headpointing system that takes the place of a mouse and allows individuals who cannot use their hands but have good head control access to the computer. A transmitting unit sits atop the monitor and sends signals to the user's headset. The user puffs into a tube connected to the headset to make selections. Typing can be done with optional on-screen keyboards. *$1195.00*

169 Ideal-Phone

IDEAMATICS
1364 Beverly Road
Suite 101
Mc Lean, VA 22101
703-903-4972
800-247-IDEA
FAX: 703-903-8949
e-mail: ideamatics@ideamatics.net
www.ideamatics.org

David L Danner, President

Integrates the personal computer and the telephone into a single, efficient workstation. It is ideal for mobility-impaired persons and others who need a hands-free operation of the phone. The Ideal-Phone includes one PC Board, a Plantronics headset, software for access and logging and complete documentation. It can be integrated into programs or pops-up over any application. MS-DOS based, version 3.0 or higher are available. *$195.00*

170 IntelliKeys (Smalle)

IntelliTools
55 Leveroni Center
Suite 9
Novato, CA 94949
707-773-2000
800-889-6687
FAX: 707-773-2001
e-mail: tech@intellitools.com
www.intellitools.com

Card and cable to create keyboard port on Apple IIe computer to allow use of IntelliKeys alternative keyboard.

171 LPB Communications

960 Brook Road
Norristown, PA 19401
610-825-4100
e-mail: lpbsales@lpbinc.com
www.lpbinc.com

John Devecka, VP Sales

Limited area AM and FM broadcast systems for hearing assistance and language translation manufacturing since 1960. Systems for small conference halls, churches and Olympic stadiums. Components or complete system. *$400.00*

172 Language, Learning & Living

Prentke Romich Company
1022 Heyl Road
Wooster, OH 44691
330-262-1984
800-262-1984
FAX: 330-263-4829
e-mail: info@prentrom.com
www.prentrom.com

A Minspeak application program designed for adolescent and adult individuals with developmental disabilities and associated learning difficulties. The software is used with Prentke Romich Company augmentative communication devices. *$355.00*

173 Large Button Speaker Phone

HARC Mercantile
PO Box 3055
Kalamazoo, MI 49003
269-324-1615
800-445-9968
FAX: 269-324-2387
e-mail: home@harcmercantile.com
www.harcmercantile.com

Ronald Slager, President

Speakerphone with or without remote control. *$395.00*

174 Large Print Telephone Dial

Maxi Aids
42 Executive Boulevard
Suite 3209
Farmingdale, NY 11735
631-752-0521
800-522-6294
FAX: 631-752-0689
e-mail: sales@maxiaids.com
www.maxiaids.com

Pressure sensitive dial with numbers that are easy to see for the disabled. *$.69*

175 **Large Print Touch-Telephone Overlays**

Maxi Aids
42 Executive Boulevard
Suite 3209
Farmingdale, NY 11735
631-752-0521
800-522-6294
FAX: 631-752-0689
e-mail: sales@maxiaids.com
www.maxiaids.com

Pressure-sensitive and easy to apply overlays that make everyday phones accessible. *$.49*

176 **Liberator**

Prentke Romich Company
1022 Heyl Road
Wooster, OH 44691
330-262-1984
800-262-1984
FAX: 330-263-4829
e-mail: info@prentrom.com
www.prentrom.com

A portable electronic communication device that uses Minspeak so that symbols are used to represent words, sentences or phrases. Liberator can be accessed by pressing keys, optical headpointing and a wide variety of switch activated scans. It can be configured with 8, 32 or 128 locations. It offers a variety of unique features to permit the most effective communication possible. $7,345-$8,575.

177 **Meroni Premiapri Press-Button Door Knob**

Meroni Locks of America
8012 NW 75th Avenue
Tamarac, FL 33321
800-749-5625
FAX: 305-556-2405

Michael Knight, Director
P Carlo Cau, VP

Door lock used in environments where barrier free access is required.

178 **Metropolitan Washington Ear**

35 University Boulevard E
Silver Spring, MD 20901
301-681-6636
FAX: 301-681-5227
e-mail: info@washear.org
www.washear.org

Nancy Knauss, Administrative Director

Multi-media reading service for blind and visually impaired. Offering 24 hour audio radio reading, dial-in newspapers and web casting, as well as audio description at theaters, museums and films.

179 **Micro IntroVoice I**

Voice Connection
2324 N Batavia Street
Suite 105
Orange, CA 92865
714-685-1066
FAX: 714-685-1070
e-mail: voicecnx@aol.com
www.voicecnx.com

Shirlee Dworak, VP Sales/Marketing

Complete voice input/output unit which provides voice recognition of 1,000 words and unlimited synthesized text-to-speech. Its small size is ideal for allowing someone to enter data into the computer when hands are busy or cannot be used. Also controlling of items can be set up. The MicroIntroVoice III allows one to control the wheelchair by voice. *$999.00*

180 **Micro IntroVoice II**

Voice Connection
2324 N Batavia Street
Suite 105
Orange, CA 92865
714-685-1066
FAX: 714-685-1070
e-mail: voicecnx@aol.com
www.voicecnx.com

Shirlea Dworak, VP Sales/Marketing

This battery powered, stand-alone voice system provides 1,000-word recognition, recorded playback, and unlimited text-to-speech synthesis. *$1295.00*

181 **Micro IntroVoice III**

Voice Connexion
10522 Covington Circle
PO Box 7065
Villa Park, CA 92861
714-685-1066
FAX: 714-628-1321
e-mail: voicecnx@aol.com
www.voicecnx.com/miv3.htm?

Voice actuated interface unit that can be installed on most existing and all new wheel wheelchair occupant to speak commands to control the motion of the chair. *$2495.00*

182 **MicroTalker B**

Voice Connection
2324 N Batavia Street
Orange, CA 92865
714-685-1066
FAX: 714-685-1070
e-mail: voicecnx@aol.com
www.voicecnx.com

The MicroTalker B announces recorded voice messages in response to ASCII text received via its serial port. *$395.00*

183 **Mini Teleloop**

HARC Mercantile
PO Box 3055
Kalamazoo, MI 49003
269-324-1615
800-445-9968
FAX: 269-324-2387
e-mail: home@harcmercantile.com
www.harcmercantile.com

Ronald Slager, President

Home induction loop amplifier for use with hearing aids equipped with T-Coil. *$159.95*

184 **Multiple Phone/Device Switch**

HARC Mercantile
PO Box 3055
Kalamazoo, MI 49003
269-324-1615
800-445-9968
FAX: 269-324-2387
e-mail: home@harcmercantile.com
www.harcmercantile.com

Ronald Slager, President

Used to switch phone lines between two devices. *$34.95*

185 **Oticon Portable Telephone Amplifier**

Hear You Are
4 Musconetcong Avenue
Stanhope, NJ 07874
800-287-EARS
FAX: 973-347-7662

Attaches to any sound source, picks up sound, amplifies it and induces it onto hearing aid telecoils. *$93.00*

186 **Outdoor Loud Bell**

Hear You Are
4 Musconetcong Avenue
Stanhope, NJ 07874

800-287-EARS
FAX: 973-347-7662

This outdoor bell with a loud mechanical ringer features an easy plug-in installation to either a modular or hook-up. *$79.16*

187 **Personal FM Systems**

HARC Mercantile
PO Box 3055
Kalamazoo, MI 49003

269-324-1615
800-445-9968
FAX: 269-324-2387
e-mail: home@harcmercantile.com
www.harcmercantile.com

Ronald Slager, President

Wireless FM systems transmit sound via a radio carrier wave. *$599.95*

188 **Personal Infrared Listening System**

HARC Mercantile
PO Box 3055
Kalamazoo, MI 49003

269-324-1615
800-445-9968
FAX: 269-324-2387
e-mail: home@harcmercantile.com
www.harcmercantile.com

Ronald Slager, President

Wireless method if listening to TV and radio with individually controlled amplification. *$199.00*

189 **Plantronics SP-04**

DQP
14167 Meadow Drive
Grass Valley, CA 95945

800-456-4979
FAX: 530-477-7122

Headset telephone for people who have a hard time grasping the telephone.

190 **Prentke Romich Company**

1022 Heyl Road
Wooster, OH 44691

330-262-1984
800-262-1984
FAX: 330-263-4829
e-mail: info@prentrom.com
www.prentrom.com

Barry Romich, Chairman
Joe Durbin, President
Cherie Weaver, Marketing Coordinator

The Prentke Romich Company is a full service company offering easy, yet powerful communication aids. The company believes in supporting customers before and after the sale by offering funding assistance, distance learning training, extended warranty, service assistance and much more. Visit our website to view our full line catalog, read about our success stories and to sign up for our online newsletter.

191 **Push to Talk Amplified Handset**

HARC Mercantile
PO Box 3055
Kalamazoo, MI 49003

269-324-1615
800-445-9968
FAX: 269-324-2387
e-mail: home@harcmercantile.com
www.harcmercantile.com

Ronald Slager, President

Replacement receiver which is hearing aid compatible and is designed for high noise conditions. *$79.95*

192 **Remote Control Speakerphone**

Ameriphone
12082 Western Avenue
Garden Grove, CA 92841

800-874-3005
FAX: 714-897-4703
e-mail: ameriphone@ameriphone.com
www.ameriphone.com

Lisa DeLeuil, Sales Manager
Michael Hartberger, President
John Koste, Product Manager

A multi-functional speaker phone specially designed to meet the needs of motion-impaired persons who are unable to use a conventional phone without assistance.

193 **Ring-a-Lite**

Tellus Business Services
1120 Samspon Road
Lee's Summit, MO 64081

816-765-3885
FAX: 816-765-3301
e-mail: telus@birch.net
www.birch.net/~telus/ring.htm

Ralph Taylor, Partner

Allows persons to see a telephone ringing, eliminating missing calls. This easy to use unit connects directly to existing telephone connections and also works to signal incoming TDD messages. *$39.95*

194 **Scanning Director II**

APT Technology
236A N Main Street
Shreve, OH 44676

330-567-2001
800-549-2001
FAX: 330-567-3073
e-mail: sales@apt-technology.com
www.apt-technology.com

Grace Miller, Office Manager

Controls all features of a TV, VCR, satellite system, etc. by means of scanning controlled by a single or dual switch. Operates also as an accessory to an ECU, also controls 16 lamps/appliances using X-10. *$795.00*

195 **Silent Call Communications**

4581 S Lapuer Road
Suite F
Lake Orion, MI 48359

800-572-5227
FAX: 248-377-4168
e-mail: silentcall@ameritech.net
www.silentcall.com

George Elwell, President
Suzie Wright, Office Manager

Alerting devices such as paging systems and smoke detectors for deaf and deaf-blind people.

196 **Silent Call: Portable Visual and/or Vibratory Alerting System**

Hear You Are
4 Musconetcong Avenue
Stanhope, NJ 07874

800-278-EARS
FAX: 973-347-7662

Small portable alerting device strobe light and vibrator announcer. Alerts to doorbell, telephone, smoke detector or sound monitors activations. Each alert is identified by a different colored light indicator. *$249.95*

197 **Sonic Alert**
Harris Communications
15155 Technology Drive
Eden Prairie, MN 55344
952-906-1180
800-825-6758
FAX: 952-906-1099
e-mail: mail@harriscomm.com
www.harriscomm.com

Bill Williams, National Sales Manager

Offers visual alerting devices that provide safety and convenience by turning vital sound into flashing light: telephone ring signalers, doorbell signalers, baby cry signalers and wake up alarms.

198 **Sonic Alert: Visual and Vibratory Alarm Clock**
Hear You Are
4 Musconetcong Avenue
Stanhope, NJ 07874
800-284-EARS
FAX: 973-347-7662

Clock features a large green LED display with extremely loud pulsating alarm. The tone and volume is adjustable so users can select their individual needs. Outlets are provided for a table lamp and a bed shaker. *$52.45*

199 **Sound Induction Receiver**
HARC Mercantile
PO Box 3055
Kalamazoo, MI 49003
269-324-1615
800-445-9968
FAX: 269-324-2387
e-mail: home@harcmercantile.com
www.harcmercantile.com

Ronald Slager, President

Sound induction receiver to be used with any loop system. *$67.00*

200 **SpeakEasy Communication Aid**
AbleNet
1081 10th Avenue SE
Minneapolis, MN 55414
800-322-0956
FAX: 612-379-9143
e-mail: customerservice@ablenetinc.com
www.ablenetinc.com

SpeakEasy is a digitalized Voice Output Communication Aid that is ideal for anyone who is beginning to develop communication skills such as making choices and identifying symbols. It holds 12 messages totaling four minutes and 20 seconds of recording time. It measures 7 1/2 inch by 1 3/4 inch and weighs only one pound. Activate messages using the built in keyboard or via external switch. *$399.00*

201 **Speakwriter 2000**
HumanWare
6140 Horseshoe Bar Road
Suite P
Loomis, CA 95650
916-652-7253

Talking typewriter.

202 **Speech Discrimination Unit**
HARC Mercantile
PO Box 3055
Kalamazoo, MI 49003
269-324-1615
800-445-9968
FAX: 269-324-2387
e-mail: home@harcmercantile.com
www.harcmercantile.com

Ronald Slager, President

Speech Adjust-A-Tone improves speech discrimination for use with telephone and/or TV and radio. *$189.95*

203 **Speechmaker-Personal Speech Amplifier**
HARC Mercantile
PO Box 3055
Kalamazoo, MI 49003
269-324-1615
800-445-9968
FAX: 269-324-2387
e-mail: home@harcmercantile.com
www.harcmercantile.com

Ronald Slager, President

Portable, body worn personal speech amplifier for people with a weak voice. *$316.00*

204 **Standard Touch Turner Sip & Puff Switch**
Access to Recreation
8 Sandra Court
Newbury Park, CA 91320
805-498-7535
800-634-4351
FAX: 805-498-8186
e-mail: dkrebs@accesstr.com
www.accesstr.com

Don Krebs, President

A page turning device.

205 **Stretch-View Wide-View Rectangular Illuminated Magnifier**
Dazor Manufacturing Corporation
4483 Duncan Avenue
Saint Louis, MO 63110
314-652-2400
800-345-9103
FAX: 314-652-2069
e-mail: info@dazor.com
www.dazor.com

Kirk Cressey, Marketing Director
Bob Smith, National Sales Manager

Provides shadow-free illumination or a highlighting effect under the magnifying lens with an 18-watt compact fluorescent light source. The magnifier is mounted on a floating arm that allows you to position the light source and lens with the touch of a finger.

206 **Strobe Light Signalers**
HARC Mercantile
PO Box 3055
Kalamazoo, MI 49003
269-324-1615
800-445-9968
FAX: 269-324-2387
e-mail: home@harcmercantile.com
www.harcmercantile.com

Ronald Slager, President

Strobe alerts. Plugs into receivers for signaling systems. *$39.95*

207 **TTY's: Telephone Device for the Deaf**
HARC Mercantile
PO Box 3055
Kalamazoo, MI 49003
269-324-1615
800-445-9968
FAX: 269-324-2387
e-mail: home@harcmercantile.com
www.harcmercantile.com

Ronald Slager, President

With or without printer. *$239.00*

208 **TalkTrac Wearable Communicator**

Ablenet
1081 10th Avenue SE
Minneapolis, MN 55414
800-322-0956
FAX: 612-379-9143
e-mail: customerservice@ablenetinc.com
www.ablenetinc.com

The TalkTrac Wearable Communicator is a personal, portable communication aid that is wearable on the wrist. TalkTrac features: simple to user, 75 seconds of recording time, four 3/4 x 1/2 message locations, rechagreable, water resistant, adjustable 9" band, Boardmaker compatible.

209 **Talkback Wireless Doorbell Intercom**

Rice International Corporation
7952 Pines Boulevard
Pmbk Pines, FL 33024
954-983-6464
FAX: 305-895-7660

Donald Van Der Laan, General Manager
Suzanne Minnick, Advertising Manager

Wireless radio frequency combined with doorbell and intercom. Outside unit uses 9 volt battery and features hands free operation. This device automatically turns off after one minute. *$ 99.95*

210 **Talking Calculators**

Assistive Device Network
2241 S Triangle X Lane
Tucson, AZ 85713
866-674-3549
FAX: 520-883-3172
e-mail: info@assistivedevices.net
employ-ability.org/erc/disabilitiesatwork6

211 **Talking Clocks**

HARC Mercantile
PO Box 3055
Kalamazoo, MI 49003
269-324-1615
800-445-9968
FAX: 269-324-2387
e-mail: home@harcmercantile.com
www.harcmercantile.com

Ronald Slager, President

Talking clocks with loud alarms, high and low volume control, choices of sound effects, hourly report options. Other languages are available. *$20.50*

212 **Talking Watches**

HARC Mercantile
PO Box 3055
Kalamazoo, MI 49003
269-324-1615
800-445-9968
FAX: 269-324-2387
e-mail: home@harcmercantile.com
www.harcmercantile.com

Ronald Slager, President

Digital display, hourly reports, alarm with rooster crow, in English or Spanish. *$20.25*

213 **Telecaption Adapter**

HARC Mercantile
PO Box 3055
Kalamazoo, MI 49003
269-324-1615
800-445-9968
FAX: 269-324-2387
e-mail: home@harcmercantile.com
www.harcmercantile.com

Ronald Slager, President

Caption opens up the world of television to hearing impaired people. Viewers can read on the screen what they may not be able to hear. Closed captions are the dialogue and sound effects of a TV program or home video printed on the screen, similar to subtitles. *$ 159.95*

214 **Touch Turner-Page Turning Devices**

Touch Turner Company
13621 103rd Avenue NE
Arlington, WA 98223
360-651-1962
FAX: 360-658-9380
e-mail: touchturner@worldnet.att.net
www.touchturner.com

Turns pages in either direction powered by flashlight batteries and holds the reading at the proper angle for sitting or reclining.

215 **Ultratec: Auto Answer TTY**

Hear You Are
4 Musconetcong Avenue
Stanhope, NJ 07874
800-278-EARS
FAX: 973-347-7662

Full featured primitive TTY with auto answering features for business or emergency services. Has direct connect or acoustic coupling with turbo communications mode, equipped with auto ID and relay Voice Announcer. Large memory buffer supports storing of conversation, memory message and directories. *$549.00*

216 **Unity**

Prentke Romich Company
1022 Heyl Road
Wooster, OH 44691
330-262-1984
800-262-1984
FAX: 330-263-4829
e-mail: info@prentrom.com
www.prentrom.com

A Minspeak application program available for the Liberator and Delta Talker communication devices. Provides single word vocabulary to people of all ages at varying stages of language development, who may be either cognitively intact or challenged. *$355.00*

217 **Vantage**

Prentke Romich Company
1022 Heyl Road
Wooster, OH 44691
330-262-1984
800-262-1984
FAX: 330-263-4829
e-mail: info@prentrom.com
www.prentrom.com

Vantage is a portable communication aid that features the Unity Enhanced vocabulary software and a large high quality dynamic display. Vantage also employs the recently upgraded 4.0 operating system that makes system settings quick and easy. Vantage has synthesized speech powered by DECtalk Software, Spelling and Word Protection software, built-in visor (flip-up protective cover), digitized speech capability and built-in computer access and ECU controls. 15 and 45 location keyguards available. *$6295.00*

218 **Vibrotactile Personal Alerting System**

HARC Mercantile
PO Box 3055
Kalamazoo, MI 49003
269-324-1615
800-445-9968
FAX: 269-324-2387
e-mail: home@harcmercantile.com
www.harcmercantile.com

Ronald Slager, President

Composed of a small wireless personal device that receives coded signals and a group of transmitters that send them. *$195.95*

219 **Viewstar**

Viewstar
15303 Ventura Boulevard
Sherman Oaks, CA 91403 **818-382-4104**

Leonard Weinstein, Technical Director

A stand-alone CCTV system for single view reading, writing and examining small objects. *$1545.00*

220 **Voice Amplified Handsets**

HARC Mercantile
PO Box 3055
Kalamazoo, MI 49003 **269-324-1615**
800-445-9968
FAX: 269-324-2387
e-mail: home@harcmercantile.com
www.harcmercantile.com

Ronald Slager, President

Designed for the person who has a weak speaking voice. Control increases the level of the user's voice and can increase as much as 30%. *$65.00*

221 **WalkerTalker**

Prentke Romich Company
1022 Heyl Road
Wooster, OH 44691 **330-262-1984**
800-262-1984
FAX: 330-263-4829
e-mail: info@prentrom.com
www.prentrom.com

A portable direct selection communication device for active persons. The 16 location keyboard and speakers are carried in a belt that straps comfortably around the waist. The keyboard can be removed from its pouch to use by activating keys. Two versions are available, standard memory and expanded memory. *$1195.00*

222 **Whisper 2000**

DQP
14167 Meadow Drive
Grass Valley, CA 95945
800-456-4979
FAX: 530-477-7122

Personal sound amplification system that features a transmitter, phone and relay system for the hard-of-hearing.

Chairs

223 **Adjustable Chair**

Bailey Manufacturing Company
118 Lee Street
PO Box 130
Lodi, OH 44254 **330-948-1080**
800-321-8372
FAX: 330-948-4439
e-mail: baileymfg@baileymfg.com
www.baileymfg.com

Adelle McClendon, Customer Service
Sandy Mooney, Customer Service
Judie Butler, Dealer Contact

The seat and footboard of this versatile chair can be adjusted to accommodate children of various sizes.

224 **Adjustable Classroom Chair**

Bailey Manufacturing Company
118 Lee Street
Suite 130
Lodi, OH 44254 **330-948-1080**
800-321-8372
FAX: 330-948-4439
e-mail: baileymfg@attmail.com
www.baileymfg.com

This adjustable classroom chair with accessory tray has a seat and footboard that can be adjusted to fit children of various sizes.

225 **Adjustable Clear Acrylic Tray**

Bailey Manufacturing Company
118 Lee Street
Suite 130
Lodi, OH 44254 **330-948-1080**
800-321-8372
FAX: 330-948-4439
e-mail: baileymfg@attmail.com
www.baileymfg.com

Adjusts for height and depth and is equipped with a spill rim for easy to clean edges.

226 **Adjustable Rigid Chair**

Kuschall of America
708 Via Alondra
Camarillo, CA 93012
800-654-4768

The Champion 3000 is a fully adjustable rigid frame chair weighing only 21 pounds with a new clamping system that adjusts seat height and angle without tools.

227 **Adjustable Tee Stool**

Bailey Manufacturing Company
118 Lee Street
Suite 130
Lodi, OH 44254 **330-948-1080**
800-321-8372
FAX: 330-948-4439
e-mail: baileymfg@attmail.com
www.baileymfg.com

May be used to encourage balance as well as develop integrative and perceptual motor skills.

228 **AirLift Toileting System from Mobility**

5726 La Jolla Boulevard #104
La Jolla, CA 92037 **858-456-8121**
866-456-8121
FAX: 858-456-8139
e-mail: info@mobilityinc.net
www.mobilityinc.net

Steve Winston, VP Sales
Eric Proffitt, VP Marketing

The Mobility AirLift toileting system makes it easy and painless to get on and off the toilet. With or without an assistant, the AirLift absorbs the user's weight, providing gentle lowering to a sitting position and smooth lifting to a standing position.

229 **BackSaver**

BackSaver Products Company
53 Jeffrey Avenue
Holliston, MA 01746 **508-429-5940**
800-251-2225
FAX: 508-429-8698
e-mail: stevek@backsaver.com
www.backsavercorp.com

Steven Kusmin, Sales Director

Eliminates slouching and extra pressure on your back and thighs which impairs circulation.

230 **Better Back**

Orthopedic Products Corporation
4100 1/2 Glencoe Avenue
Marina Del Rey, CA 90292
323-584-6977
FAX: 310-306-0177

An orthopedic multi-purpose seat.

231 **Carendo**

Arjo
50 N Gary Avenue
Roselle, IL 60172
630-307-2756
800-323-1245
FAX: 888-594-2756
e-mail: lchevrie@arjousa.com
www.arjo.com

Lorena Chverie, Marketing Communications

The Carendo hygiene chair has been designed for caregivers.

232 **Century 50/60XR Sit**

Arjo
50 N Gary Avenue
Roselle, IL 60172
630-307-2756
800-323-1245
FAX: 888-594-2756
e-mail: lchevrie@arjousa.com
www.arjo.com

Lorena Cherie, Marketing Communications

This bathing system has a built-in cleaning/disinfectant injection system with adjustable flowmeter. The incorporation of an automatic hot water alarm/shut-off system, and digital temperature monitors, helps to assure resident safety and comfort.

233 **Convert-Able Table**

Rehab and Educational Aids for Living
187 S Main Street
Dolgeville, NY 13329
800-696-7041
FAX: 315-429-3071
e-mail: rdesign@tweny.rr.com
www.realdesigninc.com

Kris Wohnsen, Sales

This table has push button height adjustment and interchangeable tops so it can become a desk, art easel or a sensory stimulation bowl.

234 **Evac + Chair Emergency Wheelchair**

Evac + Chair Corporation
PO Box 2396
New York, NY 10021
212-369-4094
FAX: 212-369-3710
e-mail: sales@evac-chair.com
www.evac-chair.com

Robert McLean, Sales Manager

Gravity driven evaluation chair allows one non-disabled person to smoothly glide a seated passenger down fire stairs and across landings to exit on a combination of wheels and track belts. Pivots in own width for tight landing turns. Aluminum; weight 18 pounds. Compactly stores on wall mount, 38 by 20 by 9 inches. Maximum capacity 300 pounds. Self braking features. No installation, works on all fire exit stairs. *$950.00*

235 **Golden Technologies**

401 Bridge Street
Old Forge, PA 18518
800-624-6374
FAX: 800-628-5165

236 **Granstand III MSS Standing System**

Prime Engineering
4202 W Sierra Madre Avenue
Fresno, CA 93722
559-276-0991
800-827-8263
FAX: 800-800-3355
e-mail: info@primeengineering.com
www.primeengineering.com

Prime Engineering is a manufacturer of adult and pediatric Standing Devices, Patient Transfer Equipment and Lift Assisted Gait Trainers. Products include the all-new Granstand III Modular Standing System, Granstand II adult standing device, Superstand Multi-Position pediatric stander, the Lift, the CindyLift and the Original Lift Walker.

237 **High-Low Chair**

Rehab and Educational Aids for Living
187 S Main Street
Dolgeville, NY 13329
800-696-7041
FAX: 315-429-3071

Kris Wohnsen, Sales

A high chair and mobile floor sitter in one. The high-low chair comes with colorful upholstered wipe clean seat and height adjustable tray. The chair has a single lever adjustment to change the seat height. Lateral and head supports are available as options. *$ 1199.00*

238 **Hygea-Chair**

TRIAID
PO Box 1364
Cumberland, MD 21501
301-759-3525
800-306-6777
FAX: 301-759-3525
e-mail: sales@triaid.com
www.triaid.com

Iain A MacDonald, Sales Director
Ann M Hutter, Sales Executive

Available in four sizes, the Hygea-Chair is an all purpose hygiene chair for children. It is supplied complete with a range of accessories fitted as standard to enhance the flexibility of the system: braked wheels, harness, footrest and seat insert comfort cover. It can be used in the shower, over the toilet or as a commode. *$950.00*

239 **Ladybug Corner Chair**

Rehab and Educational Aids for Living
187 S Main Street
Dolgeville, NY 13329
800-696-7041
FAX: 315-429-3071

For children 0-3 years. This chair is adjustable for long leg for conventional sitting.

240 **Lumex Recliner**

Graham-Field Health Products
2935 NE Parkway
Atlanta, GA 30360
800-347-5678
FAX: 800-726-0601
www.grahamfield.com

Combines therapeutic benefits of position change with attractive appearance.

241 **Mulholland Positioning Systems**

215 N Main Street
PO Box 391
Santa Paula, CA 93061
800-543-4769
FAX: 805-933-1082
e-mail: john@mulhoolandinc.com
www.mulhollandinc.com

John Oderkirk, Marketing

Provides a full line of standing aids, seating systems, adaptive components and bath aids.

242 **Multi-Use Classroom Chair**

Bailey Manufacturing Company
118 Lee Street
Suite 130
Lodi, OH 44254
330-948-1080
800-321-8372
FAX: 330-948-4439
e-mail: baileymfg@attmail.com
www.baileymfg.com

This classroom chair can be customized to meet the individual needs of any physically challenged child with the addition of easily attached accessories.

243 **Quality Lift Chair**

Mobilelectrics Company
4014 Bardstown Road
Louisville, KY 40218
800-876-6846
FAX: 502-495-2476

Come and go as you please, sit and stand when you want, without help from anyone.

244 **Roll Chair**

Bailey Manufacturing Company
118 Lee Street
Suite 130
Lodi, OH 44254
330-948-1080
800-321-8372
FAX: 330-948-4439
e-mail: baileymfg@attmail.com
www.baileymfg.com

The padded roll helps maintain proper hip abduction and prevents scissoring of the legs.

245 **Safari Tilt**

Convaid Products
PO Box 4209
Palos Verdes, CA 90274
310-618-0111
FAX: 310-618-8811
e-mail: convaid@west.net
www.convaid.com

Mervyn Watkins, President

A semi-contour seat provides positioning with 5-45 degree tilt adjustment. One step design folds compactly into a lightweight chair.

246 **Spatial Tilt Custom Chair**

Redman Powerchair
1660 S Research Loop #126
Tucson, AZ 85710
520-546-6002
800-727-6684
FAX: 520-546-5530

Custom chair designed for comfort with a solid seat and back with modifications available for seat depth, height or width.

247 **Special Needs 5**

Baby Jogger Company
PO Box 2189
Yakima, WA 98907
509-457-0925
800-241-1848
FAX: 509-453-7732
e-mail: bfetzer@babyjogger.com
www.babyjogger.com/p6.asp

Billy Fetzer, Sales Representative

Special need mobility devices give passengers smooth rides indoor and outdoors. The light weight aluminum frame supports up to 200 pounds. Modifications available.

248 **Transfer Bench with Back**

Frohock-Stewart
39400 Taylor Parkway
N Ridgeville, OH 44035
440-329-6000
FAX: 440-365-7483

This bench with air-cushioned seat sections has a full, reversible backrest for safety and comfort.

Cushions & Wedges

249 **ACU Massage Cushion**

Massage Relaxation Products
PO Box 7243
Alhambra, CA 91802
800-999-1089

Hundreds of tiny massaging beads which help relieve lower back pain through massaging your own acupressure points.

250 **Action Products**

22 N Mulberry Street
Hagerstown, MD 21740
301-797-1414
800-228-7763
FAX: 301-733-2073
e-mail: service@actionproducts.com
www.actionproducts.com

Dee Price, Customer Service Manager
Fred Nelson, Seating & Positioning Specialist
Michael Bredal, VP Sales North America

Wheelchair pads, mattress pads, positioning cushions and insoles that aid in the prevention and cure of pressure sores by reducing pressure. All products are made of Akton viscoelastic polymer that does not leak, flow or bottom out. Manufacturer of the Xact line of positioning cushions for patients with high risk of skin breakdown.

251 **Adjustable Wedge**

Bailey Manufacturing Company
118 Lee Street
Suite 130
Lodi, OH 44254
330-948-1080
800-321-8372
FAX: 330-948-4439
e-mail: baileymfg@attmail.com
www.baileymfg.com

Orthopedically and neurologically disabled children can freely move arms and hands while lying on this adjustable wedge.

252 **Back Machine**

Kingstar International America
PO Box 10157
Chicago, IL 50610
312-951-1115
FAX: 312-943-1727
www.kingstar.com

Robin Morgenstern, President

A nine position adjustable lumbar support that is compact and lightweight, portable and able to fit most chairs, adaptable for different body sizes and will not lose its shape. The inner spring design will give the spinal column over-all support to compensate for stress, fatigue and improper posture.

253 **Back-Huggar Pillow**

Bodyline Combort Systems
3730 Kori Road
Jacksonville, FL 32257
904-262-4068
800-874-7715
FAX: 904-262-2225
e-mail: info@bodyline.com
www.bodyline.com

Don Dodds, Office Manager

Exclusive design makes almost any seat more comfortable by exerting soothing pressure against back muscles and discs.

254 **BetaBed Pressure Pad**

Huntleigh Healthcare
40 Christopher Way
Eatontown, NJ 07724
732-578-9898
800-223-1218
FAX: 732-578-9889
www.huntleigh-healthcare.com

Bob Angel, President/CEO

Alternating pressure pad system automatically relieves tissue damaging pressure every 2 minutes.

255 **Bye-Bye Decubiti (BBD)**

Ken McRight Supplies
7456 S Oswego Avenue
Tulsa, OK 74136
918-492-9657
FAX: 918-492-9694

Ken McRight, President

The BBD therapeutic wheelchair cushions have been market-proven since 1951 — in the prevention and cure of pressure sores (decubiti). These natural rubber inflatable products have recently been expanded to include pediatric, sports and double-valve models. Moderately priced, they offer a viable and cost-effective alternative in the market. $84.00-$112.00

256 **Dynamic Systems**

235 Sunlight Drive
Leicester, NC 28748
828-683-3523
FAX: 828-683-3511
e-mail: dsi@sunmatecushions.com
www.sunmatecushions.com

Pamela Price, Customer Service
Ellie Brown, Executive Officer Manufacturing
Cathy Ramsey, Exec Officer FIPS/Spec Projects

SunMate orthopedic foam sheets and cushions, pudgee pads for pressure relief and skin breakdown prevention, laminar wheelchair cushions and Foam-in-Place Seating for custom molding seat inserts. Sample packs and literature available upon request.

257 **Econo-Float Water Flotation Cushion**

Jefferson Industries
1940 Rutgers University Boulevard
Lakewood, NJ 08701
732-905-9001
800-257-5145
FAX: 732-905-9899

Charles Landa, General Manager

An inexpensive, yet effective approach to the problem of pressure ulcers for patients confined to wheelchairs, geriatric chairs, etc. *$15.00*

258 **Econo-Float Water Flotation Mattress**

Jefferson Industries
1940 Rutgers University Boulevard
Lakewood, NJ 08701
732-905-9001
800-257-5145
FAX: 732-905-9899

Charles Landa, General Manager

Helps prevent and treat pressure ulcers by reducing and distributing pressure over the patient's bony prominences while supporting the body evenly over a greater surface area. *$39.00*

259 **Enhancer Cushion**

ROHO Group
100 N Florida Avenue
Belleville, IL 62221
618-277-9173
800-851-3449
FAX: 618-277-9561
e-mail: mail@therohogroup.com
www.therohogroup.com

Jackie Wiegert, Corporate Marketing

Uses AIR IN PLACE progressive positioning for enhanced midline channeling of the femurs, lateral stability and tissue protection.

260 **Flex-Air Pressure Relief System**

Relax-A-Flex
211 River Street
Bennington, VT 05201
802-447-1166
800-782-8889
FAX: 802-442-6875

Solves mattress problems.

261 **Functional Forms**

Consumer Care Products
1446 Pilgrim Road
Plymouth, WI 53073
920-893-4614
FAX: 800-977-2256
e-mail: ccpi@consumercareinc.com
www.consumercareinc.com

These blocks, wedges, rolls, cervical pillows, head and leg supports and barrel rolls in resilient high density foam covered with durable antibacterial, antistatic, flame resistant, non-absorbent vinyl are used to attain individualized support for the most difficult positioning needs for children and adults. Unique sizes allow fitting for almost any person. Use during exercise, feeding, therapy, recreation and rest at home, school and health care facilities. Packages available.

262 **GT Wheelchair Cushion**

Relax-A-Flex
211 River Street
Bennington, VT 05201
802-447-1166
800-782-8889
FAX: 802-442-6875

The specially designed gel pads in this cushion help relieve pressure on the back.

263 **Gaymar Industries**

Gaymar Industries
10 Centre Drive
Orchard Park, NY 14127
716-662-2551
800-828-7341
FAX: 716-662-6120
e-mail: pmatteliano@gaymar.com
www.gaymar.com

Steve Snyder, VP Marketing
Peggy Matteliano, Communications Specialist

Gaymar offers a complete line of support surfaces, including low-air-loss mattresses, specialty foam mattresses, turning mattresses, air overlays and fluid therapy beds. These products economically prevent and treat bedsores. Clinical and reimbursement professionals are available to answer any question related to bedsores (decubitus ulcers). Also offers a complete line of temperature control devices. The T-Pump delivers warm therapy to effectively dilate vessels and increase blood flow.

264 Geo-Matt for High Risk Patients

Span-America Medical Systems
70 Commerce Center
Greenville, SC 29615
864-288-8877
800-888-6752
FAX: 864-288-8692
www.spanamerica.com

Helps prevent pressure sores in high risk patients.

265 High Profile Single Compartment Cushion

ROHO Group
100 N Florida Avenue
Belleville, IL 62221
618-277-9173
800-851-3449
FAX: 618-277-9561
e-mail: mail@therohogroup.com
www.therohogroup.com

Jackie Wiegert, Corporate Marketing

With 4 inch cells, the HIGH PROFILE is the cushion of choice for individuals who suffer from ischemic ulcers (pressure sores) or who have a history of tissue breakdown.

266 Inflatable Back Pillow

Corflex
669 E Industrial Park Drive
Manchester, NH 03109
603-623-3344
800-426-7353
FAX: 603-623-4111
www.corflex.com

Folds flat to fit into its own carrying case, this inflatable back pillow ensures comfort while at home or traveling.

267 Jobri

520 N Division Street
Konawa, OK 74849
800-432-2225
FAX: 800-769-0520
e-mail: support@jobri.com
www.jobri.com

Mike Deaton, General Manager

268 Lumbo-Posture Back Support

Ken McRight Supplies
7456 S Oswego Avenue
Tulsa, OK 74136
918-492-9657
FAX: 918-492-9694

Ken McRight, President

Rubber inflatable back support that offers therapeutic relief to all who must sit for lengthy periods of time, whether used in a wheelchair, auto or bed. *$97.65*

269 Lumex Cushions and Mattresses

Graham-Field Health Products
2935 NE Parkway
Atlanta, GA 30360
800-347-5678
FAX: 800-726-0601
www.grahamfield.com

Line of cushions and pillows give comfort and independence to the physically challenged.

270 Medpro Static Air Chair Cushion

Medpro
1950 Rutgers University Boulevard
Lakewood, NJ 08701
800-257-5145
FAX: 732-905-9899

Jody Gorran, President

Provides a protective layer of air beneath the patient helping prevent and treat pressure ulcers. *$94.95*

271 Medpro Static Air Mattress Overlay

Medpro
1950 Rutgers University Boulevard
Lakewood, NJ 08701
800-257-5145
FAX: 732-905-9899

Jody Gorran, President

Supports the patient on a cushioned network of air designed to redistribute the patient's weight reducing tissue interface pressure. Medpro's design incorporates a series of 65 air-breather vents that maintain air circulation. Medpro effectively reduces pressure and helps prevent and treat pressure ulcers. *$164.95*

272 Mini-Max Cushion

ROHO
100 N Florida Avenue
Belleville, IL 62221
800-850-7646
FAX: 618-277-6518
e-mail: rohoinc@rohoinc.com
www.rohoinc.com

Julie Petry, Corporate Marketing

Designed for the active individual with low risk of skin breakdown. The unique air cells of the MINI-MAX provide significant shock and impact absorption, skin protection and stability.

273 NEXUS Wheelchair Cushioning System

ROHO
100 N Florida Avenue
Belleville, IL 62221
800-850-7646
FAX: 618-277-6518
e-mail: rohoinc@rohoinc.com
www.rohoinc.com

Julie Petry, Corporate Marketing

A unique modular cushion that mates a contoured polyurethane foam base with a dry flotation support pad. It is designed to give the user positioning and stability, while offering maximum protection to the ischia, sacrum and coccyx.

274 Nek-Lo, Nek-Lo Hot and Cold Pillow-Perfect, Body Buddy

Rinz-L-O Pillow Company
340 W Maplehurst Street
Ferndale, MI 48220
248-548-3993
800-594-9093
FAX: 248-548-0447
e-mail: rinzlo@aol.com

G Rick Rinz, President

Nek-Lo a U-shaped cervical pillow; Nek-Lo Hot and Cold - U-shaped pillow with hot/cold pack; Pillow-Perfect - Uses your conventional pillow to insert cover that has cervical support form piece. Magne-Aid and Magne-Systems - Magnetic therapy braces. *$12.98*

275 Pediatric Seating System

ROHO
100 N Florida Avenue
Belleville, IL 62221
800-850-7646
FAX: 618-277-6518
e-mail: rohoinc@rohoinc.com
www.rohoinc.com

Julie Petry, Corporate Marketing

ROHO Cushions for kids use individual air cells, creating the most versatile and dynamic cushioning products available. These cushions are designed to specifically fit pediatric wheelchairs.

276 **Quadtro Cushion**

ROHO
100 N Florida Avenue
Belleville, IL 62221
800-850-7646
FAX: 618-277-6518
e-mail: rohonic@rohoinc.com

Julie Petry, Corporate Marketing

For individuals who require special positioning of the pelvis or thighs and are at risk of skin breakdown, the Quadtro, with 4 inch cell height and air in place, progressive positioning is the cushion of choice.

277 **Roho Quadtro Select Cushion**

ROHO Group
100 N Florida Avenue
Belleville, IL 62221
618-277-9173
800-851-3499
FAX: 618-277-9561
e-mail: mail@therohogroup.com
www.therohogroup.com

Jackie Wiegert, Corporate Marketing

Protects against skin breakdown. 4 quadrants allow you to lock air in place.

278 **Silicone Padding**

Spenco Medical Group
PO Bos 2501
Waco, TX 76702
254-772-6000
800-433-3334

For the management of pressure sores, this padding provides a special support system which allows even distribution of pressure and cool, comfortable well-ventilated support.

279 **Soft-Touch Convertible Flotation Mattress**

Medpro
1950 Rutgers University Boulevard
Lakewood, NJ 08701
800-257-5145
FAX: 732-905-9899

Jody Gorran, President

Gives the patient the option to choose between water and gel flotation depending on the needs of the patient. The mattress helps prevent and treat pressure ulcers by spreading the patient's weight over a greater surface area. $164.95-$239.95.

280 **Soft-Touch Gel Flotation Cushion**

Medpro
1940 Rutgers University Boulevard
Lakewood, NJ 08701
732-905-9001
800-257-5145
FAX: 732-905-9899

Jody Gorran, President

Acts like an additional layer of fatty tissue beneath the patient to help prevent and treat pressure sores. *$99.95*

281 **Spenco Medical Group**

PO Box 2501
Waco, TX 76702
254-772-6000
800-433-3334
e-mail: spenco@spenco.com
www.spenco.com

Mark B Connors, VP Sales/Marketing
Patty Smith, Controller
Steven B Smith, CEO

Wheel chair cushions, Silicore mattress pads, wound dressings, second skin blister and burn pads, Polysorb insoles, elbow, knee and wrist supports and walking shoes.

282 **Stop-Leak Gel Flotation Cushion**

Jefferson Industries
1940 Rutgers University Boulevard
Lakewood, NJ 08701
732-905-9001
800-257-5145
FAX: 732-905-9899

Charles Landa, General Manager

Helps protect against pressure ulcers by functioning as an extra protective layer of fat which helps reduce and distribute pressure. *$18.00*

283 **Stop-Leak Gel Flotation Mattress**

Jefferson Industries
1940 Rutgers University Boulevard
Lakewood, NJ 08701
732-905-9001
800-257-5145
FAX: 732-905-9899

Charles Landa, General Manager

Protects persons from messy leaks while it protects from pressure ulcers. *$54.00*

284 **Sun-Mate Seat Cushions**

Dynamic Systems
235 Sunlight Drive
Leicester, NC 28748
828-683-3523
FAX: 828-683-3511
e-mail: dsi@sunmatecushions.com
www.sunmatecushions.com

Pamela Price, Customer Service
Ellie Brown, Executive Officer Manufacturing
Cathy Ramsey, Exec Officer FIPS/Spec Projects

Line of cushions, pads and accessory items for personal comfort of the disabled. SunMate Orthopedic foam cushions and sheets that contours slowly to give uniform pressure distribution and soft spring back. Liquid SunMate for Foam-in-Place Seating (FIPS) to make custom molded seat inserts.

285 **Twin-Rest Seat Cushion & Glamour Pillow**

Better Sleep
57 Industrial Road
Berkeley Heights, NJ 07922
908-464-2200
FAX: 908-464-0058

Makes any seat more comfortable because it is ingeniously designed to soothe sensitive areas while at work, in the car or at home.

Dressing Aids

286 **Button Aid**

Maxi Aids
42 Executive Boulevard
Suite 3209
Farmingdale, NY 11735
631-752-0521
800-522-6294
FAX: 631-752-0689
e-mail: sales@maxiaids.com
www.maxiaids.com

Makes buttoning possible with the use of only one hand. *$9.95*

287 **Clothing Identification Kit**

Sense-Sations
919 Walnut Street
Philadelphia, PA 19107
215-627-0600
FAX: 215-922-0692

This kit contains labels and tells you what is on the hanger. *$7.75*

288 **Deluxe Sock and Stocking Aid**

Therapro
225 Arlington Street
Framingham, MA 01702
508-872-9494
800-257-5376
FAX: 508-875-2062
e-mail: info@theraproducts.com
www.theraproducts.com

Flexible plastic, lined with blue nylon to reduce friction and outside with beige terry cloth to hold sock firmly until it is on the foot. *$12.95*

289 **Dressing Stick**

Maxi Aids
42 Executive Boulevard
Suite 3209
Farmingdale, NY 11735
631-752-0521
800-522-6294
FAX: 631-752-0689
e-mail: sales@maxiaids.com
www.maxiaids.com

Helps put on coats, sweaters and garments even when arm and shoulder movement is limited. *$7.95*

290 **Elastic Shoelaces**

Therapro
225 Arlington Street
Framingham, MA 01702
508-872-9494
800-257-5376
FAX: 508-875-2062
e-mail: info@theraproducts.com
www.theraproducts.com

The elastic laces allow the wearer to slip tied shoes on and off. *$4.25*

291 **Featherweight Reachers**

Therapro
225 Arlington Street
Framingham, MA 01702
508-872-9494
800-257-5376
FAX: 508-875-2062
e-mail: info@theraproducts.com
www.theraproducts.com

Useful in dressing or retrieving objects. *$17.95*

292 **Folding Dressing Stick**

Access with Ease
PO Box 1150
Chino Valley, AZ 86323
928-636-9469
800-531-9479
FAX: 928-636-0292
e-mail: KMJC@northlink.com

Helps the physically-challenged user put on shirts, coats and jackets easily. The dressing sticks are available 12 to 28 inches long. Folds for easy storage. *$16.95*

293 **Heavy Duty Sock Tuckers**

Sense-Sations
919 Walnut Street
Philadelphia, PA 19107
215-627-0600
FAX: 215-922-0692

This device keeps socks and hosiery paired throughout the laundering cycles. *$1.50*

294 **Mirror Go Lightly**

AbleNet
1081 10th Avenue SE
Minneapolis, MN 55414
800-322-0956
FAX: 612-379-9143
e-mail: customerservice@ablenetinc.com
www.ablenetinc.com

Framed in plastic, the mirror can be tilted to provide either a normal or magnified image or to direct its lights at, or away from, the user. *$22.00*

295 **Molded Sock and Stocking Aid**

Therapro
225 Arlington Street
Framingham, MA 01702
508-872-9494
800-257-5376
FAX: 508-875-2062
e-mail: info@theraproducts.com
www.theraproducts.com

Sock or stocking is pulled over the molded plastic and then can be put on more easily. *$13.25*

296 **Say What**

Maxi Aids
42 Executive Boulevard
Suite 3209
Farmingdale, NY 11735
631-752-0521
800-522-6294
FAX: 631-752-0689
e-mail: sales@maxiaids.com
www.maxiaids.com

Braille the tag with information that the wearer wants on the tag and place the tag on a hanger. The custom-identification program makes it easier for the user to remember and identify just the right clothes. *$4.95*

Health Aids

297 **AMI**

PO Box 808
Groton, CT 06340
860-536-3735
800-248-4031
FAX: 860-536-4362
e-mail: amiaqua@aol.com
www.amiaqua.com

David Cote, President
Dow Cote, Domestic Sales Manager

The Aqua PT provides the major benefits of Hydrotherapy, Massage Therapy and Dry Heat Therapy. 36 water jets provide continuous full body or localized massage while the client remains CLOTHED AND DRY! Adjustable water pressure, temperature and pulsation frequency can massage in either a two direction travel mode for musculoskeletal pain management or a one direction mode flowing water from head to foot for a contrast massage-relax therapy. $25,000 to $30,000.

298 **Absorbent Dressing Powder**

Baxter Healthcare Corporation
1 Baxter Parkway
Deerfield, IL 60015
847-948-2000
FAX: 847-948-3948
www.baxter.com

Powder dressing for the treatment of pressure sores and other skin ulcers.

299 American Medical Industries

330 E 3rd Street
Suite 2
Dell Rapids, SD 57022
605-428-5501
FAX: 605-428-5502
e-mail: amiusa@siouxvalley.nets
www.ezhealthcare.com

Dan Anderson, VP

EZ-Swallow, EZ-Health, EZ-Home Care, Kleen-Handz, Kleen-Scent, EZ-Irrigator, EZ-VU, Pureshark, Gobot and AMI are all trademarks of American Medical Industries. Healthcare products made easy.

300 Aud-A-Mometer

Maxi Aids
42 Executive Boulevard
Suite 3209
Farmingdale, NY 11735
631-752-0521
800-522-6294
FAX: 631-752-0689
e-mail: sales@maxiaids.com
www.maxiaids.com

Audible clinical thermometer. *$199.95*

301 BIPAP S/T Ventilatory Support System

Respironics
1010 Murry Ridge Lane
Murrysville, PA 15668
724-387-4000
FAX: 724-387-5012
e-mail: customerservice@respironics.com
www.respironics.com

James Liken, President/CEO
Gerald McGinnis, Chairman
Daniel Bevevino, VP/CFO

Respironics, a recognized resource in the medical device market, provides innovative products and unique designs to the health care provider while helping them to grow and manage their business efficiently.

302 Bath and Shower Bench 3301B

Mada Medical Products
625 Washington Avenue
Carlstadt, NJ 07072
201-460-0454
800-526-6370
FAX: 201-460-3509
e-mail: sales@madamedical.com
www.madainternational.com

The bath and shower bench is corrosion resistent, has a cross brace design and angled legs to prevent tipping, and seat height adjustments.

303 Bed Rails

Mada Medical Products
625 Washington Avenue
Carlstadt, NJ 07072
201-460-0454
800-526-6370
FAX: 201-460-3509
e-mail: sales@madamedical.com
www.madainternational.com

Chrome plated steel rails and crossbars, all welded construction, telescopic side rail length adjustable, and a standard rail height of 16 inches.

304 Coast to Coast Home Medical

3381 Fairlane Farms Road
Suite 4D
Wellington, FL 33414
800-330-6316

Home-delivered medical supplies for diabetes, respiratory, arthritis and impotence supplies.

305 Crutches

Mada Medical Products
625 Washington Avenue
Carlstadt, NJ 07072
201-460-0454
800-526-6370
FAX: 201-460-3509
e-mail: sales@madamedical.com
www.madainternational.com

All aluminum construction, underarm crutch with double pushbutton height adjustment.

306 Drew Karol Industries

PO Box 1066
Greenville, MS 38702
601-378-2188
FAX: 601-378-3188
e-mail: dki@techinfo.com

Andrew Hoszowski, President

Orally operated toothbrush and dental care system for persons with limited or complete loss of hand or arm use - wheelchair accessible. *$600.00*

307 Duraline Medical Products

324 Werner Street
PO Box 67
Leipsic, OH 95856
419-943-2044
800-654-3376
FAX: 419-943-3637
e-mail: duraline@q1.net
www.dmponline.com

An assortment of quality incontinence products for adults.

308 Duro-Med Industries

1778 W Cherry Street
Jessup, GA 31545
800-526-4753
FAX: 800-479-7968

Manufacturers of a complete line of Home Health Care products. Featured products are patient gowns, back and seat cushions, pillows and a complete line of aids for daily living.

309 Easy Ply

BioMedical Life Systems
PO Box 1360
Vista, CA 92085
800-726-8367
FAX: 760-727-4220
e-mail: information@bmls.com
www.bmls.com

This disposable electrode has a cloth backing of a super-breathable medical tape that allows for comfort and a longer life.

310 Electronic Stethoscopes

HARC Mercantile
PO Box 3055
Kalamazoo, MI 49003
269-324-1615
800-445-9968
FAX: 269-324-2387
e-mail: home@harcmercantile.com
www.harcmercantile.com

Ronald Slager, President

High production fidelity with a number volume control wheel. *$454.95*

311 **Emergency Medical Identification with Free Fax**

Merion Station Mail Order Company
PO Box 11
Jenkintown, PA 19046
800-333-8247
800-333-TAGS
FAX: 877-738-2500

Linda R Katz, President
Alex Katz, Secretary/Treasurer

Emergency medical identification tags, pendants and bracelets. *$24.95*

312 **Fold-Down 3-in-1 Commode**

Mada Medical Products
625 Washington Avenue
Carlstadt, NJ 07072
201-460-0454
800-526-6370
FAX: 201-460-3509
e-mail: sales@madamedical.com
www.madainternational.com

The Fold-Down commode is constructed of heavy duty 1 inch diameter steel tubing with X frame, has folding features convenient for storage and transport, easily removable back rest, and full length armrests.

313 **Freedom Three Wheel Walker**

Mada Medical Products
625 Washington Avenue
Carlstadt, NJ 07072
201-460-0454
800-526-6370
FAX: 201-460-3509
e-mail: sales@madamedical.com
www.madainternational.com

The freedom walker has ultra light touch locking loop brakes and sure grip hand grips.

314 **Grab Bars and Tub Rails**

Mada Medical Products
625 Washington Avenue
Carlstadt, NJ 07072
201-460-0454
800-526-6370
FAX: 201-460-3509
e-mail: sales@madamedical.com
www.madainternational.com

Several models made of heavy walled steel, available in knurled steel or white epoxy paint, various lengths and round flanges for either vertical or horizontal mounting.

315 **Healing Dressing for Pressure Sores**

Baxter Healthcare Corporation
1 Baxter Parkway
Deerfield, IL 60015
847-948-2000
FAX: 847-948-3948
www.baxter.com

A dressing specifically designed to promote healing of pressure sores and other dermal ulcers.

316 **Invacare Corporation**

One Invacare Way
Elyria, OH 44035
440-329-6000
800-333-6900
FAX: 440-329-6568
e-mail: selder@invacare.com
www.invacare.com

Susan Elder, Dir of Marketing Communications

The world's leading manufacturer and distributor of medical products which promote recovery and active lifestyles through more than 25,000 providers worldwide.

317 **Liberty Lightweight Aluminum Stroll Walker**

Mada Medical Products
625 Washington Avenue
Carlstadt, NJ 07072
201-460-0454
800-526-6370
FAX: 201-460-3509
e-mail: sales@madamedical.com
www.madainternational.com

The Liberty walker has a spring loaded push down braking system, adjustable handle height with locking system, a 12" wide fully padded seat, and a removable shopping basket.

318 **MADAMIST 50/50 PSI Air Compressor**

Mada Medical Products
625 Washington Avenue
Carlstadt, NJ 07072
201-460-0454
800-526-6370
FAX: 201-460-3509
e-mail: sales@madamedical.com
www.madainternational.com

The new compressor rated at 50 PSI is designed to drive humidifiers, nebulizers, mist tents and ideal to administer pentamidine aerosol therapy.

319 **MOMS Catalog**

24700 Avenue Rockefeller
Valencia, CA 91355
800-232-7443
FAX: 800-622-3429
e-mail: customercare@momscatalog.com
www.momscatalog.com

MOMS catalog features high quality incontinence supplies, mobility products, bath safety products urological products, aids for daily living products, ostomy supplies and many other adpative items. MOMS offers low prices, excellent customer service and convenient home delivery to your doorstep.

52 pages

320 **MedDev Corporation**

730 N Pastoria Avenue
Sunnyvale, CA 94085
408-730-9702
800-543-2789
FAX: 408-730-9732
e-mail: info@meddev-corp.com
www.meddev-corp.com

Aids to rehabilitate hands following injury or illness, including patented complementary FingerHelper, ThumbHelper and Iso HandHelper models. Med Dev also manufactures Soft Touch foam exercisers and the FiddlLink exerciser for digital dexterity. The Ultimate Hand Helper, an Ergonomically designed hand excerciser, is curved to conform to the shape of the hand.

321 **Medi-Grip**

Therapro
225 Arlington Street
Framingham, MA 01702
508-872-9494
800-257-5376
FAX: 508-875-2062
e-mail: info@theraproducts.com
www.theraproducts.com

Reasonably priced, non-skid material. This non-slip material is available in Marine Blue, Desert Sand and Burgundy rolls 12 inches x 144 inches. *$11.95*

322 **Patient Deluxe Transport Chair 3250TC**

Mada Medical Products
625 Washington Avenue
Carlstadt, NJ 07072
201-460-0454
800-526-6370
FAX: 201-460-3509
e-mail: sales@madamedical.com
www.madainternational.com

Mada's lightweight design transport chair is constructed of heavy gauge chrome-plated, steel tubing with reinforced cross braces.

323 **Patient Transport Chair 3200TC**

Mada Medical Products
625 Washington Avenue
Carlstadt, NJ 07072
201-460-0454
800-526-6370
FAX: 201-460-3509
e-mail: sales@madamedical.com
www.madainternational.com

Mada's lightweight design transport chair is constructed of heavy gauge chrome-plated, steel tubing with reinforced cross braces.

324 **Patriot Extra Wide Folding Walkers**

Mada Medical Products
625 Washington Avenue
Carlstadt, NJ 07072
201-460-0454
800-526-6370
FAX: 201-460-3509
e-mail: sales@madamedical.com
www.madainternational.com

The extra wide walkers have padded foam hand grips, two-stage push button folding mechanism, dual width adjustment, height adjustment, and non-skid tips.

325 **Patriot Folding Walker Series**

Mada Medical Products
625 Washington Avenue
Carlstadt, NJ 07072
201-460-0454
800-526-6370
FAX: 201-460-3509
e-mail: sales@madamedical.com
www.madainternational.com

The patriot walker has high density padded foam hand grips, high strength 1" lightweight anodized dull silver aluminum tube construction, adjustable height with push-button lock security, non-skid tips, and a single button folding mechanism.

326 **Patriot Reciprocal Folding Walkers**

Mada Medical Products
625 Washington Avenue
Carlstadt, NJ 07072
201-460-0454
800-526-6370
FAX: 201-460-3509
e-mail: sales@madamedical.com
www.madainternational.com

The reciprocal folding walkers have padded foam hand grips, height adjustable with snap in security, double front cross brace, and non-skid tips.

327 **Pocket Otoscope**

HARC Mercantile
PO Box 3055
Kalamazoo, MI 49003
269-324-1615
800-445-9968
FAX: 269-324-2387
e-mail: home@harcmercantile.com
www.harcmercantile.com

Ronald Slager, President

Simple, durable and dependable pocket otoscope uses standard replaceable parts. *$24.00*

328 **Quad Canes**

Mada Medical Products
625 Washington Avenue
Carlstadt, NJ 07072
201-460-0454
800-526-6370
FAX: 201-460-3509
e-mail: sales@madamedical.com
www.madainternational.com

There are large and small base quad canes with high density foam grips.

329 **Standard 3-in-1 Commode**

Mada Medical Products
625 Washington Avenue
Carlstadt, NJ 07072
201-460-0454
800-526-6370
FAX: 201-460-3509
e-mail: sales@madamedical.com
www.madainternational.com

The standard commode is constructed of a heavy duty anodized aluminum frame, seat adjustment and an easily removable back rest.

330 **Standard Wheelchair 3100DELR**

Mada Medical Products
625 Washington Avenue
Carlstadt, NJ 07072
201-460-0454
800-526-6370
FAX: 201-460-3509
e-mail: sales@madamedical.com
www.madainternational.com

Mada's standard wheelchairs are designed and built for long-lasting, reliable operation. Each wheelchair is constructed of heavy gauge chrome plated steel framework and tube in tube construction at stress points. Mada's state-of-the art engineering uses the most modern components to provide the strength needed while keeping the chair's weight down.

331 **Standard Wheelchair 3100F**

Mada Medical Products
625 Washington Avenue
Carlstadt, NJ 07072
201-460-0454
800-526-6370
FAX: 201-460-3509
e-mail: sales@madamedical.com
www.madainternational.com

Mada's standard wheelchairs are designed and built for long-lasting, reliable operation. Each wheelchair is constructed of heavy gauge chrome plated steel framework and tube in tube construction at stress points. Mada's state-of-the art engineering uses the most modern components to provide the strength needed while keeping the chair's weight down.

332 **Stick Canes**

Mada Medical Products
625 Washington Avenue
Carlstadt, NJ 07072
201-460-0454
800-526-6370
FAX: 201-460-3509
e-mail: sales@madamedical.com
www.madainternational.com

Mada's stick canes are adjustable with a locking security system.

333 Strider

Osborn Medical Corporation
100 W Main Street
PO Box 324
Utica, MN 55979
507-932-5028
800-535-5865
FAX: 507-932-5044
www.osbornmedical.com

Strider allows you to exercise in most chairs found in your home. No more small, uncomfortable bicycle seats to sit on while exercising. With Strider, your hands are free to read the paper or your favorite book while you exercise.

334 Talking Thermometers

Maxi Aids
42 Executive Boulevard
Suite 3209
Farmingdale, NY 11735
631-752-0521
800-522-6294
FAX: 631-752-0689
e-mail: sales@maxiaids.com
www.maxiaids.com

Clearly announces temperature in Fahrenheit or Celcius. *$17.95*

335 Transfer Bench

Mada Medical Products
625 Washington Avenue
Carlstadt, NJ 07072
201-460-0454
800-526-6370
FAX: 201-460-3509
e-mail: sales@madamedical.com
www.madainternational.com

The transfer bench is a one piece bench with a wide base for stability, 1" diameter aluminum framework, corrosion resistant, and an adjustable seat.

Hearing Aids

336 Battery Device Adapter

AbleNet
1081 10th Avenue SE
Minneapolis, MN 55414
800-322-0956
FAX: 612-379-9143
e-mail: customerservice@ablenetinc.com
www.ablenetinc.com

Mary Kay Walch

A cable which connects to and adapts battery-operated devices for external switch control. Two sizes are available to adapt devices with either AA or C and D size batteries. *$8.00*

337 Custom Earmolds

Lloyd Hearing Aid Corporation
128 Kishwaukee Street
PO Box 1645
Rockford, IL 61104
815-964-4191
800-323-4212
FAX: 815-964-8378
e-mail: hearingaids@inwave.com
www.lloydhearingaid.com

Andrew Palmquist, President

Hearing aid molds, custom built to the exact fit of the customer. *$29.95*

Yearly

338 Digital Hearing Aids

Lloyd Hearing Aid Corporation
128 Kishwaukee Street
Rockford, IL 61104
815-964-4191
800-323-4212
FAX: 815-964-8378
e-mail: hearingaids@inwave.com

Latest hearing technology. Huge discounts on most makes. *$7.50*

339 Discounts on Hearing Aids

Lloyd Hearing Aid Corporation
128 Kishwaukee Street
PO Box 1645
Rockford, IL 61104
815-964-4191
800-323-4212
FAX: 815-964-8378
e-mail: hearingaids@inwave.com

Andrew Palmquist, President

Hearing aids at discounts of up to 60%. Most makes and models with service to/from anywhere in the US with a 30-day home trial. Start at $300.

340 Doorbell Signalers

HARC Mercantile
PO Box 3055
Kalamazoo, MI 49003
269-324-1615
800-445-9968
FAX: 269-324-2387
e-mail: home@harcmercantile.com
www.harcmercantile.com

Ronald Slager, President

Doorbell signalers to alert with either louder chime or flashing light. *$29.99*

341 Double Gong Indoor/Outdoor Ringer

HARC Mercantile
PO Box 3055
Kalamazoo, MI 49003
269-324-1615
800-445-9968
FAX: 269-324-2387
e-mail: home@harcmercantile.com
www.harcmercantile.com

Ronald Slager, President

Loud outdoor ringer that attaches to the wall for outside applications. *$50.00*

342 Duracell & Rayovac Hearing Aid Batteries

Lloyd Hearing Aid Corporation
128 Kishwaukee Street
Rockford, IL 61104
815-964-4191
800-323-4212
FAX: 815-964-8378
e-mail: hearingaids@inwave.com

Andrew Palmquist, President

Batteries for hearing aids at discounted prices. As low as 70 cents each.

343 Harris Communications

Harris Communications
15155 Technology Drive
Eden Prairie, MN 55344
952-906-1180
800-825-6758
FAX: 952-906-1099
e-mail: mail@harriscomm.com
www.harriscomm.com

Bill Williams, National Sales Manager

A national distributor of assistive devices for the deaf and hard of hearing with many manufacturers represented. Catalog includes a wide range of assistive devices as well as a variety of books and videotapes related to deaf and hard-of-hearing issues. Products available for children, teachers, hearing professionals, interpreters and anyone interested in deaf culture, hearing loss and sign language.

180 pages Yearly

344 Hearing Aid Batteries

HARC Mercantile
PO Box 3055
Kalamazoo, MI 49003 **269-324-1615**
800-445-9968
FAX: 269-324-2387
e-mail: home@harcmercantile.com
www.harcmercantile.com

Ronald Slager, President

Hearing aid batteries in all popular sizes in mercury, zinc air, silver as well as Nicad and Varta and batteries for electrolarynx and infrared systems. $3.95-$25.00.

345 Hearing Aid Battery Testers

HARC Mercantile
PO Box 3055
Kalamazoo, MI 49003 **269-324-1615**
800-445-9968
FAX: 269-324-2387
e-mail: home@harcmercantile.com
www.harcmercantile.com

Ronald Slager, President

From pocket size to professional type battery testers which test mercury, zinc air, silver, specialty and general usage batteries. *$11.95*

346 Hearing Aid Dehumidifier

HARC Mercantile
PO Box 3055
Kalamazoo, MI 49003 **269-324-1615**
800-445-9968
FAX: 269-324-2387
e-mail: home@harcmercantile.com
www.harcmercantile.com

Ronald Slager, President

Removes moisture from hearing aids and valuables. Contains desiccant pack and humidity guide, all in a rugged, vinyl case which provides protection and is water resistant. *$6.00*

347 In the Ear Hearing Aid Battery Extractor

HARC Mercantile
PO Box 3055
Kalamazoo, MI 49003 **269-324-1615**
800-445-9968
FAX: 269-324-2387
e-mail: home@harcmercantile.com
www.harcmercantile.com

Ronald Slager, President

Ideal tool to use when battery is stuck in battery compartment in ITE and canal hearing aids. *$3.00*

348 Micro Audiometrics Corporation

655 Keller Road
Murphy, NC 28906 **828-644-0771**
800-729-9509
FAX: 828-644-0772
e-mail: sales@microaud.com
www.microaud.com

Jason Keller, VP
Lance Ralph, Marketing

Manufacturer and distributor of hearing testing instruments, including the complete line of Earscan.

349 Model E-90W Hearing Aid

Rhodes Hearing
PO Box 358
Brookport, IL 62910 **618-564-2026**

This hearing aid slips directly into the ear. *$327.00*

350 Model F-188T Hearing Aid

Rhodes Hearing
PO Box 358
Brookport, IL 62910 **618-564-2026**

Designed to fit behind your ear at the most natural hearing level for detecting both distance and sound direction. *$329.00*

351 Mushroom Inserts

Lloyd Hearing Aid Corporation
128 Kishwaukee Street
PO Box 1645
Rockford, IL 61104 **815-964-4191**
800-323-4212
FAX: 815-964-8378
e-mail: hearingaids@inwave.com

A universal earplug useful in wearing behind the ear type hearing instruments. *$2.50*

352 Oval Window Audio

33 Wildflower Court
Nederland, CO 80466 **303-447-3607**
FAX: 303-447-3607
e-mail: info@ovalwindowaudio.com
www.ovalwindowaudio.com

Norman Lederman, Director R&D
Paula Hendricks, Educational Director

Manufacturer of induction loop hearing assistance technologies compatible with hearing aids already used by many hard of hearing people. Also multisensory sound systems for use in speech and music therapy and science classes.

Kitchen & Eating Aids

353 Bagel Holder

Maxi Aids
42 Executive Boulevard
Suite 3209
Farmingdale, NY 11735 **631-752-0521**
800-522-6294
FAX: 631-752-0689
e-mail: sales@maxiaids.com
www.maxiaids.com

Holds bagels in place for easy slicing. *$3.95*

354 Big Bold Timer Low Vision

Maxi Aids
42 Executive Boulevard
Suite 3209
Farmingdale, NY 11735 **631-752-0521**
800-522-6294
FAX: 631-752-0689
e-mail: sales@maxiaids.com
www.maxiaids.com

Sixty-minute mechanical timer with large, easy-to-read numbers for the vision impaired. *$9.95*

355 Box Top Opener

Sammons Preston Rolyan
4 Sammons Court
Bolingbrook, IL 60440
630-226-1300
800-323-5547
FAX: 630-226-1389
e-mail: spr@abilityone.com
www.sammonsprestonrolyan.com

This handy device exerts the pressure on those hard-to-open boxes of laundry/dishwasher soap, rice and prepared dinners. *$2.95*

356 Capscrew

Access with Ease
PO Box 1150
Chino Valley, AZ 86323
928-636-9469
800-531-9479
FAX: 928-636-0292
e-mail: KMJC@northlink.com

Remove lids and caps easily. Can be mounted on walls or cupboards. Non-slip surface grips small and large jars. *$7.95*

357 Cool Handle

Maxi Aids
42 Executive Boulevard
Suite 3209
Farmingdale, NY 11735
631-752-0521
800-522-6294
FAX: 631-752-0689
e-mail: sales@maxiaids.com
www.maxiaids.com

A specially designed, heat-resistant handle, available in three sizes which can be affixed to the handles of most fry, sauce and saute pans. *$7.95*

358 Cordless Receiver

AbleNet
1081 10th Avenue SE
Minneapolis, MN 55414
800-322-0956
FAX: 612-379-9143
e-mail: customerservice@ablenetinc.com
www.ablenetinc.com

The Cordless Receiver in conjunction with the Cordless Big Red Switch, can be used anywhere a switch is currently used to control battery or electrically-operated toys, games or appliances; augmentative communication systems; and computers (through a computer switch interface). *$79.00*

359 Deluxe Long Ring Low Vision Timer

Maxi Aids
42 Executive Boulevard
Suite 3209
Farmingdale, NY 11735
631-752-0521
FAX: 631-752-0689
e-mail: sales@maxiaids.com
www.maxiaids.com

Bold black numerals on white background allows for easy reading at any distance. *$17.95*

360 Deluxe Roller Knife

Sammons Preston Rolyan
4 Sammons Court
Bolingbrook, IL 60440
630-226-1300
800-323-5547
FAX: 630-226-1389
e-mail: spr@abilityone.com
www.sammonsprestonrolyan.com

Stainless steel blade rolls smoothly, cutting food cleanly. *$10.95*

361 Dual Brush with Suction Base

Sammons Preston Rolyan
4 Sammons Court
Bolingbrook, IL 60440
630-226-1300
800-323-5547
FAX: 630-226-1389
e-mail: spr@abilityone.com
www.sammonsprestonrolyan.com

Two brushes clean the inside and outside of bottles and glasses at the same time using just one hand. *$14.50*

362 Easy Pour Locking Lid Pot

Maxi Aids
42 Executive Boulevard
Suite 3209
Farmingdale, NY 11735
631-752-0521
800-522-6294
FAX: 631-752-0689
e-mail: sales@maxiaids.com
www.maxiaids.com

Baked enamel and dishwasher safe, the pot comes with an easy lid that locks in place for extra safety. *$24.95*

363 Electric Can Opener & Knife Sharpener

Maxi Aids
42 Executive Boulevard
Suite 3209
Farmingdale, NY 11735
631-752-0521
800-522-6294
FAX: 631-752-0689
e-mail: sales@maxiaids.com
www.maxiaids.com

Features include a powerful magnet lid holder, the ability to open odd-shaped cans, and easy operation for the physically challenged. *$19.95*

364 Evio Plastics

310 Industrial Parkway
PO Box 2295
Sandysky, OH 44870
419-621-1105
FAX: 419-626-2183

Doug Didion, Admininstrator Director

Handi Holder is a plastic holder for 1/2 gallon paper cartons of milk or juice. It is used to pour milk or juice without spills by using the handle.

365 Food Markers/Rubberbands

Maxi Aids
42 Executive Boulevard
Suite 3209
Farmingdale, NY 11735
800-522-6294
FAX: 631-752-0689
e-mail: sales@maxiaids.com
www.maxiaids.com

These are durable plastic markers, easily identified by touch, texture, shape and form which help the visually impaired orient themselves to food location on the plate. *$11.95*

366 Funnel

Sense-Sations
919 Walnut Street
Philadelphia, PA 19107
215-627-0600
FAX: 215-922-0692

Wide mouth funnel aids in pouring liquids or dry goods from container to container. *$1.25*

367 **Good Grips Cutlery**

Therapro
225 Arlington Street
Framingham, MA 01702 **508-872-9494**
800-257-5376
FAX: 508-875-2062
e-mail: info@theraproducts.com
www.theraproducts.com

Stainless steel utensils have a special twist built into the metal to facilitate bending of a spoon or fork at any angle for right or left handed people. *$7.50*

368 **Granberg Superior Systems**

2502 Thayer Avenue
Saskatoon
Saskatchewan, CANADA, S7L5Y **306-374-9440**
FAX: 306-373-8715

Height adjustable cabinets for easy reach to food and other necessities.

369 **Guide A Knife**

Maxi Aids
42 Executive Boulevard
Suite 3209
Farmingdale, NY 11735 **631-752-0521**
800-522-6294
FAX: 631-752-0689
e-mail: sales@maxiaids.com
www.maxiaids.com

Adjustable food slicing system guides the knife for even, uniform slices while protecting the user. *$11.95*

370 **Handy-Helper Cutting Board**

Maxi Aids
42 Executive Boulevard
Suite 3209
Farmingdale, NY 11735 **631-752-0521**
800-522-6294
FAX: 631-752-0689
e-mail: sales@maxiaids.com
www.maxiaids.com

Laminated cutting board with unique features to hold food in place with corner ledge for cutting and spreading. *$19.95*

371 **Innerlip Plates**

Therapro
225 Arlington Street
Framingham, MA 01702 **508-872-9494**
800-257-5376
FAX: 508-875-2062
e-mail: info@theraproducts.com
www.theraproducts.com

Food may be pushed to the side of the plate, then scooped up with a fork and spoon. Available in beige or blue. *$5.00*

372 **Jordan's Motility Solutions: Adapt-Able Utensils**

PO Box 132772
Tyler, TX 75713 **903-526-2100**
FAX: 903-526-2103
e-mail: info@disabilityaccessories.com
www.disabilityaccessories.com

Gene Howland, President

Adapt-Able eating utensils encourage independent eating for individuals with limited mobility. Angle and reach of utensils can be adjusted to address specific needs.

373 **Long Oven Mitts**

Sammons Preston Rolyan
4 Sammons Court
Bolingbrook, IL 60440 **630-226-1300**
800-323-5547
FAX: 630-226-1389
e-mail: spr@abilityone.com
www.sammonsprestonrolyan.com

Protect hands and forearms from heat, flames and oven grates with these practical mitts that allow a longer reach and less bending. *$8.95*

374 **Magnetic Card Reader**

Maxi Aids
42 Executive Boulevard
Suite 3209
Farmingdale, NY 11735
800-522-6294
FAX: 631-752-0689
e-mail: sales@maxiaids.com
www.maxiaids.com

Produces audible labels so a recorded card can be taped on cans of food or a box of cake mix; even adding instructions for baking. *$159.95*

375 **Make-and-Shake Ice Tray**

Sense-Sations
919 Walnut Street
Philadelphia, PA 19107 **215-627-0600**
FAX: 215-922-0692

A covered ice tray that can be filled with water and then safely transported to the freezer without spilling. *$2.00*

376 **Maxi Aid Braille Timer**

Maxi Aids
42 Executive Boulevard
PO Box 3209
Farmingdale, NY 11735 **631-752-0521**
800-522-6294
FAX: 631-752-0689
e-mail: sales@maxiaids.com
www.maxiaids.com

Three raised dots at 15, 30 and 45, two raised dots at remaining five minute intervals and one raised dot at remaining two and a half minute intervals, offers ease of operation to make this a helpful aid for the visually impaired. *$12.95*

377 **Nosey Cup**

Therapro
225 Arlington Street
Framingham, MA 01702 **508-872-9494**
800-257-5376
FAX: 508-875-2062
e-mail: info@theraproducts.com
www.theraproducts.com

For those with a stiff neck or persons who can't tip their head back while drinking. *$6.00*

378 **Paring Boards**

Therapro
225 Arlington Street
Framingham, MA 01702 **508-872-9494**
800-257-5376
FAX: 508-875-2062
e-mail: info@theraproducts.com
www.theraproducts.com

Suction feet stabilize board and stainless steel prongs hold food in place for easy one-handed cutting. *$32.50*

379 **PowerLink 2 Control Unit**

AbleNet
1081 10th Avenue SE
Minneapolis, MN 55414
800-322-0956
FAX: 612-379-9143
e-mail: customerservice@ablenetinc.com
www.ablenetinc.com

The PowerLink 2 Control Unit allows switch operation of electrical appliances. It can be used to activate 1 or 2 appliances (up to 1700 watts combined). If 2 appliances are used, they will activate simultaneously. There are four modes of control on the PowerLink 2; direct mode, timed (seconds) mode, timed (minutes) mode and latch mode. Meets safety standards from Underwriters Laboratory (UL) and Canadian Standards Association (CSA) for electrical appliances. *$159.00*

380 **Sammons Preston Rolyan**

4 Sammons Court
Bolingbrook, IL 60440
630-226-1300
800-323-5547
FAX: 630-226-1389
e-mail: spr@abilityone.com
www.sammonsprestonrolyan.com

Sammons Preston Rolyan is a leading provider of rehabilitation and assistive devices to help those with disabilities meet daily physical challenges and achieve their greatest level of independence. With one of the industry's largest catalogs, Sammons Preston Rolyan offers a wide range of products available.

Annually

381 **Slicing Aid**

Snug Seat
PO Box 1739
Matthews, NC 28106
704-882-0668
800-336-7684
FAX: 704-882-0751
e-mail: sales@snugseat.com
www.snugseat.com

Earlene Hucks, Marketing Coordinator

The design of these knives allows a better working posture and makes optimal use of strength in the arms and hands.

382 **Small Appliance Receiver**

AbleNet
1081 10th Avenue SE
Minneapolis, MN 55414
800-322-0956
FAX: 612-379-9143
e-mail: customerservice@ablenetinc.com
www.ablenetinc.com

The Small Appliance Receiver, in conjunction with the Cordless Big Red Switch, allows you to control small electrical appliances in the environment without a cord. It should only be used with low-wattage appliances (under 500 watts) which have two prong plugs (ie, radios, fans, lamps, blenders, etc.). It should not be used with heat generating appliances. *$32.00*

383 **Steel Food Guard**

Maxi Aids
42 Executive Boulevard
Suite 3209
Farmingdale, NY 11735
631-752-0521
800-522-6294
FAX: 631-752-0689
e-mail: sales@maxiaids.com
www.maxiaids.com

Provides stable area to push against while eating. *$ 10.95*

384 **Thick-n-Easy**

Therapro
225 Arlington Street
Framingham, MA 01702
508-872-9494
800-257-5376
FAX: 508-875-2062
e-mail: info@theraproducts.com
www.theraproducts.com

Instant food thickener that sets in 30 seconds and will not become thicker even after refrigeration. *$6.50*

385 **Thumbs Up Cup**

Therapro
225 Arlington Street
Framingham, MA 01702
508-872-9494
800-257-5376
FAX: 508-875-2062
e-mail: info@theraproducts.com
www.theraproducts.com

This cup is designed for those with limited strength or coordination or arthritis. The two backward-tilt handles and thumb rests allow finger joints to be used to their greatest mechanical advantage. *$9.50*

386 **Un-Skru**

Multi-Marketing & Manufacturers
PO Box 1070
Littleton, CO 80160
800-506-0248
e-mail: penlane@xpert.net
www.seniorshops.com/unskru.html

Janet Lane, President

This jar and bottle opener mounts permanently to the underside of a cabinet, shelf, table or counter so it is out of sight yet always ready to use. Opens all sizes of jar lids — easily and with little strength. *$7.95*

387 **Undercounter Lid Opener**

Sammons Preston Rolyan
4 Sammons Court
Bolingbrook, IL 60440
630-226-1300
800-323-5547
FAX: 630-226-1389
e-mail: spr@abilityone.com
www.sammonsprestonrolyan.com

The gripper of this unit which installs under the counter can help unscrew any cap. *$5.75*

388 **Uni-Turner**

Sammons Preston Rolyan
4 Sammons Court
Bolingbrook, IL 60440
630-226-1300
800-323-5547
FAX: 630-226-1389
e-mail: spr@abilityone.com
www.sammonsprestonrolyan.com

Odd shaped handles can be turned easily with one handed L-shaped Uni-Turner. *$16.50*

389 **Universal Hand Cuff**

Therapro
225 Arlington Street
Framingham, MA 01702
508-872-9494
800-257-5376
FAX: 508-875-2062
e-mail: info@theraproducts.com
www.theraproducts.com

Comfortable cuff with Velcro strap holds utensils, toothbrushes, etc. *$9.95*

Lifts, Ramps & Elevators

390 Access Industries

4001 E 138th Street
Grandview, MO 64030
800-829-9760
FAX: 816-763-4467
e-mail: marketing@accessind.com
www.accessind.com

Whether you want to open your facility or stay in the home you love, Access Industries has the perfect wheelchair lift, stair lift or elevator to suit your budget and needs. Our lifts have the best warranties. Our nationwide network of dealers are close by and ready to help.

391 Accessibility Lift

Inclinator Company of America
2200 Paxton Street
Suite 1557
Harrisburg, PA 17111
717-234-8065
800-343-9007
FAX: 717-234-0941
e-mail: isaks@inclinator.com
www.inclinator.com

Dotty Keith, Sales Manager

An economical lift for restricted usage that provides barrier-free access that can be used by churches, schools, lodging halls and meeting halls to meet compliance requirements, with the dignified convenience and freedom they deserve.

392 Adjustable Incline Board

Bailey Manufacturing Company
118 Lee Street
Suite 130
Lodi, OH 44254
330-948-1080
800-321-8372
FAX: 330-948-4439
e-mail: baileymfg@attmail.com
www.baileymfg.com

Incline board for the physically challenged with a foot board with non-slip tread.

393 AlumiRamp

855 E Chicago Street
Quincy, MI 49082
517-639-8777
800-800-3864
FAX: 517-639-4314
e-mail: ramps@alumiramp.com
www.alumiramp.com

Linda Burke, President
Doug Cannon, Customer Service
Pam Kelley, Customer Service

Complete line of modular and portable ramps for both home and vehicle use. Welded construction and non-skid extruded surfaces are featured on all our ramps.

394 Area Access

8117 Ransell Road
Falls Church, VA 22042
703-573-2111
800-333-2732
FAX: 703-207-0446
e-mail: c_wenn@hotmail.com
www.areaaccess.com

Cliff Wenn, Sales Manager
Barbara Spellman, Mobility Consultant

Serving the entire Mid-Atlantic with Scooters, Stairway Lifts and Elevators. Large inventory and fully stocked showrooms.

395 Barrier Free Lifts

9230 Prince William Street
Manassas, VA 20110
703-361-6531
800-582-8732
FAX: 703-361-7861
e-mail: info@barrierfreelifts.com
www.barrierfreelifts.com

Larry Pigeon, VP of Sales
Wanda Bullock, Administrative Assistant

Barrier Free Lifts overhead track systems can be ceiling mounted, wall mounted and free standing. Mobile floor model patient lifts are also available in a variety of models. Overhead track lifts can be portable or permanently installed in track. They can be manual or fully motorized to provide state of the art equipment for lifting and transferring people. Many sling options are available to fit individual needs and a nationwide network of independent dealers is available for consultation.

396 Bruno Independent Living Aids

Bruno Independent Living Aids
1780 Executive Drive
PO Box 84
Oconomowoc, WI 53066
262-567-4990
800-882-8183
FAX: 262-567-4341
e-mail: webmaster@bruno.com
www.bruno.com

Patrick Foy, National Sales Manager
Karla Branham Shaw, Marketing

An ISO 9001 Certified Manufacturer of automotive lifts for scooter, wheelchairs, and powerchairs, three and four wheel scooters, and straight and custom curve stairlifts.

397 Butlers Wheelchair Lifts

Flinchbaugh Company
390 Eberts Lane
York, PA 17403
717-848-2418
800-326-2418
FAX: 717-843-7385

Steve Williams, President
Brian McMaster, President Sales
Greg E Ness, Sales Manager

This wheelchair lift can be equipped with an end ramp and guard. Automatically retractable, it locks firmly into place when the lift is in operation.

398 Cheney's Liberty II

Handi-Lift
1051 Paulison Avenue
Clifton, NJ 07011
845-429-0368
800-503-2003
FAX: 845-947-4522

Economical lift for straight stairways.

399 Classique

Handi-Lift
1051 Paulison Avenue
Clifton, NJ 07011
845-429-0368
800-503-2003
FAX: 845-947-4522

The Classique elevator answers access problems in churches, schools and small offices.

400 Columbus McKinnon Corporation

140 John James Audubon Parkway
Amherst, NY 14228
716-639-4224
800-888-0985
FAX: 716-696-3220

Larry Smith, Manager

Supplies various lift and transfer systems for independent or attended applications including ceiling mounted or free-standing overhead track lifts and mobile floorbase units for homes, schools and healthcare facilities. Lift Systems for transferring between bed, chair, commode or bath are available with a variety of slings, scales and accessories.

401 **Cub, SuperCub and Special Edition Scooters**

Bruno Independent Living Aids
1780 Executive Drive
PO Box 84
Oconomowoc, WI 53066
262-567-4990
800-882-8183
FAX: 262-953-5501
e-mail: webmaster@bruno.com
www.bruno.com

Patrick Foy, National Sales Manager
Karla Branham Shaw, Marketing

Bruno Independent Living Aids, Inc. has over 12 different scooter models. Bruno Cub and SuperCub scooters, has front or rear-wheel drive, in both 3 and 4-wheel versions and comes in four different colors plus a pediatric version. Each scooter can handle up to 300 pounds. Bruno Special Edition scooters resemble a fire engine, police car, Humvee and motorcycle. $2,000-$5,000

402 **Curb-Sider Super XL**

Bruno Independent Living Aids
1780 Executive Drive
PO Box 84
Oconomowoc, WI 53066
262-567-4990
800-882-8183
FAX: 262-953-5501
www.bruno.com

Michael R Bruno, Chairman of the Board/CEO

The lift of choice for storing your fully or partially assembled scooter or power chair weighing up to 400 pounds in the rear of your van or minivan, SUV, pickup truck or some station wagon applications.

403 **Custom Lift Residential Elevators**

Waupaca Elevator Company
1726 N Ballard Street
Appleton, WI 54911
920-991-9082
800-238-8739
FAX: 920-991-9087
e-mail: csr@waupacaelevator.com
www.waupacaelevator.com

Waupaca Elevator residential elevators and dumbwaiters add value, convenience and reliability to today's homes.

404 **Deluxe Convertible Exercise Staircase**

Sammons Preston Rolyan
4 Sammons Court
Bolingbrook, IL 60440
630-226-1300
800-323-5547
FAX: 630-226-1389
e-mail: spr@abilityone.com
www.sammonsprestonrolyan.com

Here's an exercise staircase to fit any department configuration. Just reposition a few nuts and bolts to change from a straight to a corner type staircase.

405 **Easy Pivot Transfer Machine**

Rand-Scot
401 Linden Center Drive
Fort Collins, CO 80524
800-467-7967
FAX: 970-467-7967
e-mail: randscot@webaccess.net
www.easypivot.com

The Easy Pivot Patient Lifting System allows for strain-free, one-caregiver transfers of the disabled individual.

406 **Easy Stand**

Altimate Medical
PO Box 180
Morton, MN 56270
507-697-6393
800-342-8969
FAX: 507-637-3024

Designed to make standing fast and simple. The easy to operate hydraulic lift system provides a controlled lifting and lowering. With the convenience of simply transferring to the chair and reaching a standing position in seconds with no straps to struggle with.

407 **Econol Elevator Lift Corporation**

2513 Center Street
Suite 854
Cedar Falls, IA 50613
800-328-2560
FAX: 319-277-4778

Sharon R Martin, President
Adrian L Martin, Sales

Offers a full line of lifts, dumbwaiters, stair riders and elevators for persons with disabilities.

408 **Econol Stairway Chair Ride**

Econol Stairway Lift Corporation
2513 Center Street
Cedar Falls, IA 50613

This chair ride unit is of sturdy steel construction and rides sideways, not backwards.

409 **Economical Liberty**

Handi-Lift
1051 Paulison Avenue
Clifton, NJ 07011
845-429-0368
800-503-2003
FAX: 845-947-4522

Installs quickly and easily on most straight stairways. It uses regular household current and mounts over the carpet or directly to the stairs without marring.

410 **Electra-Ride Elite**

Bruno Independent Living Aids
1780 Executive Drive
PO Box 84
Oconomowoc, WI 53066
262-567-4990
800-882-8183
FAX: 262-953-5501
www.bruno.com

Michael R Bruno, Chairman of the Board/CEO

The new Electra-Ride Elite installs to within 5 inches of the wall and has a 350 pound weight capacity. Bruno stairlifts can fit almost any custom curve or straight rail application and requires no structural modification to the stairway. Plus, battery power allows for uninterupted operation even during a power outage.

411 **Electra-Ride III**

Bruno Independent Living Aids
1780 Executive Drive
PO Box 84
Oconomowoc, WI 53066
262-567-4990
800-882-8183
FAX: 262-953-5501
www.bruno.com

Michael R Bruno, Chairman of the Board/CEO

Bruno stairlifts can fit almost any custom curve or straight rail application and requires no structural modification to the stairway. Plus, battery power allows for uninterrupted operation even during a power outage.

412 **Excel Stairway Lift**

Access Industries
4001 E 138th Street
Grandview, MO 64030
800-829-9760
FAX: 816-763-4467
e-mail: marketing@accessind.com
www.accessind.com

Installs easily on either side of a straight stairway for independent, step-free living. The lift fastens securely to the stairs without marring walls and is adjustable to match any stairway slope with an incline angle up to 45 degrees. Available with battery back up.

413 **Freedom Bath**

Arjo
50 N Gary Avenue
Roselle, IL 60172
630-307-2756
800-323-1245
FAX: 888-594-2756
e-mail: lchevrie@arjousa.com
www.arjo.com

Lorena Chevrie, Marketing Communications

Residents can relax on a semi-reclining seat and enjoy the soothing deluxe whirlpool system. Freedom Bath offers a revolutionary solution with its unique Roll-Door.

414 **Freedom Wheelchair Lifts**

580 TC Jester Boulevard
Houston, TX 77007
713-864-1460
FAX: 713-864-1469
e-mail: info@freedomwheels.com
www.freedomwheels.com/index.html

Sandy Patterson

Freedom Wheels, Inc. is committed to people with disabilities and personal transportation options for an independent lifestyle.

415 **Golden-Glide Stairway Lift**

Access Industries
4001 E 138th Street
Grandview, MO 64030
800-829-9760
FAX: 816-763-4467
e-mail: marketing@accessind.com
www.accessind.com

Model 95 monorail track design can be custom-made to fit virtually any stairway. The unit can carry a side rider around stairway curves and corners with 90 to 180 degree turns and one or more landings. The lift can carry a maximum of 300 pounds up to 6 feet on its roomy 17-1/2 inch seat. Call and send controls are available at top or bottom landings. A four point safety sensor is a standard security feature.

416 **Handi Home Lift**

Handi-Lift
1051 Paulison Avenue
Clifton, NJ 07011
845-429-0368
800-503-2003
FAX: 845-947-4522

An outdoor lift designed to provide access over porch stairs or other steps that impede movement.

417 **Handi Prolift**

Handi-Lift
1051 Paulison Avenue
Clifton, NJ 07011
845-429-0368
800-503-2003
FAX: 845-947-4522

Provides dependable vertical transportation for multi-level buildings.

418 **Handi-Ramp**

Handi-Ramp
510 N Avenue
Libertyville], IL 60048
847-680-7700
800-876-7267
FAX: 847-816-8866
e-mail: rampmarketing@aol.com
www.handiramp.com

Thom Disch, CEO
Doug Eickhoff, General Manager
Vicki Tumilson, Marketing Manager

Provides a complete line of economical, ADA Compliant access ramping products. Line includes Van attachable and Wheelchair Tie Downs; Aluminum or Expanded Metal Folding Portables; aluminum channels; Portable, Sectional Ramp Systems; Semi-Permanent Ramps, Platforms and Systems. All ramp series are available in varied lengths and widths in combination with platforms and optional hand railing, single or double bar construction with return ends. Special Order ramps and ramp systems. $575 and up.

419 **Homecare Products EZ-Access Portable Ramps**

15824 SE 296th Street
Kent, WA 98042
800-451-1903
FAX: 800-630-2350
e-mail: ezaccess@homecareproducts.com
www.homecareproducts.com

Don Everard, VP Marketing
Deanne Sandvold, VP Sales

EZ-ACCESS Ramps bridge gaps over curbs and steps, allowing scooters and wheelchairs to continue on a smooth, safe course. Available in several different styles and sizes, ranging from a two-foot curb ramp to a 10-foot multi-purpose ramp. All ramps are made of anodized aluminum.

420 **Homewaiter**

Inclinator Company of America
2200 Paxton Street
Suite 1557
Harrisburg, PA 17111
717-234-8065
800-343-9007
FAX: 717-234-0941
e-mail: isaks@inclinator.com
www.inclinator.com

Dotty Keith, Sales Manager

With its roller truck riding in a specially formed monorail, it is easy to install and highly adaptable to existing conditions. It can travel up to 35 feet, opening on any or all three sides at different stations, whether at counter level or floor level.

421 **Inclinette**

Inclinator Company of America
2200 Paxton Street
Suite 1557
Harrisburg, PA 17111
717-234-8065
800-343-9007
FAX: 717-234-0941
e-mail: isaks@inclinator.com
www.inclinator.com

Inclinette provides comfort and convenience in providing multi-floor access to persons who have difficulty climbing stairs.

422 **Lectra-Lift**

La-Z-Boy
1284 N Telegraph Road
Monroe, MI 48162
734-242-1444
FAX: 734-457-2005
www.lazboy.com

Gerald L Kiser, President/CEO
David M Risley, SVP/CFO
Patrick H Norton, Chairman

This power recliner has a single motor drive that operates three distinct cycles: lifting, leg elevation and full power recline.

423 **Liberty LT**

Handi-Lift
1051 Paulison Avenue
Clifton, NJ 07011
845-429-0368
800-503-2003
FAX: 845-947-4522

Stair lift with dual armrests that lock into position. The comfortable, contoured seat is designed to swivel and move forward at the bottom or top landings to facilitate transfer.

424 **Lifestand**

Independence Providers
PO Box 232171
Encinitas, CA 92023
800-782-6324
FAX: 610-586-0847
e-mail: Dallery@msn.com
www.lifestandusa.com

Jacques A Dallery, President

Lifestand offers a full line of standing wheelchairs for manual operation. Power assisted are fully motorized. *$7000.00*

425 **LiftUp**

15 Highland Road
Eastham, MA 02642
508-255-5394

Richard C Peterson, Publisher

Plans for electric transfer device, especially suitable for bathroom use, lifts user erect with unique upper-body sling. Developed by an engineer to help cope with his multiple sclerosis quadriplegia, there are many now in use. Low-cost and simple make-it-yourself. *$19.00*

426 **Lifts for Swimming Pools and Spas**

Aquatic Access
417 Dorsey Way
Louisville, KY 40223
502-425-5817
800-325-5438
FAX: 502-425-9607
e-mail: info@AquaticAccess.com
www.AquaticAccess.com

Aquatic Access manufacturers and sells water-powered lifts providing access to in-ground and above-ground swimming pools, spas, boats and docks. *$2310.00*

427 **Lizzie Lift**

Handicap Helpers
604 W Main Street
Appalachia, VA 24216
276-565-1889
FAX: 276-565-3623
e-mail: JBlevins@me.vcos.edu
www.hurtback.org

James W Blevins, President

A stable patient lift that provides independence for the disabled by allowing one caregiver to move them from bed to upright position more easily and effectively. The Lizzie Lift which can be used as a gurney bed, lounge chair or wheelchair, not only decreases back injury for caregivers but also alleviates the fear of being moved. Can be used in hospitals, nursing homes and homes. FDA listing, Patent pending. $7,000-$8,000.

428 **Mecalift Sling Lifter**

Arjo
50 N Gary Avenue
Roselle, IL 60172
630-307-2756
800-323-1245
FAX: 888-594-2756
e-mail: lchevrie@arjousa.com
www.arjo.com

Lorena Chevrie, Marketing Communications

Takes all the effort out of lifting while protecting the caregiver from the risk of backstrain.

429 **Minivator Residential Elevator**

Access Industries
4001 E 138th Street
Grandview, MO 64030
800-829-9760
FAX: 816-763-4467
e-mail: marketing@accessind.com
www.accessind.com

The perfect choice for a person who is contemplating moving from their multi-storied home because they cannot get up and down the stairs. The low cost, compact Minivator elevator can help these people live independently. The Minivator can be installed in the corner of a room without a shaft or hoistway, so the elevator doesn't have to disfigure the structure. The Minivator elevator can take a person or persons between floors in less than a minute and can accommodate a standard size wheelchair.

430 **One for All Lift All**

Amigo Mobility International
6693 Dixie Highway
Bridgeport, MI 48722
989-777-0910
800-692-6446
FAX: 989-777-8184
www.myamigo.com

Mike Galen, Comptroller
Shirley Beebe, Order/Sales Operations
Mike LeBrake, Product Manager

The Lift-All transports your wheelchair easily into the trunk of an automobile and neatly stores it for easy access.

431 **Ortho Kinetics**

W220N507 Springdale Road
Waukesha, WI 53186
800-824-1068
FAX: 262-542-4258

Anne Tyler, Director Marketing

Products to enhance people's lives through mobility. These electric three and four wheel vehicles are designed to surpass consumer expectations by providing total comfort, convenience and performance features found nowhere else. Ortho-Kinetics has a full line of vehicles for any application.

432 **Out-Sider III**

Bruno Independent Living Aids
1780 Executive Drive
PO Box 84
Oconomowoc, WI 53066
262-567-4990
800-882-8183
FAX: 262-953-5501
www.bruno.com

Michael R Bruno, Chairman of the Board/CEO

Lets you carry your scooter fully assembled and keeps your trunk space available for other things.

433 **Parker Bath**

Arjo
50 N Gary Avenue
Roselle, IL 60172 **630-307-2756**
800-323-1245
FAX: 888-594-2756
e-mail: lchevrie@arjousa.com
www.arjo.com

Lorena Chevrie, Marketing Communications

This involves no manual lifting, strain or stress for the caregiver.

434 **Pool Lifts for In-Ground Pools**

Aquatic Access
417 Dorsey Way
Louisville, KY 40223 **502-425-5817**
800-325-5438
FAX: 502-425-9607
e-mail: info@AquaticAccess.com
www.AquaticAccess.com

Provide independent or assisted access to in-ground pools. Lifts are powered with water pressure from a garden hose and are portable. Some lifts have a three-hundred pound lift capacity and others have a four-hundred pound capacity, perfect for commercial installations or home use. ADA compliant. *$3245.00*

435 **Porch-Lift Vertical Platform Lift**

Access Industries
4001 E 138th Street
Grandview, MO 64030
800-829-9760
FAX: 816-763-4467
e-mail: marketing@accessind.com
www.accessind.com

Provide stairway access indoors and out for people who use wheelchairs. Lifting heights range from 1 to 144 feet and are available for both commercial and residential applications. Easy to install and operate, the units are space and cost efficient solutions to ADA compliance.

436 **Ramplette Telescoping Ramp**

Graham-Field Health Products
2935 NE Parkway
Atlanta, GA 30360
800-347-5678
FAX: 800-726-0601
www.grahamfield.com

A multi-functional, easily moved economical ramp weighing 25 pounds.

437 **Ricon Corporation**

12450 Montague Street
Pacoima, CA 91331 **818-899-7588**
800-322-2884
FAX: 818-890-3354
www.riconcorp.com

Ricon corporation is a world leader in the manufacture of lifts and other mobility products for people with disabilities. The Ricon product line features the Activan(R) a lowered floor minivan conversion, wheelchair lifts power seat base and automatic door openers.

438 **Silver Glide Stairway Lift**

Access Industries
4001 E 138th Street
Grandview, MO 64030
800-829-9760
FAX: 816-763-4467
e-mail: marketing@accessind.com
www.accessind.com

The economical Silver-Glide easily installs on either side of a straight stairway. The seat, armrest and footrest can be folded to save stairway space when the unit is not in use. The unit plugs into an outlet at the top or bottom of the stairs and uses regular household current. Also available with battery operated system. Heavy duty steel cable drive system permits the rider to travel up to 20 feet.

439 **Smart Leg**

Invacare Corporation
899 Cleveland Street
Elyria, OH 44035 **440-329-6426**
e-mail: info@invacare.com
www.invacare.com

A Malachi Mixon III, CEO
Gerald B Blouch, President/COO
Thomas R Miklich, CFO

An ingenious elevating leg rest that automatically extends to correctly fit every outstretched leg.

440 **Smooth Mover**

Dixie EMS
385 Union Avenue
Brooklyn, NY 11211
800-347-3494
FAX: 718-387-9310
e-mail: customerSVC@dixieems.com
www.dixieems.com

Patient mover is a board designed to transfer patients from bed to stretcher or table with one or two people. *$199.95*

441 **SpectraLift**

Inclinator Company of America
2200 Paxton Street
Suite 1557
Harrisburg, PA 17111 **717-234-8065**
800-343-9007
FAX: 717-234-0941
e-mail: isaks@inclinator.com
www.inclinator.com

Dotty Keith, Sales Manager

A newly designed hydraulic wheelchair lift made of fiberglass construction suitable for commercial and residential use.

442 **Spectrum Aquatics**

7100 Spectrum Lane
Missoula, MT 59808 **406-543-5309**
800-776-5309
FAX: 406-728-7143
e-mail: info@spectrumaquatics.com
www.spectrumaquatics.com

George Bowman, VP Operations
David Murray, President
Aaron Erickson, Sales Manager

Manufacturers of swimming pool disabled access products such as lifts, ramps, railings, ladders, and stainless steel hydrotherapy tanks for the swimming pool and medical therapy markets.

443 **Stair & Glide Stairway Lift**

Access Industries
4001 E 138th Street
Grandview, MO 64030
800-829-9760
FAX: 816-763-4467
e-mail: marketing@accessind.com
www.accessind.com

Solves many multi-level accessibility problems in home. Lifts easily to install on straight or curved stairways. The rail attaches directly to steps without disturbing walls or staircase. The heavy duty drive mechanism means reliable, trouble-free operation. Public building and outdoor packages available.

444 **StairLIFT SC & SL**

Inclinator Company of America
2200 Paxton Street
Suite 1557
Harrisburg, PA 17111
717-234-8065
800-343-9007
FAX: 717-234-0941
e-mail: isaks@inclinator.com
www.inclinator.com

Simple, self-contained and efficient stair units.

445 **Stairway Elevators**

Bruno Independent Living Aids
1780 Executive Drive
Suite 84
Oconomowoc, WI 53066
262-567-4990
800-882-8183
FAX: 262-567-4341
e-mail: webmaster@bruno.com

Bruno offers a full line of stairway elevators, including the Electra-Ride II featuring access during power interruptions, convenient installation, comfort and a powerful drive system. The Electra-Ride which features battery-powered technology, a rail width of 25 inches and seat rotation for easy transfers. The Comfort-Ride AC stair lift which is battery operated, has a rail width of 7.25 inches and folded width of less than 14.5 inches.

446 **Stand Aid**

Stand Aid of Iowa
1009 Second Avenue
PO Box 386
Sheldon, IA 51201
800-831-8580
FAX: 712-324-5210
e-mail: standaid@reconnect.com
www.standaid.com

Stand Aid can help you achieve independence and mobility safely and easily. Lifts you from a chair or bed with the flick of a switch, securing the user in an upright standing position.

447 **Straight and Custom Curved Stairlifts**

Bruno Independent Living Aids
1780 Executive Drive
PO Box 84
Oconomowoc, WI 53066
262-567-4990
800-882-8183
FAX: 262-953-5501
e-mail: webmaster@bruno.com
www.bruno.com

Patrick Foy, National Sales Manager
Karla Branham Shaw, Marketing

Bruno stairlifts can fit almost any curve or straight rail application and requires little or no structural modification to the stairway. Normal rail position for a Bruno inside turn is 7 to 8 inches from the wall or obstruction which is the tightest radius of any stairlift manufacturing company in the world. The Bruno inside turn is ideal for bi-level homes or staircases with mid-level doors. Bruno's unique battery power allows for uninterrupted operation even during a power outage.

448 **SureHands Lift & Care Systems**

982 Route 1
Pine Island, NY 10969
845-258-6500
800-724-5305
FAX: 845-258-6634
e-mail: info@surehands.com
www.surehands.com

Thomas Herceg, President
Joyce Moraczewski, Marketing Coordinator

SureHands Lift & Care Systems offer a unique, patented and exlusive range of lift and transfer systems to meet private and institutional needs of individuals with motor disabilties. Includes permanent and portable models for homes, workplaces and recreation. The SureHands Body Support offers safe, easy and secure transfers for user and the opportunity for independent transfers for some. They are a back-saver for caregivers. All lifts are easily maintained and operated with mininum assistance.

449 **Swing-A-Way**

Braun Corporation
1014 S Monticello Street
Suite 310
Winamac, IN 46996
574-946-6157
800-THE-LIFT
FAX: 574-946-4670

A swing lift for transporting patients from bed to bath and more. It features a gravity-down operation made possible by a newly designed pump module package. The new, quieter module features a built-in hand pump and a plastic reservoir for easy fluid checking. This is a vehicle lift not bath lift.

450 **Turning Automotive Seating (TAS)**

Bruno Independent Living Aids
1780 Executive Drive
PO Box 84
Oconomowoc, WI 53066
262-567-4990
800-882-8183
FAX: 262-953-5501
www.bruno.com

Michael R Bruno, Chairman of the Board/CEO

Transfer in and out of a car, minivan, pickup truck and full size van without any lifting!

451 **VPL Series Vertical Wheelchair Lift**

Access Industries
4001 E 138th Street
Grandview, MO 64030
800-829-9760
FAX: 816-763-4467
e-mail: marketing@accessind.com
www.accessind.com

Provide stairway access indoors and out for people who use wheelchairs. Lifting heights from 1 to 144 feet for loads up to 750 pounds are available for both commercial and residential applications. Easy to install and operate, the units are space and cost efficient solutions to ADA access compliance. Attendant operation, toe-guard enclosure and restricted access hoistway enclosure options are available.

452 **Vangater, Vangater II, Mini-Vangater**

PO Box 310
Winamac, IN 46996
800-THE-LIFT
FAX: 574-946-7935
www.braunlift.com

Tri-fold and fold-in-half lifts represent a major innovation in the field of adapted van transportation.

453 **Vertical Home Lift Sales**
2715 Seaboard Lane
Long Beach, CA 90805
800-795-6227
FAX: 562-634-4120

Rick Pierce, Vertical Home Lift Sales
Betty Haskings, Office Manager
Jerry MacDonald, President

Sales and service of van and truck lifts. Sales and service of wheel chair lifts for vans and automobiles. Sales, installation and service of vertical home lifts, scooter lifts and pool lifts. Sales of scooters.

454 **Vestibular Board**
Bailey Manufacturing Company
118 Lee Street
Suite 130
Lodi, OH 44254
330-948-1080
800-321-8372
FAX: 330-948-4439
e-mail: baileymfg@attmail.com
www.baileymfg.com

Creates tilting in a rolling motion for reclining patients who need help developing balance.

455 **Wecolator Stairway Lift**
Access Industries
4001 E 138th Street
Grandview, MO 64030
800-829-9760
FAX: 816-763-4467
e-mail: marketing@accessind.com
www.accessind.com

Solves many multi-level accessibility problems in home. Lifts easily to install on straight or curved stairways. The rail attaches directly to steps without disturbing walls or staircase. The heavy duty drive mechanism means reliable, trouble-free operation. Public building and outdoor packages available.

456 **Wheelchair Carrier**
203 Matzinger Road
Toledo, OH 43612
419-478-4423
800-541-3213
FAX: 419-476-1324
e-mail: bDunlap@WCCAIMCO.com
www.wheelchaircarrier.com

Bob Dunlap, President
Joni Kaiser, Sales/Accounting

Wheelchair, scooter and powerchair carriers for hitch mount on vehicles, priced from $199 to $999.

457 **Ziggy Medi-Chair**
Laszlo Corporation
PO Box 1182
Florissant, MO 63031
314-830-3222
FAX: 314-830-3222
e-mail: suhayda@aol.com
mc-usa.com

Les Suhayda, President
Dale Bibko, Secretary

A lift and transfer system that maximizes time and safety for disabled and bedridden patients. A multifunctional product that benefits patients with disabilities and caregivers in a home or institutional government. A motorized system that lifts patients and saves caregivers from injury and workman's compensation claims.

Major Catalogs

458 **AMI: Accessories for Mobile Independence**
5235 Mission Oaks Boulevard
Suite 381
Camarillo, CA 93012
805-987-8653

Gay Dawson, Owner

Ponchos, tote bags, gloves, and sweat pants for wheelchair-using consumers.

459 **AbleNet**
1081 10th Avenue E
Minneapolis, MN 55414
612-379-0956
800-322-0956
FAX: 612-379-9143
e-mail: customerservice@ablenetinc.com
www.ablenetinc.com

Allison Locey, Administrative Assistant
Kara Hans O'Brien, Marketing Coordinator

Creates and markets simple technology and educational services that enhance the quality of life for people with disabilities. By developing, and supporting easy-to-use, affordable and durable assistive technology to an individual's needs, capabilities, and interests, AbleNet's products foster independence, participation, inclusion and fun throughout a lifetime.

460 **Access Store Products for Barrier Free Environments**
Access Store.Com
820 W 7th Street
Chico, CA 95928
530-879-5600
800-497-2003
FAX: 530-893-1560
e-mail: sales@accessstore.com
www.accessstore.com

Timothy Vander Heiden, President
Lisa Bantum, Sales Administrator

One of the largest online ADA Compliance Catalogs available. Offers everything from innovative barrier removal products to survey equipment, to unique specialty products.

461 **Achievement Products**
PO Box 9033
Canton, OH 44711
800-373-4699
FAX: 800-766-4303
e-mail: achievepro@aol.com
www.specialkidszone.com

Teresa Cardon
Kyle Hall, Customer Service Manager

Offer a wide range of pediatric rehabilitation equipment and special education products including foam and adult weights, weighted vests, positioning equipment, sensory integration products and ADL. Call for your free catalog.

462 **Adaptive Clothing: Adults**
Special Clothes
PO Box 333
E Harwich, MA 02645
508-896-7939
FAX: 508-896-7939
e-mail: SPECIALCLO@aol.com
www.special-clothes.com

Judith Sweeney, President

Special Clothes produces a catalogue of garments for adults with disabilities and/or incontinence. Offerings include: undergarments, snap-crotch tee shirts, sleepwear, jumpsuits, bibs and some footwear. The catalogue is available without charge. Comparable to department store prices. Special Clothes produces a catalog of adaptive clothing for children in sizes from toddler through young adults. A full line of clothing is included from undergarments through wheelchair jackets and ponchos.

463 **Adaptive Technology Catalog**

Synapse Adaptive
3095 Kerner Boulevard
Suite S
San Rafael, CA 94901
415-455-9700
800-317-9611
FAX: 415-455-9801
e-mail: info@synapseadaptive.com
www.synapseadaptive.com

Speech recognition and adaptive technology for individuals with disabilities.

464 **Adrian's Closet**

PO Box 9506
Rancho Santa Fe, CA 92067
800-831-2577
FAX: 714-364-4380
e-mail: adrians@electriciti.com

Fashions for the physically challenged child. Clothing offers Velcro closures, front pockets, concealed back openings and fashions for seated posture.

465 **Adult Long Jumpsuit with Feet**

Special Clothes
PO Box 333
E Harwich, MA 02645
508-896-7939
FAX: 508-896-7939
e-mail: specialclo@aol.com
www.special-clothes.com

Judith Sweeney, President

Line of clothing for people with disabilities. Child and adult catalog available.

466 **Adult Short Jumpsuit**

Special Clothes
PO Box 333
E Harwich, MA 02645
508-896-7939
FAX: 508-896-7939
e-mail: specialclo@aol.com
www.special-clothes.com

Judith Sweeney, President

This pull-on jumpsuit provides comfort and full coverage without bulk. Wide leg ribbing ends at mid-thigh, with snaps at the crotch. We use fine quality, comfortable cotton knit. 100% cotton knit. Made in USA. Option: long sleeves - add $3.00. Colors: white, navy, teal, light blue, light pink, red, burgundy, royal blue and black. Sm & Med: $36.50/3 for $104.00; L & XL: $39.00/3 for $111.25; and XXL: $42.00/3 for $119.25.

467 **American Discount Medical**

11124 NE Halsey #677
Portland, OR 97220
503-257-0820
800-877-9100
FAX: 503-258-8197
e-mail: adm@information44.com
www.americandiscountmed.com

Tom Ruf, General Manager

Deeply discounts every major brand medical product available.

468 **Apria Healthcare**

26220 Enterprise Court
Lake Forest, CA 92630
800-277-4288
e-mail: contact_us@apria.com
www.apria.com

Lifts, chairs, bathroom aids, bedroom aids, eating utensils and independent living aids for the physically challenged.

469 **Armstrong Medical**

575 Knightsbridge Parkway
Lincolnshire, IL 60069
847-803-4000
800-323-4220
FAX: 847-913-0138
www.armstrongmedical.com

Training aids, anatomical models, medical equipment, pediatrics equipment and rehabilitation equipment.

470 **Assistive Technology Sourcebook**

Special Needs Project
324 State Street
Suite H
Santa Barbara, CA 93101
805-962-8087
800-333-6867
FAX: 805-962-5087
e-mail: books@specialneeds.com
www.specialneeds.com

Alexandra Enders, Editor
Marian Hall, Editor

Provides you with 18 chapters of practical information on all aspects of assistive technology for individuals with functional limitations. *$60.00*

576 pages

471 **Bailey**

118 Lee Street
PO Box 130
Lodi, OH 44254
330-948-1080
800-321-8372
FAX: 330-948-4439
e-mail: baileymfg@attmail.com
www.baileymfg.com

Ambulation aids, balance aids, benches, chairs, exercise devices, tables, stools, rehabilitation and physical therapy equipment for the physically challenged.

70 pages

472 **Best 25 Catalog Resources for Making Life Easier**

Meeting Life's Challenges
9042 Aspen Grove Lane
Madison, WI 53717
608-824-0402
FAX: 608-824-0403
e-mail: help@MeetingLifesChallenges.com
www.MeetingLifesChallenges.com

Unique reference guide to locate thousands of useful and hard-to-find adaptive devices to make dressing, eating, cooking, grooming, communicating, playing, exercising, etc. easier, safer and less frustrating for people of all ages and disabilities. A comprehensive, up-do-date reference for people with disabilities, caregivers and healthcare professionals. *$8.95*

36 pages
ISBN 1-891854-03-8

473 **Bibs**

Special Clothes
PO Box 333
E Harwich, MA 02645
508-896-7939
FAX: 508-896-7939
e-mail: SPECIALCLO@aol.com
www.special-clothes.com

Judith Sweeney, President

A variety of bib styles are available to protect clothing inconspicuously.

474 **Body Suits**

Special Clothes
PO Box 333
E Harwich, MA 02645
508-896-7939
FAX: 508-896-7939
e-mail: specialclo@aol.com
www.special-clothes.com

Judith Sweeney, President

These are one piece garments that can be used to protect skin under braces, to add warmth and to shield incisions. Prices range from $18.25-22.50.

475 **Carolyn's Low Vision Products**

1415 57th Avenue W
Bradenton, FL 34207
800-648-2266
FAX: 941-739-5503
e-mail: carolynscatalog@aol.com
www.carolynscatalog.com

Carolyn Tojek, President

Free mail-order catalog of items for visually impaired people. We also have a retail store.

476 **Communication Aids for Children and Adults**

Crestwood Communication Aids
6625 N Sidney Place
Milwaukee, WI 53209
414-352-5678
FAX: 414-352-5679
e-mail: crestcomm@aol.com
www.communicationaids.com

Ruth B Leff MS CCC, Speech-Language Pathologist

A free catalog of communication aids for children and adults with disabilities. Over 300 light and high tech switches and aids, and a large selection of adapted and voice-activated toys. Talking Pictures and Passports communication boards, easy to use and moderately priced talking aids.

32 pages Yearly

477 **Danmar Products**

221 Jackson Industrial Drive
Ann Arbor, MI 48103
734-761-1990
800-783-1998
FAX: 734-761-8977
e-mail: sales@danmarproducts.com
www.danmarproducts.com

Dan Russo, Sales/Marketing
Suzanne Gubachy, Sales Manager
Amy Belleau, Sales

Manufactures adaptive equipment for persons with physical and mental disabilities, from seating and positioning equipment, flotation devices, toileting aids to hard and soft shell helmets.

478 **Dayspring Associates**

2111 Foley Road
Havre De Grace, MD 21078
410-939-5900
FAX: 410-939-6252

This publisher provides a directory of 1,000 rehabilitation aids.

479 **Enrichments Catalog**

Sammons Preston Rolyan
4 Sammons Court
Bolingbrook, IL 60440
630-226-1300
800-323-5547
FAX: 630-226-1389
e-mail: spr@abilityone.com
www.sammonsprestonrolyan.com

Provides people with physical challenges with the products they need to help live their lives to the fullest. Includes items for everyday tasks and personal care; assistive products for home use; toileting and bathing aids; grooming and dressing devices; kitchen and dining aids. Also items for range of motion, mobility and exercise such as weights, therapy putty and exercise equipment; ergonomic gloves and supports; canes, crutches, walkers and wheelchair accessories. 36-page catalog.

480 **Equipment Shop**

PO Box 33
Bedford, MA 01730
781-275-7681
800-525-7681
FAX: 781-275-4094
e-mail: info@equipmentshop.com
www.equipmentshop.com

Kenneth D Larson, Owner

Pediatric therapy equipment including pezzi Gymnastik balls, Tripp Trapp chair, airex mats, tricycle accessories, sensory integration equipment and adaptive devices.

481 **Everest & Jennings**

Division of Graham-Field
2935 NE Parkway
Atlanta, GA 30360
800-347-5678
FAX: 800-726-0601
e-mail: cs@everestjennings.com
www.everestjennings.com

Manufactures more than 200 items for persons with physical disabilities, including wheelchairs, seat cushions, shower chairs, grab bars and more.

482 **Express Medical Supply**

28 Seebold Spur
Fenton, MO 63026
800-633-2139
FAX: 800-633-9188
e-mail: sales@exmed.net
www.exmed.net

Chris Winston, Manager

Offers a full line of medical and ostomy supplies. at discounted prices. Order by phone or online.

483 **FlagHouse Rehab Resources**

601 FlagHouse Drive
Hasbrouck Heights, NJ 07604
201-288-7600
800-793-7900
FAX: 800-793-7922
e-mail: sales@flaghouse.com
www.flaghouse.com

Brigid DeLime, Clinical Product Manager

Contains over 2,000 products of interest to therapy professionals.

Bi-Annually

484 **Gem Wheelchair Scooter and Service**

176-39 Union Turnpike
Flushing, NY 11366 **718-969-8600**
800-943-3578
FAX: 718-969-8300
e-mail: wheelsu@aol.com
www.wheelchairsusa.com

Jeff Bochner, President

GEM repairs and sells all makes and models of manual and motorized wheelchairs, power scooters, ramps and stairway lifts. Clients are in all five New York City Boroughs and Nassau County. Medicare and Medicaid accepted, pick-up and delivery, loaner equipment, and while-u-wait repair services available. Gem also buys and sells used equipment.

485 **HAC Hearing Aid Centers of America: HARC Mercantile**

Hearing Center
1111 W Centre Avenue
Portage, MI 49024 **269-324-0301**
800-445-9968
FAX: 800-413-5248
TTY:800-445-9968
e-mail: home@harcmercantile.com
www.harcmercantile.com

Ronald Slager, President

Specializes in products for the hard of hearing and deaf as required under ADA including visual alerting products for fire, phone, door, wake up, phone amplification, TTY, FM and infrared listening systems.

486 **Harris Communications**

Harris Communications
15155 Technology Drive
Eden Prairie, MN 55344 **952-906-1180**
800-825-6758
FAX: 952-906-1099
e-mail: mail@harriscomm.com
www.harriscomm.com

Bill Williams, National Sales Manager

A national distributor of assistive devices for the deaf and hard of hearing with many manufacturers represented. Catalog includes a wide range of assistive devices as well as a variety of books and videotapes related to deaf and hard-of-hearing issues. Products available for children, teachers, hearing professionals, interpreters and anyone interested in deaf culture, hearing loss and sign language.

180 pages Yearly

487 **Health and Rehabilitation Products**

Luminaud
8688 Tyler Boulevard
Mentor, OH 44060 **440-255-9082**
800-255-3408
FAX: 440-255-2250
e-mail: info@luminaud.com
www.luminaud.com

Thomas Lennox, President
Dorothy Lennox, VP

Switches for limited capability, stoma and trach covers, shower protectors and thermo-stim oral motor stimulator. Personal voice amplifiers for people with weak voices. Artificial larynges for people with no voices. Small electronic communication boards. Books for laryngectomies and speech pathologists.

488 **HealthCare Solutions**

Blue Chip II
3478 Hauck Road
Cincinnati, OH 45241 **513-271-5115**
800-417-5115
FAX: 513-527-3686

LK Barker, Director
Kim Fischer, Administrative Assistant

Quality rehabilitation equipment sales and rental. Available equipment includes manual and powered mobility, positioning/seating equipment, vehicle modification, environmental controls, augmentative and alternative communication devices, adaptive computer access, ambulance aids and aids for daily living. Equipment provision is carried out through a total team approach.

489 **Hear You Are**

98 Route 46 W
Budd Lake, NJ 07828 **973-347-7662**
FAX: 973-691-0611

Dorinne S Davis, President

A large catalog of various assistive and communication devices for people who are hearing impaired. *$3.00*

42 pages

490 **Hig's Manufacturing**

2917 Anthony Lane N
Minneapolis, MN 55418 **612-638-1330**
FAX: 612-638-1341

Factory direct, lightweight aluminum, portable, 2 & 4-way folding, telescoping tracks, threshold, van, scooter and approach ramps.

491 **Huntleigh Healthcare**

40 Christopher Way
Eatontown, NJ 07724 **732-578-9898**
800-223-1218
FAX: 732-578-9889
www.huntleigh-healthcare.com

Bob Angel, President/CEO

Offers quality products including support surfaces, seating surfaces and intermittent pneumatic compression devices.

492 **Hygienics Direct Company**

3968 194th Trail
Miami, FL 33160 **305-937-0824**
800-463-7337
FAX: 305-937-0825
www.hygienics.com

Michael Brier, President

Offers a complete line of incontinence products and skin care products consisting of disposable and reuseable panties for women and pants for men. Also new line of Safe And Dry mattress pads and waterproof mattress covers.

16 pages Bi-Annual

493 **LS&S**

PO Box 673
Northbrook, IL 60065 **847-498-9777**
800-468-4789
FAX: 847-498-1482
TTY:800-317-8533
e-mail: info@LSSproducts.com
www.LSSproducts.com

Specializes in products for the blind, visually impaired, hearing impaired, and deaf. Free catalog upon request.

494 **Lighthouse Low Vision Products**

Lighthouse International
111 E 59th Street
New York, NY 10022
212-521-9200
800-829-0500
FAX: 212-821-9702
e-mail: info@lighthouse.org
www.lighthouse.org

This supplier provides vision-related products.

495 **Luminaud**

8688 Tyler Boulevard
Mentor, OH 44060
440-255-9082
800-255-3408
FAX: 440-255-2250
e-mail: info@luminaud.com
www.luminaud.com

Thomas Lennox, President
Dorothy Lennox, VP

Offers a line of artificial larynx, personal voice amplifiers, special switches, stoma covers and other communication, health and safety items.

496 **Maxi Aids**

42 Executive Boulevard
PO Box 3209
Farmingdale, NY 11735
631-752-0521
800-522-6294
FAX: 631-752-0689
e-mail: sales@maxiaids.com
www.maxiaids.com

Products specially designed for the blind, low vision, visually impaired, deaf, deaf-blind, hard of hearing, arthritic, diabetic and individuals with special needs.

497 **New Vision Store**

919 Walnut Street
Philadelphia, PA 19107
215-627-0600
FAX: 215-922-0692
e-mail: webmaster@thenewvisionstore.com
www.thenewvisionstore.com

Catalog for individuals with visual impairments, listing visual aids, magnifiers, large print books and more.

30 pages

498 **Nurion-Raycal**

Station Square
Building 2
Paoli, PA 19301
610-647-2435
FAX: 610-647-2216

Nazir A Ali, President

Electronic travel aids for the blind, deaf-blind, visually impaired persons, and those with Hemispatial neglect. Devices detect obstacles, finds clear path, landmarks. Lase Cane incorporates lasers to detect drop-off, obstacles at different heights and distances. Polaron, a hand-held or chest-mounted unit, utilizes ultrasound to detect obstacles at various distances. Wheelchair Pathfinders incorporate ultrasound and lasers to detect drop-off and obstacles on the sides and forward.

499 **Pearson Reid London House**

1 N Deerborne Street
16th Floor
Chicago, IL 60602
312-938-9200
800-922-7343
FAX: 312-242-4400
e-mail: pearsonreidlondonhouse@pearson.com
www.pearsonreidlondonhouse.com

Publishes human resource assessment instruments for employment settings. The instruments include job analysis procedures to identify important characteristics for job success and objective assessment procedures to evaluate applicants and employees on these characteristics.

500 **Potomac Technology**

1 Church Street
Suite 101
Rockville, MD 20850
301-762-4005
800-433-2838
FAX: 301-762-1892
e-mail: info@potomactech.com
www.potomactech.com

Pat Relidan, VP

This catalog offers a variety of products for the deaf and hard of hearing, such as: wake-up devices, alarm clocks, alerting systems, assistive listening devices, signalers, smoke detectors, TTY, telephones and telephone amplifiers. We also carry novelties, and educational books and videos.

24 pages

501 **Prentke Romich Company Product Catalog**

1022 Heyl Road
Wooster, OH 44691
330-262-1984
800-262-1984
FAX: 330-263-4829
e-mail: info@prentrom.com
www.prentrom.com

Cherie Weaver, Marketing Coordinator

A full line product catalog containing information on speech-output communication devices, environmental controls and computer access products.

502 **Products for People with Disabilities**

LS&S
PO Box 673
Northbrook, IL 60065
847-498-9777
800-468-4789
FAX: 847-498-1482
TTY:800-317-8533
e-mail: info@LSSproducts.com
www.LSSproducts.com

LS&S, LLC has a free catalog of products for the blind, deaf, visually and hearing impaired including: TTYs, computer adaptive devices, CCTVs, talking blood pressure, blood glucose and talking scales.

503 **Rehabilitation Engineering and Assistive Technology Society of North America (RESNA)**

1700 N Moore Street
Suite 1540
Arlington, VA 22209
703-524-6686
FAX: 703-524-6630
e-mail: membership@resna.org
www.resna.org

Shannon Marullo, Director, Professional Services
Tonya Vaughn, Professional Services Manager
Sarah Bourke, Executive Assistant

Association of rehabilitation professionals and people interested in advancing technology for people with disabilities.

504 **Sammons Preston Enrichments Catalog**

Sammons Preston Rolyan
4 Sammons Court
Bolingbrook, IL 60440 **630-226-1300**
800-323-5547
FAX: 630-226-1388
e-mail: sp@sammonspreston.com
www.sammonspreston.com

Tony Napolitano, Director Marketing Services

Our Enrichnments Catalog offers products that make the tasks and challenges of living at home— bathing, getting dressed, getting around— a little easier. Choose from personal care items to kitchen and dining aids, household helpers to mobility devices, plus a complete selection of pain-reducing products, exercise items, health monitoring equipment and more.

40 pages Yearly

505 **Special Edition for Disabled People**

Lawrence Research Group
PO Box 31039
San Francisco, CA 94131 **415-468-3805**
800-242-2823
FAX: 415-468-3912
e-mail: info@xandria.com
www.xandria.com

Marcia Jackson, Marketing Director

Sexual aids for the handicapped. A catalog of product and informational resources and quotes from the top professionals in this field. *$4.00*

32 pages

506 **Sportaid**

78 Bay Creek Road
Loganville, GA 30052 **770-979-0945**
800-743-7203
FAX: 770-554-5944
e-mail: stuffosportaid.com
www.sportaid.com

Jimmy Green

Offers an assortment of wheelchairs (everyday and racing), wheelchair sports equipment, replacement tires, hubs, spokes, pushrims, cushions and more. Call for free catalog.

68 pages Yearly

507 **Ultratec**

450 Science Drive
Madison, WI 53711 **608-238-5400**
800-482-2424
FAX: 608-238-3008
e-mail: service@ultratec.com
www.ultratec.com

Jackie Morgan, Director Marketing

The world's largest manufacturer of text telephones and amplified telephones. Products include desktop TTYs with built-in printer, memory capabilities, as well as compact portable units for cellular and cordless use. Ultratec also manufactures public TTYs for pay phone accessibility.

Yearly

508 **WCI/Weitbrecht Communications**

2716 Ocean Park Boulevard
Suite 1007
Santa Monica, CA 90405 **310-452-8613**
800-233-9130
FAX: 310-450-9918
e-mail: sales@weitbrecht.com
www.weitbrecht.com

Donna Barwald, Sales Manager

Catalog featuring a wide range of assistive devices for the deaf, hard of hearing, mobility and speech impaired.

24 pages

509 **Walgreens Home Medical Center**

7173 Cermak Road
Berwyn, IL 60402 **708-795-1295**
800-323-2828
FAX: 708-795-1308

Paul Pankros RPh, Director

Hospital supplies and home medical equipment with nationwide direct mail delivery.

510 **Walton Way Medical**

1225 Walton Way
Augusta, GA 30901 **706-722-0276**
FAX: 706-722-0279

Offers medical, therapeutic, urological, hygiene and skin care products for disabled persons.

511 **Wheelchair Batteries**

Accent Books & Products
PO Box 700
Bloomington, IL 61702 **309-378-2961**
800-787-8444
FAX: 309-378-4420
e-mail: acmtlvng@aol.com

Raymond C Cheever, Publisher
Betty Garee, Editor

Offers valuable tips for trouble-free travel at minimum cost: selecting the right battery the first time and how to use and re-charge your battery to make it last longer. *$3.50*

32 pages Paperback
ISBN 0-91570-22-1

Miscellaneous

512 **BeOK Key Lever**

Sammons Preston Rolyan
4 Sammons Court
Bolingbrook, IL 60440 **630-226-1300**
800-323-5547
FAX: 630-226-1389
e-mail: spr@abilityone.com
www.sammonsprestonrolyan.com

Handy accessory helps position key to provide maximum leverage enabling the user to work the most stubborn lock. *$11.50*

513 **Big Lamp Switch**

Maxi Aids
42 Executive Boulevard
Suite 3209
Farmingdale, NY 11735 **631-752-0521**
800-522-6294
FAX: 631-752-0689
e-mail: sales@maxiaids.com
www.maxiaids.com

This big, three-spoked knob replaces small rotating knobs which are a problem for those with arthritis or other limitations of the fingers. *$6.75*

514 Big Red Switch

AbleNet
1081 10th Avenue SE
Minneapolis, MN 55414
800-322-0956
FAX: 612-379-9143
e-mail: customerservice@ablenetinc.com
www.ablenetinc.com

Mary Kay Walch

Five inches across the top and activates no matter where on its surface it is touched. It is made of shatterproof plastic and contains a cord storage compartment. Also available in green, yellow and blue. *$42.00*

515 Book Holder

Access with Ease
PO Box 1150
Chino Valley, AZ 86323
928-636-9469
800-531-9479
FAX: 928-636-0292
e-mail: KMJC@northlink.com

This hands free reading book holder enables the user to read hands free. Moveable pegs prevent slipping, yet allow easy turning. Folds flat and has built in handle for easy carrying. *$16.95*

516 Bookholder: Roberts

Therapro
225 Arlington Street
Framingham, MA 01702
508-872-9494
800-257-5376
FAX: 508-875-2062
e-mail: info@theraproducts.com
www.theraproducts.com

Gray plastic, ideal for hand free reading, adjusts to all sizes of books and prevents pages from flipping for the physically challenged. *$27.50*

517 Brandt Industries

4461 Bronx Boulevard
Bronx, NY 10470
718-994-0800
800-221-8031
FAX: 718-325-7995
e-mail: brandtindinc@aol.com
www.brandtind.com

Neil Brandt, President
Kathy Rice, Order Expediter

518 Bus and Taxi Sign

Maxi Aids
42 Executive Boulevard
Suite 3209
Farmingdale, NY 11735
631-752-0521
800-522-6294
FAX: 631-752-0689
e-mail: sales@maxiaids.com
www.maxiaids.com

Signs that the individual with a disability can use to attract the attention of bus or taxi drivers. *$3.75*

519 Call Alarm/Switch Delay Unit

Words+
40015 Sierra Highway B-145
Palmdale, CA 93550
800-869-8521
FAX: 661-266-8969

Ginger Woltosz, VP
Tim Ross, Manager

For use with any single system. Provides loud audible attention-getting alarm that can be either a steady or pulsating tone. Once activated, the alarm must be turned off by pressing a reset button. *$299.00*

520 Care Electronics

4700 Sterling Drive
Suite D
Boulder, CO 80301
303-444-2273
888-444-8284
FAX: 303-447-3502
e-mail: tmoody@riveraisland.com
www.medicalshoponline.com

Donna Lewis, Sales Manager
Tom Moody, President

Care Electronics manufactures safety monitoring systems for caregivers, home-health care, and nursing homes. WanderCARE monitors loved ones who tend to wander away from home. Care Deluxe Occupancy systems monitor patients in bed and in wheelchairs to help prevent falls. WetSENSE provides incontinence monitors.

521 Center for Assistive Technology and Environmental Access

490 10th Street NW
Atlanta, GA 30332
404-894-4960
FAX: 404-894-9320
www.catea.org

Barbara Christopher, Administrative Coordinator
Elizabeth Bryant, Project Director II

The Center for Assistive Technology and Environmental Access (CATEA) promotes maximum function, activity and access of persons with disabilities through the use of technology. The foci of the Center includes the development, evaluation and utilization of Assistive Technology and the design and development of Accessible Environments.

522 Child Convertible Balance Beam Set

Bailey Manufacturing Company
118 Lee Street
Suite 130
Lodi, OH 44254
330-948-1080
800-321-8372
FAX: 330-948-4439
e-mail: baileymfg@attmail.com
www.baileymfg.com

This convertible set is used to develop balance in two stages.

523 Child Variable Balance Beam

Bailey Manufacturing Company
135 S Mount Zion Road
Lebanon, IN 46052
330-948-1080
800-321-8372
FAX: 330-948-4439
e-mail: baileymfg@attmail.com
www.baileymfg.com

The four walking beams can be arranged in several different ways for variable balance training.

524 Child's Mobility Crawler

Bailey Manufacturing Company
118 Lee Street
Suite 130
Lodi, OH 44254
330-948-1080
800-321-8372
FAX: 330-948-4439
e-mail: baileymfg@attmail.com
www.baileymfg.com

Neurologically delayed or orthopedically impaired small children can perform crawling and coordination exercises while being comfortably supported by the crawler.

525 **Choice Switch Latch and Timer**

AbleNet
1081 10th Avenue SE
Minneapolis, MN 55414
800-322-0956
FAX: 612-379-9143
e-mail: customerservice@ablenetinc.com
www.ablenetinc.com

A Choice Switch Latch and Timer allows one user to learn to make choices. It has two switch inputs and can control two devices. Once one device has been activated, the other will not function until the first one is turned off or completes its timed cycle. *$83.00*

526 **Cordless Big Red Switch**

AbleNet
1081 10th Avenue SE
Minneapolis, MN 55414
800-322-0956
FAX: 612-379-9143
e-mail: customerservice@ablenetinc.com
www.ablenetinc.com

The Cordless Big Red Switch, when used in conjunction with either the Cordless Receiver or the Small Appliance Receiver, gives you cordless control of toys, games, and appliances in your environment. *$89.00*

527 **DEUCE Environmental Control Unit**

APT Technology
236A N Main Street
Shreve, OH 44676
330-567-2001
888-549-2001
FAX: 330-567-3073
e-mail: sales@apt-technology.com
www.apt-technology.com

Grace Miller, Office Manager

Allows a severely disabled person to control a variety of useful devices via a dual switch. DEUCE controls phone, 4 AC powered devices such as a radio, 4 switch controlled devices such as a page turner and up to 16 lights and or appliances distributed around the environment. Starts at $1,500.

528 **Dazor Manufacturing Corporation**

4483 Duncan Avenue
Saint Louis, MO 63110
314-652-2400
800-345-9103
FAX: 314-652-2069
e-mail: info@dazor.com
www.dazor.com

Kirk Cressey, Marketion Director
Bob Smith, National Sales Manager

Dazor is a US manufacturer of quality task lighting. Products include fluorescent, incandescent and halogen lighting fixtures. Illuminated magnifiers combine light and magnification to greatly enhance activities such as reading and make hobbies more enjoyable. All lamps come in a variety of mounting options to include desk bases, clamp on, floor stands and wall tracks. $95 - $450.

529 **Digi-Flex**

Therapro
225 Arlington Street
Framingham, MA 01702
508-872-9494
800-257-5376
FAX: 508-875-2062
e-mail: info@theraproducts.com
www.theraproducts.com

This is a unique hand and finger exercise unit. Recommended for use of individuation of fingers, web space and general strengthening of work hands. Available in a variety of resistances. *$17.50*

530 **Dorma Group North America**

Dorma Drive
Drawer AC
Reamstown, PA 17567
800-523-8483
FAX: 717-336-2106
e-mail: archdw@dorma-usa.com
www.dorma-usa.com

Paul Kosakowski, President/CEO
Gary Phillips AHC, VP Regional Sales, East
Ken Theaker, VP Regional Sales, West

DORMA provides a complete line of door controls, including barrier-free units that comply with the Americans with Disabilities Act. A wide variety of surface applied and concealed closers, low energy operators, exit devices and electronic access control systems are available to address these equipments.

531 **Dual Switch Latch and Timer**

AbleNet
1081 10th Avenue SE
Minneapolis, MN 55414
800-322-0956
FAX: 612-379-9143
e-mail: customerservice@ablenetinc.com
www.ablenetinc.com

A Dual Switch Latch and Timer allows two users to activate two devices at a time in the latch. Timed seconds or timed minutes mode of control. *$88.00*

532 **Folding Reacher**

Accent Books & Products
PO Box 700
Bloomington, IL 61702
309-378-2961
800-787-8444
FAX: 309-378-4420
e-mail: acmtlvng@aol.com

Lightweight, adjustable, foldable reachers allowing one-handed operation. *$13.95*

533 **Foot Inversion Tread**

Bailey Manufacturing Company
118 Lee Street
Suite 130
Lodi, OH 44254
330-948-1080
800-321-8372
FAX: 330-948-4439
e-mail: baileymfg@attmail.com
www.baileymfg.com

Effective for correcting flat feet. These angled boards require the patient to walk on the outside of the foot instead of the arch.

534 **Foot Placement Ladder**

Bailey Manufacturing Company
118 Lee Street
Suite 130
Lodi, OH 44254
330-948-1080
800-321-8372
FAX: 330-948-4439
e-mail: baileymfg@attmail.com
www.baileymfg.com

Adjustable cross bars for different length steps. Reinforced metal crosses for easier climbing for the physically-disabled.

535 **Handy Reacher**

Access with Ease
PO Box 1150
Chino Valley, AZ 86323
928-636-9469
800-531-9479
FAX: 928-636-0292
e-mail: KMJC@northlink.com

Long handled reacher works for retrieving items off shelves, picking fruit in the garden, dusting high places, getting objects behind the couch and lots of uses. Rubber jaws that open 5 inches wide with a magnet on one tip, wooden arm that extends the reach 30 inches to a metal handle. Other model reachers are available. *$7.95*

536 **Hospital Environmental Control System**

Prentke Romich Company
1022 Heyl Road
Wooster, OH 44691
330-262-1984
800-262-1984
FAX: 330-263-4829
e-mail: info@prentrom.com
www.prentrom.com

Permits the non-ambulatory patient to operate a variety of electrical items in a single room. A large liquid crystal display is mounted in front of the user and they scan through the menu of operations and make a selection using a sip-puff switch. Options include nurse call, standard telephone functions, electric bed control, hospital television operation and electrical appliance on and off. *$3860.00*

537 **Knock Light**

HARC Mercantile
PO Box 3055
Kalamazoo, MI 49003
269-324-1615
800-445-9968
FAX: 269-324-2387
e-mail: home@harcmercantile.com
www.harcmercantile.com

Ronald Slager, President

Easily attaches to a door with velcro, portable. *$29.95*

538 **Leg Elevation Board**

Bailey Manufacturing Company
118 Lee Street
Suite 130
Lodi, OH 44254
330-948-1080
800-321-8372
FAX: 330-948-4439
e-mail: baileymfg@attmail.com
www.baileymfg.com

Includes seven positions to a 30 degree incline, three pillows with Velcro, easy carry hand slot and a natural finish.

539 **Leveron**

Lindustries
21 Shady Hill Road
Weston, MA 02493
781-237-8177

Willard H Lind, President
Louise T Lind, VP

Leveron is a doorknob lever handle for ease of operation. Leveron converts standard doorknobs to lever action without removing existing hardware. No gripping, twisting or pinching when hands are wet, arthritic or arms are full. Leveron provides convenience. Available in five colors: almond, satin brass, silver metallic, dark bronze and Hi-Glow (glows in the dark) at low cost to comply with ADA access requirements in public and private places. *$16.95*

540 **Location Finder**

Maxi Aids
42 Executive Boulevard
Suite 3209
Farmingdale, NY 11735
631-752-0521
800-522-6294
FAX: 631-752-0689
e-mail: sales@maxiaids.com
www.maxiaids.com

Helps find house, apartment, car or office. Just press the transmitter and sound will be emitted indicating the location. *$99.95*

541 **Longreach Reacher**

Therapro
225 Arlington Street
Framingham, MA 01702
508-872-9494
800-257-5376
FAX: 508-875-2062
e-mail: info@theraproducts.com
www.theraproducts.com

Reacher is useful when reaching, sitting or when standing. *$18.95*

542 **Loop Scissors**

Therapro
225 Arlington Street
Framingham, MA 01702
508-872-9494
800-257-5376
FAX: 508-875-2062
e-mail: info@theraproducts.com
www.theraproducts.com

Pliable, plastic handles that allow for easy and controlled cutting. *$14.25*

543 **Magni-Cam & Primer**

Innoventions
5921 S Middlefield Road
Suite 102
Littleton, CO 80123
800-854-6554
FAX: 303-727-4940
e-mail: magnicam@magnicam.com
www.magnicam.com/

Tom Winter, VP Marketing
Ed Bettinardi, President

Magni-Cam and Primer are hand-held, light weight, inexpensive auto-focus electronic magnification systems designed to meet the reading and writing needs of those with low vision. The systems present the image in black and white or in color with three different view modes. Connects to any TV monitor in minutes. Systems read any surface with no distortion. Two battery powered systems are available, providing total portability and flexibility.

544 **Med Covers**

Med Covers
PO Box 1527e
Garner, NC 27529
919-779-3555
800-948-8917
FAX: 919-779-3540
e-mail: medteam@medcovers.com
www.medcovers.com

Jeanie Falkie, Sales Counsultant Med Division

Manufactures cases and covers for the medical and data capture industries. Specializing in oxygen cylinder, scooter and wheelchairs covers, and accessories.

545 **Plastic Card Holder**

Therapro
225 Arlington Street
Framingham, MA 01702 **508-872-9494**
800-257-5376
FAX: 508-875-2062
e-mail: info@theraproducts.com
www.theraproducts.com

For those with reduced finger control. *$4.00*

546 **PortaPower Plus**

Words+
1220 W Avenue J
Lancaster, CA 93534 **661-266-8500**
800-869-8521
FAX: 661-266-8969

Phil Lawrence, VP
Rachel Nielsen, Customer Support

Rechargeable battery pack designed to give longer life and remote usage time to laptop computers and other portable battery-operated devices and accessories. Requires a 12 volt auto adapter. *$149.00*

547 **Power Door**

11240 Gemini Lane
Dallas, TX 75229
800-688-1758
FAX: 972-620-9875
e-mail: info@powerdoor.com
www.powerdoor.com

Jim Goldthwaite, National Sales Manager

Power door, low energy door operators.

548 **ProtectaCap, ProtectaCap+PLUS, ProtectaChin Guard and ProtectaHip**

Plum Enterprises
500 Freedom View Lane
PO Box 85
Valley Forge, PA 19481 **610-783-7377**
800-321-PLUM
FAX: 610-783-7577
www.plument.com

Janice Carrington, President

Plum Enterprises Award Wininng Exquiste, Ergonomic Protective Wear keeps you safe from the dangers of falls. ProtectCap+Plus and ProtectHips are engineered for superior shock-absorption and designed for exquiste simplicity and amazing lightweight comfort the perfect blend of style and function.

549 **Rocker Balance Square**

Bailey Manufacturing Company
118 Lee Street
Suite 130
Lodi, OH 44254 **330-948-1080**
800-321-8372
FAX: 330-948-4439
e-mail: baileymfg@attmail.com
www.baileymfg.com

The rocker is used in developing activity, balance control and coordination.

550 **Room Valet Visual-Tactile Alerting System**

HARC Mercantile
PO Box 3055
Kalamazoo, MI 49003 **269-324-1615**
800-445-9968
FAX: 269-324-2387
e-mail: home@harcmercantile.com
www.harcmercantile.com

Ronald Slager, President

ADA compliant built-in visual-tactile alerting system. The Room Valet is fully supervised and has power failure back up. Alerts to in-room smoke, building alarm, door, phone and alarm clock. Designed for permanent installation.

551 **Scott Sign Systems**

PO Box 1047
Tallevast, FL 34270 **941-355-5171**
800-237-9447
FAX: 941-351-1787
e-mail: mail@scottsigns.com
www.scottsigns.com

Call for a brochure.

552 **Series Adapter**

AbleNet
1081 10th Avenue SE
Minneapolis, MN 55414
800-322-0956
FAX: 612-379-9143
e-mail: customerservice@ablenetinc.com
www.ablenetinc.com

Allows two-switch operation of any battery-operated device or electrical devices. *$13.00*

553 **Sharp Calculator with Illuminated Numbers**

Independent Living Aids
200 Robbins Lane
Jericho, NY 11753 **516-937-1848**
800-537-2118
FAX: 516-937-3906
e-mail: can-do@independentliving.com
www.independentliving.com

A trim desktop calculator with large illuminated numbers that can be carried anywhere. *$34.95*

554 **Signaling Wake-Up Devices**

HARC Mercantile
PO Box 3055
Kalamazoo, MI 49003 **269-324-1615**
800-445-9968
FAX: 269-324-2387
e-mail: home@harcmercantile.com
www.harcmercantile.com

Ronald Slager, President

Wake up devices. Vibrating alarm clocks, available with flashing lights, louder alarm noises and more. *$29.50*

555 **Smoke Detector with Strobe**

HARC Mercantile
PO Box 3055
Kalamazoo, MI 49003 **269-324-1615**
800-445-9968
FAX: 269-324-2387
e-mail: home@harcmercantile.com
www.harcmercantile.com

Ronald Slager, President

Most of the smoke alarms are twice as loud, and have a 120+ candela strobe that will wake a person from a sound sleep. Mounting hardware for ceiling or wall. *$165.95*

556 **SteeleVest**

Steele
PO Box 7304
Kingston, WA 98346 **360-297-4555**
888-783-3538
FAX: 360-297-2816
e-mail: info@steelevest.com
www.steelevest.com

Vest developed by NASA provides an external cooling system.

557 Step-by-Step Communicator

AbleNet
1081 10th Avenue SE
Minneapolis, MN 55414
800-322-0956
FAX: 612-379-9143
e-mail: customerservice@ablenetinc.com
www.ablenetinc.com

Allows you to record a series of messages (as many as you want up to the 75 second limit). It has a 2 1/2 inches diameter switch surface and is 3 inches at its tallest point. Angled switch surface makes it easy to see and access. *$129.00*

558 TV & VCR Remote

AbleNet
1081 10th Avenue SE
Minneapolis, MN 55414
800-322-0956
FAX: 612-379-9143
e-mail: customerservice@ablenetinc.com
www.ablenetinc.com

Controls a TV, a VCR or a TV that is connected through a VCR tuner. It may be programmed to control functions such as on and off, channel up, preprogrammed TV channels and if desired, other TV functions such as mute and pause. *$82.00*

559 Tactile Thermostat

Sense-Sations
919 Walnut Street
Philadelphia, PA 19107
215-627-0600
FAX: 215-922-0692

Large embossed numbers on cover ring and raised temperature setting knob. *$31.50*

560 Talking Desktop Calculators

Maxi Aids
42 Executive Boulevard
Suite 3209
Farmingdale, NY 11735
631-752-0521
800-522-6294
FAX: 631-752-0689
e-mail: sales@maxiaids.com
www.maxiaids.com

Unique voice synthesizers call out numerals and functions as they are keyed in or read out data stored in memory. *$467.95*

561 Therapy Putty

Therapro
225 Arlington Street
Framingham, MA 01702
508-872-9494
800-257-5376
FAX: 508-875-2062
e-mail: info@theraproducts.com
www.theraproducts.com

Designed to exercise and strengthen hands, ranging from soft to firm for developing a stronger grasp. Available in two, four and six ounce sizes. Three ounce putty in unique clear fist shaped container.

562 Transcription Services

Access-USA
24 James Street
PO Box 160
Clayton, NY 13624
800-263-2750
FAX: 800-563-1687
e-mail: info@access-usa.com
www.access-usa.com

Deborah Haight, PICOE

Access-USA provides one-stop alternate format transcription services for almost any type of document-reports, schedules, menus, monthly statements, brochures, reports, etc. Items may be submitted on computer disk, hard copy or email. Alternate formats include Braille, large print, Braille and print, audio recordings, adapted disks as well as video services-open/closed captioning and video descriptions. Accessible products Braille Business Cards and ADA signage. Braille and print stickers.

563 Window-Ease

A-Solution
1332 Cobo Place NE
Albequeque, NM 87106
505-256-0115
FAX: 505-256-3756
www.windowease.com

Robert Gorrell, President
Jeff Dodd, Sales

Device adapts horizontally and vertically sliding windows to ANSI A117.1 standards. 10:1 mechanical advantage at the crank arm opens a 50lb window with 5lbs force. Price ranges from $350.00-$450.00.

Office Devices & Workstations

564 Auditech: Audioport Personal Amplifier

PO Box 821105
Vicksburg, MS 39182
800-229-8293
FAX: 800-221-8639
e-mail: info@auditechusa.com
www.auditechusa.com

Make everyday conversations more comfortable and easy to hear with the Audioport. This all-in-one unit has a powerful built-in microphone and amplifer, so no wires or separate transmitters are needed. Designed for one-on-one or small group conversations, it amplies up to eight feet away. It automatically adjusts for sharp sudden noises and allows user's voice to sound natural. All in one small, durable unit. *$189.00*

565 Auditech: Classroom Amplification Sy Focus CFM802

PO Box 821105
Vicksburg, MS 39182
800-229-8293
FAX: 800-221-8639
e-mail: info@auditechusa.com
www.auditechusa.com

The SOUNDFOCUS FM System is designed to cover background noise and compensate for distance. Students find it easier to focus their attention and not strain to be heard. Two speaker system. *$1052.00*

566 Auditech: DirectEar Transmitter and Headset

PO Box 821105
Vicksburg, MS 39182
800-229-8293
FAX: 800-221-8639
e-mail: info@auditechusa.com
www.auditechusa.com

Turn up the volume when watching TV. The headset can also be used separately in public theaters and cinemas, that have infrared transmission. Additional headset receivers can be purchased. A neckloop can also be added to the headset. *$219.00*

567 **Auditech: Personal FM Educational System**

PO Box 821105
Vicksburg, MS 39182

800-229-8293
FAX: 800-221-8639
e-mail: info@auditechusa.com
www.auditechusa.com

Personal FM Educational System is a portable system for classroom use. The teacher wears a microphone. Students use a portable receiver which works clearly and easily. For users who have a hearing problem, a switch, a necklooop telecoil coupler is available. *$679.00*

568 **Auditech: Personal PA Value Pack System**

PO Box 821105
Vicksburg, MS 39182

800-229-8293
FAX: 800-221-8639
e-mail: info@auditechusa.com
www.auditechusa.com

Reliable hearing assistance. This wireless FM system broadcasts to listeners with a hearing assistance system, helping them overcome background noise at a distance from the sound source. *$899.00*

569 **Auditech: Pocketalker Pro**

PO Box 821105
Vicksburg, MS 39182

800-229-8293
FAX: 800-221-8639
e-mail: info@auditechusa.com
www.auditechusa.com

Pocketalker Pro can help you hear virtually anywhere whether in a car, crowded restaurant or at a noisy gathering. It can work to reduce background noise and easily converts to the Telelink. *$ 140.00*

570 **Combination File/Reference Carousel**

Center for Rehabilitation Technology
490 10th Street NW
Suite 118
Atlanta, GA 30318

404-265-1650
800-457-9555
FAX: 404-875-9409
e-mail: rerc-br@scsn.net

TW Gannaway, Executive VP

Offers two reading platforms and file holders joined on one easily rotated carousel. The carousel is easily rotated by head, mouth or handstick. Page retainer adjusts to hold open a variety of books and magazines. *$299.00*

571 **Extensions for Independence**

555 Saturn Boulevard
Suite B-368
San Diego, CA 92154

619-423-7709
FAX: 619-423-7709
e-mail: info@mouthstick.net
www.mouthstick.net

Arthur Heyer, President

Develops, manufactures and markets special vocational equipment for the physically handicapped. Products: mouthsticks, computer mechanical aids: key locks and diskette loaders. Also, turntable desks, wheelchair portable desks, filing trays with slanted sides, telephone adapters, and motorized artist easel. All these products have been designed to solve the functional limitations of people with little or no use of hands and/or arms.

572 **Infogrip: AdjustaCart**

1794 E Main Street
Ventura, CA 93001

805-652-0770
800-397-0921
FAX: 805-652-0880
e-mail: sales@infogrip.com

Sit or stand while working with this easily adjustable desk. With a simple squeeze of a paddle the front surface travel range of 12 3/4. The front surface tilts 9 degrees toward and 15 degrees away from you. Anthro carts are made of 1" thick industrial grade particleboard shelves with high-pressure laminated 16 gauge steel tube legs that safely hold 150 pounds. Spring assisted mechanism. There are holes in 1: increment in the legs so that you can put the shelves and accessories where needed. *$629.00*

573 **Infogrip: BAT Personal Keyboard**

1794 E Main Street
Ventura, CA 93001

805-652-0770
800-397-0921
FAX: 805-652-0880
e-mail: sales@infogrip.com

One handed, compact input device that replicates all the functions of a full size keyboard, but with greater efficiency and convenience. Bat is easy to learn and use. Letters, numbers, commands and macros are simple key combinations, chords, that you can master in no time. BAT's unique ergonomic design reduces hand strain and fatigue for greater comfort and productivity. *$200.00*

574 **Infogrip: ErgoPOD Model 500**

1794 E Main Street
Ventura, CA 93001

805-652-0770
800-397-0921
FAX: 805-652-0880
e-mail: sales@infogrip.com

ErgoPOD Model 500 provides a workstation solution to computer users who work from a reclining position. Model 500 straddles a bed or recliner and can hold up to 21" monitors anywhere on its surface, and will securely position the monitor at angles up to 60 degrees. The adjustable keyboard mechanism and motorized height adjustment make ergonomic configuration easy — even for the most demanding cases. *$ 1895.00*

575 **Infogrip: King Keyboard**

1794 E Main Street
Ventura, CA 93001

805-652-0770
800-397-0921
FAX: 805-652-0880
e-mail: sales@infogrip.com

Giant alternative keyboard that plugs directly into a computer— no special interface is required. The keys are 1.25 inches in diameter, slightly recessed, and provide both tactile and auditory feedback. The King has a built-in keyboard so that you can rest on its surface without activating keys. This keyboard allows you to control both keyboard and mouse functions, so it's great for people who have difficulty maneuvering a standard mouse. *$130.00*

576 **Infogrip: Large Print Keyboard**

1794 E Main Street
Ventura, CA 93001

805-652-0770
800-397-0921
FAX: 805-652-0880
e-mail: sales@infogrip.com

Standard Windows keyboard with large print keys. The keyboard and its keys are the same size as a standard keyboard; however, the print has been enhanced. The characters measure .5" by .25", about 3 times larger than standard keyboard characters. *$130.00*

577 **Infogrip: Large Print/Braille Keyboard Labels**

1794 E Main Street
Ventura, CA 93001
805-652-0770
800-397-0921
FAX: 805-652-0880
e-mail: sales@infogrip.com

Makes a standard keyboard more accessible for visually impaired individuals with large print or Braille keyboard labels. Characters on the large print labels are .5" by .25", about 3 times larger than standard keyboard characters. Braille labels are available as clear labels with Braille dots or large print with Braille. Each set includes all the keys used on a standard Windows keyboard. *$29.00*

578 **Infogrip: OnScreen**

1794 E Main Street
Ventura, CA 93001
805-652-0770
800-397-0921
FAX: 805-652-0880
e-mail: sales@infogrip.com

OnScreen features word prediction/completion (with an editable dictionary), Key Dwell Timer (a timer that selects a key under the cursor), integrated Verbal Keys Feedback, Show and Hide Keys (turns on/off keys to prevent access and minimize confusion) a Smart Window (automatically re-positions the keyboard or panels off of the area in use). On Screen also offers edit, numeric, macro, calculator and Windows enhancement capabilities. *$200.00*

579 **Infogrip: OnScreen with CrossScanner**

1794 E Main Street
Ventura, CA 93001
805-652-0770
800-397-0921
FAX: 805-652-0880
e-mail: sales@infogrip.com

OnScreen features word prediction/completion (with an editable dictionary), Key Dwell Timer (a timer that selects a key under the cursor), integrated Verbal Keys Feedback, Show and Hide Keys (turns on/off keys to prevent access and minimize confusion) a Smart Window (automatically re-positions the keyboard or panels off of the area in use). On Screen also offers edit, numeric, macro, calculator and Windows enhancement cababilities. CrossScanner launches, runs and controls Windows functions. *$200.00*

580 **Liaison Computer Work Station**

APT Technology
236A N Main Street
Shreve, OH 44676
330-567-2001
888-549-2001
FAX: 330-567-3073
e-mail: sales@apt-technology.com
www.apt-technology.com

Grace Miller, Office Manager

A full function computer work station for high level (C-2 to C-5) spinal cord injured users. It transparently emulates both keyboard and mouse, using rapid direct selection which commonly yields letter by letter typing rates of 15 to 20 words per minute. The user controls it via proportional IR remote control from the DU-IT controlled power wheelchair and chin or tongue/lip controller or via a desk-mounted proportional controller as a stand alone device. Full ECU features included. *$ 4685.00*

581 **PhoneMax Amplified Telephone**

Assistive Devices Network
2241 S Triangle X Lane
Tucson, AZ 85713
866-674-3549
FAX: 520-883-3172
e-mail: info@assistivedevices.net
www.assistivedevices.net

582 **Talking Electronic Organizers**

Independent Living Aids
200 Robbins Lane
Jericho, NY 11753
516-937-1848
800-537-2118
FAX: 516-937-3906
e-mail: can-do@independentliving.com
www.independentliving.com

Marvin Sandler, President

Electronic, portable, personal organizers that talk the user through all the functions and are totally voice interactive. $199.95 and up.

583 **Television Remote Controls with Large Numbers**

Independent Living Aids
200 Robbins Lane
Jericho, NY 11753
516-937-1848
800-537-2118
FAX: 516-937-3906
e-mail: can-do@independentliving.com
www.independentliving.com

Marvin Sandler, President

Large 5 1/2 inch x 8 1/2 inch unit that has easy to see and use buttons. Can be used on nearly every TV, VCR and cable boxes. *$ 39.95*

Scooters

584 **Alante**

Golden Technologies
401 Bridge Street
Old Forge, PA 18518
570-451-7477
800-624-6374
FAX: 570-451-7494
e-mail: info@goldentech.com
www.goldentech.com

Rich Golden, CEO
Fred Kiwak, VP
Bob Smith, VP Sales

Rear-wheel-drive vehicle that represents the best in powered mobility.

585 **Amigo Centra**

Amigo Mobility International
6693 Dixie Highway
Bridgeport, MI 48722
989-777-0910
FAX: 800-334-7274

Features an adjustable handle that bends, making steering comfortable and enjoyable. The rugged construction and variable speed make it the perfect choice for indoor/outdoor mobility. *$2495.00*

586 **Amphibious ATV Distributors**

Amphibious ATV Distributors
2760 Greendale Drive
Sarasota, FL 34232
941-379-6186
800-843-2811
FAX: 941-377-8979
e-mail: CBeach1419@aol.com
www.maxsixwheel.com

Clay Beach, Owner

A two and four passenger, all-terrain vehicle that can provide you with year round activities the whole family can enjoy. Accessible and drivable for the physically disabled. Used in hunting, fishing and outdoor activities on land and in the water. Many options and accessories available. Delivery anwyhere in the US and worldwide. $5,000-$9,000.

587 **Avant Walker**

ETAC USA
12801 E Independence Boulevard
PO Box 1739
Matthews, NC 28106
800-678-7684
FAX: 704-882-0751
e-mail: info@snugseat.com
www.snugseat.com/avant.html

Elegant styling makes the Avant an attractive companion. The adjustable height seat and backrest offer comfort and security whenever or wherever you choose to stop and rest. Pressure sensitive brakes require little strength to operate. Folds easily with one hand. Lifetime warranty on frame and brake straps for original owner. $395-$50.

588 **Bravo! + Three-Wheel Scooter**

Ortho-Kinetics
PO Box 1647
Waukesha, WI 53187
262-542-6060
800-824-1068
FAX: 262-542-3990

Anne Tyler, Marketing Director

Designed to increase your mobility indoors. The Bravo! plus has extendible rear wheels for outdoor use and comes with easy to use finger tip controls and a maintenance free gel-cell battery. Available in red, blue, green or light sand gray with an optional power seat lift. Call for complete line of 3 and 4-wheel electronic vehicles.

589 **Cruiser Bus Buggy 4MB**

Convaid Products
PO Box 2458
Palos Verdes Peninsula, CA 90274
310-618-0111
FAX: 310-618-8811
www.convaid.com

Mervyn Watkins, President

In sizes from infant through young adult, this positioning buggy is crash-tested.

590 **Electric Mobility Corporation**

1 Mobility Plaza
PO Box 156
Sewell, NJ 08080
856-468-1000
800-257-7955
FAX: 856-468-3426
www.emobility.com

Manufactures Rascal Scooters.

591 **Explorer+ 4-Wheel Scooter**

Ortho-Kinetics
PO Box 1647
Waukesha, WI 53187
262-542-6060
800-824-1068
FAX: 262-542-4258
www.orthokinetics.com

Anne Tyler, Director Marketing

A tough and rugged 4-wheel, rear-wheel drive, transaxle scooter designed to take you just about anywhere you want to go. Easy to use finger-tip controls and maintenance free gel-cell batteries and an extendible, take-apart frame, make the Explorer+ a perfect fit for people seeking greater mobility. Available in red, blue, green and gray, with an optional power seat lift. $3,499-$3,999.

592 **Featherlite**

No Boundaries
12882 Valley View Street
Suite 5
Garden Grove, CA 92845
714-891-5899
800-926-8637
FAX: 714-891-0658
www.noboundaries.tv

Lightweight scooter folds in seconds without tools or bending down for hassle free travel on airplanes, cruise ships, trains, RVs, buses and more! Heaviest component weighs 27 pounds. Fits easily in almost any vehicle trunk.

593 **Invacare Fulfillment Center**

Invacare Corporation
One Invacare Way
Elyria, OH 44035
440-329-6000
800-333-6900
FAX: 440-329-6568
e-mail: info@invacare.com
www.invacare.com

Susan Elder, Dir of Marketing Communications

Invacare Corporation is the world's leading manufacturer and distributor of non-acute medical products which promote recovery and active lifestyles for people requiring home and other non-acute health care.

594 **Leisure Lift**

Leisure Lift
1800 Merriam Lane
Kansas City, KS 66106
800-255-0285
FAX: 913-722-2614
e-mail: leisure-lift@kc.rr.com
www.pacesaver.com

Leisure Lift offers light three wheel scooter models and seven power wheelchair models. *$2695.00*

595 **MVP+ 3-Wheel Scooter**

Ortho-Kinetics
PO Box 1647
Waukesha, WI 53187
262-547-1600
800-824-1068
FAX: 262-542-3990

The MVP+ is the rugged 3-wheel rear-wheel drive, tranaxle scooter with finger tip controls, and featuring an extendible, take-apart frame for a perfect fit. The MVP+ comes with maintenance free gel-cell batteries and is available in red, blue, green or light sand gray, with an optional power seat lift. $2,599-$3,099.

596 **Minova Walker**

ETAC USA
2325 Parklawn Drive
Suite J
Waukesha, WI 53186
800-678-3822
FAX: 262-796-4605
e-mail: etac1usa@execpc.com
www.execpc.com/~etac1usa

Childrens Walker shares the same basic principles as Adult Nova. The handles are adjustable for both width and height. The walker is easy to fold with a remarkable safety braking system. $498-$525.

597 **Mitsubishi Truck: FE434**

Mitsubishi Fuso Truck of America
PO Box 464
Bridgeport, NJ 08014
856-467-4500
FAX: 856-467-4695

A cab-over, turbo-charged diesel with optional four-speed automatic transmission, has wide angle front and side windows for improved visibility.

598 **Motorized Stander**

Advanced Technology Corporation
1601 Charlotte Street
Kansas City, MO 64108
816-421-6688
800-785-9108
FAX: 816-221-8371
e-mail: advancedtech@prodigy.net

Joel Poindexter

Occupant-operated motorized vehicle that offers independence, increased mobility and ease of movement to disabled people.

599 **Motovator Three-Wheel Scooter**

Motovator
22626 Normandie Avenue
Suite E
Torrance, CA 90502
310-320-5941

e-mail: gene.massey@motovator.com
www.motovator.com

This three-wheel electric wheelchair is a very maneuverable scooter with a turning radius that will get you around furniture, around a corner, through a doorway and more.

600 **Moxie**

No Boundaries
12882 Valley View Street
Suite 5
Garden Grove, CA 92845
714-891-5899
800-926-8637
FAX: 714-891-0658
www.noboundaries.tv

Disassembles into three parts in less than a minute. Heaviest component weighs 41 pounds. Portable, affordable and downright snazzy!

601 **Nova Rollators**

ETAC USA
2325 Parklawn Drive
Suite J
Waukesha, WI 53186
800-678-3822
FAX: 262-796-4605
e-mail: etac1usa@execpc.com

Light and easy to handle, fully adjustable for individual needs. Large cushioned tires allow the Nova to roll outdoors and indoors. $498-$637.

$498 - $637

602 **Outdoor Independence**

Palmer Industries
PO Box 5707
1 Heath Avenue
Endicott, NY 13763
607-754-2957
800-847-1304
FAX: 607-754-1954
e-mail: palmer@palmerind.com
www.palmerind.com

Joanne Martone, Information Specialist
Lisa Carter, Manager of Sales

The futuristic electric three-wheeler designed to take you almost anywhere.

603 **Pace Saver Plus II**

Leisure-Lift
1800 Merriam Lane
Kansas City, KS 66106
800-255-0285

e-mail: leisure-lift@kc.rr.com
www.pacesaver.com

The scooter combines outdoor ruggedness with indoor maneuverability at a low price.

604 **Palmer Independence**

Palmer Industries
PO Box 707
Endicott, NY 13760
607-748-8227
800-847-1304

Futuristic electric three wheeler designed to take the rider almost anywhere.

605 **Palmer Twosome**

Palmer Industries
1 Health Avenue
PO Box 5707
Endicott, NY 13763
607-754-2957
800-847-1304
FAX: 607-754-1954
e-mail: palmer@palmerind.com
www.palmerind.com

Joanne Martone, Information Specialist
Lisa Carter, Manager of Sales

All electric two seat vehicle for those who can't pedal.

606 **Polaris Trail Blazer**

Polaris Industries
2100 Highway 55
Medina, MN 55340
763-542-0500
800-765-2747
FAX: 763-542-0599
www.polarisindustries.com

W Hall Wendel, Chairman
Thomas Tiller, President
Micheal Malone, VP

A four-wheeler that has many engineered innovations, features such as: full floorboards for full comfort, single lever breaking with auxiliary foot brake, electronic throttle control, parking brake and adjustable handlebars.

607 **Quickie 2**

Sunrise Medical/Quickie Designs
2382 Faraday Avenue
Suite 200
Carlsbad, CA 92008
760-930-1500
FAX: 760-930-1585
www.sunrisemedical.com

This custom, ultralight, folding, everyday scooter offers portability and performance plus modular flexibility.

608 **Rascal 3-Wheeler**

Electric Mobility Corporation
1 Mobility Plaza
PO Box 156
Sewell, NJ 08080
856-468-1000
800-257-7955
FAX: 856-468-3426
www.emobility.com

For primarily outdoor use, this three wheeler provides extra strength, durability and reliability.

609 **Rascal ConvertAble**

Electric Mobility Corporation
1 Mobility Plaza
PO Box 156
Sewell, NJ 08080
856-468-1000
800-257-7955
FAX: 856-468-3426
www.emobility.com

An electric vehicle that's a compact mobile chair one minute and a rugged outdoor scooter the next. Use both indoors and outdoors. Also available with joystick controls.

610 Regal Scooters

Bruno Independent Living Aids
1780 Executive Drive
Suite 84
Oconomowoc, WI 53066
262-567-4990
800-882-8183
FAX: 262-567-4341
e-mail: webmaster@bruno.com

This line includes the Regal Standard, the Regal Large Adult, the Regal Small Adult, the Regal Pediatric, The Regal Ten models 65 and 75, and The Regal Four. These scooters offer adjustable flip-up armrests, pneumatic tires front and rear, and more.

611 Regent

Golden Technologies
401 Bridge Street
Old Forge, PA 18518
570-451-747
800-624-6324
FAX: 570-451-7974
e-mail: info@goldentech.com
www.goldentech.com

Top-rated performance scooter, with extra features and economically priced.

612 Roadster 20

ATV Solutions
4700 W 60th Avenue
Unit 4
Arvada, CO 80003
303-450-2881
866-777-9727
888-867-1159
FAX: 303-450-2880
e-mail: sales@atvsolutions.com
www.atvsolutions.com

Great for indoor or outdoor use. The powerful, quiet drive system, independent front suspension and fully reclining high-back seat make for a smooth, quiet ride. The Roadster is loaded with great features at a bargain price.

613 Safari Scooter

Ranger All Seasons Corporation
PO Box 132
George, IA 51237
712-475-2811
800-225-3811
FAX: 712-475-3320
e-mail: ranger@rconnect.com
www.rangerallseason.com

Randy Riecks, Sales Manager

Safari is Ranger's most popular scooter. Available in either a 40 inch or 43 inch frame length with an ultra-quiet, totally enclosed transacle drive. The Safari has some of the same features as the SOLO, the user-friendly take-apart and tiller adjustment, color impregnated— not painted— ABS plastic body. The most versatile Ranger Scooter, the Safari is an excellent choice for indoor use, and can take the place of most front wheel drive scooters. It is also an excellent outdoor scooter.

614 Scoota Bug

Golden Technologies
401 Bridge Street
Old Forge, PA 18518
570-451-7477
800-624-6324
FAX: 570-451-7974
e-mail: info@goldentech.com
www.goldentech.com

A lightweight, completely modular scooter, that disassembles and fits into most auto trunks.

615 Scooter Discounters

1945 Winterhaven Drive
Virginia Beach, VA 23456
757-430-2664
800-229-1317
e-mail: sales@scooterone.com
www.scooterone.com

Offers electric scooters, scooter lifts, ramps, batteries and more at excellent value without sacrificing quality or service.

616 Shuttle

Mobilelectrics Company
4014 Bardstown Road
Louisville,]Y 40218
800-876-6846
FAX: 502-495-2476

A three wheel scooter with safety features for ease of handling, comfort and maximum pleasure.

617 Sidekick Scooter

Mobilelectrics Company
4014 Bardstown Road
Louisville, KY 40218
800-876-6846
FAX: 502-495-2476

The seat and foot space provides ample comfort for the average person and the length of the scooter gives it indoor maneuverability.

618 Sierra 3000/4000

Ortho-Kinetics
PO Box 1647
Waukesha, WI 53187
262-542-6060
800-824-1068
FAX: 262-542-3990

Look to the Sierra 3000/4000 series vehicles for comfort, convenience and performance. Increased leg and foot room, adjustable seat height and arm width, as well as adjustable tiller angle provide maximum comfort. For convenience, the Sierra is equipped with integrated cargo and cup holders and thumb/finger controls with built in wrist rest. Advanced safety features such as stall and free-wheeling situation identification and correction, anti roll-back sensory device and audio/visual feedback.

619 Solo Scooter

Ranger All Seasons Corporation
PO Box 132
George, IA 51237
712-475-2811
800-225-3811
FAX: 712-475-3320
e-mail: ranger@rconnect.com
www.rangerallseason.com

Randy Riecks, Sales Manager

The SOLO is Ranger's flagship model. Introduction of the SOLO 1991 set the standard for easy disassembly of a scooter. The SOLO has a long list of user friendly features including patented take-apart and tiller adjustment mechanisms, non-rusting aluminum frame, comfortable contoured seats as standard, color impregnated-not painted-ABS plastic bodies, charger plug conveniently located on the Accelerator box and many more. Available in ultra-quiet drive and four wheel models.

620 SoloRider Industries

PO Box 371047
Denver, CO 80237
303-858-0505
800-898-3353
FAX: 303-858-0707
e-mail: info@solorider.com
www.solorider.com

Roger Pretekin, President

Manufactures and distributes the AteeA- the revolutionary single rider specifically designed to meet the needs of individuals with disabilities.

621 **Sportster 10**

ATV Solutions
4700 W 60th Avenue
Unit 4
Arvada, CO 80003
303-450-2881
866-777-9727
888-867-1159
FAX: 303-450-2880
e-mail: sales@atvsolutions.com
www.atvsolutions.com

Sportster 10 is our most maneuverable scooter, ideal for riders who must operate in tight spaces. Equipped with all of the great features of the Roadster 20, this three-wheeler is an exceptional buy.

622 **Surry Tricycloped**

National Manufacturing Company
PO Box 3268
Boise, ID 83703 **208-343-3639**

The Surry has a sleek, aerodynamic design with canted side rails and simple hand controls for gas and brakes.

623 **Systems 2000**

BioMedical Life Systems
PO Box 1360
Vista, CA 92085
800-726-8367
FAX: 760-727-4220
e-mail: information@bmls.com
www.bmls.com

This five-mode TENS device has four adjustable modulations, plus conventional settings and comes with a five-year warranty.

624 **Terra-Jet: Utility Vehicle**

TERRA-JET USA
Junction Highway 417 & 419
PO Box 918
Innis, LA 70747
225-492-2249
800-864-5000
FAX: 225-492-2249
e-mail: 207767@mcimail.com
terrajet.tripod.com

Larry Rabalaus, President
Dora Rabalaus, Secretary/Treasurer

TERRA-JET utility vehicles are unique in its ability to traverse many different types of terrain in remote areas otherwise inaccessible. It has a multitude of uses for industry, sportsmen or the whole family. Uniquely designed, industrial duty construction of low maintenance and low fuel consumption. $8,675-$21,995.

625 **Terrier Tricycle**

TRIAID
PO Box 1364
Cumberland, MD 21501
301-759-3525
800-306-6777
FAX: 301-759-3525
e-mail: sales@triaid.com
www.triaid.com

Iain A MacDonald, Sales Director
Ann M Hutter, Sales Executive

Provides fun therapy and actively encourages participation, awareness and the building of self confidence. Designed for children from about five years it features ATB styling, 16 inch wheels, adjustable steering stop and a supportive saddle. Handlebar and seat adjustments combine with a broad wheelbase to ensure the rider is in the optimum position to pedal and the tricycle gives good stability and confident handling. Support accessories are available.

626 **Trekker 40**

ATV Solutions
4700 W 60th Avenue
Unit 4
Arvada, CO 80003
866-777-9727
888-867-1159
FAX: 303-450-2880
e-mail: sales@atvsolutions.com
www.atvsolutions.com

Our biggest, toughest scooter. With a huge 450 pound capacity and five inches of ground clearance, this machine is ideal for the daily outdoor user. The high top speed means you get there fast and the four-wheel suspension makes the ride smooth and comfortable.

627 **Tri-Lo's**

TRIAID
PO Box 1364
Cumberland, MD 21501
301-759-3525
800-306-6777
FAX: 301-759-3525
e-mail: sales@triaid.com
www.triaid.com

Iain A MacDonald, Sales Director
Ann M Hutter, Sales Executive

Available in three sizes, these Tricycles provide fun therapy for children from 2-15 years. Propelled by hand cranks, the Tri-Lo's are highly recommended by therapists for Spina Bifida children and any other child where the use of the lower limbs is restricted. The Tri-Lo's feature a robust frame with allowance for growth, low foot platform for ease of transfer, padded seat and back cushion, padded armrests, two forms of braking and an anti-tipping device. *$740.00*

628 **Tri-Wheelers**

Braun Corporation
1014 S Monticello Street
Suite 310
Winamac, IN 46996
574-946-6157
800-843-5438
FAX: 574-946-4670

Provides convenience features, producing a high efficiency performance with ultra-smooth operation.

629 **Triumph 3000/4000**

Ortho-Kinetics
PO Box 1647
Waukesha, WI 53187
262-542-6060
800-824-1068
FAX: 262-542-3990

The Triumph 3000/4000 series vehicles provide unique comfort and convenience features found nowhere else. Digital Dash with soft touch keypad, deluxe seat with suspension and integral cargo and cup holders are just a few of these features. Equipped with TOPS 24 (Total Ortho Power System) ensuring maximum power, performance and reliability. Luxurious options such as velour or allante seat fabrics, stylized wheels, metallic or pearl color options and digital controls are all standard. $2,899-$3,39

630 Triumph Scooter

Ortho-Kinetics
PO Box 1647
Waukesha, WI 53187
262-547-1600
800-824-1068
FAX: 262-542-3990

The sleek rugged three-wheel, rear-wheel drive, transaxle scooter with up-top controls, designed to help increase mobility and become more active. The Triumph is designed for both indoor and outdoor use. Available in red, blue, green or gray, with an optional power seat lift. $2,899-$3,399.

631 Uno Walker

ETAC USA
2325 Parklawn Drive
Suite J
Waukesha, WI 53186
800-678-3822
FAX: 262-796-4605
e-mail: etac1usa@execpc.com
www.execpc.com/~etac1usa

A number one in any language. Elegantly designed with height adjustable handles, seat mudguards, and adjustable wheel locks are standard. Accessories include tray assemble, basket, crutch/cane holder, backrest and oxygen holder. $299-$400.

632 X10 Powerhouse

Words+
40015 Sierra Highway B-145
Palmdale, CA 93550
661-266-8500
800-869-8521
FAX: 661-266-8969

Ginger Woltosz, VP
Tim Ross, Manager

Controls AC-powered appliances with a control unit and appliance modules. Plug the appliance modules into the outlets, then plug the appliances into the modules. *$199.00*

Stationery

633 Address Book

Sense-Sations
919 Walnut Street
Philadelphia, PA 19107
215-627-0600
FAX: 215-922-0692

The big print address book is the first personal book to provide enlarged writing spaces, making it easier to write down and retrieve information. *$12.50*

634 Big Print Address Book

Access with Ease
PO Box 1150
Chino Valley, AZ 86323
928-636-9469
800-531-9479
FAX: 928-636-0292
e-mail: KMJC@northlink.com

Karen Clymer, President

Oversized organizer makes locating information easier for those with limited vision. The 7 1/2 inch by 9 1/2 inch plastic coil bound book has more than 500 listings with laminated alphabet tabs. *$16.95*

635 Bold Line Paper

Sense-Sations
919 Walnut Street
Philadelphia, PA 19107
215-627-0600
FAX: 215-922-0692

This pad consists of 100 sheets of paper with bold lines to help guide the writing of an individual with limited vision. *$2.50*

636 Braille Notebook

Maxi Aids
42 Executive Boulevard
Suite 3209
Farmingdale, NY 11735
631-752-0521
800-522-6294
FAX: 631-752-0689
e-mail: sales@maxiaids.com
www.maxiaids.com

Made of heavy-duty board, covered with waterproof imitation leather and three rings for binding, including braille paper and titles. *$12.95*

637 Braille: Greeting Cards

Sense-Sations
919 Walnut Street
Philadelphia, PA 19107
215-627-0600
FAX: 215-922-0692

Birthday, anniversary, get well, sympathy and Christmas cards offering braille print for the blind. *$.95*

638 Brailled Desk Calendar

Maxi Aids
42 Executive Boulevard
Suite 3209
Farmingdale, NY 11735
631-752-0521
800-522-6294
FAX: 631-752-0689
e-mail: sales@maxiaids.com
www.maxiaids.com

Schedule appointments, remember birthdays or write messages for a particular day. *$39.95*

639 Clip Board Notebook

Sense-Sations
919 Walnut Street
Philadelphia, PA 19107
215-627-0600
FAX: 215-922-0692

Kit includes a pack of Bold Line paper and black ink pen. *$5.95*

640 Deluxe Signature Guide

Maxi Aids
42 Executive Boulevard
Suite 3209
Farmingdale, NY 11735
631-752-0521
800-522-6294
FAX: 631-752-0689
e-mail: sales@maxiaids.com
www.maxiaids.com

Rods supported by two rubber blocks facilitate writing. *$1.25*

641 Highlighter and Note Tape

Therapro
225 Arlington Street
Framingham, MA 01702
508-872-9494
800-257-5376
FAX: 508-875-2062
e-mail: info@theraproducts.com
www.theraproducts.com

A great way to highlight and draw attention to words without damaging original. Price ranges from $4.00-$7.00.

642 **Letter Writing Guide**

Independent Living Aids
200 Robbins Lane
Jericho, NY 11753
516-937-1848
800-537-2118
FAX: 516-937-3906
e-mail: can-do@independentliving.com
www.independentliving.com

Marvin Sandler, President

Sturdy plastic sheet with 13 apertures corresponding to standard line spacing. *$3.49*

643 **Lettering Guide Value Pack**

Independent Living Aids
200 Robbins Lane
Jericho, NY 11753
516-937-1848
800-537-2118
FAX: 516-937-3906
e-mail: can-do@independentliving.com
www.independentliving.com

Included in this useful pack are four durable plastic lettering and number guides for tracing letters when the individual is unable to write letters unassisted. *$6.29*

644 **Maxi Marks**

Maxi Aids
42 Executive Boulevard
Suite 3209
Farmingdale, NY 11735
631-752-0521
800-522-6294
FAX: 631-752-0689
e-mail: sales@maxiaids.com
www.maxiaids.com

Braille writing and identification products. *$2.50*

645 **Pencil/Pen Weighted Holders**

Therapro
225 Arlington Street
Framingham, MA 01702
508-872-9494
800-257-5376
FAX: 508-875-2062
e-mail: info@theraproducts.com
www.theraproducts.com

Securely hold any pencil or pen. These weighted holders allow for more control along with proprioceptive feedback to encourage better writing skills.

646 **Raised Line Drawing Kit**

Maxi Aids
42 Executive Boulevard
Suite 3209
Farmingdale, NY 11735
631-752-0521
800-522-6294
FAX: 631-752-0689
e-mail: sales@maxiaids.com
www.maxiaids.com

For writing script or drawing graphs by the use of special plastic paper. *$24.45*

647 **Signature and Address Self-Inking Stamps**

Independent Living Aids
200 Robbins Lane
Jericho, NY 11753
516-937-1848
800-537-2118
FAX: 516-937-3906
e-mail: can-do@independentliving.com
www.independentliving.com

Gives thousands of impressions before requiring re-inking. *$11.95*

648 **Steady Write**

Maxi Aids
42 Executive Boulevard
Suite 3209
Farmingdale, NY 11735
631-752-0521
800-522-6294
FAX: 631-752-0689
e-mail: sales@maxiaids.com
www.maxiaids.com

Furnishes the writer with increased holding capacity and stabilizes the hand. *$6.95*

649 **Wings & Wheels Greeting Cards**

Wings & Wheels
5 Cleveland Avenue
Dover, NJ 07801
800-422-5309
FAX: 973-989-9072
e-mail: flyingspiritedmsn.com
www.wings-wheels.com

Nanette Courtine, Owner

Offer inclusive greeting cards. Depicts people with disabilities on the cards.

Visual Aids

650 **Aluminum Adjustable Support Canes for the Blind**

Maxi Aids
42 Executive Boulevard
Suite 3209
Farmingdale, NY 11735
631-752-0521
800-522-6294
FAX: 631-752-0689
e-mail: sales@maxiaids.com
www.maxiaids.com

Adjustable canes for the visually impaired. *$17.95*

651 **Audio Book Contractors**

PO Box 40115
Washington, DC 20016
202-363-3429
FAX: 202-363-3429
e-mail: flogibsonABC@aol.com

Flo Gibson, President

Over 950 titles of unabridged classic books on audio cassettes in sturdy vinyl covers with picture and spine windows. Discounted prices for disabled patrons.

652 **Beyond Sight**

5650 S Windermere
Littleton, CO 80120
303-795-6455
FAX: 303-795-6425
e-mail: bsistore@beyondsite.com
www.beyondsight.com

Jim Misener, President

Products for the blind and visually impaired including talking clocks, watches and calculators. They also carry a large selection of Braille products, magnifiers, reading machines and computer equipment. New products include: Accucheck Voicemate and PureFocus vision spray and GPS Talk, the first talking GPS system for the blind.

653 **Big Number Pocket Sized Calculator**

Independent Living Aids
200 Robbins Lane
Jericho, NY 11753
516-937-1848
800-537-2118
FAX: 516-937-3906
e-mail: can-do@independentliving.com
www.independentliving.com

A handy pocket size calculator with big numbers that fits easily into purse or pocket. *$14.95*

654 **Braille Compass**

Maxi Aids
42 Executive Boulevard
Suite 3209
Farmingdale, NY 11735
631-752-0521
800-522-6294
FAX: 631-752-0689
e-mail: sales@maxiaids.com
www.maxiaids.com

The visually impaired can tell the direction by using this compass. *$42.95*

655 **Braille Plates for Elevator**

Maxi Aids
42 Executive Boulevard
Suite 3209
Farmingdale, NY 11735
631-752-0521
800-522-6294
FAX: 631-752-0689
e-mail: sales@maxiaids.com
www.maxiaids.com

The plates have curing type pressure sensitive material applied for metal to metal bonding. *$79.95*

656 **Braille Touch-Time Watches**

Independent Living Aids
200 Robbins Lane
Jericho, NY 11753
516-937-1848
800-537-2118
FAX: 516-937-3906
e-mail: can-do@independentliving.com
www.independentliving.com

Marvin Sandler, President

White dial with black numerals and hands makes telling time possible quickly and easily for the visually impaired. *$44.95*

657 **Extra Loud Alarm with Lighter Plug**

HARC Mercantile
PO Box 3055
Kalamazoo, MI 49003
269-324-1615
800-445-9968
FAX: 269-324-2387
e-mail: home@harcmercantile.com
www.harcmercantile.com

Ronald Slager, President

Battery operated, easy to read, digital clock with extra loud alarm. *$45.00*

658 **Low Vision Telephones**

Assistive Devices Network
2241 S Triangle X Lane
Tucson, AZ 85713
866-674-3549
FAX: 520-883-3172
e-mail: info@assistivedevices.net
http://assistivedevices.net/about.htm

659 **Man's Low-Vision Quartz Watches**

Independent Living Aids
200 Robbins Lane
Jericho, NY 11753
516-937-1848
800-537-2118
FAX: 516-937-3906
e-mail: can-do@independentliving.com
www.independentliving.com

Marvin Sandler, President

An inexpensive, easy-to-read watch with chrome case. *$ 27.95*

660 **Men's/Women's Low Vision Watches & Clocks**

Maxi Aids
42 Executive Boulevard
Suite 3209
Farmingdale, NY 11735
631-752-0521
800-522-6294
FAX: 631-752-0689
e-mail: sales@maxiaids.com
www.maxiaids.com

Choose from a wide range of watches from braille automatic to quartz pocket watches.

661 **Rigid Aluminum Cane with Golf Grip**

Maxi Aids
42 Executive Boulevard
Suite 3209
Farmingdale, NY 11735
631-752-0521
800-522-6294
FAX: 631-752-0689
e-mail: sales@maxiaids.com
www.maxiaids.com

A straight, tubular, heavy gauge aluminum rigid cane for blind and visually impaired persons. *$12.95*

662 **TAJ Braille Typewriter**

Maxi Aids
42 Executive Boulevard
Suite 3209
Farmingdale, NY 11735
631-752-0521
800-522-6294
FAX: 631-752-0689
e-mail: sales@maxiaids.com
www.maxiaids.com

Smooth edged, simple and sturdy construction. Creates braille on 8 1/2 x 11 paper. *$495.00*

663 **Three M Brailler**

Maxi Aids
42 Executive Boulevard
Suite 3209
Farmingdale, NY 11735
631-752-0521
800-522-6294
FAX: 631-752-0689
e-mail: sales@maxiaids.com
www.maxiaids.com

For visually impaired, blind and sighted persons, produces braille on 3/8 and 1/2 inch vinyl tape. The dial has braille and regular characters. *$47.95*

664 **Three M Large Printed Labeler**

Maxi Aids
42 Executive Boulevard
Suite 3209
Farmingdale, NY 11735
631-752-0521
800-522-6294
FAX: 631-752-0689
e-mail: sales@maxiaids.com
www.maxiaids.com

Ideal for persons with low vision. Can also be read tactually by blind persons with a knowledge of the print alphabet. *$ 133.95*

665 **Timex Easy Reader**

Independent Living Aids
200 Robbins Lane
Jericho, NY 11753
516-937-1848
800-537-2118
FAX: 516-937-3906
e-mail: can-do@independentliving.com
www.independentliving.com

An easy-to-read large face watch that's water resistant. *$29.95*

666 **Unisex Low Vision Watch**

Independent Living Aids
200 Robbins Lane
Jericho, NY 11753
516-937-1848
800-537-2118
FAX: 516-937-3906
e-mail: can-do@independentliving.com
www.independentliving.com

Marvin Sandler, President

Unisex watch with large numbers and wide hands. Gold-toned case with either expansion or leather band. *$31.95*

667 **Visual Alerting Guest Room Kit**

HARC Mercantile
PO Box 3055
Kalamazoo, MI 49003
269-324-1615
800-445-9968
FAX: 269-324-2387
e-mail: home@harcmercantile.com
www.harcmercantile.com

Ronald Slager, President

ADA compliant visual alerting guest room kit for the hard of hearing and deaf. Includes visual smoke detector, phone alert, door knock sensor, tactile alarm clock and telephone amplifier. Variations include TTY.

Walking Aids: Canes, Crutches & Walkers

668 **Air Lift Oxygen Carriers**

Air Lift Unlimited
1212 Kerr Gulch Road
Evergreen, CO 80439
303-526-4700
800-776-6771
FAX: 303-526-4774
e-mail: info@airlift.com
www.airlift.com

Lori Fortier, Office Manager

Air Lift offers a full line of carriers for portable liquid and cylinder oxygen systems. These versatile carriers meet the needs of oxygen-dependent individuals and parents with oxygen-dependent children seeking more comfortable and convenient ways to transport oxygen. Carriers include backpacks, fanny packs, shoulder/hand bags and carriers for wheelchairs, scooters and walkers. All carriers feature non-flammable, washable fabric and adjustable straps; liquid carriers feature mesh pouches.

669 **Aluminum Crutches**

Arista Surgical Supply Company
67 Lexington Avenue
New York, NY 10010
212-679-3694
800-223-1984
FAX: 212-696-9046
e-mail: aristasurgical@juno.com
www.aristasurgical.com

Lightweight aluminum crutches with wood underarms and handgrips. *$25.00*

670 **Aluminum Walking Canes**

Maxi Aids
42 Executive Boulevard
Suite 3209
Farmingdale, NY 11735
631-752-0521
800-522-6294
FAX: 631-752-0689
e-mail: sales@maxiaids.com
www.maxiaids.com

Lightweight but strong, these walking canes are made of a heavy gauge aluminum tube with safety locknuts and heavy-duty rubber tips. *$10.75*

671 **Arrow Walker**

TRIAID
PO Box 1364
Cumberland, MD 21501
301-759-3525
800-306-6777
FAX: 301-759-3525
e-mail: sales@triaid.com
www.triaid.com

Iain A MacDonald, Sales Director
Ann M Hutter, Sales Executive

A weight supportive walker designed for children with cerebral palsy or other neuromuscular handicaps. Its comprehensive range of accessories and adjustments allow the Arrow Walker to be tailored to each individual user's needs. The innovative design allows these alterations to be made quickly and easily, enabling multiple daily therapy sessions to take place. The low profile shape allows easier access through doorways and around obstacles. *$957.00*

672 **Deluxe Nova Wheeled Walker & Avant Wheeled Walker**

Sammons Preston Rolyan
4 Sammons Court
Bolingbrook, IL 60440
630-226-1300
800-323-5547
FAX: 630-226-1389
e-mail: spr@abilityone.com
www.sammonsprestonrolyan.com

Lightweight and simple to handle with an easy-to-operate braking system. *$425.40*

673 **Deluxe Standard Wood Cane**

Arista Surgical Supply Company
67 Lexington Avenue
New York, NY 10010
212-679-3694
800-223-1984
FAX: 212-696-9046
e-mail: aristasurgical@juno.com
www.aristasurgical.com

A standard old-fashioned wooden cane for the physically challenged. *$10.00*

674 **Maxi Superior Cane**

Maxi Aids
42 Executive Boulevard
Suite 3209
Farmingdale, NY 11735
631-752-0521
800-522-6294
FAX: 631-752-0689
e-mail: sales@maxiaids.com
www.maxiaids.com

Convenient folding cane designed for optimum balance. Tapered joints provide rigidity when open, and are made of heavy gauge aluminum. *$17.50*

675 **Micro IntroVoice III**

Voice Connection
2324 N Batavia Street
Orange, CA 92865
714-685-1066
FAX: 714-685-1070
e-mail: voicecnx@aol.com
www.voicecnx.com

Voice actuated interface unit that can be installed on most existing and all new wheel wheelchair occupant to speak commands to control the motion of the chair. *$2295.00*

676 **Nova Walker**

ETAC USA
2325 Parklawn Drive
Suite J
Waukesha, WI 53186
800-678-3822
FAX: 262-796-4605
e-mail: etac1usa@execpc.com
www.execpc.com/~etac1usa

Elegant design that provides a comfortable, natural walking style. The seat offers security and stability wherever you go. Folds easily with one hand. Offers lifetime warranty on frame and brake straps for original user.

677 **Out-N-About American Walker**

742 Market Street
Oregon, WI 53575
608-835-9255
FAX: 608-835-5234

Luann Smith, President

The lightweight Out-N-About is easy to handle. The four wheel design provides greater support and stability than any other walking aids. Its large rubber tires move effortlessly over most surfaces, indoors and out. The small turning radius makes it ideal for getting through confined spaces and narrow doorways. The attractive, burgundy colored, tubular steel frame is extremely durable. The Out-N-About folds flat and stands alone for easy storage. Made in USA.

678 **Prone Support Walker**

Consumer Care Products
PO Box 684
Sheboygan, WI 53082
920-459-8353
FAX: 920-459-9070

Terry Grall, President
Alice Maffongelli, Customer Service

This walker, in five sizes for children to adults, facilitates semi-prone to full upright mobility and dynamic weight bearing. The walker requires the user to push off the floor teaching the user to work with the floor and achieving a more efficient gait. Options such as tray, back support, and hip pads allow adaptation to most needs. $750-$1,300.

679 **Push-Button Quad Cane**

Arista Surgical Supply Company
67 Lexington Avenue
New York, NY 10010
212-679-3694
800-223-1984
FAX: 212-696-9046
e-mail: aristasurgical.juno.com
www.aristasurgical.com

A reliable walking cane offering independence to the physically challenged user. *$25.00*

680 **Rand-Scot**

401 Linden Center Drive
Fort Collins, CO 80524
970-484-7967
800-467-7967
FAX: 970-484-3800
TTY:800-467-7967
e-mail: info@randscot.com
www.randscot.com

Joel Lerich, President
Joellen Sarmast, Business Manager

Manufactures the Easy Pivot patient lift, the BBD wheelchair cushion line and Saratoga Exercise products for the disabled. Offers a line of patient lifts and standers for the disabled. Manufactures the EasyPivot patient lift for 1 person transfers. A video is available at no charge for potential users. $800.-$3,000.

681 **Reclining Power Wheelchairs**

LaBac Systems
3535 S Kipling Street
Denver, CO 80235
303-914-9914
800-445-4402

Power recline seating systems for wheelchairs, offering more comfort and dependability for the physically challenged.

682 **Scooter & Wheelchair Battery Fuel Gauges and Motor Speed Controllers**

Curtis Instruments
200 Kisco Avenue
Mount Kisco, NY 10549
914-666-2971
FAX: 914-666-2188
e-mail: mikolaya@curtisinst.com
www.curtisinstruments.com

Provides a readable, accurate indication of battery in easy to read type of display. Innovative, efficient motor speed controllers for single or dual PM motor vehicles.

683 **Skyway**

Skyway Machine
4451 Caterpillar Road
Redding, CA 96003
800-332-3357
FAX: 530-243-5104
e-mail: sales@skywaywheels.com
www.skywaytuffwheels.com

Parrey Cremeans, Sales Manager
Bart Weems, Sales/Customer Service

For over 20 years Skyway has been the world leader in composite wheels. Supplying over 650 different wheel combinations for wheelchairs, lawn and garden products, bicycles and a large assortment of wheeled devices. Wheel sizes range from 4 inch to 24 inch diameter.

684 **StairClimber**

Martin Technology
29 N Main Street
Gloversville, NY 12078
800-800-1410
FAX: 518-725-9522

A walker-capable person can climb and descend stairs with this walker-designed StairClimber.

685 **Standing Aid Frame with Rear Entry**

Consumer Care Products
PO Box 684
Sheboygan, WI 53082 **920-459-8353**
FAX: 920-459-9070

Terry Grall, President
Alice Maffongelli, Customer Service

This rugged stander, made of natural hardwood in sizes for one to twelve year olds, allows weight bearing in an upright position. Table, upper trunk and/or head support, hip pads and casters allow individualized fitting. The new hinged rear entry option makes entry into this stander easy and quick for parents, teachers and therapists. $572-$1,800.

686 **Thomas Hardware, Parts & Fasteners**

1001 Rockland Street
Reading, PA 19604
800-634-4293
FAX: 800-634-3099

Bob Ruhe, Marketing Manager

Wheelchair restraint kits.

687 **Tilt-N-Table**

Osterguard Enterprises c/o Jim's Shop
3228 W Olive Avenue
Fresno, CA 93722 **559-275-4695**

These are lightweight tables for wheelchairs that are angle and height adjustable to your changing needs.

688 **Torso Support**

Grandmar
5675-C Landregan Street
Emeryville, CA 94608

An aid for people who are unable to maintain an upright position in an automobile or a wheelchair.

689 **Ventura Enterprises**

35 Lawton Avenue
Danville, IN 46122 **317-745-2989**
FAX: 317-745-3179
www.venturaenterprises.com

Linda Plunkett, President

Manufacturer of everyday living mobility aids. Products include carrying aids for walkers and wheelchairs and also wheelchair cushions.

690 **WCIB Heavy-Duty Folding Cane**

Maxi Aids
42 Executive Boulevard
Suite 3209
Farmingdale, NY 11735 **631-752-0521**
800-522-6294
FAX: 631-752-0689
e-mail: sales@maxiaids.com
www.maxiaids.com

A four section aluminum folding cane with a golf-type grip handle and flexible wrist loop. #1749015, 34-60 *$17.95*

691 **Walker Leg Support**

Sammons Preston Rolyan
4 Sammons Court
Bolingbrook, IL 60440 **630-226-1300**
800-323-5547
FAX: 630-226-1389
e-mail: spr@abilityone.com
www.sammonsprestonrolyan.com

For lower extremity trauma. An alternative to crutches that allows safe, stable ambulation and frees hands and arms for daily tasks. *$11.50*

692 **Wheelchair Aide**

Graham-Field
400 Rabro Drive
Hauppauge, NY 11788 **516-582-5900**

This is a heavy-duty wheelchair comfort tray which surrounds the wheelchair user and provides a large, smooth surface for dining, writing, hobbies or work. The heavy gauge plastic tray is easy to clean and attaches with two Velcro straps.

693 **Wheelchair Back Pack and Tote Bag**

Med Covers
1639 Green Street
Suite D
Raleigh, NC 27603 **919-829-5777**

Accessories are specifically designed with the wheelchair user in mind. The Back Pack has a main roomy pouch for larger items and has a full length zipper with four sliders for convenient access.

694 **Wheelchair Work Table**

Bailey Manufacturing Company
118 Lee Street
Lodi, OH 44254 **330-948-1080**
800-321-8372
FAX: 330-948-4439
e-mail: baileymfg@attmail.com
www.baileymfg.com

An adjustable height, functional, individual cut-out work table featuring a wood-grain laminate, scratch resistant top with chrome plated steel legs.

Wheelchairs: Accessories

695 **Advantage Wheelchair & Walker Bags**

Laurel Designs
5 Laurel Avenue
Belvedere, CA 94920
FAX: 415-435-1451
e-mail: laureld@ncal.verio.com

Janet Sawyer, Co-Owner
Lynn Montoya, Co-Owner

Wheelchair sport packs include: long, short, neon, multi-color and blowin' in the wind socks. Prices range from $20.00 to $60.00.

696 **Battery Operated Cushion**

DA Schulman
7701 Newton Avenue N
Brooklyn Park, MN 55444 **763-561-2908**

Battery-operated, dynamic cushion for wheelchairs.

697 **Dual-Mode Charger**

Lester Electrical
625 W A Street
Lincoln, NE 68522 **402-477-8988**
FAX: 402-474-1769
e-mail: sales@lesterelectrical.com
www.lesterelectrical.com

Edith Earnest, Sales Service Coord.
Paul Schmidt, Sales Engineer

Fully automatic battery charger.

698 **Ezback Recline Control**

APT Technology
236A N Main Street
Shreve, OH 44676 **330-567-2001**
888-549-2001
FAX: 330-567-3073
e-mail: sales@apt-technology.com
www.apt-technology.com

Helen L Thompson, Marketing Manager
David M Bayer, Rehab Engineer

A versatile, easy to install and operate motor controller intended to control power recline and similar machinery on a power wheelchair. Optional EDMA permits control of 2 motors via a single or dual switch. Accommodates limit switches, various configurations and is rugged and reliable. *$685.00*

699 **Featherspring**

712 N 34th Street
Seattle, WA 98103 **206-545-8585**
FAX: 206-547-8589
www.featherspring.com

Peter Rothschild, President

Foot supports for wheelchair users to prevent and treat cold feet, sore heels, swollen feet and weak ankles. *$199.95*

700 **George H Snyder Enterprises**

5809 NE 21st Avenue
Fort Lauderdale, FL 33308
FAX: 954-491-2886

George Snyder, President

Attachments for wheelchairs.

701 **Mat Factory**

760 W 16th Street
Building E
Costa Mesa, CA 92627 **949-645-3122**
800-628-7626
FAX: 949-645-0966
e-mail: MATFACTORY@pop3.concentric.net
www.matfactoryinc.com

Roger Maloney, President

The Safety Deck II is an interlocking grid system made from recycled rubber tires and recycled PVC. The tiles are set directly on top of the ground and permit grass to grow through the holes and cover the surface. The system provides safe, non-barrier access for wheelchairs over grass. Once the grass has covered the tiles the only maintenance required is watering and mowing. Safety Deck II also allows for beach and sand access.

702 **One Thousand FS**

Fortress
PO Box 489
Clovis, CA 93613 **559-322-5437**
FAX: 559-323-0299

Add-on power system installs in minutes, enabling the driver to relax and drive anywhere with smooth, silent electric power.

703 **Pac-All Wheelchair Carrier**

Pac-All Carriers
2321 Carolton Road
Maitland, FL 32751 **407-830-6604**
800-628-6672
FAX: 407-339-2847

LE Angel

No more lifting and no more pain wheelchair carrier. VA approved. Made in USA.

$158 - $226.40

704 **Wheel Life News**

University of Virginia, Rehab Engineering Centers
3363 University Station
Charlottesville, VA 22903 **434-924-0311**

Features tie downs and other adaptive technology for persons with disabilities.

705 **Wheelchair Accessories**

Diestco Manufacturing Company
PO Box 6504
Chico, CA 95927 **530-893-3136**
800-795-2392
FAX: 530-893-2635
e-mail: info@diestco.com
www.diestco.com

Chris Cawthon, VP Sales/Marketing

Diestco makes innovative accessories for wheelchairs, scooters and walkers. Products include canopies, backpacks, cupholders, pouches, threshhold ramps, laptrays and others.

706 **Wheelchair Rocker**

Artec
PO Box 25103-A
Greenville, SC 29616 **864-288-2111**

Randy Crew, President

The Carolina Rocker turns a wheelchair into a rocking chair for fun, relaxation and therapy for children and adults. $499

Wheelchairs: General

707 **Act Wheelchair**

Etac USA
2325 Parklawn Drive
Suite J
Waukesha, WI 53186
800-678-3822
FAX: 262-796-4605
e-mail: etac1usa@execpc.com
www.execpc.com/~etac1usa

A carefully designed Swedish wheelchair made of lightweight titanium for active users. Seat frame and upholstery are adjustable to fit each individual. Available in Frame widths from 15.5 to 18 inches. The colors available are: black, red plum teal, blue and silver. Lifetime warranty on frame for original user.

708 **Bariatric Wheelchairs Regency FL**

Gendron
Lugbill Road
Archbold, OH 43502
800-537-2521
www.gendroninc.com

Steven Cotter, VP Sales

Bariatric wheelchairs, for users weighing up to seven hundred pounds. Manual and power styles built to order for specific needs.

709 Basic Wheelchair

ETAC USA
2325 Parklawn Drive
Suite J
Waukesha, WI 53186
800-678-3822
FAX: 262-796-4605
e-mail: etac1usa@execpc.com
www.execpc.com/~etac1usa

A carefully designed crossfolding wheelchair made from extruded aluminum, the Basic is designed with the caregiver in mind and easily folds for transportation or storage. Available in widths of 14 to 20 inches, has incontinence upholstery which is easily washable with mild soap and water. Swing away, detachable legrests and footrests are standard with fixed hub rear wheels. $1,000 - $2,000

710 Big Bounder Power Wheelchair

21st Century Scientific
4915 Industrial Way
Coeur D Alene, ID 83815
208-667-8800
800-448-3680
FAX: 208-667-6600
e-mail: 21st@wheelchairs.com
www.wheelchairs.com

RD Davidson, Sales/Marketing Director
Jeanie L Saville, Sales Associate

Manufactured for the bariatric in virtually any dimension. Its powerful motors and rugged frame can accommodate users up to 1000 lb. 21st Century Scientific, Inc's unique construction can reduce the overall width of the chair. This may make the difference between using normal doorways or remodeling a home. $10,495.

711 Breezy

Sunrise Medical/Quickie Designs
2382 Faraday Avenue
Carlsbad, CA 92008
760-930-1500
FAX: 760-930-1585
www.sunrisemedical.com

This lightweight chair is durable, comfortable and flexible enough to meet the needs of a wide range of wheelchair users.

712 Champion 1000

Kuschall of America
3601 Rider Trail S
Earth City, MO 63045
314-512-7000
800-654-4768
FAX: 800-542-3567

Ultralight wheelchair designed to improve mobility. $1,689

713 Champion 2000

Kuschall of America
3601 Rider Trail S
Earth City, MO 63045
314-512-7000
800-654-4768
FAX: 800-542-3567

Rigid chair that folds side-to-side. $1,765

714 Champion 3000

Kuschall of America
3601 Rider Trail S
Earth City, MO 63045
314-512-7000
800-654-4768
FAX: 800-542-3567

The high-performance chair built for perfectionists. $1,695

715 Convaid

PO Box 4209
Palos Verdes, CA 90274
310-618-0111
888-266-8243
FAX: 310-618-2166
e-mail: convaid@convaid.com
www.convaid.com

Five different styles of wheelchairs.

716 Cross Wheelchair

ETAC USA
2325 Parklawn Drive
Suite J
Waukesha, WI 53186
800-678-3822
FAX: 262-796-4605
e-mail: etac1usa@execpc.com
www.execpc.com/~etac1usa

A carefully designed crossfolding Swedish wheelchair made of aluminum. The cross has a contouring back rest upholstery that can be adjusted as the user needs to change. Frame widths available in 14 -20 inches. Seat frame and upholstery are adjustable to fit each individual. Lifetime warranty on frame for original user. $1,295 -$2,500

717 Custom

Fortress
PO Box 489
Clovis, CA 93613
559-322-5437
FAX: 559-323-0299

Ultralight aluminum wheelchair that can be customized to customer's requests. Fifteen frame colors, eight seat widths and depths, along with thirteen rear wheel combinations are just a few of the features offered at the standard package price.

718 Custom Durable

21279 Protecta Drive
Elkhart, IN 46516
574-266-1005
800-933-0256
FAX: 574-293-0202

Wheelchairs; accessories.

719 Edge

Fortress
PO Box 489
Clovis, CA 93613
559-322-5437
FAX: 559-323-0299

An ultra lightweight aircraft aluminum wheelchair that is suitable for sports, school or the workplace.

720 Etac USA: F3 Wheelchair

2325 Parklawn Drive
Suite J
Waukesha, WI 53186
800-678-3822
FAX: 262-796-4605
e-mail: etac1usa@execpc.com
www.execpc.com/~etac1usa

A swedish wheelchair designed to provide function, comfort and flexibility. Seat frame and upholstery are adjustable to fit each individual. Swing away, detachable footrests are standard. Available in frame widths from 14, 18 and 20 inch. Numerous accessories are available in order to individualize each chair. Lifetime warranty on frame for original user.

721 **Etac USA: Sting Wheelchair**

2325 Parklawn Drive
Suite J
Waukesha, WI 53186
800-678-3822
FAX: 262-796-4605
e-mail: etac1usa@execpc.com
www.execpc.com/~etac1usa

A swedish wheelchair designed to adjust to meet the growing child's every need. Both the seat and the backrest are width, height, and angle adjustable. Footrest, adjustable in height, depth and angle, swings back under the seat. Numerous accessories available. Lifetime warranty on frame for the original user.

722 **Evacu-Trac**

Garaventa Canada
PO Box L-1
Blaine, WA 98230 **360-332-2231**
800-663-6556

This emergency evacuation chair is designed for safety and fast operation.

723 **Folding Chair with a Rigid Feel**

Kuschall of America
3601 Rider Trail S
Earth City, MO 63045 **314-512-7000**
800-654-4768
FAX: 800-542-3567

The Champion 1000 is a new concept in folding chairs. Even though it's ultra light, it has the feel and performance of a rigid chair.

724 **Formula Series Active Mobility Wheelchairs**

Everest & Jennings
3233 Mission Oaks Boulevard
Camarillo, CA 93012 **805-389-7450**

This is a new series of lightweight wheelchairs designed for the active user.

725 **Freestyle II**

Fortress
PO Box 489
Clovis, CA 93613 **559-322-5437**
FAX: 559-323-0299

Effort-sparing, ultra-lightweight aircraft aluminum construction and design allow for easy propelling over various rolling surfaces.

726 **Gadabout Wheelchairs**

Gadabout Wheelchairs
1165 Portland Avenue
Rochester, NY 14621 **585-338-1000**
800-828-4242

Enjoy independence with the wheelchair that is lightweight, portable, convenient, comfortable and sturdy.

727 **Gendron**

Lugbill Road
Archbold, OH 43502
800-537-2521
FAX: 419-446-2631

Steven Cotter, VP Sales

Manufacturer of wheelchairs for a variety of other applications, specializing in bariatric mobility products.

728 **HiRider**

Gaymar Industries
10 Centre Drive
Orchard Park, NY 14127 **716-662-2551**
800-828-7341

A wheelchair that provides mobility in both sitting and standing positions.

729 **Innovative Products**

4351 W College Avenue
Appleton, WI 54914 **269-684-5050**
800-424-3369
FAX: 920-738-9050

Wheelchairs; accessories.

730 **Liberty**

Fortress
PO Box 489
Clovis, CA 93613 **559-322-5437**
FAX: 559-323-0299

Ultra lightweight wheelchair provides a comfortable fit and leaves people able to function as normally as possible in daily activities.

731 **Lightweight Breezy**

Motion Design
2382 Faraday Avenuek Avenue
Suite 200
Carlsbad, CA 92008 **760-930-1500**
FAX: 760-930-1585
www.sunrisemedical.com

A lightweight wheelchair. *$750.00*

732 **Majors Medical Equipment**

14601 Old Lima Road
Suite 100
Fort Wayne, IN 46818 **260-637-8586**
800-611-5552
e-mail: majorsmedical@majorsmedical.com

America's largest selection of wheelchairs and homecare equipment.

733 **National Mobility Equipment Dealers Association**

11211 N Nebraska Avenue
Suite A5
Tampa, FL 33612 **813-977-6603**
800-833-0427
FAX: 813-977-6402
e-mail: nmedadroeling@aol.com
www.nmeda.org

Dana Roeling, Executive Director

Trade association that will benefit anyone that manufactures, buys, sells, installs, prescribes or needs a working knowledge of adaptive equipment for transportation for the disabled.

734 **Natural Access**

PO Box 5729
Santa Monica, CA 90409 **609-588-9830**
800-411-7789
FAX: 310-392-3874
e-mail: national@superlink.net
www.landeez.com

John Egan, Owner

Provides the Landeez all-terrain wheelchair, that can roll easily on sand, gravel and snow for outdoor fun. The entire chair can fit inside a travel bag!

735 **Posture-Glide Lounger**

Graham-Field Health Products
2935 NE Parkway
Atlanta, GA 30360
800-347-5678
FAX: 800-726-0601
www.grahamfield.com

Provides all day comfort and safe, independent mobilization with feet or hands. The ergonomically engineered seat back provides correct support.

736 **Prairie Cruiser**

Wheelchairs of Kansas
PO Box 320
Ellis, KS 67637
785-726-4950
800-537-6454
FAX: 800-337-2447
e-mail: workinfo@go2wok.com
www.wheelchairsofkansas.com

A large-frame powerchair constructed of high quality, stress tested stainless steel to insure durability and peak performance.

737 **Redman Apache**

Redman Powerchair
3840 S Palo Verde Road
Tucson, AZ 85714
800-727-6684
FAX: 520-546-5530

These ultralight, active use wheelchairs offer quick release rear wheels, adjustable arm height and detachable arm swing-away.

738 **Redman Crow Line**

Redman Powerchair
3840 S Palo Verde Road
Tucson, AZ 85714
800-727-6684
FAX: 520-546-5530

Reclining wheelchair that reclines a full 90 degrees to flat and can be stopped anywhere on the axis.

739 **Rolls 2000 Series**

Invacare Corporation
899 Cleveland Street
Elyria, OH 44035
440-329-6426
800-333-6900
e-mail: info@invacare.com

These wheelchairs are the first light-weight wheelchairs designed for rental use.

740 **Side-to-Side Folding Chair**

Kuschall of America
3601 Rider Trail S
Earth City, MO 63045
314-512-7000
800-654-4768
FAX: 800-542-3567

The Champion 2000 is a folding chair with the ride and feel of a rigid chair.

741 **Stand-Up Wheelchairs**

Lifestand
PO Box 232171
Encinitas, CA 92023
800-782-6324
FAX: 610-586-0847
e-mail: dallery@msn.com

Jacques A Dallery, President

Offers a complete line of manual, electric and stand-up wheelchairs for the disabled.

742 **Surf Chair**

2052 S Peninsula Drive
Daytona Beach, FL 32118
386-253-0986
800-841-6610
FAX: 386-253-7600

Wheelchairs; accessories.

743 **Swede Elite**

ETAC USA
2325 Parklawn Drive
Suite J
Waukesha, WI 53186
800-678-3822
FAX: 262-796-4605
e-mail: etac1usa@execpc.com

A carefully designed Swedish wheelchair made of lightweight titanium for the active user. Available in frame widths from 14-18 inches and colors available are: black, red, plum, teal-blue, and Silver. Custom colors available at additional cost and there is a lifetime warranty on the frame for original user. $1,740-$2,500

744 **Swede Sting**

ETAC USA
2325 Parklawn Drive
Suite J
Waukesha, WI 53186
800-678-3822
FAX: 262-796-4605
e-mail: etac1usa@execpc.com

A carefully designed Swedish wheelchair combining durability with individual adjustments to meet the changing needs of the growing child. Available in three widths 11, 12, and 13, and five colors: black, red, blue, teal and plum. $1595-$2,500

745 **Vista Wheelchair**

Arista Surgical Supply Company
67 Lexington Avenue
New York, NY 10010
212-679-3694
800-223-1984
FAX: 212-696-9046
e-mail: aristasurgical@juno.com
www.aristasurgical.com

Vista has a rugged cold-rolled steel frame, durable vinyl upholstery and steel bearings to assure a smooth ride. *$220.00*

746 **Wheelchair with Shock Absorbers**

Iron Horse Productions
2624 Conner Street
Port Huron, MI 48060
810-987-6700
800-426-0354

The Iron Horse is a revolutionary concept in wheelchair design that offers comfort, indoors and outdoors. *$2375.00*

Wheelchairs: Pediatric

747 **Commuter & Kid's Commuter**

Fortress
PO Box 489
Clovis, CA 93613
559-322-5437
FAX: 559-323-0299

The first of a new generation of power wheelchairs. These chairs feature direct drive power yet are foldable, transportable and affordable.

748 **Convaid**

2830 California Street
Torrance, CA 90503
888-266-8243
FAX: 310-539-3670
e-mail: convaid@earthlink.net
www.convaid.com

Merv Watkins, President
Rodolfo Restelli, Controller
Nathan Watkins, Executive VP

Convaid manufactures Mobile Positioning Systems for children. The Expedition, Safari Tilt, Cruiser, EZ Rider and Metro offer a non-institutional styling and are lightweight and compact-folding. The steel/aluminum structure is engineered for maximum comfort and durability. The mobile positioning lines come with more than 20 positioning features and a full range of positioning adaptations. All chairs have been successfully crash-tested and offer a limited lifetime warranty (except the Metro).

749 **Imp Tricycle**

TRIAID
PO Box 1364
Cumberland, MD 21501
301-759-3525
800-306-6777
FAX: 301-759-3525
e-mail: sales@triaid.com
www.triaid.com

Iain A MacDonald, Sales Director
Ann M Hutter, Sales Executive

Provides fun therapy and actively encourages participation, awareness and the building of self confidence. Designed for children from about 3 years, it features ATB styling, 12 inch wheels, adjustable steering stop and a supportive saddle. Handlebar and seat adjustments combine with a broad wheelbase to ensure the rider is in the optimum position to pedal and the tricycle gives good stability and confident handling. Support accessories are available. *$590.00*

750 **Kid's Custom**

Fortress
PO Box 489
Clovis, CA 93613
559-322-5437
FAX: 559-323-0299

Custom pediatric mobility needs. This ultra lightweight chair is tailor fit to each child, to make wheeling fun and encourages kids to be active because they feel free, safe and secure.

751 **Kid's Edge**

Fortress
PO Box 489
Clovis, CA 93613
559-322-5437
FAX: 559-323-0299

This wheelchair offers multiple options, features and modifications at no upcharge.

752 **Kid's Liberty**

Fortress
PO Box 489
Clovis, CA 93613
559-322-5437
FAX: 559-323-0299

Offers a broad range of seat heights, widths and depths, back heights and numerous other modifications to accommodate the specific and unique requirements of children.

753 **Kid-Friendly Chairs**

Vector Mobility
5030 E Jensen Avenue
Fresno, CA 93725
800-441-0358
FAX: 559-441-0359

Manual base offers the lowest available floor to seat height, growth capability, one-third the parts of a conventional chair and no welds to break. The power unit features standard shapes and personality designs from elephants to inch worms and autos to rainbows, lowest seat height, and smallest turning radius on the market.

754 **Seven Fifty-Five FS**

Fortress
PO Box 489
Clovis, CA 93613
559-322-5437
FAX: 559-323-0299

Unharness the curiosity of childhood with the modular power/base seating system that sets kids free. This device is engineered and built especially for children.

755 **TMX Tricycle**

TRIAID
PO Box 1364
Cumberland, MD 21501
301-759-3525
800-306-6777
FAX: 301-759-3525
e-mail: sales@triaid.com
www.triaid.com

Iain A MacDonald, Sales Director
Ann M Hutter, Sales Executive

Provides fun therapy and actively encourages participation, awareness and the building of self confidence. Designed for children from about eight years, it features ATB styling, 20 inch wheels, adjustable steering stop and a supportive saddle. Handlebar and seat adjustments combine with a broad wheelbase to ensure the rider is in the optimum position to pedal and the tricycle gives good stability and confident handling. Support accessories are available. *$795.00*

Wheelchairs: Powered

756 **Bounder Plus Power Wheelchair**

21st Century Scientific
4915 Industrial Way
Coeur D Alene, ID 83815
208-667-8800
800-448-3680
FAX: 208-667-6600
e-mail: 21st@wheelchairs.com
www.wheelchairs.com

RD Davidson, Sales/Marketing Director
Jeanie L Saville, Sales Associate

Available in widths of 16 to 20 inches for users up to 500 pounds with a 2 year warranty on the entire chair. It offers all the standard features of a BOUNDER, plus reinforced rear wheel mounts, reinforced caster barrels, and super duty upholstery (with double liner and web straps under every screw). The BOUNDER Plus also features tandem cross struts, middle vertical support strut, seat rails supported at five points and back upholstery attached with machine screws.

757 **Bounder Power Wheelchair**

21st Century Scientific
4915 Industrial Way
Coeur D Alene, ID 83815
208-667-8800
800-448-3680
FAX: 208-667-6600
e-mail: 21st@wheelchairs.com
www.wheelchairs.com

RD Davidson, Sales/Marketing Director
Jeanie L Saville, Sales Associate

Available in a variety of widths from 16 to 18 inches for users up to 250 pounds. The rugged frame is constructed with steel tubing. The standard 12 position Adjustable Front Forks, made of 1/4 inch thick steel, provides impact dampening and seat tilt adjustment. A Dual Group 27 Sliding Battery Box provides extended range and easy battery maintenance. *$8695.00*

758 **Damaco D90**

Damaco
20542 Plummer Street
Chatsworth, CA 91311
800-432-2434
FAX: 818-709-5282

Portable power unit that fits manual wheelchairs with large rear wheels. Weighing just 22 pounds, the power system can be removed and stored in a matter of seconds. *$2495.00*

759 **Eagle Sportschairs**

2351 Parkwood Road
Snellville, GA 30039
770-972-0763
800-932-9380
FAX: 770-985-4885
e-mail: bewing@bellsouth.net
www.eaglesportschairs.com

Barry Ewing, Owner
Alice Kirk, Customer Service
Marty Frierson, Sales

The Eagle line of custom lightweight performance chairs includes a range of options to fit all racing and sport needs including; track, baseball, quad-rugby, tennis, field events and waterskiing. Also popular for daily use. We are able to customize any chair to accommodate size and disability and all frames have a full five year warranty.

760 **Geronimo**

Redman Powerchair
3840 S Palo Verde Road
Suite 202
Tucson, AZ 85714
800-727-6684
FAX: 520-546-5530

Wheelchair offering direct drive, two year electronic guarantee and micro controls.

761 **One Thousand FS**

Fortress
PO Box 489
Clovis, CA 93613
559-322-5437
FAX: 559-323-0299

Add-on power system installs in minutes, enabling the driver to relax and drive anywhere with smooth, silent electric power.

762 **Penny & Giles Pilot**

Voice Connection
2324 N Batavia Street
Orange, CA 92865
714-685-1066
FAX: 714-685-1070
e-mail: voicecnx@aol.com
www.voicecnx.com

Motorized wheelchair that requires no special mounting or installation.

763 **Permobil Max 90**

Permobil
30 Ray Avenue
Burlington, MA 01803
781-272-7410
FAX: 781-229-9841

The power wheelchair for those needing an easily maneuverable and quiet indoor chair but who also need to use their chair outdoors.

764 **Permobil Super 90**

Permobil
30 Ray Avenue
Burlington, MA 01803
781-272-7410
FAX: 781-229-9841

The power wheelchair is designed for travel over uneven and hilly terrain outdoors and indoors.

765 **Power for Off-Pavement**

Redman Powerchair
3840 S Palo Verde Road
Suite 202
Tucson, AZ 85714
800-727-6684
FAX: 520-546-5530

Power-drive wheelchair has a solid seat and can handle safely and securely knolls and off-pavement terrain.

766 **Pride Remote Plus**

Voice Connection
2324 N Batavia Street
Orange, CA 92865
714-685-1066
FAX: 714-685-1070
e-mail: voicecnx@aol.com
www.voicecnx.com

Motorized wheelchair that requires no special mounting or installation.

767 **Quickie Qtronix**

Voice Connection
2324 N Batavia Street
Orange, CA 92865
714-685-1066
FAX: 714-685-1070
e-mail: voicecnx@aol.com
www.voicecnx.com

Motorized wheelchair that requires no special mounting or installation.

768 **Roll-Aid**

Stand Aid of Iowa
PO Box 386
Sheldon, IA 51201
800-831-8580
FAX: 712-324-5210
e-mail: standaid@connect.com

Adapts to fit all standard collapsible wheelchairs. It is convenient, portable and provides electric rollator mobility instantly. *$1748.00*

Wheelchairs: Racing

769 **Aeroedge**

Fortress
PO Box 489
Clovis, CA 93613
559-322-5437
FAX: 559-323-0299

The ultimate in racing wheelchair design. Two innovative and exclusive Fortress features make this the fastest machine on three wheels.

770 **East Penn Manufacturing Company**

East Penn Manufacturing Company
PO Box 147
Lyon Station, PA 19536 **610-682-6361**
FAX: 610-682-4781
e-mail: eastpenn@eastpenn-delu.com

Harold Eberly, VP Sales

Specially engineered for demanding deep-cycle applications Gelled electrolyte Deka Dominator Batteries provides maintenance-free operation, longer battery life and hours of reliable performance. Their excellent recharge characteristics provide quick turn around time.

771 **Invacare Top End**

4501 63rd Circle
Pinellas Park, FL 33781 **727-522-8677**
800-532-8677
FAX: 727-522-1007
www.invacare.com

Mary Carol Peterson, Marketing

Manufacturers of light weight, rigid, sport-specific wheelchairs such as the Eliminator line of racing chairs,T-3 tennis and softball chairs, and the Terminator for quad rugby and basketball. The Excelerator, XLT three-wheel hand cycle for adults and juniors. Check out our full line of wheelchairs to fit every need. $1,895-$2,495

Aging

772 **Aging in America**
1500 Pelham Parkway S
Bronx, NY 10461 **413-584-1460**
FAX: 413-586-1121
e-mail: cemoylan@aol.com

Ralph Hall, President

Research and services organization for professionals in gerontology. Objectives are: to produce, implement and share effective and affordable programs and services that improve the quality of life for the elderly community; to better prepare professionals and students interested in or currently involved with, aging and the aged. Conducts research projects, educational and training seminars, and in-service curricula for long-term and acute care facilities.

773 **Alabama Association of Homes and Services for the Aging**
Wesley Gardens
1555 Taylor Road
Montgomery, AL 36117 **334-399-8989**
FAX: 334-272-5774

774 **American Association of Homes and Services for the Aging**
2519 Connecticut Avenue NW
Washington, DC 20008 **202-783-2242**
FAX: 202-783-2255
e-mail: info@aahsa.org
www.aahsa.org

The American Association of Homes and Services for the Aging (AAHS) represents not-for-profit organizations dedicated to providing high-quality health care, housing and services to the nation's elderly. AAHSA organizations serve more than one million older persons af all income levels, creeds and races.

775 **Arizona Association of Homes and Housing for the Aging**
3839 N 3rd Street
Suite 201
Phoenix, AZ 85012 **602-230-0026**
FAX: 602-230-0563

776 **Association of Ohio Philanthropic Homes and Housing for Aging**
855 S Wall Street
Columbus, OH 43206 **614-444-2882**
FAX: 614-444-2974

777 **California Association of Homes and Services for the Aging**
7311 Greenhaven Drive
Suite 175
Sacramento, CA 95831 **916-392-5111**
FAX: 916-428-4250
e-mail: lbloxham@aging.org
www.aging.org

778 **Center for Understanding Aging**
200 Executive Boulevard
Suite 201
Southington, CT 06489 **718-824-4004**
FAX: 718-824-4242
e-mail: couper.natla@snet.net

Donna Couper, Director

Seeks to dispel myths about aging and old age, encourages communication among generations and works to create a social environment where people of all ages can live together. Also serves as a clearinghouse of information on issues of aging and intergenerational programs. Provides professional speakers and workshop leaders.

779 **Children of Aging Parents**
1609 Woodbourne Road
Suite 302A
Levittown, PA 19057 **215-945-6900**
800-227-7294
FAX: 215-945-8720
e-mail: caps4caregivers@aol.com
www.caps4caregivers.org

Nancy Harven, Administrative Assistant

A national clearinghouse for caregivers of the elderly. It provides information and referral, educational programs and materials and caregiver support groups. CAPS also produces a quarterly newsletter which is available through the organization. Individuals: $25.00. Organizational/Professional: $100.00.

780 **Colorado Association of Homes and Services for the Aging (CAHSA)**
1888 Sherman Street
#610
Denver, CO 80203 **303-837-8834**
FAX: 303-837-8836
e-mail: info@cahsa.org
www.cahsa.org

The American Association of Homes and Services for the Aging (AAHS) represents nonprofit organizations dedicated to providing high quality health care, housing and services to the nation's elderly. AAHSA organizations serve more than one million older persons af all income levels, creeds and races.

781 **Connecticut Association of Not-for-Profit Providers for the Aging**
300 Piesearch Parkway
Meriden, CT 06450 **203-237-4556**
FAX: 203-237-4908
www.canpfa.org

782 **Delaware Association of Nonprofit Homes for the Aging**
Westminister Village
1175 McKee Road
Dover, DE 19901 **302-674-8030**
FAX: 302-674-8650

783 **Florida Association of Homes for the Aging**
1812 Riggins Road
Tallahassee, FL 32308 **386-671-3700**
FAX: 386-671-3790
www.faha.org

784 **Georgia Association of Homes and Services for the Aging**
1678 Tullie Circle NE
Suite 120
Atlanta, GA 30329 **404-728-0223**
FAX: 404-636-6753

785 **Indiana Association of Homes for the Aging**
402 W Washington
Room W454
Indianapolis, IN 46204 **317-232-7020**
FAX: 317-232-7867

786 **Iowa Association of Homes and Services for the Aging**

1701 48th Street
Suite 203
West Des Moines, IA 50266
515-440-4630
FAX: 515-440-4631
e-mail: iahsa@ageiowa.org
www.ageiowa.org

Dana Petrowsky, President/CEO

787 **Kansas Association of Homes for the Aging**

217 SE Eighth Street
Suite 1106
Topeka, KS 66603
785-233-7443
FAX: 785-233-9471
e-mail: kahsainfo@kahsa.org
www.kahsa.org

John Grace, President/CEO
Tina Andres, Office Manager
Kevin McFarland, Vice President

KAHSA is a non-profit organization representing over 150 non-profit community, church and government sponsored adult care homes, retirement communities, and social service programs for the elderly.

788 **Kentucky Association of Not-for-Profit Homes and Services for the Aging**

2501 Nelson Miller Parkway
Louisville, KY 40223
502-992-4380
FAX: 502-635-9286
www.kahsanet.org

789 **Life Service Network of Illinois: Springfi eld**

2 Lawrence Square
Springfield, IL 62704
217-789-1677
FAX: 217-789-1778
e-mail: info@aahsa.org
www.aahsa.org

The American Association of Homes and Services for the Aging (AAHS) represents not-for-profit organizations dedicated to providing high-quality health care, housing and services to the nation's elderly. AAHSA organizations serve more than one million older persons af all income levels, creeds and races.

790 **Life Services Network of Illinois**

911 N Elm Street
Suite 228
Hinsdale, IL 60521
630-325-6170
FAX: 630-325-0749

791 **Louisiana Association of Homes and Service for the Aging**

5630 Bankers Avenue
PO Box 14615
Baton Rouge, LA 70808
225-928-1114
FAX: 225-928-1319

792 **Massachusetts Aging Services Association**

135 S Huntington Avenue
Boston, MA 02130
617-739-3235
FAX: 617-739-3236
www.massaging.org

793 **Michigan Association of Homes and Serivces for the Aging**

6215 W St. Joseph Highway
Lansing, MI 48917
517-886-1302
FAX: 517-886-1670

794 **Mid-Atlantic LifeSpan**

10280 Old Columbia Road
Suite 220
Columbia, MD 21046
410-381-1176
800-521-3591
FAX: 410-381-0240
www.manpha.org

Isabella Firth, President

To deliver quality housing, healthcare, and community and related services to the aging. Offers educational and research programs and statistics.

795 **Minnesota Health and Housing Alliance**

2550 University Avenue W
Suite 350 S
St Paul, MN 55114
651-645-4545
800-462-5368
FAX: 651-645-0002
www.mhha.com

796 **Mississippi Association of Homes and Services for the Aging**

Naval Home
1800 Beach Drive
Gulfport, MS 39507
601-896-3110
FAX: 228-897-4013

797 **Missouri Association of Homes for the Aging**

515 E High Street
Suite 101 W
Jefferson City, MO 65101
573-635-6244
FAX: 573-635-6618

798 **National Center for Vision and Aging**

Lighthouse
111 E 59th Street
New York, NY 10022
212-821-9200
800-829-0500
FAX: 212-821-9707
e-mail: info@lighthouse.org
www.lighthouse.org

799 **National Voluntary Organizations for Independent Living for the Aging**

409 3rd Street SW
Washington, DC 20024
202-205-6770
FAX: 202-479-0735
www.ncoa.org

Stephanie Trapp, Program Manager

Emphasizes the needs for in-home and community-based health care and social services designed to help older persons remain in or return to their homes and live independently, Works to educate and assist voluntary organizations to help develop such services. Encourages cooperation between voluntary organizations and the public, provides forum for organizations, agencies and consumer groups to share ideas and develop a network of services for the aged.

800 **Nebraska Association of Homes for the Aging**

1701 K Street
Suite B
Lincoln, NE 68508
402-436-2165
FAX: 402-434-5685

801 **New Jersey Association of Nonprofit Homes for the Aging**

13 Roszel Road
Suite B113
Princeton, NJ 08540 **609-452-1161**
FAX: 609-452-2907
e-mail: info@aahsa.org
www.aahsa.org

The American Association of Homes and Services for the Aging (AAHS) represents not-for-profit organizations dedicated to providing high-quality health care, housing and services to the nation's elderly. AAHSA organizations serve more than one million older persons af all income levels, creeds and races.

802 **New York Association of Homes and Services for the Aging**

150 State Street
Suite 301
Albany, NY 12207 **518-449-2707**
FAX: 518-455-8908
e-mail: ecs@nyahsa.org
www.nyahsa.org

803 **North Carolina Association of Nonprofits for the Aging**

3301 Woman's Club Drive
Suite 145
Raleigh, NC 27612 **919-571-8333**
FAX: 919-571-1297

804 **Northern New England Association of Homes and Services for the Aging**

345 Edward J Roy Drive
Suite 201
Manchester, NH 03104 **603-626-3479**
FAX: 603-626-3763

805 **Oklahoma Association of Homes and Services for the Aging**

OK Christian Home
906 North Boulevard
Edmondton, OK 73034 **405-341-0810**
FAX: 405-341-0976

The American Association of Homes and Services for the Aging (AAHS) represents not-for-profit organizations dedicated to providing high-quality health care, housing and services to the nation's elderly. AAHSA organizations serve more than one million older persons af all income levels, creeds and races.

806 **Oregon Association of Homes for the Aging**

7360 SW Hunziker Street
Suite 207
Tigard, OR 97223 **503-684-3788**
FAX: 503-624-0870

The American Association of Homes and Services for the Aging (AAHS) represents not-for-profit organizations dedicated to providing high-quality health care, housing and services to the nation's elderly. AAHSA organizations serve more than one million older persons af all income levels, creeds and races.

807 **Pennsylvania Association of Nonprofit Homes for the Aging**

1100 Bent Creek Boulevard
Mechanicsburg, PA 17050 **717-763-5724**
FAX: 717-763-1057
e-mail: info@panpha.org
www.panpha.org

The American Association of Homes and Services for the Aging (AAHS) represents nonprofit organizations dedicated to providing high quality health care, housing and services to the nation's elderly. AAHSA organizations serve more than one million older persons af all income levels, creeds and races.

808 **Quality Health Care Foundation of Wyoming**

PO Box 3050
Cheyenne, WY 82003 **307-637-7575**
FAX: 307-637-7575

The American Association of Homes and Services for the Aging (AAHS) represents not-for-profit organizations dedicated to providing high-quality health care, housing and services to the nation's elderly. AAHSA organizations serve more than one million older persons af all income levels, creeds and races.

809 **Rhode Island Association of Facilities for the Aging**

225 Chapman Street
Mail Box 7
Providence, RI 02905 **401-490-7610**
FAX: 401-490-7614

Kathryn Gann, Manager

The American Association of Homes and Services for the Aging (AAHS) represents nonprofit organizations dedicated to providing high-quality health care, housing and services to the nation's elderly. AAHSA organizations serve more than one million older persons af all income levels, creeds and races.

810 **South Carolina Association of Nonprofit Homes for the Aging**

Greenwood Methodist Home
1110 Marshall Road
Greenwood, SC 29646 **803-227-7231**
FAX: 803-227-7161

The American Association of Homes and Services for the Aging (AAHS) represents not-for-profit organizations dedicated to providing high-quality health care, housing and services to the nation's elderly. AAHSA organizations serve more than one million older persons af all income levels, creeds and races.

811 **Tennessee Association of Homes for the Aging**

4343 Lebanon Road
Hermitage, TN 37076 **615-871-8162**
FAX: 615-871-8164

The American Association of Homes and Services for the Aging (AAHS) represents not-for-profit organizations dedicated to providing high-quality health care, housing and services to the nation's elderly. AAHSA organizations serve more than one million older persons af all income levels, creeds and races.

812 **Texas Association of Homes and Services for the Aging**

2205 Hancock Drive
Austin, TX 78756 **512-467-2242**
FAX: 512-467-2275
www.tahsa.org

The American Association of Homes and Services for the Aging (AAHS) represents not-for-profit organizations dedicated to providing high-quality health care, housing and services to the nation's elderly. AAHSA organizations serve more than one million older persons af all income levels, creeds and races.

813 Washington Association of Housing and Services for the Aging

545 Andover Park W
Suite 211
Seattle, WA 98188
206-204-0040
FAX: 206-204-0046
e-mail: wahsa@wahsa.com
www.wahsa.com

The American Association of Homes and Services for the Aging (AAHS) represents nonprofit organizations dedicated to providing high-quality health care, housing and services to the nation's elderly. AAHSA organizations serve more than one million older persons af all income levels, creeds and races.

814 West Virginia Hospital Association

100 Association Drive
Charleston, WV 25311
304-344-9744
FAX: 304-344-9745
www.wvha.com

WVHA supports its members in achieving a strong, healthy West Virginia through advocacy, education information and technical assistance.

815 Wisconsin Association of Homes & Services for the Aging

204 S Hamilton Street
Madison, WI 53703
608-255-7060
FAX: 608-255-7064
www.wahsa.org

The American Association of Homes and Services for the Aging (AAHS) represents not-for-profit organizations dedicated to providing high-quality health care, housing and services to the nation's elderly. AAHSA organizations serve more than one million older persons af all income levels, creeds and races.

Business Support

816 Council of Better Business Bureaus' Foundation

4200 Wilson Boulevard
Suite 800
Arlington, VA 22203
703-276-0100
FAX: 703-525-8277
e-mail: @cbbb.bbb.org
www.bbb.org

Candy McIlhenny, Executive Director

Seven Title III compliance guides are available for: car sales and service; restaurants and bars; recreation and fitness centers; grocery stores; retail stores; professional offices; and travel and tour agents. *$2.50*

817 Disability Community Small Business Development Center

2568 Packard Road
Ann Arbor, MI 48104
734-971-0277
800-433-5255
FAX: 734-971-0826
e-mail: cilstaff@aacil.org
www.comnet.org/local/orgs/dcsbdc

Edward Wollmann, Coordinator

Provides business counsel and services to entrepreneurs with disabilities in the state of Michigan. Our organization conducts feasibility studies, assists business plans and works with vocational rehabilitation organizations in helping entrepreneurs start and run small businesses.

818 Fedcap Rehabilitation Services

211 W 14th Street
New York, NY 10011
212-727-4200
FAX: 212-727-4374
e-mail: info@fedcap.org
www.fedcap.org

Susan Jourad, Director Community Relations

A private nonprofit organization providing vocational rehabilitation and job placement for people with disabilities and barriers to employment.

819 Independent Visually Impaired Enterprisers

American Council of the Blind
1155 15th Street NW
Suite 1004
Washington, DC 20005
202-467-5081
800-424-8666
FAX: 202-467-5085
e-mail: info@acb.org
www.acb.org

Strives to broaden vocational opportunities in business for the visually impaired. Works to improve rehabilitation facilities for all types of business enterprises and publicizes the capabilities of blind and visually impaired business persons.

820 Industry-Labor Council

National Center for Disability Services
201 I U Willets Road
Albertson, NY 11507
516-897-2527
FAX: 516-747-2046
www.business-disability.com

Gary Kishanuk, Manager

Helps the business community develop effective, low-cost corporate policies and practices for integrating people with disabilities in the workplace.

821 International Association of Machinists

3830 S Meridian Avenue
Wichita, KS 67217
316-522-1591
FAX: 316-522-7989

Ron Eldridge, President

Placement programs for persons with disabilities.

822 Job Accommodation Network

PO Box 6080
Morgantown, WV 26506
304-293-7186
800-526-7234
FAX: 304-293-5407
e-mail: jan@jan.icdi.wvu.edu
www.jan.wvu.edu

DJ Hendricks, Director

Provides a service of the US Department of Labor's Office on Disability Employment Policy, information on practical accommodations that can be successfully utilized in business and industry. It enables businesses to communicate with others to find ways to manage and lower disability costs. JAN also collects job accommodation information and makes it available to those seeking ways to enable persons having functional limitations caused by disabilities to be productive in the work environment.

823 Life Development Institute

18001 N 79th Avenue
Suite E-71
Glendale, AZ 85308
623-773-2774
FAX: 623-773-2788

Robert Crawford, President

Serves older adolescents and adults with learning disabilities, ADD and related disorders. The purpose of the training is to enable program participants to pursue responsible independent living, enhance academic/workplace literacy skills and facilitate placement in educational/employment opportunities, commensurate with individual capabilities. Includes a stand alone, regionally accredited 2-year college.

824 **OpportunityPlus of NC**

PO Box 35481
Charlotte, NC 28235 **704-519-0600**
FAX: 704-519-0699
e-mail: info@opportunity-plus.org
www.opportunity-plus.org

Customized career path for people with physical disabilities. Operates as an employment agency for people with physical disabilities. Peer directed and staffed. Professional approach.

General Disabilities

825 **Academy of Dentistry for Persons with Disabilities**

211 E Chicago Avenue
5th Floor
Chicago, IL 60611 **312-440-2661**
FAX: 312-440-2824
e-mail: fosccdzz@worldnet.att.net
www.specialdentistry.org

James Balija CAE

A professional organization of individuals concerned with the oral health care of persons with special needs. Association publishes a bi-monthly journal entitled 'Special Care in Dentistry' and a newsletter interface.

826 **Access Unlimited**

570 Hance Road
Binghamton, NY 13903
800-849-2143
FAX: 607-669-4595
www.accessunlimited.com

Sherry Sinai, Administrative Coordinator
Sherry Lowry, Director

Assists educators, health care providers and parents in discovering how personal computers help children and adults with disabilities compensate for some of the barriers imposed by their conditions. Access Unlimited markets and offers technical support for over 500 special computer products, acts as a free information center and provides free telephone consultation to special educators, health care providers and other professionals.

827 **Accu-Chem Laboratories**

990 N Bowser Road
Suite 800-880
Richardson, TX 75081 **214-234-5412**
800-451-0116
FAX: 972-234-6095
e-mail: accuchem@accuchem.com
www.accuchem.com

828 **Acupressure Institute**

1533 Shattuck Avenue
Berkeley, CA 94709 **510-845-1059**
800-442-2232
FAX: 510-845-1496
e-mail: info@acupressure.com
www.acupressure.com

Michael Reed Gach, PhD

Information, career training and mail order catalog.

829 **Advocacy Center for Persons with Disabilities**

2671 W Executive Center
Suite 100
Tallahassee, FL 32301 **850-488-9071**
800-342-0823
FAX: 850-488-8640
e-mail: info@advocacycenter.org
www.advocacycenter.org

Marjorie Menzel, Communications Director

The mission of the Center is to advance the dignity, equality, self-determination and expressed choices of individuals with disabilities. The Center promotes, expands, protects and seeks to assure the human and legal rights of people through the provision of information and advocacy. The Center administers six federally-mandated programs in the State of Florida. It is completely independent of all state agencies providing services to persons with disabilities.

830 **Alliance for Technology Access**

2175 E Francisco Boulevard
Suite L
San Rafael, CA 94901 **415-455-4575**
800-455-7970
FAX: 415-455-0654
e-mail: atainfo@ataccess.org
www.ataccess.org

Mary Lester, Executive Director
Libbie Butler, Administrative Assistant

The Alliance for Technology Access (ATA) is a national network of technology resource centers, community-based organizations, technology vendors and individuals who are committed to increasing the use of technology by children and adults with disabilities and functional limitations.

831 **American Academy of Pediatrics**

141 NW Point Boulevard
Elk Grove Village, IL 60007 **847-228-5005**
FAX: 847-228-5097
www.aap.org

Michelle Esquivel, Project Manager

Offers policy information, referrals and treatment information for children and adolescents.

832 **American Association for the Advancement of Science**

Project on Science, Technology and Disability
1200 New York Avenue NW
Washington, DC 20005 **202-483-2101**
FAX: 202-371-9849
e-mail: vstern@aaas.org
www.aaas.org

Virginia Stern, Director

The Project on Science, Technology and Disability was founded in 1975, by the American Association for the Advancement of Science. Primarily an information center, the Project links people with disabilities, their families, professors, teachers and counselors with scientists and engineers with disabilities, who can share their education and career coping strategies in technical fields. Maintains a database of scientists and engineers with disabilities. Manages a summer internship program.

833 **American Association of Music Therapy**

8455 Colesville Road
Suite 1000
Silver Spring, MD 20910 **301-589-3300**
FAX: 301-589-5175
e-mail: info@musictherapy.org
www.musictherapy.org

Andrea H Farbman, Executive Director
Judy Simpson, Director of Government Relations

834 **American Association of People with Disabilities**

1629 K Street NW
Suite 503
Washington, DC 20006
202-457-0046
800-840-8844
FAX: 202-457-0473
e-mail: aapd@aol.com
www.aapd-dc.org

The American Association of People with Disabilities (AAPD) is a nonprofit non-partisan, cross-disability, national membership organization whose goals are unity, leadership and impact. AAPD's mission is to advance the economic and political power of all people with disabilities. AAPD Member Benefits include a quarterly newsletter, adaptive vehicleinsurance, financial services, car rental discounts and life insurance.

835 **American Board of Chelation Therapy**

1407 1/2 N Wells Street
Chicago, IL 60610
312-266-3688
800-356-2228
FAX: 312-266-3685
e-mail: jackhonk@mindspring.com
abct.info

Jack Hank, Executive Director

Certification Board.

836 **American Botanical Council**

PO Box 144345
Austin, TX 78714
512-926-4900
FAX: 512-926-2345
e-mail: tbennett@herbalgram.org
www.herbalgram.org

Offers information and HerbalGram magazine.

837 **American Camping Association**

5000 State Road 67 N
Martinsville, IN 46151
765-342-8456
800-428-2267
FAX: 765-342-2065
www.acacamps.org

Kim Bruno, Communications/Development Spec
Peg Smith, Executive Director

838 **American Chiropractic Association**

1701 Clarendon Boulevard
Arlington, VA 22209
703-276-8800
FAX: 703-243-2593
www.acatoday.com

Major source for chiropractic information.

839 **American Counseling Association**

5999 Stevenson Avenue
Alexandria, VA 22304
800-347-6647
800-473-2329
FAX: 703-823-6862
e-mail: membership@counseling.org
www.counseling.org

Richard Yep, Executive Director
Jane Goodman, President

Provides a variety of programs and services that support the personal, professional and program development goals of its members. ACA works together with 17 divisions to provide quality services to the variety of clients who use their services in college, community agencies, substance abuse, and rehabilitation.

840 **American Foundation of Traditional Chinese Medicine (AFTCM)**

2710 X Street
Suite 2A
Sacramento, CA 95818
916-455-0347
800-477-4564
888-432-5669
e-mail: office@csomaonline.org
www.csomaonline.org

The American Foundation of Traditional Chinese Medicine (AFTCM) has joined the California State Oriental Medicine Association (CSOMA).

841 **American Herbalists Guild**

1931 Gaddis Road
Canton, GA 30115
770-751-6021
FAX: 770-751-7472
e-mail: ahgoffice@earthlink.net
www.americanherbalistsguild.com

Aviva Jill Romm, President

Information on herbal therapies and a directory of schools and teachers.

842 **American Institute of Hypnotherapy American Pacific University**

615 Piikoi Street
Suite 501
Honolulu, HI 96814
808-596-7765
577-927-8
FAX: 808-596-7764
www.ampac.edu

Provides a large variety of media resources.

843 **American Massage Therapy Association**

820 Davis Street
Suite 100
Evanston, IL 60201
847-864-0123
888-843-2682
FAX: 847-864-1178
e-mail: info@amtamassage.org
www.amtamassage.org

Joseph Schlesinger, Communications Assistant

Offers comprehensive information on massage and bodywork. Offers free Find A Massage Therapist National Locator Service, toll-free 888-843-2682.

844 **American Organization for Bodywork Therapies of Asia**

1010 Haddonfield-Berlin Road
Suite 408
Voorhees, NJ 08043
856-782-1616
FAX: 856-782-1653
e-mail: aobta@prodigy.net
www.holisticmed.com/www/bodywork.html

Julie Kaplan, VP
Debra Howard, President

National not-for-profit professional association of practitioners of Bodywork Therapies of Asia. Includes acupressure, AMMA Therapy, Chi Nei Tsang, Five Element Shiatsu, Integrative Eclectic Shiatsu, Japanese Shiatsu, Macrobiotic Shiatsu, Shiatsu Anma Therapy, Jin Shin Do Bodymind Acupressure, Traditional Thai Massage, Tuina, and Zen Shiatsu.

845 American Red Cross: National Headquarters

8111 Gatehouse Road
Falls Church, VA 22042 **202-737-8300**
FAX: 202-728-6481
e-mail: info@usa.redcross.org
www.redcross.org/dc/ncc

Offers counseling, emergency relief for disaster victims, information and referrals and emergency assistance for members of the military and their families.

846 American Self-Help Clearinghouse

Saint Clare's Hospital
Denville, NJ 07834 **908-813-9603**
800-367-6274
FAX: 973-625-8848
www.selfhelpgroups.org

Edward Madara, Director

A clearinghouse that makes referrals to self-help groups and self-help clearinghouses throughout the nation. Publishes a variety of materials that are helpful to professionals and consumers who would like to start self-help groups. The Self-Help Sourcebook has listings of over 800 national, international, and model groups. Helps individuals to start needed new groups.

847 American Social Health Association

PO Box 13827
Research Triangle Park, NC 27709 **919-361-8400**
FAX: 919-361-8425
www.ashastd.org

Voluntary health agency working against STD's.

848 American Society of Teachers of the Alexander Technique

PO Box 60008
Florence, MA 01062 **413-584-2359**
800-473-0620
FAX: 413-584-3097
www.amsat.ws

Dana Ben-Yehuda, Media Relations Committee Chair

The AmSAT Mission: To define, maintain and promote the Alexander Technique at its highest standard of professional practice and conduct.

849 Association for Applied Psychophysiology and Biofeedback

10200 W Avenue
Suite 304
Wheat Ridge, CO 80033 **303-422-8436**
FAX: 303-422-8894
e-mail: aapb@resourcenter.com
www.aapb.org

Paul M Lehrer PhD BCIAC, President
Lynda P Kirk MA LPC BCIAC, President-Elect

Provides names and phone numbers of local chapters. Mission is to advance the development, dissemination and utilization of knowledge about applied psychophysiology and biofeedback to improve health and the quality of life through research, education, and practice.

850 Association for Network Care

444 N Main Street
Longmont, CO 80501 **303-678-8101**
FAX: 303-678-8089
e-mail: info@associationfornetworkcare.com
www.associationfornetworkcare.com

Supports the consciousness, advances the practice of, and promotes the public availability of Network Spinal Analysis. Supports the advancement and understanding of the relationship of the spine and nervous system to consciousness, the expression of innate intelligence, self-organization, and healing. Encourages the support of the science, art, and philosophically similar and compatible models in various healing arts through workshops, seminars, journals, newsletters and research projects.

851 Association for Persons in Supported Employment

1627 Monument Avenue
Richmond, VA 23220 **804-278-9187**
FAX: 804-278-9377
e-mail: apse@apse.org
www.apse.org

Supported employment enables people with disabilities who have not been successfully employed to work and contribute to society. Focuses on a person's abiliities and provides the supports the individual needs to be successful on a long-term basis.

852 Association of University Centers on Disabilities

AUCD
1010 Wayne Avenue
Suite 920
Silver Spring, MD 20910 **301-588-8252**
FAX: 301-588-2842
TTY:301-588-3319
e-mail: info@aucd.org
www.aucd.org

Aaron Bishop MSW, Technical Assistance
George Jesien PhD, Executive Director
Donna Meltzer, Director Legislaitve Affairs

The central office for the 61 University Centers for Excellence programs and 21 Mental Retardation and Developmental Disabilities Research Centers and is their representative to the federal government. UCEDD's are located at major universities and teaching hospitals in all 50 states, the District of Columbia and many US territories. UCCED's target their activities to support the independence, productivity and integration into the community of individuals with developmental disabilities.

853 Association on Higher Education and Disability (AHEAD)

University of Massachusetts Boston
100 Morrissey Boulevard
Boston, MA 01215 **617-287-3880**
FAX: 617-287-3881
TTY:617-287-3882
e-mail: ahead@postbox.asc.ohio-state.edu
www.ahead.org

Ed Suddath, Executive Vice President

International, multicultural organization of proessionals committed to full participation in higher education for persons with disabilities. Plans and develops training programs, workshops, publications and conferences. Founded in 1977 to address the need and concern for upgrading the quality of services and support available to persons with disabilities in higher education.

854 Bastyr University Natural Health Clinic

1307 N 45th Street
Suite 200
Seattle, WA 98103
206-834-4100
FAX: 206-834-4107
www.bastyrcenter.org

Offers naturopathic medicine visits, nutrition consultations, counseling, acupuncture treatments and Chinese herbal medicine services.

855 Beach Center on Families and Disability

University of Kansas
311 Haworth Hall
1200 Sunnyside Avenue
Lawrence, KS 66045
785-864-7600
FAX: 785-864-7605
www.beachcenter.org

A federally funded center that conducts research and training in the factors that contribute to the successful functioning of families with members who have disabilities.

856 Bio-Electro-Magnetics Institute

2490 W Moana Lane
Reno, NV 89509
775-827-9099
FAX: 775-827-9099

857 Bonnie Pruden Myotherapy

3661 N Campbell, Suite 102
PO Box 65240
Tucson, AZ 85728
520-529-3979
800-221-4634
FAX: 520-529-6679
www.bonniepruden.com

Provides a list of certified myotherapists and clinics where myotherapy is offered.

858 CAPP National Parent Resource Center Federation for Children with Special Needs

56 Temple Place
Suite 664
Boston, MA 02111
617-542-7860
800-537-0446
FAX: 617-542-7832
e-mail: pal@fcsn.org
www.ppal.net

Donna Welles, Director
Lisa Lambert, Assistant Director

A parent-run resource system designed to further the needs and goals of family-centered, community-based coordinated care for children with special health needs and their families. Offers written materials, training packages, workshops and presentations for parents and professionals on special education, health care financing and other topics.

859 CARF Rehabilitation Accreditation Commission

4891 E Grant Road
Tucson, AZ 85712
520-325-1044
FAX: 520-318-1129
www.carf.org

Brain Boon PhD, President/CEO

CARF serves as the standards-setting and accrediting body for rehabilitation and life enhancement programs and services. The independent, not-for-profit commission promotes quality, value, and optimal outcomes of services through a consultative accreditation process that centers on enhancing the lives of the persons served. At present, CARD has accredited more than 19,000 programs and services in the US, Canada, and Sweden in the areas of adult day services, behavioral health, and medical rehab.

860 Canine Companions for Independence

National Offices
2965 Dutton Avenue
PO Box 446
Santa Rosa, CA 95402
707-577-1700
800-572-2275
FAX: 707-577-1711
e-mail: info@caninecompanions.org
www.caninecompanions.org

Corey Hudson, Executive Director
Petey Rapalus, Public Relations Manager

A nonprofit organization that provides highly trained assistance dogs for people with disabilities, helping them to achieve greater independence.

861 Canine Helpers for the Handicapped

5699-5705 Ridge Road
Lockport, NY 14094
716-433-4035
FAX: 716-439-0822
e-mail: chhdogs@aol.com
caninehelpers.netfirms.com/

A nonprofit organization devoted to training dogs to assist people with disabilities to lead more independent, secure lives.

1983

862 Center Academy

6710 86th Avenue N
Pinellas Park, FL 33782
727-541-5716
FAX: 727-544-8186
e-mail: centacadpp@aol.com
www.centeracademy.com

Lisa Steller, Intake Coordinator
Robert Detweiler JD, Principal

Provides day programs for students grades 4-12 who have learning disabilities or who need motivation. Please call for more information.

863 Center for Assistive Technology

University at Buffalo
515 Kimball Tower
Buffalo, NY 14214
716-829-3141
800-628-2281
FAX: 716-829-3217
TTY:800-628-2281
e-mail: jweir@acsu.buffalo.edu
www.cat.buffalo.edu

Jennifer Murphy, Coordinator

Nonprofit organization that conducts research and provides educational and services programs to increase consumer knowledge related to assistive technology for those with disabilities. Five specific areas of work: research on assistive devices used for all aspects of daily living, education for students and clinical professionals, assistive device service provision, development and evaluation of new innovative technology ideas, and public policy analysis.

864 Center for Assistive Technology and Environmental Access

490 10th Street NW
Atlanta, GA 30332
404-894-4960
FAX: 404-894-9320
www.catea.org

Barbara Christopher, Administrative Coordinator
Elizabeth Bryant, Project Director II

The Center for Assistive Technology and Environmental Access (CATEA) promotes maximum function, activity and access of persons with disabilities through the use of technology. The foci of the Center includes the development, evaluation and utilization of Assistive Technology and the design and development of Accessible Environments.

865 **Center for Developmental Disabilities**

University of South Carolina
8301 Farrow Road
School of Medicine, Education Bldg.
Columbia, SC 29208
803-935-5231
FAX: 803-935-5059
e-mail: scsis@dccisc.edu
www.scsis.org

Denise Rivers, Project Coordinator

Information on early intervention and the elderly.

866 **Center for Mind/Body Studies**

5225 Connecticut Avenue
NW Suite 414
Washington, DC 20015
202-966-7338
FAX: 202-966-2589

867 **Center for Universal Design**

NC State University
Pullen Road, Brooks Hall, Room 200
Campus Box 8613
Raleigh, NC 27695
919-515-3082
800-647-6777
FAX: 919-515-3082
e-mail: cud@ncsu.edu
www.design.ncsu.edu/cud

A federally funded resource center that works toward improving housing for people with disabilities. Provides technical assistance, training and publications on accessible housing and universal design.

868 **Change**

1413 Park Road NW
Washington, DC 20010
202-387-3725
FAX: 202-387-3729

Andrea Dorsett, Executive Director

Offers counseling/assessment, emergency food and clothing referrals, rental assistance and job assistance to disabled persons in the District of Columbia area.

869 **Children's Alliance**

420 Capitol Avenue
Frankfort, KY 40601
502-875-3399
FAX: 502-223-4200
e-mail: melissa.lawson@childrensallianceky.org
www.childrensallianceky.org

Melissa Lawson, Director of Member Services

An association of individuals and human services organizations committed to being a voice for at-risk children and families. Interacts with the legislative and executive branches of government and assists members in developing services that most effectively meet the needs of at-risk children and families.

870 **Children's National Medical Center**

111 Michigan Avenue NW
Washington, DC 20010
202-884-2160
FAX: 202-884-4492
e-mail: cnmc.org
www.cnmc.org

Donald Brown, President

Offers diagnosis, treatment, follow-up services, outpatient services and medical services to children.

871 **College of Maharishi Vedic Medicine Health Center**

1603 N 4th Street
Building 144, 2nd Floor
Fairfield, IA 52556
641-472-8477
800-369-6480
FAX: 641-472-1179
e-mail: admissions@mum.edu
www.mum.edu/CMVM/cmvmhc.html

Provides referrals consultations to the Fairfield community and to visitors from around the world at its clinic on the Maharishi University of Management campus. Staff physicians are medical doctors with years of experience practicing Maharishi Vedic Medicine.

872 **Disabled Children's Relief Fund**

PO Box 7420
Freeport, NY 11520
516-377-1605
FAX: 516-377-3978
e-mail: dc1605@aol.com
www.dcrf.com

Jerome H Blue PhD, President

National not-for-profit organization that provides modest grants for disabled children with preference given to those with no health insurance. Grants are provided for assistive devices, equipment and rehabilitative services.

873 **Disabled and Alone/Life Services for the Handicapped**

352 Park Avenue S
11th Floor
New York, NY 10010
212-532-6740
800-995-0066
FAX: 212-532-3588
e-mail: info@disabledandalone.org
www.disabledandalone.org

Roslyn Brilliant, Executive Director

A national nonprofit humanitarian organization whose primary concern is the well-being of handicapped persons, particularly when their families can no longer care for them. Disabled and Alone 1) Helps families do sensible planning for and with their disabled children; 2) Provides advocacy and oversight when the parents cannot do so; 3) Advises families, attorneys and financial planners about life planning for a family member with a disability.

874 **Distance Education and Training Council**

1601 18th Street NW
Washington, DC 20009
202-234-5100
FAX: 202-332-1386
e-mail: detc@detc.org
www.detc.org

Michael Lambert, Executive Director

Advocates quality distance education in America. Serves as a clearinghouse of information about the field and sponsors a nationally recognized accrediting agency for distance education.

875 **Division for Physical and Health Disabilities**

1920 Association Drive
Reston, VA 20191
703-620-3660
FAX: 703-624-9494
www.cec.sped.org

Advocates for quality education for individuals with physical disabilities, multiple disabilities, and special health care needs served in schools, hospitals, or home settings. DPHD's members include classroom teachers, administrators, related service personnel, hospital/homebound teachers, and parents.

876 **Division on Mental Retardation and Developmental Disabilities**

1110 N Glebe Road
Suite 300
Arlington, VA 22201
703-620-3660
FAX: 703-264-9494
www.cec.sped.org

Janice Burdick, President

Promotes the education and general welfare of indivduals with mental retardation, developmental disabilities and intellectual challenges and those who serve them. MRDD's members include professionals and paraprofessionals interested in individuals who are mentally retarded, developmentally disabled or have related learning problems.

877 **Doctor's Data**

PO Box 111
W Chicago, IL 60186
630-377-8139
800-323-2784
FAX: 630-587-7860
e-mail: inquiries@doctorsdata.com
www.doctorsdata.com

Darrell S Hickok, Chief Operating Officer

Independent reference laboratory providing data on levels of toxic and essential elements in hair, amino acids, and metabolites in blood and urine.

878 **Dynamic Learning Center**

PO Box 1112
Ben Lomond, CA 95005
831-336-3457
FAX: 831-336-5854

879 **ERIC Clearinghouse on Disabilities and Special Education**

1110 N Glebe Road
Arlingtonn, VA 22201
800-328-0272
FAX: 703-620-4334
www.ericec.org

Provides information on federal disability legislation, funding for programs serving individuals with disabilities, and programs and services for people with disabilities on the national, state and local levels.

880 **Easter Seals**

977 Pismo Street
PO Box 1036
Solvang, CA 93464
805-543-4122
800-221-6827
FAX: 805-543-8951

Linda Lee Harry, Executive Director

A nonprofit referral agency, that maintains listings of more than 12,000 organizations and community-based resource centers for all ages and disabilities to access. Also offers a quarterly newsletter, Direct Connect.

881 **Eden Foods**

701 Tecumseh Road
Clinton, MI 49236
517-456-7424
888-447-3336
FAX: 517-456-6075
www.edenfoods.com

Network of family farms and suppliers since 1968 centered around macrobiotics.

882 **Educational Accessibility Services**

Wayne State University
583 Student Center Building
5221 Gullen Mall
Detroit, MI 48202
313-577-1851
FAX: 313-577-4898
TTY:313-577-3365
e-mail: eas@teadmin.sa.wayne.edu
www.eas.wayne.edu

Susan Neste, Director
Jane DePriester-Morandini, Learning Specialist

A powerful advocating force for students with disabilities at the university. Our purpose is to provide students with the resources they need to succeed and to support their participation in all University programs and activities with dignity and independence.

883 **Electro Medical**

18433 Armistad
Fountain Valley, CA 92708
714-964-6776
800-422-8726
FAX: 714-428-4599

884 **Environmental Health Center**

8345 Walnut Hill Lane
Suite 220
Dallas, TX 75231
214-368-4132
FAX: 214-691-8432
e-mail: contact@ehcd.com
www.ehcd.com

William J Rea MD, Staff, President
Bertie Griffiths PhD, Staff
Nancy A Didriksen PhD, Staff

Clinic providing patient care in the areas of Immunotherapy, Nutrition, Physical Therapy, Chemical Depuration, Energy Balancing, Electromagnetic Sensitivity Testing, Psychological Support Services, Family Practice Medicine and Internal Medicine.

885 **Esalen Institute**

Highway 1
Big Sur, CA 93920
831-667-3000
FAX: 831-667-2724
e-mail: info@esalen.org
www.esalen.org

Founded in 1962 as an alternative education center devoted to the exploration of the world of unrealized human capacities that lies beyond the imagination. Blends East/West philosophies, experiential/didactic workshops, and a steady influx of philosophers, psychologists, artists, and religious thinkers.

886 **Estate Planning for the Disabled**

3100 Arapahoe Avenue
Suite 112
Boulder, CO 30303
800-683-4607

Counsels and assists parents of children with special needs to develop viable estate plans, letters of intent, wills and special needs trusts. EPD will work with the appropriate professionals and agencies to help put together an effective comprehensive plan.

887 **FELDENKRAIS GUILD of North America (FGNA)**

3611 SW Hood Avenue
Suite 100
Portland, OR 97201
503-221-6612
800-775-2118
FAX: 503-221-6616
e-mail: guild@feldenkrais.com
www.feldenkrais.com

Maureen Lynch, Contact

This is the organization which sets the standards for and certifies all FELDENKRAIS practitioners in North America. In order to practice, a practitioner must be a graduate of an FGNA accredited program (a minimum of 800 instruction hours over a three to four year period), and agree to follow both the Code of Professional Conduct and the Standards of Practice. FGNA may be contacted for further information about the FELDENKRAIS METHOD or for a list of FELDENKRAIS practitioners sorted by region.

888 **Family Resource Center on Disabilities**

20 E Jackson
Suite 300
Chicago, IL 60604 **312-939-3513**
800-952-4199
FAX: 312-939-7297
TTY:312-939-3519
www.ameritech.net/users/frcdptiil/FRCD

Mary Mostissy, President
Charlotte Des Jardins, Executive Director

Not-for-profit advocacy organization dedicated to improving services for all children with disabilities by providing support and services to affected families, informing parents of their rights, and helping parents become advocates for their children. Offers family support services, training, seminars and information and referral services. Publishes monthly newsletter.

889 **Family Voices**

3411 Candelaria NE
Suite M
Albuquerque, NM 87107 **505-867-2368**
888-835-5669
FAX: 505-867-6517
e-mail: kidshealth@familyvoices.org
www.familyvoices.org

Trish Thomas, National Outreach Coordinator

Not-for-profit voluntary organization dedicated to ensuring that children's health issues are addressed as public and private healthcare systems undero change in communities, states and the nation. National grassroots clearinghouse for information and education in ways to assure and improve health care for children with disabilities and chronic conditions. Provides materials including pamphlets, a newsletter and one-page papers on important topics.

890 **Favarh/Farmington Valley ARC**

225 Commerce Drive
PO Box 1099
Canton, CT 06019 **860-693-6662**
FAX: 860-693-8662
e-mail: favarh@favarh.org
www.favarh.org

Tom Thompson, Executive Director

Provides a variety of programs and services to adults with developmental, physical or mental disabilities and their families throughout the Farmington Valley communities of Avon, Burlington and more. Favarh's programs are designed to enhance the personal, social, emotional, vocational and living capabilities of persons with disabilities.

891 **Federation for Children with Special Needs**

1135 Tremont Street
Suite 420
Boston, MA 02120 **617-236-7210**
800-331-0688
FAX: 617-572-2094
e-mail: fcsninfo@fcsn.org
www.fcsn.org

Richard J Robison, Executive Director

Provides information, support and assistance to parents of children with disabilities, their professional partners and their communities.

892 **Fragrance and Health**

Human Ecology Action League (HEAL)
PO Box 29629
Atlanta, GA 30359 **404-248-1898**
FAX: 404-248-0162
e-mail: HEALNatnl@aol.com
members.aol.com/HEALNatnl/index.html

Katherine P Collier, Membership Coordinator

$24.00

35 pages

ISBN 0-967009-50-2

893 **Friends of Disabled Adults and Children**

4900 Lewis Road
Stone Mountain, GA 30083 **770-491-9014**
FAX: 770-491-0026
e-mail: fodac@fodac.org
www.fodac.org

Chris Brand, Executive Director

Not-for-profit organization dedicated to providing necessary services and support to physically and mobility impaired people of all ages. Provides free mobility impairment, rehabilitative, and home healthcare equipment. Provides variety of brochures and pamphlets. Community reentering program.

894 **George Washington University Health Resource Center**

2121 K Street NW
Suite 220
Washington, DC 20037 **202-973-0904**
800-544-3284
FAX: 202-973-0908
e-mail: askheath@heath.gwu.edu
www.heath.gwu.edu

Dr Pamela Ekpone, Director

National clearinghouse for information about education after high school for people with disabilities. Also serves as an information exchange about educational support services, policies, procedures, adaptations and opportunities on American campuses, vocational-technical schools, adult education programs, independent living centers and other training entities after high school.

895 **Goodwill Industries International**

9200 Wisconsin Avenue
Bethesda, MD 20814 **301-530-6500**
FAX: 301-530-1516
www.goodwill.org

Strives to achieve the full participation in society of disabled persons and other individuals with special needs by expanding their opportunities and occupational capabilities through a network of 179 autonomous, nonproft, community-based organizations providing services throughout the world in response to local needs.

896 **Great Lakes Association of Clinical Medicine**

70 W Huron Street
Chicago, IL 60610 **312-266-7246**

Members practice chelation therapy.

897 **Health Action**

243 Pebble Beach
Santa Barbara, CA 93117 **805-682-3230**

898 **Health Resource Center for Women with Disabilities**

Rehabilitation Institute of Chicago
345 E Superior Street
Chicago, IL 60611 **312-238-1051**
FAX: 312-238-1205
TTY:312-908-8523
e-mail: hrcwd@rehabchicago.org
rehabchicago.org

Judy Panko Reis, Director
Kristi Kirchner, MD, Medical Director
Linda E Miller, Domestic Violence Coordinator

National, not-for-profit, general health and service center providing accessible medical services for women with disabilities. Conducts research into health issues concerning disabled women and offers educational resources for healthcare professionals and women with disabilities. Provides materials and educational opportunities through its library and resource center, newsletter, information sheets, brochures, videos and free seminars for women and their healthcare providers.

899 **Homeopathic Educational Services**

2124 Kittredge Street PMBQ
Berkeley, CA 94704 **510-649-0294**
800-359-9051
FAX: 510-649-1955
e-mail: mail@homeopathic.com
www.homeopathic.com

Dana Ullman MPH, Director and Owner

Resource center for homeopathic products and services including books, tapes, research, medicines, medicine kits, software for the general public and the health professional and correspondence courses.

900 **Human Ecologist**

Human Ecology Action League (HEAL)
PO Box 29629
Atlanta, GA 30359 **404-248-1898**
FAX: 404-248-0162
e-mail: HEALNatnl@aol.com
members.aol.com/HEALNatnl/index.html

Diane Thomas, Editor
$26.00
35 pages Quarterly

901 **Human Ecology Action League (HEAL)**

PO Box 29629
Atlanta, GA 30359 **404-248-1898**
FAX: 404-248-0162
e-mail: HEALNatnl@aol.com
members.aol.com/HEALNatnl/index.html

Katherine P Collier, Membership Coordinator

Serving people with multiple chemical sensitivities (MCS), and others concerned about the effects of chemicals on human health.

902 **IL Center: Cape Organization for Rights of the Disabled**

1019 Iyannough Road
#4
Hyannis, MA 02601 **508-775-8300**
800-541-0282
FAX: 508-775-7022
e-mail: bhcord@cape.com
www.vse.cape.com/~bhcord

Bill Henning, Executive Director

903 **Informed Birth and Parenting**

PO Box 3675
Ann Arbor, MI 48106 **313-662-6857**

Resources on pregnancy, childbirth, and parenting; refers midwives; certifies educators and assistants.

904 **Institute for Health and Disability**

University of Minnesota
420 Delaware Street SE
Box 721
Minneapolis, MN 55455 **612-624-3939**
FAX: 612-626-2134
TTY:612-624-3939
e-mail: instihd@tc.umn.edu
www.peds.umn.edu/peds-adol/ih.html

Marty Smith MA, Executive Director

905 **Institute for Music, Health and Education**

PO Box 4179
Boulder, CO 80306 **303-443-8484**

906 **Institute for Scientific Research**

33 Bonad Road
Winchester, MA 01890 **781-368-9094**
FAX: 781-368-9096

Steve Guberman, Director

Conducts research on the sociological aspects of disabilities and rehabilitation. Conducts evaluations of programs designed to train professionals and to rehabilitate individuals with disabilities.

907 **Institute of Transpersonal Psychology**

PO Box 4437
Stanford, CA 94305 **415-327-2066**

908 **InterNatural**

PO Box 489
Twin Lakes, WI 53181 **262-889-8581**
800-643-4221
FAX: 800-905-6887
e-mail: internatural@lotuspress.com
www.internatural.com

Mail order distribution of over 14,000 natural health and wellness products, books and videos.

909 **International Academy of Oral Medicine and Toxicology**

PO Box 608531
Orlando, FL 32860 **407-298-2450**
e-mail: mziff@iaomt.org
www.iaomt.org

Michael F Ziff, Executive Director

Nonprofit organization dedicated to funding solid peer-reviewed scientific research in the area of toxic substances used in dentistry as well as providing continuing education and carefully reviewed procedures, protocols, and methodologies to reduce the risk for patients and professionals.

910 **International Association of Professional Natural Hygientists**

Regency Health Resorts & Spas
2000 S Ocean Drive
Hallandale, FL 33009 **305-454-2220**

Members are physicians who specialize in therapeutic fasting.

911 **International Chiropractors Association**

1110 N Glebe Road
Suite 1000
Arlington, VA 22201
703-528-5000
800-423-4690
FAX: 703-528-5023
www.chiropractic.org

Established in 1926 to empower humanity in the expression of maximum health, wellness and human potential through the universal chiropractic expression and utilization. Strives to advance chiropractics throughout the world as a distinct health care profession predicated upon its unique philosophy, science and art.

912 **International Clinic of Biological Regeneration**

PO Box 509
Florissant, MI 63032
314-921-3997
800-826-5366
FAX: 314-921-8485
e-mail: info@icbr.com
www.icbr.com

C Tom Smith, Meical Director

International cell therapy center since 1981.

913 **International College of Applied Kinesiology**

6405 Metcalf Avenue
Suite 503
Shawnee Mission, KS 66202
913-384-5336

Referral service for applied kinesiologists.

914 **International Institute of Reflexology**

PO Box 12462
St. Petersburg, FL 33733
727-343-4811

Information, seminars, publications and referrals.

915 **International Medical and Dental Hypnotherapy Association**

4110 Edgeland
Suite 800
Royal Oak, MI 48073
313-549-5594
800-257-5467

916 **International Ozone Association**

31 Strawberry Hill Avenue
Stamford, CT 06902
203-348-3542

917 **International Women's Health Coalition**

24 E 21st Street
New York, NY 10010
212-979-8500
FAX: 212-979-9009
www.iwhc.org

Information and pamphlets on sexually transmitted diseases and other health concerns.

918 **Invincible Athletics**

PO Box 541
Lancaster, MA 01523
508-368-1818

Teaches how to incorproate Ayurvedic training principles into athletic conditioning.

919 **Kessler Institute for Rehabilitation**

1199 Pleasant Valley Way
W Orange, NJ 07052
973-414-4700
888-537-7537
888-537-7537
FAX: 973-243-6861
www.kessler-rehab.com

Kathy Lewis, VP Marketing
Maura Bergen, Public Relations Coordinator

Kessler Institute for Rehabilitation is world renowned for treating individuals with physical disabilities, resulting from spinal cord and brain injuries, stroke and amputee, sports and work-related, and other illnesses and injuries. Kessler offers comprehensive programs designed to meet each person's individual needs.

920 **Mainstream**

6930 Carroll Avenue
Suite 240
Takoma Park, MD 20912
301-749-9030
FAX: 301-839-9292
e-mail: info@mainstream.org
www.mainstreaminc.org

David A Pichette, Executive Director
Karen Morgret, National Program Director
Janet Cassidy, Dallas TX Regional Manager

Non-profit organization that works with employers and service providers around the country to increase employment opportunities for persons with disabilities.

921 **Matheny School and Hospital**

PO Box 339
Peapack, NJ 07977
908-234-0011
FAX: 908-719-2137
e-mail: info@matheny.org
www.matheny.org

Steven Proctor, President
Gabor Barabas MD, Medical Director
Gary E Eddey MD, Director of Medicine & Dentistry

A residential and outpatient facility for children and adults with physical disabilities such as Cerebral Palsy, Spina Bifida, Muscular Dystrophy and Lesch-Nyhan disease. Matheny offers medical and dental care, therapies, augmentative communication, and other allied health services as well as special education, respite care and adult medical day care.

922 **MedEscort International**

PO Box 8766
Allentown, PA 18105
610-791-3111
800-255-7182
FAX: 610-791-9189
e-mail: medescort@fast.net
www.medescort.com

Offers specially trained escorts for individuals who cannot travel alone due to age or disability.

923 **Meridian Valley Clinical Laboratory**

801 SW 16th Street
Suite 126
Renton, WA 98055
425-271-8689
800-234-6825
FAX: 425-271-8674
e-mail: meridian@meridianvalleylab.com
www.meridianvalleylab.com

A clinical test facility dedicated to providing the most accurate and informative data for patient diagnosis and therapeutic monitoring. With our current research and up-to-date information and various aspects of clinical nutritional medicine, our methodologies and capabilities include areas of analytical chemistry, heavy metal determination, microbiology, and immunology.

924 **MetaMatrix Medical Laboratory**
5000 Peachtree Street
Industrial Boulevard
Norcross, GA 30071
770-446-5483
FAX: 770-441-2237

925 **Mind-Body Clinic**
824 Boylston Street
Chestnut Hill, MA 02467
617-991-0102
FAX: 617-991-0112
e-mail: mbmi@caregroup.harvard.edu

Herbert Benson MD, President
Marilyn Wilcher, Senior VP

926 **Mind/Body Health Services**
393 Dixon Road
Boulder, CO 80302
303-440-8460

927 **Mobility International USA**
PO Box 10767
Eugene, OR 97440
541-343-1284
FAX: 541-343-6812
e-mail: info@miusa.org
www.miusa.org

Susan Sygall, Executive Director
Pamela Houston, Public Relations Coordinator
Tracy Scharn, Project Assistant

A US based national nonprofit organization dedicated to empowering people with disabilities around the world through leadership development, training and international exchange to ensure inclusion of people with disabilities in international exchange and development programs. The National Clearinghouse on Disability & Exchange, a joint project managed by MIUSA provides free information and referrals.

928 **NLP Comprehensive**
PO Box 927
Evergreen, CO 80437
303-987-2224
800-233-1657
FAX: 303-987-2228
www.nlpco.com

NLP, or Neuro-Linguistic Programming, is the science of how the brain codes learning and experience. This coding affects all communication and behavior. NLP Comprehensive helps individuals and businesses make the fullest use of their talents and resources. We teach the thought processes and communication strategies of exceptional performers through workshops, books, and tapes.

929 **National Association for Holistic Aromatherapy**
4509 Interlake Avnue N
#233
Seattle, WA 98103
206-547-2164
888-ASK-NAHA
FAX: 206-547-2680
www.naha.org

The NAHA is an educational, nonprofit organization dedicated to enhancing public awareness of the benefits of true aromatherapy. It offers aromatherapy courses and acts as a referral service.

930 **National Association of Developmental Disabilities Councils**
1234 Mass Avenue NW
Suite 103
Washington, DC 20005
202-347-1234
FAX: 202-347-4023
e-mail: naddc@naddc.org
www.naddc.org

Donna Heuneman, Executive Director

Represents Developmental Disabilities Councils in areas of public policy. Provides training and technical assistance to Councils.

931 **National Association of Retired Volunteer Program Directors**
703 Main Street
Paterson, NJ 07503
973-754-2675

Maureen Mulligan, President

Seeks to provide national visibility and advocacy to facilitate communications among membership and to act as representative for those served by RSVP before national governmental bodies. Bestows grants and awards, compiles statistics and conducts workshops.

932 **National Association of the Physically Handicapped**
1375 Dewitt Drive
Akron, OH 44313
330-724-1994
800-743-5008
e-mail: www.trumanjm@aol.com
www.naph.net

Jerry Snyder, National President

The NAPH was established in 1958 to advance the social, economic, and physical welfare of the physically handicapped in the United States. NAPH proposes and supports legislation to provide more educational and rehabilitation opportunities, tax relief, employment, and other benefits for the physically handicapped. Data and information relating to the physically handicapped are collected and studied and reported to members. NAPH supports efforts to make all public facilities accessible.

933 **National Center for Education in Maternal and Child Health**
Georgetown University
Box 571272
Washington, DC 20057
202-784-9770
FAX: 202-784-9777
e-mail: info@ncemch.org
www.ncemch.org

Dr Rochelle Mayer, Director

Provides information on children with special health needs, child health and development, adolescent health, nutrition, violence and injury prevention and other issues of maternal and child health for health professionals and the public.

934 **National Clearinghouse on Women and Girls with Disabilities**
Educational Equity Concepts
114 E 32nd Street
Room 701
New York, NY 10016
212-243-1110
FAX: 212-627-0407
TTY:212-243-1110
e-mail: information@edequity.org
www.edequity.org

Ellen Rubin, Coord. of Individuality Program

Provides information, resources and referrals. Publishes Bridging the Gap, a national directory which lists organizations that serve women and girls with disabilities and gives resource information. Also publishes curriculum on children with disabilities and programs in science for children with disabilties.

935 **National College of Naturopathic Medicine**

049 SW Porter Street
Portland, OR 97201
503-499-4343
FAX: 503-499-0027
www.ncnm.edu

Founded in 1956, and set in the beautiful Pacific Northwest city of Portland, Oregon, NCNM offers two graduate degrees, as well as a certified post-doctoral naturopathic residency program.

936 **National Council for Community Behavioral Healthcare**

12300 Twinbrook Parkway
Suite 320
Rockville, MD 20852
301-984-6200
FAX: 301-881-7159
www.nccbh.org

Jeannie Campbell, Executive VP

National organization of community-based providers of behavioral health services.

937 **National Council on Disability**

1331 F Street
Suite 850
Washington, DC 22004
202-272-2000
FAX: 202-272-2022
www.ncd.gov

Mark Quigley, Communications Director

Federal agency led by 15 members appointed by the President of the United States and confirmed by the United States Senate. The overall purpose of the National Council is to promote policies, programs, practices and procedures that guarantee equal opportunities to persons with disabilities.

938 **National Council on Independent Living**

1916 Wilson Boulevard
Suite 209
Arlington, VA 22201
703-525-3406
FAX: 703-525-3409
e-mail: ncil@ncil.org
www.ncil.org

Anne Marie Hughey, Executive Director
Kelly Buckland, NCIL VP

Advances the independent living philosophy and advocates for the human rights of and services for people with disabilities to further their full integration and participation in society. The National Council on Independent Living (NCIL) is the oldest cross disability, grassroots organization run by and for people with disabilities.

939 **National Early Childhood Technical Assistance Center**

137 E Franklin Street
Suite 500
Chapel Hill, NC 27514
919-962-2001
FAX: 919-966-7463
e-mail: nectacunc.edu
www.nectas.org

Assists states and other designated governing jurisdictions as they develop multidisciplinary, coordinated and comprehensive services for children with special needs.

940 **National Easter Seal Society**

230 W Monroe Street
Chicago, IL 60606
312-422-0600
FAX: 312-726-8628
www.seal.com

Janet D Jamieson, Communications Mgr.

The mission of the Society is to help people with disabilities achieve independence. Easter Seals provides quality rehabilitation services, technological assistance and disability prevention, advocacy and public education programs. A nationwide network of affiliate societies serving each of the 50 United States, the District of Columbia and Puerto Rico, all of which work together to serve more than 1 million people each year. There are 160 chapters offering more than 400 programs nationwide.

941 **National Endowment for the Arts: Office for AccessAbility**

1100 Pennsylvania Avenue NW
Washington, DC 20506
202-682-5532
FAX: 202-682-5715
e-mail: richards@arts.endow.gov
www.arts.endow.gov/partner

Suzanne Richard, Accessibility Specialist

Offers technical assistance on making programs accessible to older adults and individuals with various disabilities.

942 **National Guild of Hypnotists**

PO Box 308
Merrimack, NH 03054
603-429-9438
FAX: 603-424-8066
e-mail: nghreferrals@ngh.net
www.ngh.net

The National Guild of Hypnotists, Inc. is a not-for-profit, educational corporation in the State of New Hampshire. Founded in Boston, Massachusetts in 1951, the Guild is a professional organization comprised of dedicated individuals committed to advancing the field of hypnotism. We provide an open forum for the free exchange of ideas concerning hypnotism. The Guild is a resource for members and a vehicle for legal and legislative action.

943 **National Information Center for Children and Youth with Disabilities (NICHCY)**

PO Box 1492
Washington, DC 20013
202-884-8200
800-695-0285
FAX: 202-884-8441
e-mail: nichcy@aed.org
www.nichcy.org

Provides free information to assist parents, educators, caregivers, advocates and others in helping children and youth with disabilities become participating members of the community. In addition to a wealth of printed materials, the Center disseminates materials on cassette, computer disc and in Spanish. The Center can also provide personal responses to specific questions.

944 **National Information Clearinghouse**

Association for the Care of Children's Health
7910 Woodmont Avenue
Suite 300
Bethesda, MD 20814
301-654-6549
800-922-9224
FAX: 301-986-4553

A national information and referral system providing assistance to meet the information needs of caregivers and to protect the rights of infants with disabilities and life-threatening conditions.

945 **National Institute on Disability and Rehabilitation Research**

400 Maryland Avenue, SW
Washington, DC 20202 **202-205-8134**
FAX: 202-205-8515
www.ed.gov/offices/OSERS/NIDRR

Conducts comprehensive and coordinated programs of extramural research and related activities to maximize the full inclusion, social integration, employment and independent living of disabled individuals of all ages. Provides funding for programs to assist ADA compliance, including Regional Disability and Business Technical Assistance Centers, Materials Development Projects, and Peer Training Projects.

946 **National Maternal and Child Health Clearinghouse**

2070 Chain Bridge Road
Suite 450
Vienna, VA 22182 **703-730-5200**
FAX: 703-821-2098
e-mail: nmchc@circsol.com
www.nmchc.org

Linda Cramer, Director

Offers information, books and pamphlets to professionals, parents and children facing health issues or disabilities.

947 **National Mental Health Association**

2001 N Beauregard Street
12th Floor
Alexandria, VA 22311 **703-684-7722**
800-969-6642
FAX: 703-684-5968
e-mail: infoctr@nmha.org
www.nmha.org

Michael Faenza MSSW, President/CEO

Nonprofit organization addressing all issues related to mental health and mental illness. With more than 340 affiliates nationwide, NMHA works to improve the mental health of all Americans, especially the 54 million individuals with mental disorders, through advocacy, education, research and service.

1909

948 **National Organization on Disability**

910 16th Street NW
Suite 600
Washington, DC 20006 **202-293-5960**
FAX: 202-293-7999
e-mail: ability@nod.org
www.nod.org

Alan Reich, President
Brewster Thackeray, VP, Communications
John Hershey, Advice and Resource Manager

The National Organization on Disability promotes the full and equal participation of men, women and children with disabilities in all aspects of American life. Founded in 1982, NOD is the leading national disability organization concerned with all disabilites, all age groups and all disability issues.

949 **National Parent Network on Disabilities**

1130 17th Street NW
Suite 400
Washington, DC 20036 **202-463-2299**
FAX: 202-463-9405
e-mail: npnd@mindspring.com
www.npnd.org

Linda Shpeherd, Executive Director

Established to provide a presence and national voice for parents of children, youth and adults with special needs. The organization shares information and resources in order to promote parents influence on policy issues concerning the needs of people with disabilities.

950 **National Rehabilitation Association (NRA)**

633 S Washington Street
Alexandria, VA 22314 **703-836-0850**
FAX: 703-836-0848
TTY:703-836-0849
e-mail: info@nationalrehab.org
www.nationalrehab.org

Dedicated to advocating, supporting, and enhancing the lives of individuals with disabilities and their families. disseminates up-to-date information, conducts educational seminars, and provides opportunities through knowledge and diversity for professionals in the field of rehabilitation. Produces educational materials and sponsors an annual training conference with exhibits displaying the latest in rehabilitation technologies, awards, and provides access to a nationwide employment network.

951 **National Rehabilitation Information Center (NARIC)**

4200 Forbes Boulevard
Suite 202
Lanham, MD 20706 **301-459-5900**
800-346-2742
FAX: 301-459-4263
e-mail: naricinfo@heitechservices.com
www.naric.com

Tamie Pyle, Information Specialist

For 20 years, the staff of the NARIC has collected and disseminated the results of federally funded research projects. NARIC's literature collection, which also includes commercially published books, journal articles and audiovisuals, averages around 200 new documents per month. Funded by the National Institute on Disability and Rehabilitation Research to serve anyone, professional or lay person, who is interested in disability and rehabilitation.

952 **National Respite Locator Service**

800 Eastowne Drive
Suite 105
Chapel Hill, NC 27514 **919-490-5577**
800-773-5433
FAX: 919-490-4905
www.respitelocator.org

Dedicated to assisting parents, caregivers and professionals find temporary relief services in their state and local area. Provides appropriate referrals for further assistance and has a leaflet describing the organization.

953 **National Vaccine Information Center**

421 E Church Street
Vienna, VA 22180 **703-938-0342**
FAX: 703-938-5768
www.nvic.org

Kathi Williams, Director

A national nonprofit educational organization dedicated to preventing, through public education, vaccine injuries and deaths. NVIC represents vaccine consumers and health care providers, including parents whose children suffered illness or died following vaccination. NVIC supports the right of vaccine consumers to have access to the safest and most effective vaccine as well as the right to make informed, independent vaccination decisions.

954 **National Women's Health Network**

514 10th Street
Suite 400
Washington, DC 20004 **202-347-1140**
FAX: 202-347-1168
www.womenshealthnetwork.org

Publications and information packets on women's health issues. Members receive our bimonthly newsletter, Network News.

955 Native American Protection and Advocacy Project
DNA People's Legal Services
3535 E 30th Street
Suite 201
Farmington, NM 84702 **505-566-5880**
800-862-7271
FAX: 505-566-5889

Therese Yanan, Project Director

956 North America Riding for the Handicapped Association
PO Box 33150
Denver, CO 80233 **303-452-1212**
800-369-7433
FAX: 303-252-4610
e-mail: narha@narha.org
www.narha.org

William Scebbi, Executive Director

National nonprofit equestrian organization dedicated to serving individuals with disability by giving disabled individuals the opportunity to ride horses. Establishes safety standards, provides continuing education and offers networking opportunities for both its individuals and center members. Produces educational materials including fact sheets, brochures, booklets, audio-visual tapes, a directory and NARHA's magazine Strides.

957 Nurse Healers: Professional Associates International
3760 S Highland Drive
Suite 429
Salt Lake City, UT 84106 **801-273-3399**
FAX: 509-693-3537
www.therapeutic-touch.org

Rebecca Good, Coordinator
Dolores Krieger PhD RN, Advisor/Founder

Cooperative among health professionals interested in healing. Sets the standards for the practice and teaching of Therapeutic Touch. Voluntary, not-for-profit organization.

958 Pacific Institute of Aromatherapy
PO Box 6842
San Rafael, CA 94903 **415-479-9121**
FAX: 415-479-0614
pacificinstituteofaromatherapy.com

Offers courses in the practice of aromatherapy.

959 Parent Professional Advocacy League
59 Temple Place
Suite 664
Boston, MA 02111 **617-542-7860**
800-537-0446
FAX: 617-542-7832
e-mail: pal@fcsn.org
www.ppal.net

Donna Welles, Director
Lisa Lambert, Assistant Director
Jodi Merrill, Administrative Assistant

Promotes a strong voice for families of children and adolescents with mental health needs. Advocates for supports, treatments and policies that enable families to live in their communities in an environment of stability and respect.

960 Parent to Parent
2900 Woodcock Road
Atlanta, GA 30341 **770-451-5484**
800-229-2058
FAX: 770-458-4091

Dedicated to strengthening, supporting, and empowering families by establishing one to one parent to parent contacts. Enhances the ability of parents to access services and resources for children with special needs by providing information, resources, and referrals to appropriate services; supports and empowers families to participate in parent programs and disability issues. Educational materials consist of a quarterly newsletter and a fact sheet containing managed care information.

961 Parents Helping Parents (PHP)
3041 Olcott Street
Santa Clara, CA 95054 **408-727-5775**
FAX: 408-727-0182
e-mail: info@php.com
www.php.com

Dedicated to assisting children with any type of special need: mental, physical, emotional, or learning disability. Mission is to help children with special needs receive love, hope, respect, and services needed to achieve their full potential by strengthening their families and the professionals who serve them. Developed and implemented numerous programs; produce a variety of educational and support materials, including information packets, brochures, database and a quarterly newletter.

962 Parents for Residential Reform
Federation for Children with Special Needs
1135 Tremont Street
Suite 420
Boston, MA 02120 **617-236-7210**
800-672-7084
FAX: 617-572-2094
e-mail: pfrr@fcsn.org
www.pfrr.org

Andrea Watson, Founder/Project Coordinator

Parents of children with special needs, whose children require intensive residential education settings, face a myriad of unique circumstances in their efforts to provide ongoing support to their children. PFRR provides information on placement, restraint medication, IEP, standardized testing, transition, parent/peer connections, workshops, trainings and the maze of state and federal agencies. We educate on the rights of parents, and their young people who are receiving services.

963 Peak Energy Performanceer
1621 N Circle Drive
Colorado Springs, CO 80909 **719-548-1600**
800-331-2303
FAX: 719-572-8081

Information on removal of mercury fillings.

964 People First International
PO Box 12642
Salem, OR 97309 **503-362-0336**
FAX: 503-585-0287
e-mail: people1@open.org
www.people1.org

Steven Kramer, President
Ruth Morris, VP
Rodney Carver, VP

Self-advocacy organization of developmentally disabled people who have joined together to learn how to speak for themselves.

965 **People-to-People Committee for the Handicapped**
PO Box 18131
Washington, DC 20036 **301-493-5883**
FAX: 301-493-0510
e-mail: ngvb096@prodigy.com

David Brigham, Chairman

Individuals concerned about that circumstances of handicapped people throughout the world. Disseminates information, acts as a consultant in promoting exchange activities, coordinates special assistance in developing countries and more.

966 **People-to-People Committee on Disability**
PO Box 18131
Washington, DC 20036 **703-535-6011**
FAX: 703-836-0367
e-mail: ngvb096@prodigy.com
www.shrm.org

David Brigham, Chairman

Individuals concerned about the circumstances of handicapped people throughout the world. Disseminates information, acts as a consultant in promoting exchange activities, coordinates special assistance projects in developing countries and more.

967 **People-to-People International: Committee for the Handicapped**
501 E Armour Boulevard
Kansas City, MO 64109 **816-531-4701**
800-676-7874
FAX: 816-561-7502
e-mail: ptpi@ptpi.org
www.ptpi.org

Dr David Waugh, Chairman
Marc L Bright, VP Special Programs

Goals of this committee include: betterment of the handicapped through international unity; educating those with and without handicaps through technical assistance; opening access doors through sensory aids, prosthetic devices and travel tips; and coordination of major international cultural exchanges.

968 **Polarity Wellness Center**
10 Leonard Street
Suite A
New York, NY 10013 **212-334-8392**
FAX: 212-925-5675

Information, publications and referral directories.

969 **Portland Naturopathic Clinic: NCNM National Health Centers Eastside Clinic**
National College of Naturopathic Medicine
49 SW Wporter Street
Portland, OR 97201 **503-499-4343**
FAX: 503-499-0027
www.ncnm.edu

Outpatient clinic in naturopathic medicine with diagnostic services, naturopathic treatments and a natural pharmacy.

970 **Quan Yin Healing Arts Center**
455 Valencia Street
San Francisco, CA 94103 **415-861-4964**
FAX: 415-861-0579
e-mail: qyhacinfo@aol.com
www.quanyinhealingarts.com

Ruth Kierans, Operations Manager

Acupuncture, herbal medicine, yoga and massage therapy, lectures, discussion groups and nutritional information.

971 **Rehabilitation International**
25 E 21st Street
New York, NY 10010 **212-420-1500**
FAX: 212-505-0871
e-mail: Rehabintl@rehab-international.org
www.rehab-international.org

Lex Frieden, President
George Wilson, Treasurer

Worldwide network of people with disabilities, service providers and government agencies working together to improve the quality of life for the dosabled people and their families, has more than 200 member organizations in 90 nations.

972 **Rehabilitation Services Administration of the District of Columbia**
810 1st Street NE
Suite 10004
Washington, DC 20002 **202-442-8663**
FAX: 202-442-8742
e-mail: dcrsal@msn.com

Elizabeth B Parker, Administrator
Janice Williams, Chief Client Services Divsion
Melvin Joyner, Chief Vending Facility Program

Offers vocational rehabilitation services to people with disabilities.

973 **Rocky Mountain Resource & Training Institute**
6355 Ward Road
Suite 310
Arvada, CO 80004 **303-420-2942**
FAX: 303-420-8675
TTY:303-420-2942

Serves people with disabilities and provides training to the agencies that assist them. Facilitates disabled individuals' transition from school to adult life; provides information and resources concerning assistive technology, devices, and services; promotes and ensures compliance with the federal Americans with Disabilities Act (ADA) and other legislation promoting the rights and inclusion of people with disabilities; promotes supported employment, strategic planning and development.

974 **Ronald McDonald House**
500 17th Street
Huntington, WV 25701 **304-529-1122**
FAX: 304-529-2970
e-mail: margaret@mchouse.org
www.mchouse.org

A home-away-from-home, a temporary lodging facility for the families of seriously ill children being treated at nearby hospitals. Each house is run by a local nonprofit agency comprised of members of the medical community, McDonald's owners, businesses and civic organizations and parent volunteers.

975 **St. John Valley Associates**
10C 11th Avenue
Madawaska, ME 04756 **207-728-7197**
FAX: 207-728-7550
e-mail: sjva@ncil.net

Michael St John, Executive Director
Andrew McQuarrie, Board President

A nonprofit association with the mission of empowering adult citizens with mental retardation to dignify themselves. Three broad-based programs and services (Independence Plus, Job Involvements, People Now) are designed to allow each individual to upgrade learning skills, assert rights, increase independence and accept new responsibilities.
$75.00

976 **Standard Search: Oral Health Care for People with Developmental Disabilities**

National Oral Health Information Clearing House
1 NOHIC Way
Bethesda, MD 20892 **301-402-7364**
FAX: 301-907-8830
e-mail: nidr@aerie.com
www.nohic.nidcr.hih.gov

Patricia Sheridan, Project Director

Helps meet the information needs of special care patients and health care providers. Staff provides the custom or standardized services on special care topics in oral health, including developmental disabilities. Each record in the search contains a bibliographic citation and abstract including info for the user on how to obtain materials directly.

977 **TEACCH**

University of North Carolina at Chapel Hill
CB # 7180 310 Medical School
Wing E
Chapel Hill, NC 27599 **919-966-2173**
FAX: 919-966-4127
www.teacch.com

Gary B Mesibov, PhD, Professor/Director

Focus on the person with autism and the development of a program around this person's skills, interests and needs.

978 **Teacher Preparation and Special Education**

21 G Street NW
Suite 416
Washington, DC 20052 **202-994-6170**
800-449-7374
FAX: 202-994-3365
gsehd.gwu.edu/gsehd

Madeline Will, Assistant Secretary

Administers the Education of the Handicapped Act and related programs for the education of handicapped children, including grants to institutions of higher learning and fellowships to train educational personnel. Grants to states for the education of handicapped children, research and demonstration.

979 **Technology and Media Division**

Council for Exceptional Children
1110 N Glebe Road
Suite 300
Arlington, VA 22201 **703-620-3660**
FAX: 703-264-9494
www.cec.sped.org

Janice Burdick, President

Promotes the availability and effective use of technolgy and media for individuals with disabilities and/or who are gifted. Members include special education teachers, speech and language therapists, rehabilitation therapists, counselors, researchers, teacher educators and others.

980 **Thresholds Psychiatric Rehabilitation Centers**

4101 N Ravenswood Avenue
Chicago, IL 60613 **773-477-7505**
888-997-3422
FAX: 773-880-6279
e-mail: jerry@thresholds.org
www.thresholds.org

Jerry Dincin, Executive Director
Jay Forman, Associate Director

A nationally-recognized psychosocial rehabilitation agency serving persons with severe and persistent mental illness. The agency offers its programming at 22 service locations and more than 40 residential facilities throughout Chicago and Northern Illinois. Also offers specialized programming for older adults, young adults, parents, the homeless and the hearing impaired and mentally ill.

Sliding scale

981 **Trager International**

24800 Chagrin Boulevard
Suite 205
Beachwood, OH 44122 **216-896-9383**
e-mail: trager@trager.com
www.trager.com

Represents and supports Trager psychophysical integration and Mentastics movement education.

982 **Upledger Institute**

11211 Prosperity Farms Road
Suite D-325
Palm Beach Gardens, FL 33410 **561-622-4334**
800-233-5880
FAX: 561-622-4771
e-mail: upledger@upledger.com
www.upledger.com

Health resource center dedicated to the advancement of complementary and innovative techniques.

983 **Visiting Nurse Association of America**

99 Summer Street
Suite 1700
Boston, MA 02110 **617-737-3200**
FAX: 617-737-1144
e-mail: vnaa@vnaa.org
www.vnaa.org

Carolyn Markey, President/CEO
Holli Adams, Office Manager/Exec Assistant
Jeannine Berube, Manager Member Relations/Events

Serve our members through work in promoting community based home health care, through business development, national puble imaging, member services and government advocacy.

984 **Vocational Rehabilitation Center**

1062 E Lancaster Avenue
Rosemont, PA 19010 **610-525-1810**
800-221-1042
FAX: 610-520-0935
www.arcofl-n.org/backup/providors/ovr.htm

OVR is the Pennsylvania Office of Vocational Rehabilitation, a state agency that helps persons with disabilities help themselves to prepare for, start and maintain a career. OVR has fifteen offices located around the state with over 400 professional vocational rehabilitation counselors. These counselors work every year with thousands of persons who have physical, mental and emotional disabilities.

985 **Western DuPage Special Recreation Association**

116 N Schmale Road
Carol Stream, IL 60188 **630-681-0962**
FAX: 630-681-1262
e-mail: info@wdsra.com
www.wdsra.com

Peggy Wilson, Superintendent Recreation
Ron Bergquist, Assistant Superintendent

A cooperative extension of nine park districts in Chicago's western suburbs. Provides more than 1,000 recreational programs, trips and special events each year for individuals of all ages with special needs. Also offers assistance to inviduals with special needs who wish to take part in park district programs. Serves the park districts of Bloomingdale, Carol Stream, GlenEllyn, Naperville, Roselle, Warrenville, W Chicago, Wheaton and Winfield, Illnois.

986 **Western States Training Associates**

2290 E 4500 S
Suite 120
Salt Lake City, UT 84117 **801-278-1022**
FAX: 801-278-1088

987 **Wheelchair Access**

RD
PO Box 12
Glenmore, PA 19343 **610-942-3266**
FAX: 610-942-0282
e-mail: info@waccess.org
www.waccess.org

Dedicated to providing comprehensive information to individuals with disabilities concerning wheelchair accessible homes for sale or rent, vans, wheelchairs, and any other equipment they require. Produces a variety of educational materials including a regular newsletter.

988 **Women to Women**

PO Box 306
Portland, ME 04112
800-832-2342
FAX: 207-791-7869
e-mail: personalprogram@womentowomen.com
www.womentowomen.com

Combination of alternative and conventional medicine in women's health, bring science and disipline to natural and preventative methods. Publishes the Creating Health Guide, a quarterly collection of articles written by the health care professionals at Women to Women.

989 **World Institute on Disability**

510 16th Street
Suite 100
Oakland, CA 94612 **510-763-4100**
FAX: 510-763-4109
e-mail: wid@wid.org
www.wid.org

A public policy center that is run by persons with disabilities. Research, training and public policy center promoting the civil rights and the full societal inclusion of people with disabilities.

Hearing Impaired

990 **Academy of Dispensing Audiologists**

3008 Millwood Avenue
Columbia, SC 29205 **803-256-7181**
FAX: 803-765-0860
e-mail: info@audiologist.org
www.audiologist.org

Carol Davis, Executive Director

Encourages audiology training programs to include pertinent aspects of hearing aid dispensing in their curriculum.

991 **Academy of Rehabilitative Audiology**

PO Box 26532
Minneapolis, MN 55426 **952-920-0484**
FAX: 952-920-6098
e-mail: ara@incnet.com
www.audrehab.org

Jodell Newman Ryan PhD, President
Sheila Pratt PhD, President-Elect
Frances Laven MS, Executive Director

Provides professional education, research and interest in programs for hearing handicapped persons.

992 **Advocates for Hearing Impaired Youth**

PO Box 75949
Washington, DC 20013 **301-589-8444**
FAX: 202-651-5817
e-mail: spnolts@juno.com

Information on deafness, hearing impairments, child welfare and advocacy.

993 **Alexander Graham Bell Association for the Deaf and Hard of Hearing**

3417 Volta Place NW
Washington, DC 20007 **202-337-5220**
FAX: 202-337-8314
e-mail: info@agbell.org
www.agbell.org

K Todd Houston PhD, Executive Director/CEO

The Alexander Graham Bell Association for the Deaf and Hard of Hearing (AG Bell) is the world's oldest and largest membership organization promoting the use of spoken language by children and adults who are hearing impaired. Members include parents of children with hearing loss, adults who are deaf or hard of hearing, educators, audiologists, speech-language pathologists, physicians and other professionals in fields related to hearing loss and deafness.

994 **American Academy of Environmental Medicine**

7701 E Kellogg
Suite 625
Wichita, KS 67207 **316-684-5500**
FAX: 316-684-5709
e-mail: administrator@aaem.com
www.aaem.com

Training for physicians in environmental medicine.

995 **American Academy of Otolaryngology: Head and Neck Surgery**

1 Prince Street
Alexandria, VA 22314 **703-739-1316**
FAX: 703-683-5100
www.entnet.org

Charles Krause, President

Promotes the art and science of medicine related to otolaryngology-head and neck surgery, including providing continuing medical education courses and publications.

996 **American Association of Acupuncture and Oriental Medicine**

433 Front Street
Catasauqua, PA 18032 **610-266-1433**
888-500-7999
FAX: 610-264-2768
e-mail: aaom1@aol.com
www.aaom.org

National organization of acupuncturists.

997 **American Association of the Deaf-Blind**
814 Thayer Avenue
Suite 302
Silver Spring, MD 20910
301-495-4403
800-735-2258
FAX: 301-495-4404
TTY:301-495-4402
e-mail: info@addbi.org

Jauine McNamara, Executive Director

The mission of the American Association of the Deaf-Blind is to enable deaf-blind persons to achieve their mximum potential through incresed independence, productivity and intergration into the community. AADB holds biennial conferences where deaf-blind people come together fot education, support, and socialization. we provide a quarterly publication, the DEAF-BLIND AMERICAN magazine to our employees. We are also running a Mentoring Pilot involving deaf-blind youth. *$15.00*

Membership dues

998 **American Hearing Research Foundation**
55 E Washington Street
Suite 2022
Chicago, IL 60602
312-726-9670
FAX: 312-726-9695
e-mail: blederer@american-hearing.org
www.american-hearing.org

William L Lederer, Executive Director
Lorraine L Koch, Assistant Director

The purposes of the Foundation are to promote, conduct and furnish financial assistance for medical research into the cause, prevention and cure of deafness, impaired hearing and balance disorders; encourage the collaboration of clinical and laboratory research; encourage and improve teaching in the medical aspects of hearing problems; and disseminate the most reliable scientific knowledge to physicians, hearing professionals and the public.

999 **American Society for Deaf Children**
1820 Tribute Road
Suite A
Sacramento, CA 95815
916-641-6084
800-942-2732
FAX: 916-641-6085
TTY:916-641-6084
e-mail: asdcl@aol.com
www.deafchildren.org

Elaine Ocuto, President

Formerly the International Association of Parents of the Deaf, this organization offers educational materials and counseling for deaf children and parents of deaf children. The 18,000 members include parents, families, and friends of deaf children, and offers 96 local chapters.

1000 **American Society of Deaf Social Workers**
11300 US Highway 19 N
Horizon Hospital
Clearwater, FL 33764
727-541-2646
800-288-4673
FAX: 727-541-4402

1001 **American Speech-Language-Hearing Association**
10801 Rockville Pike
Rockville, MD 20852
301-897-5700
800-638-8255
FAX: 301-897-7348
e-mail: actioncenter@asha.org
www.asha.org

John E Bernthal, President
Frederick T Spahr PhD, Executive Director
Joanne Jessen, Publications Director

Provides information for both the general public and physicians in an easy-to-access manner, on speech, hearing and language disorders. Exhibits by companies specializing in alternative and augmentative communications products, publishers, software and hardware companies, and hearing aid testing equipment manufacturers.

1002 **American Tinnitus Association**
PO Box 5
Portland, OR 97207
503-248-9985
800-634-8978
FAX: 503-248-0024
e-mail: tinnitus@ata.org
www.ata.org

Cherly McGinnis MBA, Executive Director
Barbara Sanders, Director of Education
Rachel Wray, Director of Advocacy and Support

Information about tinnitus and referrals to local hearing professionals and support groups nationwide. Publishes the magazine Tinnitus Today.

1003 **Arkansas Rehabilitation Research and Training Center for the Deaf and Hard of Hearing**
University of Arkansas
4601 W Markham Street
Little Rock, AR 72205
501-686-9691
FAX: 501-686-9698
TTY:501-686-9691
e-mail: rehabres@cavern.uark.edu
www.uark.edu/deafrtc

Douglas Watson, Director

Focuses on issues affecting the employability of deaf and hard of hearing rehabilitation clients; career assessment, career mobility, and advancement. Provides information and/or databases related to the rehabilitation of deaf and hard of hearing people served by the Federal/State Vocational Rehabilitation Program.

1004 **Association of Late-Deafened Adults**
1145 Westgate Street
Suite 206
Oak Park, IL 60301
877-348-7537
FAX: 877-348-7537
e-mail: president@alda.org
www.aldra.org

Candis Shannon, Editor of ALDA News

Provides resources, information, and advocacy of the needs of deafened adults. Publishes ALDA News.

1005 **Auditory-Verbal International**
2121 Eisenhower Avenue
Suite 402
Alexandria, VA 22314
703-739-1049
FAX: 703-739-0395
TTY:703-739-0874
e-mail: audiverb@aol.com
www.auditory-verbal.org

Sara Blair Lake, Executive Director/CEO
Tom Lucches, President

To provide the choice of listening and speaking as the way of life for children and adults who are deaf or hard of hearing.

1006 Better Hearing Institute

515 King Street
Suite 420
Alexandria, VA 22314
703-684-3391
800-EAR-WELL
FAX: 703-684-6048
e-mail: mail@betterhearing.org
www.betterhearing.org

Implements national public information programs on hearing loss and medical, surgical, hearing aid, and rehabilitation assistance.

1007 Boys Town National Research Hospital

555 N 30th Street
Omaha, NE 68131
402-498-6511
FAX: 402-498-6638
e-mail: peb@boystown.org
www.boystown.org

Patrick E Brookhouser MD, Director

State-of-the-art research, diagnosis and treatment of individuals with ear diseases, hearing and balance disorders, cleft lip and palate, and speech/language problems.

1008 Caption Center

Media Access Group at WGBH
125 Western Avenue
Boston, MA 02134
617-300-3600
FAX: 617-300-1020
e-mail: caption@wgbh.org
www.wgbh.org/caption

Lori Kay, Director

Has been pioneering and delivering accessible media to disabled adults, students and their families, teachers and friends for over 30 years. Each year, the Center captions more than 10,000 hours worth of broadcast and cable programs, feature films, large-format and IMAX films, home videos, music videos, DVDs, teleconferences and CD-Roms.

1972

1009 Captioned Media Program

National Association of the Deaf
1447 E Main Street
Spartanburg, SC 29307
864-585-1778
800-237-6213
FAX: 800-538-5636
TTY:800-237-6819
e-mail: info@cfv.org
www.cfv.org

Bill Stark, Project Director

Provides open-captioned media on a free-loan basis to deaf and hard of hearing persons, parents and teachers of hard of hearing children and groups/organizations that serve deaf and hard of hearing persons. Over 4,000 titles in our collection and media is available via mail (postage paid both ways) and through Internet streaming via our website.

1010 Cochlear Implant Club International

PO Box 464
Buffalo, NY 14223
716-838-4662
FAX: 716-838-4662
TTY:716-838-4662
e-mail: 76207.3114@compuserve.com

Bev Fish, President
Craig G Carpenter, Executive Director

Not-for-profit voluntary organization dedicated to serving implant users, candidates, their families and professional supporters. Purposes are to promote opportunities afforded by the use of cochlear implants through mutual sharing of ideas and personal experiences; enhance community awareness of hearing impairment and to promote better understanding of implants; and to promote improved financial support. Publishes educational materials including a newsletter, brochures, and audiovisual aids.

1011 Communication Service for the Deaf (CSD)

102 N Krohn Place
Sioux Falls, SD 57103
605-367-5760
800-642-6410
FAX: 605-367-5958
e-mail: info@c-s-d.org
www.c-s-d.org

Benjamin J Soukup, CEO

Since 1975, CSD has provided a variety of services to deaf and hard of hearing individuals. From relay services to community interpreting, advocacy to education, CSD promotes self-actualization, professional growth, independence and greater access for our consumers across the country.

1012 Conference of Educational Administrators Serving the Deaf

PO Box 1778
St Augustine, FL 32086
904-810-5200
FAX: 904-810-5525
e-mail: email@ceasd.org
www.ceasd.org

Joe Finnegan, Executive Director
Barbara Raimondo, Government Relations Liaison
Mike Bello, Treasurer

Focuses on improvements in the education of deaf and hard of hearing people through research, personnel development, advocacy and training.

1013 Convention of American Instructors of the Deaf

CAID Membership Office
PO Box 377
Bedford, TX 76095
817-354-8414
e-mail: caid@swbell.net
www.caid.org

Carl J Kirchner, President

Promotes professional development, communication and information; publishes American Annals of the Deaf, News 'n Notes; hosts biennial convention.

1014 Davis Center for Hearing, Speech and Learning: Hearing Therapy

98 Route 46 W
Budd Lake, NJ 07828
973-347-7662
FAX: 973-691-0611
e-mail: info@daviscenter.net
www.thedaviscenter.com

Dorinne S Davis, Director

The Davis Center's Sound Therapy Programs make positive changes for children and adults with Autism, ADD/ADHD, Auditory Processing Issues, Dyslexia, Learning Disabilities and other learning challenges. Our programs adress issues such as: phonics, spelling, writing, reading comprehension, hearing only parts of words, following directions, discriminating between sounds, sound sensitivity, behavioral responses, focus, attention and more.

1015 **Deaf Artists of America**

302 Goodman Street N
Suite 205
Rochester, NY 14607
585-244-3460
800-421-1220
FAX: 585-244-3690

Tom Willard, Executive Director

Organized to bring support and recognition to deaf and hard of hearing artists. Goals are to publish information about deaf artists, provide cultural and educational opportunities, exhibit and market deaf artists' work, and collect and disseminate information about deaf artists.

1016 **Deaf Entertainment Foundation (DEF)**

Deaf Entertainment Guild (DEG)
8306 Wilshire Boulevard
Suite 906
Beverly Hills, CA 90211
323-782-1344
FAX: 323-782-1344
e-mail: deafent@aol.com
www.deo.org

Mark Brudney, Marketing & Public Relations
Eldon Greenfield, DEOnline Webmaster
Dan McClintock, DEOnline Editor

Provides information to promote and accelerate the presence of deaf and hard of hearing talents in motion pictures, television, theater, and the performing arts.

1017 **Deaf REACH**

3521 12th Street NE
Washington, DC 20017
202-832-6681
FAX: 202-832-8454
www.deaf-reach.org/jobs.html

Sarah Brown, Executive Director

Offers referral, education, advocacy, counseling, and housing services for deaf mentally ill, multihandicapped and/or low income deaf people in the metro District of Columbia area.

1018 **Deaf and Hard of Hearing Entrepreneurs Council**

814 Thayer Avenue
Suite 303
Silver Spring, MD 20910
FAX: 301-588-0390
e-mail: jmcfadden@macf.com

Jim McFadden, President

Encourages, recognizes, and promotes entrepreneurship by people who are deaf and hard of hearing. Publishes Deaf and Hard of Hearing Entrepreneurs Council (newsletter).

1019 **Deafness Research Foundation**

575 Fifth Avenue
Floor 11
New York, NY 10017
212-599-0027
800-535-3323
FAX: 212-599-0039
www.drf.org

John Wheeler, President

Nation's largest voluntary health organization for research, treatment, and prevention of all ear disorders. Provides information and referral services; publishes The Receiver.

1020 **Deafness and Communicative Disorders Branch of Rehab Services Administration Office**

Special Education and Rehab Services
Department of Education
330 C Street SW, Room 3228
Washington, DC 20202
202-205-9152
FAX: 202-205-9340

Annette Reichman MS CRC, Branch Chief

Promotes improved rehabilitation services for deaf and hard of hearing people and individuals with speech or language impairments. Provides technical assistance to public and private agencies and individuals.

1021 **Dogs for the Deaf**

10175 Wheeler Road
Central Point, OR 97502
541-826-9220
FAX: 541-826-6696
e-mail: info@dogsforthedeaf.org
www.dogsforthedeaf.org

Robin Dickson, CEO/President

Trains hearing dogs to alert deaf persons to certain sounds. Dogs are chosen from pet adoption shelters and assigned on the basis of a prioritized waiting list. Five to six months of training teaches them to alert their masters to the sounds of alarm clocks, smoke alarms, doorbells, oven timers, telephones, etc.

1022 **Ear Foundation**

1817 Patterson Street
Nashville, TN 37203
615-284-7807
800-545-4327
FAX: 615-329-7935
e-mail: ear@earfoundation.org
www.earfoundation.org

C Gary Jackson MD, President

National, nonprofit organization committed to integrating the hearing and balance impaired into the mainstream of society through public awareness and medical education. Also administers The Meniere's Network, a national network of patient support groups providing people with the opportunity to share experiences and coping strategies.

1023 **Episcopal Conference of the Deaf**

PO Box 27685
Philadelphia, PA 19118
215-247-1059
FAX: 315-449-1602
e-mail: Bmose@aol.com
www.ecdeaf.com

Rev Virginia Nagel, President
Roy Brown, Deaf Episcopalian Editor

Promotes ministry for deaf people throughout the Episcopal Church. Affiliated with approximately 65 congregations in the United States. Publishes The Deaf Episcopalian. *$10.00*

8-12 pages Quarterly

1024 **Exploring the Bible: Bible Studies for the DEAF**

LifeWay Church Resources
127 9th Avenue N
Nashville, TN 37234
800-458-2772
FAX: 615-251-5933
e-mail: ofernan@lifeway.com
www.lifeway.com/lwc

Oscar J Fernandez, Editor in Chief

Bible study lessons for every three months written by and for persons who are deaf. Based on the Family Bible Series (International Sunday School Lessons).

1025 **Gallaudet University**

800 Florida Avenue NE
Washington, DC 20002
202-651-5000
e-mail: public.relations@gallaudet.edu
www.gallaudet.edu

I King Jordan PhD, President

The world's only four year liberal arts university for students who are deaf or hard of hearing. Established in 1864 by an act of Congress, Gallaudet offers more than 50 undergraduate and graduate degree programs and numerous continuing education and summer courses.

1026 **Gallaudet University Alumni Association**

Gallaudet University
800 Florida Avenue NE
Washington, DC 20002 **202-651-5060**
FAX: 202-651-5062
e-mail: alumni.relations@gallaudet.edu
www.gallaudet.edu/alumni.htm

Sam Sonnenstrahl, Executive Director
Andrew Lange, President
Mercy Coogan, Editor Gallaudet Today

Represents more than 14,000 alumni of Gallaudet University across the United States and around the world. A liberal arts university for students who are deaf or hard of hearing. Publishes Gallaudet Today.

1027 **Georgiana Organization**

Box 2607
Westport, CT 06880 **203-454-1221**
FAX: 203-454-3788

Annabel Stehli's organization promoting Auditory Integration Training in the USA.

1028 **HEAR Center**

301 E Del Mar Boulevard
Pasadena, CA 91101 **626-796-2016**
FAX: 626-796-2320
e-mail: auditory@mindspring.com
www.hearcenter.org

Josephine Wilson, Executive Director

Auditory and verbal program designed to help hearing impaired children, infants and adults lead normal and productive lives. Seeks to develop auditory techniques to aid people who have communication problems due to deafness. Offers diagnostic evaluations for speech and hearing. Individual auditory, verbal training and speech-language therapy.

1029 **Hands Organization**

2501 W 103rd Street
Chicago, IL 60655 **773-239-6662**
FAX: 773-239-2565
e-mail: handsorg@aol.com
www.handsdeaf.org

Kate Kubey, Executive Director

A nonprofit organization of both deaf and hearing persons working together to address the needs and concerns of the deaf community. The organization is working to raise the consciousness of the hearing world to the realities of deafness, and to bridge the gap between services already in place for the deaf and the large number of deaf people who have never been reached by those services. Offers a monthly publication.

1030 **Health Resource Center**

National Council on Education
One Dupont Circle
Washington, DC 20036 **202-939-9320**
800-544-3284
FAX: 202-833-4760
e-mail: health@ace.nche.edu
www.acenet.edu

Vickie M Barr, Director

Offers publications and a telephone service of use to administrators, service providers, teachers, instructors, rehabilitation counselors, health professionals and individuals with disabilities and their families.

1031 **Hear Now**

9745 E Hampden Avenue
Suite 300
Denver, CO 80231 **303-695-7797**
800-648-4327
FAX: 303-695-7789
e-mail: jostelter@aol.com

Elaine Hansen MAA CCCA, Program Director
M Bernice Dinner PhD, President

Committed to making technology accessible to deaf and hard of hearing individuals throughout the United States. Provides hearing aids and cochlear implants for very low income, hard of hearing and deaf individuals.

1032 **Hearing Education and Awareness for Rockers**

PO Box 760847
San Francisco, CA 94146 **415-431-3277**
FAX: 415-552-4296
e-mail: hear@hearnet.com
www.hearnet.com

Kathy Peck, Executive Director

Dedicated to educating the public about the real dangers of hearing loss resulting from repeated exposure to excessive noise levels. Operates a 24-hour hotline (415-773-9590) to provide information on hearing loss and hearing protection, assistance and scientific research. Other programs include national public service announcements campaigns, outreach to schools, HEAR affiliates, hearing protection and Can't Hear You Knocking! video.

1033 **House Ear Institute**

2100 W Third Street
5th Floor
Los Angeles, CA 90057 **213-483-4431**
FAX: 213-483-8789
www.hei.org

John W House MD, President

Offers pediatric hearing tests, otologic and audiologic evaluation and treatment, rehabilitation, hearing aid dispensing, and cochlear implant services. Outreach programs focus on families with hearing impaired children.

1034 **International Catholic Deaf Association**

United States Section
1030 LaGrange Road
#9
LaGrange, IL 60525
FAX: 708-579-5847
TTY:708-579-5817
e-mail: icdaus@ameritech.com

Kathleen Kush, Director
Peter Un, President
Peter Noyes, Pastoral President

Responds to spiritual-related requests worldwide from deaf or hard of hearing Catholics.

1035 **International Hearing Dog**

5901 E 89th Avenue
Henderson, CO 80640 **303-287-3277**
FAX: 303-287-3425
e-mail: ihdi@aol.com
www.ihdi.org

Valerie Foss-Brugger, President/Director

Trains dogs to assist deaf persons by responding to telephones, doorbells, babies, etc.

1036 **International Hearing Society**
16880 Middlebelt Road
Suite 4
Livonia, MI 48154 **734-522-7200**
800-521-5247
FAX: 734-522-0200
www.hearingihs.org

Robin L Clowers, Executive Director
Cindy J Helms, Director Marketing/Comm.
Pyllis V Wilson, Associate Director

Professional association of specialists who test hearing and select, fit and dispense hearing instruments. The society conducts programs of competence qualifications, education and training.

1037 **International Lutheran Deaf Association**
1333 S Kirkwood Road
St. Louis, MO 63122 **314-965-9917**
800-433-3954
FAX: 314-965-0959

James Swalley, President

Promotes ministry for deaf people throughout the Lutheran Church.

1038 **John Tracy Clinic**
806 W Adams Boulevard
Los Angeles, CA 90007 **213-748-5481**
800-522-4582
FAX: 213-749-1651
e-mail: mmartindale@jtc.org
www.jtc.org

Barbara F Hecht PhD, President
Mary Ann Bell, VP Development & Communications

Educational facility for infants and preschool-aged children who have hearing losses and their families. In addition to on-site services, worldwide correspondence courses in English and Spanish are offered to parents whose children are preschool age and are hard of hearing, deaf, or deaf-blind. All services of JTC are free of charge to the families. The Clinic also offers on site and online Master's Degrees in Deaf Education with USC.

1039 **Junior National Association of the Deaf**
814 Thayer Avenue
Silver Spring, MD 20910 **301-587-1788**
FAX: 301-587-1791
e-mail: nadyouth@nad.org

Nancy B Rarus, Executive Director

Developes and promotes citizenship, scholarship, and leadership skills in deaf and hard of hearing students of grades 7 through 12.

1040 **League for the Hard of Hearing**
71 W 23rd Street
New York, NY 10010 **917-305-7700**
FAX: 917-305-7888
e-mail: postmaster@lhh.org
www.lhh.org

Keith D Muller, Executive Director

National diagnostic rehabilitation, human services agency founded in 1910. Offers comprehensive services for infants, children and adults with hearing loss regardeless of age or mode of communication. Clinical programs iclude Tinnitus Center and Cochlear Implant evaluation, consultation, auditory training. LHH also offers extensive public education programs, advocacy, support and publications.

1041 **Lexington School for the Deaf: Center for the Deaf**
30th Avenue and 75th Street
Jackson Heights, NY 11370 **718-899-8800**
FAX: 718-899-9846
www.lexnyc.org

Oscar Cohen, Superintendent/Director

Offers a comprehensive range of services to deaf, hard of hearing and speech impaired persons from infancy to elderly through its affiliate agencies: The Center for Mental Health Services; The Lexington Hearing and Speech Center, Lexington Vocational Services, and the Lexington School for the Deaf. The Lexington Center also provides services through its research division which houses the only federally funded Rehabilitation Engineering Center.

1042 **Michigan Association for Deaf, Hearing and Speech Services**
2929 Covington Court
Suite 200
Lansing, MI 48912 **517-487-0066**
800-968-7327
FAX: 517-487-2586
e-mail: yourear@msu.edu
www.madhs.org

Jennifer Mora, Associate Director

Substance abuse and anti violence prevention videos for deaf and hard of hearing students (alcohol, marijuana, inhalants) acted in sign language, voicing and captioning. HIV/AIDS prevention and information for the deaf and hard of hearing. Lending library books, videos and audio tapes. Accessibility in courts video and information. TTY distribution program.

1043 **NTID Center on Employment**
National Technical Institute for the Deaf
52 Lomb Memorial Drive
Rochester, NY 14623 **585-475-6219**
FAX: 585-475-7570
www.rit.edu/ntid/coops/jobs

The NTID Center on Employment is a resource for employers seeking qualified, technically trained college graduates and coops/interns who are deaf. Some 1,100 students from all over the U.S. study at NTID, one of eight colleges of Rochester Institute of Technology, in progrmas at various degree levels in Business. Computing and Information Sciences, the Graphic Arts and Science and Engineering.

1044 **National Association of the Deaf**
814 Thayer Avenue
Suite 250
Silver Spring, MD 20910 **301-587-1788**
FAX: 301-587-1791
TTY:301-587-1789
e-mail: nadinfo@nad.org
www.nad.org

Nancy J Bloch, Executive Director

Nation's largest organization safeguarding the accessability and civil rights of 28 million deaf and hard of hearing Americans in education, employment, health care, and telecommunications. Focuses on grassroots advocacy and empowerment, captioned media deafness-related information and publications, legal assistance, and policy development.

1045 **National Black Deaf Advocates**
1 Lomb Memorial Drive
Rochester, NY 14623 **585-475-2411**
800-421-1220
FAX: 585-475-6500

Promotes leadership, deaf awareness and active participation in the political, educational and economic processes that affect the lives of black deaf citizens.

1046 National Captioning Institute
1900 Gallows Road
Suite 3000
Vienna, VA 22182
703-917-7600
FAX: 703-917-9878
TTY:703-917-7600
e-mail: mail@ncicap.org
www.ncicap.org

Jack Gates, President/CEO
Karen O'Connor, National Director Sales

Formed in 1979, the nonprofit National Captioning Institute is the global captioning leader, supplying the highest quality closed-captioning services to the television, cable, and home video industries.

1047 National Captioning Institute Help Desk
1900 Gallows Road
Suite 3000
Vienna, VA 22182
703-917-7600
FAX: 703-917-9878
TTY:703-917-7686
e-mail: mail@ncicap.org
www.ncihelpdesk.org

Steve Scher, Help Desk Coordinator

A free service that is avaliable to answer questions and help solve significant, recurring progblems with captioning and described video.

1048 National Catholic Office of the Deaf
7202 Buchanan Street
Landover Hills, MD 20784
301-577-1684
FAX: 301-577-1690
TTY:301-577-4184
e-mail: ncod@erols.com
www.ncod.org

Arvilla Rank, Executive Director

Helps coordinate efforts of deaf or hard of hearing people who are involved in the ministry, acts as a resource center, assists bishops and pastors become available to the deaf and hard of hearing.

1049 National Center for Accessible Media
WGBH Educational Foundation
125 Western Avenue
Boston, MA 02134
617-300-3400
FAX: 617-300-1035
e-mail: ncam@wgbh.org
www.wgbh.org/ncam

Larry Goldberg, Director

Aims to increase access to public mass media (television, radio, print, movies, multimedia) for unserved customers, such as disabled people or speakers of other languages.

1050 National Cued Speech Association
Information Service
23970 Hermitage Road
Shaker Heights, OH 44122
FAX: 800-459-3529

Cathy Quenin PhD, Editor

Membership organization that provides advocacy and support regarding use of Cued Speech. Information available.

1051 National Deaf Education Network and Clearinghouse
Gallaudet University
KDES PAS-6
800 Florida Avenue NE
Washington, DC 20002
202-651-5051
FAX: 202-651-5708
e-mail: infotogo@gallaudet.edu
clerccenter.gallaudet.edu

Responds to inquiries about a diverse range of topics related to deaf and hard of hearing children in the age group of 0 to 21.

1052 National Family Association for Deaf-Blind
111 Middle Neck Road
Sands Point, NY 11050
516-944-8900
800-225-0411
FAX: 516-944-7302
e-mail: NFADB@aol.com
www.NFADB.org

Mary Fox, Administrative Assistant

A membership organization which provides resources, education, advocacy, referrals and support for families with children who are deaf-blind; professionals in the field and individuals who are deaf-blind.

1053 National Fraternal Society of the Deaf
1118 S 6th Street
Springfiel, IL 62703
217-789-7429
FAX: 217-789-7489
e-mail: thefrat@nfsd.com
www.nfsd.com

Al Van Nevel, Grand President
Ronald L Delvislo, Treasure

Work in the area of life insurance and advocacy for deaf people. Has 75 divisions across the country.

1054 National Information Center for Children and Youth with Disabilities (NICHCY)
PO Box 1492
Washington, DC 20013
202-884-8200
800-695-0285
FAX: 202-884-8441
e-mail: nichcy@aed.org
www.nichcy.org

Provides fact sheets, state resource sheets and general information to assist parents, educators, caregivers, advocates and others in helping children and youth with disabilities participate as fully as possible in their communities.

1055 National Information Clearinghouse on Children who are Deaf-Blind
Teaching Research
345 Monmouth Avenue
Monmouth, OR 97361
800-438-9376
FAX: 503-838-8150
e-mail: dblink@tr.wou.edu
www.tr.wou.edu/dblink

John Reiman PhD, Director

Collects, organizes, and disseminates information related to children and youth of ages 0 to 21 who are deaf-blind and connects consumers of deaf-blind information to the appropriate resources. Publishes a number of topical papers and publishes Deaf-Blind Perspective.

1056 National Institute on Deafness and Other Communication Disorders (NIDCD)

1 NOHIC Way
Bethesda, MD 20892
301-402-7364
FAX: 301-907-8830
TTY:800-241-1055
e-mail: nohic@nidcr.nih.gov
www.nohic.nidcr.nih.gov

Marin Allen, Project Officer
Mia Esserman, Project Manager

The NIDCD Information Clearinghouse is a national resource center for health information about hearing, balance, smell, taste, voice, speech and language for health professionals, patients, industry and the public.

1057 National Rehabilitation Information Center (NARIC)

1010 Wayne Avenue
Suite 800
Silver Spring, MD 20910
301-562-2400
800-346-2742
FAX: 301-562-2401
e-mail: naricinfo@kra.com
www.naric.com

Mark Odum, Director

Provides information and referral services on disability and rehabilitation, including quick information and referral, database searches of the bibliographic database REHABDATA, and document delivery.

1058 National Technical Institute for the Deaf

52 Lomb Memorial Drive
Rochester, NY 14623
585-424-3480
FAX: 585-475-6500
TTY:716-475-6906
e-mail: ntidmc@rit.edu
www.rit.edu/ntid

Admissions Department

Provides technological postsecondary education to deaf and hard-of-hearing students. One of seven colleges of Rochester Institute of Technology.

1059 National Theatre of the Deaf

5 W Main Street
PO Box 659
Chester, CT 06412
860-526-4971
FAX: 860-526-0066
e-mail: bookntd@aol.com
www.ntd.org

Camille L Jeter, Director

Professional development of deaf actors.

1060 Okada Specialty Guide Dogs

7509 E Saviors Path
Floral City, FL 34436
352-344-2212
FAX: 352-344-0210
e-mail: okada@hitter.net
www.okadadogs.com

Pat Putnam, Director

Trains dogs to aid deaf, hearing-impaired, Alzheimer's, seizure, amnesia and residential companion guide dogs.

Price varies

1061 Registry of Interpreters for the Deaf

333 Commerce Street
Alexandria, VA 22314
703-838-0030
FAX: 703-838-0454
TTY:703-838-0459
e-mail: 72620.3143@compuserve.com
www.rid.org

Clay Nettles, Director

A membership organization with over 7,000 members, including professional interpreters and translators, individuals who are deaf or hard of hearing, and professionals in related fields.

1062 Rehabilitation Engineering Research Center on Hearing Enhancement and Assistive Devices

Lexington School for the Deaf/Center for the Deaf
30th Avenue and 75th Street
Jackson Heights, NY 11370
718-899-8800
FAX: 718-899-9846
e-mail: info@hearingresearch.org
www.hearingresearch.org

Harry Levitt PhD, Project Director

Promotes and develops technological solutions to problems confronting individuals with hearing loss.

1063 Rehabilitation Research & Training Center for Persons Who Are Hard of Hearing or Deafened

California School of Professional Psychology
6160 Cornerstone Court E
San Diego, CA 92121
858-623-2777
800-432-7619
FAX: 858-642-0266
e-mail: rrtc@cspp.edu
www.narrtc.org/members.html

Raymond J Trybus PhD, Director

Focuses on conducting research and developing training programs related to employment and personal adjustment of individuals who are hard of hearing or late deafened.

1064 SEE Center for the Advancement of Deaf Children

PO Box 1181
Los Alamitos, CA 90720
562-430-1467
FAX: 562-795-6614
e-mail: seectr@aol.com
www.seecenter.com

Esther Zawolkow, Director

Information and referral for parents and educators of deafness-related topics and Signing Exact English (SEE).

1065 Scottish Rite Center for Childhood Language Disorders

Children's Hospital
1630 Columbia Road NW
Washington, DC 20009
202-939-4703
FAX: 202-939-4717
e-mail: trobinso@cnmc.org

Dr. Tommie L Robinson Jr, Director

Offers speech-language evaluations and treatment, hearing screening and consultations to children ages birth through adolescence. Bilingual services are also available.

1066 Self Help for Hard of Hearing People

7910 Woodmont Avenue
Suite 1200
Bethesda, MD 20814
FAX: 301-913-9413
TTY:301-657-2249
e-mail: national@shhh.org
www.shhh.org

Barbara Thomas, Meeting Planner, Board Liaison

A nonprofit, educational organization that is dedicated to the well-being of people of all ages and communication styles who do not hear well. SHHH is the largest international consumer organization of its kind.

1067 Sound, Listening, and Learning Center

301 E Bethany Home Road
Suite A107
Phoenix, AZ 85012
602-381-0086
FAX: 602-957-6741
www.soundlistening.com

Provides education, workshops, consulting, therapeutic sessions, and information on the Tomatis method.

1068 Tele-Consumer Hotline

901 Fifteenth Street NW
Suite 230
Washington, DC 20005
800-332-1124
FAX: 800-332-1124

Sylvia Rosenthal, Executive Director

Impartial consumer information service about residential telecommunication concerns.

1069 Telecommunications for the Deaf (TDI)

8630 Fenton Street
Suite 604
Silver Spring, MD 20910
301-589-3786
FAX: 301-589-3797
e-mail: info@tdi-online.org
www.tdi-online.org

Claude L Stout, Executive Director
James D House, Member Service/Public Rel. Dir.

Promoting equal access to telecommunications and media for people who are deaf, late-deafened, hard of hearing or deaf-blind through consumer education and involvement; technical assistance and consulting; applications of exisiting and emerging technologies; networking and collaboration; uniformity of standards; and national policy development and advocacy.

1070 Tripod

1727 W Burbank Boulevard
Burbank, CA 91506
818-972-2080
FAX: 818-972-2090
e-mail: tripodschool@earthlink.net

Barbara Muntan, VP Board of Directors

An educational program for deaf and hard-of-hearing students in conjunction with Burbank Unified School District. The program offers educational services from birth through 12th grade. This partnership features co-enrollment and co-teaching models.

1071 USA Deaf Sports Federation

3607 Washington Boulevard
Suite 4
Ogden, UT 84403
FAX: 801-393-7916
e-mail: homeoffice@usadsf.org
www.usadsf.org

Valerie G Kinney, Administrative Assistant

Governing body for all deaf sports and recreation in the United States.

1072 Vestibular Disorders Association

Vestibular Disorders Association
PO Box 4467
Portland, OR 97208
503-229-7705
800-837-8428
FAX: 503-229-8064
e-mail: veda@vestibular.org
www.vestibular.org

Lisa Haven, Executive Director

Provides information and support for people with inner-ear vestibular disorders and develops awareness of the issues surrounding these disorders.

1073 World Recreation Association of the Deaf

PO Box 3211
Quartz Hill, CA 93586
FAX: 805-943-6112
TTY:805-943-8879
e-mail: Brucegross@aol.com

Bruce Gross, President

Established to foster the development of innovation in recreational and cultural activities for the deaf and hard of hearing community. Quarterly newsletter.

Professional

1074 ACB Government Employees

American Council of the Blind
1155 15th Street NW
Suite 1004
Washington, DC 20005
202-467-5081
800-424-8666
FAX: 202-467-5085
e-mail: info@acb.org
www.acb.org

Members are present, former and retired employees of federal, state and local government agencies. Concerns of the organization include recruitment, placement and advancement of blind and visually impaired employees.

1075 ACB Social Service Providers

American Council of the Blind
1155 15th Street NW
Suite 1004
Washington, DC 20005
202-467-5081
800-424-8666
FAX: 202-467-5085
e-mail: info@acb.org
www.acb.org

Blind and visually impaired social workers, social service professionals, students pursuing careers in social work and other interested persons are members of this organization. ACBSSP works to promote full participation by visually impaired social services professionals in the field of social welfare.

1076 AHEAD Association

PO Box 21192
Columbus, OH 43221
617-287-3880
FAX: 617-287-3881
TTY:617-287-3882
e-mail: ahead@postbox.asc.ohio-state.edu
www.ahead.org

This is a national association of professionals working on college campuses with disabled students.

1077 American Academy of Biological Dentistry
PO Box 856
Carmel Valley, CA 93924
831-659-5385
FAX: 831-659-2417
e-mail: mail@biologicaldentistry.org
www.biologicaldentistry.org

Promotes non-toxic diagnostic and therapeutic approaches in dentistry; hosts seminars on biological diagnosis and therapy.

1078 American Academy of Environmental Medicine
7701 E Kellogg
Suite 625
Wichita, KS 67207
316-684-5500
FAX: 316-684-5709
e-mail: administrator@aaem.com
www.aaem.com

Training for physicians in environmental medicine.

1079 American Academy of Orthomolecular Medicine
Huxley Institute for Biosocial Research
900 N Federal Highway
Baca Raton, FL 33432
800-847-3802

Provides information and referrals to orthomolecular physicians.

1080 American Academy of Osteopathy
3500 DePauw Boulevard
Suite 1080
Indianapolis, IN 46268
317-879-1881
e-mail: snoone@academyofosteopathy.org
www.academyofosteopathy.org

Stephen J Noone, CAE, Executive Director

Represents osteopathic practitioners.

1081 American Academy of Physical Medicine and Rehabilitation
1 IBM Plaza
Suite 2500
Chicago, IL 60611
312-464-9700
FAX: 312-464-0227
e-mail: info@aapmr.org
www.aapmr.org

John M Wilson, Marketing & Communications

This national medical specialty society represents more than 6,500 physical medicine and rehabilitation physicians, whose patients include people with physical disabilities and chronic, disabling illnesses. The academy's mission is to maximize quality of life, minimize the incidence and prevalence of impairments and disability, promote societal health and enhance the understanding and development of the specialty. The organization offers information, referrals, and patient materials.

1082 American Association of Children's Residential Centers
51 Monroe Place
Suite 1603
Rockville, MD 20850
301-738-6460
FAX: 301-738-6461
e-mail: info@aacrc-dc.org
www.aacrc-dc.org

Bob Lieberman MA LPC, President
Elissa Malter Schwartz, Association Director
Aamy Parsley, Association Assistant

Brings professionals together to advance the frontiers of knowledge pertaining to the spectrum of therapeutic living environments for children and adolescents with behavioral health disorders.

1083 American Association of Naturopathic Physicians
8201 Greensboro Drive
Suite 300
McLean, VA 22102
703-610-9037
877-969-2267
FAX: 703-610-9005
www.naturopathic.org

Licensed naturopathic physicians.

1084 American College of Advancement in Medicine
23121 Verdugo Drive
Suite 204
Laguna Hills, CA 92653
949-583-7666
FAX: 949-455-9679
www.acam.org

Provides training and education to physicians and scientists. Also provides referrals and informational material.

1085 American College of Nurse Midwives
818 Connecticut Avenue NW
Suite 900
Washington, DC 20006
202-728-9860
FAX: 202-728-9897
e-mail: info@acnm.org
www.acnm.org

Refers local midwives.

1086 American Group Psychotherapy Association
25 E 21st Street
6th Floor
New York, NY 10010
212-477-2677
877-668-2472
FAX: 212-979-6627
e-mail: groupsinc@aol.com
www.agpa.org

Marsha S Block CAE, CEO
Jan I Vadell, Associate Executive Officer
Angela Stephens, Communations/Education Director

AGPA serves as the national voice specific to the interests of group psychotherapy. Its 4,100 members and 31 affiliate societies provide a wealth of professional, educational and social support for group psychotherapists in the United States and around the world.

1087 American Holistic Medical Association
6728 McLean Village Drive
McLean, VA 22101
610-266-1433
888-500-7999
FAX: 703-556-8729
e-mail: info@holisticmediscine.org
www.holisticmedicine.org

Professional organization for holistic practitioners.

1088 American Occupational Therapy Association
4720 Montgomery Lane
Bethesda, MD 20814
301-654-7655
800-789-2682
FAX: 301-652-7711
TTY:800-377-8555
e-mail: praota@aota.org
www.aota.org

Fred Whiting, PR Director
Anne Morris PhD, Gerontology Manager

A national professional society representing the interests and concerns of occupational therapy practitioners, and to improve the quality of occupational therapy services. The ADA Consultants Network is a listing of occupational therapists who are available to help employers comply with the provisions of the Americans with Disabilities Act.

1089 American Psychiatric Association

Psychiatric Services
1000 Wilson Boulevard
Suite 1825
Arlington, VA 22209 **703-907-7300**
FAX: 703-907-1095
e-mail: psjournal@psych.org
www.psych.org

Connie Gartner, Managing Editor
Laurie Oseran, Communications and Marketing

Works to promote the best interest of patients and those actually or potentially making use of psychiatric services.

1090 American Society of Bariatric Physicians

5433 E Evans Place
Denver, CO 80222 **303-770-2526**
FAX: 303-779-4834
e-mail: info@asbp.org
www.asbp.org

Provides referrals to bariatric physicians, the study and treatment of obesity.

1091 American Society of Clinical Hypnosis

130 E Elm Court
Suite 201
Roselle, IL 60172 **630-980-4740**
FAX: 630-351-8490
e-mail: info@asch.net
www.asch.net

Physicians and dentists trained in hypnosis for treating health conditions.

1092 American Society of Teachers of the Alexander Technique

PO Box 60008
Florence, MA 01062 **413-584-2359**
800-473-0620
FAX: 413-584-3097
www.amsat.ws

Dana Ben-Yehuda, Media Relations Committee Chair

The AmSAT Mission: To define, maintain and promote the Alexander Technique at its highest standard of professional practice and conduct.

1093 Association for the Care of Children's Health

19 Mantua Road
Mount Royal, NJ 08061 **856-423-3610**
FAX: 301-986-4553
e-mail: acch@clark.net
www.look.net

Heather Bennett-McCabe Phd, Executive Director

An international multidisciplinary organization which promotes the emotional, developmental, and psychosocial well-being of children and families in all health care settings.

1094 Behavior Therapy and Research Society

Temple University Medical School
Philadelphia, PA 19129 **352-344-2212**
FAX: 215-707-4086

This organization promotes behavior therapy by conducting and facilitating research in behavioral interventions and providing information through consultations, conferences and publications, about the use of these methods.

1095 Case Management Society of America

8201 Cantrell Raod
Suite 230
Little Rock, AR 72227 **501-225-2229**
FAX: 501-221-9068
e-mail: cmsa@cmsa.org
www.cmsa.org

1096 College of Optometrists in Vision Development

353 H Street
Suite C
Chula Vista, CA 92010 **619-425-6191**
FAX: 619-420-3010

Certifies optometrists who specialize in vision therapy.

1097 Community Enterprises

41 Mechanic Street
PO Box 176
Windsor, CT 06095 **860-688-7918**
FAX: 860-688-5599
e-mail: cehftd@aol.com
www.communityenterprises.com

Susan Cauley, VP Operations

Provide supported education services in a community college setting; supported employment including job training, placement and follow-up; transitional services from group homes and other settings to supported living within the community.

1098 Environmental Dental Association

16905 Avenida De Acacias
PO Box 2184
Rancho Santafe, CA 92067 **858-586-1208**
800-388-2184
FAX: 858-756-7843
e-mail: info@enviromentaldental.com
www.gettingwell.com/content/natural_medicine/

Organization of alternative dentists concerned about the toxic effects of dental materials and procedures.

1099 Feldenkrais Guild of North America (FGNA)

3611 SW Hood Avenue
Suite 100
Portland, OR 97201 **503-221-6612**
800-775-2118
FAX: 503-221-6616
e-mail: guild@feldenkrais.com
www.feldenkrais.com

Maureen Lynch, Contact

This is the organization which sets the standards for and certifies all FELDENKRAIS practitioners in North America. In order to practice, a practitioner must be a graduate of an FGNA accredited program (a minimum of 800 instruction hours over a three to four year period), and agree to follow both the Code of Professional Conduct and the Standards of Practice. FGNA may be contacted for further information about the FELDENKRAIS METHOD or for a list of FELDENKRAIS practitioners sorted by region.

1100 Gallaudet University

800 Florida Avenue NE
Washington, DC 20002 **202-651-5050**
FAX: 202-651-5704
e-mail: public.relations@gallaudet.edu
www.gallaudet.edu

1101 International Association of Yoga Therapists

2400A County Center Drive
PO Box 2418
Santa Rosa, CA 95403 **707-928-9898**
e-mail: mail@yrec.org
www.yrec.org

Larry Payne PhD, Director
Jamie Shaw, MPT, Associate Director

Champions the cause of yoga through annual conferences, annual journals and newsletters. Serves the growing number of yoga teachers, especially those who use yoga therapeutically.

1102 Job Accommodation Network

PO Box 6080
Morgantown, WV 26506 **304-293-7186**
800-526-7234
FAX: 304-293-5407
e-mail: jan@jan.icdi.wvu.edu
www.jan.wvu.edu

DJ Hendricks, Director

The JAN is an international information service for people with disabilities and their employers. They have information about implementation of workplace accommodations, as well as resources to promote an awareness of functional limitations associated with disability.

1103 Maharishi Ayur-Veda Medical Center

PO Box 282
Fairfield, IA 52556 **641-472-8477**

Provides referrals to health centers, also training and information to the lay public.

1104 National Association of Blind Educators

National Federation of the Blind
1800 Johnson Street
Baltimore, MD 21230 **410-659-9314**
FAX: 410-685-5653
e-mail: nfb@nfb.org
www.nfb.org

Mary Willows, President

Membership organization of blind teachers, professors and instructors in all levels of education. Provides support and information regarding professional responsibilities, classroom techniques, national testing methods and career obstacles. Publishes The Blind Educator, national magazine specifically for blind educators.

1105 National Association of Blind Lawyers

National Federation of the Blind
1800 Johnson Street
Baltimore, MD 21230 **410-659-9314**
FAX: 410-685-5653
e-mail: nfb@nfb.org
www.nfb.org

Scott LaBarre, President

Membership organization of blind attorneys, law students, judges and others in the law field. Provides support and information regarding employment, techniques used by the blind, advocacy, laws affecting the blind, current information about the American Bar Association and other issues for blind lawyers.

1106 National Association of Blind Secretaries and Transcribers

National Federation of the Blind
1800 Johnson Street
Baltimore, MD 21230 **410-659-9314**
FAX: 410-685-5653
e-mail: nfb@iamdigex.net
www.nfb.org

Membership organization of blind secretaries and transcribers at all levels, including medical and paralegal transcription, office workers, customer-service personnel and many other similar fields. Addresses issues such as technology, accomodation, career planning and job training.

1107 National Association of Blind Teachers

American Council of the Blind
1155 15th Street NW
Suite 1004
Washington, DC 20005 **202-467-5081**
800-424-8666
FAX: 202-467-5085
e-mail: info@acb.org
www.acb.org

Works to advance the teaching profession for blind and visually impaired people, protects the interest of teachers, presents discussions and solutions for special problems encountered by blind teachers and publishes a directory of blind teachers in the US.

1108 National Association of Protection and Advocacy Systems

900 2nd Street NE
Suite 211
Washington, DC 20002 **202-408-9514**
FAX: 202-408-9520
e-mail: info@napas.org
www.napas.org

Curtis Decker, Executive Director
Eugenia Wheeler, Receptionist
Nachama Wilker, Executive Director of Training

The membership association of the directors of three federally funded programs: the Protection & Advocacy Systems for persons with developmental disabilities and the P&A's for persons with mental illness, which provide legal advocacy for clients; and the Client Assistance Program, which assists clients of vocational rehabilitation services with eligibility and legal problems.

1109 National Association of State Directors of Developmental Disabilities Services (NASDDDS)

113 Oronoco Street
Alexandria, VA 22314 **703-683-4202**
FAX: 703-684-1395
e-mail: rgettings@nasddds.com
www.nasddds.org/index.shtml

Robert Gettings, Executive Director
Karol Snyder, Manager Membership Services

A nonprofit organization devoted to improving and expanding services to persons with developmental disabilities. The primary aims of the association are to: facilitate an exchange of information regarding the most advanced and efficacious methods of providing care and training to this population and represent the interests of state programs for persons with mental retardation/developmental disabilities in the development and implementation of federal programs.

1110 National Clearinghouse of Rehabilitation Training Materials

Oklahoma State University
5202 N Richmond Hill Road
Stillwater, OK 74078
405-624-7650
800-223-5219
FAX: 405-624-0695
www.nchrtm.okstate.edu

Judy Seefeldt, Director
Carolyn Cash, Information Coordinator

Offers reference materials on vocational rehabilitation for professionals and the disabled.

1111 National Deaf Education Network and Clearinghouse

KDES PAS-6
800 Florida Avenue NE
Washington, DC 20002
202-651-5051
FAX: 202-651-5054
e-mail: clearinghouse.infotogo@gallaudet.edu
http://clerccenter.gallaudet.edu

1112 National Federation of the Blind in Computer Science

National Federation of the Blind
1800 Johnson Street
Baltimore, MD 21230
410-659-9314
FAX: 410-685-5653
e-mail: nfb@iamdigex.net
www.nfb.org

Curtis Chong, Director Technology

National organization of blind persons knowledgeable in the computer science and technology fields. Works to develop new technologies, to secure access to current technology and to develop new ways of using current or new technologies by the blind.

1113 National Federation of the Blind: Merchants Division

National Federation of the Blind
1800 Johnson Street
Baltimore, MD 21230
410-659-9314
FAX: 410-685-5653
e-mail: nfb@iamdigex.net
www.nfb.org

Membership organization of blind persons employed in either self-employment work or the Randolph-Sheppard vending program. Provides information regarding rehabilitation, social security, tax and other issues which directly affect blind merchants. Serves as advocacy and support group.

1114 National Federation of the Blind: Blind Industrial Workers of America

National Federation of the Blind
2757 N Pine Grove Avenue
Suite 313
Chicago, IL 60614
773-472-3085
e-mail: nfb@nfb.org
www.nfb.org

Kenneth Staley, President

Membership organization of blind persons employed in industrial and manufacturing work or in government job programs for the blind. Dedicated to protecting the rights of blind workers in salary, job stability, advancement, and labor issues.

1115 National Federation of the Blind: Public Employees Division

National Federation of the Blind
1800 Johnson Street
Baltimore, MD 21230
410-659-9314
FAX: 410-685-5653
e-mail: nfb@iamdigex.net
www.nfb.org

Organization of blind persons holding local, state or federal jobs. Focuses on issues such as changes in governmental hiring and retention practices, new job skills needed for the future, government employment downsizing, new electronic means of finding public sector jobs, self-advocacy and career planning strategies.

1116 National Federation of the Blind: Science and Engineering Division

National Federation of the Blind
1800 Johnson Street
Baltimore, MD 21230
410-659-9314
FAX: 410-685-5653
e-mail: nfb@iamdigex.net
www.nfb.org

Blind persons with expertise and experience in fields such as genetics, telecommunications, biology, chemistry, physics and nuclear physics or mechanical, electronic and chemical engineering. This is a strong support group to encourage blind persons in pursuit of these careers, many of which have been considered not possible for the blind in the past.

1117 National Federation of the Blind: Writers Division

National Federation of the Blind
1800 Johnson Street
Baltimore, MD 21230
410-659-9314
FAX: 410-685-5653
e-mail: nfb@iamdigex.net
www.nfb.org

Blind writers in all styles, including poetry, short story, fiction, non-fiction, magazine writing and theatrical work offer encouragement and support to blind writers and authors. Issues cover various aspects of this business, including selling your work, publishing, technology, motivation and discovering writing and publishing resources.

1118 Opportunities Unlimited and Brain Injury Services of Village Northwest

3407 Glen Oaks Boulevard
Sioux City, IA 51104
712-252-7135
FAX: 712-277-8602

We provide eight transitional rehabilitation services to individuals with brain injury, spinal cord injury and physical disabilities. Community inclusion is the cornerstone of both agencies. Therapies include: physical, occupational, speech, cognitive as well as vocational, recreational and nursing services.

1119 Project RSVP

5201 Leesburg Pike
Suite 600
Falls Church, VA 22041
888-606-7787
FAX: 304-292-2278

Project RSVP supports the SSA's initiative to expand operations vocational rehabilitation services through a national network of private providers. Rehabilitation companies interested in gaining access to a new client base, acquiring a new funding stream, and developing creative service delivery and entrepreneurial partnerships, may benefit from such a program.

1120 **Rolf Institute**
205 Canyon Boulevard
Suite 200
Boulder, CO 80302 **303-449-5903**
800-530-8875
FAX: 303-449-5978
e-mail: info@rolf.org
www.rolf.org

Chrisanna Gordon, Administrative Liasion

Offers information, practitioner directory, training and certification.

1121 **Teacher Education Division**
1110 N Glebe Road
Suite 300
Arlington, VA 22201 **703-620-3660**
FAX: 703-264-9494
www.cec.sped.org

Janice Burdick, President

Promotes the preparation and continuing professional development of effective professionals in special education and related fields. TED's members include persons involved in the education and continuing development of professionals in special education and related fields, such as general education, allied health, speech and language pathology, rehabilitation, legal services and more.

1122 **United Educational Services**
PO Box 1099
Buffalo, NY 14224
800-458-7900
FAX: 716-668-7875

David L Slosson, VP
Cathy A Rajca, Customer Service

Publisher and distributor of Curricular Materials, Tests, Developmental Resource and Collaborative Materials for Speech-Language Pathologists, special educators, and classroom teachers. United also sponsors professional workshops for special educators, classroom teachers, counselors, administrators and parents.

1123 **Universal Institute: Rehab & Fitness Center**
15-17 Microlab Road
Suite 101
Livingston, NJ 07039 **973-992-8181**
FAX: 973-992-9797

Universal institute is a 15,000 square foot, state of the art rehabilitation facility that specializes in neurological disorders such as brain injuries, spinal cord injury, strokes, etc. We offer PT, OT, speech patholgy, cognitive remediation, aqua therapy and EMG biofeedback.

1124 **Universal Pediatric Services**
475 S 50th Street
Suite 700
W Des Moines, IA **515-224-1122**
FAX: 515-224-0630

Universal Pediatric Services, provides high tech care to medically fragile children and adults in the home setting. Emphasis is placed on the provision of services in the rural areas, the ability to service high tech needs and the promotion of primary nurse concept.

1125 **Victorian Acres Premier**
1529 34th Avenue SW
Altoona, IA 50009 **515-967-0103**
FAX: 515-967-0101

VAP is a quality provider of rehabilitation, vocational, residential and community-based treatment programs for persons with acquired brain injury. Services are offered to a broad range of ages, acquities and funding resources. Res-Care Premier currently operates programs in Illinois, Missouri, Iowa, Texas and Florida, with plans for program development across the US.

1126 **Visually Impaired Data Processors**
American Council of the Blind
1155 15th Street NW
Suite 1004
Washington, DC 20005 **202-467-5081**
800-424-8666
FAX: 202-467-5085
e-mail: info@acb.org
www.acb.org

Advocates for higher standards in the training of qualified blind students, creates a healthy environment for more employment opportunities in government, provides for the exchange of work technique ideas and works with agencies to increase the availability of braille and recorded materials.

1127 **World Chiropractic Alliance**
2950 N Dobson Road
Suite 1
Chandler, AZ 85224
800-347-1011
FAX: 480-732-9313
www.worldchiropracticalliance.org

Cindy Rondberg, Chief Financial Officer
David Jackson DC, CEO
Jack Masche DC, COO

Dedicated to protecting and strengthening chiropractic around the world. Serving as a watchdog and advocacy organization, we place our emphasis on education and political action.

1989

Specific Disabilities

1128 **ARRISE**
9238 Parklane Avenue
Franklin Park, IL 60131 **847-451-2740**
FAX: 847-451-4008

Provides information about autism.

1129 **Acid Maltase Deficiency Association (AMDA)**
PO Box 700248
San Antonio, TX 78270 **210-494-6144**
FAX: 210-490-7161
e-mail: tianrama@aol.com
www.amda-pompe.org

Marylyn House

Offers a newletter, informational materials, networking, referrals to local resources, national advocacy efforts, and also maintains a research registry.

1994

1130 **Alzheimer's Disease Education and Referral Center (ADEAR)**

ADEAR Center
PO Box 8250
Silver Spring, MD 20907
800-438-4380
FAX: 301-495-3334
e-mail: adear@alzheimers.org
www.alzheimers.org

The Alzheimer's Disease Education and Referral (ADEAR) center provides information about Alzheimer's disease and related disorders to health professionals, patients and their families and the public. Most of the publications are provided at no charge as a service of the National Institute on Aging (NIA), one of the Federal Government's National Institutes of Health.

1990

1131 **American Academy for Cerebral Palsy and Developmental Medicine**

6300 N River Road
Suite 727
Rosemont, IL 60018
847-698-1635
FAX: 847-823-0536
e-mail: raymond@aaos.org
www.aacpdm.org

Sheril King, Executive Director

Multidisciplinary scientific society devoted to the study of cerebral palsy and other childhood onset disabilities, to promoting professional education for the treatment and management of these conditions and to improving the quality of life for people with these disabilities.

September

1132 **American Academy of Allergy, Asthma and Immunology**

611 E Wells Street
Milwaukee, WI 53202
414-272-6071
800-822-2762
FAX: 414-272-6070
e-mail: info@aaaai.org
www.aaaai.org

Lanny J Rosenwasser MD FAAAAI, President

Nonprofit association representing allergists, clinical immunologists, asthma specialists, allied health professionals, and others with a special interest in allergy and asthma. The AAAAI's mission is to advance the knowledge, education and practice of allergy, asthma and immunology.

1133 **American Academy of Child and Adolescent Psychiatry**

3615 Wisconsin Avenue NW
Washington, DC 20016
202-628-1816
FAX: 202-966-2891
e-mail: webmaster@aacap.org
www.aacap.org

Richard M Sarles MD, President

A 501 (C)(3) nonprofit membership organization composed of over 6,500 child and adolescent psychiatrists. Members actively research, evaluate, diagnose and treat psychiatric disorders and pride themselves on giving direction to and responding quickly to new developments in addressing the health care needs of children and their families.

53 pages

1134 **American Amputee Foundation**

PO Box 250218
Little Rock, AR 72225
501-666-2523
FAX: 501-666-8367
e-mail: american_amputee_foundation@hotmail.com

Amanda Erickson, Research Asiastant
CJ Walden, Executive Director
Kim McIntyre, Office Manager

Serves primarily as a national information clearinghouse and referral center assisting mainly amputees and their families. AAF researches and gathers information including studies, product information, services, self-help publications and review articles written within the field. AAF has helped with claims, justification letters to payers, testimony and life care planning. Free information packet for phone or letter inquiries.

1975

1135 **American Association of Naturopathic Physicians**

3201 New Mexico Avenue NW
Suite 350
Washington, DC 20016
202-895-1392
877-969-2267
FAX: 202-274-1992
e-mail: memberservices@Naturopathic.org
www.naturopathic.org

Michael Traub ND DHANP CCH, President
Nancy Dunne Boggs ND, VP/Chair Professional Affairs
Corey Resnick ND, Treasurer

National professional society representing naturopathic physicians who are licensed or eligible for licensing as primary care providers.

1985

1136 **American Association of Naturopathic Physicians**

8201 Greensboro Drive
Suite 300
McLean, VA 22102
703-610-9037
877-969-2267
FAX: 703-610-9005
www.naturopathic.org

Michael Traub ND DHANP CCH, President
Nancy Dunne Boggs ND, VP/Chair Professional Affairs
Corey Resnick ND, Treasurer

National professional society representing naturopathic physicians who are licensed or eligible for licensing as primary care providers.

1985

1137 **American Association of Spinal Cord Injury Nurses**

7520 Astoria Boulevard
Jackson Heights, NY 11370
718-803-3782
FAX: 718-803-0414
www.aascin.org

Sara Lerman MPH, Program Manager

A nonprofit organization dedicated to promoting quality care for individuals with spinal cord impairment. The AASCIN is a membership organization of registered and licensed practical nurses in the US and Canada who practice in diverse SCI settings. The AASCIN Nursing Research Program funds research in the area of spinal cord impairment and nursing practice. There is an annual educational conference sponsored by AASCIN. In addition, 'SCI Nursing' is published by AASCIN.

1983

1138 American Association of Spinal Cord Injury Psychologists & Social Workers

7520 Astoria Boulevard
Jackson Heights, NY 11370 **718-803-3782**
FAX: 718-803-0414
e-mail: ssofer@epva.org
www.aascipsw.org

Vivian Beyda PhD, Associate Executive Director
Stephen Sofer PhD, Program Manager

Organized and operated for scientific and educational purposes to advance and improve the psychosocial care of persons with spinal cord impairment, develop and promote education and research related to the psychosocial care of persons with spinal cord injury, recognize psychologists and social workers whose careers are devoted to the problems of spinal cord impairment.

1139 American Back Society

2647 International Boulevard
Suite 401
Oakland, CA 94601 **510-536-9929**
FAX: 510-536-1812
e-mail: info@americanbacksoc.org
www.americanbacksoc.org

Philip E Greenman DO FAAO, President

A membership organization dedicated to relieving the pain and impairment caused by back problems. Sponsors symposia for presenting research findings.

1140 American Board for Certification in Orthotics & Prosthetics

330 John Carlyle Street
Suite 210
Alexandria, VA 22314 **703-836-7114**
FAX: 703-836-0838
e-mail: info@abcop.org
www.abcop.org

Frank E Riddle Jr CO, President
Lance Hoxie, Executive Director

The organization for the orthotic and prosthetic profession for over 50 years the ABC accredits and certifies practitioners in accordance with established professional standards to help ensure quality care for the physically challenged.

1141 American Cancer Society

1599 Clifton Road NE
Atlanta, GA 30329 **404-320-2424**
800-ACS-2345
FAX: 404-325-2217
e-mail: bjubb@cancer.org
www.cancer.org

Cynthia Currence, Marketing Director

Offers counseling, seminars, conferences, support groups and transportation, providing 58 divisions and approximately 3,100 chapters.

1142 American Chemical Society Committee on Chemists with Disabilities

1155 16th Street NW
Washington, DC 20036 **202-872-4600**
800-227-5558
FAX: 202-776-8299
TTY:202-872-6355
e-mail: cwd@acs.org
membership.acs.org/C/CWD

Kathleen Thompson, Staff Liaison

Strives to inform chemistry educators and employers of scientific and technical personnel about the capabilities and contributions of chemical professionals who happen to have physical, sensory or learning disabilities. Mission is to promote opportunities—educational and professional—for persons with disabilities interested in pursuing careers in chemistry and in fields requiring knowledge of chemistry, and to demonstrate the capabilities of those persons to educators, employers and peers.

1143 American Cleft Palate/Craniofacial Association

104 S Estes Drive
Suite 204
Chapel Hill, NC 27514 **919-933-9044**
FAX: 919-933-9604
e-mail: info@cleftline.org
www.cleftline.org

Michael P Karnell, President
A Michael Sadove, VP

International nonprofit medical society of health care professionals who treat and/or perform research on birth defects of the head and face. Publishes Cleft Palate-Craniofacial Journal. Affiliated with Cleft Palate Foundation.

1144 American Diabetes Association

National Call Center
1701 N Beauregard Street
Alexandria, VA 22311
800-342-2383
e-mail: askADA@diabetes.org
www.diabetes.org

Mission is to prevent and cure diabetes, and to improve the lives of all people affected by diabetes.

1145 American Foundation for Urologic Disease

1100 Corporate Boulevard
Linthicum, MD 21090
800-242-2383
FAX: 410-468-1808
e-mail: admin@afud.org
www.afud.org

Jodi L Miller, Director Education

The AFUD is a 501(c)(3) organization dedicated to the prevention of urologic diseases through the expansion of patient education, research, public awareness and advocacy.

1146 American Heart Association: National Center

7272 Greenville Avenue
Dallas, TX 75231 **972-735-8501**
800-242-8721
FAX: 214-706-5233
www.americanheart.org

Barbra Jackson, Director

Fifty-five state affiliates monitoring local chapters offering educational materials, seminars, conferences and transportation for members nationwide. Maintains a listing of over 1,000 stroke support groups across the nation for referral to stroke survivors, their families, caregivers and interested professionals.

1147 American Juvenile Arthritis Organization (AJAO)

Arthritis Foundation
1330 W Peachtree Street
PO Box 7669
Atlanta, GA 30357 **404-872-7100**
800-283-7800
FAX: 404-872-9559
e-mail: help@arthritis.org
www.arthritis.org

Beverly Simmons-Johnson, Director

Devoted to serving the special needs of children, teens and young adults with childhood rheumatic diseases and their families. Members are parents, family members, doctors, nurses, occupational and physical therapists, social workers, young adults and anyone with an interest in arthritis in young people.

1148 American Lung Association

61 Broadway
6th Floor
New York, NY 10006
212-315-8700
800-586-4872
FAX: 212-315-8870
e-mail: info@lungusa.org
www.lungusa.org

Elizabeth Margulies, Corporate Communications

Voluntary health organization with a national office and constituent and affiliate associations around the country. Fights lung disease in all its forms, with special emphasis on asthma, tobacco control and environmental health.

1904

1149 American Network of Community Options and Resources

1101 King Street
Suite 380
Alexandria, VA 22314
703-535-7850
FAX: 703-535-7860
e-mail: cramos@ancor.org
www.ancor.org

Renee L Pietrangelo, CEO
Suellen R Galbraith, Director of Public Policy
Jerri McCandless, Director Member Services

Nonprofit trade association representing private providers who provide supports and services to people with disabilities.

1150 American Orthotic and Prosthetic Association

330 John Carlyle Street
Suite 200
Alexandria, VA 22314
571-431-0876
FAX: 571-431-0899
e-mail: info@aopanet.org
www.aopanet.org

Keith D Cornell CP BOCO FAAOP, President
Michael E Harmontree, VP

A national trade association representing patient care facilities and manufacturers of prosthetic and orthotic devices. A major focus is to provide industry companies with information about reimbursement, insurance and government regulations and other business management issues.

1917

1151 American Osteopathic Association

142 E Ontario Street
Chicago, IL 60611
312-202-8000
800-621-1773
FAX: 312-202-8200
e-mail: info@aoa-net.org
www.aoa-net.org

Darryl A Beehler DO, President

National organization for the advancement of osteopathic medicine in the US, and the professional association for over 48,000 physicians. The AOA accredits the Colleges of Osteopathic Medicine, osteopathic internship and residency programs and health care facilities.

1152 American Paraplegia Society

Journal of Spinal Cord Medicine
75-20 Astoria Boulevard
Jackson Heights, NY 11370
718-803-3782
FAX: 718-803-0414
www.apssci.org

Todd A Linsenmeyer MD, President

Organized and operated for scientific and educational purposes to advance and improve health care of persons with spinal cord impairment, develop and promote education and research related to spinal cord impairment, recognize physicians and doctoral level researchers whose careers are devoted to the problems of spinal cord impairment.

1153 American Sleep Disorders Association

1 Westbrook Corporate Center
Suite 920
Westchester, IL 60154
708-492-0930
FAX: 708-492-0943
e-mail: lbrink@aasmnet.org
www.aasmnet.org

Jerome Barrett, Executive Director
Sara Norstad, Executive Secretary
Pat Aldrich, Asst Dir Finance/Office Services

Dedicated to improving sleep health and promoting the highest quality education and research within the field of sleep medicine.

1154 American Spinal Injury Association

Rehabilitation Institute of Chicago
345 E Superior Street, Room 1436
Chicago, IL 60011
312-238-6207
FAX: 312-238-0869
e-mail: mars@northwestern.edu
www.asia-spinalinjury.org

Marcia L Sipski MD, President/Director

Professional association for physicans and other health professionals working in all aspects of spinal cord injury. Conducts annual scientific meeting to survey latest advancements in the field. See website for full details.

1973

1155 American Stroke Association

National Center
7272 Greenville Avenue
Dallas, TX 75231
888-478-7653
FAX: 214-706-5231
e-mail: strokeconnection@heart.org
www.strokeassociation.org

Barbra Jackson, Director

Fifty-five state affiliates monitoring local chapters offering educational materials, seminars, conferences and transportation for members nationwide. Maintains a listing of over 1,000 stroke support groups across the nation for referral to stroke survivors, their families, caregivers and interested professionals.

1156 Amytrophic Lateral Sclerosis Association

27001 Agoura Road
Suite 150
Calabasas Hills, CA 91301
818-880-9007
800-782-4747
FAX: 818-880-9006
e-mail: alsinfo@alsa-national.org
www.alsa.org

Mary Lyon RN MN, VP Patient Services

National not-for-profit voluntary health organization dedicated solely to the fight against ALS. Purpose is to encourage, identify and fund quality research into the cause, means of prevention and possible cures of ALS and improve living with ALS.

1157 Arthritis Consulting Services

2787 E Oakland Park Boulevard
Suite 204
Fort Lauderdale, FL 33306 **954-739-3202**
800-327-3027
FAX: 954-337-2887
e-mail: acs@stoparthritis.com
www.stoparthritis.com

Donna Pinorsky RN, Administrator

Provides information on holistic approaches to the treatment of arthritis.

1158 Arthritis Foundation

1330 W Peachtree Street NW
PO Box 7669
Atlanta, GA 30357 **404-872-7100**
800-283-7800
FAX: 404-872-9559
e-mail: help@arthritis.org
www.arthritis.org

Eileen M Rose, Administrative Assistant

Offers information and referrals regarding educational materials and programs, fund-raising, support groups, seminars and conferences offered by 55 local chapters across the United States.

1159 Association for Children with Down Syndrome

4 Fern Place
Plainview, NY 11779 **516-933-4700**
FAX: 516-933-9524
e-mail: information@acds.org
www.acds.org

Sebastian J Muzio, Executive Director

A leader in early intervention and preschool education. Services are provided to children who have a wide variety of developmental delays.

1966

1160 Association of Birth Defect Children

930 Woodcock Road
Suite 225
Orlando, FL 32803
800-313-2232
www.birthdefects.org

Beth Mekdeci, President

National not-for-profit organization that functinos as a clearinghouse, providing parents and professionals with information about birth defects and services for children with disabilities. Studies the links between drugs, radiation, alcohol, chemicals, lead, mercury, dioxin, and birth defects. Publishes newsletters and publications for parents, professionals, and interested organizations.

1161 Association of Children's Prosthetic/Orthotic Clinics

6300 N River Road
Suite 727
Rosemont, IL 60018 **847-698-1637**
FAX: 847-823-0536
e-mail: raymond@aaos.org
www.acpoc.org

Sheril King, Executive Director

Established for the purpose of supporting clinical teams that treat children with prosthetic or orthotic devices. Goals are achieved through programs of professional education and clinical research.

1162 Asthma and Allergy Foundation of America

1233 20th Street NW
Suite 402
Washington, DC 20036 **202-466-7643**
800-727-8462
FAX: 202-466-8940
e-mail: info@aafa.org
www.aafa.org

C Ben Hadden, President
Jean McCoy, VP

Not-for-profit organization dedicated to improving the quality of life for people with asthma and allergies and their caregivers through education, advocacy and research. Provides practical information, community based services, support and referrals through a national network of chapters and educational support groups. Also raises funds for asthma care and research.

1953

1163 Ataxia-Telangiectasia Children's Project (A-T Children's Project)

668 S Military Trail
Deerfield Beach, FL 33442 **954-481-6611**
800-543-5728
FAX: 954-725-1153
e-mail: info@atcp.org
www.atcp.org

Brad A Margus, President
Jennifer Thornton, Executive Director
Rosa Fernandez, Family Support/Communications

A public, tax-exempt, nonprofit organization formed to raise funds through events and contributions from corporations, foundations and friends. Funds are used to accelerate first-rate, international scientific research aimed at finding a cure and improving the lives of all children with ataxia-telangiectasia.

1164 Attention Deficit Disorder Association

1788 Second Street
Suite 200
Highland Park, IL 60035 **847-432-2332**
FAX: 847-432-5874
e-mail: michelenovotni@yahoo.com
www.add.org

Michele Novotni, PhD, President
Terry Matlen MSW ACSW, VP
Mary Jane Johnson PCC ACT, Secretary

Mission is to help people with AD/HD lead happier, more successful lives through education, research and public advocacy. Whether you have AD/HD yourself, someone special in your life does, or you treat, counsel or teach those who do, ADDA is an organization for you. ADDA focuses especially on the needs of AD/HD adults and young adults with AD/HD. Parents of children with AD/HD are also welcome.

1165 Attention Deficit Disorders Association: Southern Region

12345 Jones Road
Suite 287-7
Houston, TX 77070 **281-897-0982**
FAX: 281-894-6883
e-mail: addaoffice@pdq.net
www.adda-sr.org

Pam Esser, Executive Director
Marian Bryant, President

Mission is to: provide a resource network; to support individuals impacted by attention deficit disorders; to advocate for the development of community resources and services that meet the educational, social, and health care needs of all individuals with ADD/ADHD; to keep the public informed on the disorder through the media, an association newsletter, referral service, monthly chapter meetings, educational programs, parent and adult services as well as conferences and workshops.

1166 Attention Deficit Information Network

58 Prince Street
Needham, MA 02492 **781-455-9895**
FAX: 781-444-5466
e-mail: adin@gis.net
www.addinfonetwork.org

Libby Ostrofoky, President

A nonprofit volunteer organization that offers support and information to families of children and adults with ADD, and to professionals through a network of AD-IN chapters. AD-IN was founded in 1988 by several parent support group leaders on the premise of parents helping parents deal with their children with ADD. Network has parent and adult support group chapters throughout the country.

1167 Autism Services Center

605 9th Street
PO Box 507
Huntington, WV 25710 **304-525-8014**
FAX: 304-525-8026

Ruth C Sullivan PhD, Executive Director
Sue McClelland, Director Office Administration

Service agency for individuals with autism and other developmental disabilities and their families. Assists families and agencies attempting to meet the unique needs of individuals with autism and other developmental disabilities: makes available technical assistance in designing programs. Provides supervised apartments, groups homes, respite services, independent living programs and job-coached employment. Provides case management services for a four-county area in West Virginia.

1168 Autism Society of America

7910 Woodmont Avenue
Suite 300
Bethesda, MD 20814 **301-657-0881**
800-3AU-TISM
FAX: 301-657-0869
www.autism-society.org

ASA is the largest and oldest grassroots organization within the autism community, with more than 200 chapters and over 20,000 members and supporters nationwide. ASA is the leading source of education, information and referral about autism and has been the leader in advocacy and legislative initiatives for more than three decades.

1169 Autism Treatment Center of America

2080 S Undermountain Road
Sheffield, MA 01257 **413-229-2100**
800-714-2779
FAX: 413-229-8931
e-mail: information@son-rise.org
www.son-rise.org

Sean Fitzgerald, Assistant Director

Since 1983, the Autism Treatment Center of America has provided innovative training programs for parents and professionals caring for children challenged by Autism, Autism Spectrum Disorders, Pervasive Developmental Disorder (PDD) and other developmental difficulties. The Son-Rise Program teaches a specific yet comprehensive system of treatment and education designed to help families and caregivers enable their children to dramatically improve in all areas of learning.

1170 Autism Treatment Center of America: The Son-Rise Program

2080 S Undermountain Road
Sheffield, MA 01257 **413-229-2100**
800-714-2779
FAX: 413-229-3202
e-mail: correspondence@option.org
www.son-rise.org

Since 1983, the Autism Treatment Center of America has provided innovative training programs for parents and professionals caring for children challenged by Autism, Autism Spectrum Disorders, Pervasive Developmental Disorder (PDD) and other developmental difficulties. The Son-Rise Program teaches a specific yet comprehensive system of treatment and education designed to help families and caregivers enable their children to dramatically improve in all areas of learning.

1171 Batten Disease Support and Research Association

120 Humphries Drive
Suite 2
Reynoldsburg, OH 43068 **740-927-4298**
800-448-4570
e-mail: bdsral@bdsra.org
www.bdsra.org

George Maxim, President
Lance Johnston, Executive Director

An international support and research networking organization for families of children and young adults with an inherited neurological degenerative disorder known as Batten Disease.

1986

1172 Birth Defect Research for Children

930 Woodcock Road
Suite 225
Orlando, FL 32803 **407-245-7035**
800-313-2232
FAX: 407-245-7087
www.birthdefects.org

A nonprofit organization that provides information about birth defects of all kinds to parents and professionals. Offers a library of medical books and files of information on less common categories of birth defects and is involved in research to discover possible links between environmental exposures and birth defects.

1173 Brain Injury Association of New York State

10 Colvin Avenue
Albany, NY 12206 **518-459-7911**
800-228-8201
FAX: 518-482-5285
e-mail: info@bianys.org
www.bianys.org

Michael V Kaplen Esq, President
Judith Avner, Executive Director
Judith Sandman, Membership/Development Director

Statewide nonprofit membership organization that advocates on behalf of individuals with brain injury and their families and promotes prevention.

1982

1174 Brain Injury Association of Texas

1339 Lamar Square Drive
Suite C
Austin, TX 78704 **512-326-1212**
800-392-0040
512-326-8088
e-mail: infobox@BIATx.org

Chip Howe, Representative

Strives to meet the urgent need to develop programs for public awareness and education, to support research and rehabilitation and to provide family guidance.

1982

1175 **Breast Cancer Action**

55 New Montgomery Street
Suite 323
San Francisco, CA 94105
415-243-9301
877-278-6722
FAX: 415-243-3996
e-mail: info@bcaction.org
www.bcaction.org

Jo Ann Madigan, President
Renetia Martin, VP

Carries the voices of people affected by breast cancer to inspire and compel the changes necessary to end the breast cancer epidemic. Holds monthly meetings and publishes a bimonthly newsletter on topics related to breast cancer. Works closely with California Breast Cancer Organization and the National Cancer Coalition.

1990

1176 **Bristol Association for Retarded Citizens**

621 Jerome Avenue
PO Box 726
Bristol, CT 06011
860-582-9102
FAX: 860-582-8280
e-mail: brstl.assoc.rtrddol@snet.net
www.geocities.com/bristolarc

Rosemarie Cassin, Executive Director
Marcia Lada, Program Coordinator

The Bristol Association for Retarded Citizens is a private, nonprofit, CARF accredited, United Way organization made up of parents, educators, professionals in the field, and volunteers who are dedicated to providing services to and improving the quality of life for people with disabilities in the greater Bristol area.

1957

1177 **Cancer Care: National Office**

275 7th Avenue
New York, NY 10001
212-221-3300
800-813-HOPE
FAX: 212-719-0263
e-mail: cancercareinc.org
www.cancercare.org

Diane Blum, Executive Director
Priscilla Hartung, Director Social Services

Cancer Care is a national nonprofit organization whose mission is to provide free professional help to people with all cancers through counseling, education, information and referral and direct financial assistance.

1178 **Cancer Control Society**

2043 N Berendo Street
Los Angeles, CA 90027
323-663-7801
FAX: 323-663-7757
e-mail: cfwintner@aol.com
www.cancercontrolsociety.com

Norman Fitz, President
Frank Cousineau, VP

To prevent and control cancer and other degenerative diseases through nutrition and nontoxic therapies.

1179 **Child Neurology Service**

Inova Fairfax Hospital
3300 Gallows Road
Falls Church, VA 22042
703-698-1110
FAX: 703-204-6588
www.inova.org

Offers infants and children to age 21 with neurological problems diagnosis, consultation, recommendations for therapy and more services. We also care for adults with cerebral palsy.

1180 **Children and Adults with Attention Deficit Disorders (CHADD)**

8181 Professional Place
Suite 150
Landover, MD 20785
301-306-7070
800-233-4050
FAX: 301-306-6788
www.chadd.org

Clarke Ross, CEO
Karen White, Director Natl Resource Center

National nonprofit organization founded in 1987 in response to the frustration and sense of isolation experienced by parents and their children with AD/HD.

1181 **Christopher Reeve Paralysis Foundation**

500 Morris Avenue
Springfield, NJ 07081
973-379-6299
800-225-0292
FAX: 973-912-9433
e-mail: info@crpf.org
www.crpf.org

Christopher Reeve, Chairman
Joel M Faden, Secretary

Committed to funding research that develops treatments and cures for paralysis caused by spinal cord injury and other central nervous system disorders. The Foundation also vigorously works to improve the quality of life for people living with disabilities through its grants program, paralysis resource center and advocacy efforts.

1182 **Citizens Alliance for Venereal Disease Awareness**

800 W Central Road
Mt. Prospect, IL 60056
847-398-3378

Offers information on symptoms, treatment and prevention of STDs.

1183 **Cleft Palate Foundation**

104 S Estes Drive
Suite 204
Chapel Hill, NC 27514
919-933-9044
800-242-5338
FAX: 919-933-9604
e-mail: info@cleftline.org
www.cleftline.org

Earl J Seaver, PhD, President
Kerry F Callahan, MA CCC-SLP, Secretary

A nonprofit organization dedicated to optimizing the quality of life for individuals affected by facial birth defects. It was founded by the American Cleft Palate-Craniofacial Association to be the public service arm of the professional Association. Produces free publications.

1973

1184 **College of Syntonic Optometry**

322 N Aurora Street
Ithaca, NY 14850 **607-277-4749**
FAX: 607-277-5216
www.syntonicphototherapy.com

Dr Larry Wallace, President
Dr Cathy Stern, VP

An active and growing post-graduate educational organization.

1185 **Community Services for Autistic Adults and Children**

751 Twinbrook Parkway
Rockville, MD 20851 **301-762-1650**
FAX: 301-762-5230
TTY:800-735-2258
e-mail: csaac@csaac.com
www.csaac.org

Patricia D Juhrs, Executive Director

1186 **Connecticut Association for Children and Adults with Learning Disabilities (CACLD)**

25 Van Zant Street
Suite 15-5
E Norwalk, CT 06855 **203-838-5010**
FAX: 203-866-6108
e-mail: cacld@optonline.net
www.cacld.org

Beryl Kaufman, Executive Director

CACLD is a regional nonprofit organization providing information and support to benefit children and adults with LD and ADD. CACLD is a resource for families and professionals.

1187 **Cranial Academy**

8202 Clearvista Parkway
Suite 9D
Indianapolis, IN 46256 **317-594-0411**
www.cranialacademy.com

John L Baumeier DO, President
Therese M Scott DO, VP

Not-for-profit group comprised of physicians dedicated to promote and safeguard the health of their patients.

1947

1188 **DB-Link**

Teaching Research
345 N Monmouth Avenue
Monmouth, OR 97361
800-438-9376
FAX: 503-838-8150
TTY:800-854-7013
e-mail: dblink@tr.wou.edu
www.tr.wou.edu/dblink

Dr John Reiman, Executive Director

Federally funded information and referral service that identifies, coordinates and disseminates (at no cost) information related to children and youth who are deaf-blind (ages 0-21 years).

1189 **Dental Amalgam Syndrome (DAMS)**

725-9 Tramway Lane NE
Albuquerque, NM 87122 **505-291-8239**
FAX: 505-294-3339

Offers information dedicated to enlightening the public on the potential risks of mercury in dental amalgam fillings.

1190 **Epilepsy Foundation**

4351 Garden City Drive
Landover, MD 20785 **301-459-3700**
800-332-1000
FAX: 301-577-2684
e-mail: postmaster@efa.com
www.epilepsyfoundation.org

William E Braunlich, President

National charitable organization, wholly dedicated to the welfare of people with epilepsy. Mission is to work for children and adults affected by seizures through research, education, advocacy and service.

1968

1191 **Exceptional Cancer Patients**

522 Jackson Park Drive
Meadville, PA 16335 **814-337-8192**
FAX: 814-337-0699
e-mail: info@mind-body.org
www.ecap-online.org

Provides exceptional resources, comprehensive professional training programs and extraordinary interdisciplinary retreats that help people facing the challenges of cancer and other chronic illnesses discover their inner healing resources.

1192 **Extensions for Independence**

555 Saturn Boulevard
#B-368
San Diego, CA 92154 **619-423-7709**
866-632-7149
e-mail: info@mouthstick.net
www.mouthstick.net

Arthur Heyer, President/Designer

Designer and manufacturer of home and office related equipment for the disabled.

1976

1193 **Families of Spinal Muscular Atrophy**

PO Box 196
Libertyville, IL 60048 **847-367-7620**
800-886-1762
FAX: 847-367-7623
e-mail: sma@fsma.org
www.fsma.org

Audrey Lewis, Executive Director
Colleen McCarthy, Youth Director

Volunteer-driven, nonprofit organization raises funds to promote research to find a cure for the Spinal Muscular Atrophies, and to support families affected by SMA.

1984

1194 **Federation of Families for Children's Mental Health**

2001 N Beauregard Street
12th Floor
Alexandria, VA 22311 **703-684-7722**
800-969-6642
FAX: 703-684-5968
e-mail: ffcmh@ffcmh.org
www.nmha.org

Barbara Huff, Executive Director
Elaine Scaton, Technical Assistance Coordinator

A national parent-run organization focused on the needs of children with emotional, behavioral or mental disorders and their families. Call national office for local chapter referral. Sliding scale membership.

1195 Feingold Association of the US

127 E Main Street
Suite 106
Riverhead, NY 11901
631-369-9340
800-321-3287
FAX: 631-369-2988
e-mail: Help@feingold.org
www.feingold.org

Nonprofit public 501 (C)3 charity dedicated to helping children and adults apply proven dietary techniques for better behavior, learning and health.

1196 Gazette International Networking Institute

4207 Lindell Boulevard
Suite 110
Saint Louis, MO 63108
314-53404-75

1197 Health Education AIDS Liason (HEAL)

PO Box 1103
Old Chelsea Station
New York, NY 10113
212-674-HOPE
www.healaids.com

Michael Ellner, President
Tom DiFerdinando, Executive Director
Barnett J Weiss, Board Member

Nonprofit, community-based educational organization providing information, hope, and support to people who are HIV positive or living with AIDS. The men and women at HEAL are health professionals, people living with life threatening diseases, and concerned volunteers.

1198 Herpes Resource Center

PO Box 13827
Research Triangle Park, NC 27709
919-361-8400
FAX: 919-361-8425
www.ashastd.org/hrc/

Support and information for those with recurring genital herpes infections.

1199 International Association for Cancer Victors: Northern California Chapter

5336 Harwood Road
San Jose, CA 95124
408-448-4094
FAX: 408-264-9659
www.cancervictors.org

Volunteer community service organization to inform and support interested persons who want to learn more about natural, nontoxic remedies and practices.

1962

1200 International Rett Syndrome Association

9121 Piscataway Road
Clinton, MD 20735
301-856-3334
800-818-7388
FAX: 301-856-3336
e-mail: irsa@rettsyndrome.org
www.rettsyndrome.org

Kathy Hunter, President
Kathryn Kissam, Secretary

Nonprofit voluntary organization dedicated to serving as an information and referral center for physicians and families of children with Rett Syndrome. The Association's mission includes supporting and promoting research into the prevention, control, and cure of the disorder; increasing public awareness; and providing emotional support for affected families. Engages in patient advocacy; promotes family and professional education; and provides referrals to support groups.

1985

1201 Joni and Friends

PO Box 3333
Agoura Hills, CA 91376
818-707-5664
FAX: 818-707-2391
TTY:818-707-9707
e-mail: jafmin@joniandfriends.org
www.joniandfriends.org

N Douglas Mazza, Executive Vice President
John Wern, Director-Wheels for the World
Steve Appelerg, Director Communication

A nonprofit organization seeking to accelerate Christian ministry with people affected by disabilities. JAF educates churches and the community worldwide concerning the needs of the disabled and how those needs can be met. We sponsor family retreats for families with disabled members. Wheels for the World collects, restores and distributes used wheelchairs to disadvantaged populations around the world.

1979

1202 Judge David L Bazelon Center for Mental Health Law

1101 15th Street NW
Suite 1212
Washington, DC 20005
202-467-5730
FAX: 202-223-0409
e-mail: info@bazelon.org
www.bazelon.org

Robert Bernstein, Executive Director

A national nonprofit public interest organization, advocates for public policies that can enable people with mental disabilities to live in freedom and with dignity. Website offers resources on health care, fair housing, special education and enforcement of Americans with Disabilities Act. Publications list available.

1203 Juvenile Diabetes Foundation International

120 Wall Street
New York, NY 10005
212-789-9500
800-533-2873
FAX: 212-785-9595
e-mail: info@jdfcom
www.jdf.org

Shira Kandel, Manager Public Information

The world's leading nonprofit, nongovernmental funder of diabetes research. It was founded in 1970 by parents of children with diabetes. JDF's mission is to find a cure for diabetes and its complications through the support of research. JDF also sponsors international workshops and conferences for biomedical researchers, individual chapters offer support groups and other activities for families affected by diabetes. JDF has more than 110 chapters and affiliates worldwide. Quarterly newsletter.

1204 Leukemia & Lymphoma Society

1311 Mamaroneck Avenue
White Plains, NY 10605
914-949-5213
FAX: 914-949-6691
www.leukemia.org

Norbert J Seiber, Chairman
Frank T Short, Vice Chairman
Alan M Gerwitz MD, Vice Chairman Med./Sci. Affairs

Mission is to cure leukemia, lymphoma, Hodgkin's disease and myeloma, and to improve the quality of life of patients and their families.

1949

1205 **Lighthouse International**

Hudson Valley Region
170 Hamilton Avenue
White Plains, NY 10601
914-683-7500
888-222-9320
FAX: 914-686-5866
e-mail: visionrehab@lighthouse.org
www.lighthouse.org

Barbara Silverstone DSW, President/CEO
Judith Millman ACSW MBA, VP Hudson Valley Region
James P O'Toole, Chair Regional Advisory Board

A leading resource worldwide on vision impairment and rehabilitation. Through its pioneering work in vision rehabilitation services, education, research and advocacy, Lighthouse International enables people of all ages who are blind or partially sighted to lead independent and productive lives. Founded in 1905 and headquartered in New York, Lighthouse International is a not-for-profit organization, depending on the support of individuals, foundations and corporations.

1206 **Little People of America**

PO Box 65030
Lubbock, TX 79464
888-572-2001
e-mail: LPADataBase@juno.com
www.lpaonline.org

Matt Roloff, President
Randy Bradford, Senior VP
Craig Holloway, Finance VP

Assists dwarfs with their physical and developmental concerns resulting from short stature, usually no taller then 4' 10". Provides medical, environmental, educational, vocational, and parental guidance, so that short-statured individuals and their families may enhance their lives and lifestyles with minimal limitations.

1957

1207 **March of Dimes Birth Defects Foundation**

1275 Mamaroneck Avenue
White Plains, NY 10605
914-428-7100
FAX: 914-997-4763
e-mail: askus@marchofdimes.com
www.marchofdimes.com

The mission of the March of Dimes is to improve the health of babies by preventing birth defects and infant mortality. The MOD Resource Center provides information and referral services to the public from 9:00 am to 8:00 pm EST.

1208 **Mississippi Society for Disabilities**

3226 N State Street
Jackson, MS 39216
601-982-7051
601-982-1951
e-mail: msclinic@bellsouth.net
www.msdisabilities.com

Kim J Gonzales MS CCC/SLP, Clinic Director

Nonprofit outpatient and contract therapy provider of speech/therapy, occupational therapy and physical therapy services from birth through geriatrics.

1209 **Multiple Sclerosis Center of Oregon**

Oregon Health & Sciences University
3181 SW Sam Jackson Park Road
Portland, OR 97201
503-494-5759

www.ohsu.edu/som-ms

Dennis Bourdette, Director

Committed to Multiple Sclerosis research and patient and community education.

1210 **Multiple Sclerosis Foundation**

6350 N Andrews Avenue
Fort Lauderdale, FL 33309
954-776-6805
800-225-6495
FAX: 954-938-8708
e-mail: admin@msfocus.org
www.msfocus.org

Tammi Robinson, Director Program Services
Tea Barbaris, Special Event Coordinator

Contemporary national, nonprofit organization that provides free support services and public education for persons with Multiple Sclerosis, newsletters, toll-free phone support, information, referrals, home care, assitive technology, and support groups.

1211 **Muscular Dystrophy Association**

3300 E Sunrise Drive
Tucson, AZ 85718
520-529-2000
800-572-1717
FAX: 520-529-5300
e-mail: mda@mdausa.org
www.mdausa.org

Bob Mackle, Director Public Information

MDA provides comprehensive medical services to tens of thousands of people with neuromuscular diseases at some 230 hospital-affiliated clinics across the country. The Association's worldwide research program, which funds over 400 individual scientific investigations annually, represents the largest single effort to advance knowledge of neuromuscular diseases and to find cures and treatments for them. In addition, MDA conducts far-reaching educational programs for the public and professionals.

1212 **NIH Osteoporosis and Related Bone Diseases National Resource Center**

1232 22nd Street NW
Washington, DC 20037
202-223-0344
800-624-BONE
FAX: 202-293-2356
e-mail: orbdnrc@nof.org
www.osteo.org

Distributes information to patients, health professionals and the public on osteoporosis, Paget's disease of bone, osteogenesis imperfecta, and other metabolic bone diseases. Information on prevention, early detection and treatment of these diseases is available.

1213 **National AIDS Fund**

1030 15th Street NW
Suite 860
Washington, DC 20005
202-408-4848
FAX: 202-408-1818
www.aidsfund.org

Kandy Ferree, President/CEO

Dedicated to eliminating HIV/AIDS as a major health and social problem.

1214 **National Amputation Foundation**

40 Church Street
Malverne, NY 11565
516-887-3600
FAX: 516-887-3667
e-mail: amps76@aol.com
www.nationalamputation.org

Al Pennacchia, President
Donald A Sioss, Executive Secretary

Helps people who have had amputations to adjust to society. Members are military veterans with service connected amputations, as well as civilian amputees, who help show new amputees how to cope. It provides legal, vocational and psychological services and facilitates self help groups. 2,000 members. Publishes a veteran newsletter for amputees.

Quarterly 1919

1215 **National Association for Continence**

PO Box 176
Charleston, SC 29402 **843-377-0900**
800-252-3337
FAX: 843-377-0905
e-mail: memberservices@nafc.org
www.nafc.org

Nancy Muller, Executive Director
Rachel Coker, Publicity/Publications Associate
Nikki Dean, Health Educator/Member Services

NAFC is the world's largest and most prolific consumer advocacy organization dedicated to helping people who struggle with incontinence and related voiding dysfunction.

1216 **National Association for Down Syndrome**

PO Box 4542
Oak Brook, IL 60522 **630-325-9112**
FAX: 630-325-8842
www.nads.org

Kim Xidas, Family Support Coordinator

Works for a strong network of support systems within their own organization and with medical, educational and school service professionals who work with children and adults with Down Syndrome. NADS serves the Chicago Metropolitan area.

1217 **National Association to Aid Fat Americans**

PO Box 188620
Sacramento, CA 95818 **916-443-0303**

Support and education for overweight people.

1218 **National Ataxia Foundation**

2600 Fernbrook Lane
Suite 119
Minneapolis, MN 55447 **763-553-0020**
FAX: 763-553-0167
e-mail: naf@ataxia.org
www.ataxia.org

Donna Gruetzmacher, Executive Director
Karla Brown, Administrative Assistant

Combats all types of hereditary Ataxia through education, service and research programs.

1957

1219 **National Brachial Plexus/Erb's Palsy Association**

PO Box 23
Larsen, WI 54947 **920-836-2151**
FAX: 209-644-5813
e-mail: nationalbpi@powernetonline.com
www.delphi.com/nationalbpi

Brenda Copeland-Moore, President
Kris Kiesow, Treasurer
Cheryl Pratt, VP

To educate, inform, and assist those affected by Brachial Plexus Palsy by offering information, contacts, resources, parent matching, and assistance developing chapters or support groups throughout the United States.

1220 **National Center for Learning Disabilities**

381 Park Avenue S
Suite 1401
New York, NY 10016 **212-545-9665**
888-575-7373
FAX: 212-545-9665
www.ncld.org

John G Gantz Jr, Chairman

National, nonprofit organization dedicated to increasing opportunities for all individuals with learning disabilities to achieve their potential. Services include national information and resources, public outreach and communications and legislative advocacy and public policy. Free online newsletters available through the website.

1977

1221 **National Council for Community Behavioral Healthcare**

12300 Twinbrook Parkway
Suite 320
Rockville, MD 20852 **301-984-6200**
FAX: 301-881-7159
www.nccbh.org

Marilyn LaCelle ACSW, Chair

National organization of community-based providers of behavioral health services. Mission is to champion opportunities that advance our members' ability to deliver proactive and holistic health care services.

1222 **National Council on Spinal Cord Injury**

151 Tremont Street
Boston, MA 02111 **617-451-5757**
FAX: 617-338-4266
e-mail: neuro@jiac.net

Arthur D Vllian, President

A membership organization for agencies and individuals. Fosters communication among members of the spinal cord injury community and the general public. Supports research and works for the integration of individuals with spinal cord injury into the general community.

1223 **National Diabetes Information Clearinghouse**

1 Information Way
Bethesda, MD 20892 **301-654-3327**
800-860-8747
FAX: 301-907-8906
e-mail: ndic@info.niddk.nih.gov
www.niddk.nih.gov

Barbara Gordon, Co-Project Manager
Ruth Ann Spier, Co-Project Manager

An information and referral service of the National Institute of Diabetes and Digestive and Kidney Diseases, one of the National Institutes of Health. The clearinghouse responds to written inquiries, develops and distributes publications about diabetes, and provides referrals to diabetes organizations, including support groups. The NDIC maintains a database of patient and professional education materials, from which literature searches are generated.

1978

1224 **National Digestive Diseases Information Clearinghouse**

2 Information Way
Bethesda, MD 20892 **301-654-3810**
800-891-5389
FAX: 301-907-8906
e-mail: nddic@info.niddk.nih.gov
www.niddk.nih.gov

Kathy Kranzfeider, Director

Information and referral service of the National Institute of Diabetes and Digestive and Kidney Diseases. A central information resource on the prevention and management of digestive diseases, the clearinghouse responds to written inquiries, develops and distributes publications about digestive diseases, provides referrals to digestive disease organizations and support groups, and maintains a database of patient and professional education materials from which literature searches are generated.

1225 **National Down Syndrome Society**

666 Broadway
New York, NY 10012
212-460-9330
800-221-4602
FAX: 212-979-2873
e-mail: info@ndss.org
www.ndss.org

Thomas J O'Neill, President
Stephen Riggio, VP

Not-for-profit organization increases public awareness about Down syndrome and works to discover its underlying causes through research, education and advocacy. Distributes timely and informative materials, encourages and supports the activities of local parent support groups, sponsors sonferences and scientific symposia and undertakes major advocacy efforts—all to increase awareness and acceptance of people with Down syndrome.

1979

1226 **National Hemophilia Foundation**

116 W 32nd Street
11th Floor
New York, NY 10001
212-328-3700
800-424-2634
FAX: 212-328-3777
e-mail: info@hemophilia.org
www.hemophilia.org

Richard T Hellner, Chief Executive Officer

Offers counseling, educational materials, fundraising, loans, seminars and support groups with over 40 local chapters.

1227 **National Institute of Arthritis and Musculoskeletal and Skin Diseases**

1 AMS Circle
Bethesda, MD 20892
301-495-4484
877-226-4267
FAX: 301-718-6366
e-mail: niamsinfo@mail.nih.gov
www.nih.gov/niams

Dr Stephen Katz, Director
Dr Steven J Hausman, Deputy Director

Mission is to support research into the causes, treatment and prevention of arthritis and musculoskeletal and skin diseases, the training of basic and clinical scientists to carry out this research, and the dissemination of information on research progress in these diseases.

1228 **National Institute of Neurological Disorders and Stroke**

NIH Neurological Institute
PO Box 5801
Bethesda, MD 20824
301-496-5751
800-352-9424
FAX: 301-402-2186
www.ninds.nih.gov

Marian Emr, Director Communications

America's focal point for support of research on brain and nervous system disorders. Its active public information program provides physicians, patients and the public with educational materials and research highlights. Materials provided by the public information program include brochures, fact sheets, information packets and special reports. All publications are free of charge.

1229 **National Kidney and Urologic Diseases Information Clearinghouse**

3 Information Way
Bethesda, MD 20892
301-654-4415
800-891-5390
FAX: 301-907-8906
e-mail: nkudic@info.niddk.nih.gov
www.niddk.nih.gov

Kathy Kranzfeldop, Director

Increases knowledge and understanding about diseases of the kidneys and urologic system among people with these conditions and their families, health care professionals and the general public.

1987

1230 **National Mental Health Association**

2001 N Beauregard Street
12th Floor
Alexandria, VA 22311
703-684-7722
800-969-6642
FAX: 703-684-5968
e-mail: infoctr@nmha.org
www.nmha.org

Michael Faenza MSSW, President/CEO

Nonprofit organization addressing all issues related to mental health and mental illness. With more than 340 affiliates nationwide, NMHA works to improve the mental health of all Americans, especially the 54 million individuals with mental disorders, through advocacy, education, research and service.

1909

1231 **National Mental Health Consumers' Self-Help Clearinghouse**

1211 Chestnut Street
Suite 1207
Philadelphia, PA 19107
215-751-1810
800-553-4539
FAX: 215-636-6312
e-mail: info@mhselfhelp.org
www.mhselfhelp.org

Karena Bayruns, Information/Referral
Mimi Rose, Program Director

Consumer-run national technical assistance center serving the mental health consumer movement. We help connect individuals to self-help and advocacy resources, and we offer expertise to self-help groups and other peer-run services for mental health consumers.

1232 **National Multiple Sclerosis Society**

733 3rd Avenue
New York, NY 10017
800-344-4867
FAX: 212-986-7981
e-mail: nat@nmss.org
www.nationalmssociety.org

Thomas Kuhn, President

Mission is to end the devastating effects of MS. Provides professional and public education; information and referral; and supports research. One hundred and forty local chapters and branches offer counseling services, advocacy, discount prescription and health care products program, and assistance in obtaining adaptive equipment.

1233 **National Organization for Rare Disorders**

NORD
55 Kenosia Avenue
PO Box 1968
Danbury, CT 06813
203-744-0100
800-999-6673
FAX: 203-798-2291
TTY:203-797-9590
e-mail: orphan@rarediseases.org
www.rarediseases.org

James Broatch, Chair
Carolyn Asbury PhD, Vice Chair

Unique federation of voluntary health organizations dedicated to helping people with rare orphan diseases and assisting the organizations that serve them. NORD is committed to the identification, treatment and cure of rare disorders through programs of education, advocacy, research and service.

1234 **National Parkinson Foundation**

Bob Hope Parkinson Research Center
1501 NW 9th Avenue, Bob Hope Road
Miami, FL 33136
305-547-6666
800-327-4545
FAX: 305-243-4403
e-mail: mailbox@parkinson.org
www.parkinson.org

Daniel Arty, President
Alan M Slewett Esq, Secretary

The purpose of this Foundation is to find the cause and cure for Parkinson's Disease and related neurodegenerative disorders through research, to educate general medical practitioners to detect the early warning signs of Parkinson's Disease and to improve the quality of life for both patients and their caregivers. Provides current information to patients, caregivers and families. Publishes quarterly newsletter.

1957

1235 **National Stroke Association**

96 Inverness Drive E
Suite I
Englewood, CO 80112
303-649-9299
800-787-6537
FAX: 303-771-1886
e-mail: info@stroke.org
www.stroke.org

Thelma Edwards RN, Director Exhibits

The only national health organization solely committed to stroke prevention, treatment, rehabilitation and community reintegration. Provides packaged training programs, on-site assistance, physician, patient and family education materials to acute and rehab hospitals. Develops workshops; operates the Stroke Information & Referral Center and produces professional publications such as Stroke: Clinical Updates and the Journal of Stroke and Cerebrovascular Diseases.

1236 **Overeaters Anonymous World Services Office**

6075 Zenith Court NE
Rio Rancho, NM 87124
505-891-2664
FAX: 505-891-4320
e-mail: info@overeatersanonymous.org
www.overeatersanonymous.org

Support groups and a twelve-step method of healing for compulsive eaters.

1237 **Pacer Center (Parent Advocacy Coalition for Educational Rights)**

8161 Normandale Boulevard
Minneapolis, MN 55437
952-838-9000
800-537-2237
FAX: 952-838-0199
TTY:612-827-7770
e-mail: pacer@pacer.org
www.pacer.org

Paula F Goldberg, Executive Director

Mission is to expand opportunities and enhance the quality of life of children and young adults with disabilities and their families based on the concept of parents helping parents. Offers workshops, individual assistance and written information. Provides programs and materials that assist multicultural families, programs for students, schools and professionals with disability awareness puppet and child abuse prevention programs. Computer Resource Center/Software Lending Library available.

1238 **Paralyzed Veterans of America**

801 18th Street NW
Washington, DC 20006
202-872-1300
800-424-8200
e-mail: info@pva.org
www.pva.org

Joseph L Fox Sr, National President
Tom Wheaton, Senior VP
Gene A Crayton, National VP

A congressionally chartered veterans service organization, has developed a unique expertise on a wide variety of issues involving the special needs of our members— veterans of the armed forces who have experienced spinal cord injury or dysfunction.

1946

1239 **Parents of Children with Down Syndrome**

11600 Nebel Street
Rockville, MD 20852
301-984-5781
FAX: 301-816-2429

Karen O'Connor, President

Activities include formal and informal meetings; parent-to-parent counseling; contacting new parents of Down Syndrome children to offer support and information on community resources; providing information on doctors, hospitals and professionals.

1240 **People Against Cancer**

604 East Street
PO Box 10
Otho, IA 50569
515-972-4444
FAX: 515-972-4415
e-mail: info@PeopleAgainstCancer.net
www.peopleagainstcancer.com

A nonprofit, grassroots public benefit organization dedicated to 'New Directions in the War on Cancer.' We are a democratic organization of people with cancer, their loved ones and citizens working together to protect and enhance medical freedom of choice.

1241 **Polio Connection of America**

PO Box 182
Howard Beach, NY 11414
718-835-5536
FAX: 718-738-1509
e-mail: w1066@msn.com
www.geocities.com/w1066w

George Cook, Executive Director

This is a voluntary nonprofit organization dedicated to locating polio survivors and providing them with information concerning Post-Polio Syndrome. Committed to locating, informing and supporting polio survivors affected with Post-Polio Syndrome to help them receive appropriate treatment. Provides appropriate referrals, as well as educational materials including a newsletter, brochures and booklets. Also an advocate for Post-Polio Syndrome research.

8 pages Quarterly

1242 **Polio Society**

PO Box 106273
Washington, DC 20016 **301-897-8180**
FAX: 202-466-1911
www.polio.org/

Ed Grebenstein, President
Jessica Scheer PhD, Executive Director

National not-for-profit voluntary organziation created to provide education resources and support group services to people who had polio and are now experiencing the late effects of polio. Activities include maintenance of a national membership database of polio survivors and health care professionals; sponsorship of major national UPDATE conferences about post-polio issues; and publication of Options, quarterly newsletter.

1243 **Post-Polio Health International**

4207 Lindell Boulevard
Suite 110
Saint Louis, MO 63108 **314-534-0475**
FAX: 314-534-5070
TTY:800-735-2966
e-mail: info@post-polio.org
www.post-polio.org

Joan L Headly, Executive Director

To enhance the lives and independence of polio survivors and home mechanical ventilator users by promoting education, networking and advocacy among these individuals and healthcare providers.

1244 **Prader-Willi Alliance of New York**

267 Oxford Street
Rochester, NY 14607 **716-442-1655**
800-442-1655
FAX: 716-271-2782
e-mail: balleregballer@aol.com
www.prader-willi.org

Elinor G Baller, Secretary

The Prader-Willi Foundation is a national, nonprofit public charity that works for the benefit of individuals with Prader-Willi syndrome and their families.

1245 **Prader-Willi Syndrome Association USA**

5700 Midnight Pass Road
Sarasota, FL 34242 **941-312-0400**
800-926-4797
FAX: 941-312-0142
www.pwsausa.org

National, nonprofit public charity that works for the benefit of individuals with Prader-Willi syndrome and their families.

1246 **Rasmussen's Syndrome and Hemispherectomy Support Network**

8235 Lethbridge Road
Millersville, MD 21108 **410-987-5221**
FAX: 410-987-521
e-mail: rssnlynn@aol.com

Al & Lynn Miller, Founders

National not-for-profit organization dedicated to providing information and support to individuals affected by Rasmussen's Syndrome and Hemispherectomy. Publishes a periodic newsletter and disseminates reprints of medical journal articles concerning Rasmussen's Syndrome and its treatments. Maintains a support network that provides encouragement and information to individuals affected by Rasmussen's Syndrome and their families.

1247 **Shake-A-Leg**

PO Box 1264
Newport, RI 02840 **401-849-8898**
FAX: 401-848-9072
e-mail: shake@shakealeg.org
www.shakealeg.org

Paul Callahan, CEO
Eileen Callahan, Bookkeeper
Sarah Everhart, Program Director

Nonprofit charitable organization founded to serve people with disabilities, with an emphasis placed on spinal cord and related nervous system impairments. Mission is to provide mainstream, complimentary and recreational therapeutic services that develop independent living skills for individuals who have experienced spinal cord injury and related nervous system disorders.

1982

1248 **Simonton Cancer Center**

PO Box 890
Pacific Palisades, CA 90272 **310-457-3811**
800-459-3424
FAX: 310-457-0421
e-mail: ocsimonton@mindspring.com
www.simontoncenter.com

O Carl Simonton MD, Medical Director

A model of emotional support for the treatment of cancer patients, an approach that introduces the concept that one's state of mind could influence their ability to survive cancer. Offers patient program and self-help literature, audio and video materials.

1249 **Society for Progressive Supranuclear Palsy (SPSP)**

Woodholme Medical Building #515
1838 Greene Tree Road
Baltimore, MD 21208 **410-486-3330**
800-457-4777
FAX: 410-486-4283
e-mail: spsp@psp.org
www.psp.org

Elizabeth Brisson, President
Stephen Hamer, VP
Kelley Harrison PhD, Secretary

Mission is to promote and fund research into finding the cause and cure for progressive supranuclear palsy (PSP). Provides information, support and advocacy to persons diagnosed with PSP, their families and caregivers. Educates physicians and allied health professionals on PSP and how to improve patient care.

1250 **Spina Bifida Association of America**

4590 Macarthur Boulevard NW
Suite 250
Washington, DC 20007 **202-944-3285**
800-621-3141
FAX: 202-944-3295
e-mail: sbaa@sbaa.org
www.sbaa.org

Alex Brodrick, Chair
Tim Yoder, Vice Chair

Nonprofit organization. Mission is to promote the prevention of spina bifida and to enhance the lives of all affected. Addresses the specific needs of the spina bifida community and serves as the national representative of almost 60 chapters. Toll free 800 information and referral service. Legislative updates.

1973

1251 **Spinal Cord Society (SCS)**

19051 County Highway 1
Fergus Falls, MN 56537 **218-739-5252**
FAX: 218-739-5262
www.members.aol.com/scsweb

International organization for cure research and treatment of spinal cord injury paralysis and related problems.

1978

1252 **Support Group for Brachial Plexus Injury**

18 Staci Lane
Webster, NY 14580 **585-787-0197**
FAX: 585-872-6158
e-mail: jdebryne@aol.com

Jeff DeBryne, President

The Support Group for Brachial Plexus Injury was established to provide resources and emotional support to families impacted by Erb's Palsy and other brachial plexus injuries by advising on how best to receive and obtain insurance and treatment for this disorder.

1253 **Texas Speech-Language-Hearing Association**

PO Box 140647
Austin, TX 78714 **512-452-4636**
888-729-8742
FAX: 512-454-3036
e-mail: donise@callier.utdallas.edu
www.txsha.org

Donise Pearson, President

Mission is to encourage and promote the role of the speech-language pathologist and audiologist as a professional in the delivery of clinical services to persons with communications disorders. Encourages basic scientific study of processes of individual human communication with reference to speech, hearing and language.

1254 **Tourette Syndrome Association**

42-40 Bell Boulevard
Bayside, NY 11361 **718-224-2999**
800-237-0717
FAX: 718-279-9596
e-mail: ts@tsa-usa.org
www.tsa-usa.org

Fred Cook, Chair
Judit Ungar, President

National, nonprofit membership organization. Mission is to identify the cause of, find the cure for, and control the effects of this disorder. A growing number of local chapters nationwide provide educational materials, seminars, conferences and support groups for over 35,000 members. Publishes brochures, flyers, educational materials and papers on treatment and research. Offers videos for purchase through a catalog of publications.

1972

1255 **United Cerebral Palsy Association**

1660 L Street NW
Suite 700
Washington, DC 20036 **202-776-0406**
800-872-5827
FAX: 202-776-0414
TTY:202-973-7197
e-mail: webmaster@ucp.org
www.ucpa.org

Stephen Bennett, President/CEO

National not-for-profit self-help organization dedicated to providing information and support to individuals with Cerebral Palsy and other disabilities, and their families. Supports more than 160 local affiliates; these affiliates provide a variety of programs and services for affected families, including support groups. Offers several educational and support materials, including a quarterly magazine, regular newsletters, and research reports.

1256 **United Cerebral Palsy Association of New York State**

330 W 34th Street
New York, NY 10001 **212-947-5770**
FAX: 212-594-4538
e-mail: info@cerebralpalsynys.org
www.cerebralpalsynys.org

Susan Constantino, Associate Executive Director
Cheryl Bradway, Administrative Assistant
Barbara Crosier, Legislative Affairs Director

Mission is to advocate and provide direct services with and for individuals with cerebral palsy and other significant disabilities, and their families, throughout New York State, in order to promote lifelong opportunities and choices for independence, inclusion and enhanced quality of life. Provides services and programs for more than 40,000 individuals with cerebral palsy and developmental disabilities and their families.

1257 **United Cerebral Palsy Association of New York State**

90 State Street
Suite 929
Albany, NY 12207 **518-436-0178**
FAX: 518-436-8619
e-mail: info@cerebralpalsynys.org
www.cerebralpalsynys.org

Susan Constantino, Associate Executive Director
Cheryl Bradway, Administrative Assistant
Barbara Crosier, Legislative Affairs Director

Mission is to advocate and provide direct services with and for individuals with cerebral palsy and other significant disabilities, and their families, throughout New York State, in order to promote lifelong opportunities and choices for independence, inclusion and enhanced quality of life. Provides services and programs for more than 40,000 individuals with cerebral palsy and developmental disabilities and their families.

1258 **Vermont Back Research Center**

1 S Prospect Street
Burlington, VT 05401 **802-656-0015**
800-527-7320
FAX: 802-660-9243
e-mail: backtalk@salus.med.uvm.edu
www.ncddr.org/du/researchexchange/v04n03/real

Martin Krag MD, Director

Conducts research aimed at reducing back-related disability following injury or acute pain episodes. Current research includes studies of posture, seating, vibration, materials handling, and exercise. The Center develops and tests assistive devices, and promotes employment of people with back disorders and rapid return to work after injury. The staff provides a variety of information services, including bibliographic searches and fact finding.

1259 **World's Best Books from the Diabetes Experts: Publications Catalog**

American Diabetes Association
1701 N Beauregard Street
Alexandria, VA 22311
703-549-1500
800-232-6733
FAX: 770-442-9742
e-mail: bookorders@diabetes.org
www.diabetes.org

John Fedor, Associate Director
Janel Chrobot, Marketing Specialist

A 24 page, full-color catalog of more than 80 books and products for people with diabetes. Titles of categories of books include: cookbooks, meal planning and nutrition, new books and self-care.

1260 **YAI: National Institute for People with Disabilities**

460 W 34th Street
New York, NY 10001
212-273-6100
FAX: 212-947-7524
www.yai.org

Joel Levy DSW, CEO
Phil Levy, COO

A not-for-profit professional organization serving developmentally disabled children and adults in many programs throughout the New York metropolitan area. Provides over 200 program sites for thousands of participants. Services include residential, day, outpatient, clinical, early childhood, respite and family support, camping, employment training, case management and recreation opportunities.

1957

Visually Impaired

1261 **ACB Radio Amateurs**

American Council of the Blind
1155 15th Street NW
Suite 1004
Washington, DC 20005
202-467-5081
800-424-8666
FAX: 202-467-5085
e-mail: info@acb.org
www.acb.org

A radio amateur network of blind, visually impaired and sighted members who gather and share common problems and solutions to help members improve radio amateurs in getting started, provides access to educational materials in special media and publishes a directory for the visually impaired.

1262 **Achromatopsia Network**

PO Box 214
Berkeley, CA 94701
510-540-4700
FAX: 510-540-4767
e-mail: futterman@achromat.org
www.achromat.org

Frances Futterman, Facilitator

The Achromatopsia Network is a nonprofit organization for individuals concerned with acrhomatopsia. It is committed to sharing information about achromatopsia and providing resources to meet the special needs of those affected by this eye condition; helping individuals and families concerned with achromatopsia to connect with one another; and promoting awareness and educating with a special emphasis on accomplishing this goal among those who provides services to the visually impaired.

1263 **American Academy of Ophthalmology**

Public Education Program
655 Beach Street
PO Box 7424
San Francisco, CA 94120
415-561-8500
FAX: 415-561-8533
e-mail: federal@aao.org
www.aao.org

To advance the lifelong learning and professional interests of Eye MDs to ensure that the public can obtain the best possible eye care.

1264 **American Action Fund for Blind Children and Adults**

1800 Johnson Street
Suite 100
Baltimore, MD 21230
410-659-9315
e-mail: actionfund@nfb.org
www.actionfund.org

Jean Dyon Norris, Director Operations

A service agency which specializes in providing to blind people help which is not readily available to them from government programs or other existing service systems. Planned especially to meet the needs of blind children, the elderly blind, and the deaf-blind.

1919

1265 **American Association of the Deaf-Blind**

814 Thayer Avenue
Room 302
Silver Spring, MD 20910
301-495-4403
FAX: 301-495-4404
TTY:301-495-4402
e-mail: info@aadb.org
www.aadb.org

Harry Anderson, President
Arthur Roehrig, VP
Marilyn Fernandez-Trader, Secretary

National consumer organization, of, by and for deaf-blind Americans. Deaf-blind does not necessarily mean totally deaf and totally blind. It is a broad term that describes people who have varying degrees and types of both vision and hearing loss together. Mission is to endeavor to enable deaf-blind persons to achieve their maximum potential through increased independence, productivity and integration into the community.

1266 **American Council of Blind Lions**

American Council of the Blind
1155 15th Street NW
Suite 1004
Washington, DC 20005
202-467-5081
800-424-8666
FAX: 202-467-5085
e-mail: info@acb.org
www.acb.org

Educates Lions Club members about the needs and capabilities of blind people, exchanges information concerning Club activities in the field of work for the blind and encourages blind people to join Lions Clubs and other civic activities.

1267 **American Council of the Blind**

1155 15th Street NW
Suite 720
Washington, DC 20005
202-347-2693
800-424-8666
FAX: 202-467-5085
e-mail: info@acb.org
www.acb.org

Paul Edwards, President

A national membership organization whose members are visually impaired and fully sighted individuals who are concerned about the dignity and well-being of blind people throughout America. Formed in 1961, the Council has become the largest organization of blind people in the US with over 70 state affiliates and special interest chapters.

1268 **American Foundation for the Blind**

11 Penn Plaza
Suite 300
New York, NY 10001
212-502-7600
800-232-5463
FAX: 212-502-7777
e-mail: afbinfo@afb.net
www.afb.org

Carl R Augusto, President

Eliminating barriers that prevent people who are blind or visually impaired from reaching their potential. Dedicated to addressing the critical issues of literacy, independent living, employment, and access through technology for ten million Americans who are blind or visually impaired.

1921

1269 **American Optometric Association**

243 N Lindbergh Boulevard
St. Louis, MO 63141
314-991-4100
FAX: 314-991-4101
www.aoanet.org

Wesley E Pittman, President

A federation of state, student and armed forces optometric associations with 32,000 members. Mission is to improve the quality and availability of eye and vision care everywhere. Founded in 1898.

1270 **American Printing House for the Blind**

1839 Frankfort Avenue
PO Box 6085
Louisville, KY 40206
502-895-2405
800-223-1839
FAX: 502-899-2274
e-mail: info@aph.org
www.aph.org

Fred Gissoni, Customer Support

Devoted solely to producing products for people who are visually impaired. We manufacture books and magazines in braille, large type, recorded and computer disk form. We also make a wide range of educational and daily living aids, such as braille paper and styluses, talking book equipment, and synthetic speech computer products. APH also offers CARL ET AL, an electronic database that lists accessible books in all formats.

1271 **Associated Blind**

110 William Street
9th Floor
New York, NY 10038
212-766-6800
FAX: 212-766-6809
e-mail: memberservices@esight.org
www.tabinc.org

Ruth-Ellen Simmonds, Executive Director

Organization dedicated to fostering economic and social independence among individuals who are blind or visually impaired. Services include adaptive computer education, information and referral and life enrichment programs.

1272 **Associated Services for the Blind**

919 Walnut Street
Philadelphia, PA 19107
215-627-0600
FAX: 215-922-0692
e-mail: asbinfo@asb.org
www.asb.org

Patricia C Johnson, CEO
Ron Hughes, Senior Development Officer

Established to promote self-esteem, independence, and self-determination in blind and visually impaired people. Accomplishes this by providing support through education, training, and materials. Also serves as a voice and advocate for the rights of the people served by removing barriers through community action and education.

1273 **Association for Education & Rehabilitation of the Blind & Visually Impaired**

1703 N Beauregard Street
Suite 440
Alexandria, VA 22311
703-671-4500
FAX: 703-671-6391
e-mail: markr@aerbvi.org

Greg Goodrich, President
Mark Richert, Executive Director

Dedicated to rendering support and assistance to the professionals who work in all phases of education and rehabilitation of blind and visually impaired children and adults.

1984

1274 **Association for Macular Diseases**

210 E 64th Street
8th Floor
New York, NY 10021
212-605-3719
FAX: 212-605-3795
e-mail: association@retinal-research.org
www.macula.org

Nikolai Stevenson, President
Walter Ross, Editor in Chief
Joan Daly, Treasurer

Not-for-profit organization promotes education and research in this scarcely explored field. Acts as a nationwide support group for individuals and their families endeavoring to adjust to the restrictions and changes brought about by macular disease. Offers hotline, educational materials, quarterly newsletter, support groups, referrals and seminars for persons and families affected by macular disease.

1978

1275 **Blind Children's Center**

4120 Marathon Street
Los Angeles, CA 90029
323-664-2153
800-222-3567
FAX: 323-665-3828
e-mail: info@blindchildrenscenter.org
www.blindchildrenscenter.org

A family-centered agency which serves children with visual impairments from birth to school-age. The center-based and home-based services help the children to acquire skills and build their independence. The Center utilizes its expertise and experience to serve families and professionals worldwide through support services, education and research.

1276 **Blinded Veterans Association**

477 H Street NW
Washington, DC 20001
202-371-8880
800-669-7079
FAX: 202-371-8258
e-mail: bva@bva.org
www.bva.org

Thomas H Miller, Executive Director
George E Brummell, Natl. Dir. Field Service Program

Helps veterans and their families meet the challenges of blindness.Offers two main service programs without cost to blinded veterans. Field service program provides counseling o veterans and families and information on benefits and re - habilitation.

1945

1277 **Books for Blind and Physically Handicapped Individuals**

Library of Congress
1291 Taylor Street NW
Washington, DC 20011
202-707-5100
800-424-8567
FAX: 202-707-0712
TTY:202-707-0744
e-mail: nls@loc.gov
www.loc.gov/nls

Frank Kurt Cylke, Director

Administers a national library service that provides braille and recorded books and magazines on free loan to anyone who cannot read standard print because of visual or physical disabilities who are eligible residents of the United States or American citizens living abroad. Computerized version available online at www.loc.gov/nls/reference/facts.html.

1931

1278 **Braille Institute of America**

741 N Vermont Avenue
Los Angeles, CA 90029
323-663-1111
800-272-4553
FAX: 323-666-5881
e-mail: media@brailleinstitute.org
www.brailleinstitute.org

Fortune Zuckerman, Director Special Projects

Over 200 educational classes are offered in independent living skills, mobility, reading and writing Braille, art and music. Also offered are adult counseling, career services, access technology training and subsidies, child development and youth services, low vision services, braille press, braille publications, talking book library services, retail store for adaptive items, tours, speakers, and educational materials. Programs and services are offered at five regional centers, and all are free.

1279 **Braille Revival League**

American Council of the Blind
1155 15th Street NW
Suite 1004
Washington, DC 20005
202-467-5081
800-424-8666
FAX: 202-467-5085
e-mail: info@acb.org
www.acb.org

Encourages blind people to read and write in braille, advocates for mandatory braille instruction in educational facilities for the blind, strives to make available a supply of braille materials from libraries and printing houses and more.

1280 **Canine Helpers for the Handicapped**

5699 Ridge Road
Suite 5705
Lockport, NY 14094
716-433-4035
FAX: 716-439-0822
e-mail: chhdogs@aol.com

Beverly Underwood, Executive Director
Rich Godfrey, Training Director

A non-profit organization devoted to training assistance dogs to assist people with disabilities to lead more independent, secure lives. We train hearing dogs, service dogs, multi-service dogs, seizure alert dogs and therapy dogs. All dogs in the program are rescued or donated, so the program has the double mission of saving dogs' lives and helping people. The program operates through the generous financial support of many caring people, organizations, and businesses. Application Fee $150.00.

1281 **Caption Center**

Media Access Group at WGBH
125 Western Avenue
Boston, MA 02134
617-300-3600
FAX: 617-300-1020
e-mail: caption@wgbh.org
www.wgbh.org/caption

Lori Kay, Director

Has been pioneering and delivering accessible media to disabled adults, students and their families, teachers and friends for over 30 years. Each year, the Center captions more than 10,000 hours worth of broadcast and cable programs, feature films, large-format and IMAX films, home videos, music videos, DVDs, teleconferences and CD-Roms.

1972

1282 **Chicago Lighthouse for People who are Blind or Visually Impaired**

1850 W Roosevelt Road
Chicago, IL 60608
312-666-1331
FAX: 312-243-8539
www.thechicagolighthouse.org

James Kesteloot, Executive Director
Terrence Longo, Assistant Director

The Chicago Lighthouse provides quality educational, clinical, vocational and rehabilitational services to people of all ages who are blind or visually impaired.

1283 **Christian Record Services/National Camps for Blind Children**

4444 S 52nd Street
Lincoln, NE 68516
402-488-0981
FAX: 402-488-7582
e-mail: info@christianrecord.org
www.christianrecord.org

Larry Pitcher, President

Provides free Christian publications and programs, as well as new opportunities for people with visual impairments. Free services include subscription magazines available in braille, large print and audio cassette, full-vision books combining braille and print, lending library, gift bibles and study guides in braille, large print and audio cassette, national camps for blind children and scholarship assistance for blind young people trying to obtain a college education.

1284 **Collier County Public Library**

2385 Orange Blossom Drive
Naples, FL 34109
239-593-3511

Bill Bailey, President

Systematically collect, organize and disseminate in a timely and cost effective manner, a select collection of print and non-print materials and services for the informational, educational, recreational and cultural needs of the residents of Collier County.

1285 **Columbia Lighthouse for the Blind**

1120 20th Street NW
Suite 750 S
Washington, DC 20036
202-454-6400
877-324-5252
FAX: 202-454-6401
e-mail: info@clb.org
www.clb.org

Dale Otto, President
Tammy Koger, VP

Private not-for-profit 501 (c)(3) organization offers programs that enable individuals who are blind or visually impaired to obtain and maintain independence at home, school, work and in the community. Programs and services include early intervention services, training and consultation in assistive technology, career placement services, comprehensive low vision care and a wide range of rehabilitation services.

1286 **Council of Families with Visual Impairments**

American Council of the Blind
1155 15th Street NW
Suite 1004
Washington, DC 20005
202-467-5081
800-424-8666
FAX: 202-467-5085
e-mail: info@acb.org
www.acb.org

A network of parents with blind or visually impaired children that offers support and outreach, shares experiences in parent/child relationships, exchanges educational, cultural and medicaa information about child development and more.

1287 **Dallas Lighthouse for the Blind**

4245 Office Parkway
Dallas, TX 75204
214-821-2375
800-735-2989
FAX: 214-824-4612
www.dallaslighthouse.org

Gary M Matesic, Chair
Michael Orfinik, President

Mission is to provide opportunities leading toward independence for virtually all people with vision disabilities, regardless of age.

1931

1288 **Deaf-Blind Division of the National Federation of the Blind**

National Federation of the Blind
1800 Johnson Street
Baltimore, MD 21230
410-659-9314
FAX: 410-685-5653
e-mail: nfb@iamdigex.net
www.nfb.org

Purpose is to help blind persons achieve self-confidence and self-respect and to act as a vehicle for collective self-expression by the blind.

1940

1289 **Eye Bank Association of America**

1015 18th Street NW
Suite 1010
Washington, DC 20036
202-775-4999
FAX: 202-429-6036
e-mail: sightebaa@aol.com
www.restoresight.org

Patricia Acken-O'Neil Esq, President/CEO

Not-for-profit organization dedicated to the restoration of sight through the promotion and advancement of eye banking. Promotes research and professional education with a newsletter, brochures and pamphlets.

1961

1290 **Fidelco Guide Dog Foundation**

PO Box 142
Bloomfield, CT 06002
860-243-5200
FAX: 860-243-7215
e-mail: admissions@fidelco.org
www.fidelco.org

Roberta C Kaman, President

Purpose is to breed, train and place Fidelco German shepherd guide dogs with blind persons throughout the Northeast. Provides training services to blind persons, reviews performance of the guide dog teams to see that satisfactory level of achievement is maintained, utilizes genetic processes and clinical methods to improve and refine the breed and maintains an ongoing program for development and improvement of training methods.

1961

1291 **Fight for Sight**

381 Park Avenue S
Suite 809
New York, NY 10013
212-679-6060
FAX: 212-679-4466

Voluntary health organization that works to conquer defective sight and blindness. Provides grants to accredited medical colleges and institutions to help supply equipment, technical assistance and materials for research projects and a limited number of clinical service projects.

1292 **Greater Boston Aid to the Blind**

1980 Center Street
W Roxbury, MA 02132
617-323-5111
FAX: 617-323-6687
e-mail: eyeinfo@gbab.org
www.gbab.org

Nancy Deehan, President

Dedicated exclusively to the rehabilitation and support of visually impaired people aged 50 and over.

1912

1293 **Guide Dog Users**

American Council of the Blind
1155 15th Street NW
Suite 1004
Washington, DC 20005
202-467-5081
800-424-8666
FAX: 202-467-5085
e-mail: info@acb.org
www.acb.org

Promotes the acceptance of blind people and their dogs, works for enforcement and expansion of laws admitting guide dogs into public places, advocates for quality training and follow-up services.

1294 **Guide Dogs for the Blind**

PO Box 151200
San Rafael, CA 94915
415-499-4000
800-295-4050
FAX: 415-499-4035
e-mail: information@guidedogs.com
www.guidedogs.com

Sue Sullivan, Admissions Manager

Offers dog guides for qualified visually impaired people in the United States and Canada. No charge for dog or training.

1942

1295 Guiding Eyes for the Blind

611 Granite Springs Road
Yorktown Heights, NY 10598
914-245-4024
800-942-0149
FAX: 914-245-1609
e-mail: info@guidingeyes.org
www.guidingeyes.org

William D Badger, President and CEO
Bev Klayman, Manager of Admissions Services

Provides the means for blind and visually impaired individuals to achieve mobility, independence and companionship through the use of our professionally bred and trained guide dogs. Each month Guiding Eyes graduates approximately 12 guide dog/student teams from all over the US, Canada, and internationally. The guide dogs, 26 day residential training program, special needs program and lifetime follow-up services are offered at no cost to the students. Also provides at home training at no cost.

1954

1296 Guiding Eyes for the Blind: Breeding and Placement Center

Guiding Eyes for the Blind
361 Route 164
Patterson, NY 12563
845-878-3867
FAX: 845-878-3749
e-mail: info@guidingeyes.org
www.guidingeyes.org

William D Badger, President and CEO
Bev Klayman, Manager of Admissions Services

Provides the means for blind and visually impaired individuals to achieve mobility, independence and companionship through the use of our professionally bred and trained guide dogs. Each month Guiding Eyes graduates approximately 12 guide dog/student teams from all over the US, Canada, and internationally. The guide dogs, 26 day residential training program, special needs program and lifetime follow-up services are offered at no cost to the students. Also provides at home training at no cost.

1954

1297 Helen Keller National Center

111 Middle Neck Road
Sands Point, NY 11050
516-944-8900
800-225-0411
FAX: 516-944-7302
e-mail: hkncdir@aol.com
www.helenkeller.org/national

Joseph McNulty, Executive Director

Provides evaluation and training in vocational skills, adaptive technology and computer skills, orientation and mobility, independent living, communication, speech-language skills, creative arts, fitness and leisure activities.

1298 Horizons for the Blind

2 N Williams Street
Crystal Lake, IL 60014
815-444-8800
FAX: 815-444-8830
e-mail: mail@horizons-blind.org
www.horizons-blind.org

Mission is to improve the quality of life for people who are blind or visually impaired by increasing accessibility to culture, education, recreation and consumer information on a national basis.

1977

1299 Information Access Project: National Federation of the Blind

1800 Johnson Street
Baltimore, MD 21230
410-659-9314
FAX: 410-685-5653
e-mail: nfb@nfb.org
www.nfb.org

Marc Maurer, President

Assists entities covered by the ADA in finding methods for converting visually displayed information, such as flyers, brochures and pamphlets, to formats accessible to individuals who are visually impaired.

1300 Institute for Families of Blind Children

1300 N Vermont, Suite 305
PO Box 54700
Los Angeles, CA 90054
323-669-4649
FAX: 323-665-7869
www.instituteforfamilies.org

Nancy Mansfield MA, Executive Director

Offers counseling and support to families facing the devastating diagnosis of blindness in their child. Provides skilled professional assistance to help a family to cope. A clearinghouse of information for these families and their physicians through the publication of medical journal articles, books, videotapes and other training materials.

1987

1301 International Agency for the Prevention of Blindness

National Eye Institute
2020 Vision Place
Bethesda, MD 20892
301-496-5248
800-869-2020
FAX: 301-402-1065
www.nei.nih.gov

Hannah B Faal MD, President
Suzanne Gilbert, VP

This agency was established in 1975 as a coordinating, umbrella organization to lead an international effort in mobilizing resources for blindness prevention activities.

1975

1302 International Association of Audio Information Services (IAAIS)

1102 W International Airport Road
Anchorage, AK 99518
412-434-6023
800-280-5325
e-mail: aiblink@ak.net
www.iaais.org

Ben Martin, President
Lori Miller, Administrative Assistant

Encourages and supports the establishment and maintenance of services that provide access to printed information for individuals who cannot read conventional print because of blindness or any other visual, physical or learning disability.

1977

1303 Jewish Braille Institute of America

110 E 30th Street
New York, NY 10016
212-889-2525
800-433-1531
FAX: 212-689-3692
e-mail: admin@jbilibrary.org
www.jbilibrary.org

Ellen Isler MD, Executive VP
Israel A Taub, Associate Director

Seeks the integration of Jews who are blind, visually impaired and reading disabled into the Jewish community and society in general. More than 20,000 men, women and children in 50 countries receive a broad variety of JBI services.

1931

1304 John Milton Society for the Blind

475 Riverside Drive
Suite 455
New York, NY 10115 **212-870-3335**
FAX: 212-870-3229
e-mail: order@jmsblind.org
www.careministries.org/jmsfb.html

Darcy Quigley, Executive Director

Publishes free magazines and Bible studies in Braille, cassette and large print for blind and visually impaired youth and adults.

1305 Library Users of America

American Council of the Blind
1155 15th Street NW
Suite 1004
Washington, DC 20005 **202-467-5081**
800-424-8666
FAX: 202-467-5085
e-mail: info@acb.org
www.acb.org

Sharon Strzalkowski, President

Dedicated to the improvement of information access for blind and visually impaired people. Provides for chapters in states through the US to encourage the development, acquisition and use of technology which enables blind and visually impaired persons to use printed material independently in library settings and elsewhere.

1306 Lighthouse International

111 E 59th Street
New York, NY 10022 **212-821-9200**
800-829-0500
FAX: 212-821-9707
e-mail: info@lighthouse.org
www.lighthouse.org

Barbara Silverstone MD, President/CEO

Mission is to overcome vision impairment for people of all ages through worldwide leadership in rehabilitation services, education, research, prevention and advocacy.

1905

1307 Lighthouse National Center for Vision and Child Development

111 E 59th Street
New York, NY 10022 **212-821-9200**
800-821-9713
FAX: 212-821-9705
e-mail: info@lighthouse.org
www.lighthouse.org

Mary Ann Lang

Provides for the needs of children who are visually impaired and their families through professional training, technical assisance, and research. Yearly newsletter.

1308 Lions Clubs International

300 W 22nd Street
Oak Brook, IL 60523 **630-571-5466**
FAX: 630-571-8890
www.lionsclubs.org

Kay K Fukushima, International President
Dr. Tae Sup Lee, VP

1917

1309 Mobile Association for the Blind

2440 Gordon Smith Drive
Mobile, AL 36617 **251-473-3585**
877-292-5463
FAX: 251-470-8622

Mahlon McCracken, Executive Director

Offers work adjustment training, job placement, activities of daily living, mobility, communication skills and sheltered employment for adults who are visually impaired and for persons with other disabilities.

1924

1310 National Alliance of Blind Students NABS Liaison

American Council of the Blind
1155 15th Street NW
Suite 1004
Washington, DC 20005 **202-467-5081**
800-424-8666
FAX: 202-467-5085
e-mail: info@acb.org
www.acb.org

Works to facilitate progress toward full accessibility of college programs and facilities, provides opportunities for discussion of issues important to students and assists with National Student Seminars.

1311 National Association for Parents of Children with Visual Impairments (NAPVI)

PO Box 317
Watertown, MA 02472 **617-972-7441**
800-562-6265
FAX: 617-972-7444
e-mail: napvi@perkins.org
www.napvi.org

Susan LaVenture, Executive Director
Mary Zabelski, President
Kate Aldrich, VP

A partnership organization with the National Eye Health Education Program and the National Agenda for the Education of Children and Youths with Visual Impairments including those with multiple disabilities. Information and support network for parents of children with visual impairments.

1312 National Association for Visually Handicapped

22 W 21st Street
6th Floor
New York, NY 10010 **212-889-3141**
FAX: 212-727-2931
e-mail: staff@navh.org
www.navh.org

Lorraine Marchi LHD, Founder/CEO

Serves the partially seeing (not the totally blind), providing visual aid counseling and distribution, large print— including a free by mail loan library, informational literature, a quarterly newsletter, educational outreach, referrals, emotional support, and advocacy. Works with eye care professionals and the business community regarding low vision resources and accommodations.

1313 National Association for Visually Handicap ped

3201 Balboa Street
San Francisco, CA 94121 **415-221-3201**
415-221-8754
FAX: 212-727-2931
e-mail: staff@navh.org
www.navh.org

Lorraine Marchi LHD, Founder/CEO

Serves the partially seeing (not the totally blind), providing visual aid counseling and distribution, large print— including a free by mail loan library, informational literature, a quarterly newsletter, educational outreach, referrals, emotional support, and advocacy. Works with eye care professionals and the business community regarding low vision resources and accommodations.

1314 National Association of Blind Students

National Federation of the Blind
1800 Johnson Street
Baltimore, MD 21230 **410-659-9314**
FAX: 410-685-5653
e-mail: sassywolf@ev1.net
www.nfbstudents.org

Angela Wolf, President

For over 30 years, this national organization of blind students has provided support, information and encouragement to blind college and university students. Leads the way in offering resources in isues such as national testing, accessible textbooks and materials, overcoming negative attitudes about blindness from school personnels. Offers strong advocacy and motivational support.

1967

1315 National Association of Guide Dog Users

National Federation of the Blind
1800 Johnson Street
Baltimore, MD 21230 **410-659-9314**
FAX: 410-685-5653
e-mail: nfb@iamdigex.net
www.nfb.org

Provides information and support for guide dog users and works to secure high standards in guide dog training. Addresses issues of discrimination of guide dog users and offers public education about guide dog use.

1316 National Association to Promote the Use of Braille

National Federation of the Blind
5805 Kellogg Avenue
Edina, MN 55424 **952-927-7694**
e-mail: nadine.jacobson@visi.com
www.nfb.org

Nadine Jacobson, President

Dedicated to securing improved Braille instruction, increasing the number of Braille materials available to the blind and providing information about the importance of Braille in securing independence, education and employment for the blind.

1317 National Braille Association

3 Townline Circle
Rochester, NY 14623 **585-427-8260**
FAX: 585-427-0263
e-mail: nbaoffice@compuserve.com
www.nationalbraille.org

Providing continuing education to those who prepare Braille, and provides Braille materials to persons who are visually impaired. Maintains collection of Braille textbooks, music, technical tables, and general interest items. Catalogs of the Braille collection in print or Braille are free on request.

1318 National Braille Press

88 St. Stephen Street
Boston, MA 02115 **617-266-6160**
888-965-8965
FAX: 617-437-0456
e-mail: orders@nbp.org
www.nbp.org

Tony Grima, Marketing Manager

A nonprofit braille printing and publishing house.

1927

1319 National Center for Vision and Child Development

Lighthouse
111 E 59th Street
New York, NY 10022 **212-821-9200**
800-829-0500
FAX: 212-821-9707
e-mail: info@lighthouse.org
www.lighthouse.org

1320 National Diabetes Action Network for the Blind

National Federation of the Blind
1412 I-70 Drive SW
Suite C
Columbia, MO 65203 **573-875-8911**
e-mail: ebryant@socket.net
www.nfb.org/diabetes.htm

Leading support and information organization of persons losing vision due to diabetes. Provides personal contact and resource information with other blind diabetics about non-visual techniques of independently managing diabetes, monitoring glucose levels, measuring insulin and other matters concerning diabetes. Publishes Voice of the Diabetic, the leading publication about diabetes and blindness.

1321 National Eye Institute: National Institute of Health

2020 Vision Place
Bethesda, MD 20892 **301-496-5248**
800-869-2020
FAX: 301-402-1065
e-mail: 2020@nei.nih.gov
www.nei.nih.gov

Protects and prolongs the vision of the American people. Conducts and supports research that helps prevent and treat eye diseases and other disorders of vision.

1968

1322 National Federation of the Blind

1800 Johnson Street
Baltimore, MD 21230 **410-659-9314**
FAX: 410-685-5653
e-mail: nfb@access.digex.net
www.nfb.org

Marc Maurer, President

The largest membership organization of blind people in the nation, with chapters in every state and approximately 50,000 individual members. It seeks to integrate the blind into society on the basis of equality with the sighted so that the blind are seen as normal, participating citizens. Has 700 local chapters.

1323 National Federation of the Blind: Human Services Division

6656 S Lincoln
Littleton, CO 80121 **303-703-8198**
800-401-4632
e-mail: jdeden@ccb-denver.org
www.nfb.org

Julie Deden, President

Membership organization of blind persons working in counseling, personnel, psychology, social work, psychiatry, rehabilitation and other social science and human resource fields. Dedicated to improving employment opportunities and advancement for blind persons and provides resources regarding blindness-related techniques and methods used in these fields.

1324 National Federation of the Blind: Masonic Square Club

46 Powderock Place
Baltimore, MD 21236
410-598-0155
FAX: 410-685-5653
e-mail: nfb@iamdigex.net
www.nfb.org

Fred Flowers, President

Blind individuals committed to sharing of Masonic experiences, goals and history.

1325 National Federation of the Blind: Music Division

National Association of Blind Musicians
1740 Tamarack Lane
Janesville, WI 53545
608-752-8749
e-mail: lmentink@tds.net
www.nfb.org

Linda Mentink, President

Blind persons dedicated to advancing employment and entertainment opportunities in various music fields. Offers support and information regarding copyright, publishing, promotion and other career details.

1326 National Industries for the Blind

1901 N Beauregard Street
Suite 200
Alexandria, VA 22311
703-998-0770
FAX: 703-998-8268
www.nib.org

Jim Gibbons, President/CEO
Angela Jackson, VP/Corporate Communications

A nonprofit organization that represents over 100 associated industries serving people who are blind in thirty-six states. These agencies serve people who are blind or visually impaired and help them to reach their full potential. Services include job and family counseling, job skills training, instruction in Braille and other communication skills, children's programs and more.

1327 National Organization of Parents of Blind Children

National Federation of the Blind
1800 Johnson Street
Baltimore, MD 21230
410-659-9314
FAX: 410-685-5653
e-mail: bcheadle@nfb.org
www.nfb.org/nopbc.htm

Barbara Cheadle, President

Support, information and advocacy organization of parents of blind or visually impaired children. Addresses issues ranging from help to parents of a newborn blind infant, mobility and Braille instruction, education, social and community participation, development of self-confidence and other vital factors involved in the growth of a blind child. Strong national network of contacts with other parents offers encouragement and positive philosophical support. Publishes Future Reflections.

1328 National Organization of the Senior Blind

111 Marquette Avenue
Apartment 503
Minneapolis, MN 55401
612-375-1625
FAX: 410-685-5653
e-mail: judysanders@usfamily.net
www.nfb.org

Judy Sanders, President

Membership organization of elderly blind persons providing support and information to other blind seniors. Issues include concerns such as remaining active in community and social life, maintaining private homes or living in retirement communities or nursing homes, learning the techniques used by the blind, independently caring for oneself and maintaining a positive approach to vision loss.

1329 New Eyes for the Needy

549 Milburn Avenue
PO Box 332
Short Hills, NJ 07078
973-376-4903
FAX: 973-376-3807

Carl DeBell, Executive Director

Nonprofit, nonsectarian volunteer organization provides new glasses for those who cannot afford to buy them.

1330 Prevent Blindness America

500 E Remington Road
Schaumburg, IL 60173
708-843-2020
800-331-2020
FAX: 847-843-8458
e-mail: info@preventblindness.org
www.preventblindness.org

Ronald J Anderson, VP/General Manager

Dedicated to fighting blindness and saving sight. Nationwide affiliates, divisions, and chapters serves millions of people each year through public and professional education, community and patient service programs, and research. The organization produces educational materials including brochures. Program activities include patient advocacy, referrals and a toll-free help line.

1908

1331 Recording for the Blind & Dyslexic

20 Roszel Road
Princeton, NJ 08540
609-452-0606
800-221-4792
FAX: 609-987-8116
e-mail: info@rfbd.org
www.rfbd.org

Susan Garber, Consumer Publications Admin.

Provides recorded and computerized textbooks, library services and other educational resources to people who cannot effectively read standard print because of a visual impairment, dyslexia or other physical disability. RFB&D also provides bibliographic reference services and acts as a recording service for additional titles. RFB&D has two membership programs—individual and institutional (school).

1332 Seeing Eye

Washington Valley Road
PO Box 375
Morristown, NJ 07963
973-539-4425
FAX: 973-539-0922
e-mail: info@seeingeye.org
www.seeingeye.org

Judy Deuschle, Director Student Services

The Seeing Eye breeds, raises and trains dogs to guide blind and visually impaired people and instructs qualified individuals in the use and care of their Seeing Eye dogs.

1333 Services for the Visually Impaired

8720 Georgia Avenue
Suite 210
Silver Spring, MD 20910
301-589-0894
FAX: 301-589-7281
e-mail: judyras@tidalwave.net
www.servicesvi.org

Judy Rasmussen, Executive Director

Offers services for the totally blind, legally blind, visually impaired, and more with counseling, educational, recreational, rehabilitation and computer training services. Braille transcription services for businesses. Audio cassette and quarterly newsletter. Provides volunteer readers/shoppers.

1334 Special Technologies Alternative Resources

210 McMorran Boulevard
Port Huron, MI 48068
810-982-3600
800-272-8570
FAX: 810-987-6768
TTY:877-472-7840
e-mail: star@sccl.lib.mi.us
www.sccl.lib.mi.us/star.html

Mary JoKoch, Coordinator

Addresses the needs of a very unique diverse group of people by offering a full range of library services for people who cannot read standard print. Provides reading material in specialized formats that permit individuals with disabilities to have access to the written word, delivering to customer's mailboxes free of charge. Talking Book Machines, recorded books and magazines, descriptive videos, large print editions and braille books and magazines.

1335 Taping for the Blind

3935 Essex Lane
Houston, TX 77027
713-622-2767
FAX: 713-622-2772
www.tapingfortheblind.org

Cynthia Franzetti, Executive Director

Broadcasts on HTBR, Houston's Taping For The Blind radio, a free 24-hour radio reading service and custom records reading material on audiotape, copied onto cassettes, for use by blind and physically handicapped persons. Promotes increased interest in and use of, free audio materials.

1336 United States Association of Blind Athletes

33 N Institute Brown Hall
Colorado Springs, CO 80903
719-333-4195
FAX: 719-630-0616
e-mail: media@usaba.org
www.usaba.org

Mark Lucas, Acting Executive Director
Nicole Jamentas, Communications Officer

Athletic association for blind athletes, this association is the national governing body for the United States visually impaired athletes. Quarterly newsletter.

1337 Vermont Association for the Blind and Visually Impaired

37 Elmwood Avenue
Burlington, VT 05401
802-863-1358
800-639-5861
FAX: 802-863-1481
e-mail: vabvi@aol.com
www.vabvi.org

Stephen Pouliot, Executive Director

Information and referral services.

1338 Vision Foundation

818 Mount Auburn Street
Watertown, MA 02472
781-926-4232
800-852-3029
FAX: 781-926-1412

Barbara Kibler, Executive Director

Offers peer counseling, support groups, seminars, information and referral and services for persons with vision loss, AIDS project, rehabilitation services for elders with vision loss.

1339 Vision World Wide

UN Printing
5707 Brockton Drive
Suite 302
Indianaplis, IN 46220
317-254-1332
800-431-1739
FAX: 317-251-6588
e-mail: info@visionww.org
www.visionww.org

Patricia L Price, President/Managing Editor

Believing there is hope when vision fails, Vision World Wide provides relevant information on a variety of topics through its Information and referral Helpline, Website, E-Mail Announce Lists, Information Packets, and Journal, Vision Enhancement -all designed to encourage and support individuals with vision loss, family members, and professionals who serve them. Journal available in large print, audiocassette, computer disc and enhanced letter format. Also provides consumer protection services.

1340 Visions/Services for the Blind & Visually Impaired

500 Greenwich Street
3rd Floor
New York, NY 10013
212-625-1616
888-245-8333
FAX: 212-219-4078
e-mail: info@visionsvcb.org
www.visionsvcb.org

Diane Weiss, Director Rehabilitation
Betsy Fabricant, Director Programs
Nancy D Miller, Executive Director

Offers rehabilitation services for blind persons of all ages in New York City; self study kits on audio cassette for blind and visually impaired persons in the areas of personal management, mobility training and sensory development.Vacation camp for the Blind offers year round residential recreation and rehabilitation programs located in Rockland county. Community center for blind persons.

1341 Visually Impaired Veterans of America

American Council of the Blind
1155 15th Street NW
Suite 1004
Washington, DC 20005
202-467-5081
800-424-8666
FAX: 202-467-5085
e-mail: info@acb.org
www.acb.org

Directs members to resources, promotes the rights of visually impaired veterans to receive all benefits, encourages research and development of new products for blind people.

1342 Washington Ear

35 University Boulevard E
Silver Spring, MD 20901
301-681-6636
FAX: 301-681-5227
e-mail: info@washear.org
www.washear.org

Nancy Knauss, Administrative Director

A nonprofit organization providing reading and information services for the blind, visually impaired and physically disabled persons who cannot effectively read print, see plays, watch television programs or view museum exhibits. This organization provides radio reading services, dial-in telephone newspaper service, National Symphony Orchestra program notes on audio cassette and raised line and large print atlases and books.

Alabama

1343 **ASCCA**

Alabama Easter Seal Society
Camp ASCCA
PO Box 21
Jacksons Gap, AL 36861 **256-825-9226**
800-843-2267
FAX: 256-825-8332
e-mail: ascca@webshoppe.net
www.campascca.org

Jerry Bynam, Director

Programs for campers with asthma/respiratory ailments, blood disorders, diabetes, epilepsy and spina bifida. Coed, ages 6-99. One-week sessions June-August.

1344 **Adventure Program**

Lakeshore Foundation
4000 Ridgeway Drive
Birmingham, AL 35209 **205-313-7474**
888-868-2303
FAX: 205-313-7475
e-mail: information@lakeshore.org
www.lakeshore.org

The Lakeshore Foundation Adverunture Program is a community resource, not only for individuals, but also for other organizations that serve people with disabilities. They organize adventures, assist with equipment, and make every effort to increase the accessibility of the outdoors. Certified Therapeutic recreation specialists coordinate the program.

1345 **Basketball School**

Alabama School for Deaf and Blind
PO Box 698
Talladega, AL 35161 **256-761-3222**
FAX: 256-761-3278
www.aidb.state.al.us

1346 **Camp Candlelight**

Eplilepsy Foundation of North & Central Alabama
701 37th Street S
Suite 2
Birmingham, AL 35222 **205-324-4222**
800-950-6662
FAX: 205-324-4338
www.efa.org/ncalabama

Every summer, the Epilepsy Foundation offers a week-long camp for children ages 6 to 18. Activities are held on the 230 wooded acres of Camp ASCCA. Trained counselors, program staff and three registered nurses supervise the campers.

1347 **Camp Rap-A-Hope**

PO Box 161413
Mobile, AL 36616 **251-343-3042**
FAX: 251-343-3004
e-mail: msmc@ddyne.com

Sheree LaCoste, Executive Director

Camp is located in Citronelle, Alabama. Offers one-week camping sessions to children with cancer at no charge. Coed, ages 7-17.

1348 **Camp Smile-A-Mile**

PO Box 550155
Birmingham, AL 35255 **205-323-8427**
FAX: 205-323-6220
e-mail: campsam@mindspring.com
www.campsam.org

Camp Smile-A-Mile is a non-profit organization for children who have or had cancer in Alabama.

1349 **Camp Sugar Falls**

Shades Crest Building
200 Montgomery Highway, Suite 205
Birmingham, AL 35209 **205-802-6996**
FAX: 205-802-6991
e-mail: joye.taylor@tenethealth.com
www.bwmc.com

Joye Taylor
Judy Baker

1350 **Liz Moore Low Vision Center**

Low Vision Center
50 Medical Park E Drive
Birmingham, AL 35235 **205-838-3162**
FAX: 205-838-3515
e-mail: mcjones@ehs.com

Madelyn Jones, Educator Coordinator

1351 **Summer Camp for Children with Muscular Dystrophy**

700 Century Park S
Birmingham, AL 35226 **205-823-8191**
FAX: 205-823-1057

Melanie Walters, Health Care Services

Alaska

1352 **American Diabetes Summer Camp**

American Diabetes Association
801 W Fireweed Lane
Suite 103
Anchorage, AK 99503 **907-272-1424**
800-342-2383
FAX: 907-272-1428
e-mail: askADA@diabetes.org
www.diabetes.org

Eileen Stenkavich

A camp for children with diabetes.

1353 **Camp Alpine**

Skaggs Foundation
2217 E Tudor Road
Suite 1
Anchorage, AK 99507 **907-562-7372**
FAX: 907-562-0545
TTY:907-563-8284
www.sesa.org

1354 **Camp Wheeze Away**

American Lung Association
2217 E Tudor Road
Suite 1
Anchorage, AK 99507 **907-562-7372**
FAX: 907-562-0545
TTY:907-563-8284
www.sesa.org

1355 **Champ Camp**

American Lung Association
PO Box 40407
Indianapolis, IN 46240 **317-415-5530**
FAX: 317-415-5595
e-mail: admin@champcamp.org
www.champcamp.org

Provides outdoor activities and enrichment experiences for children and adolescents with tracheostomies and those requiring ventilator assistance.

1356 **Kushtaka**

Camp Fire Boys & Girls Alaska
3745 Community Park Drive 104
Anchorage, AK 99508 **907-279-3551**
FAX: 907-278-9829

Tara Markley, Camp Director

Camp is located in Cooper Landing, Alaska. Specializes in programs for campers with asthma/respiratory ailments and diabetes. Coed, ages 6-18.

1357 **Muscular Dystrophy Association Free Camp**

Muscular Dystrophy Association
2217 E Tudor Road
Suite 1
Anchorage, AK 99507 **907-562-7372**
800-478-5683
FAX: 907-562-0545
TTY:907-563-8284
www.sesa.org

1358 **Outdoor Recreation and Community Accesss**

2217 E Tudor Road
Suite 1
Anchorage, AK 99507 **907-790-2218**
FAX: 907-562-0545
TTY:907-563-8284
www.sesa.org

Arizona

1359 **Arizona Camp Sunrise**

American Cancer Society SW
2929 E Thomas Road
Phoenix, AZ 85016 **602-553-7129**
FAX: 602-224-7466

Barbara Nicholas, Manager/Programs

Camp is in Payson, Arizona. Provides one-week summer camping sessions at no charge to children aged 8-18 who have had, or currently have, cancer.

1360 **Camp Civitan**

Civitan Foundation of Arizona/Southern Nevada
444 W Camelback Road
Suite 307
Phoenix, AZ 85013 **602-264-0435**
FAX: 602-264-0628
e-mail: info@campcivitan.com

Marianne Beram, Camp Director

Camp for the physically and/or mentally challenged. Ages 12 and up. Week long summer sessions offered near Williams, Arizona. Activities include arts and crafts, hikes, sports, sing-a-longs, dances etc. $250 per week.

1361 **Camp Honor**

Hemophilia Association
4001 N 24th Street
Phoenix, AZ 85016 **602-955-3947**
FAX: 602-955-1962
e-mail: mike@hemophiliaz.org
www.hemophiliaz.org

Michael Rosenthal, Executive Director

Camp is located in Prescott, Arizona. One-week sessions for children with hemophilia or HIV and their siblings, as well as children of hemophiliacs. Coed, ages 7-17.

1362 **Camp Rainbow**

Pheonix Children's Hospital
1919 E Thomas Road
Phoenix, AZ 85016 **602-546-1000**
www.phxchildrens.com

Camp is located in Prescott, Arizona. Offers one-week sessions for children who have had, or currently have, cancer. Boys and girls ages 7-17.

1363 **Easter Seals Arizona**

903 N Second Street
Phoenix, AZ 85004 **602-252-6061**
800-626-6061
FAX: 602-252-6065
www.azseals.org

1364 **Lions Camp Tatiyee**

1016 N 32nd Street
Suite 5
Phoenix, AZ 85008 **602-244-9756**
800-246-9771
FAX: 602-244-8667
e-mail: lionscamp@aol.com
www.geocities.com/lionscampt

Pamela Swanson, Executive Director

Camp is located in Lakeside, Arizona. Provides one-week sessions for campers with a wide variety of disabilities. May-August. Coed, ages 7-17 and seniors.

Arkansas

1365 **Camp Aldersgate**

Med Camps Coordinator
2000 Aldersgate Road
Little Rock, AR 72205 **501-225-1444**
FAX: 501-225-2019
e-mail: arkcamp@aol.com

Sarah M Spencer, Director

A private nonprofit social service agency allied with the United Methodist Church which co-sponsors a series of summer medical camps with Med Camps of Arkansas, Inc., and thirteen various health agencies. The camps allow children and youth, ages 6-16, who have various medical conditions and physical disabilities to enjoy traditional camping experiences adapted to their abilities. The Camp also offers respite care, senior citizens programs, West Side Clinic and the Children's Center. Coed.

California

1366 **Ability First**

2555 E Colorado Boulevard
Pasadena, CA 91107 **626-396-1010**
877-768-4600
FAX: 626-396-1021
e-mail: mail@abilityfirst.org
www.abilityfirst.org

Brenda Starkins, Social Service Coordinator

Services include residential camping programs, aquatics and infant through adult recreational and enrichment programs and housing, adapted sports including martial arts.

1367 **All Nations Camp**
PO Box 1958
Wrightwood, CA 92397 **760-249-3822**
FAX: 760-249-4492

Ismael Nieto

Camp for children with disabilities, ages 8 to 18.

1368 **Bar 717 Ranch/Camp Trinity**
Star Route
Box 150
Hayfork, CA 96041 **530-628-5992**
FAX: 530-628-9392
e-mail: camptrinity@bar717.com
www.bar717.com

Kent Collard, Director

Offers two, three and four-week camping sessions May-September. Accepts campers with diabetes and mobility limitation. Coed, ages 8-16. Also families, single adults and seniors.

1369 **Camp Bloomfield/Foundation for the Junior Blind**
5300 Angeles Vista Boulevard
Los Angeles, CA 90043 **323-295-4555**
FAX: 323-296-0424
e-mail: info@fjb.org
www.fjb.org

Mark Vrbka, Sr Director of Programs

Camp is located in Malibu. Offers one and two-week camping sessions June-August for blind and visually impaired campers. Coed, ages 5-18. Also families and single adults.

1370 **Camp Conrad Chinnock**
Diabetic Youth Services
6300 Willshire Boulevard 100
Los Angeles, CA 90048 **323-966-2890**
FAX: 323-966-2790
www.dys.org

Tamara Smith, Director Program Services

Offers one and two-week sessions for campers with diabetes. Coed, ages 7-16. Also families.

1371 **Camp Del Corazon**
11615 Hesby Street
N Hollywood, CA 91601 **818-754-0312**
888-621-4800
FAX: 818-754-0842
www.campdelcorazon.org

Lisa Knight, Executive Director
Kevin Shannon, Medical Director
Glenn Knight, CEO

Active camping program for campers with heart defects.

1372 **Camp El Camino Pines**
Lutheran Retreats
11900 Frontier Road
Frazier Park, CA 93225 **661-245-3519**
FAX: 661-245-2047
e-mail: elcamino@lrccsca.org
www.lrccsca.org

Dianne Eller, Co-Site Director
Gene Eller, Co-Site Director
Rich Gregory, Associate Director

Camp is located in Frazier Park, California. Christian camp offering half-week and one-week sessions for hearing impaired campers. Coed, ages 8-18. Also families.

1373 **Camp Esperanza-Arthritis Foundation**
Camp Harold F Whittle
Big Bear Lake, CA 90010
800-954-2873
www.arthritis.org

A one-week camp in August that allows children suffering from arthritis to participate in such activities as horseback riding, swimming, etc. in a fun-filled environment.

1374 **Camp Forrest**
Angel View
2400 N Palm Canyon Drive
Suite A4
Palm Springs, CA 92262 **760-366-8129**
FAX: 760-366-0146
e-mail: angelviewcamp@aol.com
www.angelview.org

"Buck" Prentiss, Camp Director

Camp is located in Joshua Tree, California. Offers to one-week sessions June-August to both able-bodied campers and those with a wide variety of disabilities. Coed, ages 10-25.

1375 **Camp Joan Mier**
Ability First
2555 E Colorado Boulevard
Pasadena, CA 91107 **626-396-1010**
FAX: 310-457-6374
e-mail: mail@abilityfirst.org
www.abilityfirst.org

Kelly Privitt, Director

Camp is located in Malibu. Offers one-week sessions June-August to campers with a wide variety of disabilities.

1376 **Camp Krem**
PO Box 207740
El Sobrante, CA 94820 **510-222-6662**
FAX: 510-223-3046
e-mail: campkrem@campingunlimited.com
www.campingunlimited.com

Frances Perry, Executive Director

Camp Krem offers an traditional camping program for children and adults with developmental disabilities, encouraging choice and decision-making. Activities include swimming, hiking, backpacking, independent living, and joint programs with camps for normal campers. Six travel camps that enables campers to experience adventure and self-sufficiency is also available. Tuition $550 for 2 weeks.

1377 **Camp Laurel**
PO Box 93204
Los Angeles, CA 90093 **323-653-5005**
FAX: 323-653-0558
e-mail: info@camplaurel.org
www.camplaurel.org

Margot Andrew, Director

Provides half-week to one-week sessions for children with HIV/AIDS. Coed, ages 6-16. Also families.

1378 **Camp Okizu**
8 Digital Drive #102
Novato, CA 94949 **415-382-9083**
FAX: 415-382-8384
e-mail: okizu@aol.com
www.okizu.org

Suzanne Randall, Executive Director

Camp is located in Berry Creek, California. Offers one-week sessions June-August for children who have cancer. Coed, ages 6-17. Also siblings.

1379 Camp Paivika

Ability First
2555 E Colorado Boulevard
Pasadena, CA 91107 **626-396-1010**
FAX: 909-338-2502
e-mail: mail@abilityfirst.org
www.abilityfirst.org

Kelly Kunsek, Camp Director

Camp is located in Crestline, California. A nonprofit camp owned and operated by Ability First to provide outdoor, recreational camping services for children and adults with physical and/or developmental disabilities. Located in the San Bernadino mountains, the camp has a dining lodge and rec room, four cabins, infirmary, program building and pool that are all fully accessible. Camp is available to rent during winter/spring for up to 80 people. Coed, ages 7-70.

1380 Camp Rainbow

Amie Karen Cancer Fund
6535 Wilshire Boulevard 120
Los Angeles, CA 90048 **323-655-5977**
FAX: 310-967-1141
e-mail: joanne.borromeo@cshs.org

Joanne Borromeo, Director

Camp is located in Glendale, California. One-week sessions in August for campers with HIV and cancer. Coed, ages 7-17.

1381 Camp Ronald McDonald at Eagle Lake

PO Box 172
Susanville, CA 96130 **530-825-3158**
FAX: 530-825-3158
www2.kidscamps.com

1382 Camp Ronald McDonald for Good Times

1954 Cotner Avenue
Los Angeles, CA 90024 **310-268-8488**
FAX: 310-473-3338
e-mail: info@campronaldmcdonald.org
www.campronaldmcdonald.org

Brian Crater, Director

Camp is located in Mountain Center, California. Year-round camping sessions at no charge for children who have cancer. Coed, ages 7-18. Also families.

1383 Camp-A-Lot

ARC of San Diego
9285 Chesapeake Drive
Suite 0
San Diego, CA 92123 **858-874-3243**
800-748-5575
FAX: 858-874-3250
e-mail: palsarc@pacbell.net

Lin Taylor, Director

Offers one-week sessions for campers with attention deficit disorder, autism, mobility limitation and developmental disabilities.

1384 Camping Unlimited

Camping Unlimited for Children
PO Box 20774
El Sobrante, CA 94820 **510-222-6662**
FAX: 510-223-3046
e-mail: campkern@campingunlimited.com

Frances Perry, Executive Director

Camp is located in Boulder Creek, California. Offers one and two-week sessions June-August to campers with a variety of disabilities. Coed, ages 5-50. Camping unlimited also weekend programs and travel camps, year round progams and recreation.

1385 Camps for Children & Teens with Diabetes Diabetes Society of Santa Clara Valley

1165 Lincoln Avenue
Suite 300
San Jose, CA 95125 **408-287-3785**
800-989-1165
FAX: 408-287-2701
e-mail: camp@diabetesscv.org
www.diabetesscv.org

Sharon Ogbor, Executive Director
Barbara Latady, Development Director

Since 1974, sponsered up to 20 day camps, family camps and resident camps for children four through 17. These camps provide an opportunity for children with diabetes to go to camp, meet other children and gain a better understanding of their diabetes. The total experience can help campers develop mroe confidence in their abilities to control their diabetes effectively while enjoying the traditional camp experience. Camps are located throughout CA and parts of Nevada.

1386 Costanoan

VIA Rehabilitation Services
2851 Park Avenue
Santa Clara, CA 95050 **408-243-7861**
FAX: 408-867-4817
e-mail: sberry@viaservices.org
www.viaservices.org

Susan Berry, Camp Director

Camp is located in Cupertino, California. Serves a wide range of disabilities with half-week to one-week sessions June-August. Coed, ages 5-90.

1387 Diabetic Youth Foundation

5167 Clayton Road
Suite F
Concord, CA 94521 **925-680-4994**
FAX: 925-680-4863
e-mail: info@dyf.org
www.dyf.org

Mats Wallin, Executive Director
Janet Cooper, Camp Director
Jeff Heiser, Program Director

We offer summer residential camp programs (Bearskin Meadow Camp) and year-round educational and recreational programs for children, teens and families affected by diabetes.

1388 Easter Seal Camp Harmon

Easter Seals for Central California
9010 Soquel Drive
Suite 1
Aptos, CA 95003 **831-684-2166**
FAX: 831-338-0200
e-mail: mmooney@scruznet.com

Mike Mooney, Director Camping

Camp is located in Boulder Creek, California. One and two-week sessions for children and adults with diabetes and epilepsy. Coed, ages 6-70.

1389 Easter Seal Summer Camp Programs

2645 Pleasant Hill Road
Pleasant Hill, CA 94523 **925-689-1777**

Beverly Mayhall

Offers education, adventure and the experience and enjoyment of living-out-of-doors in a striking and challenging wilderness environment. Serves ages 6 to 60, male and female.

1390 **Enchanted Hills Camp for the Blind**
Lighthouse for the Blind
214 Van Ness Avenue
San Francisco, CA 94102 **415-431-1481**
FAX: 415-863-7568
e-mail: afletcher@lighthouse-sf.org

Tony Fletcher, Director

Camp is located in Napa, California. Half-week, one and two-week sessions for blind, deaf/blind children and adults, ages 5 and up. This program offers a basic camping experience. Activities include music, art, dance, hiking and riding. Camperships are available to California residents.

1391 **Gloriana Opera Company**
721 N Franklin Street
Fort Bragg, CA 95437 **707-964-7469**
FAX: 707-964-9653

Since 1977 superlative music theater productions all year long, plus concert, childrens workshops and classes.

1392 **Junior Wheelchair Sports Camp**
Santa Barbara Parks and Recreation Department
PO Box 1990
Santa Barbara, CA 93102 **805-564-5324**
FAX: 805-965-0500

This five-day camp is for children 5-19 years old that are physically disabled. Sports instruction in aquatics, tennis, track and field, basketball, archery and new sports activities introduced each year. The camp counselors and instructors are also physically disabled to provide the children with a role model. Fee based on fundraising efforts.

1393 **Lazy J Ranch Camp**
12220 Cotharin Road
Malibu, CA 90265 **310-457-5572**
FAX: 310-457-8882
e-mail: crazzycraig@earthlink.net
www.LazyJRanchCamp.com

Craig Johnson, Executive Director

Offers one, two and nine-week sessions for campers with ADD. Coed, ages 5-15. Also families.

1394 **Pilgrim Pines Camp**
United Church of Christ
39570 Glen Road
Yucaipa, CA 92399 **909-797-1821**
800-616-6612
FAX: 909-797-2691
www.pilgrimpinescamp.org

Mickey Stone, Executive Director

Christian camp offering one-week sessions for campers with developmental disabilities. Coed, ages 10-Adult. Also families.

1395 **Quest Camp**
2333 San Ramon Valley Boulevard
Suite 200
San Ramon, CA 94583 **925-743-1370**
FAX: 925-743-1937
e-mail: bfield12@aol.com
www.questcamps.com

Robert Field PhD, Director

Camp is located in Alamo, California. Day camp offering three to eight-week sessions including psychological treatment for children with ADD and other mild to moderate psychological disorders. Coed, ages 6-15.

1396 **Quickie Sports Camps**
Quickie Designs
2382 Faraday Avenue
Suite 200
Carlsbad, CA 92008 **760-930-1500**
800-456-8168
FAX: 760-930-1585
www.sunrisemedical.com

Tennis and basketball camps for the wheelchair bound.

1397 **Reach for the Sky**
American Cancer Society
2655 Camino del Rio N
Suite 100
San Diego, CA 92108 **619-682-7427**
FAX: 619-296-0928
www.cancer.org

Rocco Diubaldi, Director

One-week sessions for children who have had, or currently have, cancer. Coed, ages 8-18.

1398 **Reach for the Sky Day Camp**
American Cancer Society
2655 Camino del Rio N
Suite 100
San Diego, CA 92108 **619-682-7427**
FAX: 619-296-0928
www.cancer.org

Barbara Wiggins, Director

One-week sessions for children who have cancer and their siblings. Coed, ages 4-10.

1399 **Summer Day Camp**
Yorba Linda Placentia Farm YMCA
18333 Lemon Drive
Yorba Linda, CA 92887 **714-777-9622**
FAX: 714-777-1903

Clare McKenna, Program Director

One-week sessions for children with ADD and speech/communication impairment. Coed, ages 5-14.

Colorado

1400 **Breckenridge Outdoor Education Center**
PO Box 697
Breckenridge, CO 80424 **970-453-6422**
FAX: 970-453-4676
e-mail: boec@boec.org
www.boec.org

Rich Cook, Executive Director

Provides year-round adventure based wilderness and adaptive ski programs for people with disabilities. The Center excels in offering challenging, rewarding outdoor experiences individually designed to the abilities and needs of participants.

1401 **Camp Paha-City of Lakewood**
City of Lakewood Rise Above!
12100 W Alameda Parkway
Lakewood, CO 80228 **303-987-4866**
FAX: 303-987-4863
e-mail: joabur@lakewood.org
www.lakewood.org

Jo Burns, RISE Above! Coordinator
Dinah Sherrill, Camp Paha Camp Director

Three and seven-week sessions June-August for campers with all disabilities ages 6-25. Coed, ages 6-25.

1402 Camp Shady Brook
207 N Nevada
Colorado Springs, CO 80903
719-532-1539
FAX: 719-272-7026
e-mail: campinfo@ppymca.org
www.ppymca.org

Chris Pierce, Director

Camp is located in Sedalia, Colorado. One-week sessions for campers with HIV. Boys and girls 7-16. Also families, seniors and single adults.

1403 Challenge Aspen
PO Box M
Aspen, CO 81612
970-923-0578
800-530-3907
FAX: 970-923-7338
e-mail: possibilities@challengeaspen.com
www.challengeaspen.com

Sarah Williams, Program Director
Stacey Degen, Program Coordinator
Allison Bartholomeus, Volunteer Coordinator

1404 Colorado Lions Camp
Lions of Colorado
PO Box 9043
Woodland Park, CO 80866
719-687-2087
FAX: 719-687-7435
e-mail: lionscamp@aol.com
www.lionscamp.com

Jeff Rice, Executive Director
Glenn Scofield, Program Supervisor

Outdoor recreational camping for the handicapped. All normal camp activities offered. 1 to 4 staff supervision with a nurse or doctor in attendance.

1405 Easter Seals Colorado Rocky Mountain Villa ge
5755 W Alameda Avenue
Lakewood, CO 80226
303-233-1666
FAX: 303-569-3857
e-mail: campinfo@cess.org

Melissa Huber, Director

Camp is located in Empire, Colorado. One-week sessions June-August for children and adults with a wide variety of disabilities. Coed, ages 7-70. Single adults, families.

1406 Glacier View Ranch
Rocky Mountain Conference
2520 S Downing
Denver, CO 80210
303-733-3771
FAX: 303-459-3325
e-mail: vajewett@juno.com

Vern Jewett, Ranch Manager

Camp is located in Ward, Colorado. One-week sessions June and July. Programs for campers with asthma/respiratory aliments. Coed, ages 7-17.

1407 Magic of Music and Dance
PO Box M
Aspen, CO 81612
970-923-0578
800-530-3901
FAX: 970-923-7338
www2.kidscamps.com

Camp activities focus on music and performing arts for children with disabilities.

1408 Rocky Mountain Village
Easter Seals Colorado
PO Box 115
Empire, CO 80438
313-569-2333
FAX: 303-569-3857
e-mail: campinfo@cess.org
www.eastersealsco.org

Roman Kratczyk, Director

Sessions are conducted for both developmentally and physically disabled children and adults. Activities include swimming, horseback riding, outdoor education, zigline challenge course elements.

1409 Sky Ranch Lutheran Camp
161 E Saturn Drive
Suite 2
Fort Collins, CO 80525
970-493-5258
FAX: 970-493-7960

Ralph Yernberg, Director

Daily Bible study and worship for disabled campers.

Connecticut

1410 Camp Harkness
301 Great Neck Road
Waterford, CT 06385
860-443-7818
FAX: 860-443-7818
e-mail:
www.sbac.org/camp_harkness_spring_campout.htn

In 1991 a group of parents and adults with spina bifida, were brought together with the mission: to educate the public about spina bifida and issues affecting people who have this disability. To provide support and information and to promote programs that will help people with spina bifida. Since then SBAC has worked hard to support parents, adults with spina bifida and families

1411 Camp Horizons
PO Box 323
S Windham, CT 06266
860-456-1032
FAX: 860-456-4721
e-mail: lauren.perrotti@camphorizons.org
www.camphorizons.org

Lauren Perrotti, Director of Operations

Two, four, six and eight-week sessions June-August for campers with developmental disabilities and autism. Coed, ages 8-40.

1412 Camp Jewell YMCA Outdoor Center
YMCA of Greater Hartford
160 Jewell Street
Camping Services
Hartford, CT 06103
860-522-4183
FAX: 860-379-2782
e-mail: camp.jewell@ghymca.org

Paul Kamin, Camp Director

Camp is located in Colebrook, Connecticut. Two-week sessions for children with cancer. Coed, ages 8-16. Also families.

1413 **Easter Seal Camp Hemlocks**
Easter Seals of Connecticut
PO Box 100
Amston, CT 06231 **860-228-9438**
800-221-6827
FAX: 860-228-2091
e-mail: helenm@eastersealsofct.org
www.eastersealsofct.org

Sharon Nichols, Director

Camp is located in Hebron, Connecticut. One and two-week sessions June-August for campers with a variety of disabilities. Coed, ages 6-80. Families, seniors, single adults.

1414 **Hole in the Wall Gang Camp**
565 Ashford Center Road
PO Box 156
Ashford, CT 06278 **860-429-3444**
FAX: 860-429-7295
e-mail: kijico@aaol.com
www.holeinthewallgang.org

Jim Canton, Director

Low-cost eight-week sessions June-August for children with cancer and HIV. Coed, ages 7-15.

1415 **Isola Bella**
American School for the Deaf
139 N Main Street
W Hartford, CT 06107 **860-520-2300**
FAX: 860-824-4276
www.asd-1817.org

Hearing-impaired children, ages 6-19, blend educational instruction in communications with recreational activities. Qualified deaf and hearing staff members with experience in education, child care and counseling are employed at the camp.

1416 **Mansfield's Holiday Hill**
41 Chaffeeville Road
Mansfield Center, CT 06250 **860-423-1375**
FAX: 860-456-2444

Dudley Hamlin

A home not far from home where beautiful fields, forests, facilities and a caring staff support the activities and relationships of our camp families. The camp offers many programs such as: Outdoor Adventure; Tumbling; Dance; Adventure Ropes Course; Swimming; Arts & Crafts; Archery; Tennis and more to thirty boys and girls.

1417 **Marvelwood Summer**
Marvelwood School
476 Skiff Mountain Road
PO Box 3001
Kent, CT 06757 **860-927-0047**
FAX: 860-927-5325
e-mail: marvelwood.school@snet.net
www.themarvelwoodschool.com

Anne Davidson, Head of School

The emphasis in this summer program is on diagnosis and remediation of individual reading, spelling, writing, mathematics and study problems. Offered to ages 12-16.

1418 **Shadybrook Learning Center**
PO Box 365
Moodus, CT 06469 **860-873-8800**
800-666-4752
FAX: 860-873-1849

Les Kershnar

Up to seven week summer residential, individualized program incorporating educational, recreational and vocational programs. This disguised learning environment promotes independence, friendships, and social appropriateness where learning is fun and fun is learning.

1419 **Tourette Syndrome Association of CT Camp**
Sunrise Resort
Moodus, CT 06469 **203-234-0508**

www2.kidscamps.com

Delaware

1420 **Childrens Beach House**
100 W 10th Street
Suite 411
Wilmington, DE 19801 **302-655-4288**
FAX: 302-645-9467
e-mail: childrens.beach.house@dol.net
www.cbhinc.org

Diane B O'Hara, Program Director

Camp is located in Lewes, Delaware. Four-week sessions June-August for Delaware children with hearing impairment or speech/communication impairment. Coed, ages 6-12.

District of Columbia

1421 **Columbia Lighthouse for the Blind Summer Camp**
1120 20th Street NW
Suite 750 S
Washington, DC 20036 **202-454-6400**
877-324-5252
FAX: 202-454-6401
e-mail: info@clb.org
www.clb.org

Dale Otto, President
Tammy Koger, VP

Helps enable the blind or visually impaired to obtain and maintain independence at home, school, work and in the community. Programs and services include early intervention services, training and consultation in assistive technology, career placement services, comprehensive low vision care and a wide range of rehabilitation services. Highly acclaimed summer camp, picnics and holiday activities encourage blind and visualy impaired children to make new friends and experience the joys of childhood.

1422 **Lab School of Washington**
4759 Reservoir Road NW
Washington, DC 20007 **202-965-6600**
FAX: 202-965-5106
www.labschool.org

Sally Smith, Founder
Susan Feeley, Admissions Director

The Lab School six week summer session includes individualized reading, spelling, writing, study skills and math programs. A multisensory approach addresses the needs of bright learning disabled children. Related services such as speech/language therapy and occupational therapy are integrated into the curriculum. Elementary/Intermediate; Junior High/High School.

Florida

1423 **Boggy Creek Gang Camp**
30500 Brantley Branch Road
Eustis, FL 32736 **352-483-4200**
FAX: 352-483-0589
e-mail: info@boggycreek.org
www.boggycreek.org

Dorcas Tomasek, Camp Director
Roger Murtie, President/CEO
Dr Joe Chiaro, Medical Director

Year-round sessions for children with a variety of chronic or life-threatening illnesses including cancer, hemophila, epilepsy, heart defects, HIV, spina bifida and asthma/respiratory ailments. Coed, ages 7-16.

1424 **Camp Challenge**
31600 Camp Challenge Road
Sorrento, FL 32776 **352-383-4711**
FAX: 352-383-0744
e-mail: camp@fl.easter-seals.org

Melissa Guinta, Director

One and two-week sessions for campers with developmental and or physical disabilities, hearing impairment and the blind/visually impaired. Ages 6-99 and families.

1425 **Camp Thunderbird**
Florida Fund for Special Children
Camp Thunderbird
PO Box 1300
Apopka, FL 32704 **407-889-8088**
FAX: 407-889-8072
e-mail: canpthunderbird@questions.org
www.questinc.com

Shirley O'Brien, Director

Residential summer camping program for children and adults with a developmental disability. Campers enjoy swimming, sports, nature hikes, canoeing, etc. One and two-week sessions June-August. Coed, ages 8-80.

1426 **Developmental Center**
6710 86th Avenue N
Pinellas Park, FL 33780 **727-546-9681**
FAX: 727-546-8186

Dr. Eric Larson

Specifically designed for the learning disabled child and other children with difficulties in concentration, strategy, social skills, impulsivity, distractibility and study strategies. Programs offered include: attention training, visual-motor remediation, socialization skills training, relaxation training, horseback riding and more. The day camp meets weekdays from 9-3 for 3,4 or 5 week sessions.

1427 **Florida Camp for Children and Youth with Diabetes**
PO Box 14136
Gainesville, FL 32604 **352-334-1323**
FAX: 352-334-1326

Rhonda Rogers

An adventure camp for children and youth with diabetes.

1428 **Florida Diabetes Camp**
University Station
PO Box 14136
Gainesville, FL 32604 **352-334-1323**
FAX: 352-334-1326
e-mail: fccyd@hotmail.com
www.floridadiabetescamp.org

Rosalie Bandyopadhyay, Director

Camp is located in De Leon Springs, Florida. One and two-week sessions June-August for children with diabetes. Coed, ages 6-18 and families.

1429 **Florida Lions Camp**
Lions of Multiple District 35
2819 Tiger Lake Road
Lake Wales, FL 33853 **863-696-1948**
FAX: 863-692-2398
e-mail: flc@gtc.net
www.lionscampfl.org

Barbara Cage, Director

One-week sessions June-August for children with a variety of disabilities. Coed, ages 5-21.

1430 **Florida School-Deaf and Blind**
207 N San Marco Avenue
St. Augustine, FL 32084 **904-827-2200**
800-344-3732
www.fsdb.k12.fl.us

Jerry Stewart, Principal

1431 **Florida Sheriffs Caruth Camp**
Florida Sheriffs Youth Ranches
1170 Youth Camp Road
Barberville, FL 32105 **386-749-9999**
FAX: 352-447-0400
e-mail: meneli@xtalwind.net

Jodi Saks, Camp Director

Camp is located in Inglis, Florida. One-week sessions for children with ADD. Coed, ages 10-15.

1432 **Florida WMU Camps**
Florida Baptist Convention
1230 Hendricks Avenue
Jacksonville, FL 32207
800-226-8584
FAX: 904-396-6470
e-mail: vcornaire@flbaptist.org

Dr. Sharon Thompson, Camp Director

Camp is located in Marianna, Florida. One-week sessions June-July for girls with ADD. Ages 8-18.

1433 **Indian Acres Camp for Boys**
2914 Medinah
Weston, FL 33332 **954-385-3545**
FAX: 954-349-7812
e-mail: geoff@indianacres.com
www.indianacres.com

Lisa Newman, Director
Geoffrey Newman, Director

Camp is located in Fryeburg, Florida. Four and seven-week sessions June-August for boys with ADD ages 7-16.

1434 **VACC Camp**
Miami Children's Hospital
3200 SW 60th Court
Suite 203
Miami, FL 33155 **305-662-8222**
FAX: 305-663-8417
e-mail: bela.florentin@mch.com
www.vacccamp.com

Dr Moises Simpser, Director
Bela Florentin, VACC Camp Coordinator

Free week-long overnight camp for ventilation assisted children and their families.

Georgia

1435 **Camp Breathe Easy**
American Lung Association
2452 Spring Road
Smyrna, GA 30080 **770-434-5864**
FAX: 770-319-0349
e-mail: cmobley@alaga.org
www.alaga.org

Chanda Mobley, Director

One-week sessions for children with asthma/respiratory ailments and ADD. Coed, ages 8-13.

1436 **Camp Independence**
1655 Tullie Circle
Suite 111
Atlanta, GA 30329 **404-248-1315**

1437 **Camp Lookout**
Holston Conference Camping
3130 Highway 157
Rising Fawn, GA 30738 **706-820-1163**
FAX: 706-820-9911
e-mail: info@camplookout.com
www.camplookout.com

Don Washburn, Director

Offering a variety of educational opportunities for students in 1st through 12th grades. Offerings of 1/2 to 5 day programs are available

1438 **Camp Twin Lakes**
5909 Peachtree Dunwoody Road 802
Atlanta, GA 30328 **404-231-9887**
FAX: 770-351-0475
e-mail: camptwinlakes@mindspring.com
camptwinlakes.org

Larry Melnick, Director

One-week sessions June-August for children with a variety of medical problems. Coed, ages 8-18.

1439 **Squirrel Hollow Summer Camp**
Bedford School
5665 Milam Road
Fairburn, GA 30123 **770-774-8001**
FAX: 770-774-8005
e-mail: bedfordschool@aol.com
www.thebedfordschool.org

Betsy E Box, Director
Jeff James, Assistant Director
Bonnie Sides, Administrative Secretary

For ages 7-16, held on the campus of Atlanta Christian College. This camp provides remediation of reading, math and learning disabilities. A one-week camping trip to Unicoi State Park in the North Georgia Mountains supplements the academic program with field trips, hikes, swimming and other recreational activities. Camp is held during June and July.

Hawaii

1440 **Camp Erdman YMCA**
69-385 Farrington Highway
Waialua, HI 96791 **808-637-4615**
FAX: 808-637-8874
www.camperdman.net

Josh Hermowitz, Executive Director

A specialized youth camp serving the needs of the disabled.

1441 **Camp Mokuleia**
68-729 Farrington Highway
The Episcopal Church in Hawaii
Waialua, HI 96791 **808-637-6241**
FAX: 808-637-5505
e-mail: mokuleia@pixi.com
www.campmokuleia.com

David Close, Director

One and two-week sessions for children with cancer. Boys and girls, ages 7-17.

Idaho

1442 **Camp Hodia**
2875 Mountain View Drive
Boise, ID 83704 **208-375-4333**
FAX: 208-322-0402
e-mail: info@hodia.com
www.hodia.com

Don Scott, Director

Camp is located in Alturas Lake, Idaho. One-week sessions for children with diabetes. Coed, ages 8-18. Ski Camp in Sun Valley in January, ages 12-18.

Illinois

1443 **ADA Northern Illinois Area Day Camps**
30 N Michigan Avenue
Suite 2015
Chicago, IL 60602 **312-346-1805**
FAX: 312-346-5342
e-mail: sapsey@diabetes.org

Suzanne Apsey, Program Director

One-week sessions June-August for children with diabetes. Coed, ages 4-8.

1444 **American Diabetes Association: Camp Grenada**
2580 Federal Drive
Suite 403
Decatur, IL 62526 **217-875-9011**
800-445-1667
FAX: 217-875-6849
e-mail: dscott@diabetes.org

Donna Scott, Executive Director

Camp is located in Monticello, Illinois. One-week sessions for children with diabetes. Boys and girls 8-17.

1445 **Camp Little Giant**

Southern Illinois University
Mailcode 6888
Touch of Nature Environmental
Carbondale, IL 62901 **618-453-1121**
FAX: 618-453-1188
e-mail: tonec@siu.edu
www.pso.siu.edu/tonec

Randwick Osborn, Director
Amanda Young, Assistant Camp Director

One and two week sessions for campers with a variety of disabilities. Coed, ages 8-80.

1446 **Camp New Hope**

PO Box 764
Mattoon, IL 61938 **217-895-2341**
FAX: 217-895-3658
e-mail: cnhinc@rri.net
www.campnewhope.com

Kim Carmack, Executive Director
Terri Taylor, Program Coordinator

Offers advocacy services, social and recreational services and a summer camp for the disabled.

1447 **Easter Seals Camp: Illinois**

11285A Fox Road
Yorkville, IL 60560 **630-553-7361**
FAX: 630-896-6257
www2.kidscamps.com

1448 **Easter Seals: UCP Timber Pointe Outdor Center**

20 Timber Pointe Lane
Hudson, IL 61748 **309-365-8021**
FAX: 309-365-8934
e-mail: kpodeszw@easterseals-ucp.org
www.easterseals-ucp.org

Kurt R Podeszwa, Director Camping

One and two-week sessions for campers with a wide variety of disabilities. Coed, ages 6-99.

1449 **JCYS Camp Red Leaf**

26710 W Nippersink Road
Ingleside, IL 60041 **847-740-5010**
FAX: 847-740-5014
e-mail: awilson@jcys.org
www.jcys.org

Ashley Wilson, Director

For campers with developmental disabilities and mobility limitation.

1450 **Jewish Council for Youth Services**

JCYS Camp Red Leaf
PO Box 297
Ingleside, IL 60041 **847-740-5010**
FAX: 847-740-5014
e-mail: cmiller@jcys.org
www.campredleaf.bunkl.com

Carissa Miller CTRS, Director
Diane Gould LCSW, Director Special Services

Overnight summer camp for youth and adults with developmental disabilites. Family Camps, respite weekends, trips, and other special events are offered throughout the year.

1451 **Olympia**

Southern Illinois University
Mail Code 6519
Southern Illinois University
Carbondale, IL 62901 **618-453-1423**
FAX: 618-453-1445

Craig Dittmar

Located on 6,500 acres of forests and meadows on the shores of Little Grassy Lake, Olympia Camp is for mentally and physically handicapped children and adults. Among the activities offered are arts and crafts, hay wagon rides, canoeing and swimming.

1452 **Rimland Services for Autistic Citizens**

Hoover Outdoor Education Center
11285A Fox Road
Evanston, IL 60560 **847-328-4090**
FAX: 847-328-8364

Tom Ewan, Director
Alan Kromanaker, Outdoor Education

An accessible camp facility that can be utilized by groups for day use or overnight camping experiences. Six winterized cabins, a meeting facility, indoor pool, full food service, and an excellent staff are available. Educational programs can be arranged or you can utilize the facility to manage your own programs.

1453 **Shady Oaks Camp**

16300 Parker Road
Homer Glen, IL 60491 **708-301-0816**
FAX: 208-730-4127
e-mail: soc16300@aol.com
www.shadyoakscamp.org

Scott Steele, Executive Director

Shady Oaks is a nonprofit summer camp for people with various disabilities.

1454 **Summer Wheelchair Sports Camp**

University of Illinois/Division of Rehab Education
1207 S Oak Street
Champaign, IL 61860 **217-333-4606**
FAX: 217-333-0248
www.rehab.uiuc.edu/events/campbrochure.html

Rigorous camps designed for individuals with lower extremity physical disabilities. Camp attndees will spend an average of 8-9 hours a day, focusing on development and refinement of fitness, techniques and strategies. Strength training, nutrition and mental training sessions will also be included in all camps. The camp staff is comprised of athletic staff and faculty fromt the Division of Rehabilitation Education Services and local wheelchair athltes with coaching experience

1455 **Touch of Nature Environmental Center**

Southern Illinois University
Suite 6888
Carbondale, IL 62901 **618-453-1121**
FAX: 618-453-1188
www.pso.siu.edu

Randy Osborn, Camp Director
Chilang Lawless, Camp Registrant

Providing a traditional camping experience for non-traditional campers, including recreational and outdoor programs for adults and children with various developmental, mental and physical disabilities as well as learning and behavioral disorders.

1456 **Tourette Syndrome Association of IL Camp**

5102 Oakton Street
Suite 115
Skokie, IL 60077 **847-675-2121**
FAX: 847-675-2147
www.tourettenowwhat.tripod.com/tscamp.htm

1457 **Triangle D Camp for Children with Diabetes**

Northern Illinois ADA
30 N Michigan Avenue
Suite 2015
Chicago, IL 60602 **312-346-1805**
FAX: 312-346-5342
e-mail: sapsey@ddiabetes.org

Sue Apsey, Director

Camp is located in Ingleside, Illinois. One-week sessions in August. Coed, ages 8-13.

1458 **Twin Lakes Camp**

3523 Ridge Roadeet
Lansing, IL 60438 **708-889-0986**
FAX: 708-889-0994
e-mail: twinlakescamping@aol.com
kevin.lynch.students.noctrl.edu

Pete Rekitzke, President

Provides a summer camp program for special needs children and young adults. Campers suffer from a wide range of maladies including crippling accidents, Spina Bifida, epilepsy, Cerebral Palsy, Muscular Dystrophy, Quadriplegia, Paraplegia, and other disabling diseases. Campers range in age from 8 to 27.

Indiana

1459 **Bradford Woods/Camp Riley**

Indiana University
5040 State Road 67 N
Bradford Woods
Martinsville, IN 46151 **765-342-2915**
FAX: 765-349-1086
e-mail: castone@indiana.edu
www.indiana.edu/~bradwood

Gary Robb, Director

One and two-week sessions for children with a variety of disabilities. Coed, ages 8-18.

1460 **Camp Crosley YMCA**

Muncie Family YMCA
500 S Mulberry Street
Muncie, IN 47305 **765-288-4448**
FAX: 574-834-3313
e-mail: info@campcrosley.org

Richard Armstrong, Director

Camp is located in North Webster, Indiana. Half-week, one, two and three-week sessions for campers with asthma/respiratory ailments and diabetes. Coed, ages 7-17. Also families and seniors.

1461 **Camp John Warvel**

American Diabetes Association
7363 E 21st Street
Indianapolis, IN 46219 **317-352-9226**
800-228-2897
FAX: 317-357-4288
www.diabetes.org

Elaine McClane, Director Programs

Camp is located in North Webster, Indiana. Provides an enjoyable, safe and educational out-of-doors experience for children with insulin-dependent diabetes. A unique learning atmosphere for children to acquire new skills in caring for their disease. The camp experience instills confidence for the child's self-management of diabetes. Offers one-week sessions and can accommodate 200 campers, boys and girls aged 7-16.

1462 **Camp Millhouse**

25600 Kelly Road
South Bend, IN 46614 **574-233-2202**
FAX: 574-233-2511
www2.kidscamps.com

Lea Anne Pitcher, Director

One-week sessions for campers with a variety of disabilities. Coed, ages 5-99.

1463 **Easter Seal Crossroads Rehabilitation Cent er**

4740 Kinsway Drive
Indianapolis, IN 46205 **317-466-1000**
FAX: 317-466-2000
TTY:3174793239
e-mail: info@a-roads.org
www.x-roads.org

Syndie Sorensen, Marketing & Communications

A community resource working in partnership with children and adults with disabilities or special needs and their families to promote growth, independence and dignity.

1464 **Easter Seal Society: Fort Wayne**

2542 Thompson Avenue
Fort Wayne, IN 46807 **260-456-4534**
800-234-7811
FAX: 260-745-5200
e-mail: shinkle@arc-nei.org
www.esarc.org

Steve Hinkle, CEO

Offers camp respite for adults, camp respite for children, day camping for adults, recreational services for adults, and vacation get-away program.

1465 **Easter Seals Wayne & Union Counties, IN**

5632 US Highway 40 E
PO Box 86
Centerville, IN 47330 **765-855-2482**
FAX: 765-855-2482
e-mail: easterseals@juno.com

Pat Bowers, Executive Director

Providing programs and services for youth and adults with disabilities in Wayne and Union Counties, Indiana. Limited to our service area.

1466 **Easter Seals of Bartholomew County**

1531 13th Street
Suite 1110
Columbus, IN 47201 **812-314-2899**
FAX: 812-376-0019
e-mail: www.easterseals@uwbarthco.org
www.easter-seals.org

1467 **Englishton Park Academic Remediation**

Englishton Park Presbyterian
201 N Elm
Batesville, IN 47006 **812-889-2046**

e-mail: tbarnet@venus.net
www.englishtonpark.org

Lisa Barnett, Director

Camp is located in Lexington, Indiana. Two-week sessions for children with ADD. Boys and girls, ages 7-12.

1468 Happiness Bag

3833 Union Road
Terre Haute, IN 47802 **812-234-8867**
FAX: 812-234-8867

Jodi Moan, Program Director
Patricia Porter, Executive Director

Serves developmentally disabled age 5-adult; day and residential camp program; after school program; scouting; Special Olympic anticipation (basketball, athletics, bowling, softball and aquatics); and a bowling league.

1469 Happy Hollow Children's Camp

615 N Alabama
Suite 225
Indianapolis, IN 46204 **317-638-3849**
FAX: 812-988-7505
e-mail: hhcdir@aol.com

Bernard Schrader, Director

Camp is located in Nashville, Indiana. One week sessions for under-privileged, asthmatics and burn survivors. Coed, ages 7-15.

1470 Isanogel Center

7601 W Isanogel Road 50 N
Muncie, IN 47304 **765-288-1073**
FAX: 765-288-3103
e-mail: isanogel@iquest.net
www.isanogelcenter.org

Monica Sauter, Director

One and two-week sessions June-August for special needs children through adults. Coed, ages 5-99.

Iowa

1471 ADA Camp Hertko Hollow

American Diabetes Association
6200 Aurora Avenue 504W
Des Moines, IA 50322 **515-276-2237**
FAX: 515-276-2662
e-mail: srolfe@diabetes.org
www.diabetes.org

Vivian Murray, Director

Half-week and one-week sessions for children with diabetes. Coed, ages 6-16.

1472 Camp Courageous of Iowa

12007 190th Street
PO Box 418
Monticello, IA 52310 **319-465-5916**
FAX: 319-465-5919
e-mail: jmuellerleile@campcourageous.org
www.campcourageous.org

Jeanne Muellerleile, Camp Director

A year round residential and respite care facility for individuals with special needs. Campers range in age from 3-99 years old. Activities include traditional activities like canoeing, hiking, swimming, nature and crafts plus adventure activities like caving, rock climbing, etc. Campers with disabilities have opportunities to succeed at challenging activities. This feeling of self-worth can transfer to home, work or school environments.

1473 Camp Tanager

1614 W Mount Vernon Road
Mount Vernon, IA 52314 **319-363-0681**
FAX: 319-365-6411

Robin Butler

Offers camp experiences for children 7 to 12 whose special social, economic or medical needs might not otherwise allow them to enjoy a summer camp experience. This private, non-profit camp serves over 600 children each summer with the staff-camper ratio being 1:6.

1474 Camp Wyoming

9106 42nd Avenue
Wyoming, IA 52362 **563-488-3893**
FAX: 563-488-3895
e-mail: campwyo@netins.net
www.netins.net/showcase/campwyoming

Dean E Nelson, Administrator

Mainstreaming available June through August. Youth and adults with mild to moderate mental and physical disabilities can take part in a one week experience of fun and fellowship in early July.

1475 Des Moines YMCA Camp

YMCA of Greater Des Moines
101 Locust Street
Des Moines, IA 50309 **515-471-8519**
FAX: 515-432-5414
e-mail: ycamp@dmymca.org
www.y-camp.org

David Sherry, Director

Camp is located in Boone, Iowa. Year-round one and two-week sessions for boys and girls with cancer, diabetes, asthma, cystic fibrosis, hearing impaired and other disabilities. Coed, ages 6-16 and families.

1476 Easter Seals Camp Sunnyside

Easter Seals Iowa
401 NE 66th Avenue
Des Moines, IA 50313 **515-289-1933**
FAX: 515-289-1281
e-mail: pthorne@easterseals.org
www.easterseals.org

Paul Thorne, Director Camping/Recreation

Each summer from June through August, campers with disabilities ages five and up, take part in one week camping sessions, gaining skills and independence by participating in activities like swimming, horseback riding, canoeing, fishing, camping and more. Coed, ages 4-95. Accepts seniors and single adults. Financial assistance available.

1477 L-Kee-Ta

Girl Scouts of Shining Trail
1308 Broadway
W Burlington, IA 52655 **319-752-3639**
FAX: 319-753-1410
e-mail: camplkeeta@yahoo.com

Becky Godfrey, Director

Camp is located in Danville, Iowa. Half-week and one-week sessions June-August for children with asthma/respiratory ailments. Girls, ages 7-18 and families.

1478 Riverside Lutheran Bible Camp

3001 Riverside Road
Story City, IA 50248 **515-733-5271**
FAX: 515-733-5096
www.riversidelbc.org

James Cherry

Helps disabled people to develop, renew and nurture their relationship with Jesus Christ in a unique Christian environment.

1479 **University of Iowa: Wendell Johnson Speech and Hearing Clinic**

Iowa City, IA 52242 **319-335-1845**
FAX: 319-335-8851

Richard Hurtig, Professor/Chair
Ann L Michael, Clinic Director

The clinic offers assessment and remediation for communication disorders in adults and children. The clinic also offers a Intensive Summer Residential Clinic for school age children needing intervention services because of speech, language, hearing and/or reading problems.

1480 **Wesley Woods Camp & Retired Center**

Iowa Conference United Methodist
500 E Court Avenue
Suite C
Des Moines, IA 50309 **515-283-1991**
FAX: 515-961-4162
e-mail: WesleyWoods.camp@iaymc.org
www.iaumc.org

Art & Nan Allen, Co-Directors
Heidi Holmes, Retreat/Volunteer Coordinator

Camp is located in Indianola, Iowa. Half-week and one-week sessions June-August for campers with developmental disabilities. Coed, ages 18-99.

Kansas

1481 **Camp Discovery**

American Diabetes Association
837 S Hillside
Wichita, KS 67211 **316-684-6091**
888-342-2838
FAX: 316-684-5675
e-mail: ssanders@diabetes.org
www.diabetes.org

Susan Sanders, Area Manager

Camp is located in Junction City, Kansas. Offers young people with diabetes a week of fun at rock springs 4-H Center. Special attention to diabetes makes Camp Discovery a safe environment for active youth while providing valuable diabetes managment education. Call the American Diabetes Association Kansas area office for more information. Coed, ages 8-18.

1482 **Campfire USA, Heartland Council**

G Housel
7930 State Line Road
Prairie Village, KS 66208 **913-648-2121**
FAX: 913-648-2197
e-mail: tina@kc-campfire.org
www.kc-campfire.org

Tina Jinkens, Program Coordinator

Camp is located in Waldron, Missouri. Sessions for campers with diabetes and HIV. Coed, ages 5-18, families, seniors, single adults. All campfire programs are open to young people with disabilities. Specialized fitness program for blind children and youth.

1483 **Kansas Jaycees' Cerebral Palsy Ranch**

6411 SW 50th Street
El Dorado, KS 67042 **316-775-2421**
FAX: 316-775-2421
www2.kidscamps.com

Kentucky

1484 **Bethel Mennonite Camp**

2952 Bethel Church Road
Clayhole, KY 41317 **606-666-4911**
FAX: 606-666-4911
www2.kidscamps.com

1485 **Cedar Ridge**

4010 Routt Road
Louisville, KY 40299 **502-267-5848**
FAX: 502-267-0116
e-mail: cedrrdg@aol.com

Lane Mahaffey, Director

Half-week, one and two-week sessions for children with diabetes, developmental disabilities and muscular dystrophy. Coed, ages 6-17.

1486 **Easter Seal Camp Kysoc**

Kentucky ESS
2050 Versailles Road
Lexington, KY 40504 **859-254-5701**
800-888-5377
FAX: 502-732-0783
e-mail: fun@kysoc.org
www.cardinalhill.org

Sallie Price, Director Camping/Recreation

Camp is located in Carrollton, Kentucky. Half-week, one and two-week sessions May-August, designed for the fullest camping experience for children or adults with physical disabilities, blind, deaf, behavior disorders, mental retardation, diabetes and multiple handicaps, ages 7 to 99. Coed.

1487 **Life Adventure Camp**

Susan Ownby
1122 Oak Hill Drive
Lexington, KY 40505 **859-252-4733**
FAX: 859-225-5115
e-mail: lac@lifeadventurecamp.org
www.lifeadventurecamp.org

Susan Ownby, Program Director

Wilderness camp for children, male and female, ages 9-18, with emotional and behavioral problems. Half week and one week sessions June-August.

Louisiana

1488 **Camp Bon Coeur**

PO Box 53765
Lafayette, LA 70501 **337-233-8437**
FAX: 337-233-4160
e-mail: susannah@heartcamp.com
www.heartcamp.com

Susannah Craig, Director

Two-week sessions June-July for children with heart defects. Coed, ages 8-16.

1489 **Camp Challenge**

PO Box 641253
Kenner, LA 70064 **504-347-2267**
e-mail: campersrule@aol.com

Cathy Allain, Director

Camp is located in Harvey, Louisiana. One-week sessions for boys and girls aged 6-18 who have cancer.

1490 **LA Lions LPDCI Camp Pelican**

1835 Saint Roch Avenue
New Orleans, LA 70117 **504-944-0166**
FAX: 504-948-9555
e-mail: teebone333@aol.com

Rev. R Tony Ricard, Director

Camp is located in Leesville, Louisiana. One-week residential camp for children with lung disorders. Coed, ages 5-17.

1491 **Louisiana Lions Camps: Disabled/Diabetic Youth**

LA Lions League Crippled Child
292 L Beauford Drive
Leesville, LA 71496 **337-239-6567**
FAX: 337-239-9975
e-mail: lalions@lionscamp.org

Raymond Cecil III, Director

One-week sessions June-August for disabled children. Coed, ages 7-25.

1492 **Med-Camps of Louisiana**

102 Thomas Road
Suite 615
W Monroe, LA 71291 **337-329-8405**
FAX: 337-329-8407
www2.kidscamps.com

Maine

1493 **Agassiz Village**

238 Bedford Street
Suite 8
Lexington, MA 02420 **781-860-0200**
FAX: 781-860-0352
www.agassizvillage.com

Latasha Harris, Director

Camp is located in Poland, Maine. Camp is located in Poland, Maine. Offers two and three-week sessions June-August for children with cerebral palsy, mobility limitation and spina bifida. Coed, ages 7-14.

1494 **Bancroft Camp**

Lighthouse Road
Owls Head, ME 04854
FAX: 207-729-1603
www.bancroft.org

Joseph Kuhn, Director

Has served as a summer camp for children and adults enrolled in Bancroft programs. The camp recognizes the need for individuals with developmental disabilities to vacation with their families. The camp offers a resort program for people wishing to explore the fascinating coast of Maine or to relax in the clean New England air. Accommodations include accessible rustic cabins and bayfront cottages.

1495 **Bishopswood**

Diocese of Maine Episcopal
143 State Street
Portland, ME 04101 **207-772-1953**
FAX: 207-773-0095
e-mail: gkoch@diomaine.org
www.diomaine.org

Georgia L Koch, Director

Camp is located in Hope, Maine. One to seven-week sessions for hearing impaired children June-August. Coed, ages 7-15.

1496 **Camp Lawroweld**

Northern New England Conference
91 Allen Avenue
Portland, ME 04103 **207-797-3760**
FAX: 207-797-2851
e-mail: ldayen@nnec.org
www.lawroweld.org

Harry Sabnani, Director
Linda Dayen, Camp Secretary

Camp is located in Weld, Maine. Week sessions July for campers who are blind or visually impaired, all ages. Other camps coed, ages 9-16 and families, seniors, single adults, June - September.

1497 **Camp Waban**

5 Dunaway Drive
Sanford, ME 04073 **207-324-7955**
FAX: 207-324-6050
www2.kidscamps.com

1498 **Capella**

103 Texas Avenue
Bangor, ME 04401 **207-941-2885**
FAX: 207-941-2884
www2.kidscamps.com

1499 **Pine Tree Camp Children: Adults**

114 Pine Tree Camp Road
Rome, ME 04963 **207-397-2141**
FAX: 207-397-5324
e-mail: ptcamp@pinetreesociety.org
www.pinetreesociety.org

Peter D Phair, Director Services
Harvey Chesley, Director Operations

Maryland

1500 **Camp Glyndon**

American Diabetes Association
3120 Timanus Lane
Suite 106
Baltimore, MD 21244 **410-265-0075**
FAX: 410-663-6789
e-mail: jkakacek@diabetes.org
www.diabetes.org

Robert Rainey, Director

Camp is located in Nanjemoy, Maryland. ne and two-week sessions July-August for children with diabetes and their families. Coed, ages 8-16.

1501 **Camp Greentop**

League Serving People with Disabilities
1111 E Cold Spring Lane
Baltimore, MD 21239 **410-323-0500**
FAX: 410-323-3298
e-mail: agieser.league@erols.com
www.campgreentop.org

Cisco Nochera, Camp Director

Camp is located in Sabillasville, Maryland. Summer residential camp located in the Catoctin Mountain National Park. Since 1937, Greentop has been serving children and adults with physical and multiple disabilities in a completely accessible camp setting. Campers enjoy a traditional camping program. Medical facilities staffed 24 hours a day. Half-week/one/two-week sessions June-August. ACA/MD Youth Camp.

1502 **Camp JCC**

JCC of Greater Washington
6125 Montrose Road
Rockville, MD 20852 **301-230-3759**
FAX: 301-881-6549
e-mail: jcccamp@jccgw.org
www.jccgw.org

Diane Kendall, Camp Administrator

Camp JCC serves children with disabilities alongside their neighbors anf friends. The American Camping Association has presented a National award to Camp JCC for its extraordinary model inclusion program. We also offer a program designed especially for 13-21 year olds with severe to profound disabilities. In order for us to afford to do these things, we count on contributions to our Inclusion Fund. Four and eight-week sessions general day camp program offering June-August for children.

1503 **Camp Sunrise**

American Cancer Society Maryland
8219 Town Center Drive
Baltimore, MD 21236 **410-931-6850**
FAX: 410-931-6875
e-mail: csharp1@cancer.org

Carole Sharp, Director

Camp is located in Port Deposit, Maryland. One-week sessions free of charge to children who have had, or currently have, cancer. Coed, ages 4-18.

1504 **Fairlee Manor**

Easter Seals DE/MD Eastern Shore
22242 Bay Shore Road
Chestertown, MD 21620 **410-778-0566**
FAX: 410-778-0567
e-mail: fairlee@dmv.com
www.fairleemanor.org

Sean Proa, Director

One-week sessions June-August for campers with disabilities. Coed, ages 8-99, families, seniors, single adults.

1505 **Kamp A-Komp-plish**

Melwood Horticultural Training
5606 Dower House Road
Upper Marlboro, MD 20772 **301-599-8000**
FAX: 310-870-2620
e-mail: haldous@melwood.com
www2.kidscamps.com

Heidi Aldous, Director

Camp is located in Nanjemoy, Maryland. Half-week, one-week and two-week sessions for blind/visually impaired children and those with developmental disabilities and mobility limitation. Coed, ages 8-16.

1506 **Lions Camp Merrick**

PO Box 56
Nanjemoy, MD 20662 **301-870-5858**

e-mail: RJRainey@aol.com

Robert J Rainey, Director

Programs offered April-January for children who are blind/visually impaired, hearing impaired or diabetic. Coed, ages 6-15.

1507 **Lions Camp for the Deaf**

3261 Old Wash Road
Suite 2020
Waldrof, MD 20602 **301-893-8898**

www.lionscampmerrick.org

Rev. Edward Helm, Executive Director

This recreational camp for deaf children offers a complete waterfront program including swimming, canoeing and fishing, for ages 6-14.

1508 **Maryland National Capital Park and Planning Commission**

Special Populations Division
6611 Kenilworth Avenue
Suite 205
Riverdale, MD 20737 **301-864-0420**

Offers year round and seasonal activities and programs for individuals with disabilities and families including day camps, horseback riding, beep ball, aquatics, special events and much more.

1509 **Milldale Camp**

JCC of Baltimore
3506 Gwynnbrook Avenue
Owings Mills, MD 21117 **410-542-4900**
FAX: 410-581-0561
e-mail: rblonkchtein@jcc.org
www.campmilldale.org

Rachel Blankchtein, Special Needs Director

Camp is located in Reisterstown, MD. Four and eight week sessions, June - August. Inclusion program for children entering grades 5-13 with learning, developmental, social, emotional and physical disabilities. Self-contained program for teenagers with disabilities ages 14-21 focusing on recreational and vocational activities, including weekly field trips.

1510 **Raven Rock Lutheran Camp**

17912 Harbaugh Valley Road
Sabillasville, MD 21780 **717-794-2667**
800-321-5824
FAX: 717-794-5883
e-mail: ravenrock@innernet.net
www.ravenrock.org

Lee Sodowsky

Christ-centered program for youth and mentally retarded adults.

1511 **Youth Leadership Camp**

National Association of the Deaf
814 Thayer Avenue
Silver Spring, MD 20910 **301-587-1788**
FAX: 301-587-1791
TTY:301-587-1789
e-mail: nadinfo@nad.org
www.nad.org

Elizabeth Pollard, President
Kent Kennedy, VP
Dan Brubaker, Secretary

Sponsored by the National Association of the Deaf, this camp emphasizes leadership training for deaf teenagers and young adults. In addition to many recreational activities and sports, there are academic offerings and camp projects.

Massachusetts

1512 **AU Kamp for Kids**

Abilities Unlimited
61 Union Street
Westfield, MA 01085 **413-562-5678**
FAX: 413-562-1239

Debby Clarke, Director

Two-week sessions July-August for children and young adults with a variety of disabilities. Coed, ages 3-22.

1513 Becket Chimney Corners YMCA Outdoor Center

748 Hamilton Road
Becket, MA 01223 **413-623-8991**
FAX: 413-623-5890
e-mail: egrimes@bccymca.org
www.bccymca.org

Eric Grimes, Outdoor Education Director

Half-week and one-week sessions for campers with asthma/respiratory ailments. Coed, ages 1-99, families, seniors, single adults.

1514 CNS Camp New Connections

McLean Hospital/CNS
115 Mill Street
Belmont, MA 02478 **781-855-2736**
FAX: 781-855-3691
e-mail: cnsserve@mcleanpo.mclean.org
www.mcleanhospital.org

Liana P Morgens, Director

Six-week sessions June-August for children with autism. Coed, ages 6-14.

1515 Camp Joslin

1 Joslin Place
Boston, MA 02215 **617-732-2455**
FAX: 617-735-1925
e-mail: camp@joslin.harvard.edu
www.joslin.org

Brad MacDougal, Director
Sarah Gorman, Camp Coordinator

Camp is located in Charlton, Massachusetts. For boys, ages 7-16, with diabetes. This program offers active summer sports and activities, supplemented by medical treatment and diabetes education. Coed Winter Camp and Coed Weekend Retreats are offered during the school year.

1516 Camp Ramah in New England (Summer)

39 Bennett Street
Palmer, MA 01069 **413-283-9771**
FAX: 413-283-6661
www.campramahNE.org

Howard Blas, Director

8 week sleep-away camp for Jewish adolescents with developmental disabilities. Full camping program includes swimming, Hebrew singing and dancing, sports, arts and crafts, daily services, Kosher food and Jewish studies classes. Some mainstreaming and vocational opportunities.

1517 Camp Ramah in New England (Winter)

35 Highland Circle
Needham Heights, MA 02494 **781-449-7090**
FAX: 781-449-6331
www.campramahne.org

Howard Blas, Director

8 week sleep-away camp for Jewish adolescents with developmental disabilities. Full camping program includes swimming, Hebrew singing and dancing, sports, arts and crafts, daily services, Kosher food and Jewish studies classes. Vocational program for select group of former campers.

1518 Camp Waziyatah

19 Vose Lane
E Walpole, MA 02032 **508-668-9758**
FAX: 508-668-2665
e-mail: info@wazi.com
www.wazi.com

Penny Kerns, Director
Peter Kerns, Director

Camp is located in Waterford, Massachusetts. Three, four and seven-week sessions June-August for campers with cancer and diabetes. Coed, ages 8-15 and families, single adults.

1519 Carroll School Summer Programs

25 Baker Bridge Road
Lincoln, MA 01773 **781-259-8342**
FAX: 781-259-8852
www.carrollschool.org

C Spilhaus, Director

Academic and recreational programs designed to improve learning skills and build self-confidence. The school is a tutorial program for students not achieving their potential due to poor skills in reading, writing and math. The summer camp complements the summer school offering outdoor activities in a supportive, non-competitive environment.

1520 Clara Barton Diabetes Camp

Clara Barton for Girls with Diabetes
PO Box 356
North Oxford, MA 01537 **508-987-2056**
FAX: 508-987-2002
e-mail: bcdecamp@aol.com
www.bartoncenter.org

Brooke Beverly, Resident Camp Director
Kerry Packard, Day Camp Director
Beth Sayers, Adventure Camp Director

Girls, ages 3-17, with diabetes participate in a well-rounded camp program with special education in diabetes, health and safety. Activities include swimming, boating, sports, dance, music and arts and crafts. Two week adventure camp for high school girls offering camping, hiking, canoeing, etc. Also a minicamp (one week) for girls 6-12. Day camps are offered in Worcester, Boston, and New York City.

1521 Eagle Hill School: Summer Program

242 Old Petersham Road
Hardwick, MA 01037 **413-477-6000**
FAX: 413-477-6837
e-mail: admission@ehs1.org
www.ehs1.org

Erin E Wynne, Dean of Admission

For children ages 9-19 with specific learing (dis)abilities and/or Attention Deficit Disorder, this summer program is designed to remediate academic and social deficits while maintaining progress achieved during the school year. Electives and sports activities are combined with the academic courses to address the needs of the whole person in a camp-like atmosphere.

1522 Easter Seals Massachusetts-Agassiz Village

484 Main Street
6th Floor
Worcester, MA 01608 **508-757-2756**
FAX: 508-751-6444
e-mail: camp@eastersealsma.org
www.eastersealsma.org

Ruz Fisher, Camp Manager

1523 Four-H Camp Howe

PO Box 326
Goshen, MA 01032 **413-549-3969**
FAX: 413-268-8206
e-mail: info@camphowe.com
www.camphowe.com

Terrie Campbell, Executive Director

One and two-week sessions June-August for children with a variety of disabilities. Coed, ages 7-17.

1524 **Handi-Kids**

470 Pine Street
Bridgewater, MA 02324 **508-697-7557**
FAX: 508-697-1529
e-mail: denise@handikids.com
www.handikids.org

Mary L Gallant, Program Director

A therapeutic recreational facility in Bridgewater, Massachusetts offering after-school programs, special events, school vacation full-week and summer day camp programs. Every individual is welcome. Two-week sessions July-August.

Sliding Scale

1525 **Kolburne School**

343 NM Southfield Road
New Marlborough, MA 01230 **413-229-8787**
FAX: 413-229-4165
e-mail: ks01230@aol.com

Jeane K Weinstein MA, Executive Director
Kathleen Greco LICSW, Admissions Director

A family owned residential treatment center offering psychiatric and clinical services, special education programs, K-12, vocational programs and speech/occupational therapy to mentally challenged children and adolescents.

1526 **Madden Open Hearts Camp**

Monument Valley Road
Graet Barrington, MA 01230 **413-528-2229**
888-611-1113
FAX: 413-528-6553
e-mail: info@openheartscamp.org
www.openheartscamp.org

Eight week program for children who have had and are fully recovered from open heart surgery or a heart transplant. Four two week sessions by age group. Small camp - 25 campers per session.

1527 **Tower Program at Regis College**

Regis College
235 Wellesley Street
Weston, MA 02493 **781-768-7000**
FAX: 781-768-8339

S Marilyn MacGregor

Helps average and above average college-bound students, ages 16-17, having a diagnosed dyslexic learning disability, to adjust to a college setting. Emphasis is on instruction and academic reinforcement, affective support, awareness of support services available on most college campuses and strategy training.

1528 **Winnekeag**

Southern New England Conference
PO Box 1169
South Lancaster, MA 01561 **978-365-4551**
FAX: 978-365-3838

Bob Saunders, Director

Camp is located in Ashburnham, Massachusetts. Camping sessions for blind/visually impaired children. Coed, ages 8-16.

Michigan

1529 **ADA Teen Camp at Covenant Point**

Northern Illinois ADA
30 N Michigan Ave
Suite 2015
Chicago, IL 60602 **312-346-1805**
FAX: 312-346-5342
e-mail: sapsey@diabetes.org

Suzanne Apsey, Director

Camp is located in Iron River, Michigan. Camp is located in Iron River, Michigan. One-week sessions for children and teenagers with diabetes. Coed, ages 14-18.

1530 **Adventure Learning Center at Eagle Village**

4507 170th Avenue
Hersey, MI 49639 **231-832-2234**
800-748-0061
FAX: 231-832-1468
e-mail: alc@eaglevillage.org
www.eaglevillage.org

Suzy Colins, Camp Director

This program accepts youth, ages 5-17, who are high risk or special needs - behavioral problems, emotionally unstable or Attention Deficit. The camping experience includes canoeing, hiking, swimming and high adventure activities. Half-week, one-week, and two-week sessions June-August. Coed.

1531 **Anchor Point Camp**

RBM Ministries
PO Box 128
Plainwell, MI 49080 **269-342-9879**

Accepts mentally and physically handicapped children ages 13 and up.

1532 **Camp Barakel**

PO Box 159
Fairview, MI 48621 **989-848-2279**
FAX: 989-848-2280

Lee Brown, Program Director

Five-day Christian camp experience in mid-August for campers ages 13-55 who are physically disabled, visually impaired, upper trainable mentally impaired or educable mentally impaired, bus transportation provided from locations in Lansing, Flint and Bay City, Michigan.

1533 **Camp Catch-a-Rainbow**

American Cancer Society
1755 Abbey Road
E Lansing, MI 48823 **517-332-2222**
800-723-0360
FAX: 517-664-1497
e-mail: deb.dillingham@cancer.org
www.gl.cancer.org

Debra Dillingham, Director
Michelle Kincaid, Administrative Assistant

Camp is located in Montague, Michigan. One-week sessions for children with cancer. Co-ed ages 7-15.

1534 **Camp Niobe**

4580 S Mill Road
Dryden, MI 48428 **810-796-2480**

Joanne Mandel, Director

A six week summer resident camp program for boys and girls whose learning and behavior styles have made successful participation in the traditional camp program difficult. All camp activities have a special emphasis on building self-esteem and peer relationships. Strong in waterfront, nature, campcrafts and a special arts program.

1535 Camp O'Fair Winds

Girlscouts Fair Winds Council
2029-C S Elms Road
PO Box 349
Swartz Creek, MI 48473
810-230-0244
800-482-6734
FAX: 810-230-0955
e-mail: tplotz@fwgsc.org
www.gsfwc.org

Therese Plotz, Camp Director

Accepts diabetic and learning disabled girls ages 6-12. Also accepts girls with other physical disabilities. Please call for more information.

1536 Camp Roger

8356 Belding Road NE
Rockford, MI 49341
616-874-7286
FAX: 616-874-5734
e-mail: camproger@juno.com
www.camproger.org

Robert Heetderks

Disabled campers.

1537 Camp Tall Turf

Christian Camps/Inner City Youth
935 Baxter Street SE
Grand Rapids, MI 49506
616-459-7206
FAX: 616-456-8595
e-mail: tallturf@iserv.net
www.tallturf.org

Denise Fase, Director

Camp is located in Walkerville, Michigan. Summer camping sessions for youth with asthma/respiratory ailments and ADD. Coed, ages 8-16.

1538 Central Michigan University Summer Clinics

444 Moore
Mount Pleasant, MI 48859
989-774-3803
FAX: 989-779-2799

Designed for children, ages 6 and up, with speech, language and hearing disorders who can benefit from intensive clinical work. A wide range of recreational and social activities form part of the clinical program and promote the social use of skills learned in class.

1539 Fowler Center

2315 Harmon Lake Road
Mayville, MI 48744
989-673-2050
FAX: 989-635-6355
e-mail: info@thefowlercenter.org
www.thefowlercenter.org

Thomas Hussmann, Director

Half-week, one-week and two-week sessions June-August for campers with disabilities. Coed, ages 6-99, families, seniors.

1540 Indian Trails Camp

01859 Lake Michigan Drive NW
Grand Rapids, MI 49544
616-677-5251
FAX: 616-677-2955
e-mail: lynngust@indiantrailscamp.org
www.indiantrailscamp.org

Lynn Gust, Executive Director

Year round residential camping program for children and adults with physical disabilities. One and two-week sessions. Coed, ages 6-70.

1541 Midicha

4205 Hollenbeck Road
Columbiaville, MI 48421
313-882-0658

Judy Boelstler

Disabled campers.

1542 Salvation Army Echo Grove Camp

1101 Camp Road
Leonard, MI 48367
248-628-3108
FAX: 248-628-7055
e-mail: echogrovecamp@hotmail.com

Scott R Barger Sr, Director

Camping sessions for those who are blind/visually impaired. Coed, ages 6-18 and families, seniors.

1543 Sherman Lake YMCA Outdoor Center

6225 N 39th St
Augusta, MI 49012
269-731-3021
FAX: 269-731-3020
e-mail: RobertC@ymcaSL.org

Luke Austenfeld, Director

Summer camping sessions for campers with ADD and spina bifida. Coed, ages 6-15 and families, seniors.

1544 YMCA Camp Copneconic

Flint Michigan YMCA
10407 N Fenton Road
Fenton, MI 48430
810-629-9622
FAX: 810-629-2128
e-mail: fritzcheek@campcopneconic.org
www.campcopneconic.org

Fritz Cheek, Executive Director
John Carlson, Associate Executive Director
Jim Delp, Senior Program Director

Camp is located in Fenton, Michigan. Summer sessions for campers with diabetes. Coed, ages 3-16 and seniors.

Minnesota

1545 Camp Buckskin

PO Box 389
Ely, MN 55731
218-365-2121
FAX: 218-365-2880
e-mail: buckskin@spacestar.net
www.campbuckskin.com

Thomas R Bauer CCD, Camp Director

Camp is located in Ely, Minnesota. Buckskin assists LD and ADD/ADHD individuals to realize and develop the potentials and abilities which they possess. Teaches a combination of academic and camp activities, so the campers experience success in many areas. 1:3 staff ratio ensures the program is individualized to meet each camper's needs.

1546 **Camp Friendship**

Friendship Ventures
10509 108th Avenue NW
Annandale, MN 55302
952-852-0101
800-450-8376
FAX: 952-852-0123
e-mail: fv@friendshipventures.org
www.friendshipventures.org

Laurie Tschetter, Director

Camp Friendship offers resident camp programs for children, teenagers and adults with developmental, physical or multiple disabilities, special medical conditions, Down Syndrome, Williams Syndrome, autism or other conditions. Summer camp offers archery, sailing, horseback riding, biking, fishing, creative arts, adventure challenge programs and other activities. Weekend camps and longer available. Other services available throughout the year. Coed, ages 5-90, families, seniors.

1547 **Camp Knutson**

11169 Whitefish Avenue
Crosslake, MN 56442
218-543-4232
e-mail: rcarlson@lssmn.org
www.lssmn.org

Robert Larson

Provides a camping program for mentally and physically disabled and emotionally disturbed children and adults. Campers must come with an established group that brings its own counselors. Swimming, sailing, archery, nature study and hiking are among the non-competitive activities.

1548 **Camp New Hope**

53035 Lake Avenue
McGregor, MN 55760
218-426-3560
FAX: 218-426-3560
e-mail: cnewhope@lcp2.net
www.campnewhopemn.org

Lori Bittner, Director

CNH is a private, non-profit organization which provides quality educational, recreational and leisure opportunities to children and adults with mental, physical and other developmental disabilities. Stimulating programs and quality care. Half-week and one-week sessions June-September. Coed, ages 6-99, families, seniors, single adults.

1549 **Camp Winnebago**

19708 Camp Winnebago Road
Caledonia, MN 55921
507-724-2351
FAX: 507-724-3786
e-mail: campwinn@means.net

Cathy Greeley, Executive Director

Offers one week summer sessions for children and adults with developmental disabilities. Also, integrated youth sessions to allow friends and siblings to attend with traditional campers. Respite week-ends are offered monthly throughout the year. Travel vacations are also offered as an option. Publishes a newsletter and makes a video available. Coed, ages 6-99, families, seniors, singles adults.

1550 **Courage Center I**

3915 Golden Valley Road
Golden Valley, MN 55422
763-566-0811
FAX: 612-520-0577
e-mail: camping@mtn.org
www.courage.org

Roger Upcraft, Director

Camp is located in Maple Lake, Minnesota. Summer sessions for campers with a variety of disabilities. Coed, ages 6-99, families, seniors.

1551 **Courage Center II**

3915 Golden Valley Road
Golden Valley, MN 55422
612-520-0504
FAX: 612-520-0577
e-mail: camping@mtn.org
www.courage.org

Diane Casey, Camping Department

Summer camping sessions for children who have cerebral palsy, hearing impairment, mobility limitation, speech/comminication impairment or are blind/visually impaired. Coed, ages 5-14.

1552 **Courage North**

Courage Center
3915 Golden Valley Road
Golden Valley, MN 55422
763-566-0811
FAX: 218-266-3458

Tom Fogarty, Director

Camp is located in Lake George, Minnesota. Summer sessions for campers who have blood disorders, hearing impairment, mobility limitation or are blind/visually impaired. Coed, ages 7-70.

1553 **Eden Wood Center**

Friendship Ventures
6350 Indian Chief Road
Eden Prairie, MN 55346
952-852-0101
FAX: 952-852-0123
e-mail: fv@friendshipventures.org
www.friendshipventures.org

Georgann Rumsey, President & CEO
Laurie Tschetter, Program Director

Camp is located in Eden Prairie, Minnesota. Offers resident camp programs for children, teenagers and adults with developmental, physical or multiple disabilities, Down Syndrome, special medical conditions, Williams Syndrome, autism and/or other conditions. Fishing, creative arts, golf, sports and other activities are available. Respite care weekend camps year round for children, teenagers and adults. Guided vacations for teens and adults with developmental disabilities or other unique needs.

1554 **Professional Development Programs**

14524 61st Street N
Stillwater, MN 55082
651-439-8865
FAX: 651-439-0421
e-mail: programs@pdppro.com
www.pdppro.com

Sponsors cutting edge and popular continuing education workshops and symposia of interest to professionals who provide services to children and adults with special needs.

1555 **Search Beyond Adventures**

4603 Bloomington Avenue
Minneapolis, MN 55407
612-721-2800
800-800-9979
FAX: 612-721-3409
e-mail: travel@searchbeyond.com
www.searchbeyond.com

Tours for mentally retarded adults. A catalog of 135 tours in North America, Europe and the Caribbean is available.

1556 **St. Paul Academy and Summit School**

1712 Randolph Avenue
Saint Paul, MN 55105
651-698-2451
FAX: 651-698-6787
www.spa.edu

Marlene Odahlen-Hinz, Assistant Director

Individualized instruction in basic skills, reading, math, composition, and study skills.

1557 **Wilderness Canoe Base**
Plymouth Christian Youth Center
2301 Oliver Ave N
Minneapolis, MN 55411 **612-522-6501**
FAX: 218-388-2241
www.wildernesscanoebase.org

Jim Wiinanen, Director

Camp is located in Grand Marais, Minnesota. Summer sessions for campers with substance abuse problems. Coed to age 99, families, seniors, single adults.

1558 **YMCA Camp Ihduhapi**
Minneapolis YMCA Camping Services
4 W Rustic Lodge
Minneapolis, MN 55409 **612-821-2910**
FAX: 763-479-1333
e-mail: ymcaihd@mtn.org

Erik Dussault, Director

Camp is located in Loretto, Minnesota. Summer sessions for campers with asthma/respiratory ailments and epilepsy. Coed, ages 8-14.

Mississippi

1559 **Tik-A-Witha**
PO Box 126
Van Vleet, MS 38877 **662-844-7577**
FAX: 662-680-3164
e-mail: shine@girlscoutsnems.org
www.acacamps.org

Resident camp, camp season begins in June and ends in July sessions are one week, two weeks. Campers include girls ages 6 to 17. Capacity is 100. Financial aid is available. Activities include Arts/Crafts, Camping Skills/Outdoor Living, Canoeing/Rope Courses, Counselor Training, Drama, Hiking, Horseback Western, Kayaking, Leadership Development, Nature/Eviroment Studies, Swimming-Recreational, Team Building.

Missouri

1560 **Camp Black Hawk**
16795 Highway E
Rolla, MO 65401 **573-458-2125**
e-mail: Director@BearRiverRanch.com
www.bearriverranch.com

Coed summer camp for children and adults with developmental disabilites.

1561 **Camp Carpe Diem**
Bear River Ranch
16795 Highway E
Rolla, MO 65401 **573-458-2125**
e-mail: bugbite@mail.usmo.com
www.bearriverranch.com

Coed summer camp for children and adults with developmental disablitites who need high support.

1562 **Camp MITIOG**
Share
600 Broadway
Suite 430
Kansas City, MO 64105 **816-221-6268**
FAX: 816-221-1420

Brenda O'Dell, Director

Camp is located in Excelsior Springs, Missouri. One-week summer sessions for children with spina bifida. Coed, ages 6-16.

1563 **Camp Wee-Y**
RR 2
Potosi, MO 63664 **573-438-2724**
800-323-7300

Jean Jencks

The YMCA day camp for children ages 6-8. Children are under the direction and supervision of their counselors and engage in small group and camp-wide activities and work on developing their skills and self-confidence.

1564 **Concerned Care Recreation Day Camp**
320 Armour Road
Suite 101
North Kansas City, MO 64116 **816-474-3026**
FAX: 816-474-3029

John Whalen, Director

Summer sessions for campers with developmental disabilities. Coed, ages 7-16.

1565 **Council for Extended Care of Mentally Retarded Citizens**
5227 Shaw Avenue
Suite 100a
Saint Louis, MO 63110 **314-781-4950**
FAX: 314-781-3850
e-mail: cecmrc@aol.com

Cynthia Compton, Executive Director
Marge Lindhorst, Supported Living Director
Angela Jackson, Development Director Camp

Services are provided to adults and children with developmental disabilities. Supported living arrangements are located in St. Louis city and St. Charles County. Group home and camp services are located in Dittmer, MO. Travel program also available.

1566 **EDI**
600 Kiwanis Drive
Eureka, MO 63025 **636-938-5245**
FAX: 236-938-5289
www.wymancenter.org

Fred Schaljo

Youngsters with diabetes learn how to care for themselves while participating in a wide variety of outdoor activities and trips. The camp, managed and financed by the American Diabetes Association Greater St. Louis Affiliate, offers camperships to children from the Greater St. Louis area, ages 7-16, but nonresidents may also apply.

1567 **Hickory Hill**
PO Box 1942
Columbia, MO 65205 **573-445-9146**
FAX: 573-445-5196
e-mail: camphickoryhill@juno.com
www.camphickoryhill.com

Charles Ferguson, Camp Director

Educates diabetic children concerning diabetes and its care. In addition to daily educational sessions on some aspects of diabetes, campers participate in swimming, sailing, arts and crafts and overnight camping. Coed, ages 8-17.

1568 **Kiwanis Camp Wyman**

Wyman Center
600 Kiwanis Drive
Eureka, MO 63025
636-938-5245
FAX: 636-938-5289
e-mail: kenk@wymancenter.org
www.wymancenter.org

Ken Keusenrothen, Program Director/Education
Bethany Kjellesvik, Communications Assistant

Summer sessions for youth with diabetes. Coed, ages 8-16, run in conjunction with the American Diabetes Association. Call for program description.

1569 **Lions Den Outdoor Learning Center**

3602 Lion's Den Road
Imperial, MO 63052
636-296-4480
FAX: 636-296-4476
e-mail: wyamnld@stlouis.missouri.org
stlouis.missouri.org/501c/wyman/ldoptio1.htm

Cris Rodriguez

Varied programs for mentally retarded children, ages 6 and up, includes daily living, socialization and language skills. Sports, tent camping, crafts, and nature study are also offered. Sliding scale tuition for 2 weeks.

1570 **Sidney R Baer Day Camp**

2 Millstone Drive
St Louis, MO 63146
314-432-5700
FAX: 314-432-5825
www.acacamps.org

Astrid Balzer, Special Needs
Andy Brown, Camp Director

Co-ed day camp serving campers ages 5-12 years old.

1571 **Sunnyhill Adventure Center**

Council for Extended Care
6555 Sunlit Way
Dittmer, MO 63023
636-274-9044
FAX: 636-285-1305
e-mail: cecmrc@aol.com
www.sunnyhilladventures.org

Rob Darroch, Director

Camp is located in Dittmer, Missouri. Summer sessions for campers with developmental disabilities and autism. Coed, ages 8-99.

1572 **Wonderland Camp Foundation**

18591 Miller Circle
Rocky Mount, MO 65072
573-392-1000
FAX: 573-392-3605
e-mail: amoore@advertis.net
www.wonderlandcamp.org

Allen Moore, CEO

One-week sessions May-January for mentally/physically challenged campers and respite care. Coed, ages 6-80, families, seniors, single adults.

1573 **YMCA Camp Lakewood**

YMCA of the Ozarks
Route 2
Box 240
Potosi, MO 63664
888-386-9622
FAX: 314-438-3913
e-mail: rhall@ymcastlouis.org
www.ymcastlouis.org

Nelson Bagnardi, Director

Summer sessions for campers with asthma/respiratory ailments. Coed, ages 6-18.

Nebraska

1574 **Camp Comeca**

NE Annual Conference
Box 4553
Lincoln, NE 68503
402-464-5994
FAX: 308-784-4208

Mary Garner, Manager

Camp is located in Cozad, Nebraska. Summer sessions for campers with diabetes and hearing impairment. Coed, ages 6-19, families, seniors, single adults.

1575 **Camp Easter Seals**

Easter Seals Nebraska
7171 Mercy Road
Suite 102
Omaha, NE 68106
402-345-2200
800-650-9880
FAX: 402-345-2500
e-mail: mail@ne.easter-seals.org
www.ne.easter-seals.org

Karen Ginder, President/CEO
Val McPherson, Development Director
Sheryl Fratt, Camp, Respite & Rec Director

1576 **Camp Floyd Rogers**

Floyd Rogers Foundation
PO Box 31536
Omaha, NE 68131
402-341-0866
FAX: 402-341-0866
e-mail: unclesherman@campfloydrogers.com
http://campfloydrogers.com

Sherman Poska
Micheal Nuss, Associate Director
Sally Nuss, Medical Director

A camp for diabetic children. Coed, ages 8-18.

1577 **Christian Record Services/National Camps for Blind Children**

4444 S 52nd Street
Lincoln, NE 68516
402-488-0981
FAX: 402-488-7582
e-mail: info@christianrecord.org
www.christianrecord.org

Larry Pitcher, President

Provides free Christian publications and programs, as well as new opportunities for people with visual impairments. Free services include subscription magazines available in braille, large print and audio cassette, full-vision books combining braille and print, lending library, gift bibles and study guides in braille, large print and audio cassette, national camps for blind children and scholarship assistance for blind young people trying to obtain a college education.

1578 **Eastern Nebraska 4-H Center**

21520 W Highway 31
Gretna, NE 68028
402-332-4496
FAX: 402-332-2580
e-mail: 4hcampea@unl.edu
www.ianr.unl.edu/ianr/4h

Kelly Krambeck, Camp Director

Beautiful modern facilities overlooking Platte River for the disabled campers.

1579 Kamp Kaleo
Nebraska Conference of the UCC
825 M Street
Suite 201
Lincoln, NE 68508 **402-477-4131**
FAX: 308-346-5083
e-mail: kamp@micrord.com
www.uccnebraska.org

Judie L Luther, Director

Camp is located in Burwell, Nebraska. Summer sessions for campers who are blind/visually impaired or have developmental disabilities. Coed, ages 9-18 and families, seniors, single adults.

1580 National Camps for Blind Children
Christian Record
4444 S 52nd Street
Lincoln, NE 68506 **402-488-0981**
FAX: 402-488-7582
e-mail: info@christianrecord.org
www.christianrecord.org

Arturo Grayman, Director National

Over 50 camps throughout the US and Canada are offered at no cost to legally blind children, ages 9-19. Activities include archery, beeper basketball, water sports, hiking and rock climbing and horseback riding.

1581 YMCA Camp Kitaki
Lincoln YMCA
6000 Cornhusker Highway
Lincoln, NE 68507 **402-434-9205**
FAX: 402-434-9226
e-mail: campkitaki@aol.com
www.ymcalincoln.org

Chris Klingenberg, Executive Director

Camp is located in Louisville, Nebraska. Summer sessions for children with cystic fibrosis. Coed, ages 7-17 and families.

New Hampshire

1582 Camp Allen
56 Camp Allen Road
Bedford, NH 03110 **603-622-8471**
FAX: 603-626-4295
e-mail: campallenne@aol.com

Debbie Schulte, Office Manager

A residential summer camp for individuals with disabilities. All of the activities are conducted by individual coordinators under the supervision of Program Director. Some of the activities include, aquatics, arts, crafts, games and nature programs. All camp events, special events, evening programs, and field trips are scheduled throughout the summer and are structured to meet the individual abilities and needs of each camper.

1583 Camp Dartmouth-Hitchcock
Dartmouth-Hitchcock Medical Center Pediatrics
1 Medical Center Drive
Lebanon, NH 03756 **603-650-7708**
www2.kidscamps.com

1584 Camp Fatima
Diocese of Manchester Camping
PO Box 206
Gilmanton IW, NH 03837 **603-364-5851**
FAX: 603-364-5038
e-mail: mdrumm@diocamps.org
www.diocamps.org

Dave Coffey, Resident Director

Summer sessions for children with developmental disabilities, mobility limitation and speech/communication impairment.

1585 Camp Kaleidoscope
City of Lebanon, New Hampshire
51 N Park Street
Lebanon, NH 03766 **603-448-5121**
FAX: 603-448-4891
e-mail: recreation@lebcity.com

Jennifer Letter, Director

Summer sessions for campers with ADD. Coed, ages 5-12.

1586 Carefree
PO Box 463
Reedfield, ME 04355 **603-859-3266**

Camp is located in Wolfeboro, New Hampshire. Sessions for campers with diabetes.

1587 Easter Seal Camp: New Hampshire
260 Griswold Road
Gilmanton Iron Works, NH 03837 **603-364-5818**
FAX: 603-364-0230
e-mail: dgordon@eseals.org
nh.easter-seals.org

Douglas Gordon, Director Camping/Recreation

1588 Easter Seals NH Camp Sno-Mo
260 Grlswald Lane
Box 623
Gilmanton, NH 03837 **603-364-5818**
FAX: 603-364-0230
e-mail: dgordon@eastersealsNH.org
www.easterSealsNH.org/services/camping

Douglas Gordon, Director Camping/Recreation

Easteer Seals Camp Sno-Mo is an intergrated camp, bringing together disabled invidual ages (1-24) with able bodied boy scouts. Our emphasis is on positive social interaction while finding an individual level of sucess in all passes of the camping process.

New Jersey

1589 Aldersgate Center
PO Box 122
Swartswood, NJ 07877 **973-383-5978**
FAX: 973-383-4428
e-mail: aldersgate@garden.net
www.aldersgatenj.com

Declan Thompson, Director

Camp is located in Newton, New Jersey. Summer sessions for campers with developmental disabilities. Coed, ages 6-18 and families, single adults.

1590 Camp Chatterbox
150 New Providence Road
Mountainside, NJ 07092 **908-233-3720**
www2.kidscamps.com

1591 Camp Jotoni
ARC of Somerset
141 S Main Street
Warren, NJ 08835 **908-725-8544**

Chris Reagan, Director

Camping sessions for children and adults with mobility limitation. Coed, ages 5-99.

1592 Camp Merry Heart
Easter Seals NJ
RD 21 O'Brien Road
Hackettstown, NJ 07840 **908-852-3896**
FAX: 908-852-9263
e-mail: A.Humanick@eastersealsnj.org
www.eastersealsnj.org

Alex Humanick, Director

An organized program of swimming, arts and crafts, boating, nature study and travel offered to campers with a variety of disabilities. Coed, ages 5-80, families, seniors. Fall and spring travel programs for adults.

1593 Camp Oakhurst
NY Service for the Handicapped
853 Broadway
Suite 605
New York, NY 10003 **212-533-4020**
FAX: 212-533-4023
e-mail: oakhurst06@aol.com
www.campchannel.com/campoakhurst

James Grande, Director

Camp is located in Oakhurst, New Jersey. Summer sessions for campers with cerebral palsy, mobility limitation and spina bifida. Coed, age 8-18.

1594 Camp Sun N Fun
Arc Gloucester
1555 Gateway Boulevard
Woodbury, NJ 08096 **856-848-8648**
FAX: 856-848-7753
e-mail: bpowell.homan@thearcgloucester.org
www.thearcgloucester.org

Brenda Powell, Team Leader

Camp is located in Williamstown, New Jersey. Summer sessions for campers with developmental disabilities. Coed, ages 8-88. Activities include swimming, arts & crafts, nature, sports, games, music, dance and drama.

1595 Camp Vacamas
256 Macopin Road
W Milford, NJ 07480 **973-838-1394**
877-428-8222
FAX: 973-838-7534
e-mail: michael@vacamas.org
www.vacamas.org

Michael Friedman, Executive Director
Sandi Friedman, Associate Executive Director

Disadvantaged children with asthma or sickle cell anemia, ages 8-16, are offered special programs in canoeing, backpacking, camping, music and leadership training. Sliding scale tuition. Year round programs for youth at risk groups.

1596 Cerebral Palsy Center Summer Program
7 Sanford Avenue
Belleville, NJ 07109 **973-751-0200**
FAX: 973-751-4635
www2.kidscamps.com

1597 Cross Roads Outdoor Ministries
29 Pleasant Grove Road
Port Murray, NJ 07865 **908-832-7264**
FAX: 908-832-6593
e-mail: crossroadsom@mindspring.com
www.crossroadsoutdoorministries.org

Todd Garmer, Special Education Director
Peggy Mellors, Executive Director

Program for ages 6-15 offers Bible study, worship, swimming, crafts, hiking, canoeing and campfires. Special education program for those with developmental disabilities.

1598 Easter Seals Camp Merry Heart
21 O'Brian Road
Hackettstown, NJ 07840 **908-852-3896**
FAX: 908-852-9263

Mary Ellen Ross, Director Camping

An organized program of swimming, arts and crafts, boating, nature study and travel offered to the physically disabled, developmentally disabled, cerebral palsied, brain damaged and head injured children, ages 5-18, adults 19-75+. Fall and spring travel programs for adults, Respite Weekends, call for rates.

1599 Handi Camp
PO Box 249
Akron, PA 17501 **717-859-6404**
FAX: 717-859-6914
e-mail: handi-camp@juno.com

Brian Robinson, Handi Camp Director

Christian, overnight camping program for people with disabilities, ages 7-50, in Eastern PA and Southern NJ. Sponsored by Handi Vangelism and BCM International.

1600 Happiness is Camping
2169 Grand Concourse
Bronx, NY 10453 **718-295-3100**
FAX: 908-362-5197
e-mail: hicamping@nac.net
www.happinessiscamping.org

Keely Gibbs, Director

Camp is located in Blairstown, New Jersey. Camping sessions for children with cancer. Coed, ages 7-15.

1601 Lou Henry Hoover
Washington Rock GSC
201 Grove Street
E Westfield, NJ 07090 **908-232-3236**
FAX: 908-232-2140

Deborah Hooker, Director

Camp is located in Middleville, New Jersey. Sessions for girls who are blind/visually impaired, ages 7-18.

1602 Nejeda
Camp Nejeda Foundation
910 Saddleback Road
Stillwater, NJ 07875 **973-383-2611**
FAX: 973-383-9891
e-mail: nejeda@nac.net
www.campnejeda.com

James Daschbach, Director

For children with diabetes, ages 7-15. Provides an active and safe camping experience which enables the children to learn about and understand diabetes. Activities include boating, swimming, fishing, archery, as well as camping skills.

1603 **Oak Spring Program**

Delaware Raritan GSC
108 Church Lane
E Brunswick, NJ 08816 **732-821-9090**
FAX: 732-821-4211
www.gsofdr.org/camping/Day%20Camp/oak_spring_

Maryann Polefka, Director

Camp is located in Somerset, New Jersey. Sessions for girls with mobility limitation, ages 6-16.

1604 **Round Lake Camp**

21 Plymouth Street
Fairfield, NJ 07004 **973-575-3333**
FAX: 973-575-4188
e-mail: rlc@njycamps.org
www.njycamps.org

Sheira Director, Assistant Director

For ages 7-18, this camp provides individualized academics in reading, language development and math for children with mild learning disabilities, Round Lake also offers therapeutic recreation and Jewish cultural values to its participants.

New Mexico

1605 **Camp Challenge, Event of ADA**

American Diabetes Association
2625 Pennsylvania NE
Suite 225
Albuquerque, NM 87110 **505-266-5716**
800-342-2383
FAX: 505-268-4533
e-mail: crocha@diabetes.org
www.diabetes.org

Helen Pino, Camp Director
Christine Rocha, Area Manager

One-week camping session for children with diabetes. Coed, ages 8-13. Camp will be held at Manzano Mountain Retreat, one hour from Albuquerque, New Mexico. Please call for exact dates.

1606 **Camp Enchantment**

American Cancer Society
5800 Lomas Boulevard NE
Albuquerque, NM 87110 **505-260-2105**
FAX: 505-266-9513
e-mail: gesquive@cancer.org

Geraldine Esquivel, Director

Camp is located in Alamogordo, New Mexico. One-week camping sessions for children who have or have had cancer. Coed, ages 7-17.

1607 **Santa Fe Mountain Center**

PO Box 449
Tesuque, NM 87574 **505-983-6158**
FAX: 505-983-0460

Skye Gray, Director

Camp sessions offered to disabled campers from the ages of 1-20.

New York

1608 **Advocacy Center**

277 Alexander Street
Suite 500
Rochester, NY 14607 **585-546-1700**
800-650-4967
FAX: 585-546-7069
TTY:585-546-1700
e-mail: advocacycenter.com
www.advocacycenter.com

Paul Shew, Executive Director

1609 **Advocates for Children of New York**

151 W 30th Street
5th Floor
New York, NY 10001 **212-947-9779**
e-mail: info@advocatesforchildren.org
www.advocatesforchildren.org

Jill Chaifetz, Executive Director

1610 **American Diabetes Association**

1701 N Beauregard Street
Alexandria, VA 22311
800-342-2383
www.diabetes.org

The American Diabetes Association is the nation's leading nonprofit health organization providing diabetes research, information and advocacy. Founded in 1940, the American Diabetes Association conducts programs in all 50 states and the District of Columbia, reaching more than 800 communities. The mission of the organization is to prevent and cure diabetes and to improve the lives of all people affected by diabetes.

1611 **American Diabetes Association Summer Camp**

American Diabetes Association
20 Ramona Street
Rochester, NY 14613 **585-458-3040**
FAX: 585-458-3138
e-mail: bgaines@diabetes.org

Shawna Pierce, Area Associate
Trish Donahue, Camp Director

Camp is located in Rush, New York. Sessions for children with diabetes. Coed, ages 8-16.

1612 **Association for Neurologically Impaired Brain Injured Children**

212-12 26th Avenue
Bayside, NY 11360 **718-423-9550**
FAX: 718-423-9838
e-mail: info@anibic.org

Jeanne Parisi, Executive Director
Christine Fisher, Intake Coordinator

ANIBIc is a voluntary, multi-service organization that is dedicated to serving individuals with severe learning disabilities, neurological impairments and other developmental disabilities. Services include: residential, vocational, family support services, recreation (children and adults), respite (adult), in home support services, counseling and tramatic brain injury services (adults).

1613 **Camp Huntington**

56 Brunesville Street
High Falls, NY 12440 **845-687-7840**
FAX: 845-687-7211
e-mail: camphtgn@aol.com

Bruria K Falik PhD

A co-ed residential camp for the learning disabled, ADD, neurologically impaired and mild-moderate mental retardation.

1614 Camp Jened

United Cerebral Palsy Association NY
330 W 34th Street
13th Floor
New York, NY 10001 **212-947-5770**
FAX: 845-434-2253
e-mail: jened@catskill.net

Michael Branam, Camp Director

Camp is located in Rock Hill, New York. Sessions for adults with severe developmental and physical disabilities. Coed, ages 18-99.

1615 Camp Mark Seven

Mark Seven Deaf Foundation
144 Mohawk Hotel Road
Old Forge, NY 13420 **315-357-6089**
FAX: 315-357-6403
e-mail: execdir@campmark7.org
www.campmark7.org

Dave Staehle, Execute Director

Adirondack Mountain camp for hard-of-hearing, deaf and hearing people. Coed, ages 1-99, families, seniors and single adults.

1616 Camp Northwood

G Felt
132 State Route 365
Remsen, NY 13438 **315-831-3621**
FAX: 315-831-5867
e-mail: gfelt@nwood.com

Gordon W Felt, Director

Summer sessions for children with ADD. Coed, ages 8-18.

1617 Camp Sisol: JCC

JCC of Greater Rochester
1200 Edgewood Avenue
Rochester, NY 14618 **585-461-2000**
FAX: 585-461-0805
e-mail: jcc@eznet.net
www.jccrochester.org

Rachel Rosner, Director

Camp is located in Honeoye Falls, New York. Summer sessions for children with autism. Coed, ages 5-16.

1618 Camp Venture

100 Convent Road
PO Box 402
Nanuet, NY 10954 **845-624-3860**
FAX: 845-624-7064
www.campventure.org

In more than a dozen Rockland neighborhoods, residential, employment, rehabilitation or recreation programs have arisen to help people with disabilities contribute to the life of the community. There are, for instance, more than a dozen Community Residential Facilities, Venture Industries, Venture Day Treatment, Day Habilitation, Venture Chorus, after school programs and more.

1619 Camp Whitman on Seneca Lake

89 Main Street
PO Box 278
Dresden, NY 14441 **315-536-7753**
FAX: 315-536-2128
e-mail: presgen@eznet.net
www.campwhitman.org

Thomas D Montgomery, Director

Summer sessions for young people and adults with developmental disabilities. Coed, ages 10-adult.

1620 Casowasco Camp, Conference and Retreat Center

158 Casowasco Drive
Moravia, NY 13118 **315-364-8756**
800-699-8715
FAX: 315-364-7636
e-mail: info@casowasco.org
www.casowasco.org

Michael D Huber, Director/Manager

Camp is located in Moravia, New York. Summer sessions for children with ADD. Coed, ages 6-18 and families.

1621 Chingachgook on Lake George

Capital District YMCA
1872 Pilot Knob Road
Kattskill Bay, NY 12844 **518-656-9462**
FAX: 518-656-9362
e-mail: gpainter@cdymca.org
www.chingachgook.org

George Painter, Executive Director

Sessions for campers with asthma/respiratory ailments or who are blind/visually impaired. Coed, ages 7-16, families, seniors and single adults. Sailing programs for people with disabilities.

1622 Client Assistance Program

401 State Street
Schenectady, NY 12305 **518-388-2892**
FAX: 518-388-2890
e-mail: michaelp@cqc.state.ny.us
www.cqc.state.ny.us

Michael Peluso, CAP Director

1623 Clover Patch Camp

55 Helping Hand Lane
Glenville, NY 12302 **518-384-3080**
FAX: 518-384-3001
e-mail: cloverpatchcamp@cftd.org
www.cloverpatchcamp.org

Chris Schelin, Director
Laura Taylor, Assistant Director

Camp is located in Scotia, NY. Summer sessions for campers with a variety of disabilities. Coed, ages 5-85.

1624 Deaf or Hard of Hearing Services

One Commerce Plaza
Suite 1601
Albany, NY 12234 **518-474-5652**
800-222-5627
FAX: 518-473-6073
e-mail: dsteele@mail.nysed.gov
www.nysed.gov

Dorothy Steele, Coordinator

1625 Father Drumgoole CYO Camp

Catholic Youth Organization
6581 Hylan Boulevard
Staten Island, NY 10309 **718-317-2754**
FAX: 718-273-8361

Julia Larsen, Director

Summer sessions for children with epilepsy, hearing impairment and developmental disabilities. Coed, ages 5-13.

1626 **Freedom Camp**

PO Box 2134
Auburn, NY 13021
315-253-5465
FAX: 315-253-5465
www.cayuganet.org

Mary Ellen Perry, Executive Director

A summer day camp for youths with disabilities sponsored by Freedom Recreational Services. Freedom Camp is offered in two-week sessions at Casey Park in Auburn, New York.

1627 **Friends Academy Summer Camps**

Duck Pond Road
Locust Valley, NY 11560
516-676-0393
FAX: 516-465-1720
e-mail: camp@fa.org
www.fa.org

Matthew Bradley, Director

Summer sessions for children with diabetes. Coed, ages 3-14, families.

1628 **Gow School Summer Programs**

2491 Emery Road
South Wales, NY 14139
585-655-2900
FAX: 585-652-3457
e-mail: admissions@gow.org
www.gow.org

Brett Marcoux, Director of Summer Program
Robert Garcia, Director of Admissions

Co-ed summer programs for students ages 8-16 with dyslexia or similar learning disabilities offer a balanced blend of morning academics, afternoon/evening traditional camp activities and weekend overnights. The primary purpose of these programs is to provide a positive experience while balancing these three elements. Committed to the creation of a positive and enjoyable experience for each participant by defining and merging the goals of the camp and the school, with those of camper students.

1629 **Henry Kaufmann Campgrounds Staten Island**

667 Blauvelt Road
Pearl River, NY 10965
845-735-2718
FAX: 845-735-3544

Jeffrey Alan Coopersmith, Director

Disabled campers.

1630 **Huntington**

B Falik
PO Box 368
Woodstock, NY 12498
845-679-4903
FAX: 845-679-4903
e-mail: camphtgtn@aol.com
www.camphuntington.com

Bururia Falik PhD, Director

Camp is located in High Falls, New York. Summer sessions for children and young adults with a variety of disabilities. Coed, ages 6-21.

1631 **Kamp Kiwanis**

9020 Kiwanis Road
Taberg, NY 13471
315-336-4568
FAX: 315-336-3845
e-mail: kampkiwanis@mybizz.net
www.kiwanis-ny.org/kamp/

Nancy Ann Nowak, Executive Director

Kamp Kiwanis is a mainstream camp for underprivileged youth with and without special needs. 20 campers with disabilities are integrated into weekly sessions. Coed, ages 8-14, seniors and single adults.

1632 **Maplebrook School**

5142 Route 22
Amenia, NY 12501
845-373-8191
FAX: 845-373-7029
e-mail: mbsecho@aol.com

Donna M Konkolios, Head of School
Jennifer Scully, Director Admissions

A coeductional boarding school which offers a six week camp for children with learning differences and ADD.

1633 **Marist Brothers Mid-Hudson Valley Camp**

Route 9W - Esopus
PO Box 197
Esopus, NY 12429
845-384-6620
FAX: 845-384-6479

Bro Don Nugent, Administrator
Bro Damian Novello, Director MIV Children
Michelle Fleming, Director Special Children

Serves special people: children who have cancer or who are HIV positive, deaf or mentally retarded.

1634 **Ninety-Second Street Y Camps**

1395 Lexington Avenue
New York, NY 10128
212-415-5600
FAX: 212-415-5637
e-mail: camps@92y.org
www.92y.org

Alan Saltz, Director
Steve Levin, Associate Director

Camp is located in Rockland County, New York. Summer sessions for children with ADD, autism and speech/communication impairment. Coed, ages 5-13.

1635 **Presbyterian Center at Holmes**

60 Dantan Lake Road
Holmes, NY 12531
845-878-6383
FAX: 845-878-7824
www.presbyteriancenter.org

Peter Surgerior, Executive Director
Diane Ball, Administration Assistant

Disabled campers.

1636 **Programs for Children with Disabilities: Ages 3 through 5**

1 Commerce Plaza
Suite 1624
Albany, NY 12234
518-473-6108
FAX: 518-473-5387
e-mail: erejino@mail.nysed.gov
www.nichcy.org/stateshe/ny.htm

Erlinda Rejino, Manager

1637 **Programs for Children with Special Health Care Needs**

Department of Health
Tower Building
Suite 208
Albany, NY 12237
518-474-2084
FAX: 518-474-5445
e-mail: nhro2@health.state.ny.us
www.nichy.org/state/ny.htm

Marta Riser, Acting Director

1638 Programs for Infants and Toddlers with Disabilities: Ages Birth Through 2

Empire State Plaza
Corning Tower Building, Suite 287
Albany, NY 12237 **518-473-7016**
FAX: 518-486-1090
e-mail: dmn02@health.state.ny.us
www.nichcy.org/stateshe/ny.htm

Donna M Noyes PhD, Director

1639 Radalbek

RR 1 Box 28K
Hancock, NY 13783 **607-467-2159**
FAX: 607-467-2159

Grace Kinzer

A year-round residential program, for ages 14-18, to educate and train the mentally retarded, emotionally disturbed and learning disabled in self-help skills. The program curriculum is educational, vocational and recreational, with special workshops and programs for all ages.

1640 Ramapo Anchorage Camp

PO Box 266
Rhinebeck, NY 12572 **845-876-8403**
FAX: 845-876-8414
e-mail: office@ramapoanchorage.org
www.ramapoanchorage.org

Bernie Kosberg, Executive Director
Mike Kunin, Associate Director

Residential program which serves children, ages 4-16, with a wide range of emotional, behavioral and learning problems. A one-to-one ratio of counselors-to-campers enables children to build healthy relationships, increase self-esteem and improve learning skills. Character values such as honesty, concern for others, responsibility and the courage to do one's best are encouraged. Campers demonstrate significant gains in their ability to maintain relationships, control impulses and adjust.

1641 Rochester Rotary Sunshine Camp

125 E Main
Rochester, NY 14604 **585-546-7435**
FAX: 585-546-8675
e-mail: sknipper@rochesterrotary.org

Sheila Knipper, Director

Camp is located in Rush, New York. Camping sessions for children and young adults with a variety of disabilities. Ages 7-21.

1642 Rolling Hills Country Day Camp

A Engelberg
PO Box 837
Coram, NY 11727 **631-736-3696**
FAX: 631-736-7316
e-mail: rhdcamy@unix.asb.com

Amy Engelberg, Director

Summer sessions for children with ADD. Coed, ages 3-12.

1643 Town N Country Day Camp

Foothills GSC
33 Jewett Place
Utica, NY 13501 **315-733-2391**
FAX: 315-733-1909
e-mail: jreilly@borg.com

Judith H Reilly, Program Manager

Camp is located in Camden, New York. Summer sessions for girls 5-17 with ADD or asthma/respiratory ailments.

1644 VISIONS' Vacation Camp for the Blind

111 Summit Park Road
Spring Valley, NY 10977 **845-354-3003**
FAX: 845-354-3003

Pamela Schneider, Camp Director

Respite services offered to 18 years or older visually impaired persons.

1645 Wagon Road Camp

Childrens Aid Society
PO Box 47
Chappaqua, NY 10514 **914-238-4761**
FAX: 914-238-0714
e-mail: caswrc@aol.com
www.childrensaidsociety.org

Lukas Weinstein, Director

Camping for children with a variety of disabilities. Coed, ages 6-17.

1646 YMCA Camp Weona

YMCA of Greater Buffalo
280 Cayuga Road
Buffalo, NY 14225 **716-565-6008**
FAX: 716-565-6007
www.wnybiz.com/campweona

Robert W Walker, Director

Camp is located in Gainesville, New York. Camping sessions for children and adults with epilepsy. Coed, ages 7-16, families and single adults.

North Carolina

1647 Camp Carolina Trails for Children

American Diabetes Association
434 Fayetteville St Mall
2 Hanover Square, Suite 1600
Raleigh, NC 27601 **336-766-7436**
FAX: 704-373-9113

Rick Bridges, Director

Camp for children with diabetes is located in Clemmons, North Carolina.

1648 Camp Royall

250 Bill Ash Road
Moncure, NC 27569 **919-542-1033**
FAX: 919-542-1033
e-mail: dyell@autismsociety-nc.org
www.autismsociety-nc.org

David Yell, Director

Camping sessions for children and adults with autism. Coed, ages 4-99.

1649 Camp Sky Ranch

634 Sky Ranch Road
Blowing Rock, NC 28605 **828-264-8600**
FAX: 828-265-2339
e-mail: jsharp1@triad.rr.com
www.campskyranch.com

Jack Sharp, Director

A private, residential camp for the handicapped. This season is the camp's 55th year of providing a real camping experience for the handicapped. Camp Sky Ranch was the first private camp for the handicapped in the Southeast. Activities include: swimming, boating, horseback riding, and more. Campers must be able to walk, dress and feed themselves, and take care of their toilet needs.

1650 **Camp Tekoa UMC**
United Methodist Camp Tekoa
PO Box 160
Hendersonville, NC 28793 **828-692-6516**
FAX: 828-697-3288
e-mail: director@camptekoa.org

James S Johnson, Director

Camping for children with asthma/respiratory ailments, hearing impairment and developmental disabilities. Coed, ages 6-17.

1651 **Cullowhee Experience**
Western Carolina University
Culowhee, NC 28723 **828-227-7353**
FAX: 828-227-7353
e-mail: EBEAVER@WCU.EDU
www.wcu.edu/cullowhee_exp

1652 **Mount Shepherd Retreat Center**
1045 Mount Shepherd Road Ext
Asheboro, NC 27203 **336-629-4085**
FAX: 336-629-4880
e-mail: mtsheph@asheboro.com
www.asheboro.com/mtshepherd

Rev. Kent L Shrader, Director

Camping for children with developmental disabilities. Coed, ages 7-17.

1653 **SOAR Summer Adventures**
PO Box 388
Balsam, NC 28707 **828-456-3435**
FAX: 708-456-3449

John Willson, Dir. of LD/ADD Prg.
Jonathan Jones, Executive Director

A nonprofit adventure program working with disadvantaged youth diagnosed with learning disabilities in an outdoor, challenge based environment. Focuses on esteem building and social skills development through rock climbing, backpacking, whitewater rafting, mountaineering, sailing, snorkeling, and much more. Offers two week, one month, and semester programs available. SOAR programs utilize North Carolina, Florida, Colorado, American Southwest, Alaska, and Jamaica as program areas.

1654 **Stone Mountain School**
Talisman Schools
601 Camp Elliott Road
Black Mountain, NC 28711 **828-669-8639**
FAX: 828-669-2521
e-mail: info@stonemountainschool.com
www.stonemountainschool.com

Catherine Jennings, Director
Paige Thomas, Admissions

Year round therapeutic wilderness school for emotionally disturbed boys grades 6-12. Certified mental health program, licensed by the department of facility services and certified special education school.

1655 **Talisman Summer Camp**
Aspen Youth Services
17100 Pioneer Road
Cerritos, CA 90701 **562-467-5500**
FAX: 704-669-2521
e-mail: summer@stonemountainschool.org
www.stonemountainschool.org

Linda Tatsapaugh, Director

Camp is located in Black Mountain, North Carolina. Offers a program of hiking, rafting, climbing, and caving for learning disabled ADD/ADHD and autistic young people. Coed, ages 9-18.

North Dakota

1656 **Camp Sioux**
L Dickson
314 N 4th Street
Grand Forks, ND 58203 **701-746-4427**
FAX: 701-746-9337
e-mail: ldickson@diabetes.org

Lynette Dickson, Camp Director

Camp is located in Arvilla, North Dakota. Summer camping for children with diabetes. Coed, ages 8-14.

Ohio

1657 **Agape Resident Camp**
Catholic Charities Services
1111 Superior Avenue
Cleveland, OH 44114 **216-696-6525**
FAX: 216-344-9962
e-mail: jimg@ccd.cle.dioc.org

James E Gepperth, Director

Camping for children and adults with various disabilities. Coed, ages 21-75.

1658 **Akron Rotary Camp**
263 Millcreek Drive
Akron, OH 44307 **330-374-9232**
FAX: 330-644-1013
e-mail: danr@akronymca.org
www.akronymca.org

Dan Reynolds, Director

Summer camping for children with a variety of disabilities. Coed, ages 6-17.

1659 **Beech Brook**
3737 Lander Road
Cleveland, OH 44124 **216-831-2255**
FAX: 216-831-0436
www.beechbrook.org

Mario Tonti DSW, President/CEO

Residential and day treatment center. Treatment center for emotionally disturbed children, including residential and day treatment; foster care; adoption; adn community based programs.

1660 **Breezewood Acres**
Franklin Co Cncl for Retarded Citizens
2344 E 5th Avenue
Columbus, OH 43219 **614-252-4900**
FAX: 614-252-4901

Garnett Steele, Executive VP

Camp is located Sunbury, Ohio. Camping sessions for children and adults with mobility limitation or speech/communication impairment. Ages 6-99.

1661 **CHAMP Camp**
Achievement Centers for Children
15000 Cheerful Lane
Strongsville, OH 44136 **440-238-6200**

www.achievementcentersforchildren.org

Nicole Bilkins, Director

Camp in Cleveland, Ohio for children with hearing impairment, developmental disabilities, speech/communication impairment and visual impairment/blindness.

1662 Camp Allyn

Stepping Stones Center
5650 Given Road
Cincinnati, OH 45243 **513-831-4660**
FAX: 513-831-4660
www.steppingstonescenter.org

Chris Brockman, Director

A camp in Batavia, Ohio for children and adults with disabilities. Coed, ages 7-60.

1663 Camp Cheerful

Achievement Centers for Children
15000 Cheerful Lane
Strongsville, OH 44136 **440-238-6200**
FAX: 440-238-1858
e-mail: tim.fox@achievementctrs.org
www.achievementcenters.org

Tim Fox, Director

Sessions for campers with developmental disabilities, mobility limitation and speech/communication impairment. Coed, ages 7-99.

1664 Camp Courageous

241 N Superior
2nd Floor
Toledo, OH 43604 **419-242-9587**
FAX: 419-242-4951
e-mail: cherylt@uhs-toledo.org
www.campcourageous.com

Cheryl Tresnan, Executive Director

Camp Courageous provides residential camping services for people with developmental disabilities form ages 7-75 years old. Our six day, 5 night programs give campers a chance to expirence activities such as: aquatics, arts and crafts, animal programs, sports skills, hiking, recreational and leisure education programs, nature studies, drama, cookouts and campfires.

1665 Camp Friendship

A Woody
5555 Frantz Road
Dublin, OH 43017 **614-718-4438**
www.cancer.org

Angela Woody, Director

Camp in Clarksville, Ohio for children and adults with cancer offers a variety of outdoor activities.

1666 Camp Libbey

Maumee Valley GSC
2244 Collingwood Boulevard
Toledo, OH 43620
800-860-4516
FAX: 419-782-9408
e-mail: clibbey@defnet.com
www.mvgsc.org

Christy Gustin, Director

Camp for girls 7-18 with asthma/respiratory ailments, diabetes, epilepsy and muscular dystrophy is located in Defiance, Ohio.

1667 Camp Nuhop

404 Hillcrest Drive
Ashland, OH 44805 **419-289-2227**
FAX: 419-289-2227
e-mail: cnuhop@bright.net
www.campnuhop.org

Jerry Dunlap, Director

A summer residential program for any youngster from 6 to 18 with a learning disability, behavior disorder or Attention Deficit Disorder. 84 campers and 41 staff members live on site in groups of to seven campers to every three counselors. Activities focus on positive self-concept and behaviors and teaches children to learn how to find their strengths, abilities and talents from a positive, yet realistic viewpoint.

1668 Camp Stepping Stone

Stepping Stones Center
5650 Given Road
Cincinnati, OH 45243 **513-831-4660**
FAX: 513-831-5918
www.steppingstonescenter.org

Dennis Carter, Director

Nonprofit United Way affiliated camp serving all disabilities and charging on a sliding scale.

1669 Echoing Hills

36272 CR 79
Warsaw, OH 43844 **740-327-2311**
FAX: 740-327-6371
e-mail: camp@echoinghillsvillage.org
www.echoinghillsvillage.org

Shaker Samuel, Director

Summer camp for children and adults with cerebral palsy. Coed, ages 7-70.

1670 Emanuel-Day

Emanuel-Day and Resident
331 Marlay Road
Dayton, OH 45405 **937-274-9908**

Nan Crawford, Camp Director

Camp for hearing impaired and normal hearing youth.

1671 Happiness Day at OLA/St Joe

Catholic Charities Services
1111 Superior Avenue
Cleveland, OH 44114 **216-696-6525**
FAX: 216-861-9795
e-mail: maworthington@dioceseofcleveland.org

Molly Worthington, Director

Summer camp for children and young adults with a variety of disabilities. Coed, ages 6-21.

1672 Happiness Day at Parmadale

Catholic Charities Services
1111 Superior Avenue
Cleveland, OH 44114 **216-696-6525**
FAX: 216-344-9962
e-mail: maworthington@dioceseofcleveland.org

Molly Worthington, Director

Camp is located in Parma, Ohio. Summer sessions for children and young adults with developmental disabilities. Coed, ages 6-21.

1673 **Happiness Day at St. Augustine Academy**
14808 Lake Avenue
Lakewood, OH 44107 **216-221-4227**

William Tighe
Serves mentally retarded campers with multiple handicaps.

1674 **Happiness Day at St. Augustine School**
Catholic Charities Services
1111 Superior Avenue
Cleveland, OH 44114 **216-696-6525**
FAX: 216-344-9962
e-mail: maworthington@dioceseofcleveland.org

Molly Worthington, Director
Camp is located in Lakewood, Ohio. Summer sessions for children and young adults with developmental disabilities. Coed, ages 6-21.

1675 **Happiness Day at the Center for Pastoral Leadership**
Catholic Charities Services
1111 Superior Avenue
Cleveland, OH 44114 **216-696-6525**
FAX: 216-861-9795
e-mail: maworthington@dioceseofcleveland.org

Molly Worthington, Director
Camp is located in Wickliffe, Ohio. Summer sessions for children and young adults with developmental disabilities. Coed, ages 6-21.

1676 **Highbrook Lodge**
Cleveland Sight Center
1909 E 101st Street
PO Box 1988
Cleveland, OH 44106 **216-791-8118**
FAX: 216-791-1101
www.clevelandsightcenter.org

Jacqueline Crayton, Director
Camp is located in Chardon, Ohio. Summer sessions for blind and disabled children, adults and families. Weekly rate: $100-$260 per week.

1677 **Ho Mita Koda**
Liberty A Wright
3601 S Green Road
Suite 100
Cleveland, OH 44122 **216-591-0800**
FAX: 216-591-0320
e-mail: lwright@dagc.org
www.camphomitakoda.org

Liberty A Wright, Camp Administrator
Camp is located in Newbury, Ohio. Summer sessions for children with type 1 diabetes. Coed, ages 6-15. Type 2 diabetes, coed, ages 12-17. Bicycle adventure, coed, ages 13-19. Mini-day camp, ages 4-7, coed.

1678 **Ko-Man-She**
Diabetes Association Dayton Area
120 Zeigler Street
Dayton, OH 45402 **937-220-6611**
FAX: 937-220-6609
e-mail: glester@core.com

Geri Lester, Director
Camp is located in Hamilton, Ohio. Summer sessions for children with diabetes. Coed, ages 8-17.

1679 **Leo Yassenoff JCC Day Camps**
1125 College Avenue
Columbus, OH 43209 **614-231-2731**
FAX: 614-231-8222
e-mail: mgoldberg@columbusjcc.org

Martha Goldberg, Director
Summer camping sessions for children and young adults with developmental, physical, emotional, mental and learning disabilities. Coed, ages 3-25.

1680 **Recreation Unlimited**
7700 Pipe Road
Ashley, OH 43003 **740-548-7006**
FAX: 740-747-4037
e-mail: recunl@midohio.net
www.recreationunlimited.org

Lisa Ferry, Director
Camping sessions for children and adults with a variety of disabilities. Coed, ages 5-99, families, seniors and single adults.

1681 **YMCA Outdoor Center Campbell Gard**
PO Box 122
Overpeck, OH 45011 **513-867-0600**
FAX: 513-867-0127
e-mail: campstaff@ccgymca.org
www.ccgymca.org

Rick Taylor, Director
Camp is located in Hamilton, Ohio. Camping sessions for children with ADD, autism, developmental disabilities and blindness/visual impairment. Coed, ages 6-17 and families.

Oklahoma

1682 **Camp Classen YMCA**
YMCA of Greater Oklahoma City
500 N Broadway
Suite 150
Oklahoma City, OK 73102 **405-297-7740**
FAX: 405-297-7745
e-mail: amcwhort@mcaokc.org

Albert P McWhorter, Director
Camp is located in Davis, Oklahoma. Sessions for children and adults with diabetes. Coed, ages 8-17, families, seniors and single adults.

1683 **Easter Seals Oklahoma**
2100 NW 63rd Street
Oklahoma City, OK 73116 **405-848-2525**
FAX: 405-842-9704
e-mail: easok@ilinkusa.net

Providing services such as adult day services, child development center, OTIPT, speech therapy, reading/tutoring, vision and hearing screening.

Oregon

1684 **Camp Christmas Seal**
American Lung Association of Oregon
7420 SW Bridgeport Road 200
Tuacatin, OR 97224 **503-246-1997**
FAX: 503-246-1924
e-mail: gail@lungoregon.org
www.lungoregon.org

Dave Grieshammer, Director

Camp is located in Sisterhood, Oregon. Sessions for children with asthma/respiratory ailments. Coed, ages 8-15.

1685 Camp Latgawa

Conference of United Methodists
1505 SW 18th Avenue
Portland, OR 97201 **503-226-7931**

e-mail: camplatgawa@grrtech.com
www.gocamping.org

Eva LaBonty, Director

Camp is located at Eagle Point, Oregon. Sessions for children and adults with HIV and developmental disabilities. Coed, ages 8-18 and families, seniors.

1686 Camp Magruder

Conference of United Methodists
1505 SW 18th Avenue
Portland, OR 97201 **503-226-7931**

e-mail: campmagruder@oregoncoast.com
www.gocamping.org

Ted Hulbert, Director

Camp is located in Rockaway Beach, Oregon. Sessions for children and adults with cancer and developmental disabilities. Coed, ages 9-18, families, seniors and single adults.

1687 Camp Taloali

D Sipp
15934 N Santiam Highway
Stayton, OR 97383 **503-769-6415**

e-mail: sippd@aol.com

Dave Sipp, Director

Summer sessions for children with hearing impairment. Coed, ages 9-17.

1688 Capital Camps

Jewish Camp & Conference Services
133 Rollins Avenue
Suite 4
Rockville, MD 20852 **301-468-2267**
FAX: 301-468-1719
e-mail: info@capitalcamps.org
www.capitalcamps.org

David M Phillips MSW, Executive Director

Camp is located in Waynesboro, Pennsylvania. Sessions for children with mental retardation and mild ADHD. Coed, ages 8-18.

1689 Easter Seals Oregon Camping Program

5757 SW Macadam Avenue
Portland, OR 97239 **503-228-5108**
800-556-6020
FAX: 503-228-1352
e-mail: camp@or.easter-seals.org

Luke Kramschuster, Director

Camp is located in Corbett, Oregon. Summer sessions for children and adults with a variety of disabilities. Coed, ages 6-90.

1690 Gales Creek Diabetes Camp

Gales Creek Camp Foundation
415 N State Street #120
Lake Oswego, OR 97034 **503-699-8433**
FAX: 503-699-8457
e-mail: diabchld@aracnet.com
www.galecreekcamp.org

Patti Sadowski, Executive Director
Debby Buekeloo, Operations Manager

Camp is located in Forest Grove, Oregon. Summer sessions for children with diabetes. Coed, ages 6-16, family and pre-school family camps also available.

1691 Meadowood Springs Speech and Hearing Camp

PO Box 1025
Pendleton, OR 97801 **541-276-2752**
FAX: 541-276-7227
e-mail: meadowood@oregontrail.net
www.meadowoodsprings.org

Rhonda Hack, Executive Administrator

On 143 acres in the Blue Mountains of Eastern Oregon, this camp is designed to help young people who have diagnosed clinical disorders of speech, hearing or language. A full range of activities in recreational and clinical areas is available.

1692 Mt Hood Kiwanis Camp

9320 SW Barbur Boulevard
Suite 165
Portland, OR 97219 **503-452-7416**
FAX: 503-452-0062
e-mail: mhkc@hevanet.com

Camp is located in Government Camp, Oregon. Summer sessions for children and adults with a variety of disabilities. Coed, ages 9-35.

1693 Suttle Lake United Methodist Camp

Conference of United Methodists
1505 SW 18th Avenue
Portland, OR 97201 **503-226-7931**
FAX: 541-595-2818
e-mail: suttle@outlawnet.com
www.gocamping.org

Miranda Lovgren, Director

Camp is located in Sisters, Oregon. Camping sessions for children and adults with HIV. Coed, ages 6-18, families, seniors and single adults.

1694 Upward Bound Camp: Evans Creek

PO Box C
Staylon, OR 97383 **503-897-2447**
FAX: 503-897-4116
e-mail: ubc@open.org
www.upwardboundcamp.org

Jerry Pierce, Co-Director
Laura Pierce, Co-Director

Camping Christian for children and adults with a variety of disabilities. Ages 12-99, seniors and single adults.

1695 YWCA Camp Westwind

YWCA of Greater Portland
1111 SW 10th Avenue
Portland, OR 97205 **503-294-7472**
FAX: 503-294-7399
e-mail: kims@ywca-pdx.org
www.ywca-pdx.org

Kim Summers, Director

Camp is located in Neotsu, Oregon. Sessions for children with hearing impairment. Coed, ages 7-17 and families.

Pennsylvania

1696 **Achieva**
711 Bingham Street
Pittsburgh, PA 15203 **412-995-5000**
FAX: 412-995-5001
www.achieva.info

Marsha Blanco, CEO
Camping program for the mentally and physically disabled.

1697 **Briarwood Day Camp**
1380 Creek Road
Wycombe, PA 18925 **215-598-7143**
FAX: 215-602-1060

Ted Levin
A comprehensive day camp providing lunch and transportation for children with disabilities.

1698 **Camp AIM**
51 McMurray Road
Pittsburgh, PA 15241 **412-833-5600**
FAX: 412-833-9754

Martin Brocco, Director
Disabled campers.

1699 **Camp ARC Spencer**
ARC of Beaver
3582 Broadhead Road
Suite 202
Monaca, PA 15061 **724-775-1602**
FAX: 724-775-2905
e-mail: arcbeaver@achieva.info

Drew Grivna, Executive Director
Camp is located in Fombell, Pennsylvania. Summer sessions for children and adults with developmental disabilities. Coed, ages 5-99.

1700 **Camp Can Do**
Easter Seals of Southeastern PA
468 N Middletown Road
Media, PA 19063 **610-565-2353**
FAX: 215-368-1199
www.easterseals-sepa.org

Katherine Tobias, Director
Camp is located in Kulpsville, Pennsylvania. Summer sessions for children and young adults with a variety of disabilities. Coed, ages 5-21

1701 **Camp Carefree**
Easter Seals of Southeastern PA
468 N Middletown Road
Media, PA 19063 **610-565-2353**
FAX: 610-873-3992
www.easterseals-sepa.org

Andrew Serdich, Director
Camp is located in Coatesville, Pennsylvania. Summer sessions for children and young adults with a variety of disabilities. Coed, ages 5-21.

1702 **Camp Dunmore**
Easter Seals of Southeastern PA
468 N Middletown Road
Media, PA 19063 **610-565-2353**
FAX: 610-565-5256
www.easterseals-sepa.org

Frances Carmen, Director
Summer sessions for children and young adults with a variety of disabilities. Coed, ages 5-21.

1703 **Camp Joy**
3325 Swamp Creek Road
Schwenksville, PA 19473 **610-754-6878**
FAX: 610-754-7880
e-mail: campjoy@fast.net
www.campjoy.com

Angus Murray, Camp Director
A year round residential camping program for children and adults with mental retardation and physical disabilities. Brochure, video and application available upon request.

1704 **Camp Keystone**
RR#1
Box 1515
Gouldsboro, PA 18424 **570-207-3210**
FAX: 570-842-2158
e-mail: glance@keycommresp.com
www.campkey.com

Gloria J Lance MS, Director
Keystone serves both children and adults with a variety of disabilities in various residential settings. Support services include 24 hour supervision, on site nursing services, special and therapeutic recreation programs and psychological and psychiatric services. Ages 6-66, seniors and single adults.

1705 **Camp Lee Mar**
805 Redgate Road
Dresher, PA 19025 **215-658-1708**

Seven week summer camp for children and young adults with mild to moderate developmental disabilities. 5-21 years of age

1706 **Camp Setebaid**
Setebaid Services
PO Box 196
Winfield, PA 17889 **570-524-9090**
FAX: 570-523-0769
e-mail: info@setebaidservices.org
www.setebaidservices.org

Mark Moyer, Executive Director
Diane Facer, Office Assistant
Camping sessions for children with diabetes. Coed, ages 3-13 years. Family retreat for children with diabetes and their families.

1707 **Camp Surefoot**
Easter Seals of Southeastern PA
468 N Middletown Road
Media, PA 19063 **610-565-2353**
FAX: 215-945-4073
www.easterseals-sepa.org

Bill Barnes, Director
Camp is located in Levittown, Pennsylvania. Sessions for children and young adults with a variety of disabilities. Coed, ages 5-21.

1708 **Crestfield Camp & Conference Center**

Pittsburgh Presbytery
801 Union Place
Pittsburgh, PA 15212
724-794-4022
800-794-1948
FAX: 724-794-1665
e-mail: programs@crestfield.net
www.childrenwithdiabetes.com/camps

Carolyn Dierckesen, Director

Camp is located at 195 Taggart Road, Slippery Rock, Pennsylvania. Summer sessions for children with diabetes. Coed, ages 9-18 and families.

1709 **Elling Camps**

RR 1 Box 54
Thompson, PA 18465
FAX: 717-756-3306

Lloyd E Elling, Director

For youth ages 6-21 with learning disabilities and accompanying difficulties. This camp allows them to learn to adjust socially in a community atmosphere. The structured camp program includes land and water sports, nature and forestry, industrial arts, construction and work programs, and arts and crafts.

1710 **Helping Hands**

415 Hoffmansville Road
Bechtelsville, PA 19505
610-754-6491
FAX: 610-754-7157
e-mail: handsinc@aol.com

Bruce McWaters, Director

Provides vocational and recreational programs for individuals with developmental disabilities. Offers support and information to parents, caregivers, and individuals impacted by disabilities.

1711 **Innabah**

712 Pughtown Road
Spring City, PA 19475
610-469-6111
877-UMC-CAMP
FAX: 610-469-0330
e-mail: innabah@juno.com
www.epaumc.org/camping

Christy Heflin, Director

Sessions for children and young adults with developmental disabilities. Ages 4-18, families and seniors.

1712 **Ken-Crest Services**

502 W Germantown Pike
Suite 200
Plymouth Meeting, PA 19462
610-825-9360
FAX: 610-825-4127
e-mail: kencrest@kencrest.org
www.kencrest.org

James McFalls, Executive Director
Mary Ellen Caffrey, Director Children's Services

Ken-Crest provides services and supports for people who have developmental disability or who are at risk for disability across southeastern Pennsylvania and Delaware. Ken-Crest's community-based programs span the entire age continuum. Services for children include assessment, early intervention, therapies and parent education. For adults, Ken-Crest provides a full range of residential, employment, healthcare and therapy services.

1713 **Kweebec**

814 Woodbine Avenue
Box 511
Penn Valley, PA 19072
800-543-9830
FAX: 610-667-6376
e-mail: ckweebec@aol.com

Les Weiser, Director

Camp is located in Schwenksville, Pennsylvania. Sessions for children and adults with diabetes. Coed, ages 6-16, families, seniors and single adults.

1714 **Living Waters**

Penn West Conference UCC
320 S Maple Avenue
Greensburg, PA 15601
724-834-0344
FAX: 724-834-0324
e-mail: pennwest@westol.com
www.pennwest.org

Carl Hancock, Director

Camp is located in Schellsburg, Pennsylvania. Sessions for children and adults with developmental disabilities, ages 6-96 and families.

1715 **Make-a-Friend**

3975 Conshohocken Avenue
Philadelphia, PA 19131
215-879-1000
FAX: 215-879-8424

Specialized day camp.

1716 **New Jersey Camp Jaycee**

33 Lake Drive
Hightstown, NJ 08520
609-443-1200
FAX: 609-443-1202
e-mail: campjaycee@aol.com
www.campjaycee.org

Joan Travis, Administrative Director

Camp is located in Effort, Pennsylvania. Sessions for children and adults with autism and developmental disabilities. Coed, ages 7-85, seniors and single adults.

1717 **New Jersey YMHA/YWHA Camps Milford**

21 Plymouth Street
Fairfield, NJ 07004
973-575-3333
FAX: 973-575-4188
e-mail: info@njycamps.org
www.njycamps.org

Leonard M Robinson, Director

Camp is located in Milford, Pennsylvania. Summer sessions for children with ADD. Coed, ages 6-17 and families.

1718 **Outside in School**

303 Center Avenue
Greensburg, PA 15601
724-837-1518
FAX: 724-837-0801
e-mail: outside@icubed.com
www.outsideinschool.com

Michael C Henkel, Director

Camp is located in Bolivar, Pennsylvania. Sessions for children with ADD and substance abuse problems. Boys 11-18 and girls 13-18.

1719 **Phelps School Summer School**

Paoli Pike & Sugartown Roads
Malvern, PA 19355 **610-644-1754**
FAX: 610-644-6679
e-mail: adms@phelpsschool.org
www.phelpsschool.org

Jim Spiro, Director Admissions
Bob Aherns, Director Summer School

Open for grades 7-11 to make up academic deficiencies or complete studies in English, math and reading. Sports include riding, tennis and swimming. A program is also available to a limited number of international students in English as a Second Language.

1720 **Ramah in the Poconos**

261 Old York Road, The Pavilion
Suite 734
Jenkintown, PA 19046 **215-885-8556**
FAX: 215-885-8905
e-mail: mcbnyc@aol.com
www.RamahPoconos.org

Marla Berkowits, Kesher Director

Camp is located in Lake Como, Pennsylvania. Summer sessions for children and adults with hearing impairment. Coed, ages 10-16, families and seniors.

1721 **Sequanota**

Lutheran Camp Association
Box 245
Jennerstown, PA 15547 **814-629-6627**
FAX: 814-629-0128
e-mail: campsequanota@aol.com
www.sequanota.net

Rev John Timm, Executive Director

Summer sessions for adults with developmental disabilities and speech/communication impairment.

1722 **Souderton Special Needs Day Camp**

149 Cherry Lane
Souderton, PA 18964 **215-723-8555**

Donna Huff

Field trips and special events for disabled campers.

1723 **Summit Camp**

339 N Broadway
Upper Nyack, NY **845-358-7565**
FAX: 718-268-0671
e-mail: summitinst@aol.com
www.summitcamp.com

Mayer A Stiskin, Director

Camp is located in Honesdale, Pennsylvania. Summer sessions for children with ADD. Coed, ages 8-17.

1724 **Variety Club Camp & Developmental Center**

Valley Forge and Potshop Roads
PO Box 609
Worcester, PA 19490 **610-584-4366**
FAX: 610-584-5586
e-mail: varietyclubcamp@hotmail.com

Ralph Townsend, Director

Year-round camping and recreation facility for children with special needs and their families. Includes summer camping, aquatics, weekend retreats and other specialty programs. Coed, ages 5-21.

1725 **Wesley Woods**

1 Fiddlegreen Road
Rural Route 1 Box 155
Grand Valley, PA 16420 **814-436-7802**
FAX: 814-436-7669

Herb West

Exceptional children's camp for children with emotional and intellectual handicaps.

1726 **Woodlands**

134 Shenot Road
Wexford, PA 15090 **724-935-6533**
FAX: 724-934-9610
e-mail: pclakeley@woodlandsfoundation.org
www.woodlandsfoundation.org

Peter Clakeley, Executive Director
Beth Snyder, Director Development/Marketing

Summer camping sessions and collaborative opportunities with charities serving individuals with disability and chronic illness. Year-round weekend retreats and aquatic programs for children and young adults with a variety of disabilities. Coed, ages 7-21.

1727 **YMCA Camp Fitch**

Youngstown YMCA
17 N Champion Street
Youngstown, OH 44501 **330-744-8411**
FAX: 330-744-8416
www.campfitch.com

William L Lyder, Director

Camp is located in North Springfield, Pennsylvania. Camping sessions for children and adults with diabetes, hearing impairment, developmental disabilities, mobility limitation and speech/communication impairment. Ages 8-16, families and seniors.

Rhode Island

1728 **Aldersgate Center**

1043 Snake Hill Road
North Scituate, RI 02857 **401-568-4350**
FAX: 401-568-1840
e-mail: Aldersgate@juno.com
www.campaldersgate.com

Jeffrey Thomas, Director

Summer sessions for children and adults with asthma/respiratory ailments. Coed, ages 7-99 and families.

1729 **Camp Ruggles**

133 Stone Dam Road
North Scituate, RI 02857 **401-647-5508**

George M Jacques, Director

Camp is located in Glocester, Rhode Island. Summer sessions for children with ADD. Coed, ages 6-12.

1730 **Canonicus Camp and Conference Center**

American Baptist Churches RI
PO Box 330
Exeter, RI 02822 **401-294-6318**
e-mail: camp@canonicus.org
www.canonicus.org

Melanie Towle, Director

Summer sessions for children with asthma/respiratory ailments. Coed, ages 4-18.

South Carolina

1731 **Burnt Gin Camp**
SC Department of Health and Environmental Control
Box 101106
Columbia, SC 29211 **803-898-0455**
FAX: 803-898-0613
e-mail: aimonemi@columb60.dhec.state.sc.us
www.state.sc.us

Marie I Aimone, Camp Director

A residental camp for children who have physical disabilities and/or chronic illnesses. Camper/staff ratio is 2:1. Five seven-day sessions for 7-15 year olds and one six-day sesssion for 16-19 year olds. Limited to residents of South Carolina.

1732 **Camp Gravatt**
1006 Camp Gravatt Road
Aiken, SC 29805 **803-648-1817**
FAX: 803-648-7453
e-mail: gravatt@groupz.net

Project adventure includes swimming, fishing, music and art and more in which disabled campers participate. Enjoy the fun and adventure of exploring a river in a canoe in the new canoe program.

South Dakota

1733 **NeSoDak Bible Camp/Klein Ranch**
Lutherans Outdoors South Dakota
2001 S Summit Avenue
Augustana College
Sioux Falls, SD 57197 **605-274-5326**
FAX: 605-947-4379
e-mail: nsdlo@itctel.com
www.lutheransoutdoors.org

Neil Sorenson, Director

Camp is located in Waubay, South Dakota. Sessions for children with diabetes. Coed, ages 8-18.

Tennessee

1734 **Camp Discovery**
Tennessee Jaycee Fund
651 E 4th Street
Suite 600
Chattanooga, TN 37403 **423-267-9718**
e-mail: campdirector2000@aol.com

Shanna Howell, Director

Camp is located in Gainesboro, Tennessee. Sessions for children and adults with developmental disabilities, mobility limitation, multiple sclerosis and muscular dystrophy, ages 7-65.

1735 **Easter Seals Camp Lindahl**
6300 Benders Ferry Road
Mount Juliet, TN 37122 **615-444-2829**
FAX: 615-444-8576
e-mail: escamp@bellsouth.net

Rob Ogden, Director

Summer sessions for children and adults with various disabilities, ages 6-99.

1736 **Indian Creek Camp**
Kentucky Tennessee Conference
PO Box 1088
Goodlettsville, TN 37070 **615-859-1391**
FAX: 615-859-2120
e-mail: darlenebee@aol.com

Jerry Mahn, Director

Camp is located in Liberty, Tennessee. Summer sessions for children and adults who are blind/visually impaired. Coed, ages 7-17, families and seniors.

Texas

1737 **American Diabetes Association**
Rural Route 2 Box 915
New Bloomfield, PA 17068 **717-852-3802**
FAX: 717-582-3402
e-mail: mknight@diabetes.org

Michelle Knight, Director

Summer camping sessions for children with diabetes. Coed, ages 4-18.

1738 **Camp CAMP**
Childrens Association Max Potential
PO Box 27086
San Antonio, TX 78227 **210-292-3566**
FAX: 210-292-3577
e-mail: campmail@sprynet.com

Brad Gilbert, Director

Camp is located in Center Point, Texas. Camping for children and young adults with a variety of disabilities. Coed, ages 5-21.

1739 **Camp John Marc**
Special Camps for Special Kids
8111 Preston Road
Suite 807
Dallas, TX 75225 **214-360-0056**
FAX: 214-368-2003
e-mail: mail@campjohnmarc.org

Vance Gilmore, Director

Camp is located in Meridian, Texas. Year-round camping for children with a variety of disabilities. Coed, ages 6-16 and families.

1740 **Camp Summit**
2915 LBJ Freeway
Suite 185
Dallas, TX 75234 **972-484-8900**
FAX: 972-620-1945
e-mail: L.BRAZIEL@campsummittx.org
www.campsummittx.org

Lura J Hammond, Director

Camp is located in Argyle, Texas. Camping for children and adults with a variety of disabilities. Coed, ages 6-99.

1741 **Camp Sweeney**
Southwestern Diabetic Fund
101 S Culberson
Gainesville, TX 76241 **940-665-9502**
FAX: 940-665-7467
e-mail: info@campsweeney.org

Ernie Fernandez MD, Camp Director
Marlene Gray, CFRE, Developmental Director

Teaches self-care and self-reliance to children ages 7-18 with diabetes. Campers participate in such activities such as swimming, fishing, horseback riding and arts and crafts while learning about how to self manage their diabetes.

1742 Camp for All

Vicki LaRue
10500 NW Freeway
Suite 145
Houston, TX 77092 **713-686-5666**
FAX: 713-686-1242
www.campforall.org

Janet Johnson, Director

Fully-accessible year round camp facility is located in Burton, Texas. Camping for children and adults with a variety of disabilities. Coed, ages 5-35 and up and families.

1743 Dallas Academy

950 Tiffany Way
Dallas, TX 75218 **214-324-1481**
FAX: 214-327-8537
e-mail: mail@dallas-academy.com
www.dallas-academy.com

Jim Richardson, Director

7-week summer session for students who are having difficulty in regular school classes.

1744 Gilmont Program Center

PO Box 254
Route 6
Gilmer, TX 75644 **903-797-3639**
FAX: 903-797-6400
e-mail: cgilmonttpc@aol.com

Tom Truitt, Director

Outdoor adventures for disabled campers which makes use of the center's twin lakes.

1745 Growing Together Diabetes Camp

E Texas Medical Center Rose City
PO Box 6400 Kiwanis
Tyler, TX 75711 **903-535-6354**
FAX: 903-535-6783

Marie Taylor, Director

Camping for children with diabetes. Coed, ages 6-14.

1746 Hill School of Fort Worth

4817 Odessa Avenue
Fort Worth, TX 76133 **817-923-9482**
FAX: 817-923-4894
e-mail: admission@hillschool.org
www.hillschool.org

Lucille H Helton, Principal
Cathy Allen, Admissions Director
Grey Owens, Principal

Provides an alternative learning environment for students having average or above-average intelligence with learning differences. Hill school is an established leader in North Texas with a 25 year history of effectively serving LD children. Beginning in 1961 as a tutorial service, Hill became a formal school in 1973. Our mission is to help those who learn differently develop skills and strategies to succeed. We do this by developing academic/study skills, and self-discipline.

1747 Hughen Center

2849 9th Avenue
Port Arthur, TX 77642 **409-983-6659**
FAX: 409-983-6408

Jeff Kuchar, Executive Director

The Center provides a therapeutic, educational, and recreational program for children with physical disabilities. Physical and occupational therapy are featured. Day and residential.

1748 Texas 4-H Center

RR 1 Box 527
Brownwood, TX 76801 **325-784-5482**
FAX: 325-784-6486

K Scott Cross, Director
Cheryl A Newberry, Extension Program Specialist

Leadership activities and personal growth.

1749 Texas Lions Camp

4100 San Antonio Highway
PO Box 290247
Kerrville, TX 78029 **830-896-8500**
FAX: 830-896-3666
e-mail: tlc@ktc.com
www.lionscamp.com

Stephen S Mabry, Executive Director

The primary purpose of the League shall be to provide, without charge, a camp for physically disabled, hearing/vision impaired and diabetic children from the State of Texas, regardless of race, religion, or national origin. Our goal is to create an atmosphere wherein campers will learn the can do philosophy and be allowed to achieve maximum personal growth and self-esteem. The camp welcomes boys and girls ages 7-16.

Utah

1750 Camp Hobe

American Cancer Society
941 E 3300 S
Salt Lake City, UT 84106 **801-483-1500**
FAX: 801-483-1558
www.camphobe.com

Jill Jackstien, Director

Camping for children with cancer ages 6-19 and their siblings.

1751 FCYD Camp

Foundation for Children & Youth
8925 S 2700 W
W Jordan, UT 84088 **801-566-6913**
www.FCYD-Inc.org

David Okubo, Director

Camping for children with diabetes. Coed, ages 1-18 and families.

1752 Kostopulos Dream Foundation/Camp Kostopulos

2500 Emigration Canyon
Salt Lake City, UT 84108 **801-582-0700**
FAX: 801-583-5176
e-mail: gethington@campk.org

Gary Ethington, Director

Summer camping for children and adults ages 7-65 with a variety of disabilities. Year round recreation on site and community based activities.

Vermont

1753 **Bennington School**
992 Fairview Street
Bennington, VT 05201 **802-447-1557**
800-639-3156
FAX: 802-447-3234

Patrick Ramsay, Admissions Director
Jeff LaBonte, Executive Director

A 115 bed residential treatment center serving emotionally and behaviorally disordered adolescent male and female students. Offer a fully accredited on-grounds educational program in addition to comprehensive clinical and residential components. The beautiful rural setting provides many recreational opportunities as well as cultural experiences.

1754 **Betsey Cox**
349 S Mountain Road
Northfield, MA 01360 **888-345-9193**
e-mail: betcoxvt@aol.com

Mike Byrom, Associate Director

Camp is located in Pittsford, Vermont. Summer sessions for girls aged 9-15 with ADD.

1755 **Farm and Wilderness Camps**
263 Farm & Wilderness Road
Plymouth, VT 05056 **802-422-3761**
FAX: 802-422-8660
e-mail: fandw@fandw.org
www2.kidscamps.com

Robert Schultz, Executive Director
Linda Berryhill, Registrar

1756 **Silver Towers Camp**
Goshen Road
Ripton, VT 05766 **802-442-0979**
FAX: 802-442-4675
e-mail: graymgt@sover.net
www.silvertowers.com

Dr. Valeri Allen, Camp Director
Brenda Metcalf, Office Manager

1757 **Thorpe Camp**
Rural Route 3 Box 3314
Goshen, VT 05733 **802-247-6611**
e-mail: mjet@sover.net
www2.kidscamps.com

Virginia

1758 **Adventure Day Camp**
Early Years Academy
13817 Spriggs Road
Manassas, VA 20112 **703-590-3659**

Camping for children with asthma/respiratory ailments and cancer. Coed, ages 2-13.

1759 **Camp Baker**
Richmond Association for Retarded Citizens
1901 Westwood Avenue
Richmond, VA 23227 **804-748-4789**
FAX: 804-796-6880
e-mail: camp.baker.arc@erols.com

Melissa Walters, Director

Summer camping for children and adults with developmental disabilities, ADD and autism. Coed, ages 5-99, seniors and single adults.

1760 **Camp Dickenson**
Holsten Conference Camping
PO Box 1178
Johnson City, TN 37605 **423-928-2156**
FAX: 276-744-7241
e-mail: ousley@tcia.net

John W Ousley, Director

Camp is located in Fries, Virginia. Camping for children and adults with developmental disabilities. Coed, ages 5-18, families, seniors and single adults.

1761 **Camp Easter Seal: East/West**
Easter Seals Virginia
201 E Main Street
Salem, VA 24153 **540-777-7325**
FAX: 540-563-8928
www.va.easter-seals.org

Deborah Duerk, Director

Summer camp sessions for children and adults ages 5-99 with physical disabilities, cognitive disabilities and sensory impairments. Therapeutic recreation activities including swimming, fishing, sports, horseback riding, rock climbing, and more. Twenty-six-day speech therapy camp children with disabilities ages 8-16. Twelve-day Spina Bifida Self Help Skills Camp.

1762 **Camp Holiday Trails**
PO Box 5806
Charlottesville, VA 22905 **434-977-3781**
FAX: 434-977-8814
e-mail: cht@nexet.net

Mark D Andersen, Executive Director

Private, nonprofit camp for children with special health needs and various chronic illnesses. Residential, 2-week sessions are open July 1 - August 10; camperships are available. Coed 7-17, nationwide and international. Canoeing, swimming, horseback riding, arts and crafts, drama, ropes course, etc. 24-hr. medical supervision by doctor and nursing staff. Air conditioned cabins.

1763 **Camp Virginia Jaycee**
2494 Camp Jaycee Road
Blue Ridge, VA 24064 **540-947-2972**
800-865-0092
FAX: 540-947-2043
e-mail: ewerness@campvirginiajaycee.com
www.campvirginiajaycee.com

Everett M Werness, President
Lauren Lightfoot, Camp Director

Summer camping for children and adults with developmental disabilities. Coed, ages 7-70. Weekend respite camps for children and adults with mental retardation.

1764 **Civitan Acres**
Eggleston Services
2210 Cedar Road
Chesapeake, VA 23323
757-487-6062
FAX: 757-487-4143
e-mail: maried@lwe.org

Marie Dugan, Director

Camping for children and adults with developmental disabilities. Coed, ages 5-99.

1765 **Loudoun County Parks & Recreation and Community Services Special Recreation Programs**
1 Harrison Street NE
PO Box 7000
Leesburg, VA 20177
703-777-0343
FAX: 703-771-5354
e-mail: prcs@loudoun.gov
www.co.loudoun.va.us

Kate Trask, Special Recreation Coordinator

Offers and promotes integration opportunities for individuals with disabilities. Coordinates ADA issues and Very Special Arts and Special Olympics for Loudoun County. Summer camps, sports, socials and community trips.

1766 **Makemie Woods Camp/Conference Retreat**
Presbytery of Eastern Virginia
PO Box 39
Barhamsville, VA 23011
800-989-2193
FAX: 757-566-8803
www.makwoods.org

Michelle Burcher, Director

Counselors serve as teachers, friends and activity leaders. The individual is important within the small group. No camper is lost in the crowd, but is an integral partner in the group process. Residential Christian Camp and conference center. Summer camp for children 8-18 and special camp for children with diabetes.

1767 **Oakland School & Camp**
Boyd Tavern
Keswick, VA 22947
434-293-9059
FAX: 434-296-8930
e-mail: www.oaklandschool.net
oaklandschool@earthlink.net

Joanne Dondero, President
Carol Smieciuch, Director

A highly individualized program stresses improving reading ability. Subjects taught are reading, English composition, math and word analysis. Recreational activities include horseback riding, sports, swimming, tennis, crafts, archery and camping. For girls and boys, ages 8-14.

1768 **Overlook Camp**
3014 Camp Overlook Lane
Keezletown, VA 22832
540-269-2267
FAX: 540-269-2267
e-mail: overlookum@aol.com

Ronald Robey, Director

A Christian life experience for youth and children, located at the base of the scenic Massanutten Mountains.

Washington

1769 **Camp Fun in the Sun**
Inland NW Health Services
157 S Howard Street
Suite 500
Spokane, WA 99201
509-232-8138
FAX: 509-232-8355
e-mail: jamesod@cherspokane.org
www.campfuninthesun.org

Dee Jameson, Director
Ann Nesbitl, Director

Summer camping for children with diabetes. Coed, ages 6-18.

1770 **Camp Killoqua**
Camp Fire US
4312 Rucker Avenue
Everett, WA 98203
425-258-5437
FAX: 425-252-2267
e-mail: info@campfireusasnohoneish.org
www.campfireusasnohomish.org/killoqua

Carol Johnson, Director

Camp is located in Stanwood, Washington. Camping for children with developmental disabilities. Coed, ages 6-17.

1771 **Easter Seals Camp Stand by Me**
Easter Seal Society of Washington
17809 S Vaughan Road
Vaughn, WA 98394
253-884-2722
FAX: 253-884-0200
e-mail: mary@seals.org
www.seals.org

Mike Mooney, Director
Mary McIntyre, Office Manager

Camp is located in Vaughn, Washington. Summer camping for adults and children with developmental disabilities and mobility limitation. Coed, ages 7-65, seniors. Respite weekends October thru May.

1772 **Northwest Kiwanis Camp**
D Coleman
PO Box 2393
Sequim, WA 98382
360-683-9045

Tom Carrolu, Director

Camp is located in Chimacum, Washington. Summer sessions for children with a variety of disabilities. Coed, ages 6-16.

1773 **Volasuca Volunteers of America**
2802 Broadway
Everett, WA 98201
425-259-3191
FAX: 360-793-8919
e-mail: camp@voaww.org
www.voaww.org

Chris Shroy, Director

Camp is located in Sultan, Washington. Summer sessions for children and adults with a variety of disabilities. Coed, ages 6-13, families and single adults.

1774 **YMCA Camp Orkila**
YMCA of Greater Seattle
16045 25th Avenue NE
Seattle, WA 98104
206-382-5003
FAX: 360-376-2267

David Hembree, Director

Camping for children with blood disorders and diabetes, ages 8-18.

West Virginia

1775 Mountaineer Spina Bifida Camp

350 Capital Street
Suite 427
Charleston, WV 25301
304-558-7098
800-642-9704
FAX: 304-558-2866
www2.kidscamps.com

1776 Stepping Stones

15 Cottage Street
Morgantown, WV 26501
304-296-0150
800-982-8799
FAX: 304-296-0194
e-mail: abilitywv@hotmail.com
www.steppingstonescenter.net

Missy Weimex, Recreation Coordinator

Non-profit organization that serves individuals with disabilities. Programs include recreation, summer camps, technology and speech therapy.

1777 YMCA Camp Horseshoe

Ohio/W Virginia YMCA
Route 2 Box 138
St George, WV 26287
304-478-2481
FAX: 304-478-4446
e-mail: david@hi-y.org
www.hi-y.org

David King, Director

Summer camping for children with cancer, ages 7-18.

Wisconsin

1778 Bright Horizons Summer Camp

Sickle Cell Disease Association of Ilinois
200 N Michigan Avenue
Suite 605
Chicago, IL 60601
312-345-1100
FAX: 312-345-1103
www.sicklecelldisease-il.org

Valerie C Beckley, Director

Camp is located in Williams Bay, Wisconsin. Camping for children with blood disorders, ages 7-13.

1779 Easter Seal Camp Wawbeek

Easter Seals Wisconsin
101 Nob Hill Road 301
Madison, WI 53713
608-277-8288
800-422-2324
FAX: 608-277-8333
e-mail: ksaville@wi-easterseals.org
www.wi-easterseals.org

Chris Hollar, Director

Disabled campers. Offers adventure programs, camp sessions for other health agencies, family camp opportunities and year round respite sessions. Coed, ages 8-99.

1780 Lutherdale Bible Camp

N7891 US Highway 12
Elkhorn, WI 53121
262-742-2352
FAX: 262-742-3169
www.lutherdale.org

Jeffrey A Bluhm, Director

Summer camping for people with developmental disabilities. Coed, ages 9-18 and families, seniors.

1781 Needlepoint Daypoint

American Diabetes Association
715 Florida Avenue S
Suite 307
Minneapolis, MN 55426
763-593-5333
FAX: 763-593-1520
e-mail: thaglund@diabetes.org
www.diabetes.org

Becky Martin, Director

Camping for children who have type 1 diabetes. Coed, ages 5-16.

1782 Phantom Lake YMCA Camp

PO Box 228
Mukwonago, WI 53186
262-363-4386
FAX: 262-363-4351
e-mail: office@phantomlakeymca.com
www.phantomlakeymca.com

Dave Lee, Director

Summer camping for children with epilepsy, ages 7-15.

1783 Timbertop Nature Adventure Camp

1000 Division
Stevens Point, WI 54481
715-342-2980
FAX: 715-342-2987

Pete Matthai, Timbertop Nature Adventure Camp

For children who can benefit from an individualized program of learning in a non-competitive outdoor setting under the skilled leadership of people who understand the environment and the unique potential of these children.

1784 Triangle Y Ranch YMCA

YMCA of Tri-County
N 84 W
17501 Menomonee Avenue
Menomonee Falls, WI 53051
262-255-9622
FAX: 262-675-4982
e-mail: YMCATRRob@aol.com

Rob Tegtmeier, Director

Camp is located in West Bend, Wisconsin. Summer camping for children with ADD. Coed, ages 5-14.

1785 Wisconsin Badger Camp

Box 723
Platteville, WI 53818
608-348-9689
FAX: 608-348-9737
e-mail: wbc@pcii.net

Brent Bowers, Camp Director

Mission is to serve people with developmental disabilities by providing quality outdoor recreational experience. All developmentally disabled individuals, regardless of the severity of their disability or inability to pay are welcome.

1786 Wisconsin Lions Camp

Wisconsin Lions Foundation
3834 County Road A
Rosholt, WI 54473

715-677-4761
FAX: 715-677-3297
e-mail: lioncamp@wi-net.com
www.wisconsinlionscamp.com

Andrea Yenter, Interim Camp Director

Serves children who have either a visual, hearing or mild cognitive disability, as well as Type I diabetes. Program activities include sailing, ropes course, hiking and canoe trips, environmental education, swimming, camping, canoeing, outdoor living skills and handicrafts. ACA accredited, located in central Wisconsin, near Stevens Point.

Dresses & Skirts

1787 Budget Cotton/Poly Open Back Gown

Buck & Buck
3111 27th Avenue S
Seattle, WA 98144
800-458-0600
FAX: 800-317-2182
e-mail: info@buckandbuck.com
www.buckandbuck.com

Short raglan sleeves, lace at neck and bodice over lapping snapback closure. *$11.00*

1788 Budget Flannel Open Back Gown

Buck & Buck
3111 27th Avenue S
Seattle, WA 98144
800-458-0600
FAX: 800-317-2182
e-mail: info@buckandbuck.com
www.buckandbuck.com

3/4 raglan sleeve, lace at neck and bodice. *$13.00*

1789 Cotton/Poly Nancy Frocks

Buck & Buck
3111 27th Avenue S
Seattle, WA 98144
800-458-0600
FAX: 800-317-2182
e-mail: info@buckandbuck.com
www.buckandbuck.com

Comes in short and long sleeves, assorted florals and plaids. *$35.00*

1790 Dusters

Buck & Buck
3111 27th Avenue S
Seattle, WA 98144
800-458-0600
FAX: 800-317-2182
e-mail: info@buckandbuck.com
www.buckandbuck.com

Three types: Floral, Budget Better. Snap front styles and gathered yokes, flannel $16.00-$24.00.

1791 Flannel Gowns

Buck & Buck
3111 27th Avenue S
Seattle, WA 98144
800-458-0600
FAX: 800-317-2182
e-mail: info@buckandbuck.com
www.buckandbuck.com

Comes in long or short with a deep button-front opening for ease of slipping on. Shorter long length. *$16.50*

1792 Fleece Cape/Poncho

Laurel Designs
5 Laurel Avenue
Belvedere, CA 94920
FAX: 415-435-1451
e-mail: laureld@ncal.verio.com

Janet Sawyer, Co-Owner
Lynn Montoya, Co-Owner

Warm and cozy high insulated cape with hood for wheelchair users, zip front, velcro side closure, self belt. All sizes and a variety of colors. *$53.00*

1793 Float Dress

Buck & Buck
3111 27th Avenue S
Seattle, WA 98144
800-458-0600
FAX: 800-317-2182
e-mail: info@buckandbuck.com
www.buckandbuck.com

A safe bet for everyone from a size medium to a 6X. Gathered yoke front and back and literally yards of fabric for fullness. Comes in cotton or polyester. *$34.00*

1794 Muu Muu

Buck & Buck
3111 27th Avenue S
Seattle, WA 98144
800-458-0600
FAX: 800-317-2182
e-mail: info@buckandbuck.com
www.buckandbuck.com

Comes in long and short styles, assorted bright floral prints. $20.00-$22.00.

1795 Polyester Nancy Frocks

Buck & Buck
3111 27th Avenue S
Seattle, WA 98144
800-458-0600
FAX: 800-317-2182
e-mail: info@buckandbuck.com
www.buckandbuck.com

Comes in short and long sleeves, assorted florals. *$ 35.00*

Footwear

1796 Acrylic Leg Warmers

Buck & Buck
3111 27th Avenue S
Seattle, WA 98144
800-458-0600
FAX: 800-317-2182
e-mail: info@buckandbuck.com
www.buckandbuck.com

Recommended for large or swollen legs where knee socks are too restrictive. *$7.00*

1797 Adult Acorn Polartec Socks

Special Clothes
PO Box 333
E Harwich, MA 02645
508-896-7939
FAX: 508-896-7939
e-mail: specialclo@aol.com
www.special-clothes.com

Judith Sweeney, President

These plush socks are made of Polartec fleece for unparalleled softness and comfort. The mid-calf length keeps feet and lower legs warmer than any conventional sock and the fabric has 2 way stretch to minimize binding. Polartec fleece is a remarkable light-weight fabric which breathes and insulates. Machine washable, of course. 100% Polartec fleece. Made in USA. Colors: solid black or charcoal print. *$18.00*

Per pair

1798 **Adult Acorn Slippers**

Special Clothes
PO Box 333
E Harwich, MA 02645
508-896-7939
FAX: 508-896-7939
e-mail: specialclo@aol.com
www.special-clothes.com

Judith Sweeney, President

These great looking, beautifully made slipper shoes keep chilly feet warm and comfortable. The sole is cut of fine suede leather, and the uppers and insoles are soft, plush Polartec fleece. The knit cuff at the ankle opens wide to slip on easily, yet is snug enough to keep the slippers in place. Machine washable. Polartec fleece, suede sole, acrylic cuff. Made in USA. Colors: burgundy with navy cuff or dark green with navy cuff. *$30.00*

Per pair

1799 **Booties with Non-Skid Soles**

Buck & Buck
3111 27th Avenue S
Seattle, WA 98144
800-458-0600
FAX: 800-317-2182
e-mail: info@buckandbuck.com
www.buckandbuck.com

Acrylic knit or quilted cotton/poly and shearling inner. *$17.00*

1800 **Foot Snugglers**

Buck & Buck
3111 27th Avenue S
Seattle, WA 98144
800-458-0600
FAX: 800-317-2182
e-mail: info@buckandbuck.com
www.buckandbuck.com

Quilted poly/cotton outers lined with plush shearling pile, provide a thick comfortable cushion which helps minimize the pressure points on tender areas. *$23.00*

1801 **Lok-Tie Shoe Laces**

Laurel Designs
5 Laurel Avenue
Belvedere, CA 94920
FAX: 415-435-1451
e-mail: laureld@ncal.verio.com

Janet Sawyer, Co-Owner
Lynn Montoya, Co-Owner

Specially designed slide locks laces in place. Can be used with one hand. Stretch laces allow maximum comfort. *$4.00*

1802 **TRU-Mold Shoes**

42 Breckenridge Street
Buffalo, NY 14213
716-881-4484
800-843-6653
FAX: 716-881-0406

Husain Syed, Production Manager

Custom made fully molded shoes, relieve pressure in sensitive areas by taking all of the weight off the painful areas.

1803 **Terrycloth Slippers**

Buck & Buck
3111 27th Avenue S
Seattle, WA 98144
800-458-0600
FAX: 800-317-2182
e-mail: info@buckandbuck.com
www.buckandbuck.com

Lines cotton/poly terrycloth upper with sewn-on, non-skid sole. *$18.00*

1804 **Velcro Booties**

Buck & Buck
3111 27th Avenue S
Seattle, WA 98144
800-458-0600
FAX: 800-317-2182
e-mail: info@buckandbuck.com
www.buckandbuck.com

The high-domed toe, and extra-wide, non-skid sole design accommodates virtually every foot related problem. *$18.00*

1805 **Velcro Sneaker**

Buck & Buck
3111 27th Avenue S
Seattle, WA 98144
800-458-0600
FAX: 800-317-2182
e-mail: info@buckandbuck.com
www.buckandbuck.com

Two velcro straps, nylon upper, rubber sole. *$22.00*

1806 **Washable Shoes**

Buck & Buck
3111 27th Avenue S
Seattle, WA 98144
800-458-0600
FAX: 800-317-2182
e-mail: info@buckandbuck.com
www.buckandbuck.com

Vinyl upper with velcro closure, Non skid sole. *$18.00*

Jackets

1807 **Fleece Bed Jacket**

Buck & Buck
3111 27th Avenue S
Seattle, WA 98144
800-458-0600
FAX: 800-317-2182
e-mail: info@buckandbuck.com
www.buckandbuck.com

Full snap front opening and collar. Assorted bright colors and pastel prints. *$22.00*

1808 **Jackets**

Special Clothes
PO Box 333
E Harwich, MA 02645
508-896-7939
FAX: 508-896-7939
e-mail: specialclo@aol.com
www.special-clothes.com

Judith Sweeney, President

Available styles include a unique back opening jacket designed to fit easily over contractures and for wheelchair comfort. Prices range from $72.00-$89.00.

1809 **Rain Poncho**

Laurel Designs
5 Laurel Avenue
Belvedere, CA 94920
FAX: 415-435-1451
e-mail: laureld@ncal.verio.com

Janet Sawyer, Co-Owner
Lynn Montoya, Co-Owner

A favorite, this rain poncho slips on in a hurry to keep you dry. All sizes and a variety of colors. *$39.00*

1810 Wheelchair Ponchos

Special Clothes
PO Box 333
E Harwich, MA 02645
508-896-7939
FAX: 508-896-7939
e-mail: specialclo@aol.com
www.special-clothes.com

Judith Sweeney, President

These ponchos are cut shorter in the back for wheelchair comfort. Prices range from $76.00-$95.00.

Miscellaneous & Catalogs

1811 AMI: Accessories for Mobile Independence

5235 Mission Oaks Boulevard
Suite 381
Camarillo, CA 93012
FAX: 805-987-8653

Gay Dawson, Owner

Ponchos, tote bags, gloves, and sweat pants for wheelchair-using consumers.

1812 Adaptive Clothing: Adults

Special Clothes
PO Box 333
E Harwich, MA 02645
508-896-7939
FAX: 508-896-7939
e-mail: specialslo@aol.com
www.special-clothes.com

Judith Sweeney, President

Special Clothes produces a catalogue of garments for adults with disabilities and/or incontinence. Offerings include: undergarments, snap-crotch tee shirts, sleepwear, jumpsuits, bibs and some footwear. The catalogue is available without charge. Comparable to department store prices. Special Clothes produces a catalog of adaptive clothing for children in sizes from toddler through young adults. A full line of clothing is included from undergarments through wheelchair jackets and ponchos.

1813 Adrian's Closet

PO Box 9506
Rancho Santa Fe, CA 92067
800-831-2577
FAX: 858-759-0578
e-mail: adrians@electriciti.com

Fashions for the physically challenged child. Clothing offers Velcro closures, front pockets, concealed back openings and fashions for seated posture.

1814 Adult Long Jumpsuit with Feet

Special Clothes
PO Box 333
E Harwich, MA 02645
508-896-7939
FAX: 508-896-7939
e-mail: specialclo@aol.com
www.special-clothes.com

Judith Sweeney, President

A full snap crotch for full access. For safety, feet have non-skid bottoms. 100% cotton knit. Made in USA. Also, identical in style, but are made of fleece for extra warmth. Fleece fabric is soft 100% cotton, and is available in Medium Blue only. Made in USA. Options on fleece jumpsuits available for additional charge. Long knit jumpsuit with feet: #A2051; Long fleece jumpsuit: #A2032; Long fleece jumpsuit with feet: #A2052.

1815 Adult Short Jumpsuit

Special Clothes
PO Box 333
E Harwich, MA 02645
508-896-7939
FAX: 508-896-7939
e-mail: specialclo@aol.com
www.special-clothes.com

Judith Sweeney, President

This pull-on jumpsuit provides comfort and full coverage without bulk. Wide leg ribbing ends at mid-thigh, with snaps at the crotch. We use fine quality, comfortable cotton knit. 100% cotton knit. Made in USA. Option: long sleeves - add $3.00. Colors: white, navy, teal, light blue, light pink, red, burgundy, royal blue and black. Sm & Med: $36.50/3 for $104.00; L & XL: $39.00/3 for $111.25; and XXL: $42.00/3 for $119.25.

1816 Bibs

Special Clothes
PO Box 333
E Harwich, MA 02645
508-896-7939
FAX: 508-896-7939
e-mail: specialclo@aol.com
www.special-clothes.com

Judith Sweeney, President

A variety of bib styles are available to protect clothing inconspicuously.

1817 Body Suits

Special Clothes
PO Box 333
E Harwich, MA 02645
508-896-7939
FAX: 508-896-7939
e-mail: specialclo@aol.com
www.special-clothes.com

Judith Sweeney, President

These are one piece garments that can be used to protect skin under braces, to add warmth and to shield incisions. Prices range from $18.25-22.50.

1818 Buck and Buck Clothing

3111 27th Avenue S
Seattle, WA 98144
206-722-4196
800-458-0600
FAX: 206-722-1144
e-mail: julie@buckandbuck.com
www.buckandbuck.com

Julie & Bill Buck, Co-Owners

Clothing for the disabled and elderly.

88 pages Yearly 1981

1819 Caring Concepts Clothing Solutions

1525 W Alton Avenue
Santa Ana, CA 92704
800-336-2660
FAX: 800-683-6510
e-mail: info@clothingsolutions.com
www.caringconcepts.com

The nations leading designer and manufacturer of assistive clothing for men and women. Free 56 page catalog available by calling 800-500-0260. 100% guarantee on all products.

1820 Carolyn's Catalog

PO Box 468
Egg Harbor, WI 54209
920-868-1050
800-648-2266
e-mail: sales@carolynscatalog.com
www.carolynscatalog.com

Carolyn Tojek, President

Free mail-order catalog of items for visually impaired people.

1821 **Cotton Stockings**

Buck & Buck
3111 27th Avenue S
Seattle, WA 98144

800-458-0600
FAX: 800-317-2182
e-mail: info@buckandbuck.com
www.buckandbuck.com

Come in regular and snug-fit, cover leg to mid-thigh and work well for swollen legs.

1822 **Easy Dressing Fashions: JC Penney**

6501 Legacy Drive
Plano, TX 75024
972-431-8676
FAX: 972-431-9103

Natalie Torre, Marketing Manager

This is an entire collection of women's and men's fashions that are designed for easy wear, easy care and complete comfort. Plus, a selection of women's apparel with velcro brand wavelock fasteners.

1823 **Exquisite Egronomic Protective Wear**

Plum Enterprises
PO Box 85
Valley Forge, PA 19481
610-783-7377
FAX: 610-783-7577
e-mail: lynn@plument.com
www.plument.com

Janice Carrington, President

Egronomic Protective Wear; ProtectaCap custom-fitting headgear has earned an unparalleled reputation for quality, safety, and comfort. ProtectaCap+Plus technologically-advanced protective headgear closes the gap between hard and soft helmets. Comes with optional ProtectaChin Guard and new sporty design. Protecthip protective undergarment is the intelligent, innovative solution to the problem of hip injuries for both men and women. Ladies' styles are covered with attractive stretch lace.

1824 **Fashion Ease**

1541 60th Street
Brooklyn, NY 11219
718-871-8188
800-221-8929
FAX: 718-436-2067
e-mail: fashionease.com@aol
www.fashionease.com

Stacey Samuels, Customer Service Agent

Adaptive apparel and footwear for people who require ease in dressing. Free catalogue.

64 pages Yearly

1825 **Forde's Functional Fashions**

8020 E Drive
Suite 317
North Bay Village, FL 33141
305-754-4457
800-531-7705
FAX: 305-757-5447
e-mail: fashions@fordes.com
www.fordes.com

Patricia Forde, President

A fashion forward line of easy to wear clothing and accessories for men, women and children. Items include, sportswear, outerwear, ponchos, robes, sleepwear, dresses, wheelchair bags, walker bags and more. Hard to find specialty items for many special needs. Designs for people who use wheelchairs. Velcro closures if buttons are a problem. Fun clothing protectors too. Choose from our terrific assortment of fabrics and colors to suit all your fashion needs in simply functional style.

1826 **Headliner**

Designs for Comfort
4310 Highborne Drive
Marietta, GA 30066
770-565-8246
800-443-9226
FAX: 877-350-0501
e-mail: headliner@mindspring.com

Curt Maurer, President
Lynne Davis, VP Marketing

A patented cap and hairpiece combination, the Headliner is both a quick, stylish coverup and an upbeat wig alternative for women experiencing hair care problems or hair loss. Ideal for social gatherings and outdoor activities as well as for sleeping and hospital stays. *$ 25.00*

1827 **Knee Socks**

Buck & Buck
3111 27th Avenue S
Seattle, WA 98144

800-458-0600
FAX: 800-317-2182
e-mail: info@buckandbuck.com
www.buckandbuck.com

Comes in regular and large size. *$3.50*

1828 **Laurel Designs Catalog**

Laurel Designs
5 Laurel Avenue
Belvedere, CA 94920
415-435-1891
FAX: 415-435-1451
e-mail: laureld@ncal.verio.com

Janet Sawyer, Owner
Lynn Montoya, Owner

Clothing for wheelchair users including rain wear, panchos and fleece capes. Other items include quality carrying bags for wheelchairs, walkers, crutches, accessories, and cookbooks of four ingredients only recipes. Home remodeling video 'Building & Remodeling for Accessibility', reacher and large print dictionary.

8 pages BiAnnual

1829 **M&M Health Care Apparel Company**

Fashion Collection
1541 60th Street
Brooklyn, NY 11219
718-871-8188
800-221-8929
FAX: 718-436-2067
e-mail: fashionease@aol.com

Stacey Samuels, Customer Service Agent

Specialized clothing for disabled people.

1830 **No-Run Nylon Stockings**

Buck & Buck
3111 27th Avenue S
Seattle, WA 98144

800-458-0600
FAX: 800-317-2182
e-mail: info@buckandbuck.com
www.buckandbuck.com

A full-length, heavy-weight stocking. *$2.25*

1831 **Professional Fit Clothing**
831 N Lake Street
Suite 1
Burbank, CA 91502
818-563-1975
800-422-2348
FAX: 818-563-1834
e-mail: kurt@professionalfit.com
www.professionalfit.com

Tom Pirruccello, President
Kurt Rieback, CFO

Professional fit clothing caters to homes that care for people with developmental disabilities and individuals who are physically challenged. Our clothing is fashionable, affordable and can be adapted to each persons special need. There is a free catalog.

20 pages

1832 **Quilted Waterproof Bib**
Buck & Buck
3111 27th Avenue S
Seattle, WA 98144
800-458-0600
FAX: 800-317-2182
e-mail: info@buckandbuck.com
www.buckandbuck.com

Made with a nylon backing, these attractive bibs will not soak through like most others, protecting clothing from stains. *$15.00*

1833 **Rolli Moden Catalog**
12225 World Trade Drive
Suite T
San Diego, CA 92128
858-676-1825
800-707-2395
FAX: 858-676-0820
e-mail: rm@rolli-moden.com
www.rolli-moden.com

Karen Turley, General Manager

A line of fashionable clothing and accessories for adult wheelchair users available.

16-24 pages Quarterly

1834 **Special Clothes Adult Catalogue**
Special Clothes
PO Box 333
E Harwich, MA 02645
508-896-7939
FAX: 508-896-7939
e-mail: specialclo@aol.com
www.special-clothes.com

Judith Sweeney, President

Produces a catalogue of adaptive clothing for adults with disabilities. Offers include undergarments, casual bottoms, jumpsuits, sleepwear, swimwear, footwear and bibs. Prices are comparable to deparment store prices. The catalogue is free.

1-14 pages

1835 **Special Clothes for Special Children**
Special Clothes
PO Box 333
E Harwich, MA 02645
508-896-7939
FAX: 508-896-7939
e-mail: specialclo@aol.com
www.special-clothes.com

Judith Sweeney, President

Offers a variety of clothes for disabled children ranging from casual unisex clothes to undergarments. Clothing offers velcro closures, adjustable waistbands, drop-front briefs, wheelchair ponchos and more.

1836 **Specialty Care Shoppe**
16126 E 161st Street S
Bixby, OK 74008
918-366-1208
FAX: 918-366-9445
e-mail: deb@specialtycareshoppe.com
www.specialtycareshoppe.com

Deb Marshall, Owner

Catalog of attractive, affordable clothing and accessories for adults with special needs. Includes items for edema, incontinence, Alzheimers, limited mobility, and hand impairment.

1837 **Super Stretch Socks**
Buck & Buck
3111 27th Avenue S
Seattle, WA 98144
800-458-0600
FAX: 800-317-2182
e-mail: info@buckandbuck.com
www.buckandbuck.com

This sock has been improved to stretch laterally throughout the foot area as well as at the top. *$3.75*

1838 **Swimwear**
Special Clothes
PO Box 333
E Harwich, MA 02645
508-896-7939
FAX: 508-896-7939
e-mail: specialclo@aol.com
www.special-clothes.com

Judith Sweeney, President

Cotton lycra swimsuits are available in boys and girls styles from size toddler-teen. One piece, designed to completely cover a diaper.

1839 **Trisha's of Acton**
PO Box 599
Acton, MA 01720
978-263-9318
877-955-5551
FAX: 978-263-4555
e-mail: trishas@tiac.net
www.trishasofacton.com

K Julie McCarthy, President

Clothing and accessories that provide dignity, freedom of movement and independence for the physically challenged.

1840 **Wishing Wells Clothing Collection**
11684 Ventura Boulevard
Suite 965
Studio City, CA 91604
818-840-6919
FAX: 818-760-3878
e-mail: FABC@dawnwells.com
www.dawnwells.com

Dawn Wells, Owner
Lorraine Parker, General Manager

Features designs full of back overlap construction and all velcro closures clothing.

Robes & Sleepwear

1841 **Adult Snap Front Sleeper**
Special Clothes
PO Box 333
E Harwich, MA 02645
508-896-7939
FAX: 508-896-7939
e-mail: specialclo@aol.com
www.special-clothes.com

Judith Sweeney, President

This soft, comfortable one piece garment is designed for easy dressing and full access. The top fastens down the front with snaps. The bottom section folds up from the back, and snaps to the waist. 100% cotton knit. Made in USA. Option, short sleeves - add $1.00. Colors: white, navy, teal, light blue, light pink, red, burgudy, royal blue and black. Sm & Med: $36.50/ 3 for $104.00; L & XL: $39.00/ 3 for $111.25; XXL: $42.00/3 for $119.75.

1842 Chamois Shower Robe

Buck & Buck
3111 27th Avenue S
Seattle, WA 98144
800-458-0600
FAX: 800-317-2182
e-mail: info@buckandbuck.com
www.buckandbuck.com

Totally covers a man or woman being wheeled to and from the shower or bath. Having test washed several fabrics, the chamois beat terry cloth for comfort, durability and faster drying time in the laundry. *$34.00*

1843 Creative Designs

Barbara Arnold
3704 Carlisle Court
Modesto, CA 95356
209-523-3166
800-335-4852
FAX: 209-523-5893
e-mail: robes4you@aol.com
www.robes4you.com

Barbara Arnold, Owner

Designer of the original Change-A-Robe and the new Handi-Robe, which allows the wearer to put it on without having to stand up. Robes are designed especially for physically challenged, disabled individuals, and wheelchair users.

1844 Flannel Pajamas

Buck & Buck
3111 27th Avenue S
Seattle, WA 98144
800-458-0600
FAX: 800-317-2182
e-mail: info@buckandbuck.com
www.buckandbuck.com

$18.00

1845 Fleece Robe

Buck & Buck
3111 27th Avenue S
Seattle, WA 98144
800-458-0600
FAX: 800-317-2182
e-mail: info@buckandbuck.com
www.buckandbuck.com

All with full-length, snap-front opening, patch pockets, short and long. Short: $39.00.

1846 His & Hers

Wishing Wells Collection
11684 Ventura Boulevard
Suite 965
Studio City, CA 91604
818-840-6919
FAX: 818-760-3878
e-mail: FABC@dawnwells.com
www.dawnwells.com

Dawn Wells, Owner

This sleep shirt is designed for him or her.

1847 Nightshirts

Buck & Buck
3111 27th Avenue S
Seattle, WA 98144
800-458-0600
FAX: 800-317-2182
e-mail: info@buckandbuck.com
www.buckandbuck.com

Come in flannel or cotton patterns and prints in sizes S-XL, of men. *$16.00*

1848 Open Back Nightshirts

Buck & Buck
3111 27th Avenue S
Seattle, WA 98144
800-458-0600
FAX: 800-317-2182
e-mail: info@buckandbuck.com
www.buckandbuck.com

Come in cotton or flannel (sizes S-XL). *$18.00*

1849 Terrycloth Robes

Buck & Buck
3111 27th Avenue S
Seattle, WA 98144
800-458-0600
FAX: 800-317-2182
e-mail: info@buckandbuck.com
www.buckandbuck.com

Two pockets, sash belts, assorted colors. *$36.00*

Shirts & Tops

1850 Adult Pull-On Feeding Bib

Special Clothes
PO Box 333
E Harwich, MA 02645
508-896-7939
FAX: 508-896-7939
e-mail: specialclo@aol.com
www.special-clothes.com

Judith Sweeney, President

This basic bib does a great job of protecting clothing from messy food and drink spills. It is constructed of sturdy, rib knit neckband which slips on comfortably. The front pocket catches food particles and is fastened at both sides with Velcro for easy cleaning. 100% nylon with neckband of 100% cotton rib. Made in USA. Colors: white or light blue. One size: 17 inches wide, & 23 inches from shoulder to bottom. *$15.00*

1851 Avoid Eye Strain, Feel it T-Shirt

Sense-Sations
919 Walnut Street
Philadelphia, PA 19107
215-627-0600
FAX: 215-922-0692

This slogan is printed in raised writing boldly across the front of our T-shirt. *$5.95*

1852 Basic Rear Closure Sweat Top

Buck & Buck
3111 27th Avenue S
Seattle, WA 98144
800-458-0600
FAX: 800-317-2182
e-mail: info@buckandbuck.com
www.buckandbuck.com

Top opens completely down the back for ease of dressing with velcro tab closures. *$20.50*

1853 **Cotton Full-Back Vest**

Buck & Buck
3111 27th Avenue S
Seattle, WA 98144
800-458-0600
FAX: 800-317-2182
e-mail: info@buckandbuck.com
www.buckandbuck.com

Wide shoulder straps that don't slide off shoulders. *$ 4.50*

1854 **Dutch Neck T-Shirt**

Buck & Buck
3111 27th Avenue S
Seattle, WA 98144
800-458-0600
FAX: 800-317-2182
e-mail: info@buckandbuck.com
www.buckandbuck.com

Stretchy neck makes it easy to get over the head. *$5.50*

1855 **Open Back T-Shirts**

Buck & Buck
3111 27th Avenue S
Seattle, WA 98144
800-458-0600
FAX: 800-317-2182
e-mail: info@buckandbuck.com
www.buckandbuck.com

Velcro tabs down the back. *$8.00*

1856 **Printed Rear Closure Sweat Top**

Buck & Buck
3111 27th Avenue S
Seattle, WA 98144
800-458-0600
FAX: 800-317-2182
e-mail: info@buckandbuck.com
www.buckandbuck.com

Comes in assorted colors, plain or with animal motifs. *$33.00*

1857 **Rear Closure Shirts**

Buck & Buck
3111 27th Avenue S
Seattle, WA 98144
800-458-0600
FAX: 800-317-2182
e-mail: info@buckandbuck.com
www.buckandbuck.com

Velcro tabs down the back on T-shirts and dress shirts. *$24.00*

1858 **Rear Closure T-Shirt**

Buck & Buck
3111 27th Avenue S
Seattle, WA 98144
800-458-0600
FAX: 800-317-2182
e-mail: info@buckandbuck.com
www.buckandbuck.com

Closes down the back with velcro tabs. *$8.50*

1859 **Serape**

Laurel Designs
5 Laurel Avenue
Belvedere, CA 94920
FAX: 415-435-1451
e-mail: laureld@ncal.verio.com

Janet Sawyer, Co-Owner
Lynn Montoyo, Co-Owner

This unique sleeveless thermal vest is designed for active wheelchair persons. Multi-colored, one size fits all. *$30.00*

1860 **T Shirt is Done in Braille: Read Gently**

Sense-Sations
919 Walnut Street
Philadelphia, PA 19107
215-627-0600
FAX: 215-922-0692

This slogan is printed in raised writing and braille dots. *$5.95*

Slacks & Pants

1861 **Comanche Pants**

Wheelies Bentwear
333 NE Jackson Street
Roseburg, OR 97470
541-673-8726
FAX: 541-673-8719

Alice King, Store Manager
Leslie Bozovich, Customer Service

An innovative answer to dressing a person who cannot stand. These pants are sculptured to provide total coverage. A new freedom in dressing; easy for attendant or for self-dressing. They can be put on a seated person right in the chair with no lifting or standing. *$35.00*

1862 **Jumpsuits**

Special Clothes
PO Box 333
E Harwich, MA 02645
508-896-7939
FAX: 508-896-7939
e-mail: specialclo@aol.com
www.special-clothes.com

Judith Sweeney, President

Several styles of one-piece garments are available for dressing ease. Front opening styles are designed for easy access. Prices range from $32.20-$44.00.

1863 **Knit Pants**

Special Clothes
PO Box 333
E Harwich, MA 02645
508-896-7939
FAX: 508-896-7939
TTY:508-896-7939
e-mail: specialclo@aol.com
www.special-clothes.com

Judith Sweeney, President

Offers the best in comfort and convience. Designed with a longer crotch and wider seat for a great fit. The elasticized waistband contains a hidden drawstring for size adjustments, and pockets are placed low for easy access while sitting. Order a full Snap Crotch (Option #1), for full access. Available in soft, 100% cotton knit. Made in USA. Colors: Light blue, teal, light pink, burgundy, navy and black. Sm & Med: $41.00; L & XL $45.00; XXL $48.00. Add full snap crotch.

1864 **Pants & Slacks**

Special Clothes
PO Box 333
E Harwich, MA 02645
508-896-7939
FAX: 508-896-7939
e-mail: specialclo@aol.com
www.special-clothes.com

Judith Sweeney, President

A variety of pant and skirt styles is available in sizes 2 toddler - 18 teen. These include straight leg and baggy jeans, drop front pleated dress pants, knit pants, shorts and skirted leggings. Prices range from $16.50-$44.00.

1865 **Side Velcro Slacks**

Buck & Buck
3111 27th Avenue S
Seattle, WA 98144
800-458-0600
FAX: 800-317-2182
e-mail: info@buckandbuck.com
www.buckandbuck.com

Slacks open down both sides from waist to hip with velcro tab closures at sides. *$25.00*

1866 **Side-Zip Sweat Pants**

Buck & Buck
3111 27th Avenue S
Seattle, WA 98144
800-458-0600
FAX: 800-317-2182
e-mail: info@buckandbuck.com
www.buckandbuck.com

Out-seam zippers un-zip 3/4 of the way down the sides to enable dressing a resident with severe leg contractures. *$32.00*

1867 **Trunks**

Buck & Buck
3111 27th Avenue S
Seattle, WA 98144
800-458-0600
FAX: 800-317-2182
e-mail: info@buckandbuck.com
www.buckandbuck.com

Come in cotton or nylon, flare leg, full cut. *$4.00*

Undergarments

1868 **Adult Absorbent Briefs**

Special Clothes
PO Box 333
E Harwich, MA 02645
508-896-7939
FAX: 508-896-7939
e-mail: specialclo@aol.com
www.special-clothes.com

Judith Sweeney, President

Soft, comfortable, 100% cotton knit brief is seven layers thick at the crotch. Sides of the brief are a non-bulky single layer. The waistband elastic is enclosed in a soft cotton knit casing and does not touch the skin. Comfortable cotton rib knit bands circle the leg. This brief will not replace a diaper, but provides absorbency for light incontinence.

1869 **Adult Lap Shoulder Bodysuit**

Special Clothes
PO Box 333
E Harwich, MA 02645
508-896-7939
FAX: 508-893-7939
TTY:508-896-7939
e-mail: specialclo@aol.com
www.special-clothes.com

Bodysuit styles fasten at the crotch with sturdy snaps to stay neatly tucked. All are made of soft, absorbent 100% cotton knit for maximum comfort. They are cut wide at the hip and seat for full coverage, and will accomodate a diaper if necessary. Soft knit rib circles the neck and leg. This cool tank style slips on easily. Deep armholes are banded with rib knit. all styles: Small/Medium $33.00/3 for $94.00; Large/X Large $38.00/3 for $108.00; XX Large $41.00/3 for $116.00. A chioce of 9 colors.

1870 **Adult Sleeveless Bodysuit**

Special Clothes
PO Box 333
E Harwich, MA 02645
508-896-7939
FAX: 508-896-7939
e-mail: specialclo@aol.com
www.special-clothes.com

Judith Sweeney, President

Bodysuit styles fasten at the crotch with sturdy snaps to stay neatly tucked. All are made of soft, absorbent 100% cotton knit for maximum comfort. They are cut wide at the hip and seat for full coverage, and will accomodate a diaper if necessary. Soft knit rib circles the neck and leg. This cool tank style slips on easily. Deep armholes are banded with rib knit. All styles: Small/Medium $33.00/3 for $94.00; Large/X-Large $38.00/3 for $108.00; XX Large $41.00/3 for $116.00. A choice of 9 colors.

1871 **Adult Swim Diaper**

Special Clothes
PO Box 333
E Harwich, MA 02645
508-896-7939
FAX: 508-896-7939
e-mail: specialclo@aol.com
www.special-clothes.com

Judith Sweeney, President

This pant is made of soft, silent, light-weight, impermeable fabric- waterproof and secure. It is a containment brief, designed to be used in the pool in place of cloth or disposable diapers, which can become waterlogged or disintegrate in the water. Waist and legbands should be snug for proper fit, so please consult sizing chart before ordering. Darlex with lining of 100% cotton knit. Lycra waist and legbands. Made in USA.

1872 **Adult Tee Shoulder Bodysuit**

Special Clothes
PO Box 333
E Harwich, MA 02645
508-896-7939
FAX: 508-893-7939
TTY:508-896-7939
e-mail: specialclo@aol.com
www.special-clothes.com

Styles fasten at the crotch with sturdy snaps to stay neatly tucked. All are made of soft, absorbent 100% cotton knit for maximum comfot. They are cut wide at the hip and seat for full coverage, and will accommodate a diaper if necessary. Soft knit rib circles the neck and leg. This bodysuit looks like a regular tee shirt, but snaps at the crotch for a neat appearance. Small/Medium $33.00/3 for $94.00; Large/X Large $38.00/3 fpr $108.00; XX Large $41.00/3 for $116.00. Choice of 9 colors.

1873 **Adult Waterproof Overpant**

Special Clothes
PO Box 333
E Harwich, MA 02645
508-896-7939
FAX: 508-896-7939
e-mail: specialclo@aol.com
www.special-clothes.com

Judith Sweeney, President

Overpants are made of a soft, silent, lightweight fabric which is waterproof and very secure. It is designed to be used over our Adult Absorbent Brief, or cloth diapers. It is completely latex-free and is an excellent non-allergenic substitute for rubber or vinyl pants. Waist and legbands should be snug to minimize leakage, so please consult the sizing chart before ordering. Darlex with lining of 100% cotton. Lycra waist and legbands. Made in USA.

1874 **Adult Wet Wrap Swim Vest**

Special Clothes
PO Box 333
E Harwich, MA 02645
508-896-7939
FAX: 508-896-7939
e-mail: specialclo@aol.com
www.special-clothes.com

Judith Sweeney, President

This vest is made of neoprene - the same material used in wet suits - and it effectively insulates the torso to retain body heat. Muscles relax, enhancing the quality of recreational swimming or water therapy. The wrap design allows full freedom of movement. Made of Neoprene in the USA. Note: Vest provides warmth ony. It is not a flotation device. Wet wrap sizes: Adult small, Adult Medium and Adult Large.

1875 **Briefs**

Special Clothes
PO Box 333
E Harwich, MA 02645
508-896-7939
FAX: 508-896-7939
e-mail: specialclo@aol.com
www.special-clothes.com

Judith Sweeney, President

A variety of unique brief styles available for easy access and practicality.

1876 **Cloth Diapers**

Angel Fluff Diaper Company
PO Box 1131
Lewisburg, TN 37091
931-359-9604
FAX: 931-359-8420
e-mail: afdc@angelfluff.com
www.angelfluff.com

Top quality cloth diapers.

1877 **Nylon Snip Slip**

Buck & Buck
3111 27th Avenue S
Seattle, WA 98144
800-458-0600
FAX: 800-317-2182
e-mail: info@buckandbuck.com
www.buckandbuck.com

Just snip with scissors at the appropriate hem length and it's ready to wear. *$12.00*

1878 **Nylon Stretch Bra**

Buck & Buck
3111 27th Avenue S
Seattle, WA 98144
800-458-0600
FAX: 800-317-2182
e-mail: info@buckandbuck.com
www.buckandbuck.com

Front hook closure with built-up shoulder straps. *$ 16.00*

1879 **Panties**

Buck & Buck
3111 27th Avenue S
Seattle, WA 98144
800-458-0600
FAX: 800-317-2182
e-mail: info@buckandbuck.com
www.buckandbuck.com

Come in nylon or cotton, band leg for comfort. *$4.00*

1880 **Safe and Dry-Feel and Sure-Toddler Dry**

Hygienics Direct Company
100 Pine Avenue
Holmes, PA 19043
888-463-7337
e-mail: mbrier1930@aol.com
www.hygenics.com

Michael Brier, President

A variety of stress incontinence disposable liners which absorb 8-10 oz. of fluid packaged in 20 and 40 counts. Also available are patented knit nylon panties in medium, large and extra large sizes. All products are priced for the mass market.

1881 **Support Plus**

99 W Street
Suite 500
Medfield, MA 02052
508-359-2910
800-229-2910
FAX: 508-359-0139
www.supportplus.com

Offers a selection of support undergarments, braces and shoes for the physically challenged and medical professionals.

Assistive Devices

1882 **Ability Research**

PO Box 721
Minnetonka, MN 55345
952-939-0121
FAX: 952-890-8393
e-mail: ability@skypoint.com
www.abilityresearch.com

John Severson, President

Manufacturers and marketers of assistive technology equipment.

1883 **Adaptivation**

2225 W 59th Street
Suite 100
Sioux Falls, SD 57105
605-335-4445
800-723-2783
FAX: 605-335-4446
e-mail: info@adaptivation.com
www.adaptiveation.com

Don Kehoe, Marketing Director

Manufacturers of environmental control switches, auditory paging systems, a mouse emulator program, and communication devices.

1884 **Adaptive Device Locator System**

Academic Software
3504 Tates Creek Road
Lexington, KY 40517
859-552-1020
FAX: 859-273-1943
e-mail: asistaff@acsw.com
www.acsw.com

Warren E Lacefield PhD, President
Penelope Ellis, Marketing Director
Sylvia P Lacefield, Graphic Artist

Employs a unique, goal-oriented approach to aid individuals in identifying adaptive devices with potential to support various physical limitations. Devices are categorized in seven database: Existence, Travel, In-situ Motion, Environmental Adaptation, Communication, and Sports & recreation. ADLS provides its users with device descriptions, pictures and lists of sources for locating products and product information. *$ 200.00*

1885 **Analog Switch Pad**

Academic Software
331 W 2nd Street
Lexington, KY 40507
859-233-2332
800-842-2357
FAX: 859-231-0725

Warren E Lacefield PhD, President
Penelope Ellis, Marketing Director

A touch-activated, force-adjustable, low-voltage DC, electronic switch designed to control battery-operated toys, environmental controls, and computer access interfaces. This device features a large activation area that is soft and compliant to the touch. Force sensitivity is adjusted by a small dial from approximately 1 ounce to 32 ounces activation pressure, applied over an area ranging from the size of a fingertip to the size of the entire switch surface. *$149.00*

1886 **Arkenstone: The Benetech Initiative**

480 S California Avenue
Palo Alto, CA 94306
800-444-4443
FAX: 727-803-8001
e-mail: jane@benetech.org
www.benetech.org/arkenstone.html

Jane Simchuk, Donor Information

Offers various models of personal ready-to-read personal computers for the disabled.

1887 **Assistive Software Products**

Innovation Management Group
22311 Ventura Boulevard
Suite 104
Woodland Hills, CA 91364
818-346-3581
800-889-0987
FAX: 818-346-3973
e-mail: cs@imgpresents.com
www.imgpresents.com

Jerry Hussong, VP Sales/Marketing

IMG is the producer of My-T-Mouse, My-T-Mouse for Kids, Onscreen and Onscreen with CrossScanner programmable 3D Onscreen Keyboards and Macro Utilities with optional Switch scanning and Word Prediction/Completion features. It also produces the Magnifier-a magnification software program with a cursor tracker and Joystick-To-Mouse-software that enables any joystick or gamepad to run Windows and Windows Applications, just like a mouse. $19.95-$199.95 US.

1888 **Augmentative Communiation Systems (AAC)**

ZYGO Industries
PO Box 1008
Portland, OR 97207
503-684-6006
800-234-6006
FAX: 503-684-6011
e-mail: zygo@zygo-usa.com
www.zygo-usa.com

Lawrence Weiss, President

Full range of AAC systems and assistive technology including computer-based systems and computer access programs and devices.

1889 **Away We Ride IntelliKeys Overlay**

Soft Touch
4300 Stine Road
Suite 401
Bakersfield, CA 93313
877-763-8868
FAX: 661-396-8760
e-mail: softtouch@funsoftware.com
www.funsoftware.com

Roxanne Butterfield

Four full color preprinted overlays to use with Away We Ride. Just put them on an IntelliKeys keyboard and you are ready to go.

1890 **BIGmack Communication Aid**

AbleNet
1081 10th Avenue SE
Minneapolis, MN 55414
800-322-0956
FAX: 612-379-9143
e-mail: customerservice@ablenetinc.com
www.ablenetinc.com

A single message communication aid, BIGmack has 20 seconds of memory and has a 5 inches in diameter switch surface. *$86.00*

1891 **C2ILMAX**

Image Systems
6103 Blue Circle Drive
Minnetonka, MN 55343
952-935-1171
FAX: 952-935-1386
e-mail: martav@imagesystemscorp.com
www.imagesystemscorp.com

Marta Volbrecht, Sales

LCD or CRT displays designed for applications requiring a larger viewing area and high to ultrahigh resolution.

1892 **Close-Up 6.5**

Norton-Lambert Corporation
PO Box 4085
Santa Barbara, CA 93140
805-964-6767
FAX: 805-683-5679
e-mail: sales@norton-lambert.com
www.norton-lambert.com

Jeannie Vesely, Marketing Coordinator

Remotely controls PC's via modem. Telecommute from your home or laptop PC to your office PC. Run applications, update spreadsheets, print documents remotely and access networks on remote PCs. Features: fast screen and file transfers, synchronize files, unattended transfers, multi-level security, transaction logs, automated installation. *$199.00*

1893 **Computer Switch Interface**

AbleNet
1081 10th Avenue SE
Minneapolis, MN 55414
800-322-0956
FAX: 612-379-9143
e-mail: customerservice@ablenetinc.com

Allows single switch access to an Apple computer. *$36.00*

1894 **Concepts on the Move Advanced Overlay CD**

Soft Touch
4300 Stine Road
Suite 401
Bakersfield, CA 93313
877-763-8868
FAX: 661-396-8760
e-mail: softtouch@funsoftware.com
www.funsoftware.com

Roxanne Butterfield

Use this overlay CD with Concepts on the Move Advanced Preacademics. Overlays match the concepts and graphics in the program. Includes standard overlays with all the choices and SoftTouch's changeable format overlays. Print and laminate the blank templates. Then print and laminate the picture keys in all three sizes - small, medium and large. Includes Overlay Printer by IntelliTools for easy printing.

1895 **Concepts on the Move Basic Overlay CD**

Soft Touch
4300 Stine Road
Suite 401
Bakersfield, CA 93313
877-763-8868
FAX: 661-396-8760
e-mail: softtouch@funsoftware.com
www.funsoftware.com

Roxanne Butterfield

Use this Overlay CD with Concepts on the Move Basic Preacademics. Overlays match the conepts and graphics in the program. Includes standard overlays with all the choices and SoftTouch's changeable format overlays. Print and laminate the blank templates. Then print and laminate the picture keys in all three sizes - small, medium and large. It is easy and fast to place the images on the blank templates.

1896 **Darci Too**

WesTest Engineering Corporation
810 Shepard Lane
Farmington, UT 84025
801-451-9191
FAX: 801-298-7102

Mary L Lynds, Manager

A universal device which allows people with physical disabilities to replace the keyboard and mouse on a personal computer with a device that matches their physical capabilities. DARCI TOO works with almost any personal computer and provides access to all computer functions. *$995.00*

1897 **Don Johnston**

26799 N Commerce Drive
Volo, IL 60073
847-740-0749
800-999-4660
FAX: 847-740-7326
e-mail: info@donjohnston.com
www.donjohnston.com

A provider of quality products and services that enable people with special needs to discover their potential and experience success. Products are developed for the areas of Physical Access, Augmentative Communication and for those who struggle with reading and writing.

1898 **EZ Touch Panel**

Words+
40015 Sierra Highway B-145
Palmdale, CA 93550
800-869-8521
FAX: 661-266-8969

Ginger Woltosz, VP
Tim Ross, Manager

Touch screen input is the most direct and intuitive method for picture-based communication for those with the required motor skills. *$399.00*

1899 **Expanded Keyboard Emulator**

Words+
40015 Sierra Highway B-145
Palmdale, CA 93550
800-869-8521
FAX: 661-266-8969

Ginger Woltosz, VP
Tim Ross, Manager

Provides DUAl word prediction, abbreviation expansion (macrocapability), five different methods of voice output, keyboard control, RAM-resident and the ability to run in graphics mode and access to commercial software applications.

1900 **Eyegaze Computer System**

LC Technologies
4415 Glen Rose Street
Fairfax, VA 22032
800-733-5284
FAX: 703-425-7677

Nancy Cleveland, Medical Coordinator

Enables people with physical disabilities to do many things with their eyes that they would otherwise do with their hands.

1901 Fall Fun IntelliKeys Overlay

Soft Touch
4300 Stine Road
Suite 401
Bakersfield, CA 93313
877-763-8868
FAX: 661-396-8760
e-mail: softtouch@funsoftware.com
www.funsoftware.com

Roxanne Butterfield

Seven full color preprinted overlays to use with Fall Fun. Just put them on an IntelliKeys keyboard and you are ready to go.

1902 FingerFoniks

Words+
40015 Sierra Highway B-145
Palmdale, CA 93550
800-869-8521
FAX: 661-266-8969

Ginger Woltosz, VP
Tim Ross, Manager

One-pound, hand-held, communicator incorporating synthesized and recorded speech. The user makes words and sentences by pressing sound (phoneme) keys on a membrane keyboard. *$995.00*

1903 Five Green & Speckled Frogs IntelliKeys Overlay

Soft Touch
4300 Stine Road
Suite 401
Bakersfield, CA 93313
877-763-8868
FAX: 661-396-8760
e-mail: softtouch@funsoftware.com
www.funsoftware.com

Roxanne Butterfield

Seven full color preprinted overlays to use with Five Green and Speckled Frogs. Just put them on an IntelliKeys keyboard and you are ready to go.

1904 Florida New Concepts Marketing

Florida New Concepts Marketing
PO Box 261
Port Richey, FL 34673
727-842-3231
800-456-7097
FAX: 727-845-7544
e-mail: compulnz@ate.net
www.gulfside.com/compulenz

Alan Lezark, Market Representative

Compu-Lenz, a combination fresnel magnifier and glass glare filter in an adjustable hood. When placed on the front of a PC monitor it magnifies the character size, reduces glare and enhances contrast. *$ 204.95*

1905 GW Micro

725 Airport N Office Park
Fort Wayne, IN 46825
260-489-3671
FAX: 260-489-2608
e-mail: webmaster@gwmicro.com
www.gwmicro.com

Computer hardware and software products for people with disabilities.

1906 Goals and Objectives

JE Stewart Teaching Tools
PO Box 15308
Seattle, WA 98115
206-262-9538
FAX: 206-262-9538

J E Stewart, Owner

Goals and Objectives software helps teachers make student plans including IEP's, IPP's and IHP's. The system provides curricula for all students and programs to develop and evaluate plans, print reports and make data forms. Systems are available for Windows and Macintosh for $139.

1907 I KNOW American History Overlay CD

Soft Touch
4300 Stine Road
Suite 401
Bakersfield, CA 93313
877-763-8868
FAX: 661-396-8760
e-mail: softtouch@funsoftware.com
www.funsoftware.com

Roxanne Butterfield

Use this Overlay CD with I KNOW American History program. Includes standard overlays and SoftTouch's changeable overlays. Includes Overlay Printer by IntelliTools. Use Overlay Maker by IntelliTools (not included) to modify the overlays or to make additional learning materials.

1908 Jelly Bean Switch

AbleNet
1081 10th Avenue SE
Minneapolis, MN 55414
800-322-0956
FAX: 612-379-9143
e-mail: customerservice@ablenetinc.com
www.ablenetinc.com

A momentary touch switch made of shatterproof plastic, small and sensitive to 2-3 ounces of pressure, this switch is provided audible feedback when activated and is a compact version of the Big Red Switch. *$42.00*

1909 KeyWiz

Words+
1220 W Avenue J
Lancaster, CA 93534
800-869-8521
FAX: 661-266-8969

Phil Lawrence, VP
Rachel Nielsen, Customer Support

A software and hardware product designed to operate on an IBM compatible PC. The software provides word prediction, abbreviation expansion and access to commercial software applications. *$695.00*

1910 LinkPower 50

Words+
40015 Sierra Highway B-145
Palmdale, CA 93550
800-869-8521
FAX: 661-266-8969

Ginger Woltosz, VP
Tim Ross, Manager

DC-to-DC switching power converter provides a continuous, independent multi-output, multi-voltage power supply to any augcom device, laptop computer, pointing device, voice synthesizer, cellular phone, or other battery-operated device directly from a wheelchair. *$449.00*

1911 MessageMate

Words+
1220 W Avenue J
Lancaster, CA 93534
800-869-8521
FAX: 661-266-8969

Rachel Nielsen, Customer Support

Lightweight, hand-held communicator providing high-quality analog recording capability using either direct select keyboards or 1 to 2 switch access. Price ranges from $549.00 to $999.00.

1912 Monkeys Jumping on the Bed IntelliKeys Overlay

Soft Touch
4300 Stine Road
Suite 401
Bakersfield, CA 93313
877-763-8868
FAX: 661-396-8760
e-mail: softtouch@funsoftware.com
www.funsoftware.com

Roxanne Butterfield

Seven full color preprinted overlays to use with Monkeys Jumping. Just put them on an IntelliKeys keyboard and you are ready to go.

1913 Morse Code Equalizer

Words+
40015 Sierra Highway B-145
Palmdale, CA 93550
800-869-8521
FAX: 661-266-8969

Ginger Woltosz, VP
Tim Ross, Manager

Provides complete word processing and voice output communications with single or dual switch Morse code inputs. Originally designed for a blind user with only eyelid movement. The system can be used by both sighted and visually impaired persons. *$1395.00*

1914 Mouthsticks

Sammons Preston Rolyan
4 Sammons Court
Bolingbrook, IL 60440
630-226-1300
800-323-5547
FAX: 630-226-1389
e-mail: spr@abilityone.com
www.sammonsprestonrolyan.com

Wide offering of mouthsticks featuring various functions (BK 5380, 5381, 5383, 5385, 6002, or BK 5370 series).

1915 Multi-Scan Single Switch Activity Center

Academic Software
331 W 2nd Street
Lexington, KY 40507
859-233-2332
800-842-2357
FAX: 859-231-0725

Warren E Lacefield PhD, President
Penelope Ellis, Marketing Director

A single switch activity center containing four educational games: Match, Maze, Dot-to-Dot, and Concentration, along with six graphics libraries; Dinosaurs, Sports, Animals, Independent Living, Vocations, and Cosmetology. MULTI-SCAN allows you to select a graphic library, choose games for each user, and adjust the difficulty level and other settings for each game. Other features allow you to save the game setups under each user's name and print out individual performance reports after sessions. *$154.00*

1916 Old MacDonald's Farm IntelliKeys Overlay

Soft Touch
4300 Stine Road
Suite 401
Bakersfield, CA 93313
877-763-8868
FAX: 661-396-8760
e-mail: softtouch@funsoftware.com
www.funsoftware.com

Roxanne Butterfield

Extend your students' learning with more than 45 pre-made overlays that support all of the skills learned at the farm. Use with the IntelliKeys keyboard. Simply print and use. Print an extra set to make off computer activities, too. Note: Requires Overlay Maker or Overlay Printer by IntelliTools.

1917 Perfect Solutions

15950 Schweizer Court
W Palm Beach, FL 33414
561-790-1070
800-726-7086
FAX: 561-790-0108
e-mail: perfect@gate.net
www.perfectsolutions.com

Andrew Kramer, President

A computer for every student and it speaks! Wireless laptop computers starting at $290.00 are ideal for students to carry with them all day. Text-to-speech and web browsing are available. *$290.00*

1918 Phillip Roy

PO Box 130
Indian Rocks Beach, FL 33785
727-593-2700
800-255-9085
FAX: 727-595-2685
e-mail: info@philliproy.com
www.philliproy.com

Ruth Bragman PhD, President

Offers multimedia materials appropriate for use with individuals with disabilities. Programs range from preschool through the adult level. Many of the programs are high interest topics/low vocabulary, ideal for transition and employability skills. Materials are also available which focus on social and personal development. Call for a free catalog.

1919 Phone-TTY

1246 US Highway 46 W
Parsippany, NJ 07054
973-299-6627
888-332-3889
FAX: 973-299-7768
e-mail: phonetty@aol.com
www.phone-tty.com

Anna M Terrazzino, Executive Director

Develops and promotes better communications for the deaf using ordinary telephone equipment and current technology. Installs computerized phone-television equipment in the homes of individuals who are deaf, enabling these individuals to communicate with local police, hospitals, answering services and news services.

1920 Rodeo IntelliKeys Overlay

Soft Touch
4300 Stine Road
Suite 401
Bakersfield, CA 93313
877-763-8868
FAX: 661-396-8760
e-mail: softtouch@funsoftware.com
www.funsoftware.com

Roxanne Butterfield

Four full color preprinted overlays to use with The Rodeo. Just put them on an IntelliKeys keyboard and you are ready to go.

1921 SS-Access Single Switch Interface for PC's with MS-DOS

Academic Software
331 W 2nd Street
Lexington, KY 40507
859-233-2332
800-842-2357
FAX: 859-231-0725

Warren E Lacefield PhD, President
Penelope Ellis, Marketing Director

A general purpose single switch hardware and software interface for DOS and the IBM and compatible PC family. It is designed to be easy to install, simple to use, and compatible with the widest possible range of computers and application software programs. SS-ACCESS! connects to one of the PC serial ports and provides a jack to connect an external switch. The DOS version of the software works by sending a user defined keystroke to the PC keyboard buffer whenever the switch is pressed. *$ 90.00*

1922 Simplicity

Words+
1220 W Avenue J
Lancaster, CA 93534
661-266-8500
800-869-8521
FAX: 661-266-8969

Phil Lawrence, VP
Rachel Nielsen, Customer Support

Swing-down mount for portable computers and other devices is made from high-quality aircraft aluminum. Simplicity contains very few moving parts and installs in minutes, providing a positive, secure support for computer/device in both the stored and overlap position. *$595.00*

1923 Slim Armstrong Mounting System

AbleNet
1081 10th Avenue SE
Minneapolis, MN 55414
800-322-0956
FAX: 612-379-9143
e-mail: customerservice@ablenetinc.com
www.ablenetinc.com

Slim Armstrong is a mounting system strong enough to hold up to five pounds in any position. Mix and match parts to create the system length you desire. *$188.00*

1924 Smart Modem

HARC Mercantile
PO Box 3055
Kalamazoo, MI 49003
269-324-1615
800-445-9968
FAX: 269-324-2387
e-mail: home@harcmercantile.com
www.harcmercantile.com

Ronald Slager, President

Smart modem makes your computer accessible to a TTY. *$ 349.00*

1925 SoftTouch Favorites IntelliKeys Overlay

Soft Touch
4300 Stine Road
Suite 401
Bakersfield, CA 93313
877-763-8868
FAX: 661-396-8760
e-mail: softtouch@funsoftware.com
www.funsoftware.com

Roxanne Butterfield

Four full color preprinted overlays to use with SoftTouch Favorites. Just put them on an IntelliKeys keyboard and you are ready to go.

1926 Songs I Sing at Preschool IntelliKeys Over lay

Soft Touch
4300 Stine Road
Suite 401
Bakersfield, CA 93313
877-763-8868
FAX: 661-396-8760
e-mail: softtouch@funsoftware.com
www.funsoftware.com

Roxanne Butterfield

Pre-made overlays for use with Songs I Sing at Preschool. Simply print and use with an IntelliKeys keyboard. Print an extra set to make off computer activities, too.

1927 String Switch

AbleNet
1081 10th Avenue SE
Minneapolis, MN 55414
800-322-0956
FAX: 612-379-9143
e-mail: customerservice@ablenetinc.com
www.ablenetinc.com

An activated switch beneficial for users with limited active movement or minimal strength. *$28.00*

1928 Switch Basics IntelliKeys Overlay

Soft Touch
4300 Stine Road
Suite 401
Bakersfield, CA 93313
877-763-8868
FAX: 661-396-8760
e-mail: softtouch@funsoftware.com
www.funsoftware.com

Roxanne Butterfield

Four preprinted overlays to use with Switch Basics. Just put them on an IntelliKeys keyboard and you're ready to go.

1929 Symbi-Key Computer Switch Interface

AbleNet
1081 10th Avenue SE
Minneapolis, MN 55414
800-322-0956
FAX: 612-379-9143
e-mail: customerservice@ablenetinc.com
www.ablenetinc.com

The Symbi-Key can be programmed to simulate any key stroke or a series of keystrokes (up to 5 per key) for single switch access to software programs whether or not it was designed for switch access. Works well in DOS and all versions of Windows providing access to any IBM program. *$299.00*

1930 Teach Me Phonemics Blends Overlay CD

Soft Touch
4300 Stine Road
Suite 401
Bakersfield, CA 93313
877-763-8868
FAX: 661-396-8760
e-mail: softtouch@funsoftware.com
www.funsoftware.com

Roxanne Butterfield

Teach Me Phonemics Blends Overlay CD contains over 40 IntelliKeys overlays for use with Teach Me Phonemics - Blends program. Choose either 4-item or 9-item layout to match the presentation you use in the program. Print extra copies of the overlays for off computer activites, too.

1931 Teach Me Phonemics Medial Overlay CD

Soft Touch
4300 Stine Road
Suite 401
Bakersfield, CA 93313
877-763-8868
FAX: 661-396-8760
e-mail: softtouch@funsoftware.com
www.funsoftware.com

Roxanne Butterfield

Teach Me Phonemics Medial Overlay CD contains over 40 IntelliKeys overlays for use with Teach Me Phonemics - Medial program. Choose either 4-item or 9-item layout to match the presentation you use in the program. Print extra copies of the overlays for off computer activites, too.

1932 **Teach Me Phonemics Overlay Series Bundle**

Soft Touch
4300 Stine Road
Suite 401
Bakersfield, CA 93313
877-763-8868
FAX: 661-396-8760
e-mail: softtouch@funsoftware.com
www.funsoftware.com

Roxanne Butterfield

Teach Me Phonemics Overlay Series Bundle includes one copy of each Teach Me Phonemics Overlay CD - Initial, Medial, Final and - four CD's in all.

1933 **Teach Me to Talk Overlay CD**

Soft Touch
4300 Stine Road
Suite 401
Bakersfield, CA 93313
877-763-8868
FAX: 661-396-8760
e-mail: softtouch@funsoftware.com
www.funsoftware.com

Roxanne Butterfield

For older version of Teach Me to Talk. Mac only version with red label and PC only version with yellow label. More than 48 pre-made overlays that match the activities on Teach Me to Talk. Simply print and use with an IntelliKeys keyboard. Print an extra set to make off computer activities, too.

1934 **Teach Me to Talk: USB-Overlay CD**

Soft Touch
4300 Stine Road
Suite 401
Bakersfield, CA 93313
877-763-8868
FAX: 661-396-8760
e-mail: softtouch@funsoftware.com
www.funsoftware.com

Roxanne Butterfield

Revised version of Teach Me to Talk Overlays for the newest version that is USB IntelliKeys compatible. This CD contains more than 48 overlays that match the activities and updated graphics of Teach Me to Talk. Includes Overlay Printer by IntelliTools for easy printing.

1935 **Teen Tunes Plus IntelliKeys Overlay**

Soft Touch
4300 Stine Road
Suite 401
Bakersfield, CA 93313
877-763-8868
FAX: 661-396-8760
e-mail: softtouch@funsoftware.com
www.funsoftware.com

Roxanne Butterfield

Seven full color, preprinted overlays to use with Teen Tunes Plus. Just put them on an IntelliKeys keyboard and you're ready to go.

1936 **TouchCorders Holder**

Soft Touch
4300 Stine Road
Suite 401
Bakersfield, CA 93313
877-763-8868
FAX: 661-396-8760
e-mail: softtouch@funsoftware.com
www.funsoftware.com

Roxanne Butterfield

The TouchCorders Holder enables you to position up to 4 TouchCorders for sequencing, spelling, communication, story telling and more. The TouchCorders Holder holds TouchCorders snugly and keeps them in place even when you are offering multiple choices to students in a group setting. The sturdy triangular shape presents TouchCorders at a 30-degree angle for better visual and physical access.

1937 **Turtle Teasers IntelliKeys Overlay**

Soft Touch
4300 Stine Road
Suite 401
Bakersfield, CA 93313
877-763-8868
FAX: 661-396-8760
e-mail: softtouch@funsoftware.com
www.funsoftware.com

Roxanne Butterfield

Seven full color preprinted overlays to use with Turtle Teasers. Just put them on the IntelliKeys keyboard and you're ready to go.

1938 **U-Control II**

Words+
1220 W Avenue J
Lancaster, CA 93534
800-869-8521
FAX: 661-266-8969

Phil Lawrence, VP
Rachel Nielsen, Customer Support

Works with the Words+ system (EX Keys, Morse WSKE, Scanning WSKE, Talking Screen) to provide wireless, portable control of items which are already infrared-controlled such as a TV, VCR, CD player, etc. *$ 395.00*

1939 **Universal Switch Mounting System**

AbleNet
1081 10th Avenue SE
Minneapolis, MN 55414
800-322-0956
FAX: 612-379-9143
e-mail: customerservice@ablenetinc.com
www.ablenetinc.com

Mounting system that allows switch placement in any position. A single lever locks all joints securely in place. Extends to 20 1/2 inches and holds up to five pounds. A mounting system for quick and easy positioning. *$189.00*

1940 **VISION**

Artic Technologies
1000 John R Roadrive
Suite 108
Troy, MI 48083
248-588-7370
FAX: 248-588-2650
e-mail: info@artictech.com
www.artictech.com

The premier access system for blind users of IBM personal computers.

1941 **WinSCAN: The Single Switch Interface for PC's with Windows**

Academic Software
331 W 2nd Street
Lexington, KY 40507
859-233-2332
800-842-2357
FAX: 859-231-0725

Warren E Lacefield PhD, President
Penelope Ellis, Marketing Director

A general purpose single-switch control interface for Windows. It provides single-switch users independent control access to educational and productivity software, multimedia programs, and recreational activities that run under Windows 3.1 and higher versions on IBM and compatible PC's. The user can navigate through Windows; choose program icons and run programs, games, and CD's; even surf the Internet with WinSCAN and his or her adaptive switch. *$349.00*

1942 **Words+ Equalizer**

Words+
40015 Sierra Highway B-145
Palmdale, CA 93550
800-869-8521
FAX: 661-266-8969

Ginger Woltosz, VP
Tim Ross, Manager

A hardware/software product designed to operate on an IBM compatible PC. The software provides an intelligent word prediction scheme, a calculator, music, plus ability to draw and play games. Equalizer is a dedicated augmentative communication system designed for use by individuals with severe motor disability. *$1395.00*

1943 **Words+ IST (Infrared, Sound, Touch)**

Words+
1220 W Avenue J
Lancaster, CA 93534
661-266-8500
800-869-8521
FAX: 661-266-8969

Phil Lawrence, VP
Rachel Nielsen, Customer Support

A unique switch that is activated by slight movement or faint sound. The switch provides user control when connected to a device driven by a single switch. Individuals are currently accessing a wide variety of communication and computer systems with movement using the IST switch. Price ranges from $295.00 to $495.00.

Braille Products

1944 **Access Systems International**

415 English Avenue
Monterey, CA 93940
831-373-6291
FAX: 831-375-5313

Developers of Braille printers.

1945 **Braille Blazer**

Blazie Engineering
11800 31st Court N
St. Petersburg, FL 33716
800-444-4443
FAX: 727-803-8001

Braille printer.

1946 **Braille N' Speak**

Blazie Engineering
11800 31st Court N
St. Petersburg, FL 33716
800-444-4443
FAX: 727-803-8001

A compact, portable talking device with a seven-key Braille keyboard, may be used as a talking computer terminal, a braille to print transcriber and a word processor.

1947 **Brailon Thermoform Duplicator**

American Thermoform Corporation
1758 Brackett Street
La Verne, CA 91750
909-593-6711
FAX: 909-593-8001
e-mail: atc@atcbrleqp.com
www.atcbrleqp.com

Ruth Haggen, VP

This copy machine, for producing tactile images copies, any Brailled or embossed original, by a vacuum forming process. This model is for the reproduction of teaching aids and mobility maps.

1948 **Computer Paper for Brailling**

Maxi Aids
42 Executive Boulevard
Suite 3209
Farmingdale, NY 11735
631-752-0521
800-522-6294
FAX: 631-752-0689
e-mail: sales@maxiaids.com
www.maxiaids.com

Specially made paper for braille printing. 1,000 sheets/case *$69.95*

1949 **Duxbury Braille Translator**

Duxbury Systems
270 Littleton Road
Suite 6
Westford, MA 01886
978-692-3000
FAX: 978-692-7912
e-mail: info@duxsys.com
www.duxburysystems.com

Dan Thibert, Director of Sales

A complete line of easy to use word processing and Braille translation software available for Windows (including NT) and Macintosh. Applications for anyone wanting to produce or communicate with Braille; signs, note cards, textbooks, business communications and forms, telephone bills, etc. Simple to use, FREE technical support. Free one year upgrades. DBT is for producing Braille in English, Spanish, French, Portuguese, Italian, Latin, Greek, German and other languages. *$600.00*

1950 **Enabling Technologies Company**

1601 NE Braille Place
Jensen Beach, FL 34957
772-225-3687
800-777-3687
FAX: 772-225-3299
e-mail: enabling@brailler.com
www.brailler.com

Kate Schenk, Marketing Department
Charlie Kiefer, Marketing Department

Manufactures the most complete line of American made Braille embossers, including desk top or portable models capable of producing high quality single sided or interpoint Braille. Also carries a complete line of adaptive technology aids for the blind community at affordable prices.

1951 **Eye Relief Word Processing Software**

SkiSoft Publishing Corporation
PO Box 364
Lexington, MA 02420
781-863-1876
FAX: 781-861-0086
e-mail: info@skisoft.com
www.skisoft.com

Ken Skier, President
Cynthia Skier, CFO

Large-type word processing program for visually-impaired PC users. *$295.00*

1952 **Freedom Scientific Blind/ Low Vision Group**

11800 31st Court N
St Petersberg, FL 33716 **727-803-8000**
800-444-4443
FAX: 727-803-8001
e-mail: info@hj.com
www.freedomscientific.com

Brian J Blazie, VP

Developer and manufacturer of assistive technology products for blind and visually impaired individuals. Software: JANS for Windows, ScreenReader, Magic Screen Magnifier, Open Book Scanning and Reading Software. Hardware: Braille wireless, personal note takers: Braille 'n Speak, BrailleLite, Type 'n Speak, Type Lite, Braille Embossers, Computer Braille Displays. Training and tutorials availible. *$16.95*

1953 **MegaDots**

Raised Dot Computing
408 S Baldwin Street
Madison, WI 53703 **608-257-9595**
800-347-9594
FAX: 608-257-4143
e-mail: info@rdcbraille.com
www.rdcbraille.com

Theresa Wantuch, Sales Manager
Caryn Navy, VP Technical Support
David Holladay, President

A revolutionary new braille translator for the PC that lets you finish projects quickly and easily. Intelligent document importation recognizes what word processor your text is from, and guesses that appropriate format for each paragraph, yielding high quality braille. *$540.00*

1954 **Raised Dot Computing**

Duxbury Systems
270 Littleton Road
Suite 6
Westford, MA 01886 **978-692-3000**
FAX: 978-692-7912
e-mail: info@duxsys.com
www.duxburysystems.com

Dan Thibert, Director of Sales

Software for the visually impaired.

Information Centers & Databases

1955 **ABLEDATA**

8630 Fenton Street
Suite 930
Silver Spring, MD 20910 **301-608-8998**
800-227-0216
FAX: 301-608-8958
TTY:301-608-8912
e-mail: ABLEDATA@macroint.com
www.abledata.com

Katherine Belknap, Director
Susan Carey, Information Specialist
David Johnson, Publications Director

ABLEDATA is an electronic database of assistive technology and rehabilitation equipment products for children and adults with physical, cognitive and sensory disabilities. ABLEDATA staff can perform database searches or the database can be searched on the ABLEDATA website database printouts, informer consumer guides and fact website sheets are available at cost from the office or free from the website.

1956 **ATTAIN**

Division of Disability, Aging & Rehab Services
32 E Washington Street
Suite 1400
Indianapolis, IN 46204 **317-486-8808**
FAX: 317-486-8809
e-mail: attain@attaininc.org
www.attaininc.org

Gary R Hand, Executive Director

Nonprofit organization that creates system change by expanding the availability of community-based technology-related activities, outreach services, empowerment and advocacy activities through the development of a comprehensive, consumer-responsive, statewide program to serve individuals with disabilities, of all ages and all disabilities, their families, caregivers, educators and service providers. Provides trainings, information and referral, system change and assessments for equipment needs.

1957 **Aloha Special Technology Access Center**

710 Green Street
Honolulu, HI 96813 **808-523-5547**
FAX: 808-536-3765
e-mail: stachi@aol.com
www.geocities.com/astachi

Computer technology center.

1958 **Audiogram/Clinical Records Manager**

David Center
98 Route 46 W
Budd Lake, NJ 07828 **973-347-0006**
FAX: 973-691-0611

Keeps track of client audiogram history and can print or view client with audiogram. The company no longer works with hearing aids. *$414.75*

1959 **Birmingham Alliance for Technology Access Center**

Birmingham Independent Living Center
206 13th Street S
Birmingham, AL 35233 **256-722-0122**
FAX: 205-251-0605
TTY:205-251-2223
e-mail: bhamilc@bellsouth.net
www.birminghamilc.org

Computer technology center.

1960 **Bluegrass Technology Center**

169 N Limestone Street
Lexington, KY 40507 **859-255-9951**
800-209-7767
FAX: 859-255-0059
TTY:606-491-8700
e-mail: office@bluegrass-tech.org
www.bluegrass-tech.org

Bob Glass, Executive Director

Provides assistive technology information, consulting and training for education, health professionals, consumers and parents of consumers. Maintains extensive lending library of assistive devices and adapted toys. Statewide training such as; AAC, how to obtain funding for assistive technology, augmentative and alternate communication, equipment implementation strategies, specific to hardware and software, etc.

1961 **CHID Combined Health Information Database**

National Institute of Health
Box CHID 9000 Rockville Pike
Rockville, MD 20892 **301-402-8714**
FAX: 301-770-5164

Richard Pike

A computerized bibliographic database, developed and managed by health-related agencies of the federal government.

1962 Carolina Computer Access Center

Metro School
700 E 2nd Street
Charlotte, NC 28202
704-342-3004
FAX: 701-342-1513
e-mail: ccacnc@aol.com
http://ccac.ataccess.org

Linda Schilling, Executive Director

Nonprofit community-based technology resource center for people with disabilities, providing information about and demonstration of the technology tools that enable individuals with disabilities to control and direct their own lives. Services and programs include: assessments, demonstrations, resource information, lending library, workshops and outreach.

1963 Center for Accessible Technology

2547 8th Street
Suite 12-A
Berkeley, CA 94710
510-841-3224
FAX: 510-841-7956
e-mail: info@cforat.org
www.cforat.org

Dmitri Belser, Executive Director
Eric Smith, Administrative Director

The Center is a grassroots consumer-based agency with programs that connect people with all types of disabilities, family members, educators, therapists and others with computer-based tools. Services include assessment, ongoing training, curriculum adaption, classes, demonstrations and a newsletter.

1964 Center for Applied Special Technology

39 Cross Street
Peabody, MA 01960
978-531-8555
FAX: 978-531-0192
www.cast.org

Bart Pisha, Director Research
Chuck Hitchcock, Director Product Development

Expands opportunities for individuals with special needs through innovative use of computers and related technology. We pursue this mission through research and product development that further universal design for learning.

1965 Center for Enabling Technology

622 Route 10
Suite 22B
Whippany, NJ 07981
973-428-1455
FAX: 973-560-9751

Carmela Balacco, Office Manager

Computer technology center offering resource time, workshops, technology, training and evaluations.

1966 Center on Evaluation of Assistive Technology

National Rehabilitation Hospital
102 Irving Street NW
Washington, DC 20010
202-877-1932
FAX: 202-723-0628
TTY:202-726-3996
e-mail: justin.m.carter@medstar.net
www.atnrc.org

The center develops ways of collecting, producing and distributing information to help users, prescribers and third-party payers make intelligent selections of devices.

1967 Compuserve: Handicapped Users' Database

5000 Arlington Centre Boulevard
Columbus, OH 43220
614-457-8600
FAX: 614-538-4023
www.compuserve.com

Audrey Weil, General Manager

This nationwide database with bulletin boards provides information for persons with disabilities and the issues and technologies that are of interest to them.

1968 Computer & Web Resources for People With Disabilities

Alliance for Technology Access
2175 E Francisco Boulevard
Suite L
San Rafael, CA 94901
415-455-4575
800-455-7970
FAX: 415-455-0654
e-mail: ataininfo@ataaccess.org
www.ataccess.org

A guide to maneuvering the growing world of computers, both the mainstream and the assistive technology.

ISBN 0-897933-00-1

1969 Computer Access Center

6234 W 87th Street
Los Angeles, CA 90045
310-338-1597
FAX: 310-338-9318
e-mail: cac@cac.org
www.cac.org

Computer technology center.

1970 Computer CITE

215 E New Hampshire Street
Orlando, FL 32804
407-896-3177
FAX: 407-895-5255
e-mail: comcite@aol.com

Lee Nasehi, Interim Director

Computer technology center.

1971 Computer Center for Viasually Impaired People: Division of Continuing Studies

17 Lexington Avenue
PO Box H-648
New York, NY 10010
212-802-2140
FAX: 212-802-2103
e-mail: spkbb@cunyvm.cuny.edu
www.baruch.cuny.edu/ccvip

Offers courses, tutors, equipment and assistance.

1972 Computer-Enabling Drafting for People with Physical Disabilities

County College of Morris
214 Center Grove Road
Randolph, NJ 07869
973-328-5000
888-226-8001
FAX: 973-328-5286
www.ccm.edu

Joe Robinson

Computer service.

1973 **Computers to Help People**

825 E Johnson Street
Madison, WI 53703
608-257-5917
FAX: 608-257-3480
e-mail: techorlochpi.org
www.chpi.org

Carl Durocher, Assistive Technologies Manager
Johnny R Lee, Operations Manager
John J Boyer, Executive Director

A center for assistive technology, assessment, consulting and training, specializing in computer access products for persons with sensory or mobility impairments. Also provides a print-to-braille service with a specialty in technical writing.

1974 **DIRLINE**

National Library of Medicine
8600 Rockville Pike
Bethesda, MD 20894
301-496-6193
888-346-3656
FAX: 301-480-3537
e-mail: custserv@nml.nih.gov
www.nlm.nih.gov/

18,000 listings of organizations that serve as information resources, including libraries, professional associations and government agencies.

1975 **Developmental Disabilities Council**

200 Lafayette Street
PO Box 3455
Baton Rouge, LA 70821
225-342-6804
FAX: 225-342-1970
www.laddc.org

Sandee Winchell, Director

Computer technology center.

1976 **Employment Resources Program**

426 W Jefferson Street
Springfield, IL 62702
217-523-2587
800-447-4221
FAX: 217-523-0427

Ceceilia Haasis, Program Manager

An information and referral service that encourages inquiries from professionals, individuals with disabilities, family members, organizations or anyone requesting information pertaining to disabilities. The staff at DRN uses both computer listings and in-house library files to provide the programs services. The DRN program is funded by a grant from the Illinois Department of Rehabilitation Services.

1977 **Functional Skills Screening Inventory**

Functional Resources
3905 Huntington Drive
Amarillo, TX 79104
806-353-1114
FAX: 806-353-1114
e-mail: webmaster@winfssi.comnhsc.edu
www.winfssi.com

Ed Hammer PhD, Owner
Heather Becker PhD, Owner

Assesses the individuals and level of functional skills and identifies supports needed by educational, rehabilitation and residential programs serving moderately and severely disabled persons. Includes enviromental assessments as well as profiles of jobs and training sites.

1978 **High Tech Center**

Cal State University
6000 J Street
Sacramento, CA 95819
916-278-6011
FAX: 916-278-7825

The Center offers Augumentative Communication Training modules: videotapes featuring clients participating in assessment and training to demonstrate procedures for selecting and using augmentative communication systems.

1979 **Increasing Capabilities Access Network**

2201 Brookwood Drive
Suite 117
Little Rock, AR 72202
501-666-8868
800-828-2799
FAX: 501-666-5319
www.arkansas-ican.org

Barbara Gullett, Project Director

A consumer responsive statewide systems change program promoting assistive technology for persons of all ages with disabilities. The program provides information on new and existing technology and maintains an equipment exchange free of charge. Training on assistive technology is also provided.

1980 **International Center for the Disabled**

340 E 24th Street
New York, NY 10010
212-585-6250
FAX: 212-585-6161
www.icdrehab.org

Les Halpert PhD, CEO
Sondra Segal, Development Officer, PR

The ICD is a comprehensive outpatient rehabilitation facility, providing medical rehabilitation, behavioral health and vocational services to children and adults with a broad range of physical, communication, emotional and cognitive disabilities.

1981 **Kentucky Assistive Technology Service Network**

8412 Westport Road
Louisville, KY 40242
502-327-0022
800-327-5287
FAX: 502-327-9974
e-mail: katsnet@iglow.com
www.katsnet.org

Ronji Dearborn, Info. & Referral Specialist

Statewide network of four regional assistive technology centers with a central coordinating office in Louisville and two regional centers in eastern Kentucky. Network services include but are not limited to assistive technology of services, loan of assistive devices, funding information and referral, assessment and evaluations, consultations on appropriate technologies, training, and technical assistance.

1982 **Learning Independence Through Computers**

1001 Eastern Avenue
Baltimore, MD 21202
410-659-5462
FAX: 410-659-5472
e-mail: lincmd@aol.com
www.linc.org

Susan Pompa, Associate Director

Computer technology center.

1983 **MEDLINE**

Dialog Corporation
2440 W El Camino Real
Mountain View, CA 94040
800-334-2564
FAX: 650-254-7070
www.dialog.com

Bibliographic citations to biomedical literature.

1984 **Maine CITE**
University of Maine at Augusta
46 University Drive
Suite 195 Jewell Hall
Augusta, ME 04330 **207-621-3022**
FAX: 207-621-3293
www.uma.maine.edu/cs/

Dave Beaulieu, Telecommunications Manager
Lauren DuBois, Director Computer Services

Computer technology center.

1985 **Maryland Technology Assistance Program**
Governor's Off. for Individuals with Disabilities
2301 Argonne Drive
Suite T-17
Baltimore, MD 21218 **410-554-9230**
800-832-4827
FAX: 410-554-9237
e-mail: mdtap@mdtap.org
www.mdtap.org

Paul Rasinski, Executive Director
Jessica Vallmer, Secretary

Assistive technology center. Information and referral, equipment display loans and demonstration, funding sources, alternative media, training, workshops and seminars. Rural outreach for individuals with disability in Maryland.

1986 **Minnesota STAR Program**
50 Sherburne Avenue
Suite 309
St Paul, MN 55155 **651-296-2771**
800-657-3862
FAX: 651-282-6671
e-mail: star.program@state.mn.us
www.admin.state.mn.us/assistivetechnology

Chuck Rassbach, Executive Director

STAR works at the state and national level on legislation and policy for AT; informs and advocates for AT through training, information and referral; works to identify solutions for barriers to acquisition of AT; and works collaboratively with state and local partners in AT service and advocacy.

1987 **Mississippi Project START**
PO Box 1698
Jackson, MS 39215 **601-987-4872**
800-852-8328
FAX: 601-364-2349
e-mail: contactus@msprojectstart.org
www.msprojectstart.org

Stephen Power, Project Director

Project START is a Tech Act project established to bring about systems change in the field of assistive technology in the state of Mississippi. Activities include providing training opportunities for consumers and service providers on subjects such as state-of-the-art AT devices, their application and funding resources; referral information on AT evaluation centers; technical assistance to AT users; establishment of an AT equipment loan program and an Information and Referral Service.

1988 **National Lekotek Center**
2100 Ridge Avenue
Evanston, IL 60201 **847-328-0001**
800-366-PLAY
FAX: 847-328-5514
TTY:800-573-4446
e-mail: lekotek@lekotek.org
www.lekotek.org

Helen McCarthy, Executive Director
Madelyn James, Programs/Training Director
Clarice Brown, Programs/Training Asst Director

Maximizes the development of children with special needs through play. Supports families through nationwide family play centers, toy lending libraries and computer play programs. Publishes six-page newsletter three times per year.

1989 **National Technology Database**
American Foundation for the Blind/AFB Press
11 Penn Plaza
Suite 300
New York, NY 10001 **212-502-7600**
800-232-3044
FAX: 412-741-0609
www.afb.org

This database includes resources for visually impaired persons. *$99.00*

1990 **New Jersey Department of Labor**
Office of the Commissioner
PO Box 110
Trenton, NJ 08625 **609-292-2323**
FAX: 609-633-9271
e-mail: cmycoff@dol.state.nj.us
www.state.nj.us/labor

Albert G Kroll, Commissioner

Computer technology center.

1991 **New Mexico Technology Assistance Program**
New Mexico State Department of Education
Division /Vocational Rehabilitation
435 Saint Michaels Drive, Bldg D
Santa Fe, NM 87505 **505-954-8533**
800-866-2253
FAX: 505-954-8562
TTY:800-659-4915
e-mail: aklaus@state.nm.us
www.nmtap.com

Alan Klaus, Project Director
Caroll Cadena, Public Contact

Examines and works to eliminate barriers to obtaining assistive technology in New Mexico. Has established a statewide program for coordinating assistive technology services; is designed to assist people with disabilities to locate, secure, and maintain assistive technology.

1992 **North Carolina Assistive Technology Project**
1110 Navaho Drive
Suite 101
Raleigh, NC 27609 **919-676-2288**
FAX: 919-850-2792
e-mail: ncatp@minespring.com
www.ncatp.org

Ricki Cook, Project Director
Annette Lauber, Funding Specialist
Jacquelyne Gordon, Consumer Resource Specialist

The North Carolina Assistive Technology Project exists to create a statewide, consumer-responsive system of assistive technology services for all North Carolinians with disabilities. The project's activities impact children and adults with disabilities across all aspects of their lives.

1993 **Northern Illinois Center for Adaptive Technology**
3615 Louisiana Road
Rockford, IL 61108 **815-229-2163**

e-mail: davegrass@earthlink.net
http://nicat.ataccess.org.nicat1.html

Computer technology center.

1994 **OCCK**

1710 W Schilling Road
Salina, KS 67401
785-827-9383
800-526-9731
FAX: 785-823-2015
e-mail: occk@occk.com
www.occk.com

Phyllis Anderson, Director Community Resource Dev.
Kathy Reed, Coordinator-Personal Supports

Computer technology center; training center for employment and independent living for people with disabilities; family support center.

1995 **Ohio Rehabilitation Services Commission**

400 E Campus View Boulevard-SW5F
Columbus, OH 43235
614-438-1200
FAX: 614-438-1257
www.state.oh.us/rsc

John M Connelly, Executive Director

State agency responsible for assisting people who have disabilities to obtain employment or to live independently in their community.

1996 **PAM Assistance Center**

Physically Impaired Association of Michigan
601 W Maple Street
Lansing, MI 48906
800-274-7426
FAX: 517-371-5898

Arselia S Ensign, Director, PAM Centre
Barbara Warren, Administrative Asst.

One of three state-supported technology and media information centers in Michigan, all under the Physically Impaired Association of Michigan. Offers resources, booklets and pamphlets listing information on devices and resources helpful in addressing basic needs of persons with disabilities.

1997 **Parents, Let's Unite for Kids**

1500 N 30th Street
Billings, MT 59101
800-222-7585
FAX: 406-657-2061
TTY:406-657-2055
e-mail: plukmt@aol.com

Computer technology center. Parents, Let's Unite for Kids offers an assistive technology lab that is open to people of all ages. The lab is a computer and assistive technology demonstration site. There is no charge for services.

1998 **Pathfinder Parent Training and Information Center**

1600 2nd Avenue SW
Minot, ND 58701
701-837-7500
800-245-5840
FAX: 701-837-7548
e-mail: ndpath01@minot.ndek.net
www.pathfinder.minot.com

Katherine Erickson, Executive Director

A member of the National Parent Training and Information Program which helps parents to better understand their child's disability and to obtain information about the programs, services and resources available. The center provides referrals through their program, support for educational programs for children with disabilities and helps parents learn to communicate more effectively with those involved in their child's program.

1999 **Pennsylvania's Initiative on Assistive Technology**

Temple University Institute on Disabilities
1301 Cecil B Moore Avenue
Philadelphia, PA 19122
215-204-1356
800-204-7428
FAX: 215-204-9371
TTY:800-750-7428
e-mail: piat@temple.edu
http://disabilities.temple.edu

Amy Goldman, Project Director

Assistive technology related information and advocacy for Pennsylvanians with disabilities; assistance with funding; short-term equipment loan and used equipment exchange programs.

2000 **Pre-Injury/Post-Injury Analysis**

CAPCO Capability Corporation
E 5805 Sharp
Suite 103
Spokane, WA 99212
800-541-5006
FAX: 509-535-1011

Used by vocational experts and attorneys in litigated cases including personal injury, product liability, medical malpractice and workers compensation.

2001 **Quick Reading Test, Phonics Based Reading, Reading SOS (Strategies for Older Students)**

Lexia Learning Systems
PO Box 466
Lincoln, MA 01773
781-259-8752
800-435-3942
FAX: 781-259-1349
e-mail: info@lexialearning.com
www.lexialearning.com

Jon Bower, President
Bob Baker, Sales Representative

Lexia's software helps children and adults with learning disabilities master their core reading skills. Based on the Orton Gillingham method, Phonics Based Reading and S.O.S. (Strategies for the Older Student) apply phonics principles to help students learn essential sound-symbol correspondence and decoding skills. The Quick Reading Tests generate detailed phonemic skills reports in only 5-8 minutes per student to provide teachers with accurate data to focus their instruction. Price: $67-$500.

2002 **Rehabilitation Engineering & Assistive Technology Society of North America (RESNA)**

1700 N Moore Street
Suite 1540
Arlington, VA 22209
703-524-6686
FAX: 703-524-6630
e-mail: membership@resna.org
www.resna.org

Larry Pencak, Executive Director
Shannon Marullo, Director, Professional Services
Tonya Vaughn, Professional Services Manager

An information center to address research, development, dissemination, integration and utilization of knowledge in rehabilitation and assistive technology.

2003 **SACC Assistive Technoloy Center**

Simi Valley Hospital N Campus
PO Box 1325
Simi Valley, CA 93062
805-582-1881
FAX: 805-582-2855
e-mail: dssaccca@aol.com

Debi Schultze, Chief Executive Officer

SACC connects children, adults and seniors with special needs to computers, technologies and resources. We provide information and referral, assessments, tutoring, presentations and outreach awareness.

2004 South Dakota Department of Human Services: Computer Technology Services

E Highway 34 500, Hillsview Plaza
500 E Capital
Pierre, SD 57501
605-773-5990
800-265-9684
FAX: 605-773-5483
TTY:605-773-3195
e-mail: davem@dhs.state.sd.us

David Miller, Division Director

Computer technology center.

2005 Star Center

60 Lynoak Cove
Jackson, TN 38305
731-668-3888
800-464-5619
FAX: 731-668-1666
e-mail: infostar@starcenter.tn.org
www.starcenter.tn.org

Judy Duke, Outreach Manager

Nation's largest assistive technology center dedicated to helping children and adults with disabilities achieve their goals for competitive employment, effective learning, returning to or starting school and independent living. Programs include: high-tech training, music therapy, art therapy, low vision evaluation, orientation and mobility evaluation and training, augmentative communication evaluation, vocational evaluations, assistive technology, job placement services and job skills training.

2006 Students with Disabilities Office

University of Texas at Austin
1 University Station A5800
Austin, TX 78712
512-471-6259
FAX: 512-475-7730
www.utexas.edu/depts/dos/ssd

Jennifer Maedgen, Assistant Dean of Students

2007 TASK Team of Advocates for Special Kids

100 W Cerritos Avenue
Anaheim, CA 92805
714-533-8275
FAX: 714-533-2533
e-mail: taskca@aol.com

Computer technology center.

2008 Target Teach

Evans Newton
15941 N 77th Street
Scottsdale, AZ 85260
480-998-2777
FAX: 480-951-2895

Aligns and monitors Special Education Instructional Materials to tests that are used to measure the effectiveness of Special Education Instructional Programs.

2009 Tech Connection

35 Haddon Avenue
Shrewsbury, NJ 07702
732-747-5310
FAX: 732-747-1896
e-mail: tecconn@aol.com
www.techconnection.org

Joanne Castellano, Center Director

Offers a noncommercial center to examine and try computers, adapted equipment, alternative input devices, and a variety of software. Program of Family Resource Associates and a member of the Alliance for Technology Access (ATA), a growing national coalition of computer resource centers, professionals, technology developers and vendors, interacting with new technology to enrich the lives of people with disabilities. Tech Connection offers evaluations, for computer technology.

2010 Tech-Able

1114 Brett Drive
Suite 100
Conyers, GA 30094
770-922-6768
FAX: 770-922-6769
e-mail: techable@techable.org
www.techable.org

Carolyn McGonagill, Director
Pat Hanus, Executive Assistant
Joe Tedesco, Assistive Tech Practitioner

Provide assistive technology to individuals with disabilities, toy-lending and software libraries, product demonstration, access to technology devices and fabrication of keyguards for keyboards. Low vision consultant on Thursdays; computer training for persons with disabilities.

2011 Technical Aids & Assistance for the Disabled Center

1950 W Roosevelt Road
Chicago, IL 60608
708-867-6060
800-346-2939
FAX: 312-421-3464
TTY:312-421-3373

Andres Hernandez, Executive Director
Robert Kaige, Technologist

Provides consultation and technical advice on adaptive aids, software and hardware.

2012 Technology Access Center of Tucson

4710 E 29th Street
PO Box 13178
Tuscon, AZ 85711
520-745-5588
FAX: 520-790-7637
e-mail: tactaz@aol.com
www.ed.arizona.edu/tact

Linda Bishop, Director of Services
Sonia Rameriez, Service Coordinator

A resource center that provides assistive technology services for people with disabilities. Center personnel develop, provide and coordinate those services in communities throughout Middle Tennessee. Services are designed to assist people with disabilities to learn about, choose, acquire and use assistive technology devices. Services are offered to any child or adult with sensory, motor or cognitive disabilities, their family members, and professionals who serve them and employ them.

2013 Technology Assistance for Special Consumers

915 Monroe Street
PO Box 443
Huntsville, AL 35804
256-532-5336
FAX: 256-532-2355
e-mail: tasc@hiwaay.net
www.ataccess.org

Linda Rags, Executive Director

T.A.S.C. is a computer resource center with 10 computers, which are equipped with special adaptations for those who are blind, visually impaired, or severely physically disabled. Our staff demonstrates and trains individuals on this equipment so that they can become more independent at home, school, and work. Over 2,500 pieces of educational software are available for individuals who are learning disabled, mentally retarded or who have developmental delays.

2014 Techspress

Resource Center for Independent Living
401-409 Columbia Street
Suite 409
Utica, NY 13502
315-797-4642
FAX: 315-797-4247
e-mail: lana.gossin@rcil.com

Lana Gossin, Director

Services include consultation and training in computer based technology for consumers, family members, and service providers as a means of fostering personal, recreational, educational and vocational independence and integration.

2015 Tenessee Technology Access Project Department of Mental Health

400 Deadrick Street
Citizens Plaza Building
Nashville, TN 37248
615-532-3122
800-732-5059
FAX: 615-532-4685
TTY:615-741-4566
e-mail: ttap@mail.state.tn.us
www.state.tn.us/humanserv/ttap_index.htm

Provides Tennesseans who have disabilities with comprehensive information related to assistive technology including resources for assistive technology devices and services, information about the funding of devices and services, resources for advocacy services, statewide systems change initiatives/activities, and assistive technology centers.

2016 Tidewater Center for Technology Access Special Education Annex

960 Windsor Oaks Boulevard
Virginia Beach, VA 23462
757-474-8455
FAX: 757-474-8648
TTY:757-474-8650
e-mail: tcta@aol.com

Marlayne Castelluzzo, Speech/Lang Pathologist
Jane Quenneville, OT/Registered
Victoria Wilson, Speech/Lang Pathologist

Nonprofit organization providing persons with disabilities access, support, and knowledge—re: technology; organization contracts for consultations, workshops and training, or conventional and assistive technologies including computers, augmented communication devices and software; resources: extensive lending library of educational software; books and videotape library; yearly individual membership and corporate membership fees; working/presentation and evaluation fees available upon request.

2017 University of Idaho Center on Disabilities and Human Development

Idaho Assistive Technology Project
129 W 3rd Street
Moscow, ID 83843
208-885-3559
800-IDA-TECH
FAX: 208-885-3628
e-mail: rseiler@uidaho.edu
www.educ.uidaho.edu/idatech

Michelle Doty, Training Coordinator
Ron Seiler, Project Coordinator
Sue House, Information and Referral

A University affiliated project (UAP) dedicated to the implementation of a comprehensive system for the delivery of assistive technology devices and services to Idaho citizens with disabilities, their families or representatives in a timely cost efficient manner. Our goals are to: provide training and technical assistance; to promote public awareness of assistive technology and to increase the capacity of public agencies and private entities to serve people with disabilities.

2018 Vermont Assistive Technology Project: Department of Aging & Disabilities

Agency of Human Services
103 S Main Street
Weeks Building
Waterbury, VT 05671
802-241-2620
FAX: 802-241-2174
e-mail: jtucker@dad.state.vt.us
www.dad.state.vt.us/

Julie Tucker, Information and Referral
Betsy Ross, Administration
Dan Gilman, AT Access Specialist

Computer technology center.

2019 Washington Technology Access Center

8705 232nd Place SW
Edmonds, WA 98026
425-883-4141
FAX: 425-776-3663

Grant Lord, Founder

The center was formed as a nonprofit organization to demonstrate how computer technology can transform limitations into opportunities for those with special needs. WTAC's mission is to increase the awareness, understanding and implementation of computer technology for persons with special needs, their friends, families, educators, rehabilitation and health professionals, public officials and employees.

2020 Xerox Imaging Systems/Adaptive Products Department

Personal Reader Department
9 Centennial Drive
Peabody, MA 01960
978-977-2000
800-248-6550
FAX: 978-977-2409

Offers information on new services, assistive devices and technology for blind, visually impaired, learning disabled and other print disabled individuals.

2021 Your Voice Village

171 River Drive
Hadley, MA 01035
800-637-8720
FAX: 413-585-1137

Michael Oestreicher, Director

A politically and socially interactive full-service computer on line service serving 43,000,000 people with disabilities. Make a difference. Be involved. Take part in polls. Let Washington know how you feel. The database also allows participants to make air line reservations, car rentals and more. *$19.95*

Keyboards, Mouses & Joysticks

2022 A4 Tech (USA) Corporation

20256 Paseo Robles
Walnut, CA 91789
909-468-0071
FAX: 909-468-2231

Manufacturers of a cordless mouse, trackballs and joysticks that emulate mouse controls, flatbed scanners, modified keyboards, and other specialty mouses.

2023 Abacus

5370 52nd Street SE
Grand Rapids, MI 49512
800-451-4319
FAX: 616-698-0325

Designs a mouse software program that permits programs written for one computer to be run on another computer.

2024 Ability Center of Greater Toledo

5605 Monroe Street
Sylvania, OH 43560 **419-885-5733**
FAX: 419-882-4813

Manufactures keyboard wrist supports to help prevent repetitive motion disorders.

2025 Step on It! Computer Control Pedals

BILBO Innovations
1290 Carmead Parkway
Suite 118
Sunnyvale, CA 94086 **408-736-6086**
800-203-0092
FAX: 408-736-6083
www.bilbo.com

Sergei Burkov, President
Katie Sheinin, Manager

BILBO Innovations, Inc. manufactures and sells Step On It keyboard control pedals. Ergonomic foot switches to emulate keystrokes and mouse clicks. Designed for victims of Repetitive Strain Injury (RSI), Carpal Tunnel Syndrome (CTS), handicapped and disabled. *$99.00*

Scanners

2026 Scanmaster

Howtek
21 Park Avenue
Hudson, NH 03051 **603-882-5200**
FAX: 603-880-3843

A digital color scanner for desktop scanning. It allows the user to digitalize, modify, enhance and store images in color or black and white.

2027 Scanning WSKE

Words+
40015 Sierra Highway B-145
Palmdale, CA 93550
800-869-8521
FAX: 661-266-8969

Ginger Woltosz, VP
Tim Ross, Manager

A software and a hardware product designed to operate on an IBM compatible PC. The software provides dual word prediction, abbreviation expansion, five different methods of voice output, and access to commercial software applications.

2028 System 2000/Versa

Words+
40015 Sierra Highway B-145
Palmdale, CA 93550
800-869-8521
FAX: 661-266-8969

Ginger Woltosz, VP
Tim Ross, Manager

Provides all of the strategies currently being used in AAC, from dynamic display color pictographic language, to dual-word prediction text language, in a single system.

2029 Zygo Industries

ZYGO Industries
PO Box 1008
Portland, OR 97207 **503-684-6006**
800-234-6006
FAX: 503-684-6011
e-mail: zygo@zygo-usa.com
www.zygo-usa.com

Lawrence Weiss, President

Screen Enhancement

2030 Beamscope II

Florida New Concepts Marketing
PO Box 261
Port Richey, FL 34673 **727-842-3231**
800-456-7097
FAX: 727-845-7544
e-mail: compulnz@gte.net

Alan Lezark, President

Meets the needs of low vision individuals in the recreational area. All models utilize a diamond cut freznel lens that can double the size of a TV screen.

$25 - $74

2031 Boxlight

Boxlight Corporation
19332 Powder Hill Place
Poulsbo, WA 98370 **360-779-7901**
800-762-5757
FAX: 888-353-4242
e-mail: sales@boxlight.com
www.boxlight.com

Joanne Luttrell, Marketing

BOXLIGHT is a global presentation solutions partner for trainers, educators and professional speakers. Solutions include projector sales, national rental service, technical support, repair, and presentation peripherals. For more information visit us online.

2032 Compu-Lenz

Florida New Concepts Marketing
PO Box 261
Port Richey, FL 34673 **727-842-3231**
800-456-7097
FAX: 727-845-7544
e-mail: compulnz@gte.net
www.gulfside.com/compulenz

Alan Lezark, President

A fresnel lens, doubles the size of computer screen characters without distortion or light refraction and reduces glare. For use on 9-15 monitors. *$204.95*

2033 FDR Series of Low Vision Reading Aids

Optelec US
6 Lyberty Way
Westford, MA 01886
800-828-1056
FAX: 978-692-6073
e-mail: chrish@optelec.com
www.optelec.com

Chris Harris, Customer Service

The Low Vision Reading Aids features; high resolution, positive and negative display, a high-quality zoom lens, versatile swivel and a 12 inch or 19 inch high-resolution monitor, color or black and white, computer compatible, or portable.

2034 IBM Independence Series: Screen Reader

IBM Corporation Special Needs Systems
PO Box 1328
Boca Raton, FL 33429
800-426-2133

A screen to text speech conversion tool.

2035 **InFocus**

AI Squared
PO Box 669
Manchester Center, VT 05255 **802-362-3612**
FAX: 802-362-1670
e-mail: zoomtext@alsquared.com

A memory-resident program that magnifies text and graphics - the entire screen, a single line or a portion of the screen.

2036 **Portable Large Print Computer**

HumanWare
175 Mason Circle
Concord, CA 94520
800-722-3393
FAX: 925-681-4630

Jim Halliday, President/CEO

A portable large print computer which magnifies up to 64 times. It is linked to a PC and has a hand-held camera.

2037 **ZoomText**

AI Squared
PO Box 669
Manchester Center, VT 05255 **802-362-3612**
FAX: 802-362-1670
e-mail: zoomtext@alsquared.com
www.aisquared.com

Scott Moore, Product Manager

A RAM-resident program that enlarges screen characters up to eight times. It runs on IBM PC, XT, AT and PS/2.

Speech Synthesizers

2038 **Artic Business Vision (for DOS) and Artic WinVision (for Windows 95)**

Artic Technologies
1000 John R Road
Suite 108
Troy, MI 48083 **248-588-7370**
FAX: 248-588-2650
e-mail: info@artictech.com
www.artictech.com

Dale McDaniel, VP Marketing
Kathy Gargagliano, VP Operations

A speech processor for blind computer users featuring true interactive speech with spread sheets, word processors, database managers, etc. Now available with both Windows 3.1 and Windows 95 access. *$ 495.00*

2039 **Audapter Speech System**

Personal Data Systems
638 Sobrato Lane
Campbell, CA 95008 **408-866-1126**
FAX: 408-866-1128
e-mail: info@personaldatasystems.com
www.personaldatasystems.com

A speech synthesizer. Its features include: intelligibility over 93 percent on the industry standard MRT test, fast response, 700-word-per-minute speech rate, speech halt control, compact unit with built-in speaker and serial interface.

2040 **Digital Voice for Talking Database**

Hy-Tek Manufacturing Company
1980 Route 30
Sugar Grove, IL 60554 **630-466-7664**
FAX: 630-466-7678

This product adds speech to PC files. Uses include personnel identification and security, multilingual training, assembly instructions and reminders.

2041 **DynaVox Devices & Software**

DynaVox Systems
2100 Wharton Street
Suite 400
Pittsburgh, PA 15203 **412-381-4883**
800-344-1778
FAX: 412-381-5241
e-mail: sales@dynavoxsys.com
www.dynavoxsys.com

Allow non-speaking individuals to communicate their thoughts, ideas and feelings easily. The devices' built-in infrared technology also provides users with more independence, allowing them to access TVs, VCRs, and computers. DynaVox software helps turn Macintosh and Windows and computers into communication devices so clinicians can use their computers to conduct training and assessments.

2042 **Electronic Speech Assistance Devices**

Luminaud
8688 Tyler Boulevard
Mentor, OH 44060 **440-255-9082**
800-255-3408
FAX: 440-255-2250
e-mail: info@luminaud.com
www.luminaud.com

Thomas Lennox, President
Dorothy Lennox, VP

Offers a full line of speech aids, voice amplifiers, mini-vox amplifiers, laryngectomec products.

2043 **Hawk Communication Device**

Wayne County Regional Educational Service Agency
33500 Van Born Road
Wayne, MI 48184 **734-334-1300**
FAX: 734-334-1432

Kimberly Kaminski, Internal Operations

The Hawk employs digital voice technology for high quality, natural voice output. The touch panel is divided into a three by three matrix for a total of nine selection areas. A bulletin microphone allows the recording of up to five seconds worth of digital speech into each of the nine selection areas. *$250.00*

2044 **In Cube Pro Voice Command**

Command Corporation
11080 Old Roswell Road
Suite 200
Alpharetta, GA 30004 **770-360-1230**
e-mail: webmaster@commandcorp.com
www.commandcorp.com

Continuous speech recognition system which can be used by people with disabilities. IN CUBE provides greatly increased capability, enhanced computer control and access. Blind and low-vision users gain voice access to the graphic user interface. Mobility-impaired people, including quadriplegics, benefit from voice window navigation and voice macro command input. Victims of various repetitive strain injuries RSI use IN CUBE to replace and eliminate repetitive keyboard and mouse operations. *$395.00*

2045 **Keywi**

Consultants for Communication Technology
508 Bellevue Terrace
Pittsburgh, PA 15202 **412-761-6062**
FAX: 412-761-7336
e-mail: cct@concommtech.com
www.concommtech.com

Kathleen H Miller PhD, Partner

Keywi enables a laptop computer to become a complete communication device. Create entire conversations, call a friend on the telephone, manage your business or personal affairs. Requires minimal training. Multiple access methods-switch, mouse, joystick, keyboard. Custom vocabulary. Powerful word prediction abilities. *$495.00*

2046 **Laptalker**

Automated Functions
7700 Irberge Pike
Suite 420
Falls Church, VA 22043 **703-883-9797**
FAX: 703-883-9798

A portable talking computer that gives visually impaired people complete desk top PC compatibility.

2047 **Mega Wolf Communication Device**

Wayne County Regional Educational Service Agency
33500 Van Born Road
Wayne, MI 48184 **734-334-1300**
FAX: 734-334-1432

Kimberly Kaminski, Internal Operations

A low cost voice output communication device which is primarily intended to provide the power of speech to those individuals who are most severely challenged mentally and/or physically. The WOLF device is User programmable and uses the Texas Instruments' Touch and Tell case and touch panel; ADAMLAB electronics with synthesized (robotic) voice. For users able to point with approximately 6 ounces of pressure. *$400.00*

2048 **One-Step Communicator**

AbleNet
1081 10th Avenue SE
Minneapolis, MN 55414
800-322-0956
FAX: 612-379-9143
e-mail: customerservice@ablenetinc.com
www.ablenetinc.com

The One-Step Communicator has 20 seconds of memory and has an angled switch surface making it easy to see and access. The switch surface is 2 1/2 inches in diameter. Detachable mounting base makes it easy to position a single unit in a variety of locations. *$129.00*

2049 **Phone Manager**

Consultants for Communication Technology
508 Bellevue Terrace
Pittsburgh, PA 15202 **412-761-6062**
FAX: 412-761-7336
e-mail: cct@concommtech.com
www.concommtech.com

Kathleen H Miller PhD, Partner

Software that allows the user to dial an outgoing call directly from the computer, even with a single switch. Synthesized speech is sent through the phone line. The synthesizer then turns into a speaker phone enabling hands free, two way conversations. *$300.00*

2050 **Talking Screen**

Words+
1220 W Avenue J
Lancaster, CA 93534
800-869-8521
FAX: 661-266-8969

Phil Lawrence, VP
Rachel Nielsen, Customer Support

An augmentative communication program that allows the user to select graphic symbols on the display to produce speech output. Symbols can be used either singly or in sequence as picture abbreviations. *$ 1395.00*

2051 **Turnkey Computer Systems for the Visually, Physically, and Hearing Impaired**

EVAS
PO Box 371
Westerly, RI 02891 **401-596-3155**
FAX: 401-596-3979
e-mail: contact@evas.com
www.evas.com

Sara Swerdlick, Customer Service Manager

Offers clear speech with pleasant inflection and tonal quality as well as variable pitch, intonation and voices.

2052 **Voice-It**

VXI Corporation
One Front Street
Rollinsford, NH 03869 **603-742-2888**
800-742-8588
FAX: 603-742-5065
e-mail: info@vxicorp.com
www.vxicorp.com

Adds voice to popular spreadsheet and word processing applications on IBM PCs and compatibles, turning spreadsheets and word processing documents into talking documents.

2053 **Window-Eyes**

GW Micro
725 Airport N Office Park
Fort Wayne, IN 46825 **260-489-3671**
FAX: 260-489-2608
e-mail: sales@gwmicro.com
www.gwmicro.com

Provides access to available software automatically reading information important to the user while ignoring the rest. A screen reader for the windows operative system.

Software: Math

2054 **AIMS Multimedia**

9710 Desoto Avenue
Chatsworth, CA 91311 **818-773-4300**
800-367-2467
FAX: 818-341-6700
e-mail: info@multimedia.com
www.aimsmultimedia.com

Wynn Sherman, President
Don Lukenbill, Communications Director

AIMS Multimedia is a leader in the production and distribution of trinaing and educational programs for the business and K-12 communities via YHS, interactive CD-ROM, DVD and Internet streaming video.

2055 **Access to Math**

Don Johnston
26799 N Commerce Drive
Volo, IL 60073 **847-740-0749**
800-999-4660
FAX: 847-740-7326
e-mail: info@donjohnston.com
www.donjohnston.com

This macintosh math worksheet program is tow products in one. For teachers, it makes customized worksheets in a snap. For students who struggle, it provides individualized on-screen lessons that contribute to success. *$79.00*

2056 Basic Math Competency Skill Building

Educational Activities Software
PO Box 754
Baldwin, NY 11510 **516-867-7878**
800-645-2796
FAX: 516-379-7429
e-mail: achieve@ea-software.com

Alan Stern, Sales Director

Comprehensive MATH SKILLS software tutorials teach concepts ranging from rounding and tables to measuring area. MAC/WIN compatible. *$369.00*

Per Unit

2057 Basic Math: Detecting Special Needs

Allyn & Bacon
75 Arlington Street
Suite 300
Boston, MA 02116 **617-848-6000**
800-852-8024
FAX: 617-848-7490
www.adlongman.com

Describes special mathematics needs of special learners.

180 pages 1989
ISBN 0-205116-35-3

2058 Campaign Math

Mindplay
3130 N Dodge Boulevard
Tucson, AZ 85716 **520-323-1303**
800-221-7911
FAX: 520-322-0363

A complete program on the electoral process as well as a math package which teaches ratios, fractions and percentages.

2059 Elements of Mathematics

Electronic Courseware Systems
1713 S State Street
Champaign, IL 61820 **217-359-7099**
800-832-4965
FAX: 217-359-6578
e-mail: sales@ecsmedia.com
www.ecsmedia.com

Jodie Varner, Manager
David Peters, President

Includes two lessons and a test in addition of simple and complex fractions. The first lesson deals with the reduction and addition of fractions and mixed numbers having common denominators, using graphics (pie slices) for illustration. The second lesson moves to problems having unlike denominators. Test results are stored in a file which is accessible to both the student and the instructor. Computer/software.

2060 Fraction Factory

Queue
1450 Barnum Avenue
Suite 207
Bridgeport, CT 06610 **203-335-0906**
800-232-2224
FAX: 203-336-2481
e-mail: QUEUEINC@aol.com
www.queueinc.com

2061 King's Rule

WINGS for Learning
1600 Green Hills Road
Scotts Valley, CA 95066 **831-464-3600**
FAX: 831-464-3600

A software mathematical problem solving game. Students discover mathematical rules as they work their way through a castle and generate and test a working hypothesis by asking questions.

2062 Learning About Numbers

C&C Software
5713 Kentford Circle
Wichita, KS 67220 **316-683-6056**
800-752-2086

Carol Clark, President

Three programs use the power of computer graphics to provide young children with a variety of experiences in working with numbers. *$50.00*

2063 Math Rabbit

Learning Company
6493 Kaiser Drive
Fremont, CA 94555 **510-490-7311**
800-825-4420
FAX: 408-263-3358
www.learningcompanyschool.com

Teaches early math concepts by matching objects to numbers, then adding and subtracting up to 18.

2064 Math for Everyday Living

Educational Activities Software
PO Box 754
Baldwin, NY 11510 **516-867-7878**
800-645-2796
FAX: 516-379-7429
e-mail: learn@ea-software.com

Al Harris, President
Alan Stern, VP

Real life math skills are taught with this tutorial and practice software program. Examples include Paying for a Meal (addition and subtraction), Working with Sales Slips (multiplication), Unit Pricing (division), Sales Tax (percent), Earning with Overtime (fractions) plus more. Software: CD-Rom, Windows, MAC, and DOS. *$159.00*

2065 Math for Successful Living

Siboney Learning Group
PO Box 220520
St Louis, MO 63122 **314-909-1760**
800-351-1404
FAX: 314-984-8063
e-mail: kculleton@siboneylg.com
www.ea-software.com

Kim Culleton, Sales Manager

These programs include managing a checking account, budgeting, shopping strategies and buying on credit.

2066 Optimum Resource Educational Software

Optimum Resource
18 Hunter Road
Hilton Head Island, SC 29926 **843-689-8000**
FAX: 843-689-8008
e-mail: sticky@stickybear.com
www.stickybear.com

Chris Gintz, VP Marketing

A complete topical curriculum of reading, math, keyboard skills and science programs that are age and skill specific. *$59.95*

2067 Piece of Cake Math

Queue
1450 Barnum Avenue
Suite 207
Bridgeport, CT 06610
203-335-0906
800-232-2224
FAX: 203-336-2481
e-mail: QUEUEINC@aol.com
www.queueinc.com

Color, sound and animation combine forces in a program of five games focusing on basic mathematical operations.

2068 Puzzle Tanks

WINGS for Learning
1600 Green Hills Road
Scotts Valley, CA 95066
831-464-3600
FAX: 831-464-3600

A mathematical problem solving game that involves multi-step problems.

2069 Right Turn

WINGS for Learning
1600 Green Hills Road
Scotts Valley, CA 95066
831-464-3600
FAX: 831-464-3600

Requires students to predict, experiment and learn about the mathematical concepts of rotation and transformation.

2070 RoboMath

Mindplay
3130 N Dodge Boulevard
Tucson, AZ 85716
520-323-1303
800-221-7911
FAX: 520-322-0363

Players learn multiplication and division using a game paddle.

2071 Stickybear Math

Optimum Resource
18 Hunter Road
Hilton Head Island, SC 29926
843-689-8000
FAX: 843-689-8008
e-mail: sticky@stickybear.com
www.stickybear.com

Chris Gintz, VP Marketing Director

Sharpen basic addition and subtraction skills with this captivating series of math exercises. *$59.95*

2072 Stickybear Numbers

Optimum Resource
18 Hunter Road
Hilton Head Island, SC 29926
843-689-8000
FAX: 843-689-8008
e-mail: sticky@stickybear.com
www.stickybear.com

Chris Gintz, VP Marketing

Counting and number recognition are as easy as 1-2-3 with this award-winning program. *$59.95*

2073 Stickybear Word Problems

Optimum Resource
18 Hunter Road
Hilton Head Island, SC 29926
843-689-8000
FAX: 843-689-8008
e-mail: sticky@stickybear.com
www.stickybear.com

Chris Gintz, VP Marketing

Hundreds of different word problems make it easy for students to practice basic math skills. *$59.95*

2074 Stickybear's Math Splash

Optimum Resource
18 Hunter Road
Hilton Head Island, SC 29926
843-689-8000
FAX: 843-689-8008
e-mail: sticky@stickybear.com
www.stickybear.com

Chris Gintz, VP Marketing

Unique multiple activities keep the learning level high while children acquire skills in addition, subtraction, multiplication and division. *$59.95*

2075 Stickybear's Math Town

Optimum Resource
18 Hunter Road
Hilton Head Island, SC 29926
843-689-8000
FAX: 843-689-8008
e-mail: sticky@stickybear.com
www.stickybear.com

Chris Gintz, VP Marketing

Children ages 5-10 gain proficiency in addition, subtraction, multiplication and division, as well as life skills and word problems. In English and Spanish, children sharpen skills both vertically and horizontally, clear crisp graphics and sound enable teachers to monitor and access skills and development. *$59.95*

2076 Tomorrow's Promise: Mathematics

9920 Pacific Heights Boulevard
San Diego, CA 92121
858-587-0087
800-247-1380
FAX: 619-622-7873
www.compasslearning.com

Steve Allen, Alternate Channels Manager

By integrating interdisciplinary content and real-world application of skills, this product emphasizes the practical value of fundamental math skills. It helps your students develop a problem-solving aptitude for ongoing mathematics achievement.

Software: Miscellaneous

2077 Adaptive Computer Systems

1835 Hafor Drive
Iowa City, IA 52246
319-338-1449
FAX: 319-338-8184

Designers of web page creation software and on-screen keyboard programs.

2078 Adventures in Musicland

Electronic Courseware Systems
1713 S State Street
Champaign, IL 61820
217-352-5510
800-832-4965
FAX: 217-359-6578
e-mail: sales@ecsmedia.com
www.ecsmedia.com

G David Peters, President
Jodie Varner, Marketing Manager

This unique set of music games features characters from Lewis Carroll's, Alice in Wonderland. Players learn through pictures, sounds, and animation which help develop understanding of musical tones, composers, and musical symbols. Games include MusicMatch, Melody Mixup, Picture Perfect and Sound Concentration. *$49.95*

2079 Ai Squared

PO Box 669
Manchester Center, VT 05255 **802-362-3612**
FAX: 802-362-1670
e-mail: zoomtext@aisquared.com
www.aisquared.com

Developers of software for the visually impaired.

2080 All About You: Appropriate Special Interactions and Self-Esteem

PCI Educational Publishing
PO Box 34270
San Antonio, TX 78212
800-594-4263
FAX: 888-259-8284
www.pcicatalog.com

This game offers parents and game players a new line of communication when discussing various issues such as learning to be thoughtful, respecting the rights and feelings of others, how to make and keep friends and more. *$49.95*

2081 All Star Review

Tom Snyder Productions
80 Coolidge Hill Road
Watertown, MA 02472 **781-926-6000**
800-342-0236
FAX: 800-304-1254
e-mail: ask@tomsnyder.com
www.tomsnyder.com

This package turns group review into a baseball game for small and large groups.

2082 At Home with Stickybear

Optimum Resource
18 Hunter Road
Hilton Head Island, SC 29926 **843-689-8000**
FAX: 843-689-8008
e-mail: sticky@stickybear.com
www.stickybear.com

Chris Gintz, VP Marketing

This dynamic new multifaceted program covers a wide range of preschool skills that go far beyond the strictly academic! At Stickybear's house, children discover the alphabet, numbers, shapes, colors; plus social skills, important safety messages and delightful off-screen activities that foster creativity. *$59.95*

2083 Attainment Company/IEP Resources

504 Commerce Parkway
PO Box 930160
Verona, WI 53593 **608-845-7880**
800-327-4269
FAX: 800-942-3865
e-mail: info@attainmentcompany.com
www.attainmentcompany.com

Brent Denu, Marketing Coordinator
Julie Denu, Technical Support
Theresa O'Connor, Office Manager

Augmentative/Alternative communication, software, videos, print and hands-on materials for developmental and cognitive disabilities.

2084 Attention Getter

Soft Touch
4300 Stine Road
Suite 401
Bakersfield, CA 93313
877-763-8868
FAX: 661-396-8760
e-mail: softtouch@funsoftware.com
www.funsoftware.com

Roxanne Butterfield

The whimsical photos morph to another photo and then to a third photo in categories. Paired with interesting sounds and music, the photo animations are so engaging that the student is motivated to activate the computer to see and hear the next one. This is a perfect vehicle to achieve goals aimed at attention getting, activating a switch or intentionality. Compatible with USB IntelliKeys keyboards.

2085 Attention Teens

Soft Touch
4300 Stine Road
Suite 401
Bakersfield, CA 93313
877-763-8868
FAX: 661-396-8760
e-mail: softtouch@funsoftware.com
www.funsoftware.com

Roxanne Butterfield

Attention Teens (formerly known as Loony Teens) is a program for teens with disabilities who need powerful input to get their attention. Attention Teens is a computer program to do just this. Paired with interesting sounds and music, the photo animations are so engaging that the student is motivated to activate the computer to see and hear the next one. Compatible with USB IntelliKeys keyboards.

2086 Away We Ride

Soft Touch
4300 Stine Road
Suite 401
Bakersfield, CA 93313
877-763-8868
FAX: 661-396-8760
e-mail: softtouch@funsoftware.com
www.funsoftware.com

Roxanne Butterfield

Software for children and teens. For Macintosh and PC.

2087 Bailey's Book House

Edmark Corporation
PO Box 97021
Redmond, WA 98073 **425-556-8400**
800-691-2986
www.edmark.com

Software for children.

2088 Battenberg & Associates

11135 Rolling Springs Drive
Carmel, IN 46033 **317-843-2208**

Offers various software programs that develop the user's visual memory, sequencing skills, word recognition, hand-eye coordination and more.

2089 Behavior Skills: Learning How People Should Act

Programming Concepts
PO Box 12428
San Antonio, TX 78212
800-594-4263
FAX: 218-248-055

Janie Haugen, Program Director
Jeff McLane, President/CEO

Helps players learn what behavior is acceptable and what behavior is not acceptable in the real world. *$49.95*

2090 Blocks in Motion

Don Johnston
26799 N Commerce Drive
Volo, IL 60073
847-740-0749
800-999-4660
FAX: 847-740-7326
e-mail: info@donjohnston.com
www.donjohnston.com

This unique art and motion program makes drawing, creating and animating fun and educational for all users. Based on the Piagetian Theory for motor-sensory development, this program promotes the concept that the process is as educational and as much fun as the end result. *$79.00*

2091 CINTEX: Speak to Your Appliances

NanoPac
4823 S Sheridan Road
Suite 302
Tulsa, OK 74145
918-665-0329
800-580-6086
FAX: 918-665-0361
e-mail: info@nanopac.com
www.nanopac.com

Silvio V Cianfrone CCSP, President

CINTEX, with a voice recognition program, will control up to 256 off/on appliances, dial and answer the phone, flash for call waiting, dial from a directory, control TV's, VCR's, stereos and more — all with your voice. CINTEX2 includes the necessary hardware and voice macros which you can use to immediately control your environment. You can tailor these macros to your personal needs and add new macros. Pops-up over current application allowing instant access. $695-$2,000.

2092 Car Builder

Optimum Resource
18 Hunter Road
Hilton Head Island, SC 29926
843-689-8000
FAX: 843-689-8008
e-mail: sticky@stickybear.com
www.stickybear.com

Chris Gintz, VP Marketing

As design engineers, users build cars on screen, specifying chassis length, wheelbase, engine type, transmission, fuel tank size, suspension, steering, tires and brakes. All functional choices are interrelated and will affect the performance of the final design. *$ 59.99*

2093 Center for Best Practices in Early Childhood

27 Horrabin Hall
Macomb, IL 61455
309-298-1634
FAX: 309-298-2305
e-mail: l_robinson1@wiu.edu
www.wiu.edu/thecenter/

Linda Robinson, Assistant Director

A group of early childhood projects which focus on children ages birth to 8 with disabilities and their families. Services include technology training, curricula, books, software and other products.

2094 Clock

9920 Pacific Heights Boulevard
San Diego, CA 92121
858-587-0087
800-247-1380
FAX: 619-622-7873
www.compasslearning.com

Steve Allen, Alternate Channels Manager

An extremely simple, easy-to-use program for children who are learning how to read the time of day from clocks and digital displays. Apple and MS-DOS and Mac available. *$39.95*

2095 Co:Writer

Don Johnston
26799 N Commerce Drive
Volo, IL 60073
847-740-0749
800-999-4660
FAX: 847-740-7326
e-mail: info@donjohnston.com
www.donjohnston.com

A writing description program that helps construct sentences. This is an easy-to-use intelligent word prediction program that works in conjunction with any word processor or text application program to reduce the number of keystrokes necessary to complete an intended word or sentence. This invaluable program can help make the writing process easier, faster and even better for writers of all ages and ability levels. *$290.00*

2096 Community Skills: Learning to Function in Your Neighborhood

Programming Concepts
PO Box 12428
San Antonio, TX 78212
800-594-4263
FAX: 218-248-055

Janie Haugen, Program Director
Jeff McLane, President/CEO

Offers parents and educators a functional way to teach community life skills. *$49.95*

2097 Companion Activities

Soft Touch
4300 Stine Road
Suite 401
Bakersfield, CA 93313
877-763-8868
FAX: 661-396-8760
e-mail: softtouch@funsoftware.com
www.funsoftware.com

Roxanne Butterfield

Print your own books, worksheets, flash cards, board games, matching games, bingo games, card games and many more. This CD offers numerous companion activities to different SoftTouch software titles. Activities range from very easy to difficult. Companion activities are great tools to reinforce learning. Use the work sheets - black and white and color - in the inclusion class for students with special needs.

2098 Computerized Speech Lab

Kay Elemetrics Corporation
2 Bridgewater Lane
Lincoln Park, NJ 07035
973-628-6200
FAX: 973-628-6363
www.kayelemetrics.com

Hardware/software for the acquisition, analysis/display, playback and storage of speech signals.

2099 Concepts on the Move Advanced Preacademics

Soft Touch
4300 Stine Road
Suite 401
Bakersfield, CA 93313
877-763-8868
FAX: 661-396-8760
e-mail: softtouch@funsoftware.com
www.funsoftware.com

Roxanne Butterfield

Choose from five concepts groups: categories, occupations, functions, goes with and prepositions. Use our Steps to Learning Design to choose how many concepts to present at one time and where to place each one in the scan array, on screen keyboard or IntelliKeys keyboard. Watch and listen as the concept morphs or changes and music plays. The words are also shown to reinforce emerging literacy skills. Compatible with USB IntelliKeys.

2100 Cooking Class: Learning About Food Preparation

Programming Concepts
PO Box 12428
San Antonio, TX 78212
800-594-4263
FAX: 218-248-055

Janie Haugen, Program Director
Jeff McLane, President/CEO

This game offers parents and educators a new way to teach basic preparation skills. Kitchen safety and sanitation are stressed throughout the game. *$49.95*

2101 Dilemma

Educational Activities Software
PO Box 754
Baldwin, NY 11510
516-867-7878
800-645-2796
FAX: 516-379-7429
e-mail: achieve@ea-software.com

Alan Stern, Sales Director

Realistic stories with a choice of different gripping endings, color graphics, a built-in dictionary and a user controlled reading rate make these computer programs compelling enough to interest all students. Comprehension and vocabulary questions follow each story. *$159.00*

2102 Dino-Games

Academic Software
331 W 2nd Street
Lexington, KY 40507
859-233-2332
800-842-2357
FAX: 859-231-0725

Warren E Lacefield PhD, President
Penelope Ellis, Marketing Director

Dino-Games are single switch software programs for early switch practice. Dinosaur games provide practice in pattern recognition, cause and effect demonstration, directionality training, number concepts and problem solving. They are compatible with most popular switch interfaces and alternate keyboards. For Macintosh, IBM and compatibles. DINO-LINK is a matching game; DINO-MAZE is a series of maze games; DINO-FIND is a game of concentration; and DINO-DOT is a collection of dot-to-dot games.

$39.95 per game

2103 Directions: Technology in Special Education

DREAMMS for Kids
273 Ringwood Road
Freeville, NY 13068
607-539-3027
FAX: 607-539-9930
www.dreamms.org

A CD containing all of 'Directions' past articles and information gathered from their newsletter which lists resources for assistive and adaptive computer tehnologies in the home, school and community. *$24.95*

2104 ESI Master Resource Guide

Educational Software Institute
4213 S 94th Street
Omaha, NE 68127
402-592-3300
800-955-5570
FAX: 402-592-2017
e-mail: info@edsoft.com
www.edsoft.com

Lee Myers, President
Kathy Cavanaugh, Catalog Manager

Educational Software Institute (ESI) provides a one-stop shop to purchase software titles by all of the best publishers. The ESI Master Gold Book catalog and CD-ROM represents more than 400 software publishers, with information on more than 8,000 software titles. Take the confusion out of software selection by calling ESI for all of your software needs - including competitive prices, software previews, knowledgeable assistance, and the largest selection available all in one place.

Yearly

2105 EZ Keys

Words+
40015 Sierra Highway B-145
Palmdale, CA 93550
661-266-5800
800-869-8521
FAX: 661-266-8969

Ginger Woltosz, VP
Tim Ross, Manager

A software and hardware product designed to operate on an IBM compatible PC. The software provides dual word prediction, abbreviation expansion, five different methods of voice output and access to commercial software applications. *$1395.00*

2106 Early Games for Young Children

Queue
1450 Barnum Avenue
Suite 207
Bridgeport, CT 06610
203-335-0906
800-232-2224
FAX: 203-336-2481
e-mail: QUEUEINC@aol.com
www.queueinc.com

Software that includes nine activities that entertain preschoolers in honing basic math and language skills.

2107 Early Music Skills

Electronic Courseware Systems
1713 S State Street
Champaign, IL 61820
217-352-5510
800-832-4965
FAX: 217-359-6578
e-mail: sales@ecsmedia.com
www.ecsmedia.com

G David Peters, President
Jodie Varner, Marketing Manager

A tutorial and drill program designed for the beginning music student. It covers four basic music reading skills: recognition of line and space notes; comprehension of the numbering system for the musical staff; visual and aural identification of notes moving up and down; and recognition of notes stepping and skipping up and down. *$ 39.95*

2108 Eating Skills: Learning Basic Table Manners

Programming Concepts
PO Box 12428
San Antonio, TX 78212
800-594-4263
FAX: 218-248-055

Janie Haugen, Program Director
Jeff McLane, President/CEO

Offers parents and educators a functional way to teach and reinforce basic table manners. *$49.95*

2109 Electronic Courseware Systems

1713 S State Street
Champaign, IL 61820
217-359-7099
800-832-4965
FAX: 217-359-6578
e-mail: sales@ecsmedia.com
www.ecsmedia.com

Jodie Varner, Manager
David Peters, President

Offers a complete library of instructional software for music, math, science and social studies.

2110 Fall Fun

Soft Touch
4300 Stine Road
Suite 401
Bakersfield, CA 93313
877-763-8868
FAX: 661-396-8760
e-mail: softtouch@funsoftware.com
www.funsoftware.com

Roxanne Butterfield

Your students can begin their day with the Pledge of Allegiance, Pumpkins, Owls, and Cats. Witches adorn Five Pumpkins Sitting on the Gate. Five Fat Turkeys out smart the pilgrims with song and antics. The owl and cat have songs of their own. A variety of activities reinforce concepts such as short, tall, first, second, third, same and different. Fall Fun includes cause and effect and easy to more difficult levels. Eight songs in all.

2111 Five Green & Speckled Frogs

Soft Touch
4300 Stine Road
Suite 401
Bakersfield, CA 93313
877-763-8868
FAX: 661-396-8760
e-mail: softtouch@funsoftware.com
www.funsoftware.com

Roxanne Butterfield

Laugh, Learn and Sing with Five Humorous Frogs. Activities start with cause and effect and progress to teach directionality and simple subtraction. This classic song makes learning numbers and number worlds easy. Selections can be set to 2, 3, 4, 5, or 6 on-screen choices. Two games are included. One teaches direction on a number line. If the child moves the frog in the correct direction, the frog gets a point. The other game teaches beginning subtraction.

2112 GoalView Performance Information System for Special Education

Learning Tools International
2391 Circadian Way
Santa Rosa, CA 95407
707-521-3530
800-333-9954
FAX: 707-521-3535
e-mail: info@ltools.com
www.goalview.com

Cathy Zier, VP

An Internet information system for students, educators and parents that enables accountability and achievement tracking; prepares IDEA compliant IEP's in minutes; provides over 250,000 Education Standards and Special Education goals and objectives in English and Spanish; generates Federal compliance reports; and creates IDEA GoalCard progress reports for students, schools and districts for every reporting period.

2113 HELP

VORT Corporation
PO Box 60132
Palo Alto, CA 94306
650-322-8282
FAX: 650-327-0747
e-mail: sales@vort.com
www.vort.com

A software version of HELP, covers over 650 skills in 6 developmental areas; cognitive, motor skills, language, gross motor, social and self-help.

2114 Handbook of Adaptive Switches and Augmentative Communication Devices

Academic Software
331 W 2nd Street
Lexington, KY 40507
859-233-2332
800-842-2357
FAX: 859-231-0725

Warren E Lacefield PhD, President/Author
Penelope Ellis, Marketing Director
Cindy L George, Author

This second edition contains physical descriptions and laboratory test data for a variety of commercially available pressure switches and augmentative communication devices and chapters on physical interaction, seating and positioning, and control access. It is an essential tool for assistive technology professionals and therapists who make decisions concerning physical access. *$60.00*

300 pages Hardcover

2115 HandiWARE

Microsystems Software
600 Worcester Road
Framingham, MA 01702
508-626-8511
800-828-2600
FAX: 508-879-1069
e-mail: infor@microsys.com
www.handiware.com

Terri McGrath, Sales/Marketing
Bill Kilroy, Product Manager

Adapted access software, assists persons with physical, hearing and visual impairments in accessing computers running DOS and Windows. HandiWARE is a suite of 8 software programs which provide users with screen magnification, alternate keyboard access, word prediction, augmentative communication, hands free telephone access, a visual beep. $20.00-$595.00.

2116 How to Write for Everyday Living

Educational Activities Software
PO Box 754
Baldwin, NY 11510
516-867-7878
800-645-2796
FAX: 516-379-7429
e-mail: achieve@ea-software.com

Alan Stern, Sales

An individualized Life Skills WRITING Software program emphasizing the reading, writing, communication and reference skills needed for real-life tasks: preparing a resume, an employment form, a business letter and envelope, a learner's permit, a social security application and banking forms. *$159.00*

2117 I KNOW American History

Soft Touch
4300 Stine Road
Suite 401
Bakersfield, CA 93313
877-763-8868
FAX: 661-396-8760
e-mail: softtouch@funsoftware.com
www.funsoftware.com

Roxanne Butterfield

The new I KNOW programs is the way students practice attending, choice making and turn-taking while uncovering learning puzzles. Each press reveals more of the image while the narrator reads the text on the screen. Offers three levels of language: short phrases, short sentences and longer sentences to match the student's learning level. Choose from the five topic areas: American Symbols, Westward Movement, Early Colonial Americans, Industrial Revolution and Biographies.

2118 **IntelliPics Studio 3**

IntelliTools
1720 Corporate Circle
Petaluma, CA 94954
707-773-2000
800-899-6687
FAX: 707-773-2001
e-mail: info@intellitools.com
www.intellitools.com

Caroline Van Howe, Marketing Director
Paula Irons, Director Mktg Communications

Multimedia authoring tool for both students and teachers to create activities, games, quizzes, slide shows, reports and presentations. *$395.00*

2119 **KIDS (Keyboard Introductory Development Series)**

Electronic Courseware Systems
1713 S State Street
Champaign, IL 61820
217-352-5510
800-832-4965
FAX: 217-359-6578
e-mail: sales@ecsmedia.com
www.ecsmedia.com

G David Peters, President
Jodie Varner, Marketing Manager

A four disk series for the very young. Zoo Puppet Theater reinforces learning correct finger numbers for piano playing; Race Car Keys teaches keyboard geography by recognizing syllables or note names; Dinosaurs Lunch teaches placement of the notes on the treble staff; and Follow Me asks the student to play notes that have been presented aurally. *$49.95*

2120 **Katie's Farm**

Lawrence Productions
1800 S 53th Street
Galesburg, MI 49053
800-556-6195
www.voyager.net/lawrence

Software for children ages four through eight.

2121 **Keyboard Tutor, Music Software**

Electronic Courseware Systems
1713 S State Street
Champaign, IL 61820
217-352-5510
800-832-4965
FAX: 217-359-6578
e-mail: sales@ecsmedia.com
www.ecsmedia.com

G David Peters, President
Jodie Varner, Marketing Manager

Presents exercises for learning elementary keyboard skills including knowledge of names of the keys, piano keys matched to notes, notes matched to piano keys, whole steps and half steps. Each lesson allows unlimited practice of the skills. The program may be used with or without a midi keyboard attached to the computer. *$39.95*

2122 **Keyboarding by Ability**

Teachers' Institute for Special Education
9933 NW 45th Street
Sunrise, FL 33351
954-572-6220
FAX: 954-572-6220
e-mail: TISE@special-education-soft.com
www.special-education-soft.com

Gary Byowitz, Director

Allows the learning diabled or dyslexic student to acquire keyboarding skills through visually cued alphabetical approach designed and tested to meet the specific learning style needs of this unique population at every grade level. Package contains: IBM software, a set of lesson plans and instructional goals; supplamental graded Data input exercises. *$148.95*

2123 **Keyboarding for the Physically Handicapped**

Teachers' Institute for Special Education
4 Gabalin Center
Huntington Station, NY 11763
631-549-1715
FAX: 516-549-1715
e-mail: jackheller@aol.com
www.users.aol.com/jackheller

Jack Heller, Director

Customed designed touch typing programs for any student. A person needs order by the number of usable fingers on each hand (not counting the thumb), and whether or not a one finger or a head-pointer edition is wanted. Package includes IBM software; a complete set of lesson plans and instructional goals. *$149.95*

2124 **Keyboarding with One Hand**

Teachers' Institute for Special Education
PO Box 2300
Wantagh, NY 11793
FAX: 516-781-4070
e-mail: jackheller@aol.com
www.users.aol.com/jackheller

Jack Heller, Director

This 22 lesson tutorial developed through 25 years of research, testing and teaching allows a student with one hand to aqure employable keyboarding skills using a touch system designed for the standard IBM PC keyboard. *$79.95*

2125 **LPDOS Deluxe**

Optelec US
6 Lyberty Way
Westford, MA 01886
800-828-1056
FAX: 978-692-6073
e-mail: chrish@optelec.com
www.optelec@optelec.com

Large print software programs. *$595.00*

2126 **Large Print DOS**

Optelec US
PO Box 796
Westford, MA 01886
978-692-9496
800-828-1056
FAX: 978-692-6073
e-mail: chrish@optelec.com
www.optelec@optelec.com

2127 **Laureate Learning Systems**

110 E Spring Street
Winooski, VT 05404
802-655-4755
800-562-6801
FAX: 802-655-4757
e-mail: info@llsys.com
www.laureatelearning.com

Michelle L Oakes, Administrative Assistant
Kathy Hollandsworth, Office Manager

Laureate publishes award-winning talking software for children and adults with disabilities. Programs cover cause and effect, language development, cognitive processing, and reading. High-quality speech, colorful graphics and amusing animation make learning fun. Accessible with TouchWindow, single switch, keyboard and mouse. No reading required. Available for windows, macintosh, DOS, AppleII and IGS computers. Call for a free catalog.

2128 Learning Company

1 Martha's Way
Hiawatha, IA 52233
319-395-9626
800-752-3777
FAX: 319-378-7392
e-mail: Linda.Talcott@learningco.com
www.learningco.com

Linda Talcott, Asst Credit/Collections

Software for children. For Macintosh or Windows (3.1 DOS or Windows 95, Windows 98 required).

2129 Little Red Hen

9920 Pacific Heights Boulevard
San Diego, CA 92121
858-587-0087
800-247-1380
FAX: 619-622-7873
www.compasslearning.com

Steve Allen, Alternate Channels Manager

Children learn about the rewards of hard work when they discover who the Little Red Hen's friends miss out on freshly baked bread. Puzzles, rhymes, story writing and other interactive exercises enhance the creative learning process. *$34.95*

2130 Looking Good: Learning to Improve Your Appearance

Programming Concepts
PO Box 12428
San Antonio, TX 78212
800-594-4263
FAX: 218-248-055

Janie Haugen, Program Director
Jeff McLane, President/CEO

This game offers a creative way to discuss all areas of grooming. *$49.95*

2131 Monkeys Jumping on the Bed

Soft Touch
4300 Stine Road
Suite 401
Bakersfield, CA 93313
877-763-8868
FAX: 661-396-8760
e-mail: softtouch@funsoftware.com
www.funsoftware.com

Roxanne Butterfield

This program combines a favorite preschool song with number and color activities. Children and adults will enjoy engaging music and delightful animation. Students with cognitive delays respond to upbeat music and interesting sounds. Large graphics help learners focus on the action. Several important concepts are presented in enjoyable activity formats. Students learn cause and effect in Let's Play and Just for Fun.

2132 Morse Code WSKE

Words+
40015 Sierra Highway B-145
Palmdale, CA 93550
800-869-8521
FAX: 661-266-8969

Ginger Woltosz, VP
Tim Ross, Manager

A software and hardware product designed to operate on an IBM compatible PC.

2133 Muppet Learning Keys

WINGS for Learning
1600 Green Hills Road
Scotts Valley, CA 95066
831-464-3600
FAX: 831-464-3600

Designed to introduce children to the world of the computer as they become familiar with letters, numbers and colors.

2134 My Own Pain

Soft Touch
4300 Stine Road
Suite 401
Bakersfield, CA 93313
877-763-8868
FAX: 661-396-8760
e-mail: softtouch@funsoftware.com
www.funsoftware.com

Roxanne Butterfield

Three Activities - Three Levels. Press the switch and the paint brush chooses the color and paints the vehicle. Music reinforces the sounds when the picture is complete. A second activity allows the student to choose the color and paint the vehicle parts any color he or she wants. The third activity is a blueprint. Print the color that matches the one in the wire drawing. Color the drawing to complete the picture.

2135 Old MacDonald's Farm Deluxe

Soft Touch
4300 Stine Road
Suite 401
Bakersfield, CA 93313
877-763-8868
FAX: 661-396-8760
e-mail: softtouch@funsoftware.com
www.funsoftware.com

Roxanne Butterfield

Toddlers, preschoolers and early elementary students will be entertained and captivated by the six major activities and animations in the delightful program. Includes 18 real animation images or 9 cartoon like characters. The teacher or child can choose which animals they want to sing about. Some activities are designed for children within the normal population, others are designed for students with moderate and severe disabilities.

2136 Please Understand Me: Software Program and Books

Cambridge Educational
PO Box 931
Monmouth Junction, NJ 08852
800-468-4227
FAX: 800-329-6687
e-mail: lisa.schmuclei@films.com
www.cambridgeeducational.com

Lisa Schmuclei, Marketing

Promotes self understanding while helping each student understand they are different from others. *$69.00*

209 pages BiAnnual
ISBN 0-927368-56-x

2137 Pond

WINGS for Learning
1600 Green Hills Road
Scotts Valley, CA 95066
831-464-3600
FAX: 831-464-3600

Software game that teaches pattern recognition and encourages observation, trial and error and the interpretation of data.

2138 Print, Play & Learn #1 Old Mac's Farm

Soft Touch
4300 Stine Road
Suite 401
Bakersfield, CA 93313
877-763-8868
FAX: 661-396-8760
e-mail: softtouch@funsoftware.com
www.funsoftware.com

Roxanne Butterfield

Once your students have completed Old Mac's Farm, let them use the fun off-computer activities to continue learning. Over 25 activites with 250 sheets you print. Board games, dot-to-dot drawings, word puzzles, make a scene, flash cards. Concentration, sentence strips, worksheets and much more are availablefor techers to expand their teaching goals. This CD is full of activites to print and use.

2139 Print, Play & Learn #7: Sampler

Soft Touch
4300 Stine Road
Suite 401
Bakersfield, CA 93313
877-763-8868
FAX: 661-396-8760
e-mail: softtouch@funsoftware.com
www.funsoftware.com

Roxanne Butterfield

Print, Play and Learn Sampler gives you over 200 activites organized by Training, Easy, Medium and Hard levels so you can ready to help your student advance. Activites cover a wide range of basic knowledge, including colors, shapes, numbers, letters and much, much more. Note: Requires Overlay Maker or Overlay Printer by IntelliTools and a color printer.

2140 Puzzle Power: Sampler

Soft Touch
4300 Stine Road
Suite 401
Bakersfield, CA 93313
877-763-8868
FAX: 661-396-8760
e-mail: softtouch@funsoftware.com
www.funsoftware.com

Roxanne Butterfield

Puzzle Power - Sampler offers a variety of puzzles in different themes. Each theme puzzle is followed by a puzzle of one item in this category. For example, first solve a puzzle for Occupations. Then, solve a puzzle that is a baker. The pictures are large, clear and easily identifiable.

2141 Puzzle Power: Zoo & School Days

Soft Touch
4300 Stine Road
Suite 401
Bakersfield, CA 93313
877-763-8868
FAX: 661-396-8760
e-mail: softtouch@funsoftware.com
www.funsoftware.com

Roxanne Butterfield

Here is a program for all of our students who need puzzle skills, but cannot access commercial puzzles. Puzzle Power puzzles start with just two pieces and progress to 16 pieces. The pictures are large, clear and easily identifiable. Four different activites enable all students to be successful. Automatic Placement: the student just presses the switch or keyboard to place the pieces. Magnet Mouse: all the student needs to do is move the mouse and it drops into place.

2142 Rodeo

Soft Touch
4300 Stine Road
Suite 401
Bakersfield, CA 93313
877-763-8868
FAX: 661-396-8760
e-mail: softtouch@funsoftware.com
www.funsoftware.com

Roxanne Butterfield

Rodeo action and familiar tunes for teens and preteens. Four activities invite students to learn, laugh, and sing as they go to the rodeo with up to six age-peer friends. Age-appropriate graphics with surprising animations reinforce the learning. The graphics are large and coorful, the melodies familiar, and the words descriptive of the action on the screen.

2143 Shop Til You Drop

Soft Touch
4300 Stine Road
Suite 401
Bakersfield, CA 93313
877-763-8868
FAX: 661-396-8760
e-mail: softtouch@funsoftware.com
www.funsoftware.com

Roxanne Butterfield

Designed specifically for preteens and teens with moderate and severe disabilities, this program will become a staple for the classroom. The student goes shopping and can choose which outfits to put together. They may choose to purchase the outfit - of course, with Mom's credit card. Another activity is a video arcade game about money. Shop 'Til You Drop can be adjusted from a single switch cause-and-effect program to row-and-column scanning to direct choice.

2144 Songs I Sing at Preschool

Soft Touch
4300 Stine Road
Suite 401
Bakersfield, CA 93313
877-763-8868
FAX: 661-396-8760
e-mail: softtouch@funsoftware.com
www.funsoftware.com

Roxanne Butterfield

Songs I Sing at Preschool offers many options for the teacher and the student. Over the years, our software has used music because our students really respond to the sounds and rhythms of songs. Teachers select which songs to present, how many to present at one time and where to place each song on the overlay, keyboard or scan array.

2145 Stickybear Town Builder

Optimum Resource
18 Hunter Road
Hilton Head Island, SC 29926 **843-689-8000**
FAX: 843-689-8008
e-mail: sticky@stickybear.com
www.stickybear.com

Chris Gintz, VP Marketing

Children learn to read maps, build towns, take trips and use a compass in this simulation program. *$59.95*

2146 Stickybear Typing

Optimum Resource
18 Hunter Road
Hilton Head Island, SC 29926 **843-689-8000**
FAX: 843-689-8008
e-mail: sticky@stickybear.com
www.stickybear.com

Chris Gintz, VP Marketing

Sharpen typing skills with three challenging activities: Stickybear Keypress, Stickybear Thump and Stickybear Stories. *$59.95*

2147 **Stickybear's Early Learning Activities**

Optimum Resource
18 Hunter Road
Hilton Head Island, SC 29926 **843-689-8000**
FAX: 843-689-8008
e-mail: sticky@stickybear.com
www.stickybear.com

Chris Gintz, VP Marketing

Two modes of play, structure and non-structured, allow youngsters to learn through prompted direction or by the discovery method. Lively animation and sound keep attention levels high and Stickybear's Early Learning Activities is bilingual, so youngsters can build skills in both English and Spanish. *$59.95*

2148 **Stickybear's Kindergarden Activities**

Optimum Resource
18 Hunter Road
Hilton Head Island, SC 29926 **843-689-8000**
FAX: 843-689-8008
e-mail: sticky@stickybear.com
www.stickybear.com

Chris Gintz, VP Marketing

This dynamic new multifaceted program covers a wide range of preschool skills that go far beyond the stricktly academic! At Stickybear's house, children discover the alphabet, numbers, shapes, colors, plus - social skills, important safety messages and delightful off-screen activities that foster creativity. Over three hours of original music can be compose by a chid and saved for future use. *$59.95*

2149 **Stickybear's Science Fair: Light**

Optimum Resource
18 Hunter Road
Hilton Head Island, SC 29926 **843-689-8000**
FAX: 843-689-8008
e-mail: sticky@stickybear.com
www.stickybear.com

Chris Gintz, VP Marketing

The first in the new series of science-based programs Stickybear Science Fair: Light presents a content rich environment which allows students, ages 7-12 to explore, experiment with and understand light and it's properties. The program presents experiments, both structured and free-form, which allow users to work with prisms, lenses, color mixing, optical illusions and more. *$59.95*

2150 **Storybook Maker Deluxe**

9920 Pacific Heights Boulevard
San Diego, CA 92121 **858-587-0087**
800-247-1380
FAX: 619-622-7873
www.compasslearning.com

Steve Allen, Alternate Channels Manager

Using Storybook Maker Deluxe and their imaginations, students can create and publish stories filled with exciting graphics. Students can write stories and watch as the text appears in the setting they've chosen. Engaging sounds and music, plus lively animations, provide positive learning reinforcement throughout the program. *$44.95*

2151 **Super Challenger**

Electronic Courseware Systems
1713 S State Street
Champaign, IL 61820 **217-352-5510**
800-832-4965
FAX: 217-359-6587
e-mail: sales@ecsmedia.com
www.ecsmedia.com

Jodie Varner, Manager
David Peters, President

An aural-visual musical game that increases the player's ability to remember a series of pitches as they are played by the computer. The game is based on a 12-note chromatic scale, a major scale, and a minor scale. Each pitch is reinforced visually with a color representation of a keyboard on the display screen. Computer/software. *$39.95*

2152 **Switch Basics**

Soft Touch
4300 Stine Road
Suite 401
Bakersfield, CA 93313
877-763-8868
FAX: 661-396-8760
e-mail: softtouch@funsoftware.com
www.funsoftware.com

Roxanne Butterfield

Discover whimsical animations and real life pictures while learning switch operations. Intriguing and humorous, nine different programs offer a multitude of learning experiences for all ages. Program options include: cause and effect, scanning, step scanning, row and column activites for one or two players. Watch the clouds roll away revealing African animals; visit the beauty salon or barber shop; work two to sixteen piece puzzles; or add swimming fish to a huge aquarium.

2153 **Teach Me Phonemics Series Bundle**

Soft Touch
4300 Stine Road
Suite 401
Bakersfield, CA 93313
877-763-8868
FAX: 661-396-8760
e-mail: softtouch@funsoftware.com
www.funsoftware.com

Roxanne Butterfield

The Teach Me Phonemics Series Bundle includes one copy of each Teach Me Phonemics program - Initial, Medial, Final and Blends - four CD's in all.

2154 **Teach Me Phonemics Super Bundle**

Soft Touch
4300 Stine Road
Suite 401
Bakersfield, CA 93313
877-763-8868
FAX: 661-396-8760
e-mail: softtouch@funsoftware.com
www.funsoftware.com

Roxanne Butterfield

Teach Me Phonemics Super Bundle includes all 4 Teach Me Phonemics programs and all 4 Teach Me Phonemics Overlay CD's - eight CD's in all.

2155 **Teach Me Phonemics: Blends**

Soft Touch
4300 Stine Road
Suite 401
Bakersfield, CA 93313
877-763-8868
FAX: 661-396-8760
e-mail: softtouch@funsoftware.com
www.funsoftware.com

Roxanne Butterfield

Teach Me Phonemics - Blends helps students explore words and hear the initial blend sounds. It features musical interludes and movement to engage the student. Teachers select the best combination options to motivate and engage the student. Options turn off and on the fly so you can quickly make changes to keep the student engaged.

2156 **Teach Me Phonemics: Final**

Soft Touch
4300 Stine Road
Suite 401
Bakersfield, CA 93313
877-763-8868
FAX: 661-396-8760
e-mail: softtouch@funsoftware.com
www.funsoftware.com

Roxanne Butterfield

Teach me Phonemics - Final helps students explore words and hear the final sounds. It features musical interludes and movement to engage the student. Options turn off and on the fly so you can quickly make changes to keep the student engaged.

2157 **Teach Me Phonemics: Initial**

Soft Touch
4300 Stine Road
Suite 401
Bakersfield, CA 93313
877-763-8868
FAX: 661-396-8760
e-mail: softtouch@funsoftware.com
www.funsoftware.com

Roxanne Butterfield

Teach Me Phonemics - Initial helps students explore the words and hear the initial sounds. It features musical interludes and movement to engage the student. Teachers select the best combination options to motivate and engage the student. Options turn off and on the fly so you can quickly make changes to keep the student engaged.

2158 **Teach Me Phonemics: Medial**

Soft Touch
4300 Stine Road
Suite 401
Bakersfield, CA 93313
877-763-8868
FAX: 661-396-8760
e-mail: softtouch@funsoftware.com
www.funsoftware.com

Roxanne Butterfield

Teach Me Phonemics - Medial helps students explore the words and hear the medial sounds. It features musical interludes and movement to engage the student. Teachers select the best combination options to motivate and engage the student. Options turn off and on the fly so you can quickly make changes to keep the student engaged.

2159 **Teach Me to Talk**

Soft Touch
4300 Stine Road
Suite 401
Bakersfield, CA 93313
877-763-8868
FAX: 661-396-8760
e-mail: softtouch@funsoftware.com
www.funsoftware.com

Roxanne Butterfield

The first activity Teach Me to Talk is used as a springboard for the student to learn to speak the word. There are 150 real pictures. When a picture is chosen, it appears on a clear background with musical interludes, movement, written word and spoken word. It culminates by morphing to the corresponding black and white Mayer-Johnson symbol. The second activity Story Time, takes some of these nouns and puts them in four line poetry. This helps student hear the word in the midst of a sentence.

2160 **Teen Tunes Plus**

Soft Touch
4300 Stine Road
Suite 401
Bakersfield, CA 93313
877-763-8868
FAX: 661-396-8760
e-mail: softtouch@funsoftware.com
www.funsoftware.com

Roxanne Butterfield

Introduce switch use to older students with disabilities. Large intersting graphics, a variety of musical interludes, and surprising animations are combined with calm soothing music and beautiful pictures in the software specifically designed for preteens and teens with severe cognitive delays and/or physical disabilities, and older students learning to use a switch.

2161 **There are Tyrannosaurs Trying on Pants in My Bedroom**

9920 Pacific Heights Boulevard
San Diego, CA 92121
858-587-0087
800-247-1380
FAX: 619-622-7873
www.compasslearning.com

Steve Allen, Alternate Channels Manager

In this popular story, Saturday chores turn into fun-filled frolicking when dinosaurs come for a visit. Sounds, music and animation make learning about phonics and vocabulary dyno-mite. *$34.95*

2162 **Three Billy Goats Gruff**

9920 Pacific Heights Boulevard
San Diego, CA 92121
858-587-0087
800-247-1380
FAX: 619-622-7873
www.compasslearning.com

Steve Allen, Alternate Channels Manager

Motivating exercises and creative activities provide hours of learning fun while young students follow the adventure of The Three Billy Goats Gruff in this animated version of the timeless tale. *$ 34.95*

2163 **Three Little Pigs**

9920 Pacific Heights Boulevard
San Diego, CA 92121
858-587-0087
800-247-1380
FAX: 619-622-7873
www.compasslearning.com

Steve Allen, Alternate Channels Manager

Help young students build reading comprehension and writing skills with this interactive version of the children's classic, The Three Little Pigs. Animated storytelling and creative activities inspire children to read, write and rhyme. *$34.95*

2164 TouchCorders

Soft Touch
4300 Stine Road
Suite 401
Bakersfield, CA 93313
877-763-8868
FAX: 661-396-8760
e-mail: softtouch@funsoftware.com
www.funsoftware.com

Roxanne Butterfield

TouchCorders are the flexible and easty-to-use communicator designed by Jo Meyer and Linda Bidabe for reach classroom use. TouchCorders are sensitive to touch at every angle and give the student kinesthetic feedback. With the unique Add 'n Touch system, Jo connects the puzzles bases of 2 or more. TouchCorders on the fly to present vocabulary, sequencing, story telling, social stories, concepts and other curriculum and communication opportunities.

2165 TouchWindow touch screen

Edmark Corporation
PO Box 97021
Redmond, WA 98073
425-556-8400
FAX: 425-556-8430
e-mail: edmarkteam@edmark.com
www.edmark.com

Software for children. *$335.00*

2166 Turtle Teasers

Soft Touch
4300 Stine Road
Suite 401
Bakersfield, CA 93313
877-763-8868
FAX: 661-396-8760
e-mail: softtouch@funsoftware.com
www.funsoftware.com

Roxanne Butterfield

Three Games, Three Levels from Easy, Medium to Hard. The Shell Game - easy: Watch one of the three turles get the tomato. Then watch carefully as they switch positions and pop shut. Choose incorrectly and the frog disappears until the correct one is displayed. The Pond - medium: Watch the tomato disappear somewhere in the pond scene. Tomato Dump - hard: Hit the shell and it turns into the tomato, giving a score. There are different difficulty levels to equalize all students.

2167 Volcanoes

Earthware Computer Services
2386 Spring Boulevard
Eugene, OR 97403
FAX: 541-342-3416

Simulation of volcano in which children play the role of the scientists. *$49.50*

2168 What Was That!

9920 Pacific Heights Boulevard
San Diego, CA 92121
858-587-0087
800-247-1380
FAX: 619-622-7873
www.compasslearning.com

Steve Allen, Alternate Channels Manager

In this bedtime story, noises in the night send three brother bears scurrying out of bed. Thoughtful questions test young readers' comprehension, while games, voice recording, writing practice and other playful activities stimulate their creativity.

2169 Wivik 3

Prentke Romich Company
1022 Heyl Road
Wooster, OH 44691
330-262-1984
800-262-1984
FAX: 330-263-4829
e-mail: info@prentrom.com
www.prentrom.com

On-screen keyboard provides access to any application in the latest Windows operating systems. Selections are made by clicking, dwelling or switch scanning. Enhancements include word prediction and abbreviation expansion.

2170 You Tell Me: Learning Basic Information

Programming Concepts
PO Box 12428
San Antonio, TX 78212
800-594-4263
FAX: 218-248-055

Janie Haugen, Program Director
Jeff McLane, President/CEO

This game teaches and reinforces basic information all individuals need to know. Questions asked in this game help prepare people to communicate personal identification information important to community survival. *$49.95*

Software: Professional

2171 Acrontech International

5500 Main Street
Williamsville, NY 14221
FAX: 716-854-4014

This company supplies software, audio mixers, and closed-caption televisions.

2172 DME VI

Dezine Associates
2625 Cumberland Parkway
Suite 310
Atlanta, GA 30339
800-441-2331
800-447-7370
800-254-9872
www.carecentric.com

This full-featured software package specific to the health care industry includes accounts receivable, order entry, inventory control and sale management in an easy-to-use format.

2173 DPS with BCP

VORT Corporation
PO Box 60132
Palo Alto, CA 94306
650-322-8282
FAX: 650-327-0747
e-mail: sales@vort.com
www.vort.com

This program uses unique DPS branching techniques to access goals and objectives.

2174 **Diagnostic Report Writer**

Parrot Software
190 Sandy Ridge Road
State College, PA 16803
800-727-7681
FAX: 814-237-7282

Fred Weiner, Owner

Creates a three page single-spaced diagnostic report for a child with a communication disorder from a list of questions; sections of the report include developmental and background history, oral peripheral exam, speech and language analysis, summary and recommendations.

2175 **Discriptive Language Arts Development**

Educational Activities Software
PO Box 754
Baldwin, NY 11510
516-867-7878
800-645-2796
FAX: 516-379-7429
e-mail: achieve@ea-software.com

Alan Stern, Sales

This multimedia language arts development program provides instruction and application of fundamental English skills and concepts. *$395.00*

2176 **EZ Dot**

CAPCO Capability Corporation
1522 N Washington Street
Suite 200
Spokane, WA 99201
FAX: 509-535-1011

A critical software tool used in vocational counseling, job restructuring, recruitment and placement, better utilization of workers, and safety issues. This software offers occupational data by title, code, industry, GEO, DPT, or OGA. *$295.00*

2177 **EZ Keys for Windows**

Words+
1220 W Avenue J
Lancaster, CA 93534
800-869-8521
FAX: 661-266-8969

Phil Lawrence, VP
Rachel Nielsen, Customer Support

A software and hardware product designed to operate on an IBM compatible PC. The software provides dual word prediction, abbreviation expansion, five different methods of voice output and access to commercial software applications. *$1395.00*

2178 **Goals and Objectives IEP Program**

Curriculum Associates
PO Box 2001
N Billerica, MA 01862
978-667-8000
800-225-0248
FAX: 800-366-1158
e-mail: info@curriculumassociates.com
www.curriculumassociates.com

BRIGANCE CIBS-R standardized scoring conversion software, is a teacher's tool that prints goal and objective pages of the IEP. In less than two minutes per student, a teacher types student data into the computer.

2179 **Nasometer**

Kay Elemetrics Corporation
2 Bridgewater Lane
Lincoln Park, NJ 07035
973-628-6200
FAX: 973-628-6363
www.kayelemetrics.com

Measures the ratio of acoustic energy for the nasal and real-time visual cueing during therapy. Used clinically in the areas of cleft palate, motor speach disorders, hearing impairment and palatal prosthetic fittings.

2180 **PSS CogRehab software**

Psychological Software Services
6555 Carrollton Avenue
Indianapolis, IN 46220
317-257-9672
FAX: 317-257-9674
e-mail: obracy@inctdirect.net
www.neuroscience.cnter.com

Nancy Bracy, Sales/Production

PSS CogRehab Software is a comprehensive and easy-to-use multimedia cognitive rehabilitation software available, for clinical and educational use with head injury, stroke LD/ADD and other brain compromises. The packages include 64 computerized therapy tasks which contain modifiable parameters that will accomodate most requirements. Exercises include attention and executive skills, multiple modalities of visuopatial and memory skills, simple, complex, proble-solving skills.

$260 - $2500

2181 **Parrot Easy Language Simple Anaylsis**

Parrot Software
190 Sandy Ridge Road
State College, PA 16803
800-727-7681
FAX: 814-237-7103

Fred Weiner, Owner

Designed for grammatical analysis of language samples. The user types and translates language samples of up to 100 utterances.

2182 **TOVA**

Universal Attention Disorders
4281 Katella Avenue
Suite 215
Los Alamitos, CA 90720
714-229-8770
800-PAY-ATTN
FAX: 714-229-8782

Dr. Lawrence Greenberg, Developer

A computerized assessment which, in conjunction with classroom behavior ratings, is a highly effective screening tool for ADD. TOVA includes software, complete instructions, and supporting data including norms.

2183 **TTAP Outreach: Technology Team Assessment Process**

27 Horrabin Hall
Macomb, IL 61455
309-298-1634
FAX: 309-298-2305
e-mail: l_robinsonl@wiu.edu
www.mprojects.wiu.edu

Linda Robinson, Coordinator

Provides training to early childhood personnel and families on a team-based model for technology assessment. TTAP's procedures are designed to assess children's ability to use technology as a tool for achieving IEP/IFSP goals. Training and written materials are available.

2184 Visi-Pitch III

Kay Elemetrics Corporation
2 Bridgewater Lane
Lincoln Park, NJ 07035 973-628-6200
FAX: 973-628-6363
www.kayelemetrics.com

Assits the speech/voice clinician in assessment and treatment tasks across an expansive range of disorders.

Software: Reading & Language Arts

2185 Choices, Choices 5.0

Tom Snyder Productions
80 Coolidge Hill Road
Watertown, MA 02472 781-926-6000
800-342-0236
FAX: 800-304-1254
www.tomsnyder.com

Teaches students to take responsibility for their behavior. Helps students develop the skills and awareness they need to make wise choices and to think through the consequences of their actions.

2186 Circletime Tales Deluxe

Don Johnston
26799 N Commerce Drive
Volo, IL 60073 847-740-0749
800-999-4660
FAX: 847-740-7326
e-mail: info@donjohnston.com
www.donjohnston.com

This interactive CD-ROM introduces and reinforces pre-literacy concepts using nursery rhymes and songs familiar to many children. This English/Spanish program emphasizes listening to and learning basic concepts such as opposites, directionality, colors and counting. *$59.00*

2187 Community Exploration

9920 Pacific Heights Boulevard
San Diego, CA 92121 858-587-0087
800-247-1380
FAX: 619-622-7873
www.compasslearning.com

Steve Allen, Alternate Channels Manager

An award-winning learning adventure takes students who are learning English as a second language on a field trip to the make-believe town of Cornerstone. More than 50 community locations come to life with sound and animation. While exploring places in this typical American community where people live, work and play, students also enhance important English language skills. Offers an exciting approach for any age student who needs to improve their English language proficiency. 4-12. *$19.95*

2188 Conversations

Educational Activities Software
PO Box 754
Baldwin, NY 11510 516-867-7878
800-645-2796
FAX: 516-379-7429
e-mail: achieve@ea-software.com

Alan Stern, Sales

Using American digitalized voices, CONVERSATIONS provides 14 different dialogues in which the student can participate. The topics offer learners important information about American culture and the workplace. Available for DOS. *$195.00*

2189 Core-Reading and Vocabulary Development

Educational Activities
PO Box 392
Freeport, NY 11520 516-623-9282
800-645-3739
e-mail: learn@edact.com
www.edact.com

Al Harris, President
Alan Stern, VP

Students begin with 36 basic words and progress to more than 200. Reading and writing activities are coordinated and integrated throughout the program for more substantial permanent learning. Five units covering readability levels from pre-primer to grade three.

Full Program

2190 Day at Play: A IKanDu Little Book

Don Johnston
26799 N Commerce Drive
Volo, IL 60073 847-740-0749
800-999-4660
FAX: 847-740-7326
e-mail: info@donjohnston.com
www.donjohnston.com

One of the products in the UKanDu Little Book Series. This early literacy program consists of several four-page animated stories that help build language experience for emergent and early readers. Children fill-in-the-blank to complete a sentence on each page and then watch the page come alive with animation and sound. After completion, it can be printed to make a book. All children can be successful as there are no wrong answers. *$45.00*

2191 Friday Afternoon

9920 Pacific Heights Boulevard
San Diego, CA 92121 858-587-0087
800-247-1380
FAX: 619-622-7873
www.compasslearning.com

Steve Allen, Alternate Channels Manager

Save hours of preparation time and dazzle your students with interesting new activities to supplement their classroom learning. With Friday afternoon, you'll produce flash cards, word puzzles, even customized bingo cards and more, all at the click of a mouse. MacIntosh diskette. *$99.95*

2192 How to Read for Everyday Living

Educational Activities Software
PO Box 754
Baldwin, NY 11510 516-867-7878
800-645-2796
FAX: 516-379-7429
e-mail: achieve@ea-software.com

Alan Stern, Sales

Basic vocabulary and key words are taught and, when need, retaught using alternative teaching strategies. Passages that students read help put the vocabulary into context. Each lesson is followed by crossword and other puzzles check comprehension.

2193 Learning English: Primary

9920 Pacific Heights Boulevard
San Diego, CA 92121 858-587-0087
800-247-1380
FAX: 619-622-7873
www.compasslearning.com

Steve Allen, Alternate Channels Manager

Four stories and rhymes help students familiarize themselves with essential English language concepts, recognize patterns in language and associate words with objects. *$49.95*

2194 Learning English: Rhyme Time

9920 Pacific Heights Boulevard
San Diego, CA 92121
858-587-0087
800-247-1380
FAX: 619-622-7873
www.compasslearning.com

Steve Allen, Alternate Channels Manager

Using classic children's rhymes in an animated multimedia program, students work on language skills, vocabulary and comprehension.

2195 Lexia I, II and III Reading Series

Lexia Learning Systems
PO Box 466
Lincoln, MA 01773
781-259-8752
800-435-3942
FAX: 781-259-1349
e-mail: info@lexialearning.com
www.lexialearning.com

Jon Bower, President
Heidi Brown, Marketing Director

Lexia's software helps children and adults with learning disabilities master their core reading skills. Based on the Orton Gillingham method, Lexia Early Reading, Phonics Based Reading and SOS (Strategies for Older Students) apply phonics principles to help students learn essential sound-symbol correspondence and decoding skills. The Quick Reading Tests generate detailed skill reports in only 5-8 minutes per student to provide data for further instruction. Price: $40-400 per workstation.

2196 Memory Castle

WINGS for Learning
1600 Green Hills Road
Scotts Valley, CA 95066
831-464-3600
FAX: 831-464-3600

Introduces a strategy to increase memory skills via an adventure game. Set in a castle, the game requires memory, reading, spelling skills and more to win.

2197 On a Green Bus: A UKanDu Little Book

Don Johnston
26799 N Commerce Drive
Volo, IL 60073
847-740-0749
800-999-4660
FAX: 847-740-7326
e-mail: info@donjohnston.com
www.donjohnston.com

This early literacy program that consists of several create-your-own 4-page animated stories that help build language experience on each page and then watch the page come alive with animation and sound. After completing the story, students can print it out to make a book which can be read over and over again. Because there are no wrong answers, all children can have a successful literacy experience. *$ 45.00*

2198 Open Book

Freedom Scientific
11800 31st Court N
St. Petersburg, FL 33716
727-803-8000
800-444-4443
FAX: 727-803-8001
e-mail: info@freedomscientific.com
www.freedomscientific.com

Software that reads scanned text allowed and includes other features that aid the vision-impaired. *$995.00*

2199 Optimum Resource Software

18 Hunter Road
Hilton Head, SC 29926
843-689-8000
FAX: 843-689-8008
e-mail: sticky@stickybear.com
www.optimumlearning.com

Chris Gintz, VP Marketing

Optimum Resource publishes over 100 K-12 education curriculum software titles under its varietal brands, StickyBear, MiddleWare, High School and Tools for Teachers.

2200 Out and About: A UKanDu Little Book

Don Johnston
26799 N Commerce Drive
Volo, IL 60073
847-740-0749
800-999-4660
FAX: 847-740-7326
e-mail: info@donjohnston.com
www.donjohnston.com

One of the products in the UKanDu Little Book Series. This early literacy program consists of several four-page animated stories that help build language experience for emergent and early readers. Children fill-in-the-blank to complete a sentence on each page and then watch the page come alive with animation and sound. After completion, it can be printed to make a book. *$45.00*

2201 Programs for Aphasia and Cognitive Disorders

Parrot Software
190 Sandy Ridge Road
State College, PA 16803
800-727-7681
FAX: 814-237-7103

Fred Weiner, Owner

Over 50 different computer programs that facilitate language, memory and attention training. Programs are available for MS DOS, WINDOWS and Apple II.

2202 Punctuation Rules

Optimum Resource
18 Hunter Road
Hilton Head Island, SC 29926
843-689-8000
FAX: 843-689-8008
e-mail: sticky@stickybear.com
www.stickybear.com

Chris Gintz, VP Marketing

Punctuation Rules is designed to help students improve their punctuation skills. Students work with appropriate level sentences which follow common rules of punctuation. The program covers material ranging from categories of sentences to forming possessives and allows students to gain strength in their ability to correctly use periods, commas, apostrophes, question marks, colons, hyphens, quotation marks, exclamation points and more. *$59.95*

2203 Quick Talk

Educational Activities Software
PO Box 754
Baldwin, NY 11510
516-867-7878
800-645-2796
FAX: 516-379-7429
e-mail: achieve@ea-software.com

Alan Stern, Sales

Students will learn and use new vocabulary immediately: high-frequency, everyday vocabulary words are introduced and used contextually using human speech, graphics and text. Voice-interactive program (MS-DOS). *$65.00*

2204 **Race the Clock**

Mindplay
3130 N Dodge Boulevard
Tucson, AZ 85716
520-323-1303
800-221-7911
FAX: 520-322-0363

A matching game, uses the animation capabilities to teach verbs. The player chooses a matching game from a menu.

2205 **Reader Rabbit**

Learning Company
500 Redwood Boulevard
Novato, CA 94947
800-825-4420
FAX: 877-278-7456
e-mail: SchoolCustomerService@riverdeep.net
www.learningcompanyschool.com

Supports young students in building fundamental reading readiness skills in a playful, multi-sensory environment.

2206 **Reading Comprehension Series**

Optimum Resource
18 Hunter Road
Hilton Head Island, SC 29926
843-689-8000
FAX: 843-689-8008
e-mail: sticky@stickybear.com
www.stickybear.com

Chris Gintz, VP Marketing

The Reading Comprehension Series, includes six volumes for Windows, MacIntosh, DOS or Apple II computers. Packed with intriguing multi-level stories, each volume will capture the interest of children ages 8-14 while teaching them crucial reading comprehension skills. These open-ended programs are versatile and easy to use. *$59.95*

2207 **Simon Sounds it Out**

Don Johnston
26799 N Commerce Drive
Volo, IL 60073
847-740-0749
800-999-4660
FAX: 847-740-7326
e-mail: info@donjohnston.com
www.donjohnston.com

This interactive phonics program enables students to learn and practice letter sounds with an instructional and nonthreatening on-screen tutor. This phonics program was designed by leading learning authorities and extensively tested in classrooms. Colorful graphics, digitalized sound and amusing animations reward students and motivate them to continue learning. *$59.00*

1998

2208 **Simon Spells**

Don Johnston
26799 N Commerce Drive
Volo, IL 60073
847-740-0749
800-999-4660
FAX: 847-740-7326
e-mail: info@donjohnston.com
www.donjohnston.com

This innovative spelling program guides students through individualized instruction presented in a way that enables them to work at their own pace. Words are phonemically presented, as well as placed in the context of sentences so as to help increase vocabulary comprehension and spelling skills. Student progress is tracked and results are stored. *$59.00*

2209 **Sound Sentences**

Educational Activities Software
PO Box 754
Baldwin, NY 11510
516-867-7878
800-645-2796
FAX: 516-379-7429
e-mail: achieve@ea-software.com

Alan Stern, Sales

This sound-interactive program breaks away from traditional language instruction. Instead of formal concentration on verb and basic vocabulary, students meet everyday English with colloquialisms they will hear in real life situations. They reinforce their knowledge of sentence structure while acquiring the ability to communicate in daily settings. (For MAC, MS-DOS and Windows). *$65.00*

2210 **Spelling Rules**

Optimum Resource
18 Hunter Road
Hilton Head Island, SC 29926
843-689-8000
FAX: 843-689-8008
e-mail: sticky@stickybear.com
www.stickybear.com

Chris Gintz, VP Marketing

A curriculum based, easy-to-use program that provides students with the practice they need to build strong spelling skills. *$59.95*

2211 **Spelling Test Generator**

Optimum Resource
18 Hunter Road
Hilton Head Island, SC 29926
843-689-8000
FAX: 843-689-8008
e-mail: sticky@stickybear.com
www.stickybear.com

Chris Gintz, VP Marketing

Using more than 3000 of the most commonly encountered words in the English language, the Spelling Test Generator prepares spelling lists on the basis of difficulty, grade level, vowels, diphthongs, word origins and starting/ending letters or sounds. *$59.95*

2212 **Stickybear Parts of Speech**

Optimum Resource
18 Hunter Road
Hilton Head Island, SC 29926
843-689-8000
FAX: 843-689-8008
e-mail: sticky@stickybear.com
www.stickybear.com

Chris Gintz, VP Marketing

Children learn parts of speech with this exciting new program. *$59.95*

2213 **Stickybear Reading**

Optimum Resource
18 Hunter Road
Hilton Head Island, SC 29926
843-689-8000
FAX: 843-689-8008
e-mail: sticky@stickybear.com
www.stickybear.com

Chris Gintz, VP Marketing

Children build vocabulary and reading comprehension skills using hundreds of word/picture sets and thousands of put-together sentence parts. *$49.95*

2214 **Stickybear Reading Comprehension**
Optimum Resource
18 Hunter Road
Hilton Head Island, SC 29926 **843-689-8000**
FAX: 843-689-8008
e-mail: sticky@stickybear.com
www.stickybear.com

Chris Gintz, VP Marketing

This multi-level reading comprehension program helps children improve reading skills with 30 high-interest stories and question sets created by the Weekly Reader editors. *$59.95*

2215 **Stickybear Spellgrabber**
Optimum Resource
18 Hunter Road
Hilton Head Island, SC 29926 **843-689-8000**
FAX: 843-689-8008
e-mail: sticky@stickybear.com
www.stickybear.com

Chris Gintz, VP Marketing

Build spelling and vocabulary skills with three different activities: Picture Spell, Word Spell and Bear Dunk. *$59.95*

2216 **Stickybear Spelling**
Optimum Resource
18 Hunter Road
Hilton Head Island, SC 29926 **843-689-8000**
FAX: 843-689-8008
e-mail: sticky@stickybear.com
www.stickybear.com

Chris Gintz, VP Marketing

Children ages 6 and up discover and practice critical spelling skills as they work with three unique action-packed activities, each with four graded levels of difficulty. The program is open-ended and teachers may add, change and modify the word lists for each individual. Stickybear Spelling contains more than 2000 recorded words. Levels may be set to allow students of different ages or abilities to compete effectively. *$59.95*

2217 **Stickybear Spelling Rules**
Optimum Resource
18 Hunter Road
Hilton Head Island, SC 29926 **843-689-8000**
FAX: 843-689-8008
e-mail: sticky@stickybear.com
www.stickybear.com

Chris Gintz, VP Marketing

Spelling Rules is designed to help students improve spelling accuracy and master the fundamentals - forming plurals (adding s, adding es, f, fe, to ves) and compound words I before E rule, capitalization and many others.. *$59.95*

2218 **Stickybear's Reading Fun Park**
Optimum Resource
18 Hunter Road
Hilton Head Island, SC 29926 **843-689-8000**
FAX: 843-689-8008
e-mail: sticky@stickybear.com
www.stickybear.com

Chris Gintz, VP Marketing

Children ages 4-8 discover and practice critical reading skills as the famous stickybear family guides users through unique, action-packed activities, each with multiple levels of difficulty and skills that address both the auditory and visual needs of budding readers. *$59.95*

2219 **Stickybear's Reading Room**
Optimum Resource
18 Hunter Road
Hilton Head Island, SC 29926 **843-689-8000**
FAX: 843-689-8008
e-mail: sticky@stickybear
www.stickybear.com

Chris Gintz, VP Marketing

The perfect combination of learning and fun, our award winning Stickybear's Reading Room provides colorful motivating thinking skills practice for children ages 4-8 with four unique bilingual learning activities. *$59.95*

2220 **Tomorrow's Promise: Language Arts**
9920 Pacific Heights Boulevard
San Diego, CA 92121 **858-587-0087**
800-247-1380
FAX: 619-622-7873
www.compasslearning.com

Steve Allen, Alternate Channels Manager

You'll strengthen students' grammar, usage and vocabulary skills promote higher order thinking skills with this comprehensive Language Arts curriculum. It utilizes cross-curricular, thematic instruction engaging multimedia learning exercises that encourage writing, speaking and listening proficiency. Promotes higher order thinking skills. *$279.95*

2221 **Tomorrow's Promise: Reading**
9920 Pacific Heights Boulevard
San Diego, CA 92121 **858-587-0087**
800-247-1380
FAX: 619-622-7873
www.compasslearning.com

Steve Allen, Alternate Channels Manager

This multimedia curriculum balances thematic, interactive exploration with core skills development, increasing your students' early reading proficiency, building a solid literacy foundation and fostering a lifelong love for reading. *$279.95*

2222 **Tomorrow's Promise: Spelling**
9920 Pacific Heights Boulevard
San Diego, CA 92121 **858-587-0087**
800-247-1380
FAX: 619-622-7873
www.compasslearning.com

Steve Allen, Alternate Channels Manager

Lovable characters and engaging multimedia effects put young students on a fast-track to early spelling proficiency with fourteen activities and three games. A full year's instruction on each CD includes 30 world lists per grade, in story context, or create word lists to suit your needs. This program addresses students' multiple learning styles and rewards students as they progress through each stage of spelling skill acquisition. *$99.95*

2223 **Vocabulary Development**
Optimum Resource
18 Hunter Road
Hilton Head Island, SC 29926 **843-689-8000**
FAX: 843-689-8008
e-mail: sticky@stickybear.com
www.stickybear.com

Chris Gintz, VP Marketing

A featured program in the middle school series. Vocabulary Development is designed to help students increase vocabulary as they strengthen reading skills. Students relate their current knowledge of vocabulary to the context in which they discover an unfamiliar word. Utilizing a variety of contextual aids, this program illustrates synonyms, antonyms, prefixes, suffixes, homophones, multiple meanings and context clues, allowing students to apply experience and context. *$59.95*

2224 Whoops

Cornucopia Software
626 San Carlos Avenue
Albany, CA 94706
FAX: 510-528-7000
e-mail: support@practicemagic.com
www.practicemagic.com

Phillip Manfield

Checks spelling three ways. It checks words as they are typed, it checks an entire screen and highlights the errors and it reads ASCII text files from a disk and lists errors.

2225 Writer

K-12 Micro Media Publishing
16 McKee Drive
Mahwah, NJ 07430
201-529-4500
800-292-1997
FAX: 201-529-5282
e-mail: sales@k12mmp.com
www.k12mmp.com

Ryan Galloway, Sales

Assistive keyboard for writing. Wireless transfer of text may be downloaded into any computer application (Word, Excel, Powerpoint). Also can be used as a real-time wireless keyboard. Includes batteries, receiver and cables. Includes complete keyboard instruction, thesaurus, self-editing checklist. *$1.99*

Software: Vocational

2226 Functional Literacy System

Conover Company
2926 Hidden Hollow Road
Oshkosh, WI 54904
920-231-4667
800-933-1933
FAX: 920-231-4809
e-mail: conover@execpc.com
www.conovercompany.com

Terry Schmitz, President

Assessment and skill building for basic functional literacy. This multimedia software program is adult in format and uses live action video taken in actual community settings to help learners become more capable of functioning independently. Twenty different programs are currently available. *$99.00*

2227 Learning Activity Packets

Conover Company
2926 Hidden Hollow Road
Oshkosh, WI 54904
920-231-4667
800-933-1933
FAX: 920-231-4809
e-mail: conover@execpc.com
www.conovercompany.com

Terry Schmitz, President

Demonstrates how basic academic skills relate to 30 major career areas. LAPs provide valuable diagnostics in applied academic applications and demonstrates to users the importance of academics as they relate to the workplace. Software. *$99.00*

2228 Microcomputer Evaluation of Careers & Academics (MECA)

Conover Company
2926 Hidden Hollow Road
Oshkosh, WI 54904
920-231-4667
800-933-1933
FAX: 920-231-4809
e-mail: conover@execpc.com
www.conovercompany.com

Terry Schmitz, President

A cost-effective, technology-based career development system which provides users with opportunities to get their hands dirty. The MECA system utilizes work simulations and is built around common occupational clusters. Each cluster, or career area, consists of hands-on WORK SAMPLES which provide a variety of career exploration and assessment experiences, linked to LEARNING ACTIVITY PACKETS, which integrate basic academic skills into the career planning and placement process. $580-$1,070.

2229 OASYS

Vertek
12835 Bel-Red Road
Suite 112
Bellevue, WA 98005
425-455-9921
800-220-4409
FAX: 425-454-7264
e-mail: marketing@vertekinc.com
www.vertekinc.com

Gale Gibson, President

A software system that matches a person's skills and abilities to occupations and employers.

2230 Reading in the Workplace

Educational Activities Software
PO Box 754
Baldwin, NY 11510
516-867-7878
800-645-2796
FAX: 516-379-7429
e-mail: achieve@ea-software.com

Alan Stern, Sales

A job-based reading software program using real-life problems and solutions to capture students' attention and improve their vocabulary and comprehension skills. Units include: automotive, clerical, health care and construction. *$295.00*

2231 Stickybear Typing

Optimum Resource
18 Hunter Road
Hilton Head Island, SC 29926
843-689-8000
FAX: 843-689-8008
e-mail: sticky@stickybear.com
www.stickybear.com

Chris Gintz, VP Marketing

The award winning Stickybear Typing program allows users to sharpen typing skills and achieve keyboard mastery with three engaging and amusing multi-level activities. *$59.95*

2232 Vocational Interest Profile Report

Cambridge Educational
90 Maccorkle Avenue SW
South Charleston, WV 25303
304-744-2055
800-468-4227
FAX: 800-329-6687
e-mail: melindab@citynet.net
www.cambridgeol.com

Melinda Ball, Marketing Director

Software that is designed to allow students to systematically define broad work categories that are of most interest. *$64.86*

ISBN 0-927368-59-5

2233 **Work-Related Vocational Assessment Systems**

Valpar International
12778 W N Avenue
Building A
Brookfield, AZ 53005
262-797-0840
800-633-3321
FAX: 262-797-8488
e-mail: sales@valparint.com
www.valparint.com

Neil Gunderson, President
Patricia L Rastaller, VP Operations

Criterion-referenced to Department of Labor standards. Evaluate academic levels for reading, spelling, math and language, and various other aptitudes.

2234 **Workplace Skills: Learning How to Function on the Job**

Programming Concepts
PO Box 12428
San Antonio, TX 78212
800-594-4263
FAX: 218-248-055

Janie Haugen, Program Director
Jeff McLane, President/CEO

Offers parents and educators a functional means by which to discuss all aspects of finding and keeping a job. *$49.95*

Word Processors

2235 **Braille Keyboard Labels**

Hooleon Corporation
417A S 6th Street
Cottonwood, AZ 86326
928-634-7515
800-937-1337
FAX: 928-634-4620
e-mail: sales@hooleon.com
www.hooleon.com

Barry Green, Sales Manager
Joan Crozier, President/Sales

Also large print keyboard lables and large print with Braille.

2236 **DARCI**

WesTest Engineering Corporation
810 Shepard Lane
Farmington, UT 84025
801-451-9191
FAX: 801-451-9393

Provides transparent access to all computer functions by replacing the computer's keyboard with a smart joystick. *$975.00*

2237 **Dreamer**

TS Micro Tech
1209 John Reed Court
City of Industry, CA 91745
626-330-0086
FAX: 626-330-6018
e-mail: sales@fanca.com

An intelligent, add-on function keyboard providing single-keystroke access to multiple-keystroke functions.

2238 **EasyKey Visual Keyboard**

Inkwell Systems
PO Box 1318
Talent, OR 97540
541-535-1210

An on-screen keyboard that floats ontop of the program in any Windows application and allows the user to type via alternative input device. *$99.00*

2239 **FlexShield Keyboard Protectors**

Hooleon Corporation
417A S 6th Street
Cottonwood, AZ 86326
928-634-7515
800-937-1337
FAX: 928-634-4620
e-mail: sales@hooleon.com
www.hooleon.com

Barry Green, Sales Manager
Joan Crozier, President/Sales

Transparent keyboard protectors allowing instant recognition of keytop legends. They have a matte finish to reduce glare.

2240 **Hooleon Corporation**

417A S 6th Street
Cottonwood, AZ 86326
928-634-7515
800-937-1337
FAX: 928-634-4620
e-mail: sales@hooleon.com
www.hooleon.com

Barry Green, Sales Manager
Joan Crozier, President/Sales

Large print and combination Braille adhesive keytop labels for computer keyboards. Helps visually impaired computer users access correct key strokes either by sight or by touch. Raised Braille meets ADA specifications and large print fills key top surface.

2241 **IntelliKeys**

IntelliTools
1720 Corporate Circle
Petaluma, CA 94954
707-773-2000
800-899-6687
FAX: 707-773-2001
e-mail: info@intellitools.com
www.intellitools.com

Caroline Van Howe, Marketing Director

Alternative, touch-sensitive keyboards; plugs into any Macintosh or Windows computer. *$395.00*

2242 **IntelliKeys IIe**

IntelliTools
1720 Corporate Center
Petaluma, CA 94954
707-773-2000
800-899-6687
FAX: 707-773-2001
e-mail: info@intellitools.com
www.intellitools.com

Caroline Van Howe, Marketing Director

Card and cable to create keyboard port on Apple IIe computer to allow use of IntelliKeys alternative keyboard. *$129.95*

2243 **IntelliKeys USB**

IntelliTools
1720 Corporate Circle
Petaluma, CA 94954
707-773-2000
800-899-6687
FAX: 707-773-2001
e-mail: tech@intellitools.com
www.intellitools.com

Paula Irons, Director Mktg Communications

IntelliKeys alternative keyboard for USB computers and Windows 2000, Mac OSX. *$69.95*

2244 **IntelliTalk**

IntelliTools
1720 Corporate Circle
Petaluma, CA 94954
707-773-2000
800-899-6687
FAX: 707-773-2001
e-mail: tech@intellitools.com
www.intellitools.com

Paula Irons, Director Mktg Communications

Talking word-processing program available for MacIntosh, Apple IIe, IBM compatible and Windows computers. *$39.95*

2245 **Internal I/O Port Adapter**

AbleNet
1081 10th Avenue SE
Minneapolis, MN 55414
800-322-0956
FAX: 612-379-9143
e-mail: customerservice@ablenetinc.com

Mary Kay Walch

A converting cable designed to provide a 9-pin joystick port for Apple II+ and older model computers. *$18.00*

2246 **Jouse**

Prentke Romich Company
1022 Heyl Road
Wooster, OH 44691
330-262-1984
800-262-1984
FAX: 330-263-4829
e-mail: info@prentrom.com
www.prentrom.com

A joystick-operated mouse that is controlled with the mouth. Moving the joystick moves the cursor. Mouse button activations can be made with the sip and puff switch that is built into the joystick. Typing can be achieved through an on-screen keyboard. Nothing is attached to the operator. The adjustable Jouse arm mounts on a table or desktop and swings away when bumped. *$995.00*

2247 **Key Tronic KB 5153 Touch Pad Keyboard**

KeyTronic
PO Box 14687
Spokane, WA 99214
800-262-6006

Integrates a regular full-function keyboard, a numeric keypad with a cursor key capability and a touch pad into one unit.

2248 **Keyguards for IntelliKeys**

IntelliTools
1720 Corporate Circle
Petaluma, CA 94954
707-773-2000
800-899-6687
FAX: 707-773-2001
e-mail: info@intellitools.com
www.intellitools.com

Caroline Van Howe, Marketing Director

Acrylic keyguards for each of IntelliKeys six standard overlays. *$250.00*

2249 **Large Print Keyboard Labels**

Hooleon Corporation
417A S 6th Street
Cottonwood, AZ 86326
928-634-7515
800-937-1337
FAX: 928-634-4620
e-mail: sales@hooleon.com
www.hooleon.com

Barry Green, Sales Manager
Joan Crozier, President/Sales

Pressure sensitive labels.

2250 **Large Type**

National Institute for Rehab Engineering
PO Box 1088
Hewitt, NJ 07421
973-853-6585
800-736-2216
FAX: 928-832-2894

Donald Selwyn, Director

Display enlargement programs for visually impaired users consist of a variety of programs for different needs, ranging from basic to full-featured.

2251 **Magic Wand Keyboard**

In Touch Systems
11 Westview Road
Spring Valley, NY 10977
845-354-7431
800-332-6244
www.magicwandkeyboard.com

Susan Crouch, VP

The magic wand keyboard allows your child to use a keyboard and mouse easily-no light beams, microphones, or sensors to wear of position. This miniature computer keyboard has zero-force keys that work with the slightest touch of a wand (hand-held of mouthstick). No strength required.

2252 **McKey Mouse**

In Touch Systems
11 Westview Road
Spring Valley, NY 10977
845-354-7431
800-332-6244

Susan Crouch, VP

Microsoft compatible mouse for persons with little or no hand/arm movement; it's an option for the Magic Wand Keyboard and adds full mouse function without adding any extra devices.

2253 **Pegasus LITE**

Words+
1220 W Avenue J
Lancaster, CA 93534
800-869-8521
FAX: 661-266-8969

Phil Lawrence, VP
Rachel Nielsen, Customer Support

Provides all of the strategies currently being used in AAC, from dynamic display color pictographic language, to dual-word prediction text language, in a single system. *$6995.00*

2254 **SuperKey**

Corland International
1800 Green Hills Road
Scotts Valley, CA 95066
831-430-0455

A keyboard enhancement program that allows the user to store frequently-used commands and retrieve them with two keystrokes and to cut and paste text between applications programs and create single-page help screens for each set of macros created.

2255 **Touchdown Keytop/Keyfront Kits**

Hooleon Corporation
417A S 6th Street
Cottonwood, AZ 86326
928-634-9578
800-937-1337
FAX: 928-634-4620
e-mail: sales@hooleon.com
www.hooleon.com

Barry Green, Sales Manager
Joan Crozier, President/Sales

These kits enlarge the key legends of a computer and include Braille for easy recognition.

2256 **Unicorn Keyboards**

IntelliTools
1720 Corporate Circle
Petaluma, CA 94954
707-773-2000
800-899-6687
FAX: 707-773-2001
e-mail: info@intellitools.com
www.intellitools.com

Caroline Van Howe, Marketing Director

Alternative keyboards with membrane surface and large, user-defined keys. Large and small sizes are available. *$250.00*

2257 **Up and Running**

IntelliTools
5221 Central Avenue
Suite 205
Richmond, CA 94804
800-899-6687
FAX: 510-528-2225
e-mail: info@intellitools.com

Instantly use hundreds of popular commercial software programs with this custom collection of setups and overlays. *$69.95*

2258 **Write This Way**

9920 Pacific Heights Boulevard
San Diego, CA 92121
858-587-0087
800-247-1380
FAX: 619-622-7873
www.compasslearning.com

Steve Allen, Alternate Channels Manager

An easy-to-use, versatile word processor designed with learning disabled or hearing-impaired individuals in mind category score fewer points. Apple or Mac available. *$99.95*

2259 **Write: OutLoud**

Don Johnston
26799 N Commerce Drive
Volo, IL 60073
847-740-0749
800-999-4660
FAX: 847-740-7326
e-mail: info@donjohnston.com
www.donjohnston.com

The award-winning feasible and user friendly talking word processor with talking spell checker. Text-to-speech technology provides multi-sensory learning and positive reinforcements for writers of all ages and ability levels. *$99.00*

General

2260 ABDA/ABMPP Workshop: The Art of Courtroom Testifying

American Board of Disability Analysts
342 24th Avenue N
Suite 200
Nashville, TN 37203 **615-327-2984**
FAX: 615-327-9235
e-mail: americanbd@aol.com

February workshop. Workshop leader: Dr. William Tsushima.

2261 APSE Conference: Revitalizing Supported Employment, Climbing to the Future

Association for Persons in Supported Employment
1627 Monument Avenue
Richmond, VA 23220 **804-278-9187**
FAX: 804-278-9377
e-mail: apse@apse.com
www.apse.org

Mary Callender, Conference Planner

A major conference on Supported Employment. The conference includes 130 sessions presented by nationally recognized leaders in the field. Conference attendees come from all 50 states, Canada and several foreign countries and include professionals in supported employment, occupational therapy, rehabilitation technology and other related fields.

July

2262 Abilities Expo

Advanstar Communications
440 Wheelers Farm Road
Suite 101
Milford, CT 06460 **203-882-1300**
FAX: 203-882-1800
e-mail: abilities@advanstar.com
www.abilitiesexpo.com

Diane Waltersdorf, Show Director

The one show for assisted and independent living products and services in the US.

2263 Alexander Graham Bell Association for the Deaf and Hard of Hearing Annual Conference

3417 Volta Place NW
Washington, DC 20007 **202-337-5220**
FAX: 202-337-8314
e-mail: info@agbell.org
www.agbell.org

Over 60 booths offering information on resources and technology for the deaf and hard of hearing.

June

2264 American Academy for Cerebral Palsy and Developmental Medicine Annual Conference

6300 N River Road
Suite 727
Rosemont, IL 60018 **847-698-1635**
FAX: 847-823-0536
e-mail: raymond@aaos.org
www.aacpdm.org

Sheril King, Executive Director

Holds annual conference in September with instructional courses such as: the fundamentals of normal walking, management of drooling in the developmentally disabled, technology dependent children, evaluation and treatment of feeding, nutritional and growth problems in the child with disabilities, Spina Bifida care, spasticity, measurement, sexual behavior and problems of the young disabled adult, grant seeking programs that care for the special needs child, etc.

September

2265 American Academy of Ophthalmology Annual Meeting

655 Beach Street
PO Box 7424
San Francisco, CA 94120 **415-561-8500**
FAX: 415-561-8533
e-mail: federal@aao.org
www.aao.org

Mission is to advance the lifelong learning and professional interests of Eye MDs to ensure that the public can obtain the best possible eye care.

November

2266 American Association of the Deaf-Blind National Conference

814 Thayer Avenue
Room 302
Silver Spring, MD 20910 **301-495-4403**
FAX: 301-495-4404
TTY:301-495-4402
e-mail: info@aadb.org
www.aadb.org

Harry Anderson, President

A week of workshops, exhibits, networking, socializing and more.

July

2267 American Association on Mental Retardation AAMR Annual Meeting

444 N Capitol Street NW
Washington, DC 20001 **202-783-1535**
800-424-3688
FAX: 202-387-2193
e-mail: anam@aamr.org
www.aamr.org

Paula A Hirt, Director Programs & Services
Malene S Ward, Meetings Coordinator

At The Crossroads: Ethics, Genetics, Leadership and Self-Determination, the annual meeting offers a full compliment of workshops, symposia, and multiperspective sessions that fill four days including social events.

May/June

2268 American Board of Disability Analysts

Disability Analyst
345 24th Avenue N
Suite 200
Nashville, TN 37203 **615-327-2984**
FAX: 615-327-9235
e-mail: americanbd@aol.com

Alexander E Horwitz MD, Executive Officer
Kenneth N Anchor PhD, Administrative Officer/Editor
Gabriel Sella MD, Continuing Education Coordinator

2269 **American Council of the Blind Annual Convention**

1155 15th Street NW
Suite 1004
Washington, DC 20005 **202-467-5081**
800-424-8666
FAX: 202-467-5085
e-mail: info@acb.org
www.acb.org

Charles Crawford, Executive Director

Offers 50-75 booths of information for the blind.

June/July

2270 **American Diabetes Association Annual Conference**

1701 N Beauregard Street
Alexandria, VA 22311 **703-379-7755**
800-342-2383
www.diabetes.org/main/application/commercewf

Christina Pappas, Marketing Planner

Trade show featuring exhibits of equipment and supplies used by professionals involved in the treatment of diabetes.

2271 **American Physical Therapy Association**

1111 N Fairfax Street
Alexandria, VA 22314 **703-684-2782**
FAX: 703-706-8519

Jane Mathews, President

National Physical Therapy Week in October hosts a variety of activities promoting healthy living. The theme for the week is Pro-Active Health Care. The Association celebration will feature fitness clinics, fun runs, athletic competitions, open houses and seminars on health and fitness topics. The APTA is a national professional organization representing more than 50,000 physical therapists, physical therapist assistants, and students. Goals are the improvement of physical therapy.

2272 **American Rehabilitation Counseling Association**

American Counseling Association
5999 Stevenson Avenue
Alexandria, VA 22304 **800-347-6647**
800-473-2329
FAX: 703-823-6862
www.counseling.org

Steve Brooke, Marketing Director

March/April

2273 **American Speech-Language-Hearing Association**

10801 Rockville Pike
Rockville, MD 20852 **301-897-5700**
800-638-8255
FAX: 301-897-7348
e-mail: actioncenter@asha.org
www.asha.org

John E Bernthal, President
Frederick T Spahr PhD, Executive Director
Joanne Jessen, Publications Director

Exhibits by companies specializing in alternative and augmentative communication products, publishers, software and hardware companies, and hearing aid testing equipment manufacturers.

2274 **American Spinal Injury Association Annual Scientific Meeting**

Rehabilitation Institute of Chicago
345 E Superior Street
Room 1436
Chicago, IL 60011 **312-238-6207**
FAX: 312-238-0869
e-mail: mars@northwestern.edu
www.asia-spinalinjury.org

Marcia L Sipski MD, President/Director

Professional association for physicans and other health professionals working in all aspects of spinal cord injury. Annual scientific meeting surveys latest advancements in the field. See website for full details.

2275 **Annual Santa Barbara Sports Festival**

PO Box 50001
Santa Barbara, CA 93150 **805-897-2680**
www.semananautica.com

A non-profit organization that seeks to promote athletic and recreational activity in Santa Barbara for all ages and abilities.

June/July

2276 **Association for Education & Rehabilitation of the Blind & Visually Impaired Intl. Conference**

1703 N Beauregard Street
Suite 440
Alexandria, VA 22311 **703-671-4500**
FAX: 703-671-6391

Greg Goodrich, President

Dedicated to rendering support and assistance to the professionals who work in all phases of education and rehabilitation of blind and visually impaired children and adults.

July 1984

2277 **Attention Deficit Disorders Association, Southern Region: Annual Conference**

12345 Jones Road
Suite 287-7
Houston, TX 77070 **281-897-0982**
FAX: 281-894-6883
e-mail: addaoffice@pdq.net
www.adda-sr.org

Pam Esser, Executive Director
Marian Bryant, President

Mission is to: provide a resource network; to support individuals impacted by attention deficit disorders; to advocate for the development of community resources and services that meet the educational, social, and health care needs of all individuals with ADD/ADHD.

February

2278 **Blazing Toward a Cure Annual Conference**

National Parkinson Foundation
Bob Hope Parkinson Research Center
1501 NW 9th Avenue, Bob Hope Road
Miami, FL 33136 **305-547-6666**
800-327-4545
FAX: 305-243-4403
e-mail: mailbox@parkinson.org
www.parkinson.org

Daniel Arty, President
Alan M Slewett Esq, Secretary

Purpose is find the cause and cure for Parkinson's Disease and related neurodegenerative disorders through research, education and dissemination of current information to patients, caregivers and families.

2279 Blind Childrens Center Annual Meeting

4120 Marathon Street
Los Angeles, CA 90029
323-664-2153
800-222-3567
FAX: 323-665-3828
e-mail: info@blindchildrenscenter.org
www.blindchildrenscenter.org

A family-centered agency which serves children with visual impairments from birth to school-age. The center-based and home-based services help the children to acquire skills and build their independence. The Center utilizes its expertise and experience to serve families and professionals worldwide through support services, education and research.

September

2280 Blinded Veterans Association National Convention

477 H Street NW
Washington, DC 20001
202-371-8880
800-669-7079
FAX: 202-371-8258
e-mail: bva@bva.org
www.bva.org

Thomas H Miller, Executive Director
George E Brummell, Natl. Dir. Field Service Program

Helps veterans and their families meet the challenges of blindness.Offers two main service programs without cost to blinded veterans. Field service program provides counseling o veterans and families and information on benefits and re - habilitation.

August

2281 Children and Adolescents with Emotional and Behavioral Disorders

Virginia Commonwealth University, Medical College
PO Box 980489
Richmond, VA 23298
804-741-7057
FAX: 804-828-2645

Cynthia R Eillis MD, Program Chair

October

2282 Closing the Gap's Annual Conference

PO Box 68
Henderson, MN 56044
507-248-3294
FAX: 507-248-3810
e-mail: info@closingthegap.com
www.closingthegap.com

International conference held annually on adaptive technology for people with disabilities.

2283 Contemporary Issues in Behavioral Health Care

American Assn. of Children's Residential Centers
440 1st Street NW
3rd Floor
Washington, DC 20001
202-628-1816
FAX: 202-638-4004
e-mail: aacrc@dc.net
www.aacrc-dc.org

Richard Biolsi ACSW, President
Elissa Malter Schwartz, Association Director

One-day program will address accreditation as it relates to current behavioral health care challenges. Four Points Sheraton Hotel in San Diego, California.

July

2284 Council for Exceptional Children Annual Convention and Expo

1110 N Glebe Road
Suite 300
Arlington, VA 22201
703-620-3660
FAX: 703-264-9494
www.cec.sped.org

Nancy Safer, Executive Director

Meet leaders and innovators in special education, their products works and services for the exceptional and gifted child.

April

2285 Eye Bank Association of America Annual Meeting

1015 18th Street NW
Suite 1010
Washington, DC 20036
202-775-4999
FAX: 202-429-6036
e-mail: sightebaa@aol.com
www.restoresight.org

Patricia Acken-O'Neil Esq, President/CEO

Not-for-profit organization dedicated to the restoration of sight through the promotion and advancement of eye banking. Promotes research and professional education with a newsletter, brochures and pamphlets.

June 1961

2286 Handicapped Student Program Postsecondary Education Association

PO Box 21192
Columbus, OH 43221
614-488-4972
FAX: 614-488-1774
e-mail: ahead@postbox.acs.ohio-state.edu
www.ahead.org

Ed Suddeth, Executive Director

July

2287 International Symposium on Parkinson's Disease Research

National Parkinson Foundation
Bob Hope Parkinson Research Center
1501 NW 9th Avenue, Bob Hope Road
Miami, FL 33136
305-547-6666
800-327-4545
FAX: 305-243-4403
e-mail: mailbox@parkinson.org
www.parkinson.org

Daniel Arty, President
Alan M Slewett Esq, Secretary

Purpose is to find the cause and cure for Parkinson's Disease and related neurodegenerative disorders through research, education and dissemination of current information to patients, caregivers and families.

Annual

2288 Joint Conference with ABMPP Annual Conference

American Board of Disability Analysts
345 24th Avenue N
Suite 200
Nashville, TN 37203
615-327-2984
FAX: 615-327-9235
e-mail: americanbd@aol.com

Joint Conference with ABMPP Annual Conference Charleston, South Carolina.

May

2289 Journal of Rehabilitation and Annual Conference

National Rehabilitation Association (NRA)
633 S Washington Street
Alexandria, VA 22314 **703-836-0850**
FAX: 703-836-0848
e-mail: info@nationalrehab.org
www.nationalrehab.org

Carol Jaafar, Director Program Services
Michelle Vaughan, Executive Director

The annual conference exhibits of companies that provide services and products to rehab professionals and persons with disabilities. Journal of Rehabilitation: Articles are written by professionals in the fields of rehabilitation and are peer reviewed. Editorial content reflects the broad perspectives of the association's memberhsip.

2290 Lowe's Syndrome Association Conference

222 Lincoln Street
W Lafayette, IN 47906 **765-743-3634**

e-mail: info@lowesyndrome.org
www.lowesyndrome.org

Jane Gallery, President
Kaye McSpadden, Public/Scienific Affairs Dir.
Nancy Lewis, Secretary

Conference held every 2 years. Provides information, newsletter, publications, parent directory, medical research and more.

June

2291 MedTrade/Comtrade, FutureShow

SEMCO Productions
1130 Hightower Trail
Atlanta, GA 30350
FAX: 770-642-4715

Mark Simmering, Executive VP/COO
Beth Lange

A showplace for more than 250,000 healthcare products and services, including respiratory, rehab, home healthcare, long-term care/alternate site, wound care/skin care, med/surg, sports medicine, IV therapy, computer and automation technology, and telecommunications. Attendees include hospitals, physicians, RNs, HMOs, insurance companies, long-term care providers, medical device manufacturers, pharmacists, therapists and more.

October

2292 National Braille Association National Conference

3 Townline Circle
Rochester, NY 14623 **585-427-8260**
FAX: 585-427-0263
e-mail: nbaoffice@compuserve.com
www.nationalbraille.org

Providing continuing education to those who prepare Braille, and provides Braille materials to persons who are visually impaired. Maintains collection of Braille textbooks, music, technical tables, and general interest items. Catalogs of the Braille collection in print or Braille are free on request.

April

2293 National Council on the Aging Conference

Conference Department
409 3rd Street SW
Washington, DC 20024 **202-205-6770**
800-424-9046
FAX: 202-479-0735
www.ncoa.com

Offers ideas and programs to increase your program and administrative skills through NCOA's professional development tracks and the offering of continuing education units.

May

2294 National Managed Health Care Congress

71 2nd Avenue
3rd Floor
Waltham, MA 02451 **781-663-6000**
FAX: 781-663-6422
www.nmhcc.org

Attracts nearly 7,000 delegates, thereby reinforcing its status as the nation's largest conferences for all managed care constituencies.

2295 Prader-Willi Alliance of New York Annual Conference

267 Oxford Street
Rochester, NY 14607 **716-442-1655**
800-442-1655
FAX: 716-271-2782
e-mail: balleregballer@aol.com
www.prader-willi.org

Elinor G Baller, Secretary

The Prader-Willi Foundation is a national, nonprofit public charity that works for the benefit of individuals with Prader-Willi syndrome and their families.

2296 RESNA Annual Conference

1700 N Moore Street
Suite 1540
Arlington, VA 22209 **703-524-6686**
FAX: 703-524-6630
e-mail: conference@resna.org
www.resna.org

Shannon Marullo, Director, Professional Services

A multidisciplinary association for the advancement of rehabilitation and assistive technologies, holds an annual conference in June. The conference brings together a large number of rehabilitation professionals, products and services from around the world and has something to offer for both professionals and consumers. The conference provides an informative and thought provoking forum for anyone with interests in rehabilitation technology.

June

2297 Rehabilitation International

25 E 21st Street
New York, NY 10010 **212-420-1500**
FAX: 212-505-0871
e-mail: Rehabintl@rehab-international.org
www.rehab-international.org

Lex Frieden, President
George Wilson, Treasurer

Worldwide network of people with disabilities, service providers and government agencies working together to improve the quality of life for the dosabled people and their families, has more than 200 member organizations in 90 nations. World Congress and Exposition on Disabilities is held in September.

2298 Rehabilitation Technology Association Conference

PO Box 1004
Institute, WV 25112 **304-766-4602**
800-624-8284
FAX: 304-766-2689
e-mail: wvrrtc@rtc2.icdi.wvu.edu

Betty Jo Tyler, RTA Coordinator
Dave Whipp, Information Manager

Holds annual conference in the spring. Publishes a quarterly newsletter and houses the Project Enable computerized bulletin board system.

2299 Santa Barbara Wheelchair Sports Conference

Santa Barbara Parks and Recreation Department
PO Box 1990
Santa Barbara, CA 93102
805-564-5324
FAX: 564-548-0

Mariana de Sena RT CTRS, Recreation Supervisor
Richard Johns

Offers a yearly conference, offers programs and services for individuals with a physically disabling condition, head injured individuals that may be visually and hearing impaired. Offers excursions, outings, competition, recreation, etc.

2300 SubAcute Care: American SubAcute Care Association Annual Convention/Expo

PO Box 17413
Washington, DC 20041
FAX: 703-318-7568

Sherlyn Remley, Exhibit Sales
Jim Wasson, Exhibit Sales

Totally dedicated to servicing the subacute arena and its major entities. Features 100+ booths and over 75 exhibitors.

March

2301 Tourette Syndrome Association Conference

42-40 Bell Boulevard
Bayside, NY 11361
718-224-2999
800-237-0717
FAX: 718-279-9596
e-mail: ts@tsa-usa.org
www.tsa-usa.org

Fred Cook, Chair
Judit Ungar, President
Trudy Colletti-Flynn, Manager, Public Relations & Comm

National, nonprofit membership organization that sponsors an annual conference for its more than 35,000 members.

Spring

2302 United Cerebral Palsy Association Development Conference

1660 L Street NW
Suite 700
Washington, DC 20036
202-776-0406
800-872-5827
FAX: 202-776-0414
TTY:202-973-7197
e-mail: webmaster@ucp.org
www.ucpa.org

Stephen Bennett, President/CEO

National not-for-profit self-help organization dedicated to providing information and support to individuals with Cerebral Palsy and other disabilities, and their families. Supports more than 160 local affiliates; these affiliates provide a variety of programs and services for affected families, including support groups. Offers several educational and support materials, including a quarterly magazine, regular newsletters, and research reports.

2303 United Cerebral Palsy Association Annual Conference

1660 L Street NW
Suite 700
Washington, DC 20036
202-776-0406
800-872-5827
FAX: 202-776-0414
TTY:202-973-7197
e-mail: webmaster@ucp.org
www.ucpa.org

Stephen Bennett, President/CEO

National not-for-profit self-help organization dedicated to providing information and support to individuals with Cerebral Palsy and other disabilities, and their families. Supports more than 160 local affiliates; these affiliates provide a variety of programs and services for affected families, including support groups. Offers several educational and support materials, including a quarterly magazine, regular newsletters, and research reports.

2304 United Cerebral Palsy Association of New York State Annual Conference

90 State Street
Suite 929
Albany, NY 12207
518-436-0178
FAX: 518-436-8619
e-mail: info@cerebralpalsynys.org
www.cerebralpalsynys.org

Susan Constantino, Associate Executive Director
Cheryl Bradway, Administrative Assistant
Barbara Crosier, Legislative Affairs Director

Mission is to advocate and provide direct services with and for individuals with cerebral palsy and other significant disabilities, and their families, throughout New York State, in order to promote lifelong opportunities and choices for independence, inclusion and enhanced quality of life. Provides services and programs for more than 40,000 individuals with cerebral palsy and developmental disabilities and their families.

October

2305 Winter Conference

American Board of Disability Analysts
345 24th Avenue N
Suite 200
Nashville, TN 37203
615-327-2984
FAX: 615-327-9235
e-mail: americanbd@aol.com

Joint Conference: American Board of Disability.

February

2306 Young Onset Parkinson Conference

National Parkinson Foundation
Bob Hope Parkinson Research Center
1501 NW 9th Avenue, Bob Hope Road
Miami, FL 33136
305-547-6666
800-327-4545
FAX: 305-243-4403
e-mail: mailbox@parkinson.org
www.parkinson.org

Daniel Arty, President
Alan M Slewett Esq, Secretary

Purpose is to find the cause and cure for Parkinson's Desease and related neurodegenerative disorders through research, education and dissemination of current information to patients, caregivers and families.

Annual

Organizations

2307 Adaptive Environments Center

374 Congress Street
Suite 301
Boston, MA 02210
617-695-1225
FAX: 617-482-8099
e-mail: adaptive@adaptenv.org
www.adaptenv.org

Valerie Fletcher, Executive Director
Lenie Kuit, Marketing Communications Coord.
Kathy Gips, Director Training

Develops educational programs and materials on universal design, Americans with Disabilities Act, home adaptation, and more. Central Adaptive Environments publication list also available.

2308 American Institute of Architects (AIA)

Information Center
1735 New York Avenue NW
Washington, DC 20006
202-783-6500
FAX: 202-626-7547
e-mail: library@aiamail.aia.org
www.aia.org

Carole Twombly, Reference Librarian
Jenni Woolums, Reference Librarian

Research service in print and online information. Large collection of books and periodicals on the building/architectural environments.

2309 Building Owners and Managers Association International

1201 New York Avenue NW
Suite 300
Washington, DC 20005
202-408-2662
FAX: 202-371-0181
e-mail: ada@bomg.org
www.boma.org

Marco A Giamberardino MPA, Director, Codes & Standards

Conducts seminars nationwide and publishes resource guidebooks for building owners and managers on ADA requirements for commercial facilities and places of public accommodation.

2310 Challenges Unlimited

171 River Drive
Hadley, MA 01035
800-637-8720
FAX: 413-585-1137

Michael Oestreicher, President

A multi-disciplined design firm founded in 1984 by concerned design professionals. The team includes architects, engineers, designers and landscape architects specializing in accessible corporate, municipal and private facilities.

2311 Mark Elmore Associates Architects

42 E Street
Crystal Lake, IL 60014
815-455-7260
FAX: 815-455-2238
e-mail: mark@elmore-architects.com
www.elmore-architects.com

Mark Elmore, AIA

Architectural designs for accessible residential and commercial buildings. ADA compliance reviews.

2312 National Conference on Building Codes and Standards

505 Huntmar Park Drive
Suite 210
Herndon, VA 20170
703-437-1011
FAX: 703-481-3596

Barbara Divver, Director Services & Membership

In conjunction with Paralyzed Veterans of America, this agency will promote the certification of State codes for equivalency with ADA standards, and encourage the development of alternative dispute resolution procedures within the existing State regulatory framework.

2313 National Legal Center for the Medically Dependent and Disabled

50 S Meridian Street
Suite 605
Indianapolis, IN 46204
317-638-1700
FAX: 812-232-0620
e-mail: nlcmdd@juno.com
www.tmarzon@aol.com

Litigation and support center for the disabled specializing in medical treatment lights/attendant care issues. *$49.00*

2314 Overcoming Mobility Barriers International

1022 S 41st Street
Omaha, NE 68105
402-342-5731
FAX: 402-342-5731

Kay Neil, Executive Director

Members are government officials, service consumers and providers, and other persons interested in removing mobility barriers for elderly, handicapped and disadvantaged persons. Advises and works in conjunction with other groups and government agencies to establish safety standards for special equipment used in retrofitting vehicles and works to retrain drivers in the use of nonconventional driving controls. Addresses such problems as possible allocation of fuel to social service agencies.

2315 Paradigm Design Group

Paralyzed Veterans of America
801 18th Street NW
Washington, DC 20006
202-872-1300
800-424-8200
FAX: 202-416-7647
e-mail: info@pva.org
www.pva.org

Kim Beasley, Managing Principal
Thomas Davies Jr, Principal

Specialized firm providing architectural consulting services related to accessible designs. Experience includes product design and building codes and standards.

2316 United States Access Board

1331 F Street NW
Suite 1000
Washington, DC 20004
202-331-1252
800-872-2253
FAX: 202-272-5447
e-mail: info@access-board.gov
www.access-board.gov

Dave Yanchulis, Public Affairs Specialist

Offers information and referrals on architectural accessibility for architects, designers, government agencies, building owners and consumers. A list of free publications is available on request. The Access Board also enforces the Architectural Barriers Act, which covers buildings and facilities designed, built or altered since 1968 with certain federal funds or leased by federal agencies. Publications: Access Currents, bi-monthly newsletter.

Publications & Videos

2317 Access Equals Opportunity

Council of BBB's Foundation
4200 Wilson Boulevard
Suite 800
Arlington, VA 22203
703-247-9301
FAX: 703-525-8277
www.bbb.org

Barbara Bate, VP
Jennifer Ley, Special Assistant

These six Title III compliance guides for existing small businesses offer creative cheap and easy suggestions for complying with the public accommodations section of the ADA. Each guide is industry specific for: retail stores, car sales/service, restaurants/bars, medical offices and fun/fitness centers. They include suggestions for readily achievable removal of architectural barriers; effective communication; and guidance for nondiscriminatory policies or procedures. *$2.50*

2318 Access House

Northside Mental Health Center
1109 E 139th Avenue
Tampa, FL 33613
813-264-1811
FAX: 813-632-0933

Cecil Woodside, Director

Barrier free regulations for design and construction.

2319 Access for All

Hospital Audiences
220 W 42nd Street
New York, NY 10036
212-575-7678
FAX: 212-575-7669
www.hospitalaudiences.org

Tricia Hennessey, Access Director

Provides physical and program accessibility information for people with disabilities to New York City cultural institutions including theaters, museums, galleries, etc.

2320 Accessible Home of Your Own

Accent Books & Products
PO Box 700
Bloomington, IL 61702
309-378-2961
800-787-8444
FAX: 309-378-4420
e-mail: acmtlvng@aol.com
www.accentonliving.com

Raymond C Cheever, Publisher
Betty Garee, Editor

This guide includes 14 articles that have appeared in the magazine on the popular subject of how to make a disabled persons home more accessible. *$5.95*

52 pages Paperback
ISBN 0-91570 -29-9

2321 Adaptable Housing: A Technical Manual for Implementing Adaptable Dwelling

HUD USER
PO Box 6091
Rockville, MD 20849
301-251-5154
800-245-2691
FAX: 202-708-4213
www.huduser.org

An illustrated manual describing methods for implementing adaptability in housing. *$3.00*

2322 Adaptive Environments Center Home Assessment Form

374 Congress Street
Suite 301
Boston, MA 02210
617-695-1225
FAX: 617-482-8099
e-mail: adaptive@adaptenv.org
www.adaptenv.org

A handy checklist for evaluating a disabled person's abilities and his/her home limitations to determine what accessibility modifications will be most effective. *$5.00*

2323 Besign for Acessibility

National Endowment for the Arts Office
1100 Pennsylvania Avenue NW
Washington, DC 20506
202-682-5532
FAX: 202-682-5715
e-mail: nasaa@nasaa-arts.org
www.arts.gov

Frank Hodsoll, Designer

A handbook for compliance with Section 504 of the Rehabilitation Act of 1973 and the Americans with Disablities Act of 1990 including technical assistance on making arts programs accessible to staff, performers and audience.

101 pages 1987
ISBN 0-160042-83-6

2324 Consumer's Guide to Home Adaptation

Adaptive Environments Center
374 Congress Street
Suite 301
Boston, MA 02210
617-695-1225
FAX: 617-482-8099
e-mail: adaptive@adaptenv.org
www.adaptenv.org

Valerie Fletcher, Executive Director
Gabriela Bonome-Simms, Director Admissions
Mike DiLorenzo, Publications Coordinator

A workbook that enables people with disabilities to plan the modifications necessary to adapt their homes. Describes how to widen doorways, lower countertops, etc. *$12.00*

52 pages Paperback

2325 Directory of Accessible Building Products

NAHB Research Center
400 Prince Georges Boulevard
Upper Marlboro, MD 20774
800-638-8556
FAX: 301-430-6180
e-mail: nahbrc.org
www.nahbrc.org

Taria Singleton, Publication Department

Contains descriptions of more than 200 commercially available products designed for use by people with disabilities and age-related limitations. Paperback. *$5.00*

104 pages Yearly

2326 Do-Able Renewable Home

AARP Fulfillment
601 E Street NW
Washington, DC 20049
202-434-2277
800-424-3410
FAX: 202-434-3443
e-mail: member@aarp.org
www.aarp.org

Describes how individuals with disabilities can modify their homes for independent living. Room-by-room modifications are accompanied by illustrations.

2327 **ECHO Housing: Recommended Construction and Installation Standards**

American Association of Retired Persons
601 E Street NW
Washington, DC 20049
800-424-3410
FAX: 202-434-6483
www.aarp.org

Illustrated design, construction, and installation standards for temporary dwelling units for elderly people on single family residential property.

2328 **EPVA Action**

Eastern Paralyzed Veterans Association
75-20 Astoria Boulevard
Flushing, NY 11370
718-397-4181
800-444-0120
FAX: 718-803-0414
e-mail: info@epva.org
www.epva.org

Association news and articles on architecture and barrier-free design, legislation and other current events affecting veterans.

Monthly

2329 **Electronic House: Enhanced Lifestyles with Electronics**

Electronic House
526 Boston Post Road
Suite 150
Wayland, MA 01778
508-358-3400
800-375-8015
FAX: 508-358-5195
e-mail: kmoyes@ehpub.com
www.electronichouse.com

Ken Moyes, Publisher

Dedicated to home automation. Featuring both extravagant and affordable smart homes that can be controlled with one touch. EH covers electronic systems that give homeowners more security, entertainment, convenience, and fun. Articles cover whole house control and subsystems like residential lighting, security, home theater, energy management and telecommunications. *$23.95*

84 pages BiMonthly
ISSN 0886-66 3

2330 **Fair Housing Design Guide for Accessibility**

National Council on Multifamily Housing Industry
15th & M Street NW
Washington, DC 20005
202-862-1600
FAX: 202-785-1255
e-mail: info@nahb.com
www.nahb.com

Thomas D Davies Jr, Author/Editor

Specifically tailored to address the needs of architects and builders. The book includes a detailed technical analysis of the legislation's impact on multifamily design, highlights potential construction problems, and identifies possible solutions. *$29.95*

2331 **Ideas for Making Your Home Accessible**

Accent Books & Products
PO Box 700
Bloomington, IL 61702
309-378-2961
800-787-8444
FAX: 309-378-4420
e-mail: acmtlvng@aol.com
www.accentonliving.com

Raymond C Cheever, Publisher
Betty Garee, Editor

Offers over 100 pages of tips and ideas to help build or remodel a home. Includes many special devices and where to get them. *$7.50*

94 pages Paperback
ISBN 0-91570 -08-6

2332 **NHeLP**

National Health Law Program
2639 S La Cienega Boulevard
Los Angeles, CA 90034
310-204-6010
FAX: 310-204-0891
e-mail: nhelp@healthlaw.org
www.healthlaw.org

Helps ensure equity and non-discrimination in federal, state, local and private health care programs by assisting local legal service attorneys, paralegal and non-LSC attorneys representing LSC-eligible clients. NHeLP provides advice, co-counsel and other litigation assistance and trainings. *$85.00*

30-32 pages Quarterly

2333 **North Carolina Accessibility Code**

North Carolina Department of Insurance
PO Box 26387
Raleigh, NC 27611
919-733-3901
FAX: 919-733-9171
e-mail: lwright@ncdoi.net

Laurel W Wright, Chief Acessiability Section

Making buildings and facilities accessible to and usable by the physically handicapped. *$20.00*

678 pages Triannually

2334 **Planner's Guide to Barrier Free Meetings**

Barrier Free Environments
PO Box 30634
Raleigh, NC 27622
919-781-0959
FAX: 919-544-4494

An illustrated guide to both temporary and permanent modifications to hotel rooms and meeting spaces to accommodate disabled people. Also includes practical advice on including disabled people in all types of meeting activities. *$22.95*

2335 **Removing the Barriers: Accessibility Guidelines and Specifications**

APPA
1643 Prince Street
Alexandria, VA 22314
703-684-1446
FAX: 703-549-2772
e-mail: webmaster@appa.org
www.appa.org

Wayne Leroy, Executive VP
Steve Glazner, Communications Director

Offers site accessibility, building entrances, doors, interior circulation, restrooms and bathing facilities, drinking fountains and additional resources. *$45.00*

125 pages
ISBN 0-91335 -59-9

2336 **Smart Kitchen/How to Design a Comfortable, Safe & Friendly Workplace**

Ceres Press
PO Box 87
Woodstock, NY 12498
845-679-5573
FAX: 845-679-5573
e-mail: cem620@aol.com
www.healthiestdiet.com

This book provides information about designing kitchens that may be helpful to people with disabilities as well as safe and energy efficient. *$16.95*

132 pages Paperback

General

2337 Accessibility Consultants

12542 Riva Ridge Lane
Houston, TX 77071 **713-728-0924**
FAX: 713-728-4857

Joe Bontke, VP

Focuses on the integration of people with disabilities into everyday life. Areas of concentration include adaptation of public facilities, preconstruction planning, corporate policies and training, job description seminars and workplace modifications.

2338 American Board of Professional Disability Consultants

1350 Beverly Road
Suite 115-327
Mc Lean, VA 22101 **703-952-0024**
FAX: 703-952-0028

Taras Cerkevitch, Operations Director
Mark Long, Development Director

Certifies physicians, psychologists, attorneys, and counselors as specialists in disability and personal injury.

2339 Augmentative Communication Consultants

280-B Moon Clinton Road
Moon Township, PA 15108
800-982-2248
FAX: 412-269-0923
e-mail: acci@usaor.net
www.acciinc.com

Millie Telega Horner CCC SLP, President

ACCI is owned by the mother of a multiple handicapped son who is non-verbal. ACCI specializes in communication devices, educational software, provocational training materials, computer access, environmental controls, switches, resource books and in-service training. Offers a wide range of products, so that ACCI can help one make the right choice. Price Range $24 - $6,500.

2340 Behavior Service Consultants

16 Lakeside Drive
Suite 97
Greenbelt, MD 20770 **301-474-2146**
301-474-1544

Leopold Walder

Offers consultative services regarding behavior modification techniques, neurological testing, therapy for individuals, families and groups.

2341 Community Alternatives Unlimited

8700 W Bryn Mawr Avenue
Suite 500
Chicago, IL 60631 **773-867-4000**
FAX: 773-867-4168

Joanell Voigt, Executive Director
Steve Zider PhD, Associate Director

Provides freestanding case management to individuals with developmental disabilities and mental illness. Provides services throughout the North Side of Chicago, and additionally, the Northern Suburbs of Cook and Lake counties.

2342 National Business & Disability Council

201 IU Willets Road
Albertson, NY 11507 **516-465-1518**
e-mail: info@business-disability.com
www.nbdc.org

Dedicated to increasing the employment of people with disabilities through a coordinated effort of N America's largest employers. Believing that people with disabilities bring value to the workplace. Provides the leadership necessary to infuse effective employment practices for workers with disabilities in our global economy.

2343 Rehab Assist

Case Management Company
6250 N River Road
Suite 3000
Rosemont, IL 60018 **847-292-4444**
FAX: 847-292-7424

Henry P Brennan MS, Director
Thomas J Kleinhenz RN, Director

Medical and catastrophic intervention consultants providing objective independent evaluations and recommendations. Services include assessments, on-site evaluations, life care planning, file and chart review, billing audits, medical and worker's compensation case management, and medical/legal consultations.

2344 RehabTech Associates

3640 Dry Creek Center
Ellicott City, MD 21043
FAX: 410-465-4072

Lynn Bryant, President

A disability consulting firm that conducts research and other projects related to disability. It also publishes and distributes publications on disability.

Aids for the Classroom

2345 AEPS Child Progress Record: For Children Ages Three to Six

Brookes Publishing
PO Box 10624
Baltimore, MD 21285 **410-337-9580**
800-638-3775
FAX: 410-337-8539
e-mail: custserv@brookespublishing.com
www.brookespublishing.com

This chart helps monitor change by visually displaying current abilities, intervention targets, and child progress. In packages of 30. *$21.00*

8 pages Gate-fold
ISBN 1-557662-51-7

2346 AEPS Curriculum for Three to Six Years

Brookes Publishing
PO Box 10624
Baltimore, MD 21285 **410-337-9580**
800-638-3775
FAX: 410-337-8539
e-mail: custserv@brookespublishing.com
www.brookespublishing.com

$49.00

304 pages Spiral-bound
ISBN 1-557661-88-X

2347 AEPS Data Recording Forms: For Children Ages Three to Six

Brookes Publishing
PO Box 10624
Baltimore, MD 21285 **410-337-9580**
800-638-3775
FAX: 410-337-8539
e-mail: custserv@brookespublishing.com
www.brookespublishing.com

These forms can be used by child development professionals on four separate occasions to pinpoint and then monitor a child's strengths and needs in the six key areas of skill development measured by the AEPS Test. Packages of 10. *$24.00*

36 pages Saddle-stiched
ISBN 1-557662-49-5

2348 AEPS Family Interest Survey

Brookes Publishing
PO Box 10624
Baltimore, MD 21285 **410-337-9580**
800-638-3775
FAX: 410-337-8539
e-mail: custserv@brookespublishing.com
www.brookespublishing.com

This is a 30-item checklist that helps families to identify interests and concerns to address in a child's IEP/IFSP. Comes in packages of 30. *$15.00*

8 pages Saddle-stiched
ISBN 1-557660-98-0

2349 AEPS Family Report: For Children Ages Birth to Three

Brookes Publishing
PO Box 10624
Baltimore, MD 21285 **410-337-9580**
800-638-3775
FAX: 410-337-8539
e-mail: custserv@brookespublishing.com
www.brookespublishing.com

This is a 64-item questionnaire that asks parents to rank their child's abilities on specific skills. In packages of 10. *$17.00*

20 pages Saddle-stiched
ISBN 1-557660-99-9

2350 Advanced Language Tool Kit

Educators Publishing Service
31 Smith Place
Cambridge, MA 02138 **617-547-6706**
800-225-5750
FAX: 617-547-0412
www.epsbooks.com

Provides an overview of the structure, organization, and sound units that are needed to develop skills for advanced reading and spelling. The kit contains a teacher's manual and threee packs of cards. *$60.00*

ISBN 0-838885-48-9

2351 Affix & Root Cards

Educators Publishing Service
31 Smith Place
Cambridge, MA 02138 **617-367-2700**
800-225-5750
FAX: 617-547-0412
www.epsbooks.com

These cards are specially designed to reinforce the adolescent's knowledge of reading, spelling and vocabulary and should be used in conjunction with language-training materials found in the Alphabetic Phonics and Gillingham curricula. Color-coded cards present word parts, definitions, and example words. *$29.70*

140 Cards
ISBN 0-838803-24-5

2352 All Kinds of Minds

Educators Publishing Service
31 Smith Place
Cambridge, MA 02138 **617-367-2700**
800-225-5750
FAX: 617-547-0412
www.epsbooks.com

A Young Student's Book about Learning Abilities and Learning Disorders is mainly a fictitious account of five appealing and realistic characters, each of whom has one or more learning disorders. Young readers will easily identify with the experiences of the characters as they appear in a variety of situations, and, at the level, there are suggestions for overcoming the effects of learning disorders. *$24.75*

296 pages
ISBN 0-838820-90-5

2353 American Sign Language Handshape Cards

TJ Publishers
817 Silver Spring Avenue
Suite 206
Silver Spring, MD 20910 **301-585-4440**
800-999-1168
FAX: 301-585-5930
e-mail: TJPubinc@aol.com

Angela K Thames, President
Jerald A Murphy, VP

Durable flashcards illustrate basic handshapes, classifiers and the American manual alphabet. An instructional booklet describes games for differing skill levels to improve vocabulary, increase hand and eye coordination, sign recognition and usage. *$16.95*

ISBN 0-960080-91-5

2354 Asthma Action Cards: Child Care Asthma/Allergy Action Card

Asthma and Allergy Foundation of America
1125 15th Street NW
Suite 502
Washington, DC 20005 **202-466-7643**
FAX: 202-466-8940
e-mail: info@aafa.org
www.aafa.org

Includes necessary information a provider needs to care for a young child who has asthma and allergies. The card includes a medication plan, a list of the child's specific signs and symptoms that indicate the child is having trouble breathing, and steps on how to handle an emergency situation.

2355 Asthma Action Cards: Student Asthma Action Card

Asthma and Allergy Foundation of America
1125 15th Street NW
Suite 502
Washington, DC 20005 **202-466-7643**
FAX: 202-466-8940
e-mail: info@aafa.org
www.aafa.org

Tool for communicating school aged children's and teen's asthma managment plan to school personnel. Includes sections for asthma triggers, daily medications, and emergency directions.

2356 Auditory-Verbal Therapy for Parents and Professionals

Alexander Graham Bell Association
3417 Volta Place NW
Washington, DC 20007 **202-337-5220**
FAX: 202-337-8314
e-mail: info@agbell.org
www.agbell.org

To teach children to listen, process spoken language and talk, auditory-verbal therapy develops language and speech through listening with effective use of hearing aids and partnership of parents, children and professionals. *$39.95*

313 pages Paperback

2357 Barrier Free Education

Center for Assistive Technology & Env Access
490 10th Street NW
Atlanta, GA 30332 **404-894-4960**
FAX: 404-894-9320
www.catea.org

Barbara Christopher, Administrative Coordinator
Elizabeth Bryant, Project Director II

Math and science activities pose unique accommodation challenges for students with disabilities. The Barrier Free Education resource on accessible science experiments was developed for high school chemistry and physics students with physical or visual disabilities under the National Science Foundation's Program for Persons with Disabilities.

2358 Basic Course in American Sign Language Package

TJ Publishers
817 Silver Spring Avenue
Suite 206
Silver Spring, MD 20910 **301-585-4440**
800-999-1168
FAX: 301-585-5930
e-mail: TJPubinc@aol.com

Angela K Thames, President
Jerald A Murphy, VP

Accompanying videotapes and textbooks will include voice translations. Hearing students can analyze sound for initial instruction, or opt to turn off the sound to sharpen visual acuity. Package includes the A Basic Course in American Sign Language text, Student Study Guide, the original four 1-hour videotapes plus the ABCASL Vocabulary Videotape. *$139.95*

280 pages

2359 Beginning Reasoning and Reading

Educators Publishing Service
31 Smith Place
Cambridge, MA 02138 **617-547-6706**
800-225-5750
FAX: 617-547-0412
www.epsbooks.com

This workbook develops basic language and thinkink skills that build the foundation for reading comprehension. Workbook exercises reingorce reading as a critical activity. *$10.45*

ISBN 0-838830-01-3

2360 Board Games for Play and Say

Pro-Ed
8700 Shoal Creek Boulevard
Austin, TX 78757 **512-451-3246**
800-897-3202
FAX: 512-451-8542
e-mail: info@proedinc.com
www.proedinc.com

Designed to make therapy more fun and enhance simple words and the production of speech sounds in isolation, phrases and sentences. *$59.00*

8 Games

2361 Book of Possibilities: Elementary Edition

AbleNet
1081 10th Avenue SE
Minneapolis, MN 55414
800-322-0956
FAX: 612-379-9143
e-mail: customerservice@ablenetinc.com
www.ablenetinc.com

Helen Canfield MA CCC/SLP, Author/Editor
Peggy Locke PhD, Author/Editor

Activity ideas for all elementary age switch users to be included in a variety of math, science, language arts, social studies, spelling and reading activities. A valuable how to resource for every educator that serves students with severe disabilities. *$27.00*

2362 Book of Possibilities: Secondary Edition

AbleNet
1081 10th Avenue SE
Minneapolis, MN 55414
800-322-0956
FAX: 612-379-9143
e-mail: customerservice@ablenetinc.com
www.ablenetinc.com

Helen Canfield MA CCC/SLP, Author/Editor
Peggy Locke PhD, Author/Editor

Suggestions for including secondary age switch users in a variety of school experiences throughout the day. Includes sections on secondary academics, general classroom activities like giving tests or reports and non-curricular activities like school plays and sports events. A valuable how to resource for educators that serve students with severe disabilities. *$27.00*

2363 Buy!

JE Stewart Teaching Tools
PO Box 15308
Seattle, WA 98115 **206-262-9538**
FAX: 206-262-9538

J E Stewart, Owner

Teaches 50 words as they appear in commercial and community situations such as clinic, sale, receipt, price and cleaner. These words are functional at school, on the job and shopping. *$32.50*

116 pages
ISBN 1-877866-05-9

2364 Catalog for Teaching Life Skills to Persons with Development Disability

PCI Educational Publishing
PO Box 34270
San Antonio, TX 78264 **210-377-1999**
800-594-4263
FAX: 888-259-8284
www.pcicatalog.com

Janie Haugen, VP
Jeff McLane, President
Leslie Boulet, Senior Marketing Manager

Over 200 educational products that help individuals learn and maintain the life skills they need to succeed in an inclusive society.

2365 Childs Spelling System: The Rules

Educators Publishing Service
31 Smith Place
Cambridge, MA 02138 **617-367-2700**
800-225-5750
FAX: 617-547-0412
www.epsbooks.com

This book presents reasonable explanations of spelling rules, makes suggestions for more effective teaching and provides lists of examples and exceptions. Basic spelling rules are listed on inside front cover. *$7.15*

32 pages
ISBN 0-838801-12-9

2366 Classroom GOAL: Guide for Optimizing Auditory Learning Skills

Alexander Graham Bell Association
3417 Volta Place NW
Washington, DC 20007 **202-337-5220**
FAX: 202-337-8314
e-mail: info@agbell.org
www.agbell.org

This reader-friendly teacher's guide filled with tips, source materials and sample charts and plans is designed for educators who have yearned for a resource that explains how to incorporate auditory goals into academic learning for students with different degrees of hearing loss. *$34.95*

Paperback

2367 Classroom Notetaker: How to Organize a Program Serving Students with Hearing Impairments

Alexander Graham Bell Association
3417 Volta Place NW
Washington, DC 20007 **202-337-5220**
FAX: 202-337-8314
e-mail: info@agbell.org
www.agbell.org

This detailed manual for instructors, administrators and staff notetakers promotes classroom notetaking within long-term educational programs as absolutely vital for students who are deaf and hard of hearing from elementary school to college. *$24.95*

127 pages Paperback

2368 Community Services for the Blind and Partially Sighted Store: Sight Connection

9709 3rd Avenue NE
Suite 100
Seattle, WA 98115 **206-525-5556**
800-458-4888
FAX: 206-525-0422
e-mail: csbstore@csbps.com
www.sightconnection.com

Over more than 3200 practical products for living with vision loss selected by certified vision rehabilitation specialists from Community Services for the Blind and Partially Sighted. Easy-to-use online store features large pringt, large phontos, secure transactions, and links to other vision-related resources. Store catalog available by mail upon request in large print, Braille, audiotape or PC disk. Phone and mail orders welcome. Store open 9-5, M-F, Pacific Time.

2369 Community Signs

JE Stewart Teaching Tools
PO Box 15308
Seattle, WA 98115 **206-262-9538**
FAX: 206-262-9538

J E Stewart, Owner

Teaches 50 words like go, fire, rest room, men, women, danger and walk needed to successfully navigate our environment. *$ 32.50*

2370 Comprehensive Assessment of Spoken Language (CASL)

AGS
Publishers Building
PO Box 99
Circle Pines, MN 827-1
800-328-2560
FAX: 763-786-9007
www.agsnet.com

Robert Zaske, Market Manager

CASL is an individually and orally administered research-based, theory-drive oral language assessment battery for ages 3 through 21. Fifteen tests measure language processing skills - comprehension, expression, and retrieval - in four language structure categories: Lexical/Semantic, Syntactic, Supralinguistic and Pragmatic. *$299.95*

2371 Creative Arts Therapy and Catalog

MMB Music
3526 Washington Avenue
Saint Louis, MO 63103 **314-531-9635**
800-543-3771
FAX: 314-531-8384
e-mail: info@mmbmusic.com
www.mmbmusic.com

Marcia Lee Goldberg, VP Sales/Marketing

Catalog of books, videos, recordings for the creative arts and wellness (music, art, dance, poetry, drama, therapies, photography).

2372 **Cursive Writing Skills**

Educators Publishing Service
31 Smith Place
Cambridge, MA 02138
617-367-2700
800-225-5750
FAX: 617-547-0412
www.epsbooks.com

These two books, written by Diana King, for grades 7-Adult for right and left-handed students. Books include exercises to establish good posture; pencil grip and paper position for both lower case and upper case letters, students also practice joining letters and copying. *$ 7.15*

ISBN 0-83881 -05-

2373 **Don Johnston**

26799 N Commerce Drive
Volo, IL 60073
847-740-0749
800-999-4660
FAX: 847-740-7326
e-mail: info@donjohnston.com
www.donjohnston.com

A provider of quality products and services that enable people with special needs to discover their potential and experience success. Products are developed for the areas of Physical Access, Augmentative Communication and for those who struggle with reading and writing.

2374 **Dyslexia Training Program**

Educators Publishing Service
31 Smith Place
Cambridge, MA 02138
617-367-2700
800-225-5750
FAX: 617-547-0412
www.epsbooks.com

This program from the Texas Scottish Rite Hospital for grades 2-8 introduces reading and writing through a two-year, cumulative series of daily one-hour videotaped lessons and accompanying student's books and teacher's guides. It is presented in a structured multi-sensory sequence of alphabet, reading, spelling, cursive handwriting, listening, language history and review activities. Students are in a class of nor more than six who work with instructional tapes as teacher's guides are available.

$6.75 - $15

2375 **Exceptional Teaching Aids**

20102 Woodbine Avenue
Castro Valley, CA 94546
510-582-4859
800-549-6999
FAX: 510-582-5911
e-mail: exteaching@aol.com
www.exceptionalteaching.com

Phil Mangold, Owner/Manager
Susan Taylorolo, Order Information
Kelli Cooney, Order Information

Providing educational teaching aids for the blind and visually impaired via catalog. Price range $2-600.

2376 **Explode the Code Books 1-8**

Educators Publishing Service
31 Smith Place
Cambridge, MA 02138
617-367-2700
800-225-5750
FAX: 617-547-0412
www.epsbooks.com

A program of workbooks helps children learn to read by teaching them to use the sounds of letters. This carefully sequenced program provides experience recognizing and combining sounds in order to read words, phrases, sentences and stories, as well as to build vocabulary. A set of fifty-four illustrated cards to practice the sounds taught in books 1-3 is now available. *$6.20*

Grades K-4, 1-3
ISBN 0-83881 -60-

2377 **First Course in Phonic Reading**

Educators Publishing Service
31 Smith Place
Cambridge, MA 02138
617-367-2700
800-225-5750
FAX: 617-547-0412
www.epsbooks.com

This book provides students with a basic foundation in phonics beginning with common consonants and short vowels, syllabication and spelling rules are also taught. There is a special emphasis on auditory and kinesthetic involvement. *$10.65*

Grades 2-3
ISBN 0-838801-24-2

2378 **Food!**

JE Stewart Teaching Tools
PO Box 15308
Seattle, WA 98115
206-262-9538
FAX: 206-262-9538

J E Stewart, Owner

Teaches 50 words like salt, pepper, hamburger, fruit, milk and soup, seen commonly on menus, packages and in directions used at home and at play. *$32.50*

2379 **Fun for Everyone**

AbleNet
1081 10th Avenue SE
Minneapolis, MN 55414
800-322-0956
FAX: 612-379-9143
e-mail: customerservice@ablenetinc.com
www.ablenetinc.com

Today, simple technology allows children and adults with disabilities to participate in leisure activities they were limited or excluded from in the past. *$20.00*

2380 **Fundamentals of Autism**

Slosson Educational Publications
PO Box 280
E Aurora, NY 14052
716-625-0930
888-756-7760
FAX: 800-655-3840
e-mail: slosson@slosson.com
www.slosson.com

Peggy Meyer, Office Personnel
Leslie Foote, Office Personnel

The Fundamentals of Autism handbook provides a quick, user friendly, effective and accurate approach to help in identifying and developing educationally related program objectives for children diagnosed as Autistic. These materials have been designed to be easily and functionally used by teachers, therapists, special education/learning disability resource specialists, psychologists and others who work with children diagnosed as Autistic. *$56.00*

72 pages

2381 GO-MO Articulation Cards

Pro-Ed Publications
8700 Shoal Creek Boulevard
Austin, TX 78757
512-451-3246
800-897-3202
FAX: 512-451-8542
e-mail: info@proedinc.com
www.proedinc.com

The most popular system used for remedying defective speech articulation in children and adults. This popular card set was the first and is still the best therapy tool of its kind, as it continues to produce results and maintains the interest of students of all ages.

2382 Get Ready/Get Set/Go for the Code

Educators Publishing Service
31 Smith Place
Cambridge, MA 02138
617-367-2700
800-225-5750
FAX: 617-547-0412
www.epsbooks.com

Primers for the Explode the Code series teaches consonants through engaging activities which includes: tracking, tracing, matching, copying, and following directions. The Activities progress is difficulty, and the three-book series for grades K-1 is cumulative. A set of picture letter cards are available.

80-96 pages $4.50 - $5.50
ISBN 0-83881 -80-

2383 Gillingham Manaual

Educators Publishing Service
31 Smith Place
Cambridge, MA 02138
617-547-6706
800-225-5750
FAX: 617-547-0412
www.epsbooks.com

Basic hardcover instructional manual for multisensory, phonetic technique of teaching reading to children with specific language disability. A classic. Many associated teaching materials, including drill cards, and stories.

352 pages $17.55 - $69
ISBN 0-83880 -00-

2384 Guide to Teaching Phonics

Educators Publishing Service
31 Smith Place
Cambridge, MA 02138
617-367-2700
800-225-5750
FAX: 617-547-0412
www.epsbooks.com

This flexible teacher's guide presents multisensory procedures developed in association with the late Dr. Samuel Orton. They consist of 100 phonograms for teaching phonetic elements and their sequences in words for reading, writing and spelling. Also contains coordinated Phonics Cards. *$13.50*

96 pages
ISBN 0-838802-41-9

2385 Homemade Battery-Powered Toys

Special Needs Project
324 State Street
Suite H
Santa Barbara, CA 93101
800-333-6867
FAX: 805-962-5087
www.specialneeds.com

Describes how to make simple switches and educational devices for severely handicapped children. *$7.50*

2386 How the Student with Hearing Loss Can Succeed in College, Second Edition

Alexander Graham Bell Association
3417 Volta Place NW
Washington, DC 20007
202-337-5220
FAX: 202-337-8314
e-mail: info@agbell.org
www.agbell.org

This revised book informs student who are deaf and hard of hearing about the mutual and co-equal effort that students and professionals must exert together to achieve success for students to be successful. *$28.95*

278 pages Paperback

2387 If it is to Be, it is Up to Me

AVKO Dyslexia Research Foundation
3084 W Willard Road
Clio, MI 48420
810-686-9283
866-285-6612
FAX: 810-686-1101
e-mail: avkoemail@aol.com
www.avko.org

Don McCabe, Research Director

This book is designed for parents to use. It will prove to the student that he isn't dumb. It builds self-confidence as the student learns he can learn without studying. *$9.95*

112 pages
ISBN 1-56400 -42-1

2388 Implementing Cognitive Strategy Instruction Across the School

Brookline Books
PO Box 97
Newton Upper Falls, MA 02464
617-558-8010
800-666-2665
FAX: 617-558-8011
e-mail: milt@brooklinebooks.com
www.brooklinebooks.com

Describes basic classroom based programs planned and executed by teachers to focus and guide students with serious reading problems to be goal oriented, strategic and self-assessing. *$24.95*

ISBN 0-914797-75-1

2389 Inclusive Play People

Educational Equity Concepts
114 E 32nd Street
New York, NY 10016
212-686-2531
FAX: 212-725-0947
TTY:212-725-1803
e-mail: information@edequity.org
www.edequity.org

Six sturdy multiracial wooden figures that provide a unique variety of nonstereotyped work and family roles and are inclusive of disabled and nondisabled people of various ages. For block building and dramatic play. *$25.00*

2390 **Instruction of Persons with Severe Handicaps**

McGraw-Hill, School Publishing
220 E Danieldale Road
DeSoto, TX 75115
972-224-1111
800-442-9685
FAX: 972-228-1982
mhschool.com

A complete introduction to the status of education as it pertains to people with severe handicaps.

2391 **Integrating Transition Planning Into the IEP Process**

Council for Exceptional Children
1110 N Glebe Road
Suite 300
Arlington, VA 22201
703-620-3660
FAX: 703-264-9494
www.cec.sped.org

Janice Burdick, President

Helps students with disabilities make a smooth transition from school to adult life. *$15.70*

78 pages

2392 **International Journal of Arts Medicine**

MMB Music
3526 Washington Avenue
Saint Louis, MO 63103
314-531-9635
800-543-3771
FAX: 314-531-8384
e-mail: info@mmbmusic.com
www.mmbmusic.com

Marcia Lee Goldberg, VP Sales/Marketing

Exploration of the creative arts and healing. Presents peer-reviewed articles clearly written by educators in the creative arts, as well as internationally prominent physicians, therapists and health care professionals.

2393 **Keeping Ahead in School**

Educators Publishing Service
31 Smith Place
Cambridge, MA 02138
617-367-2700
800-225-5750
FAX: 617-547-0412
www.epsbooks.com

This book helps students not only understand their own strengths and weaknesses but also more fully appreciate their individuality. He suggests specific ways to approach work, bypass or overcome learning disorders, and manage other struggles that may beset students in school. *$24.75*

320 pages Paperback
ISBN 0-838820-69-7

2394 **KeyMath Teach and Practice**

AGS
Publishers Building
PO Box 99
Circle Pines, MN 55014
800-328-2560
FAX: 763-786-9007
www.agsnet.com

Robert Zaske, Market Manager

This set of materials provides all the tools needed to assess students' math skills...and the strategies to deal with problem areas. Three sets are available: Basic Concepts Package; Operations Package; and Applications Package. $219.95 each or $599.95 for whole set.

2395 **Kim Marshall Series in English**

Educators Publishing Service
31 Smith Place
Cambridge, MA 02138
617-367-2700
800-225-5750
FAX: 617-547-0412
www.epsbooks.com

These two books for grades 4-8 contain a total of 36 cumulative units in grammar, writing skills and word analysis. English-Part A reviews writing skills and usage, while English-Part B reviews word analysis and parts of speech. There is a teacher's manual designed to accompany each book.

104 pages $8 - $8.95

2396 **Kim Marshall Series in Math**

Educators Publishing Service
31 Smith Place
Cambridge, MA 02138
617-367-2700
800-225-5750
FAX: 617-547-0412
www.epsbooks.com

These two books for grades 4-8 contain 35 units that cover basic computation skills, Roman numerals, English and metric measurements, graphing, fractions and basic geometry. There is a teacher's manual designed to accompany each book.

104 pages $10.45 - $11.60

2397 **Kim Marshall Series in Reading**

Educators Publishing Service
31 Smith Place
Cambridge, MA 02138
617-547-6706
800-225-5750
FAX: 617-547-0412
www.epsbooks.com

These two books for grades 4-6 contain 186 interesting stories with comprehension questions that encourage careful reading and stimulate thinking. Because of the wide appeal of the stories, these books can be used to meet the needs of a variety of students. *$8.00*

104 pages Grades 4-6

2398 **Kim Marshall Series in Vocabulary**

Educators Publishing Service
31 Smith Place
Cambridge, MA 02138
617-367-2700
800-225-5750
FAX: 617-547-0412
www.epsbooks.com

This approachable vocabulary program for grades 4-8 consists of 900 words chosen to be interesting and useful and to broaden vocabulary and improve spelling. The two books in the series each contain 18 units, and every one of these units introduces 25 words followed by 5 pages of exercises and a weekly test. A teacher's manual is available for each book. *$9.75*

128 pages

2399 **Lakeshore Learning Materials**

2695 E Dominguez Street
Carson, CA 90810
310-537-8600
800-421-5354
FAX: 310-537-5403
e-mail: lakeshore@lakeshorelearning.com
www.lakeshorelearning.com

Offers books, resources, testing materials, assessment information and special education materials for the professional in the field of special education.

190 pages

2400 Language Parts Catalog

Educators Publishing Service
31 Smith Place
Cambridge, MA 02138
617-547-6706
800-225-5750
FAX: 617-547-0412
www.epsbooks.com

Informatively and numorously explains the various aspects of language and how they operate, asking students to imagine that they are reading a catalog ffeaturing defferent parts to order that can help them improve their language abilities. *$9.00*

ISBN 0-838819-80-X

2401 Language Tool Kit

Educators Publishing Service
31 Smith Place
Cambridge, MA 02138
617-367-2700
800-225-5750
FAX: 617-547-0412
www.epsbooks.com

This kit teaches reading and spelling to students in grades 1-3 with specific language disability. It contains 163-426 cards and a comprehensive 32-page teacher's manual. Also available in Spanish. *$ 30.00*

32 pages English Edition
ISBN 0-838885-20-3

2402 Learning American Sign Language

Harris Communications
15155 Technology Drive
Eden Prairie, MN 55344
952-906-1180
800-825-6758
FAX: 952-906-1099
e-mail: mail@harriscomm.com
www.harriscomm.com

Bill Williams, National Sales Manager

Offers ASL instruction book and videotape for teachers and instructors of the hearing impaired student. *$78.95*

350 pages Video & Book

2403 Learning to Listen

Educators Publishing Service
31 Smith Place
Cambridge, MA 02138
617-367-2700
800-225-5750
FAX: 617-547-0412
www.epsbooks.com

A program to improve classroom listening skills in a variety of situations. Presents students, in grades 7-9 with instruction and 33 exercises on eight basic listening skills. After reading about a particular skill, students practice it by listening to a selection and then answering questions about the selection in writing. A teachers manual is available to accompany the student book. *$6.20*

48 pages
ISBN 0-838820-61-1

2404 Learning to Sign in My Neighborhood

TJ Publishers
817 Silver Spring Avenue
Suite 206
Silver Spring, MD 20910
301-585-4440
800-999-1168
FAX: 301-585-5930
e-mail: TJPubinc@aol.com

Angela K Thames, President
Jerald A Murphy, VP

Beautifully illustrated coloring book lets children learn signs from kids just like themselves! Recommended for ages 4 and up, let children have fun while they learn signs for words typically used in day-to-day activities. *$3.50*

32 pages Softcover
ISBN 0-93266 -36-1

2405 Learning to Use Cursive Handwriting

Educators Publishing Service
31 Smith Place
Cambridge, MA 02138
617-367-2700
800-225-5750
FAX: 617-547-0412
www.epsbooks.com

This multisensory program with instructions for introducing, teaching, practicing and reviewing lower- and upper-case cursive letters; Masters, with letter forms and lined and patterned writing paper; and Wall Cards, for lower- and upper-case letters. *$ 10.60*

96 pages Manual
ISBN 0-838802-53-2

2406 Learning to Use Manuscript Handwriting

Educators Publishing Service
31 Smith Place
Cambridge, MA 02138
617-367-2700
800-225-5750
FAX: 617-547-0412
www.epsbooks.com

This multisensory program contains a manual with instructions for introducing teaching, practicing and reviewing lower- and upper-case manuscript letters; masters with letter forms and lined and patterned writing paper; and wall cards for lower- and upper-case letters. *$10.30*

76 pages Paperback
ISBN 0-838802-50-8

2407 Let's Read: A Linguistic Reading Program

Educators Publishing Service
31 Smith Place
Cambridge, MA 02138
617-367-2700
800-225-5750
FAX: 617-547-0412
www.epsbooks.com

This linguistic approach to teaching reading emphasizes the basic relationship of spelling to sound, presenting like concepts together, providing reading materials for practice, and building on previously mastered skills for grades 1-3. Word lists and Teacher's manuals are available for Let's Read books 1-4, and Let's Look workbooks accompany the texts.

$10.35 - $19.15

2408 Literacy Program

Educators Publishing Service
31 Smith Place
Cambridge, MA 02138
617-367-2700
800-225-5750
FAX: 617-547-0412
www.epsbooks.com

This one year course, developed by the Scottish Rite Hospital, consists of 160 one hour videotaped lessons accompanied by student workbooks, designed for high schoolers and adults who read below a sixth grade level. This program uses multisensory applications to teach alphabet, reading, cursive writing, spelling, math and listening comprehension with frequent new activities. This is an ideal series for a community adult reading program. Grades 1-4.

$2.25 -$18

2409 Literature Based Reading

Oryx Press
4041 N Central Avenue
Suite 700
Phoenix, AZ 85012
602-265-2651
800-279-6799
FAX: 800-279-4663

Series offering children's books and activities to enrich the K-5 curriculum.

2410 Living an Idea: Empowerment and the Evolution of an Alternative School

Brookline Books
PO Box 1046
Cambridge, MA 02238
617-868-0360
800-666-2665
FAX: 617-868-1772
e-mail: brooklinebks@delphi.com
www.brooklinebooks.com

Edison Trickett

This book is about the creation and 14 year evolution of a public alternative inner-city high school. The school lived an idea - empowerment. Students were encouraged to participate in shaping many aspects of their education, teachers were responsible for running the school, and parents invited to help govern. *$27.95*

ISBN 0-91479 -68-9

2411 Low Tech Assistive Devices: A Handbook for the School Setting

Therapro
225 Arlington Street
Framingham, MA 01702
508-872-9494
800-257-5376
FAX: 508-875-2062
e-mail: info@theraproducts.com
www.theraproducts.com

A how-to book with step by step directions and detailed illustrations for fabrication of frequently requested low-tech assistive devices. *$42.50*

312 pages Paperback

2412 MTA Readers

Educators Publishing Service
31 Smith Place
Cambridge, MA 02138
617-367-2700
800-225-5750
FAX: 617-547-0412
www.epsbooks.com

Illustrated readers for grades 1-3 that accompany the MTA Reading and Spelling Program (Multisensory Teaching Approach). Phonetic elements in a structured, but entertaining context.

48+ pages $4.65 - $11.65

ISBN 0-83882 -33-3

2413 Making School Inclusion Work: A Guide to Everyday Practice

Brookline Books
PO Box 97
Newton Upper Falls, MA 02464
617-558-8010
800-666-2665
FAX: 617-558-8011
e-mail: milt@brooklinebooks.com
www.brooklinebooks.com

This book tells the reader how to conduct a truly inclusive program, regardless of ethnic or racial background, economic level and physical or cognitive ability. *$24.95*

254 pages

ISBN 0-914791-96-4

2414 Making the Writing Process Work: Strategie s for Composition and Self-Regulation

Brookline Books
PO Box 1047
Cambridge, MA 02238
617-495-3682
800-666-2665
FAX: 617-868-0360
e-mail: brooklinebks@delphi.com
www.brooklinebooks.com

This book is geared toward students who have difficulty organizing their thoughts and developing their writing. The specific stategies teach students how to approach, organize, and produce a final written product.. *$24.95*

240 pages Paperback

ISBN 1-571290-10-9

2415 Manual Alphabet Poster

TJ Publishers
817 Silver Spring Avenue
Suite 206
Silver Spring, MD 20910
301-585-4440
800-999-1168
FAX: 301-585-5930
e-mail: TJPubinc@aol.com

Angela K Thames, President
Jerald A Murphy, VP

Poster presents the manual alphabet. *$4.50*

2416 Many Faces of Dyslexia

International Dyslexia Association
Chester Building
Suite 382
Baltimore, MD 21286
800-ABC-D123
FAX: 410-296-0232
www.interdys.org

Gives information on the teaching and rehabilitation techniques for people with dyslexia. *$16.50*

Paperback

2417 Match-Sort-Assemble Job Cards

Exceptional Education
PO Box 15308
Seattle, WA 98115
206-542-3971
FAX: 475-486-4510

JE Stewart, Owner

Teaches workers to use a series of symbolic cues to control their own production cycles. *$565.00*

Class Set

2418 Match-Sort-Assemble Pictures

Exceptional Education
PO Box 15308
Seattle, WA 98115
206-542-3971
FAX: 475-486-4510

JE Stewart, Owner

People with profound, severe and moderate mental retardation have immediate access with MSA Pictures. Students work with pictures (and if necessary a template) to match, sort, assemble and disassemble parts that vary in shape, length and diameter. *$426.00*

Class Set

2419 Match-Sort-Assemble SCHEMATICS

Exceptional Education
PO Box 15308
Seattle, WA 98115
206-542-3971
FAX: 475-486-4510

JE Stewart, Owner

Students with moderate and mild mental retardation and those who have completed MSA Pictures are ready for MSA Schematics. It increases abstraction and displacement of instruction from the work clearly and simply. *$495.00*

Class Set

2420 Match-Sort-Assemble TOOLS

Exceptional Education
PO Box 15308
Seattle, WA 98115 **206-542-3971**
FAX: 475-486-4510

JE Stewart, Owner

Students and clients learn to use the tools required for many jobs in light industry. Mastery of the production cycle with independence, endurance and the ability to learn new tasks through pictures and schematics and basic hand functions will help clients acquire and maintain employment in a competitive field. *$595.00*

Class Set

2421 Meeting-in-a-Box

Asthma and Allergy Foundation of America
1125 15th Street NW
Suite 502
Washington, DC 20005 **202-466-7643**
FAX: 202-466-8940
e-mail: info@aafa.org
www.aafa.org

A series of self contained, comprehensive kits that contain all the necessary components for a successful asthma presentation.

2422 More Food!

JE Stewart Teaching Tools
PO Box 15308
Seattle, WA 98115 **206-262-9538**
FAX: 206-262-9538

J E Stewart, Owner

Teaches 50 more words found in restaurants, grocery stores, cookbooks such as pizza, carrot, tacos, oysters and pineapple. These words are functional at home, going shopping and during leisure. *$32.50*

2423 More Work!

JE Stewart Teaching Tools
PO Box 15308
Seattle, WA 98115 **206-262-9538**
FAX: 206-262-9538

J E Stewart, Owner

Teaches 50 words as they appear on parts, tools, job instructions, signs and labels, such as fill, grasp, release, lock, search, position and select. These words are functional in school and on-the-job. *$32.50*

2424 Multisensory Teaching Approach

Educators Publishing Service
31 Smith Place
Cambridge, MA 02138 **617-367-2700**
800-225-5750
FAX: 617-547-0412
www.epsbooks.com

Comprehensive multisensory program in reading, writing, spelling, alphabet and dictionary skills for remedial and regular instruction. Based on Orton-Gillingham and Alphabetic Phonics. A complete program organized in kits, with additional classroom materials, supplementary materials, and Handwriting Programs.

$110 - $140
ISBN 0-83888 -10-9

2425 Peabody Articulation Decks

AGS
Publishers Building
PO Box 99
Circle Pines, MN 55014
800-328-2560
FAX: 763-786-9007
www.agsnet.com

Robert Zaske, Market Manager

Complete kit of playing-card sized PAD decks let students focus on the 18 most commonly misarticulated English consonants and blends. *$115.95*

ISBN 0-88671 -75-4

2426 Phonemic Awareness in Young Children: A Classroom Curriculum

Brookes Publishing
PO Box 10624
Baltimore, MD 21285 **410-337-9580**
800-638-3775
FAX: 410-337-8539
e-mail: custserv@brookespublishing.com
www.brookespublishing.com

This is a supplemental, whole-class curriculum for improving pre-literacy listening skills. It contains activities that are fun, easy to use, and proven to work in any kindergarten classroom - general, bilingual, inclusive, or special education. This program takes only 15-20 minutes a day. *$24.95*

208 pages Spiral-bound 1997
ISBN 1-557663-21-1

2427 Phonics for Thought

Educators Publishing Service
31 Smith Place
Cambridge, MA 02138 **617-367-2700**
800-225-5750
FAX: 617-547-0412
www.epsbooks.com

This multisensory approach to phonics simultaneously teaches reading, writing and spelling to grades K-2. Two illustrated workbooks are accompanied by instructional manuals that provide procedures for each lesson; the pronunciation and formation of the letters, word lists and sentences for dictation, and games and activities for further enrichment. *$8.00*

Paperback

2428 Phonological Awareness Training for Reading

Pro-Ed Publications
8700 Shoal Creek Boulevard
Austin, TX 78757 **512-451-3246**
800-897-3202
FAX: 512-451-8542
e-mail: info@proedinc.com
www.proedinc.com

Designed to increase the level of phonological awareness in young children. Can be taught individually or in small groups and takes about 12 to 14 weeks to complete if children are taught in short sessions three or four times a week. *$129.00*

2429 Play and Say Cards

Pro-Ed
8700 Shoal Creek Boulevard
Austin, TX 78757 **512-451-3246**
800-897-3202
FAX: 512-451-8542
e-mail: info@proedinc.com
www.proedinc.com

16 decks of bright, full-color playing cards, each of which carriers a frequently misarticulated speech sound. *$89.00*

2430 Play!

JE Stewart Teaching Tools
PO Box 15308
Seattle, WA 98115 **206-262-9538**
FAX: 206-262-9538

J E Stewart, Owner

Teaches 50 more words as they appear at recreation sites, on signs and labels and in newspapers and magazines, such as movie, visitor, ticket, gallery and zoo. These words are functional in school and at leisure. *$32.50*

2431 Power Breathing Program

Asthma and Allergy Foundation of America
1125 15th Street NW
Suite 502
Washington, DC 20005 **202-466-7643**
FAX: 202-466-8940
e-mail: info@aafa.org
www.aafa.org

Devoloped the only asthma education program specifically designed for and pre-tested with teens. Teens with asthma have special challenges. This interactive program covers everything from the basics of asthma to dealing with their asthma in social situations, in college, and on the job. Includes everything you need to present this three-four session program. *$295.00*

2432 Primary Phonics

Educators Publishing Service
31 Smith Place
Cambridge, MA 02138 **617-367-2700**
800-225-5750
FAX: 617-547-0412
www.epsbooks.com

A program of storybooks and coordinated workbooks that teach reading for grades K-2. A structured phonetic approach. Contains 8 student workbooks, with 8 sets of 10 coordinated storybooks; consonant workbooks; initial consonant blend workbooks; picture dictionary, and coloring book. *$3.65*

$3.65 - $26.35
ISSN 0838-83 0

2433 Programmed Phonics Books 1-2 & Cassettes

Educators Publishing Service
31 Smith Place
Cambridge, MA 02138 **617-367-2700**
800-225-5750
FAX: 617-547-0412
www.epsbooks.com

This self-instructing program is for children who are having difficulty with the word-recognition phase of reading vocabulary that exceeds their reading vocabulary. The books review consonants and all consonant blends. A teacher's guide and Script includes dictation, which is also available on cassettes. *$7.70*

88 pages $7.50 - $45
ISSN 0838-83 0

2434 Programming Concepts

PO Box 12428
San Antonio, TX 78212
800-594-4263
FAX: 210-824-8055

2435 Reading for Content

Educators Publishing Service
31 Smith Place
Cambridge, MA 02138 **617-367-2700**
800-225-5750
FAX: 617-547-0412
www.epsbooks.com

This four book series for grades 3-6 has been completely revised and updated so that the reading passages are more current and interesting. Each book contains 43 one-page reading questions. A detachable answer sheet and progress graph are involved in each book.

96 pages $7.75 each

2436 Reading from Scratch

Educators Publishing Service
31 Smith Place
Cambridge, MA 02138 **617-367-2700**
800-225-5750
FAX: 617-547-0412
www.epsbooks.com

Contains multisensory reading and spelling material and oral and written lessons and exercises in syntax, grammar, and precomposition topics. Complete set

$6.25 - $49.30
ISBN 0-83888 -75-5

2437 Reasoning and Reading Levels I and II

Educators Publishing Service
31 Smith Place
Cambridge, MA 02138 **617-547-6706**
800-225-5750
FAX: 617-547-5750
www.epsbooks.com

Three four-unit workbooks are based on the belief that reasoning, language, and reading comprehension go hand in hand. The four-units are word meaning, sentence menaing, paragraph meaning and reasoning skills. Completely revised.

$10.45 each

2438 Recipe for Reading

Educators Publishing Service
31 Smith Place
Cambridge, MA 02138 **617-367-2700**
800-225-5750
FAX: 617-547-0412
www.epsbooks.com

A basic reading manual with 21 storybooks and 7 workbooks for grades K-3. For remedial work. Multisensory, phonetically structured. program also includes sequence chart, a record progress, and writing paper of assorted sizes.

$4.50 - $56.25
ISSN 0838-84 1

2439 Resourcing: Handbook for Special Education Resource Teachers

Council for Exceptional Children
1110 N Glebe Road
Suite 300
Arlington, VA 22201 **703-620-3660**
FAX: 703-264-9494
www.cec.sped.org

Janice Burdick, President

Everything you need to know to be a resource for other teachers and support personnel who work with special education students. *$12.00*

64 pages

2440 Rewarding Speech

Speech Bin
1965 25th Avenue
Vero Beach, FL 32960
772-770-0007
800-477-3324
FAX: 772-770-0006
www.speechbin.com

Jan J Binney, Senior Editor

Reproducible reward certificates for children. *$12.95*

32 pages

2441 Rule-ette

Educators Publishing Service
31 Smith Place
Cambridge, MA 02138
617-367-2700
800-225-5750
FAX: 617-547-0412
www.epsbooks.com

A spelling card game that teaches basic spelling rules. The game was developed for grades 3-Adult. *$14.65*

Ages 3-Adult
ISBN 0-838806-72-

2442 SAYdee Posters

Speech Bin
1965 25th Avenue
Vero Beach, FL 32960
772-770-0007
800-477-3324
FAX: 772-770-0006
www.speechbin.com

Colorful speech and language posters. *$20.00*

24 pages
ISBN 0-93785 -47-5

2443 Second Course in Phonic Reading

Educators Publishing Service
31 Smith Place
Cambridge, MA 02138
617-367-2700
800-225-5750
FAX: 617-547-0412
www.epsbooks.com

Two structured phonetic workbooks to teach reading for grades 2-3 and 4-5. Book 1 focuses on sounds of the letters, phonogram combinations, word families, and spelling rules. Book 2 develops comprehension and vocabulary skills. *$10.65*

Per Book
ISSN 0838-81 6

2444 Sequential Spelling I-VII

AVKO Educational Research Foundation
3084 W Willard Road
Clio, MI 48420
810-686-9283
FAX: 810-686-1101

Don McCabe, Research Director

Spelling books for individuals to classrooms. Builds from easier words of a word family to important power words that build self-confidence. Each of the seven levels contains 180 spelling lessons that teach phonics through the backdoor of spelling. Students learn the patterns without having to learn rules or studying. Teachers have no papers to correct.

72 pages $8.95 each
ISBN 1-56400 -11-6

2445 Signing Naturally Curriculum

Harris Communications
15155 Technology Drive
Eden Prairie, MN 55344
952-906-1180
800-825-6758
FAX: 952-906-1099
e-mail: mail@harriscomm.com
www.harriscomm.com

Bill Williams, National Sales Manager

A series based on the functional approach that is the most popular and widely used sign language curriculum designed for teaching American Sign Language. Book and videotape set for level 1 & 2. Teacher's curriculum is also available.

2446 Small Wonder

AGS
Publishers Building
PO Box 99
Circle Pines, MN 55014
800-328-2560
FAX: 763-786-9007
www.agsnet.com

Robert Zaske, Market Manager

This infant through toddler program offers a delightful array of activities to teach babies about themselves, others, their surroundings and the world outside. Level One - zero to 18 months; Level Two 18-36 months. Discount price of $389.95 when both levels ordered. *$229.95*

ISBN 0-91347 -62-5

2447 Solving Language Difficulties: Remedial Routines

Educators Publishing Service
31 Smith Place
Cambridge, MA 02138
617-367-2700
800-225-5750
FAX: 617-547-0412
www.epsbooks.com

A basic workbook for children in grades 4-6 who have a specific language disability. It can be used in any corrective reading program. It deals extensively with syllables, syllable division, prefixes, suffixes, accent and other important topics. *$9.75*

176 pages
ISBN 0-838803-26-1

2448 Sound Workbook

Educators Publishing Service
31 Smith Place
Cambridge, MA 02138
617-367-2700
800-225-5750
FAX: 617-547-0412
www.epsbooks.com

This workbook for grades 1-2 reinforces the teaching of specific vowel combinations. *$5.50*

44 pages
ISBN 0-838817-08-4

2449 Sound-Off 1-5

Educators Publishing Service
31 Smith Place
Cambridge, MA 02138
617-367-2700
800-225-5750
FAX: 617-547-0412
www.epsbooks.com

These five workbooks for grades K-2 cover the introduction of consonants and final consonant blends and consonant diagraphs, vowel-consonant-e combinations, and vowel + r combinations. There is a teacher's guide for each book. *$5.50*

32-48 pages Per Book

ISBN 0-83885 -34-

2450 Speech-Language Delights

Speech Bin
1965 25th Avenue
Vero Beach, FL 32960
772-770-0007
800-477-3324
FAX: 772-770-0006
www.speechbin.com

Activities, worksheets and games to encourage practice of speech and language skills. *$25.00*

128 pages

ISBN 0-93785 -42-4

2451 Spell of Words

Educators Publishing Service
31 Smith Place
Cambridge, MA 02138
617-367-2700
800-225-5750
FAX: 617-547-0412
www.epsbooks.com

This book can be used with any student, from grade 7-Adult, who needs help in spelling. It covers syllabication, word building with prefixes, word patterns, phonograms, suffixes, plurals and possessives. Chapters contain explanations of spelling rules, exercises and suggestions for short compositions. *$9.25*

128 pages Grades 7-Adult

ISBN 0-838801-55-2

2452 Spellbinding 2

Educators Publishing Service
31 Smith Place
Cambridge, MA 02138
617-547-6706
800-225-5750
FAX: 617-547-0412
www.epsbooks.com

Spellbinding 2 adds practice exercises with more complicated spelling problems and introduces new areas of study. The manuals give answers to exercises and include a large number of new dictations. *$11.55*

96+ pages Each

ISBN 0-838814-75-1

2453 Spellbound

Educators Publishing Service
31 Smith Place
Cambridge, MA 02138
617-367-2700
800-225-5750
FAX: 617-547-0412
www.epsbooks.com

This workbook begins with teaching simple, consistent rules and then moves on to those that are more difficult. By an inductive process, students use their own observations to confirm the spelling rules they learn. Each portion of the text is followed by exercises for drill and kinesthetic reinforcement. *$8.65*

144 pages Grades 7-Adult

ISBN 0-838801-65-X

2454 Spelling Dictionary

Educators Publishing Service
31 Smith Place
Cambridge, MA 02138
617-367-2700
800-225-5750
FAX: 617-547-0412
www.epsbooks.com

This handy reference is a dictionary/thesaurus of words most frequently used by student writers in the elementary grades. Words are listed without definitions, and synonyms are offered for commonly used words like said, big, good, etc. Children can add their own words at the bottom of each page. *$4.50*

52 pages

ISBN 0-838820-56-5

2455 Spelling Workbooks Emphasizing Rules and Generalization for Corrective Drill

Educators Publishing Service
31 Smith Place
Cambridge, MA 02138
617-367-2700
800-225-5750
FAX: 617-547-0412
www.epsbooks.com

Includes exercises for children in grades 7-12 who have reading difficulties and closely associated spelling weaknesses. The material is divided into phonetic drills, spelling rules and generalizations, syllable concepts, and punctuation symbols. There are frequent review exercises. Similar programs are available for grades 4-6 ($11.70). *$12.25*

144 pages Grades 7-12

ISBN 0-838800-90-4

2456 Starting Over

Educators Publishing Service
31 Smith Place
Cambridge, MA 02138
614-547-6706
800-225-5750
FAX: 617-547-0412
www.epsbooks.com

This comprehensive program is for a student who is ready to try to learn to read again, or for those who are learning English as a second language. Employs multisensory phonics, whole words, and language experience techniques to teach the building of words, vocabulary, and sentences. *$24.00*

ISBN 0-838881-65-5

2457 Structure of Words

Educators Publishing Service
31 Smith Place
Cambridge, MA 02138
617-367-2700
800-225-5750
FAX: 617-547-0412
www.epsbooks.com

Designed to help students in grades 7-12 learn to spell by using logic as well as memorization and drill, and to help them pronounce and arrive at the meanings of unfamiliar words. The consistent theme throughout is that of spelling, gradually shifting into the analysis of word structure and the development of a rich vocabulary. *$21.15*

96 pages Grades 7-12

ISBN 0-838801-35-8

2458 Studio 49 Catalog

MMB Music
3526 Washington Avenue
Saint Louis, MO 63103
314-531-9635
800-543-3771
FAX: 314-531-8384
e-mail: info@mmbmusic.com
www.mmbmusic.com

Marcia Lee Goldberg, VP Sales/Marketing

Percussion instruments for school, therapy, church and family.

2459 **Study Power: Study Skills to Improve Your Learning and Your Grades**

Brookline Books
PO Box 97
Newton Upper Falls, MA 02464 **617-558-8010**
800-666-2665
FAX: 617-558-8011
e-mail: milt@brooklinebooks.com
www.brooklinebooks.com

The techniques in the easy-to-use, self-teaching manual have yielded remarkable success for students from elementary to medical school, at all levels of intelligence and achievement. Key skills covered include: listening, note taking, concentration, summarizing, reading comprehension, memorization, test taking, preparing papers and reports, time management and more. These abilities are vital to success throughout every stage of learning; the benefits will last a lifetime. *$15.95*

ISBN 1-571290-46-X

2460 **Syracuse Community-Referenced Curriculum Guide for Students with Disabilties**

Brookes Publishing
PO Box 10624
Baltimore, MD 21285 **410-337-9580**
800-638-3775
FAX: 410-337-8539
e-mail: custserv@brookespublishing.com
www.brookespublishing.com

Serving learners from kindergarten through age 21, this field-tested curriculum is a for professionals and parents devoted to directly preparing a student to function in the world. it examines the role of community living domains, functional academics, and embedded skills and includes practical implementation strategies and information for preparing students whose learning needs go beyond the scope of traditional academic programs. *$54.95*

416 pages Spiral-bound
ISBN 1-557660-27-1

2461 **Teaching Individuals with Physical and Multiple Disabilities**

McGraw-Hill, School Publishing
220 E Danieldale Road
DeSoto, TX 75115 **972-224-1111**
800-442-9685
FAX: 972-228-1982
mhschool.com

Focuses on the functional needs of the handicapped and the teaching skills of background teachers that they need to help them reach the highest possible level of self-sufficiency.

410 pages

2462 **Teaching Students Ways to Remember**

Brookline Books
PO Box 97
Newton Upper Falls, MA 02464 **617-558-8010**
800-666-2665
FAX: 617-558-8011
e-mail: milt@brooklinebooks.com
www.brooklinebooks.com

Teaches techniques for improving or strengthening memory. *$21.95*

ISBN 0-914797-67-0

2463 **Teaching Test-Taking Skills: Helping Students Show What They Know**

Brookline Books
PO Box 97
Newton Upper Falls, MA 02464 **617-558-8010**
800-666-2665
FAX: 617-558-8011
e-mail: milt@brooklinebooks.com
www.brooklinebooks.com

Test-taking skills that, when used effectively, contribute to test-wise performance and help students work productively with test materials. *$21.95*

ISBN 0-914797-76-X

2464 **Tools for Transition**

AGS
Publishers Building
PO Box 99
Circle Pines, MN 55014
800-328-2560
FAX: 763-786-9007
www.agsnet.com

Robert Zaske, Market Manager

This program prepares students with learning disabilities for postsecondary education. *$129.95*

2465 **VAK Tasks Workbook: Visual, Auditory and Kinesthetic**

Educational Tutorial Consortium
4400 S 44th Street
Lincoln, NE 68516 **402-489-8133**
FAX: 402-489-8160
e-mail: etc@altel.net
www.etc-ne.com

A workbook emphasizing the multisensory approach to teaching vocabulary and spelling. It is intended for middle-grade and older students working with prefixes, roots, suffixes, homonyms, and the spelling of easily confused endings. Includes spelling posters. *$7.00*

96 pages Paperback

2466 **Volunteer Transcribing Services**

205 E 3rd Avenue
Suite 200
San Mateo, CA 94401 **650-344-8664**
FAX: 650-632-3510

Alanah Hoffman, Coordinator

VTS is a non-profit California corporation that produces large print school books for visually impaired students in grades K-12.

2467 **Word Attack Manual**

Educators Publishing Service
31 Smith Place
Cambridge, MA 02138 **617-547-6706**
800-225-5750
FAX: 617-547-0412
www.epsbooks.com

This manual and test booklet are designed to develop word recognition and spelling skills for students in grades 6-10. Contents include lessons on syllables, syllabication and accent, consonants and consonant blends, diagraphs, diphthongs, prefixes, suffixes, and compound words, and using the dictionary. *$21.15*

176 pages Grades 6-10
ISBN 0-838881-00-5

2468 **Word Demons**

Educators Publishing Service
31 Smith Place
Cambridge, MA 02138
617-367-2700
800-225-5750
FAX: 617-547-0412
www.epsbooks.com

This spelling game helps students master the 86 non-phonetic words that are demons for the child in grades 2-4 with a language disability. *$14.40*

Grades 2-4
ISBN 0-838803-28-8

2469 **Word Elements: How They Work Together**

Educators Publishing Service
31 Smith Place
Cambridge, MA 02138
617-367-2700
800-225-5750
FAX: 617-547-0412
www.epsbooks.com

This vocabulary workbook teaches common word elements - prefixes, suffixes, and roots and their meanings for grades 6-8. *$ 10.65*

112 pages Grades 6-8
ISBN 0-838815-50-2

2470 **Word Mastery**

Educators Publishing Service
31 Smith Place
Cambridge, MA 02138
617-367-2700
800-225-5750
FAX: 617-547-0412
www.epsbooks.com

This phonics classic introduces over 3,500 words and supplements any reading program with its straightforward phonics instruction. It teaches students in grades 1-3 the letters of the alphabet with key words, and follows with vowels, consonants, vowel combinations, consonant diagraphs and blends, and phonetic rules. *$8.95*

124 pages Grades 1-3
ISBN 0-838820-00-X

2471 **Wordly Wise A,B,C**

Educators Publishing Service
31 Smith Place
Cambridge, MA 02138
617-367-2700
800-225-5750
FAX: 617-547-0412
www.epsbooks.com

This series of three vocabulary books for grades 2-4 presents 8-12 words in each lesson with brief definitions, illustrations and sentences using each word in context. Exercises reinforce learning by teaching students to use words precisely in a variety of situations. Keys and tests are available for each book.

64 pages $5.50 each
ISSN 0838-84 8

2472 **Work!**

JE Stewart Teaching Tools
PO Box 15308
Seattle, WA 98115
206-262-9538
FAX: 206-262-9538

J E Stewart, Owner

Teaches 50 words as they appear on parts, tools, job instructions, signs, labels such as: hard hat, assembly, clamp, cut, drill, package and schedule. These words are functional in school and on-the-job. *$32.50*

2473 **Working Together & Taking Part**

AGS
Publishers Building
PO Box 99
Circle Pines, MN 55014
800-328-2560
FAX: 763-786-9007
www.agsnet.com

Robert Zaske, Market Manager

Two programs to build children's social skills in grades 3-6 through folk literature. Has 31 activity-rich lessons, teaching skills like: following rules, accepting differences, speaking assertively and helping others. Discount price of $279.00 when ordering both. *$149.95*

2474 **Writing Skills 1 and 2**

Educators Publishing Service
31 Smith Place
Cambridge, MA 02138
617-367-2700
800-225-5750
FAX: 617-547-0412
www.epsbooks.com

Students practice writing sentences and developing paragraphs through writing about their ideas and personal experiences. A logical sequence takes students from individual sentences to basic paragraphs of 5 sentences, expanded paragraphs, and essays. *$7.50*

64 pages Grades 4-6, 7-9
ISBN 0-83882 -50-

2475 **Writing Skills for the Adolescent**

Educators Publishing Service
31 Smith Place
Cambridge, MA 02138
617-367-2700
800-225-5750
FAX: 617-547-0412
www.epsbooks.com

Teaches the writing process in a series of logical steps as students learn to write and improve sentences, they work on grammar; which is taught in terms of writing. Meanwhile, they learn to generate ideas to compose topic sentences and to use transitional words. They gradually progress from paragraph writing to essay writing. *$10.65*

96 pages Paperback
ISBN 0-838817-04-1

Associations & Organizations

2476 **AVKO Dyslexia Research Foundation**

3084 W Willard Road
Clio, MI 48420
810-686-9283
FAX: 810-686-1101
e-mail: avkoemail@aol.com
www.avko.org

Don McCabe, Research Director

Comprised of individuals interested in helping others learn to read and spell. Develops and sells materials for teaching dyslexics or others with learning disabilities using a method involving audio, visual, kinesthetic and oral (multi-sensory) techniques.

2477 Academy for Guided Imagery

PO Box 2070
Mill Valley, CA 94942 **415-389-9324**
800-726-2070
FAX: 415-383-0944
e-mail: admin@interactiveimagery.com
www.healthy.net/agi/index_ie.html

Aims to teach people to access and use the power of the mind/body connection for healing and to further understanding of the imagery process in human life and development. Also to provide systematic training and guidance to health professionals who are interested in the use of Guided Imagery in their practice.

2478 Alliance for Parental Involvement in Education

29 Kinderhook Street
PO Box 59
E Chatham, NY 12060 **518-392-6900**
FAX: 518-392-6900
e-mail: allpie@taconic.net
www.croton.com/allpie

A nonprofit organization to encourage and assist parental involvement in education, public, private and home. Offers a newsletter, a book catolog, retreats, workshops, and a lending library.

2479 Alternative Work Concepts

PO Box 11452
Eugene, OR 97440 **541-345-3043**
FAX: 541-345-9669
e-mail: awc@teleport.com
www.teleport.com

To promote individualized, integrated, and meaningful employment opportunities in the community for adults with multiple disabilities; to improve the quality of life and provide continuous opportunities for personal growth for these individuals; and to assist businesses with workforce diversification.

2480 American College Testing Program

2201 N Dodge Street
PO Box 168
Iowa City, IA 52243 **319-537-1028**
FAX: 319-537-1014
www.act.org

Richard Ferguson, President

An independent, nonprofit organization that provides a variety of educational services to students and their parents, to high schools and colleges, and to professional associations and government agencies.

2481 American Council for Headache Education

19 Mantua Road
Mount Royal, NJ 08061 **856-423-0258**
800-255-2243
FAX: 856-423-0082
e-mail: achehq@talley.com
www.achenet.org

Linda McGillicuddy, Executive Director
Cheryl Hollo, Associate Executive Director

Nonprofit patient-health professional partnership dedicated to advancing the treatment and management of headaches and to raising the public awareness of headache as valid, biologically based illness.

2482 American School Counselor Association

801 N Fairfax Street
Suite 310
Alexandria, VA 22314 **703-683-2722**
800-306-4722
FAX: 703-683-1619
e-mail: asca@schoolcounselor.org
www.schoolcounselor.org

Kwok-Sze Wong, Executive Director

ASCA focuses on providing professional devleopment, enhancing school counseling programs, and research effective school counseling practices. Mission is to promote excellence in professional school counseling and the development of all students.

2483 American School Health Association, Journal of School Health

PO Box 708
Kent, OH 44240 **330-678-1601**
FAX: 330-678-4526
e-mail: asha@ashaweb.org
www.ashaweb.org

Susan Wooley, Executive Director

This is a monthly journal which offers information to professionals and parents on school health. Membership dues, $95.00.

2484 Association on Higher Education and Disability

University of Boston
100 Morrissey Boulevard
Boston, MA 02125 **617-287-3880**
FAX: 617-287-3881
TTY:617-287-3882
www.ahead.org

Higher education for people with disabilities. A vital resource, promoting excellence through education, communication and training.

2485 Asthma & Allergy Education for Worksite Clinicians

Asthma and Allergy Foundation of America
1233 20th Street NW
Suite 402
Washington, DC 20036 **202-466-7643**
800-727-8462
FAX: 202-466-8940
e-mail: info@aafa.org
www.aafa.org

Developed to teach health professionals in the worksite about asthma and allergies and ultimately improve the health of the employees who have theses de\iseases. The program gives worksite clinicians the knowledge and tools they need to give employees guidance on how to control environmental factors both in the home and in the workplace, self-manage thier asthma and/or allergies and to determaine if ti is necessary for employees to see an allergist if symptoms persist.

2486 Asthma & Allergy Essentials for Children's Care Provider

Asthma and Allergy Foundation of America
1233 20th Street NW
Suite 402
Washington, DC 20036
202-466-7643
800-727-8462
FAX: 202-466-8940
e-mail: info@aafa.org
www.aafa.org

Course gives child care providers the tools and knowledge they need to care for children with asthma and allergies. During the interactive, three hour program, a trained health professional teaches providers how to recognize the signs and symptoms of an asthma or allergy episode, how to institute environmental control measures to prevent these episodes, and how to properly use medication and the tools for asthma management. In areas of the country serviced by AAFA's 14 chapters.

2487 Asthma Care Training for Kids (ACT)

Asthma and Allergy Foundation of America
1125 15th Street NW
Suite 502
Washington, DC 20005
202-466-7643
FAX: 202-466-8940
e-mail: info@aafa.org
www.aafa.org

Interactive program for children ages seven to 12 and their families. Children and their families attend three group sessions seperately to learn their own unique styles and then come together at the end of each session to share their knowledge.

2488 Autism Treatment Center of America

2080 S Undermountain Road
Sheffield, MA 01257
413-229-2100
800-714-2779
FAX: 413-229-8931
e-mail: www.son-rise.org
information@son-rise.org

Sean Fitzgerald, Assistant Director

Since 1983, the Autism Treatment Center of America has provided innovative training programs for parents and professionals caring for children challenged by Autism, Autism Spectrum Disorders, Pervasive Developmental Disorders (PDD) and other development difficulties. The Son-Rise Program teaches a specific yet comprehensive system of treatment and education designed to help families and caregivers enable their children to dramatically improve in all areas of learning.

2489 Ayurvedic Institute

11311 Menaul NE
Suite A
Albuquerque, NM 87112
505-291-9698
FAX: 505-294-7572
e-mail: registrar@ayurveds.com
www.ayurveda.com

Directed by Dr. Vasant Lad, trains people in Ayurveda.

2490 CARF Rehabilitation Accreditation Commission

4891 E Grant Road
Tucson, AZ 85712
520-325-1044
FAX: 520-318-1129
e-mail: postmaster@carf.org
www.carf.org

Brian Boon PhD, President/CEO

The independent, not-for-profit commission promotes quality services for people with disabilities and others in need of rehabilitation. CARF establishes customer-focused standards to help organizations measure and improve the quality of their rehabilitation programs and services. When reviewing a rehabilitation program or service, CARF applies standards that have been developed and accepted by peers in the field.CARF has more than 16,000 programs in the US, Canada, & Sweden.

2491 CEC-Division for Early Childhood

Council of Exceptional Children
1110 N Glebe Road
Suite 300
Arlington, VA 22201
703-620-3660
FAX: 703-264-9494
www.cec.sped.org

Janice Burdick, President

A division of The Council for Exceptional Children. Promotes education for young children and infants with special needs, initiates programs that cooperatively involve parents in their children's education, stimulates communication and joint activity among early childhood organizations, sponsors professional development and disseminates research findings and information addressing issues of early childhood education and more.

2492 Clearinghouse for Specialized Media and Technology

California Department of Education
1430 N Street
Room 3410
Sacramento, CA 95814
916-445-5103
FAX: 916-323-9732
e-mail: rbrawley@cde.ca.gov
www.cde.ca.gov/csmt

Rod Brawley, Consultant

Assists schools and students in the identification and acquisition of textbooks, reference books and study materials in aural media, Braille, large print and electronic media access technology.

2493 Council for Exceptional Children

1110 N Glebe Road
Suite 300
Arlington, VA 22201
703-620-3660
FAX: 703-264-9494
www.cec.sped.org

Janice Burdick, President

The largest international organization dedicated to improving educational success for individuals with exceptionalities. CEC sets professional standards, advocates for appropriate government policies, provides continual professional development and advocates for newly and historically underserved individuals with exceptionalities. Helps professionals obtain conditions and resources necessary for effective practice.

2494 East Brunswick Adult and Community Education Program: Adult Life Skills

380 Cranbury Road
E Brunswick, NJ 08816
732-613-6984
FAX: 732-613-6981
e-mail: bmethven@ebnet.org

Bernadette Methven LSW, Program Leader

Offers education, training, and social programs for adults with developmental disabilities in an integrated adult/evening school environment. Residents of Middlesex County, New Jersey, ages 18 and over are eligible to register. Limited transportation is also available. Annual enrollemnt fee $25.00.

2495 **Educational Referral Service**
Dr. Yvonne Jones and Associates
2222 Eastlake Avenue E
Seattle, WA 98102 **206-325-2600**
FAX: 206-328-9172

Yvonne Jones

Specializes in matching children with the learning environments that are best for them and works with families to help them identify concerns and establish priorities about their child's education.

2496 **Harriet & Robert Heilbrunn Guild School**
JGB Audio Library for the Blind
15 W 65th Street
New York, NY 10023 **212-769-6331**
FAX: 212-769-6266
e-mail: info@JGB.org
www.JGB.org

Peter Williamson, Director
Ken Stanley, Manager

2497 **Howard School: Central Campus**
1246 Ponce De Leon Avenue NE
Atlanta, GA 30306 **404-377-7436**
FAX: 404-377-0884

Sandra N Kleinman, Executive Director

Enrolls students whose language-learning disabilities and differences hinder their learning to their fullest potential. Goal is to help students simultaneously build basic academi skills, maximize academic progress, develop higher level thinking skills, gain self-advocacy strategies and become independent life-long learners. Average class size is less than 10 students.

2498 **Howard School: North Campus**
9415 Willeo Road
Roswell, GA 30075 **770-642-9644**
FAX: 770-998-1398
www.howardschool.org

Sandra N Kleinman, Executive Director

Enrolls students whose language-learning disabilities and differences hinder their learning to their fullest potential. Goal is to help students simultaneously build basic academi skills, maximize academic progress, develop higher level thinking skills, gain self-advocacy strategies and become independent life-long learners. Average class size is less than 10 students.

2499 **Institute on Disability/UCED**
University of New Hampshire
7 Leavitt Lane
Suite 101
Durham, NH 03824 **603-862-4320**
FAX: 603-862-0555
e-mail: institutedisability@unh.edu
www.iod.unh.edu

Jan Nisbet, Director

This mission of the Institute is to improve the knowledge, policy and practice related to the economic and social participation of persons with disabilities. The Institute provides a blend of programs that address the needs of local schools, community services and state and federal agencies. The Institute's goal is to increase the ability of the State of New Hampshire to foster inclusion of persons with disabilities into their communities.

2500 **International Association of Parents and Professionals for Safe Alternatives in Childbirth**
Route 4
Box 646
Marble Hill, MO 63764 **573-238-2010**
FAX: 573-238-2010
e-mail: napsac@clas.net
www.napsac.org

Dedicated to exploring, implementing, and establishing safe, family-centered childbirth programs that meet the social and emotional needs of families as well as provide the safe, appropriate aspects of medical science.

2501 **International Childbirth Education Association**
PO Box 20048
Minneapolis, MN 55420 **952-854-8660**
FAX: 952-854-8772
e-mail: info@icea.org
www.icea.org

Offer teaching certificates, seminars, continuing education workshops, and a mail order center.

2502 **International Dyslexia Association: South Carolina Branch**
1500 Hallbrook Drive
Columbia, SC 29209 **803-695-1400**
800-722-1213
FAX: 803-695-1214
e-mail: info@interdys.org
www.interdys.org

Anne Vickers, Head of School
Thrace Mears, Admissions Director
John W Weaver, Advancement Director

Provides free information and referral services for diagnosis and tutoring for parents, educators, physicians, and individuals with dyslexia. 48 countries. Membership includes yearly journal and quarterly newsletter. Call for conference dates.

2503 **International Organization for the Education of the Hearing Impaired**
Alexander Graham Bell Association
3417 Volta Place NW
Washington, DC 20007 **202-337-5220**
FAX: 202-337-8314
e-mail: info@agbell.org
www.agbell.org

Professional educators of the hearing impaired make up the members of this organization which promotes the excellence in teaching the hearing impaired child.

2504 **Jewish Guild for the Blind**
JGB Audio Library
15 W 65th Street
New York, NY 10023 **212-769-6331**
800-284-4422
FAX: 212-769-6266
e-mail: audiolibrary@jgb.org
www.JGB.org

Peter Williamson, Director
Ken Stanley, Manager
Victoria Kella, Public Relations Manager

Tape recordings of best-selling books in 28 subject categories for blind, visually impaired and disabled persons.

2505 **Job Accommodation Network**

W Virginia University
PO Box 6080
Morgantown, WV 26506
800-526-7234
e-mail: bloy@wvu.edu
janweb.icdi.wvu.edu/

International toll-free consulting service that provides information about job accommodations and the employability of people with disabilities. Also provides information regarding the Americans with Disabilities Act (ADA).

2506 **Mad Hatters: Theatre That Makes a World of Difference**

PO Box 50002
Kalamazoo, MI 49005
FAX: 269-385-5868

Bobbe A Luce, Executive Director

A nationally-known theater which has presented effective and innovative programs to more than 175,000 people in over 1,150 performances in the past 15 years. Our presentations and training programs are a proven method of changing attitudes and behaviors. The Mad Hatters is a leader in the field of sensitivity-training to build community and foster the inclusion of all people in society. Fees: $500-$4000 per program, depending on topic and audience.

2507 **Michigan Psychological Association**

2105 University Park Drive
Cuite 1-C
Okemos, MI 48864
517-347-1885
FAX: 517-347-1896
e-mail: mimpa@aol.com
www.michpsych.org

Marlene O'Neill, Director

Non-profit organization of over 1000 psychologists, working to advance psychology as a science and a profession and to promote the public welfare by encouraging the highest professional standards, offering public education and providing a public service, and by participating in the public policy process on behalf of the profession and health care consumers.

2508 **National Association of Colleges and Employers**

62 Highland Avenue
Bethlehem, PA 18017
610-868-1421
800-544-5272
FAX: 610-868-0208
www.naceweb.org

Marilyn F Mackes, Executive Director
Norita Rehrig, Assistant Executive Director
Sandra Dalious, Human Resources Manager

A national association with services for career planning, placement and recruitment professionals.

2509 **National Association of Private Special Education Centers**

1522 K Street NW
Suite 1032
Washington, DC 20005
202-408-3338
FAX: 202-408-3340
e-mail: napsec@aol.com
www.napsec.com

Sherry L Kolbe, Executive Director/CEO
Alison Figi, Communications Coordinator
Rebecca Kantz, Membership Services Coordinator

Membership directory offering information on NAPSEC member schools nationwide available.

2510 **National Center for Homeopathy**

801 N Fairfax Street
Suite 306
Alexandria, VA 22314
703-548-7790
877-624-0613
FAX: 703-548-7792
e-mail: info@homeopathic.org
www.homeopathic.org

Provides information, referral lists, and courses to professionals.

2511 **National Clearinghouse for Professions in Special Education**

Council for Exceptional Children
1110 N Glebe Road
Suite 300
Arlington, VA 22201
703-620-3660
FAX: 703-264-9494
www.cec.sped.org

Janice Burdick, President

Designed to encourage individuals to seek careers in the various fields related to the education of children and youth with disabilities.

2512 **National Council on Rehabilitation Education**

California State University, Fresno
School of Education and Human Dev.
5005 N Maple Avenue, MS3
Fresno, CA 93740
559-278-0325
FAX: 559-278-0016
e-mail: charlesa@csufresno.edu

Dr Charles Arokiasamy, Administrative Secretary

Members include academic institutions and organizations, professional educators, researchers, and students. Assists in the documentation of the effect of education in improving services to persons with disabilities; determines the skills and training necessary for effective rehabilitation services; develops role models, standards and uniform licensure and certification requirements for rehabilitation personnel.

2513 **National Education Association of the United States**

1201 16th Street NW
Washington, DC 20036
202-833-4000

John Wilson, Executive Director

Offers information to educational professionals.

2514 **National Society for Experiential Education**

9001 Braddock Road
Suite 380
Springfield, VA 22151
703-426-4268
800-803-4170
FAX: 703-426-8400
e-mail: info@nsee.org
www.nsee.org

Charles Walker, Executive Director

National nonprofit organization which advocates experiential learning and works with college administrators and high school and college internship programs.

2515 **Presidents Committee on Mental Retardation Administration for Children & Families**

370 L'Enfant Promenade SW
Aerospace Center, Room 701
Washington, DC 20447
202-619-0634
FAX: 202-205-9519
www.acf.hhs.gov/programs/pcmr

Sally Atwater, Executive Director
George Bouthilet PhD, Research Director
Lauerdia Roach, Special Assistant

Prepares an annual report to the president of the USA national issue an recommendation of national signifiance.

2516 Rifin Family/Daughters of Israel

JGB Audio Library for the Blind
15 W 65th Street
New York, NY 10023
212-769-6331
800-284-4422
FAX: 212-769-6266
e-mail: info@JGB.org
www.JGB.org

Peter Wiliamson, Director
Ken Stanley, Manager

2517 SSD (Services for Students with Disabilities)

College Board
45 Columbus Avenue
New York, NY 10023
212-713-8000
FAX: 212-713-8277
www.collegeboard.org

National, nonprofit membership association dedicated to preparing, inspiring and connecting students to college and opportunity. Founded in 1900, the association is composed of more than 3,800 schools, colleges, universities and other educational organizations. Services for Students with Disabilities (SSD) provides special arrangements to minimize the possible effects of disabilities on test performance through it's Admissions Testing Program (ATP).

2518 Sandhills Academy

1500 Hallbrook Drive
Columbia, SC 29209
803-695-1400
FAX: 803-695-1214
e-mail: info@sandhillsacademy.com
www.sandhillsacademy.com

Anne Vickers, Head of School
Thrace Mears, Admissions Director
John W Weaver, Advancement Director

Exists to provide educational programs and intellectual development for average to above average students, six to 15, who learn differently and to promote the development of self-awareness, joy in learning and a vision of themselves as life-long learners.

2519 Senior Program for Teens and Young Adults with Special Needs

Camp JCC
6125 Montrose Road
Rockville, MD 20852
301-230-3759
FAX: 301-881-6549
e-mail: jcccamp@jccgw.org
www.jccgw.org

The senior Program is a transitional program for teens and young adults with mental retardation, severe learning disabilities and multiple disabilities. Socialization, recreation and independent living skills are enhanced ina fun enviroment. Activities include art, music, recreational swim and more.

2520 Shema V'Ezer

Camp JCC
6125 Montrose Road
Rockville, MD 20852
301-881-0100
FAX: 301-881-6549
e-mail: jcccamp@jccgw.org
www.jccgw.org

The Shema V'Ezer Religious School program offers Judaic education to children and teens with disabilities, ages 6 to 21, who may not benefit from a traditional religious school setting. Children with mental retardation, svere learning disabilities, visual or auditory impairment, mobility impairment, behavioral disorders and or multiple disabilities particpate in Sunday morning classes at the JCC.

2521 Shema V'Ezer Post-Bar/Bat Mitzvah Confirmation Program

JCC Camp
6125 Montrose Road
Rockville, MD 20852
301-230-3759
FAX: 301-881-6549
e-mail: jcccamp@jccgw.org
www.jccgw.org

A program for teens and young adults who wish to continue their Jewish education, but need accomodation for their special learning and socialization needs. Participants meet Sunday mornings, usually from 10 a.m. to 12 noon. Classes including educational, and socialization components culminate in confirmation ceremony, which is held at a later date. In class topics include Israel and Zionism, exploring the Jewish community, tzedakah, ethics and values, prayers, Jewish holiday observance and more.

2522 United Cerebral Palsy Research and Educational Foundation

3135 8th Street NE
Washington, DC 20017
202-269-1500
800-872-5827
FAX: 202-526-0519
e-mail: webmaster@ucpdc.org
www.ucpa.org

Grants are awarded to institutions or organizations on behalf of a principal investigator in support of biomedical and bioengineering research in areas which have a significant relationship to cerebral palsy. While most research on central nervous system structure, function and disorder may be useful, the Foundation requires that research proposals address issues of relevance to cerebral palsy.

2523 Vanguard School

PO Box 730
1777 N Valley Road
Paoli, PA 19301
610-296-6700
FAX: 610-640-0132
www.vanguardschool-pa.org

Ernest Bratlstrom, Head of School
Timothy Lanshe, Education Director
Donna Annechino, Admissions Director

An Approved Private School (APS) for students aged 2.7-21 years with traumatic brain injury (TBI), social/emotional disturbance (SED) and/or autism/pervasive developmental disorder.

2524 Worthmore Academy

5220 E Fall Creek Parkway N Drive
Indianapolis, IN 46220
317-253-5367
FAX: 317-253-5824
www.familyeducation.com/IN/worthmore_academy

Brenda Jackson, Director
Sandy Foster, Assistant Director

A center for learning disabilities providing educational assessments, alternative educational programs, academic guidance and public awareness services available as follows: full-time day school, K-8th, 1 to 1 teacher student ratio; six week summer school, K-12th, 1 to 1 teacher student ratio; after school tutoring; adult tutoring, educational assessments, counseling and educational seminars.

1988

Directories

2525 **Complete Directory for Pediatric Disorders**

Sedgwick Press/Grey House Publishing
185 Millerton Road
PO Box 860
Millerton, NY 12546 **518-789-8700**
800-562-2139
FAX: 518-789-0545
e-mail: books@greyhouse.com
www.greyhouse.com

Leslie Mackenzie, Publisher

A directory that provides parents and caregivers with information about Pediatric Conditions, Disorders, Diseases and Disabilities. *$145.00*

702 pages Annual
ISBN 1-891482-41-6

2526 **Complete Directory for People with Chronic Illness**

Sedgwick Press/Grey House Publishing
185 Millerton Road
PO Box 860
Millerton, NY 12546 **518-789-8700**
800-562-2139
FAX: 518-789-0545
e-mail: books@greyhouse.com
www.greyhouse.com

Leslie Mackenzie, Publisher

This directory is structured around the ninety most prevalent chronic illnesses. It provides a comprehensive overview of the support services and information resources available for people diagnosed with chronic illness. *$165.00*

Annual

2527 **Complete Learning Disabilities Directory**

Sedgwick Press/Grey House Publishing
185 Millerton Road
PO Box 860
Millerton, NY 12546 **518-789-8700**
800-562-2139
FAX: 518-789-0545
e-mail: books@greyhouse.com
www.greyhouse.com

Leslie Mackenzie, Publisher

A comprehensive educational guide offering over 6,500 listings on associations and organizations, schools, government agencies, testing materials, camps, products, books, newsletters, legal information, classroom materials and more. *$145.00*

702 pages Annual
ISBN 1-891482-41-6

2528 **Complete Mental Health Directory**

Sedgwick Press/Grey House Publishing
185 Millerton Road
PO Box 860
Millerton, NY 12546 **518-789-8700**
800-562-2139
FAX: 518-789-0545
e-mail: books@greyhouse.com
www.greyhouse.com

Leslie Mackenzie, Publisher

Comprehensive information covering the field of behavioral health, with critical information for both the layman and the mental health professional.

Annual

2529 **Diabetes: Caring for Your Emotions as Well as Your Health**

Harper Collins Publishers/Basic Books
10 E 53rd Street
New York, NY 10022 **212-207-7042**
800-242-7737
FAX: 212-207-7203

This book offers suggestions for adaptation, relationships with medical personnel, family strategies, employment questions, technology and support groups. *$15.00*

ISBN 1-852300-47-7

2530 **Dictionary of Special Education and Rehabilitation**

Love Publishing Company
9101 E Kenyoun Avenue
Suite 2200
Denver, CO 80237
FAX: 303-221-7444
e-mail: lovepublishing@compuserve.com
www.lovepublishing.com

A valuable basic resource in the field. It incorporates hundreds of additions and changes. *$39.95*

Paperback
ISBN 0-891082-43-3

2531 **Directory for Exceptional Children**

Porter Sargent Publishers
11 Beacon Street
Suite 1400
Boston, MA 02108 **617-523-1670**
800-342-7470
FAX: 617-523-1021
e-mail: orders@portersargent.com
portersargent.com

John Yonce, General Manager
Daniel McKeever, Senior Editor
Leslie Weston, Production Manager

A comprehensive, objective survey of 3000 schools, facilities and organizations across the country serving children and young adults with developmental, emotional, physical and mental disabilities. *$75.00*

1056 pages Trienniel
ISBN 0-875581-41-2

2532 **Educators Resource Directory**

Sedgwick Press/Grey House Publishing
185 Millerton Road
PO Box 860
Millerton, NY 12546 **518-789-8700**
800-562-2139
FAX: 518-789-0545
e-mail: books@greyhouse.com
www.greyhouse.com

Leslie Mackenzie, Publisher

Gives education professionals immediate access to Associations and Organizations, Conferences and Trade Shows, Educational Research Centers, Employment Opportunities and Teaching Abroad, School Library Services, Scholarships, Financial Resources and much more. *$ 145.00*

591 pages Annual
ISBN 1-930956-48-7

2533 Enhancing Children's Communication: Research & Foundations

Paul H Brookes Publishing Company
PO Box 10624
Baltimore, MD 21285
800-638-3775
FAX: 410-337-8539
e-mail: custserv@brokespublishing.com
www.brookespublishing.com

This groundbreaking book provides helpful insights, unique perspectives, and innovative strategies that are needed to intervene successfully with children whose developmental disabilities affect their use of communication and language. *$43.00*

448 pages 1992
ISBN 1-557660-76-X

2534 Exceptional Children: An Introductory Survey of Special Education

McGraw-Hill, School Publishing
220 E Danieldale Road
DeSoto, TX 75115
972-224-1111
800-442-9685
FAX: 972-228-1982
mhschool.com

The focus of this survey is on observable characteristics of exceptional persons, and the instructional practices which foster their fullest development.

704 pages

2535 Increasing and Decreasing Behaviors of Persons with Severe Retardation

Research Press
PO Box 9177
Champaign, IL 61826
217-352-3273
800-519-2707
FAX: 217-352-1221
e-mail: rp@researchpress.com
www.researchpress.com

Russell Pence, VP Marketing

These well-organized manuals are written for teachers, aides and persons responsible for designing or evaluating behavioral programs. Offers specific guidelines for arranging and managing the learning environment as well as standards for evaluating and maintaining success. In Volume two of this series, chapters address more restrictive procedures including physical restraint, punishment, time-out and overcorrection. Set of two volumes. *$32.95*

428 pages Item 2650
ISBN 0-878222-65-0

2536 Teaching Special Students in Mainstream

Books on Special Children
PO Box 305
Congers, NY 10920
845-638-1236
FAX: 845-638-0847
e-mail: irene@boscbooks.com

Overview of mainstream, team of professionals managing classroom behavior, tips for teachers, social acceptance and handling of specific differences. *$33.00*

515 pages Softcover

2537 Young Children with Special Needs

McGraw-Hill, School Publishing
220 E Danieldale Road
DeSoto, TX 75115
972-224-1111
800-442-9685
FAX: 972-228-1982
mhschool.com

This text examines development in the critical areas of motor, self-help, cognitive, language, social, emotional and play skills.

526 pages

Educational Publishers

2538 AFB Press

American Foundation for the Blind/AFB Press
PO Box 1020
Sewickley, PA 15143
412-741-1142
800-232-3044
FAX: 412-741-0609
e-mail: afborders@abdintl.com
www.afb.org

Develops, publishes, and sells a wide variety of informative books, pamphlets, periodicals, and videos for students, professionals, and researchers in the blindess and visual impairment fields, for people professionally involved in making the mainstream community accessible, and for blind and visually impaired people and their families; publication and video orders.

2539 American Association for Counseling & Development

American Counseling Association
5999 Stevenson Avenue
Alexandria, VA 22304
800-347-6647
800-473-2329
FAX: 703-823-6862
www.counseling.org

Offers tools and books for the professional.

2540 Brookline Books

PO Box 97
Newton Upper Falls, MA 02464
617-558-8010
800-666-2665
FAX: 617-558-8011
e-mail: milt@brooklinebooks.com
www.brooklinebooks.com

Milt Budoff PhD, Publisher

Offers books for teachers and parents on law and legislation, education, integration and mainstreaming for the disabled, their families, caregivers and teachers.

2541 Brooks/Cole Publishing Company

511 Forest Lodge Road
Pacific Grove, CA 93950
831-373-0728
FAX: 831-375-6414

Offers books in Special Education for those preparing to be special educators and for in-service professionals.

2542 **Charles C Thomas Publisher**

2600 S First Street
Springfield, IL 62704
217-789-8980
800-258-8980
FAX: 217-789-9130
e-mail: books@ccthomas.com
www.ccthomas.com

Publishes specialty titles and textbooks in medicine, dentistry, nursing, and veterinary medicine, as well as a complete line in the behavioral sciences, criminal justice, education, special education, and rehabilitation. Aims to acommodate the current needs for information.

2543 **Gallaudet University Bookstore**

Gallaudet University Press
11030 S Langley Avenue
Chicago, IL 60628
202-651-5488
800-621-2736
FAX: 202-651-5489
www.gallaudet.edu

Offers informational resources for the deaf, parents of the deaf, professionals, special educators and more. Produces a yearly catalog of materials on sign language and deafness.

2544 **Greenwood Publishing Group**

88 Post Road W
Westport, CT 06880
203-226-3571
FAX: 203-222-1502
www.greenwood.com

2545 **McGraw-Hill Company**

2460 Kerper Boulevard
Dubuque, IO 52001
563-589-4666
800-553-4920
FAX: 563-588-1451
www.mcgraw-hill.com

Marc Bigelow, Director

Offers a catalog of testing resources and materials for the special educator.

2546 **National Association of School Psychologists**

4340 EW Highway
Suite 402
Bethesda, MD 20814
301-657-0270
FAX: 301-657-0275
e-mail: lnealis@naspweb.org
www.nasponline.org

Libby Kuffner Nealis, Director Public Policy

Represents over 22,500 school psychologists and related professionals. It serves its members and society by advancing the profession of school psychology and advocating for the rights, welfare, education and mental health of children, youth and their families.

2547 **Oryx Press**

4041 N Central Avenue
Suite 700
Phoenix, AZ 85012
602-265-2651
800-279-6799
FAX: 800-279-4663

2548 **Paul H Brookes Publishing Company**

PO Box 10624
Baltimore, MD 21285
410-337-9580
800-638-3775
FAX: 410-337-8539

2549 **Pro-Ed**

8700 Shoal Creek Boulevard
Austin, TX 78757
512-451-3246
800-897-3202
FAX: 512-451-8542
e-mail: info@proedinc.com
www.proedinc.com

Publishes, produces and sells books, curricular therapy materials and journals dedicated to psychology, special education and speech, language and hearing.

2550 **Ragged Edge Magazine**

Advocado Press
PO Box 145
Louisville, KY 40201
502-894-9492
FAX: 502-899-9562
e-mail: circulation@raggededgemagazine.com
www.raggededgemagazine.com

T Smith, Circulation Manager

A bi-monthly print magazine for $17.50 a year; also has a website. *$17.50*

36 pages BiMonthly

2551 **Research Press**

PO Box 9177
Champaign, IL 61826
217-352-3273
800-519-2707
FAX: 217-352-1221
e-mail: rp@researchpress.com
www.researchpress.com

Dennis Wiziecki, Marketing Department

2552 **Special Needs Project**

324 State Street
Suite H
Santa Barbara, CA 93101
800-333-6867
FAX: 805-962-5087

2553 **Waterfront Books Publishing Company**

85 Crescent Road
Burlington, VT 05401
802-658-7477

Sherrill N Musty, Owner

State Agencies: Alabama

2554 **Alabama Department of Education: Division of Special Education Services**

Gordon Persons Building
PO Box 302101
Montgomery, AL 36104
205-242-8114
FAX: 205-242-9192
www.alsde.edu

Bill East, Assistant Director

State Agencies: Alaska

2555 Alaska Department of Education: Office of Special Education

801 W 10th Street
Suite 200
Juneau, AK 99801
907-465-2971
FAX: 907-465-3396
www.eed.state.ak.us

Myrna Howe, State Director

Administers special educational programs through the Division of Education Program Support to the disabled residing in the Alaska area.

State Agencies: Arkansas

2556 Arkansas Department of Special Education

4 Capitol Mall
Suite 105-C
Little Rock, AR 72201
501-682-4221
FAX: 501-682-4313
www.arkansas.com

Dr. Diane Sydoriak, Associate Director Special Ed.

Provides oversight of all educational programs for children and youth with disabilities, ages 3 to 21. Provides technical assistance to all public agencies providing educational services to this population.

State Agencies: Arizona

2557 Arizona Department of Education

1535 W Jefferson
Phoenix, AZ 85007
602-542-3084
FAX: 602-542-5404

Kathryn A Lund, State Director Special Education

State Agencies: California

2558 California Department of Education: Special Education Division

721 Capital Mall
Sacramento, CA 95814
916-657-3567
FAX: 916-657-4770

Jack O'Connell, Superintendent
Leo Sandoval, Director Special Education

Through consultants, coordinates the establishment and operations of special public school programs for blind and partially sighted pupils. The staff includes two regionally based consultant specialists in the education of visually impaired children, and the eligible age for help is 3-21.

State Agencies: Colorado

2559 Colorado Department of Education: Special Education Service Unit

201 E Colfax Avenue
Denver, CO 80203
303-866-6694
FAX: 303-866-6811
www.cde.state.co.us

Provides consultation on materials and educational services for visually handicapped children, supervises volunteer services, transcribes textbooks for visually handicapped students.

State Agencies: Connecticut

2560 Connecticut Department of Education: Bureau of Special Education

25 Industrial Park Road
Middletown, CT 06457
203-638-4265
FAX: 203-638-4231
www.ctserc.org

Dr. Tom Gillung, Bureau Chief

Commitment is to serve as a centralized resource for professionals, families, and community members regarding education and early intervention/prevention for all of Connecticut's children and youth and their families, particularly children with special needs, at-risk learners, and diverse learners. SERC strives for the highest possible level of excellence assistance initiatives, family education and support, and information and materials dissemination.

2561 Connecticut State Board of Education and Services for the Blind

184 Windsor Avenue
Windsor, CT 06095
860-602-4000
800-842-4510
FAX: 860-602-4030
e-mail: brian.sigman@po.state.ct.us

Brian Sigman, Director Vocational Rehab

Provides consultation for the education of visually disabled children, provide Braille instruction, independent living skills training, vocational rehabilitation services and community outreach and advocacy.

State Agencies: Delaware

2562 Department of Public Instruction: Exceptional Children & Special Programs Division

PO Box 1402
Dover, DE 19903
302-736-5471
FAX: 302-739-4221

Dr. Martha Brooks, Team Leader

State Agencies: District of Columbia

2563 **District of Columbia Public Schools: Special Education Division**

825 N Capitol Street NE
7th Floor
Washington, DC 20002 **202-442-4800**
202-442-5517

Dr. Paul L Vance, Superintendent

Committed to providing a continuum of services that offers students with disabilities the opportunity to avtively participate in the learning environemtn of their neighborhood school.

2564 **National Clearinghouse on Family Support and Children's Mental Health**

1 Dupont Circle NW
Suite 800
Washington, DC 20036 **202-939-9320**
800-544-3284
FAX: 202-833-4760
e-mail: heatah@ace.nche.edu

State Agencies: Florida

2565 **Florida Department of Education: Bureau of Education for Exceptional Students**

325 W Gaines Street
Suite 614
Tallahassee, FL 32399 **850-488-1570**
FAX: 904-922-7088

Jim Horne, Commissioner
Bettye Weir, Bureau Chief

The Department of Education strives to improve educational services for students with special needs.

State Agencies: Georgia

2566 **Georgia State Department of Education: Program for Exceptional Children**

1952 Twin Towers E
205 Butler Street
Atlanta, GA 30334 **404-656-3963**
FAX: 404-651-6457

Kathy Cox, State Superintendent
Joan Jordan, Director

Provides consultation on educational services for local schools, offers psychological testing and evaluation, maintains resource rooms in district schools and more for the blind and handicapped throughout the state.

State Agencies: Hawaii

2567 **Hawaii Department of Education: Special Needs**

3430 Leahi Avenue
Honolulu, HI 96815 **808-736-3720**
FAX: 808-732-3701

Dr. Margaret Donovan, State Administrator

Provides consultation on educational services for local schools, offers psychological testing and evaluation, maintains resource rooms in district schools and more for the blind and handicapped throughout the state.

State Agencies: Idaho

2568 **Idaho Department of Education: Special Education Services**

PO Box 83720
Boise, ID 83720 **208-334-3940**
FAX: 208-334-4664

Nolene Weaver, Supervisor

State Agencies: Illinois

2569 **Illinois State Board of Education: Department of Special Education**

100 N 1st Street
Mail Code E-216
Springfield, IL 62777 **217-782-6601**
FAX: 217-782-0372
e-mail: pstadeke@spr6.isbe.il.us
www.isbe.state.il.us/

Gail Lieberman, Policy Advisor

Mission is to advance the human and civil rights of people with disabilities in Illinois. Statewide advocacy organization providing self-advocacy assistance, legal services, education and public policy initiatives. Designated to implement the federal protection and advocacy system; has broad statutory power to enforce the rights of people with physical and mental disabilities, including developmental disabilities and mental illnesses.

State Agencies: Indiana

2570 **Indiana Department of Education: Special Education Division**

State House
Room 229
Indianapolis, IN 46204 **317-232-0570**
FAX: 317-233-0586
ideanet.doe.state.in.us/

Robert Marra, Assistant State Director

Provides consultation on educational services for local schools, offers psychological testing and evaluation, maintains resource rooms in district schools and more for the blind and handicapped throughout the state.

State Agencies: Iowa

2571 **Iowa Department of Public Instruction: Bureau of Special Education**

Grimes State Office Building
Des Moines, IA 50319 **515-281-3176**
FAX: 515-242-6019

Dr. Jeananne Hagen PhD, Acting Chief

State Agencies: Kansas

2572 Kansas State Board of Education: Special Education Outcomes Team

120 E Tenth Street
Topeka, KS 66612 **913-296-3869**
FAX: 913-296-7933
e-mail: bpassman@ksde.org
www.kansped.org

Michael Remus, Team Leader

Provides consultation on educational services for local schools, offers psychological testing and evaluation, maintains resource rooms in district schools and more for the blind and handicapped throughout the state.

State Agencies: Kentucky

2573 Kentucky Department of Education: Division of Exceptional Children's Services

500 Metro Street
Room 805, 8th Floor
Frankfort, KY 40601 **502-564-4970**
FAX: 502-564-6721
e-mail: marmstro@kde.state.ky.us
www.kde.state.ky.us

Johnny Grissom, Associate Commissioner

Provides consultation on educational services for local schools, offers psychological testing and evaluation, maintains resource rooms in district schools and more for the blind and handicapped throughout the state.

State Agencies: Louisiana

2574 Louisiana Department of Education: Office of Special Education Services

PO Box 94064
Baton Rouge, LA 70804 **504-342-3633**
FAX: 504-342-5880

Dr. Leon L Borne, Assistant Superintendent

State Agencies: Massachusetts

2575 Massachusetts Department of Education: Program Quality Assurance

350 Main Street
Malden, MA 02148 **617-388-3300**
FAX: 617-388-3476

Pamela Kaufamann, Administrator

State Agencies: Maryland

2576 Maryland State Department of Education: Division of Special Education

200 W Baltimore Street
Baltimore, MD 21201 **410-333-2490**
FAX: 410-333-8165
www.msde.state.md.us

Richard Steinke, State Director

Provides consultation on educational services for local schools, offers psychological testing and evaluation, maintains resource rooms in district schools and more for the blind and handicapped throughout the state.

State Agencies: Maine

2577 Maine Department of Education and Cultural Services: Division of Special Education

Station #23
150
Augusta, ME 04333 **207-624-5959**
FAX: 207-624-5000

David Stockford, Director

Provides consultation on educational services for local schools, assessment and instruction, maintains instructional material centers and more for the blind and handicapped throughout the state.

State Agencies: Michigan

2578 Michigan Department of Education: Special Education Services

PO Box 30008
Lansing, MI 48909 **517-373-9433**
FAX: 517-373-7504
e-mail: molsen@mpas.org
www.mpas.org

Richard Baldwin, State Director

Provides consultation on educational services for local schools, offers psychological testing and evaluation, maintains resource rooms in district schools and more for the blind and handicapped throughout the state.

2579 Services for Students with Disabilities

University of Michigan
G-625 Haven Hall 505 S State
Ann Arbor, MI 48109 **734-763-3000**
FAX: 734-936-3947
e-mail: sgoodin@umich.edu
www.umich.edu/~sswd/ssd

Sam Goodin, Director

Offers information to parents and students.

State Agencies: Minnesota

2580 State Department of Education: Special Education Section

811 Capitol Square Building
550 Cedar Street
St. Paul, MN 55101 **612-296-1793**
FAX: 612-297-7368

Wayne Erickson, Director

State Agencies: Missouri

2581 **Missouri Department of Elementary and Secondary Education: Special Education Programs**

PO Box 480
Jefferson City, MO 65102 **573-751-5739**
FAX: 573-526-4404
www.dese.state.mo.us/divspeced

Sherry Rush, Director

The Division of Special Education provides assistance to public school districts in the supervision, establishment, and improvement of programs of instruction for children with disabilities. The division operates the Missouri School for the Deaf, School for the Blind and State Schools for the Severely Handicapped. The division also supports a statewide system of sheltered workshops for adults with disabilities.

State Agencies: Mississippi

2582 **Mississippi Department of Education: Office of Special Services**

359 NW Street
PO Box 771
Jackson, MS 39205 **601-359-3490**
FAX: 601-359-2198
www.mde.k12.ms.us

Carolyn Black, Director

Key priorities are: reading, early literacy, student achievement, teachers/teaching, leadership/principals, safe and orderly schools, parent relations/community involvement, and technology.

State Agencies: Montana

2583 **Department of Public Health Human Services**

PO Box 202501
Helena, MT 59620 **406-444-4429**
FAX: 406-444-3921
www.state.mt.us

Robert Runkel, Director

Provides consultation on educational services for local schools, offers psychological testing and evaluation, maintains resource rooms in district schools and more for the blind and handicapped throughout the state.

State Agencies: North Carolina

2584 **North Carolina Department of Public Instruction: Exceptional Children Division**

301 N Wilmington Street
Raleigh, NC 27601 **919-715-1565**
FAX: 919-715-1569
e-mail: lharris@dpi.state.nc.us
www.publicschools.org

Lowell Harris, Director

Provides consultation on educational services for local schools, offers psychological testing and evaluation, maintains a continuum of educational sources in local schools for disabled children.

State Agencies: North Dakota

2585 **North Dakota Department of Education: Special Education**

600 E Boulevard Avenue
Bismarck, ND 58505 **701-328-2277**
FAX: 701-328-2461
www.dpi.state.nd.us

Gary Gronberg, Director

Provides consultation on educational services for local schools, offers psychological testing and evaluation, maintains resource rooms in district schools and more for the blind and handicapped throughout the state.

State Agencies: Nebraska

2586 **Nebraska Department of Education: Special Populations Office**

301 Centennial Mall S
PO Box 94987
Lincoln, NE 68509 **402-471-2471**
FAX: 402-471-5022
www.nde.state.ne.us/SPED/sped.html

Gary Sherman, Administrator

Assists school districts in establishing and maintaining effective special education programs for children with disabilities (date of diagnosis through the school year when a child reaches 21). Major function: provide technical assistance to school districts and to parents of children with disabilities, assist programs in meeting state and federal special education regulations. Also responsible for assuring that the rights of children with disabilities and their parents are protected.

State Agencies: New Hampshire

2587 **New Hampshire Department of Education: Bureau for Special Education Services**

101 Pleasant Street
Concord, NH 03301 **603-271-6051**
FAX: 603-271-1953
e-mail: llovering@ed.state.nh.us
www.ed.state.nh.us/

Robert Kennedy, Director

Provides educational leadership and services which promote equal educational opportunites, quality practices and programs that enable NH residents to become fully productive members of society.

State Agencies: New Jersey

2588 **New Jersey Department of Education: Division of Special Education**

CN 500
Trenton, NJ 08625 **609-633-6833**
FAX: 609-984-8422

Barbara Gantwerk, Director

State Agencies: New Mexico

2589 **New Mexico State Department of Education**
300 Don Gaspar Avenue
Santa Fe, NM 87501 **505-827-6541**
FAX: 505-827-6696
www.sde.state.nm.us

Bill Trant, Assistant Director
Judy Parks, Assistant Director

Provides consultation on educational services for local schools, offers psychological testing and evaluation, maintains resource rooms in district schools and more for the blind and handicapped throughout the state.

State Agencies: Nevada

2590 **Nevada Department of Education: Special Eduction Branch**
700 E 5th Street
Suite 113
Carson City, NV 89710 **775-687-9171**
FAX: 775-687-9123
www.nde.state.nv.us

Gloria Dopf, Assistant Deputy Superintendent

The Office of Special Ed and School Improvement Program of the Nevada State Department of Education is responsible for management of state and federal programs providing educational opportunities for students with diverse learning needs. Included are such programs as: Special Education/disabled (IDEA); disadvantaged/at-risk programs (Title I/IASA); Early childhood programs (Title I/IASA); early childhood programs; Migrant education; English language learners; NRS 395 student placement program.

State Agencies: New York

2591 **New York State Education Department**
1606 One Commerce Plaza
Albany, NY 12234 **518-474-5548**
FAX: 518-473-5387
e-mail: nysed@mail.gov
www.nysed.gov

Tom Neveldine, Assistant Commissioner

Provides vocational rehabilitation and educational services for eligible individuals with disabilities throughout New York State. Services include evaluation, counseling, job placement, and referral to other agencies.

State Agencies: Ohio

2592 **Ohio Department of Education: Division of Special Education**
933 High Street
Worthington, OH 43085 **614-466-2650**
FAX: 614-728-1097

John Hemer, Director

Provides technical assistance to educational agencies for the development and implementation of educational services to meet the needs of students with disabilities and/or those who are gifted. Provides information to parents. Administers state and federal funds allocated to educational agencies for the provision of services to students with disabilities and/or those who are gifted.

State Agencies: Oklahoma

2593 **Oklahoma State Department of Education**
2500 N Lincoln Boulevard
Suite 411
Oklahoma City, OK 73105 **405-521-3351**
FAX: 405-522-3503
www.sde.state.ok.us

Darla Griffin, Executive Director

Provides consultation on educational services for local schools, offers psychological testing and evaluation, maintains resource rooms in district schools and more for the blind and handicapped throughout the state.

State Agencies: Oregon

2594 **Oregon Department of Education: Office of Special Education**
255 Capitol Street NE
Public Service Building
Salem, OR 97310 **503-378-3598**
FAX: 503-378-7968
www.ode.state.or.us/sped/index/htm

Dr. Karen Brazeau, Associate Superintendent

state agency ensuring provision of special education services to children with disabilities from birth to age 21.

State Agencies: Pennsylvania

2595 **Pennsylvania Department of Education: Bureau of Special Education**
333 Market Street
7th Floor
Harrisburg, PA 17126 **717-783-6913**
FAX: 717-783-6139
e-mail: 00specialed@psupen.psu.edu
www.pde.state.pa.us

Richard Price, Director

Provides effective and efficient administration of the Commonwealth of Pennsylvania's resources dedicated to enabling school districts to maintain high standards in the delivery of special education services and programs for all exceptional students.

State Agencies: Rhode Island

2596 **Rhode Island Department of Education: Office of Special Needs**
22 Hayes Street
Room 209
Providence, RI 02908 **401-277-3505**
FAX: 401-277-6030

Robert M Pryhoda, Director

Provides consultation on educational services for local schools, offers psychological testing and evaluation, maintains resource rooms in district schools and more for the blind and handicapped throughout the state.

State Agencies: South Carolina

2597 **South Carolina Department of Education: Office of Exceptional Children**

808 Rutledge Building
1429 Senate Street
Columbia, SC 29201 **803-734-8806**
FAX: 803-734-4821
e-mail: sdurant@sde.state.sc.us

Ora Spann, State Director

Provides consultation on educational services for local schools, offers psychological testing and evaluation, maintains resource rooms in district schools and more for the blind and handicapped throughout the state.

State Agencies: South Dakota

2598 **South Dakota Department of Education & Cultural Affairs: Office of Special Education**

700 Governors Drive
Pierre, SD 57501 **605-773-3315**
FAX: 605-773-6139

Deboarh Barnett, State Director

State Agencies: Tennessee

2599 **Tennessee Department of Education**

710 James Robertson Parkway
8th Floor, Gateway Plaza
Nashville, TN 37243 **615-741-2851**
FAX: 615-532-9412

Joseph Fisher, Executive Director

Provides consultation on educational services for local schools, offers psychological testing and evaluation, maintains resource rooms in district schools and more for the blind and handicapped throughout the state.

State Agencies: Texas

2600 **Texas Education Agency**

1701 N Congress Avenue
Austin, TX 78701 **512-463-9414**
FAX: 512-463-9434
www.tea.state.tx.us

Jill Gray, Sr. Director

Provides consultation on educational services for local schools, offers psychological testing and evaluation, maintains resource rooms in district schools and more for the blind and handicapped throughout the state.

2601 **Texas Education Agency: Special Education Unit**

1701 N Congress Avenue
Austin, TX 78701 **512-463-9414**
FAX: 512-463-9434
e-mail: wmccain@tmail.tea.state.tx.us
www.tea.state.tx.us/Cate

Jill Gray, Sr. Director

2602 **Texas School of the Deaf**

1102 S Congress Avenue
PO Box 3538
Austin, TX 78764 **512-462-5353**
800-332-3873
www.tsd.state.tx.us

Claire Bugen, Superintendent

Promote quality educational opportunities and achievement for the deaf students of Texas by providing a comprehensive educational and residential program and a complete array of consultative services for parents and professionals throughout the state.

State Agencies: Utah

2603 **Utah State Office of Education: At-Risk and Special Education Service Unit**

250 E 500th S
Salt Lake City, UT 84111 **801-538-7706**
FAX: 801-583-7991
www.usoe.k12.ut.us

Dr. Steven Kukic, Director

Provides consultation on educational services for local schools, offers psychological testing and evaluation, maintains resource rooms in district schools and more for the blind and handicapped throughout the state.

State Agencies: Vermont

2604 **Vermont Special Education: Division of Special Education**

120 State Street
State Office Building
Montpelier, VT 05620 **802-828-3141**
FAX: 802-828-3140
www.state.vt.us/educ/new/html/pgm_sped.htm

Dennis Kane, Chief, External Leader

Provides technical assistance to schools and other organizations to help ensure that schools understand and comply with federal and state laws and regulations related to providing special education services. In addition, the special education division offers a due process procedure to parents who have concerns about services offered to their children.

State Agencies: Virginia

2605 **Virginia Department of Education: Division of Pre & Early Adolescent Education**

PO Box 2120
Richmond, VA 23216 **804-225-2847**
FAX: 804-371-2456
www.pen.k12.va.us

Austin Tuning, Lead Specialist Special Ed

Provides consultation on educational services for local schools, offers psychological testing and evaluation, maintains resource rooms in district schools and more for the blind and handicapped throughout the state.

State Agencies: Washington

2606 **Superintendent of Public Instruction: Special Education Section**
Old Capitol Building
PO Box 47200
Olympia, WA 98504 **360-753-6733**
FAX: 360-586-0247

Douglas Gill, State Director

State Agencies: West Virginia

2607 **West Virginia Department of Education: Office of Special Education**
1900 Kanawha Boulevard E
Building #6, Room B-304
Charleston, WV 25305 **304-558-2696**
FAX: 304-558-0048
wvde.state.wv.us

Dr. Michael Valentine, Director

Provides consultation on educational services for local schools, offers psychological testing and evaluation, maintains resource rooms in district schools and more for the blind and handicapped throughout the state.

State Agencies: Wyoming

2608 **Wyoming Department of Education**
2300 Capitol Avenue
2nd Floor, Hathaway Building
Cheyenne, WY 82002 **307-777-7414**
FAX: 307-777-6234
www.k12.wy.us

Sharon Davarno, State Director

Mission is to lead, model, and support continuous improvement of education for everyone in Wyoming.

Magazines & Journals

2609 **Academic Acceptance of ASL**
Gallaudet University Bookstore
11030 S Langley Avenue
Chicago, IL 60628 **202-651-5488**
800-621-2736
FAX: 202-651-5489

This monograph presents a dozen articles that demonstrate clearly and convincingly that the study of ASL affords the same educational values and the same intellectual rewards as the study of any other foreign language. *$15.95*

196 pages

2610 **Adapted Physical Activity Quarterly**
Human Kinetics
PO Box 5076
Champaign, IL 61825
800-747-4457
FAX: 217-351-2674
e-mail: humank@hkusa.com
www.humankinetics.com

Linda Bump, Director Journals

This quarterly journal contains information on current opinions, legislation, regulatory concerns, and trends. It also reports on research and investigations of case studies, programming, techniques, design of equipment and facilities. *$24.00*

Quarterly
ISSN 0736-58 9

2611 **Advance for Providers of Post-Acute Care**
Merion Publications
2900 Horizon Drive
Box 61556
King of Prussia, PA 19406 **610-278-1400**
800-355-1088
FAX: 610-278-1421
www.advanceforPAC.com

A free magazine for providers of post-acute care.

2612 **CEC Catalog**
Council for Exceptional Children
1110 N Glebe Road
Suite 300
Arlington, VA 22201 **703-620-3660**
FAX: 703-264-9494
www.cec.sped.org

Janice Burdick, President

Semi-annual catalog from the Council for Exceptional Children offering books, guides, materials, products and services for the special educator.

18 pages

2613 **Case Manager Magazine**
Mosby
10801 Executive Center Drive
Suite 509
Little Rock, AR 72211 **501-223-5165**
FAX: 501-223-0519
www.mosby.com/casemgr

Nathania Sawyer, Publisher

This national magazine is for medical case managers, social workers, counselors and home health professionals who work with people with serious injury or illness. It is a membership benefit of CMSA, the national association for case managers. *$55.00*

84 pages BiMonthly

2614 **Catalyst**
Western Ctr. for Microcomputers in Special Ed.
1259 El Camino Real
Suite 275
Menlo Park, CA 94025 **650-855-8064**
FAX: 650-324-1119
e-mail: thecatalyst@mail.earthlink.net
www.thecatalyst.us

Sue Swezey, Editor

Digest of news and information on the use of computers in special education. *$15.00*

20 pages Quarterly

2615 **Clinical Connection**
American Advertising Distibutors of Northern VA
708 Pendleton Street
Alexandria, VA 22314 **703-549-5126**
FAX: 703-548-5563

Georgina Ruley, Publisher

Covers speech language pathology.

2616 College and University

AACRAO
1 Dupont Circle NW
Suite 520
Washington, DC 20036 **202-628-1816**
FAX: 202-872-8857
e-mail: info@aacrao.com
www.aacrao.org

Scholarly research journal. American Association of Collegiate Registrars and Admissions Offers (AACRAO) is a non-profit, voluntary, professional, educational association of degree-granting postsecondary institutions, government agencies, private educational organizations and education-oriented businesses in the United States and abroad. $50 per year US; $60 per year international.

30 pages Quarterly
ISSN 0010-0889

2617 Continuing Care

Stevens Publishing Corporation
5151 Beltline Road
10th Floor
Dallas, TX 75254 **972-687-6700**
FAX: 972-687-6769
e-mail: custserv@stevenspublishing.com
www.ccareonline.com

Sandra Bienkowski, Editor
Irene Fincher, Circulation/Marketing Manager

A national magazine for case management and discharge planning professionals published monthly except for December. *$119.00*

34 pages Monthly

2618 Counseling Psychologist

American Psychological Association
2455 Teller Road
Thousand Oaks, CA 91320 **805-499-9734**
800-818-7243
FAX: 805-499-0871
e-mail: info@sagepub.com
www.sagepub.com

Thematic issues in the theory, research and practice of counseling psychology. *$78.00*

Bi-Monthly

2619 Counseling and Values

American Counseling Association
5999 Stevenson Avenue
Alexandria, VA 22304 **800-347-6647**
800-473-2329
FAX: 703-823-6862
www.counseling.org

M Harry Daniels, Editor

Counseling and Values is the official journal of the Association for Spiritual, Ethical, and Religious Values in Counseling (ASERVIC), a member association of the American Counseling Association. Counseling and Values s a professional journal of theory, research, and informed opinion concerned with the relationships among psychology, philosophy, religion, social values, and counseling. *$12.00*

TriAnnual

2620 Directions: Technology in Special Education

DREAMMS for Kids
273 Ringwood Road
Freeville, NY 13068 **607-539-3027**
FAX: 607-539-9930
www.dreamms.org

Janet P Hosmer, Contact

Provides technology tips to ease home instruction and use; describes and reviews adaptive educational software and hardware; reviews pertinent literature and audio and videotapes; describes adaptive and assistive technology devices; provides on-line service information for the disabled; announces upcoming educational and technology conference; and reports on new Department of Education legislation. *$14.95*

Monthly

2621 Disability Studies Quarterly

Department of Public Management
Suffolk University
Boston, MA 02108 **617-725-8483**
FAX: 617-573-8711
e-mail: per00906@acad.suffolk.edu

David Pfeiffer, Editor
Monique Perrier, Administrative Asst.

Contains articles on aspects of disability, often focusing on one topic, such as gender and sexuality, communication technology and measurement in disability. Also includes information on books and resources available for persons with disabilities. *$35.00*

75 pages Quarterly

2622 Early Intervention

Illinois Early Childhood Intervention
830 S Spring Street
Springfield, IL 62704 **217-522-4655**
800-852-4302
FAX: 217-522-4670
e-mail: clearinghouse@eosinc.com
www.eiclearinghouse.org

Chet Brandt, Project Director
Patricia Taylor, Project Associate

Features articles, conference calendar, material reviews and news concerning early childhood intervention and disability.

4 pages Quarterly

2623 Focus on Autism and Other Developmental Disabilities

Pro-Ed
8700 Shoal Creek Boulevard
Austin, TX 78757 **512-451-3246**
800-897-3202
FAX: 512-451-8542
e-mail: info@proedinc.com
www.proedinc.com

Practical management, treatment and planning strategies; a must for persons working with individuals with autism and other developmental disabilities. *$43.00*

64 pages Quarterly

2624 Focus on Exceptional Children

Love Publishing Company
9101 E Kenyon Avenue
Suite 2200
Denver, CO 80237 **303-221-7333**
FAX: 303-221-7444
e-mail: lovepublishing@compuserve.com

Scott Thomas, Manager

Contains research and theory-based articles on special education topics, with an emphasis on application and intervention, of interest to teachers, professors and administrators. *$36.00*

Monthly 1969

2625 HomeCare Magazine

Intertec Publishing Corporation
Stuart Ranch Road
Malibu, CA 90265 **310-317-4522**
800-543-4116
FAX: 310-317-9644
e-mail: kcavallo@interec.com
www.homecaremag.com

Karen Cavallo, Publisher

The business magazine of the home medical equipment industry offering information on legislation and regulations affecting the homecare industry, monthly profiles of suppliers, operational tips, newest products in the industry, advice on sales, government regulations. *$ 65.00*

120 pages Monthly

2626 Horizons

Haras & Trebor
PO Box 985
Gambrills, MD 21054 **301-621-9332**
FAX: 410-767-5850
TTY:301-621-9332
e-mail: storrsjh@aol.com

James Storrs, Publisher

Monthly newspaper for people with disabilities serving Maryland, Virginia, and Washington DC *$17.00*

20 pages Monthly
ISSN 1064-64 4

2627 I Wonder Who Else Can Help

AARP Fulfillment
601 E Street NW
Washington, DC 20049 **202-434-2277**
800-424-3410
FAX: 202-434-3443
e-mail: member@aarp.org
www.aarp.org

Contains information about crisis counseling, needs and resources, written in lay terms.

2628 Information from HEATH Resource Center

National Clearinghouse on Postsecondary Education
1 Dupont Circle NW
Suite 800
Washington, DC 20036 **202-939-9320**
800-544-3284
FAX: 202-833-5696
e-mail: heath@ace.nche.edu
www.HEATH-resource-center.org

The HEATH Resource Center operates the national clearinghouse on postsecondary education for individuals with disabilities. Support from the US Department of Education enables the Center, a program of the America Council on Education, to serve as an information exchange on educational support services; adaptations; and opportunities at American campuses, vocational-technical schools, adult education programs, independent living centers, and other postsecondary training entities.

2629 International Rehabilitation Review

Rehabilitation International
25 E 21st Street
New York, NY 10010 **212-505-8040**
FAX: 212-505-0871
e-mail: rehabintal@aol.com

Barbara Duncan, Editor
Kathy Marchael, Editorial Assistant

International overview of activities and programs in vocational and medical rehabilitation, prosthesis and orthotics and special education. *$30.00*

TriAnnual

2630 Intervention in School and Clinic

Pro-Ed
8700 Shoal Creek Boulevard
Austin, TX 78757 **512-451-3246**
800-897-3202
FAX: 512-451-8542
e-mail: info@proedinc.com
www.proedinc.com

A hands-on, how-to resource for teachers and clinicians working with students for whom minor curriculum and environmental modifications are ineffective. *$35.00*

64 pages

2631 Journal for Vocational Special Needs Education

University of Wisconsin
Center for Education and Work
1025 W Johnson Street
Madison, WI 53706 **608-263-2724**
FAX: 608-262-3050
e-mail: jgugerty@education.wisc.edu
www.cew.wisc.edu/jvsne/

John Gugerty, Co-Editor

Articles on vocational education for special needs population, including persons with physical and mental disabilities. *$16.00*

2632 Journal of Applied School Psychology

Haworth Press
10 Alice Street
Binghamton, NY 13904 **607-722-5857**
800-429-6784
FAX: 607-722-6362
e-mail: orders@haworthpress.com
www.haworthpress.com

Charles A Maher PsyD, Editor
S Harrington-Miller, Advertising

This journal disseminates the latest and the highest quality information to all professionals who provide special services in the schools and related educational settings. *$60.00*

BiAnnually

2633 Journal of Autism and Developmental Disabilities

Plenum Publishing Corporation
233 Spring Street
New York, NY 10013 **212-229-2859**
800-221-9369
FAX: 212-463-0742
e-mail: info@plenum.com

Eric Shopler, Editor

This journal is devoted to all the severe psychopathologies in childhood, including autism and childhood schizophrenia. *$295.00*

BiMonthly
ISSN 0162-32 7

2634 Journal of Counseling & Development

American Counseling Association
5999 Stevenson Avenue
Alexandria, VA 22304 **800-347-6647**
800-633-4931
FAX: 703-823-6862
www.counseling.org

A Scott McGowan, Editor
Carolyn Baker, Publications Director

Publishes archival material, also publishes articles that have broad interest for a readership composed mostly of counselors and other mental health professionals who work in private practice, schools, colleges, community agencies, hospitals, and government. An appropriate outlet for articles that: critcally intergrate published research; examine current professional and scientific issues; report research, new techniques, innovatetive programs and practices; and examine ACA as an organization. *$140.00*

128 pages Quarterly

2635 Journal of Developmental and Physical Disabilities

Plenum Publishing Corporation
233 Spring Street
New York, NY 10013
212-229-2859
800-221-9369
FAX: 212-807-1047
e-mail: info@plenum.com
www.kluweronline.com/issn/1056-263X

Vincent B Van Hasselt, Co-editor
Michel Hersen, Co-editor

This journal serves as a unified outlet for dissemination of work with all handicapped populations. research and clinical reports from a variety of services for multihandicapped individuals discuss such concerns as the deaf-blind, cerebral-palsied deaf, blind-mentally retarded, and emotionally disturbed retarded. Case studies originate from many professional fields including psychology, rehabilitation, special education, counseling, social work, psychiatry and rehabilitation medicine. *$46.00*

Quarterly
ISSN 1056-26 0

2636 Journal of Emotional and Behavioral Disorders

Pro-Ed
8700 Shoal Creek Boulevard
Austin, TX 78757
512-451-3246
800-897-3202
FAX: 512-451-8542
e-mail: info@proedinc.com
www.proedinc.com

An international, multidisciplinary journal featuring articles on research, practice and theory related to individuals with emotional and behavioral disorders and to the professionals who serve them. *$39.00*

64 pages Quarterly

2637 Journal of Learning Disabilities

Pro-Ed
8700 Shoal Creek Boulevard
Austin, TX 78757
800-897-3202
FAX: 512-302-9129
e-mail: proed1@aol.com
www.proedinc.com

Judith K Voress PhD, Periodicals Director

An international, multidisciplinary publication containing articles on practice, research and theory related to learning disabilities. Published bi-monthly. *$49.00*

Magazine

2638 Journal of Motor Behavior

Heldref Publications
1319 18th Street NW
Washington, DC 20036
202-296-6267
800-365-9753
FAX: 202-293-6130
e-mail: subscribe@heldref.org
www.heldref.org

Francine Hamme, Marketing Manager

A professional journal aimed at psychologists, therapists and educators who work in the areas of motor behavior, psychology, neurophysiology, kinesiology, and biomechanics. Offers up-to-date information on the latest techniques, theories and developments concerning motor control. *$77.00*

115 pages Quarterly 1969

2639 Journal of Musculoskeletal Pain

Haworth Press
10 Alice Street
Binghamton, NY 13904
607-722-5857
800-429-6784
FAX: 607-722-6362
e-mail: orders@haworthpress.com
www.haworthpress.com

I Jon Russell MD, PhD, Editor
Barbara Runnells, Managing Editor
S Harrington-Miller, Advertising

This journal serves as a central resource for the dissemination of information about musculoskeletal pain. *$75.00*

110 pages Quarterly

2640 Journal of Postsecondary Education & Disability

AHEAD
100 Morrissey Boulevard
Boston, MA 02125
617-287-3880
FAX: 617-287-3881
TTY:617-287-3882
e-mail: ahead@postbox.acs.ohio_state.edu
www.ahead.org

Provides in-depth examination of research, issues, policies and programs in postsecondary education.

2641 Journal of Prosthetics and Orthotics

Orthotics and Prosthetics National Office
330 John Carlyle Street
Suite 210
Alexandria, VA 22314
703-836-7114
FAX: 703-836-0838
e-mail: info@abcop.org
www.abcop.org

Stacey L Bell, Managing Editor

Provides the latest research and clinical thinking in orthotics and prosthetics, including information on new devices, fitting techniques and patient management experiences. Each issue contains research-based information and articles reviewed and approved by a highly qualified editorial board. *$60.00*

64 pages Quarterly
ISSN 1040-88 0

2642 Journal of Reading, Writing and Learning Disabled International

Hemisphere Publishing Corporation
1900 Frost Road
Suite 101
Bristol, PA 19007
215-785-5800
FAX: 215-785-6616

Articles on reading, writing and learning disabilities, including mainstreaming issues. *$9.00*

2643 Journal of Special Education

Pro-Ed
8700 Shoal Creek Boulevard
Austin, TX 78757
800-897-3202
FAX: 512-302-9129
e-mail: proed1@aol.com
www.proedinc.com

Judith K Voress PhD, Periodicals Director

Internationally known as the prime research journal in special education. JSE provides research articles of special education for individuals with disabilities, ranging from mild to severe. Published quarterly. *$39.00*

Magazine

2644 **Journal of Vocational Behavior**

Academic Press, Journals Division
525 B Street
Suite 1900
San Diego, CA 92101 **619-231-0926**
www.academicpress.com/jvb

The Journal of Vocational Behavior publishes empirical and theoretical articles that expand knowledge of vocational behavior and career development across the life span. Research presented in the journal encompasses the general categories of career choice, implementation, and vocational adjustment and adaptation. The articles are also valuable for applications in counseling and career development programs in colleges and universities, business and industry, government, and the military. *$7.00*

2645 **Lifespan**

Nat'l Council for Community Behavioral Healthcare
12300 Twinbrook Parkway
Suite 320
Rockville, MD 20852 **301-984-6200**
FAX: 301-881-7159
www.nccbh.org

Information on tax tips, insurance, medical care, law and legislation for people with mental disabilities.

Monthly

2646 **MDA Newsmagazine**

Muscular Dystrophy Association
2900 N Swan Road # 201
Tucson, AZ 85712 **520-795-3434**
FAX: 520-795-3989
e-mail: tusconservice@mdausa.org

Kelly Larkin, District Director

Presents news related to muscular dystrophy and other neuromuscular diseases including research, personal profiles, fundraising activities and patient services.

2647 **Measurement and Evaluation in Counseling and Development**

American Association for Counseling & Development
5999 Stevenson Avenue
Alexandria, VA 22304 **800-347-6647**
800-473-2329
FAX: 703-823-6862
www.counseling.org

William D Schafer, Editor

Journal with professional articles on testing and evaluation. *$23.00*

Quarterly

2648 **Our World**

National Center for Learning Disabilities
381 Park Avenue S
Suite 1401
New York, NY 10016 **212-545-7510**
888-575-7373
FAX: 212-545-9665
ld.org

James H Wendorf, Executive Director
Pazit Algazi, Communications/Marketing Coord.

Contains features, articles, human interest news and information and information, and other practical material to benefit the millions of children and adults with learning disabilities and their families, as well as educators and other helping professionals. Magazine

Quarterly

2649 **Psychiatric Staffing Crisis in Community Mental Health**

Nat'l Council for Community Behavioral Healthcare
12300 Twinbrook Parkway
Suite 320
Rockville, MD 20852 **301-984-6200**
FAX: 301-881-7159
www.nccbh.org

Find out some of the simple, low-cost ways you can increase workplace satisfaction among staff psychiatrists and compete successfully for their talents. *$20.00*

2650 **Readings: A Journal of Reviews and Commentary in Mental Health**

American Orthopsychiatric Association
330 7th Avenue
18th Floor
New York, NY 10001 **212-268-1399**
FAX: 212-564-6180
e-mail: amerortho@aol.com

Joan Adler, Managing Editor

Reviews of recent books in mental health and allied disciplines. Includes essay reviews and brief reviews. *$25.00*

32 pages Quarterly

2651 **Rehab Pro**

Int. Association of Rehabilitation Professionals
Framingham Office Park
1661 Worcester Road, Suite 203
Framingham, MA 01701 **508-820-8889**
800-240-9059
FAX: 831-464-4881
e-mail: phawkes@ix.netcom.com
www.rehabpro.org

Raph Crystal, Journal Editor
Leona Liberty, NASPPR Section Editor

The magazine is to promote the profession and to inform the public about the activities of the national organization, its state chapter affiliates, and the work of its special interest sections.

38 pages BiMonthly

2652 **Remedial and Special Education**

Pro-Ed
8700 Shoal Creek Boulevard
Austin, TX 78757 **512-451-3246**
800-897-3202
FAX: 512-451-8542
e-mail: info@proedinc.com
www.proedinc.com

A professional journal that bridges the gap between theory and practice. Emphasis is on topical reviews, syntheses of research, field evaluation studies and recommendations for the practice of remedial and special education. Published six times a year. *$39.00*

64 pages

2653 **Teaching Exceptional Children**

Council for Exceptional Children
1110 N Glebe Road
Suite 300
Arlington, VA 22201 **703-620-3660**
FAX: 703-264-9494
www.cec.sped.org

Janice Burdick, President

Journal designed for teachers of gifted students and students with disabilities, featuring practical methods and materials for classroom use. *$58.00*

96 pages BiMonthly

2654 **Topics in Language Disorders**

Aspen Publishers
200 Orchard Ridge Drive
Gaithersburg, MD 20878 **301-698-7100**
800-234-1660
FAX: 301-695-7931
www.aspenpublishers.com

Jack Bruggeman, Publisher

Peer review journal for professionals in the field of language disorders. Published quarterly. *$86.00*

104 pages

Newsletters

2655 **Alert**

Ass'n on Handicapped Student Service Programs
PO Box 21192
Columbus, OH 43221 **614-365-5216**
FAX: 614-365-6718

Keeps members informed about Association activities, current legislative issues, innovative programs, and more. *$30.00*

2656 **Camp Virginia Jaycee Newsletter**

2494 Camp Jaycee Road
Blue Ridge, VA 24064 **540-947-2972**
800-865-0092
FAX: 540-947-2043
e-mail: ewerness@campvirginiajaycee.com
www.campvirginiajaycee.com

Everett M Werness, President
Lauren Lightfoot, Camp Director

Summer camping for children and adults with developmental disabilities. Coed, ages 7-70. Weekend respite camps for children and adults with mental retardation.

8 pages quarterly

2657 **Counseling Today**

American Counseling Association
5999 Stevenson Avenue
Alexandria, VA 22304 **800-347-6647**
800-473-2329
FAX: 703-823-6862
www.counseling.org

Jennifer L Sacks, Editor

Aims to serve individuals active in porfessional counseling, in the school and university, in the workplace and the marketplace, as well as other citizens, community leaders and policy makers who appreciate the importance of the role of professional counselors in today's society.

Monthly

2658 **Counselor Education and Supervision**

American Counseling Association
5999 Stevenson Avenue
Alexandria, VA 22304 **800-347-6647**
800-473-2329
FAX: 703-823-6862
www.counseling.org

Margaret L Fong, Editor

$18.00

Quarterly

2659 **Counterpoint**

Nat'l Assoc. of State Directors of Special Educ.
10860 Hampton Road
Fairfax Station, VA 22039 **703-239-1557**
FAX: 703-503-8627

Newspaper designed for teachers of disabled and gifted students, featuring practical methods and materials for classroom use. *$36.00*

Quarterly

2660 **Disability Compliance for Higher Education**

LRP Publications
PO Box 24668
West Palm Beach, FL 33416 **215-784-0941**
800-341-7874
FAX: 215-784-9639
e-mail: custserve@lrp.com
www.lrp.com

The only newsletter that is dedicated to the exclusive coverage of disability issues that affect colleges and universities. *$195.00*

8 pages Monthly

2661 **Disability Resources Monthly**

Disability Resources
4 Glatter Lane
Centereach, NY 11720 **631-585-0290**
FAX: 631-585-0290
e-mail: info@disabilityresources.org
www.disabilityresources.org

Avery Klauber, Director

A newsletter that monitors, reviews and reports on resources for independent living. A monthly newsletter that features short topical articles, news items and reviews of books, pamphlets, periodicals, videotapes, on-line services, organizations and other resources for and about people with disabilities. It is intended primarily for librarians, social workers, educators, rehabilitation specialists, disability advocates, ADA coordinators and other health and social service professionals. *$33.00*

4 pages Monthly 1993

ISSN 1070-72 0

2662 **Early Childhood Reporter**

LRP Publications
747 Dresher Road
Suite 980
Horsham, PA 19044
800-341-7874
FAX: 215-784-9014
e-mail: custserve@lrp.com
www.lrp.com/ed

Frank Diamond, Managing Editor

Monthly reports with information on federal, state, and local legislation affecting the implementation of early intervention and preschool programs for children with disabilities. *$145.00*

12-16 pages $10 shipping

2663 **Fact Sheets**

University of New Hampshire: Inst on Disability
7 Leavitt Lane
Suite 101
Durham, NH 03824 **603-862-4320**
FAX: 603-862-0555
e-mail: institutedisability@unh.edu
www.iod.unh.edu

The institute on Disability provides information to family consumers, community personnel and professionals through books articles, videos, newsletters, internet and press coverage, including TV, radio and consumers forums.

2664 **Forum**

Ohio Coalition for Children with Disabilities
165 W Center Street
Bank One Building, Suite 302
Marion, OH 43302 **740-382-5452**
800-374-2806
FAX: 740-383-6421
e-mail: oceed@gte.net

Forum is a newsletter reporting on legislative and other developments affecting persons with disabilities. Other books offered include (all prices include shipping and handling): How to Write an IEP ($12.95), Accessing the General Curriculum ($12.95), and It's My Turn: Board Game ($27.95).

8 pages BiMonthly

2665 **Healthline**

CV Mosby Company
11830 Westline Industrial Drive
Saint Louis, MO 63146 **314-872-8370**
800-325-4177
FAX: 314-432-1380
e-mail: journal.service@mosby.com
www.mosby.com

Paul Insel, Editor

Health and fitness information for healthcare professionals and the general public alike.

Monthly

2666 **Help Newsletter**

Learning Disabilities Assn. of Arkansas
7509 Cantrell
Suite 103C
Little Rock, AR 72207 **501-666-8777**
FAX: 501-666-4070
e-mail: LDAA@sbcglobal.net
www.ldaarkansas.org

Bobbie Boyd, President
Dama K Jackson, Executive Administrator
Kristen Joyner, Direcotr Development

Information on how to overcome obstacles and to achieve in spite of learning disabilities. *$30.00*

8 pages Quarterly

2667 **Home Health Agency Gazette**

American Federation of Home Health Agencies
1320 Fenwick Lane
Suite 500
Silver Spring, MD 20910 **301-588-1454**
FAX: 301-588-4732
e-mail: afhha@his.com
www.atf.org/healthcare/sites/homehealth.html

Joan Guberman, Editor

Focuses on regulatory and legislative issues of interest to the home health care industry.

2668 **Inside the NIDCD Information Clearinghouse Newsletter**

NIDCD Information Clearinghouse
1 NOHIC Way
Bethesda, MD 20892 **301-402-7364**
FAX: 301-907-8830
e-mail: nohic@nidcr.nih.gov
www.nohic.nidcr.nih.gov

Biannual newsletter, resource directory, professional/consumer fact sheets, brochures, information packets and reports.

BiAnnually

2669 **International Rolf Institute**

PO Box 1868
Boulder, CO 80306 **303-449-5903**

Information, practitioner training and certification.

2670 **Learning Disabilities Consultants Newsletter**

Learning Disabilities Consultants
PO Box 716
Bryn Mawr, PA 19010 **610-668-2225**
800-869-8336
FAX: 610-446-6129

Richard Cooper, Director

Newsletter providing information about learning disabilities and differences. It contains both local and national news items and includes in each issue articles about various aspects of learning problems encountered in both children and adults. *$10.00*

6 pages 5x Year

2671 **NYALD News**

New York Association for the Learning Disabled
90 S Swan Street
Albany, NY 12210 **518-432-5787**
FAX: 518-432-5902

Kelly Jarrard, Executive Director

Newsletter offering information on the learning disabled in the New York area.

Monthly

2672 **O&P Almanac**

American Orthotic & Prosthetic Association
330 John Carlyle Street
Suite 200
Alexandria, VA 22314 **571-431-0876**
FAX: 571-431-0899
e-mail: info@aopanet.org
www.aopanet.org

Lisa Gough, Editor in Chief
Carrie Parsons, Managing Editor

Offers in-depth coverage on orthotics and prosthetics to current professional, government, business and reimbursement activities affecting the orthotics and prosthetics industry. *$59.00*

80 pages Monthly

2673 **Occupational Therapy in Health Care**

Haworth Press
10 Alice Street
Binghamton, NY 13904 **607-722-5857**
800-429-6784
FAX: 607-722-6362
e-mail: orders@haworthpress.com
www.haworthpress.com

S Harrington-Miller, Advertising
Anne E Dickerson, Editor

Each issue focuses on significant practices and concerns involving occupational therapy and therapists. *$75.00*

2674 SAMHSA News

US Department of Health and Human Services
5600 Fishers Lane
Suite 13C-05
Rockville, MD 20857 **301-443-8956**
FAX: 301-443-9050
www.samhsa.gov

Mark Weber, Associate Administrator, Commun.
Deborah Goodmad, Public Affairs Specialist

This quarterly Agency newsletter reports on information on substance abuse, mental health treatment and prevention programs of the Substance Abuse and Mental Health Services Administration.

Quarterly

2675 Sibling Information Network Newsletter

AJ Pappanikou Center
249 Glenbrook Road Unit U-64
Storrs Mansfield, CT 06269 **860-486-3493**

Lisa Glidden, Coordinator

Contains information aimed at the varying interested of our membership. Program descriptions, requests for assistance, conference announcements, literature summaries and research reports. *$8.50*

2676 Sibpage

AJ Pappanikou Center
249 Glenbrook Road
Suite U-64
Storrs Mansfield, CT 06269 **860-486-3493**

Lisa Glidden, Coordinator

Developed specifically for children containing games, recipes, pen pals, and articles written by siblings relating to developmental disabilities.

4 pages

2677 Sower

Beatrice State Development Center
3000 Lincoln Boulevard
Beatrice, NE 68310 **402-223-6002**
FAX: 402-223-6073

Current programs, objectives and goals, needs and actual happenings at the institution.

12 pages

2678 Special Education Report

Capitol Publications
1101 King Street
Suite 44
Alexandria, VA 22314 **703-683-4100**
800-655-5597
FAX: 703-793-6517

Xavier Briand, Editor
Claudia Moran, Marketing Manager

Current, pertinent information about federal legislation, regulations, programs and funding for educating children with disabilities. Covers federal and state litigation on the Individuals with Disabilities Education Act and other relevant laws. Looks at innovations and research in the field. *$266.00*

8 pages BiWeekly
ISSN 0194-22 5

2679 Topics in Early Childhood Special Education

Pro-Ed
8700 Shoal Creek Boulevard
Austin, TX 78757 **512-451-3246**
800-897-3202
FAX: 512-451-8542
e-mail: info@proedinc.com
www.proedinc.com

Designed for professionals helping young children with special needs in areas such as assessment, special programs, social policies and developmental aids. *$43.00*

Quarterly

2680 Treatment Review

AIDS Treatment Data Network
611 Broadway
Suite 613
New York, NY 10012 **212-260-8868**
800-734-7104
FAX: 212-260-8869
e-mail: network@atdn.org
www.aidsinfonyc.org/network

Ken Fernataro, Executive Director
Tracy Swan, Access Project Director

Individual members recieve treatment education, counseling, referrals and case management support. Services are available in both English and Spanish. The Treatment Review newsletter includes descriptions of approved, alternative and experimental treatments, as well as announcements of seminars and forums on treatments and clinical trials.

Quarterly

Professional Texts

2681 A Teacher's Guide to Galatosemia

Arizona Department of Health Services
1740 W Adams
Office of Nutrition Services
Phoenix, AZ 85007 **602-542-1886**
FAX: 602-542-1890
www.hs.state.az.us/cfhs/ons/

Resource book for preschool teachers and school staff on PKU basics, NutraSweet warning, and classroom activities. *$2.50*

13 pages

2682 A Teacher's Guide to HCU

Arizona Department of Health Services
1740 W Adams
Office of Nutrition Services
Phoenix, AZ 85007 **602-542-1886**
FAX: 602-542-1890
www.hs.state.az.us/cfhs/ons/

Resource book for preschool teachers and school staff on Homocysteinuria basics and classroom activities. *$2.50*

2683 A Teacher's Guide to Isovaleric Acidemia

Arizona Department of Health Services
1740 W Adams
Office of Nutrition Services
Phoenix, AZ 85007 **602-542-0186**
FAX: 602-542-1890
www.hs.state.az.us/cfhs/ons/

Resource book for preschool teachers and school staff on Isovaleric Acidemia basics and classroom activities. *$2.50*

2684 A Teacher's Guide to MSUD

Arizona Department of Health Services
1740 W Adams
Office of Nutrition Services
Phoenix, AZ 85007
602-542-1886
FAX: 602-542-1890
www.hs.state.az.us/cfhs/ons/

Resource book for preschool teachers and school staff on MSUD basics and classroom activities. *$2.50*

2685 A Teacher's Guide to Methylmalonic Acidemia

Arizona Department of Health Services
1740 W Adams
Office of Nutrition Services
Phoenix, AZ 85007
602-542-1886
FAX: 602-542-1890
www.hs.state.az.us/cfhs/ons/

Resource book for preschool teachers and school staff on Methylmalonic Acidemia basics and classroom activities. *$2.50*

2686 A Teacher's Guide to PKU

Arizona Department of Health Services
1740 W Adams
Office of Nutrition Services
Phoenix, AZ 85007
602-542-1886
FAX: 602-542-1890
www.hs.state.az.us/cfhs/ons/

Resource book for preschool teachers and school staff on PKU basics, NutraSweet warning, and classroom activities. *$2.50*

13 pages

2687 A Teacher's Guide to Propionic Acidemia

Arizona Department of Health Services
1740 W Adams
Office of Nutrition Services
Phoenix, AZ 85007
602-542-1886
FAX: 602-542-1890
www.hs.state.az.us/cfhs/ons/

Resource book for preschool teachers and school staff on Propionic Acidemia basics and classroom activities. *$2.50*

2688 AEPS Curriculum for Birth to Three Years

Brookes Publishing
PO Box 10624
Baltimore, MD 21285
410-337-9580
800-638-3775
FAX: 410-337-8539
e-mail: custserv@brookespublishing.com
www.brookespublishing.com

Directly linked to IEP/IFSP goals developed for a child from the AEPS test measure, the AEPS curriculum provides a complete set of learning activities to facilitate children's acquisition of functional skills. *$59.95*

496 pages
ISBN 1-557660-96-4

2689 Access to Health Care: Number 1&2

World Institute on Disability
510 16th Street
Suite 100
Oakland, CA 94612
510-763-4100
FAX: 510-763-4109
e-mail: wid@wid.org
www.wid.org

These health policy bulletins analyze health care needs. Volume 1 focuses on a wide range of information relevant to addressing the adequacy of the health care system for persons with disabilities or chronic illness. *$6.50*

63 pages Paperback

2690 Access to Health Care: Number 3&4

World Institute on Disability
510 16th Street
Suite 100
Oakland, CA 94612
510-763-4100
FAX: 510-763-4109
e-mail: wid@wid.org
www.wid.org

These policy bulletins focus on the capacity of the private and public health insurance systems to respond to the health care needs of persons with disabilities or chronic illness. *$6.50*

91 pages Paperback

2691 Activity-Based Approach to Early Intervention: Second Edition

Brookes Publishing
PO Box 10624
Baltimore, MD 21285
410-337-9580
800-638-3775
FAX: 410-337-8539
e-mail: custserv@brookespublishing.com
www.brookespublishing.com

Activity-based intervention shows how to use natural and relevant events to teach infants and young children, of all abilities, effectively and efficiently. *$24.00*

240 pages
ISBN 1-55766 -87-5

2692 Adapting Early Childhood Curricula for Children with Special Needs

McGraw-Hill, School Publishing
220 E Danieldale Road
DeSoto, TX 75115
972-224-1111
800-442-9685
FAX: 972-228-1982
mhschool.com

Offers information on educating the disabled.

2693 Adaptive Education Strategies Building on Diversity

Paul H Brookes Publishing Company
PO Box 10624
Baltimore, MD 21285
800-638-3775
FAX: 410-337-8539

Based on more than two decades of systematic research, this comprehensive manual provides a road map to the effective implementation of adaptive education. *$35.00*

304 pages Paperback 1992
ISBN 1-557880-84-0

2694 Advanced Sign Language Vocabulary: A Resource Text for Educators

2600 S 1st Street
Springfield, IL 62704
217-789-8980
800-258-8980
FAX: 217-789-9130
e-mail: books@ccthomas.com
www.ccthomas.com

This book is a collection of advanced sign language vocabulary for use by educators, interpreters, parents or anyone wishing to enlarge their sign vocabulary. *$48.95*

202 pages Paperback 1991
ISBN 0-398057-22-2

2695 **Advances in Cardiac and Pulmonary Rehabilitation**

Haworth Press
10 Alice Street
Binghamton, NY 13904
607-722-5857
800-429-6784
FAX: 607-722-6362
e-mail: orders@haworthpress.com
www.haworthpress.com

S Harrington-Miller, Advertising

Enhance your rehabilitation program with this authoritative volume. *$34.95*

74 pages Hardcover
ISBN 0-866869-86-3

2696 **Aging Brain**

Taylor & Francis
47 Runway Drive
 # G
Levittown, PA 19057
215-269-0400
FAX: 215-625-2940

Elderly treatment.

225 pages Paperback
ISBN 0-85066 -78-0

2697 **Aging and Rehabilitation II**

Springer Publishing Company
536 Broadway
New York, NY 10012
212-431-4370
877-687-7476
FAX: 212-941-7842
e-mail: marketing@springerpub.com
www.springerpub.com

Annette Imperati, Marketing/Sales Director

Current, multidisciplinary investigations of various practice issues. Leading experts in the field use a practical perspective to provide specific comments on interventions. The scope of this work encompasses the autonomy of elderly disabled, mobility, mental health and value issues, as well as basic aspects in rehabilitation of the elderly. *$41.95*

367 pages Hardcover
ISBN 0-82617 -80-3

2698 **Alphabetic Phonics Curriculum**

Educators Publishing Service
31 Smith Place
Cambridge, MA 02138
617-367-2700
800-225-5750
FAX: 617-547-0412
www.epsbooks.com

Ungraded multisensory curriculum for teaching phonics and the structure of language. Uses Orton-Gillingham approach to teach handwriting, spelling, reading, reading comprehension, and oral and written expression. program includes basic manual, workbooks, tests, teachers' guides, drill cards and all cards. *$28.15*

ISSN 8388-42

2699 **Alternative Educational Delivery Systems**

National Association of School Psychologists
8455 Colesville Road
Suite 1000
Silver Spring, MD 20910
301-681-3223
FAX: 301-495-8804

A book offering information to the professional on how to enhance educational options for all students.

2700 **Alternative Teaching Strategies**

Special Needs Project
324 State Street
Suite H
Santa Barbara, CA 93101
800-333-6867
FAX: 805-962-5087
www.specialneeds.com

Offers help for teachers who teach behaviorally troubled students achieve.

2701 **Antecedent Control: Innovative Approaches to Behavioral Support**

Brookes Publishing
PO Box 10624
Baltimore, MD 21285
410-337-9585
800-638-3775
FAX: 410-337-8539
e-mail: custserv@brookespublishing.com
www.brookespublishing.com

This book explains the theory and methodology of antecedent control. The treatment techniques in this book are effective for both children and adults.

416 pages Paperback 1998
ISBN 1-55766 -34-3

2702 **Applied Kinesiology: Muscle Response in Diagnosis, Therapy and Preventive Medicine**

Inner Traditions
One Park Street
Rochester, VT 05767
802-767-3174
800-246-8648
FAX: 802-767-3726
e-mail: orders@innertraditions.com
www.InnerTraditions.com

Jessica Dudley, Sales Associate

$12.95

144 pages
ISBN 0-892813-28-8

2703 **Applied Rehabilitation Counseling**

Springer Publishing Company
536 Broadway
New York, NY 10012
212-431-4370
877-687-7476
FAX: 212-941-7842
e-mail: marketing@springerpub.com
www.springerpub.com

Annette Imperati, Marketing/Sales Director

This comprehensive text describes current theories, techniques, and their applications to specific disabled populations. Perspectives on varying counseling approaches such as psychodynamic, existential, gestalt, behavioral and psychoeducational orientations are systematically outlined in an easy-to-follow format. Practical applications for counseling are emphasized with attention given to strategies, goal-setting and on-going evaluations. *$29.95*

400 pages Softcover
ISBN 0-82615 -70-4

2704 **Art-Centered Education and Therapy for Children with Disabilities**

Charles C Thomas
2600 S 1st Street
Springfield, IL 62704 **217-789-8980**
800-258-8980
FAX: 217-789-9130
e-mail: books@ccthomas.com
www.ccthomas.com

This book has been written to help both the regular education, and art and special education teachers, both pre- and in-service, better understand some of the issues and realities of providing education and remediation to children with disabilities. The book is also offered as model concept that has govern the author's personal and professional career of over thirty years. *$35.95*

284 pages Paperback
ISBN 0-398060-06-1

2705 **Assessing the Handicaps/Needs of Children**

Books on Special Children
PO Box 305
Congers, NY 10920 **845-638-1236**
FAX: 845-638-0847
e-mail: irene@boscbooks.com

Papers on treatment, rehab and social support in assessing the needs of mentally retarded children. *$66.00*

260 pages Hardcover
ISBN 0-12218 -02-0

2706 **Assessment & Management of Mainstreamed Hearing-Impaired Children**

Pro-Ed Publications
8700 Shoal Creek Boulevard
Austin, TX 78757 **512-451-3246**
800-897-3202
FAX: 512-451-8542
e-mail: info@proedinc.com
www.proedinc.com

The theoretical and practical considerations of developing appropriate programming for hearing-impaired children who are being educated in mainstream educational settings are presented in this book.

2707 **Assessment Log & Developmental Progress Charts for the Carolina Curriculum-CCITSN & CCPSN**

Brookes Publishing
PO Box 10624
Baltimore, MD 21285 **410-337-9580**
800-638-3775
FAX: 410-337-8539
e-mail: custserv@brookespublishing.com
www.brookespublishing.com

This 28-page booklet allows the progress of children with skills in the 12-36 month development range to be easily recorded. Available in packages of 10. *$23.00*

28 pages Saddle-stiched
ISBN 1-557662-21-5

2708 **Assessment and Remediation of Articulatory and Phonological Disorders**

McGraw-Hill, School Publishing
220 E Danieldale Road
DeSoto, TX 75115 **972-224-1111**
800-442-9685
FAX: 972-228-1982
mhschool.com

Offers comprehensive coverage of articulation disorders.

2709 **Assessment in Mental Handicap: A Guide to Assessment Practices & Tests**

Brookline Books
PO Box 1046
Cambridge, MA 02238 **617-868-0360**
800-666-2665
FAX: 617-868-1772
e-mail: brooklinebks@delphi.com
www.brooklinebooks.com

Helps professionals understand the rationale and uses for assessment practices, and provides details of appropriate instruments within each type: adaptive behavior scales, assessment of behavioral disturbances, early development and Plagetian tests. *$20.00*

Hardcover
ISBN 0-91479 -31-X

2710 **Assessment of Children and Youth**

Longman Education/Addison Wesley
1185 Avenue of the Americas
New York, NY 10036 **212-843-0352**
800-322-1377
FAX: 800-333-3328
www.longman.awl.com

Ginny Blanford, Editor

Introductory text for preservice and in-service special educators on assessment, based on the principle that every child is unique. Comprehensive coverage of both formal and informal assessment instruments. *$50.00*

640 pages Paperback
ISBN 0-80131 -02-5

2711 **Assessment of Individuals with Severe Disabilities**

Paul H Brookes Publishing Company
PO Box 10624
Baltimore, MD 21285
800-638-3775
FAX: 410-337-8539

Karen G Radke, Marketing Director

This expanded text offers instructors guidelines to design a comprehensive educational assessment for individuals with severe disabilities. *$34.00*

432 pages Paperback 1991
ISBN 1-557660-67-0

2712 **Assessment of the Technology Needs of Vending Facilitiy Managers In Tennessee**

Mississippi State University
PO Box 6189
Mississippi State, MS 39762 **662-325-2001**
800-675-7782
FAX: 662-325-8989
www.blind.msstate.edu/

Kelly Schaefer, Publications Manager
John Maxson, Training Director

This report summarizes the results and recommendations of a survey conducted of vending facility managers throughout the state of Tennessee who participate in the Randolph-Sheppard program. *$10.00*

39 pages Paperback

2713 **Assessment: The Special Educator's Role**

Brooks/Cole Publishing Company
511 Forest Lodge Road
Pacific Grove, CA 93950 **831-373-0728**
FAX: 831-375-6414
e-mail: bc-info@brookscole.com

Aimed at students with little or no classroom experience in assessment, the book focuses on the integration of dynamic, curriculum-based and norm-referenced data for diagnostic decisions and program planning.

580 pages Casebound
ISBN 0-53421 -32-1

2714 **Asthma Management and Education**

Asthma and Allergy Foundation of America
1125 15th Street NW
Suite 502
Washington, DC 20005 **202-466-7643**
FAX: 202-466-8940
e-mail: info@aafa.org
www.aafa.org

One session, two hour program developed to educate allied health professionals about up-to-date asthma care and patient education, information and materials. Includes hands on experience with peak flow meters and demonstrations of medical devices.

2715 **Aston-Patterning**

PO Box 3568
Incline Village, NV 89450 **775-831-8228**
FAX: 775-831-8955
e-mail: info@astonenterprises.com
www.astonenterprises.com

Jane Davis, Administrative Assistant

Integrated system of movement education, body assessment, environmental modification and fitness training.

2716 **Attention Deficit Disorder in Children and Adolescents**

Charles C Thomas
2600 S 1st Street
Springfield, IL 62704 **217-789-8980**
800-258-8980
FAX: 217-789-9130
e-mail: books@ccthomas.com
www.ccthomas.com

Jack Fadely, Author
Virginia N Hosler, Author

Presents an analysis of case studies of children and adolescents with attentional deficits and hyperactivity, demonstrating causal factors in these disorders and suggesting treatment strategies both in psychological and medical practice. Written as a review and summary of twenty years of private practice. *$35.95*

292 pages Paperback
ISBN 0-39806 -12-2

2717 **Aural Habilitation**

Alexander Graham Bell Association
3417 Volta Place NW
Washington, DC 20007 **202-337-5220**
FAX: 202-337-8314
e-mail: info@agbell.org
www.agbell.org

This classic text for professionals educators and parents discusses verbal learning and aural habilitation of young children with hearing losses to ensure that each child is educated in the best setting. It discusses communication, normal development of spoken language, speech audiologic assessment, hearing aids and use of residual hearing, and program designs for individualized needs, including the assessment and planning of IEPs. *$26.95*

324 pages

2718 **Behavior Analysis in Education: Focus on Measurably Superior Instruction**

Brooks/Cole Publishing Company
511 Forest Lodge Road
Pacific Grove, CA 93950 **831-373-0728**
FAX: 831-375-6414
e-mail: bc-info@brookscole.com

Designed to disseminate measurably superior instructional strategies to those interested in advancing sound, pedagogically effective, field-tested educational practices, this book is intended for graduate-level courses and seminars in special education and/or psychology focusing on behavior analysis and instruction.

512 pages Casebound
ISBN 0-53422 -60-9

2719 **Behavior Modification**

Sage Periodicals Press
2455 Teller Road
Thousand Oaks, CA 91320 **805-499-9734**
FAX: 805-499-0871
www.sagepublications.com

Describes in detail for replication purposes assessment and modification techniques for problems in psychiatric, clinical, educational and rehabilitation settings. *$53.00*

640 pages Quarterly

2720 **Behavior Therapy for Developmentally Disabled**

Books on Special Children
PO Box 305
Congers, NY 10920 **845-638-1236**
FAX: 845-638-0847
e-mail: irene@boscbooks.com

Definitions, treatments, and behavioral approaches for language deficits, visually impaired, autistic children and adults. *$ 47.50*

416 pages Softcover

2721 **Behavioral Disorders**

Council for Exceptional Children
1110 N Glebe Road
Suite 300
Arlington, VA 22201 **703-620-3660**
FAX: 703-264-9494
www.cec.sped.org

Janice Burdick, President

Provides professionals with a means to exchange information and share ideas related to research, empirically tested educational innovations and issues and concerns relevant to students with behavioral disorders. Individual, $20; Institution, $50.

Quarterly

2722 **Behind Special Education**

Love Publishing Company
4925 E Pacific Place
 # 22353
Denver, CO 80222
303-221-7333
FAX: 303-221-7444
e-mail: lovepublishing@compuserve.com

This new work is a critical analysis of the nature of disability, special education, school organization and reform progress. *$24.95*

ISBN 0-89108 -17-4

2723 **Beyond Drill & Practice: Expanding the Computer Mainstream**

Council for Exceptional Children
1110 N Glebe Road
Suite 300
Arlington, VA 22201
703-620-3660
FAX: 703-264-9494
www.cec.sped.org

Janice Burdick, President

Explore the use of the computer for teaching and motivating children with disabilities and other problem learners. Let teachers use these programs and strategies that show you how it works. *$10.00*

120 pages

2724 **Biomedical Concerns in Persons with Down's Syndrome**

Paul H Brookes Publishing Company
PO Box 10624
Baltimore, MD 21285
800-638-3775
FAX: 410-337-8539

Karen G Radke, Marketing Director

Written by leading authorities and spanning many disciplines and specialties, this comprehensive resource provides vital information on biomedical issues concerning individuals with Down's Syndrome. *$45.00*

336 pages Hardcover 1992
ISBN 1-557660-89-1

2725 **Breaking Barriers**

AbleNet
1081 10th Avenue SE
Minneapolis, MN 55414
800-322-0956
FAX: 612-379-9143
e-mail: customerservice@ablenetinc.com
www.ablenetinc.com

A practical resource for parents, caregivers, teachers and therapists. *$15.00*

2726 **Building and Evaluating Family Support Initiatives**

Paul H Brookes Publishing Company
PO Box 10624
Baltimore, MD 21285
800-638-3775
FAX: 410-337-8539

Karen G Radke, Marketing Director

This essential sourcebook describes the conceptual framework, mythology and recent findings of a national study on the status of family support initiatives for persons with developmental disabilities. *$31.00*

336 pages Paperback 1993
ISBN 1-557661-22-7

2727 **Building the Healing Partnership: Parents, Professionals and Children**

Brookline Books
PO Box 1046
Cambridge, MA 02238
617-868-0360
800-666-2665
FAX: 617-868-1772
e-mail: brooklinebks@delphi.com
www.brooklinebooks.com

Successful programs understand that the disabled child's needs must be considered in the context of a family. This book was specifically written for practitioner's who must work with families but who have insufficient training in family systems assessment and intervention. It is a valuable blend of theory and practice with pointers for applying the principles. *$24.95*

Paperback
ISBN 0-91479 -63-8

2728 **Career Assessment Inventories Learning Disabled**

CFKR Career Materials
11860 Kemper Road
Suite 7
Auburn, CA 95603
530-889-2357
800-525-5626
FAX: 530-889-0433

Janice Allen, Operations
Ariana Tyler, Customer Service

Takes personality, ability and interest into account in pointing learning disabled students of all ages toward intelligent and realistic career choices. Contains binder with paperback teaching guide plus 50 interest inventories and 50 abilities inventories. *$50.00*

2729 **Caring for Children with Chronic Illness**

Springer Publishing Company
536 Broadway
New York, NY 10012
212-431-4370
877-687-7476
FAX: 212-941-7842
e-mail: marketing@springerpub.com
www.springerpub.com

Annette Imperati, Marketing/Sales Director

A critical look at the current medical, social, and psychological framework for providing care to children with chronic illnesses. Emphasizing the need to create integrated, interdisciplinary approaches, it discusses issues such as the roles of families, professionals, and institutions in providing health care, the impact of a child's illness on various family structures, financing care, the special problems of chronically ill children as they become adolescents and more. *$36.95*

320 pages Hardcover
ISBN 0-82615 -00-1

2730 **Carolina Curriculum for Infants and Toddlers with Special Needs, 2nd Edition**

Brookes Publishing
PO Box 10624
Baltimore, MD 21285
410-337-9580
800-638-3775
FAX: 410-337-8539
e-mail: custserv@brookespublishing.com
www.brookespublishing.com

This book includes detailed assessment and intervention sequences, daily routine integration strategies, sensorimotor adaptations, and a sample 24-page Assessment Log that shows readers how to chart a child's individual progress. *$40.00*

384 pages Spiral-bound
ISBN 1-55766 -74-3

2731 Carolina Curriculum for Preschoolers with Special Needs

Brookes Publishing
PO Box 10624
Baltimore, MD 21285 410-337-9580
800-638-3775
FAX: 410-337-8539
e-mail: custserv@brookespublishing.com
www.brookespublishing.com

This curriculum provides detailed teaching and assessment techniques, plus a sample 28-page Assessment Log that shows readers how to chart a child's individual progress. This guide is for children between 2 and 5 in their developmental stages who are considered at risk for developmental delay or who exhibit special needs. *$34.00*

352 pages Spiral-bound
ISBN 1-55766 -32-8

2732 Challenge of Educating Together Deaf and Hearing Youth: Making Manistreaming Work

Charles C Thomas
2600 S 1st Street
Springfield, IL 62704 217-789-8980
800-258-8980
FAX: 217-789-9130
e-mail: books@ccthomas.com
www.ccthomas.com

Paul Higgins

Those who have this challenge of education: teachers, administrators, other professionals, parents, and concerned individuals will benefit from this book. Also available in cloth. *$28.95*

198 pages Softcover
ISBN 0-398063-91-5

2733 Challenged Scientists: Disabilities and the Triumph of Excellence

Greenwood Publishing Group
88 Post Road W
Suite 5007
Westport, CT 06880 203-226-3571
FAX: 203-222-1502
www.greenwood.com

This volume points out how the increasing need for scientists in this country can be lessened by utilizing a long overlooked pool of scientific talent in those persons who are scientifically oriented but who happen to have physical or sensory disabilities. Hardcover. $49.95-$55.00.

208 pages
ISBN 0-275938-73-5

2734 Child with Disabling Illness

Lippincott, Williams & Wilkins
227 E Washington Square
Philadelphia, PA 19106 215-238-4200
800-777-2295
FAX: 301-824-7390
www.lpub.com

$108.50

700 pages

2735 Childhood Behavior Disorders: Applied Research & Educational Practice

Pro-Ed Publications
8700 Shoal Creek Boulevard
Austin, TX 78757 512-451-3246
800-897-3202
FAX: 512-451-8542
e-mail: info@proedinc.com
www.proedinc.com

The only comprehensive overview of childhood behavior disorders. This book gives you the how and why for helping children with behavior disorders.

2736 Childhood Disablity and Family Systems

Haworth Press
10 Alice Street
Binghamton, NY 13904 607-722-5857
800-429-6784
FAX: 607-722-6362
e-mail: orders@haworthpress.com
www.haworthpress.com

Michael Ferrari PhD, Co-Editor
Maevin B Sussman PhD, Co-Editor
S Harrington-Miller, Advertising

Focuses on what the presence of a disabled child means to a family. Those professionals involved in teaching, research, and direct care with families having disabled children will value the coverage of such topics as the contemporary context of disability, ethical issues, family effects, and care systems. *$74.95*

246 pages Hardcover
ISBN 0-866566-71-6

2737 Children with ADD: A Shared Responsibility

Council for Exceptional Children
1110 N Glebe Road
Suite 300
Arlington, VA 22201 703-620-3660
FAX: 703-264-9494
www.cec.sped.org

Janice Burdick, President

Information on meeting the educational needs of children with ADD. *$8.90*

35 pages

2738 Children's Needs Psychological Perspective

National Association of School Psychologists
8455 Colesville Road
Suite 1000
Silver Spring, MD 20910 301-681-3223
FAX: 301-608-2514

This very popular monograph was developed with the recognition that many factors beyond the classroom and the child's own personal characteristics influence school success.

637 pages

2739 Choices: A Guide to Sex Counseling for the Physically Disabled Adult

Krieger Publishing Company
PO Box 9542
Melbourne, FL 32902 321-724-9542
800-724-0025
FAX: 321-951-3671
e-mail: info@krieger-publishing.com
www.krieger-publishing.com

Provides rehabilitation professionals with the basic information necessary for limited sexuality counseling of physically disabled adults. *$14.50*

132 pages
ISBN 0-898749-03-4

2740 Choosing Options and Accommodations for Children

Brookes Publishing
PO Box 10624
Baltimore, MD 21285 **410-337-9580**
800-638-3775
FAX: 410-337-8539
e-mail: custserv@brookespublishing.com
www.brookespublishing.com

Bridging the gap between the philosophy and practice of inclusive education, this important manual provides a practical assessment and planning process for the inclusion of students with disabilities in general education classrooms. *$29.00*

192 pages
ISBN 1-55766 -06-5

2741 Civil Law Handbook on Psychiatric & Psychological Evidence & Testimony

ABA Commission on Mental & Physical Disability Law
740 15th Street NW
9th Floor
Washington, DC 20005 **202-662-1581**
800-285-2221
FAX: 202-662-1032
e-mail: hammillj@staff.abanet.org
www.abanet.org/disability

John Hammill, Publications Coordinator
Amy Allbright, Managing Editor

Provides lawyers, judges and forensic experts with comprehensive, in-depth treatment of psychiatric and psychological evidence and testimony keyed to specific mental health law standards. *$60.00*

376 pages
ISBN 1-590310-05-5

2742 Classroom Success for the LD and ADHD Child

1406 Plaza Drive
Winston Salem, NC 27103 **336-768-1374**
800-222-9796
FAX: 336-768-9194
e-mail: blairpub@aol.com
www.blairpub.com

John F Blair, Publisher

This book offers suggestions on teaching techniques, adapting texts, recognition of children with disabilities and testing, grading and mainstreaming the learning disabled and ADHD child. *$13.95*

314 pages Paperback
ISBN 0-895871-59-9

2743 Clinical Management of Childhood Stuttering, Second Edition

Pro-Ed Publications
8700 Shoal Creek Boulevard
Austin, TX 78757 **512-451-3246**
800-897-3202
FAX: 512-451-8542
e-mail: info@proedinc.com
www.proedinc.com

Updates and integrates recent findings in childhood stuttering into a broad range of therapeutic strategies for assessing and treating the young dysfluent child. *$38.00*

336 pages

2744 Cognitive Approaches to Learning Disabilities

Pro-Ed Publications
8700 Shoal Creek Boulevard
Austin, TX 78757 **512-451-3246**
800-897-3202
FAX: 512-451-8542
e-mail: info@proedinc.com
www.proedinc.com

The first to bridge the gap between cognitive psychology and information processing theory in understanding learning disabilities. *$39.00*

495 pages Hardcover

2745 Collaborating for Comprehensive Services for Young Children and Families

Paul H Brookes Publishing Company
PO Box 10624
Baltimore, MD 21285
800-638-3775
FAX: 410-337-8539

Karen G Radke, Marketing Director

Taking collaboration a step beyond basic implementation, this useful book shows agency and school leaders how to coordinate their efforts to stretch human services dollars while still providing quality programs. Provides the building blocks needed to establish a local interagency coordinating council. *$37.00*

272 pages 1992
ISBN 1-557661-03-0

2746 Collaborative Teams for Students with Severe Disabilities

Brookes Publishing
PO Box 10624
Baltimore, MD 21285 **410-337-9580**
800-638-3775
FAX: 410-337-8539
e-mail: custserv@brookespublishing.com
www.brookespublishing.com

How can educators, parents and therapists work together to ensure the best possible educational experience for students with severe disabilities? This resource describes how a collaborative team can successfully create exciting learning opportunities for students, while teaching them to participate fully at home, school, work and play. *$ 30.00*

304 pages
ISBN 1-55766 -88-3

2747 Communicating with Parents of Exceptional Children

Love Publishing Company
4925 E Pacific Place
#22353
Denver, CO 80222 **303-221-7333**
FAX: 303-221-7444
e-mail: lovepublishing@compuserve.com

This book shows how teachers can facilitate parent involvement with children's education. It presents the mirror model of parent involvement, family, dynamics, how to listen actively to parents, values and perceptions, problem-solving, parent conferences and training groups. *$19.95*

ISBN 0-89108 -67-4

2748 Communication & Language Acquisition: Discoveries from Atypical Development

Brookes Publishing
PO Box 10624
Baltimore, MD 21285 **410-337-9580**
800-638-3775
FAX: 410-337-8539
e-mail: custserv@brookespublishing.com
www.brookespublishing.com

This text demonstrates how the study of language acquisition in children with atypical development promotes advances in basic theory. *$44.00*

352 pages Hardcover 1997
ISBN 1-557662-79-7

2749 Communication Skills for Working with Elders

Springer Publishing Company
536 Broadway
New York, NY 10012 **212-431-4370**
877-687-7476
FAX: 212-941-7842
e-mail: marketing@springerpub.com
www.springerpub.com

Annette Imperati, Marketing/Sales Director

How aging and illness affects communication. *$17.95*

160 pages Softcover
ISBN 0-82615 -20-7

2750 Communication Skills in Children with Down Syndrome: A Guide for Parents

Woodbine House
6510 Bells Mill Road
Bethesda, MD 20817 **301-897-3570**
800-843-7323
FAX: 301-897-5838
www.woodbinehouse.com

An expert shares her knowledge of speech and language development in children and adolescents with Down syndrome. Parents learn what to expect as communication skills progress from infancy through early adolescence, how Down syndrome can affect those skills, and what they can do to maximize thier child's potential in this area of development. *$ 14.95*

256 pages Paperback 1994
ISBN 0-933149-53-0

2751 Communication Unbound

Teachers College Press
Columbia University
New York, NY 10027
800-575-6566
FAX: 212-678-4149
teacherscollegepress.com/special_education_se

Complete title is 'Communication Unbound: How Facilitated Communication is Challenging the Traditional Views of Autism and Ability/Disablity'. Reveals the wonder of expression by people who have therefore between trapped in silence and diminished by presumptions of their incompetence. *$18.95*

240 pages Paperback
ISBN 0-087737-21-4

2752 Complete Handbook of Children's Reading Disorders: You Can Prevent or Correct LDs

Gallery Bookshop
PO Box 270
Mendocino, CA 95460 **707-937-2665**
FAX: 707-937-3737
e-mail: info@gallerybooks.com
www.gallerybooks.com

The complete handbook of children's reading disorders. *$34.95*

732 pages Paperback
ISBN 0-80772 -83-3

2753 Comprehensive Assessment in Special Education

Charles C Thomas
2600 S First Street
Springfield, IL 62704 **217-789-8980**
800-258-8980
FAX: 217-789-9130
e-mail: books@ccthomas.com
www.ccthomas.com

J Miller, Author
R Fox, Author
D Sexton, Author

The purpose of this book is to incorporate (1) detailed approaches to assessment, (2) assessment fundamentals, (3) traditional and emerging assessment, (4) today's special assessment concerns. *$104.95*

578 pages Hardcover
ISBN 0-398056-45-5

2754 Computer Access/Computer Learning

Special Needs Project
324 State Street
Suite H
Santa Barbara, CA 93101
800-333-6867
FAX: 805-962-5087
www.specialneeds.com

A resource manual in adaptive technology and computer training. *$22.50*

2755 Consulting Psychologists Press

3803 E Bayshore Road
PO Box 10096
Palo Alto, CA 94303 **650-964-3722**
800-624-1765
FAX: 650-969-8608
www.cpp-db.com

Catalog offering job assessment software, career development reports, educational assessment information and books for the professional.

2756 Counseling Persons with Communication Disorders and Their Families

Pro-Ed Publications
8700 Shoal Creek Boulevard
Austin, TX 78757 **512-451-3246**
800-897-3202
FAX: 512-451-8542
e-mail: info@proedinc.com
www.proedinc.com

A learning manual for speech-language pathologists and audiologists on how to deal with the emotional issues facing them in their work with clients with communication disorders and their families. *$ 29.00*

187 pages

2757 **Creating Positive Classroom Environments: Strategies for Behavior Management**

Brooks/Cole Publishing Company
511 Forest Lodge Road
Pacific Grove, CA 93950 **831-373-0728**
FAX: 831-375-6414
e-mail: bc-info@brookscole.com

A hands-on text that offers an approach to classroom management that encourages situation-specific decision making. Presenting research-based information on how to establish an effective behavior management system in both regular and special education settings, the book centers on ways to help students manage their own behavior, rather than on ways their behavior can be managed by teachers, peers, parents or other adults.

448 pages Paperbound

ISBN 0-53422 -54-4

2758 **Critical Voices on Special Education**

State University of New York Press
90 State Street
Albany, NY 12207 **518-472-5000**
800-666-2211
FAX: 800-688-2877
e-mail: info@sunypress.edu
www.sunypress.edu

Problems and progress concerning the mildly handicapped. *$21.95*

265 pages Paperback

ISBN 0-79140 -20-3

2759 **Cultural Diversity, Families and the Special Education System**

Teachers College Press
Columbia University
New York, NY 10027
800-575-6566
FAX: 212-678-4149

This timely and thought-provoking book explores the quadruple disadvantage faced by the parents of poor, minority, handicapped children whose first language is not that of the school they attend. *$22.95*

296 pages Paperback

ISBN 0-807731-19-6

2760 **Curriculum Decision Making for Students with Severe Handicaps**

Teachers College Press
Columbia University
New York, NY 10027
800-575-6566
FAX: 212-678-4149

The inclusion of severely handicapped students within the scope of public education has brought about many changes for teachers in special education, this book helps the professional to distinguish which avenues are the best to take. *$17.95*

192 pages Paperback

ISBN 0-807728-61-6

2761 **Deciphering the System: A Guide for Families of Young Disabled Children**

Brookline Books
PO Box 97
Newton Upper Falls, MA 02464 **617-558-8010**
800-666-2665
FAX: 617-558-8011
e-mail: milt@brooklinebooks.com
www.brooklinebooks.com

This book informs parents of disabled children (0-5) of their rights and the service system, e.g., ways to manage the cumulating information, tips on IEP and IFSP meetings and the educational assessment process, and how parents can work with multiple service providers. It includes contributions from both parents and professionals who have experience with the service system. *$21.95*

ISBN 0-914797-87-5

2762 **Defining Rehabilitation Agency Types**

Mississippi State University
PO Box 6189
Mississippi State, MS 39762 **662-325-2001**
800-675-7782
FAX: 662-325-8989
www.blind.msstate.edu

Kelly Schaefer, Dissemination Specialist

Relationships of participant selection and cost factors of service delivery across rehabilitation agency types. A national survey of state agencies for the blind was conducted to examine factors that define the characteristics of different agencies; similar programs were grouped together. Classification criteria were developed to distinguish agencies into logical groups based on line of authority, funding and operating procedures. *$10.00*

15 pages Paperback

2763 **Designing and Using Assistive Technology: The Human Perspective**

Brookes Publishing
PO Box 10624
Baltimore, MD 21285 **410-337-9580**
800-638-3775
FAX: 410-337-8539
e-mail: custserv@brookespublishing.com
www.brookespublishing.com

Presented here is a holistic perspective on how and why people choose and use AT. Features personal insights and the latest research on design and development. *$31.00*

352 pages Paperback 1998

ISBN 1-55766 -14-9

2764 **Developing Cross-Cultural Competence:Guide to Working with Young Children & Their Families**

Brookes Publishing
PO Box 10624
Baltimore, MD 21285 **410-337-9580**
800-638-3775
FAX: 410-337-8539
e-mail: custserv@brookespublishing.com
www.brookespublishing.com

This enlightening book perceptively and sensitively explores cultural, ethnic, and language diversity in human services. For those who work with families whose infants and young children may have or be at risk for a disability or chronic illness. (Second Edition) *$ 32.00*

448 pages Paperback

ISBN 1-55766 -31-9

2765 **Developing Individualized Family Support Plans: A Training Manual**

Brookline Books
PO Box 97
Newton Upper Falls, MA 02464 **617-558-8010**
800-666-2665
FAX: 617-558-8011
e-mail: milt@brooklinebooks.com
www.brooklinebooks.com

This manual provides in-service training coordinators, administrators, supervisors and university personnel with a compact package of functional and practical methods to train professionals about implementing family-centered individualized family support plans (IFSP'S). Also, case studies provide concrete examples to aid in learning to write IFSP's. *$24.95*

ISBN 0-914797-69-7

2766 **Developing Staff Competencies for Supporting People with Disabilities**

Brookes Publishing
PO Box 10624
Baltimore, MD 21285 **410-337-9580**
800-638-3775
FAX: 410-337-8539
e-mail: custserv@brookesopublishing.com
www.brookespublishing.com

This timely second edition, now in a new easier to read format, gives service providers helpful strategies for increasing effectiveness and maintaining well-being while working in the rewarding yet challenging field of human services. *$34.00*

480 pages Paperback
ISBN 1-55766 -07-3

2767 **Development of Language**

McGraw-Hill, School Publishing
220 E Danieldale Road
DeSoto, TX 75115 **972-224-1111**
800-442-9685
FAX: 972-228-1982
mhschool.com

An organizational book based on the developmental stages of language.

464 pages

2768 **Developmental Diagnosis Treatment**

Books on Special Children
PO Box 305
Congers, NY 10920 **845-638-1236**
FAX: 845-638-0847
e-mail: irene@boscbooks.com

Account of diagnosis and treatment of severely handicapped people of Japan. *$30.50*

209 pages Hardcover

2769 **Developmental Disabilities of Learning**

Gallery Bookshop
PO Box 270
Mendocino, CA 95460 **707-937-2665**
FAX: 707-937-3737
e-mail: info@gallerybooks.com
www.gallerybooks.com

Manual for professionals on developmental and learning disabilities in the growing child. *$25.00*

224 pages Illustrated

2770 **Developmental Disabilities: A Handbook for Occupational Therapists**

Haworth Press
10 Alice Street
Binghamton, NY 13904 **607-722-5857**
800-429-6784
FAX: 607-722-6362
e-mail: orders@haworthpress.com
www.haworthpress.com

S Harrington-Miller, Advertising

Provides broad coverage of the spectrum of problems confronted by patients with developmental disabilities and the many kinds of occupational therapy services these individuals need. Experts identify exemplary institutional and community service programs for treating patients with autism, cerebral palsy, epilepsy, and mental retardation. *$74.95*

268 pages Hardcover
ISBN 0-866569-59-6

2771 **Developmental Disabilities: A Handbook for Interdisciplinary Practice**

Brookline Books
PO Box 97
Newton Upper Falls, MA 02464 **617-558-8010**
800-666-2665
FAX: 617-558-8011
e-mail: milt@brooklinebooks.com
www.brooklinebooks.com

Successful interdisciplinary team practice for persons with developmental disabilities that require each team member to understand and respect the contributions of the others. This handbook explains the professions most often represented on interdisciplinary teams: their natures, concerns and roles in the interdisciplinary context. *$29.95*

256 pages
ISBN 1-571290-03-6

2772 **Developmental Variation and Learning Disorders**

Educators Publishing Service
31 Smith Pl
Cambridge, MA 02138 **617-367-2700**
800-225-5750
FAX: 617-547-0412
www.epsbooks.com

Discusses seven major areas of development and four major areas of academic proficiency and then ties this information together by examining factors that predispose a child to dysfunction and disability, offering guidelines to assessment and management, and analyzing long-range outcomes and factors that promote resiliency for parents, educators and clinicians. *$69.00*

640 pages Cloth
ISBN 0-838819-92-3

2773 **Diagnosis and Treatment of Old Age**

S Karger Publishers
26 W Avon Road
 # 529
Farmington, CT 06085 **860-675-7834**
FAX: 860-675-7302

These papers furnish a concise update on the diagnosis and treatment of Alzheimer's disease. *$57.75*

112 pages Hardcover
ISBN 3-80554 -44-3

2774 Digest of Neurology and Psychiatry

Institute of Living: Hartford Hospital
200 Retreat Avenue
Hartford, CT 06106
860-545-5555
800-673-2411
e-mail: fishe@harthosp.org

Harold I Schwartz MD, Editor
Elizabeth A Fishe, Asssociate Editor

Abstracts and reviews of selected current literature in psychiatry, neurology and related fields.

2775 Disability Funding News

CD Publications
8204 Fenton Street
Silver Spring, MD 20910
301-588-6380
800-666-6380
FAX: 301-588-6385
e-mail: dfn@cdpublications.com
www.cdpublications.com

Martha McPartlin, Editor

Grantseeking tips and strategies for nonprofit, government administrators, plus proved fundraising ideas. Includes grant application critiques, ho-to advice, and private and public funding updates. *$ 199.00*

8 pages Monthly

2776 Disability and Rehabilitation

Taylor & Francis
47 Runway Drive
 # G
Levittown, PA 19057
800-821-8312
FAX: 215-785-5515

Mike Hunninghake, Journals Representative

An international, multidisciplinary journal seeking to encourage a better understanding of all aspects of disability, and to promote the rehabilitation process. *$395.00*

Monthly
ISSN 0963-82 8

2777 Divided Legacy: A History of the Schism in Medical Thought, The Bacteriological Era

North Atlantic Books
1456 4th Street
Berkeley, CA 94710
510-559-8277
FAX: 510-559-8279

Concluding volume of Coulter's history of medical philosophy, from ancient times to today. Covers the orgins of bacteriology and immunology in world medicine; describes the clash between orthodox and alternative medicine.

1993

2778 Dual Relationships in Counseling

American Counseling Association
5999 Stevenson Avenue
Alexandria, VA 22304
800-347-6647
800-473-2329
FAX: 703-823-6862
www.counseling.org

Covers topics such as whether to accept a client, whether to reveal information, whether to refer a case, whether to consider factors you might not otherwise consider, and how to deal with gifts, invitations and social situations. *$23.95*

244 pages paperback 1992
ISBN 1-556200-90-0

2779 Early Intervention, Implementing Child & Family Services for At-Risk Infants

Pro-Ed Publications
8700 Shoal Creek Boulevard
Austin, TX 78757
512-451-3246
800-897-3202
FAX: 512-451-8542
e-mail: info@proedinc.com
www.proedinc.com

New directions and recent legislation have produced a need for this guide which is designed for professionals facing the challenge of program development for disabled and at-risk infants, toddlers and their families. *$36.00*

394 pages
ISBN 0-890796-21-1

2780 Ecology of Troubled Children

Brookline Books
PO Box 97
Newton Upper Falls, MA 02464
617-558-8010
800-666-2665
FAX: 617-558-8011
e-mail: milt@brooklinebooks.com
www.brooklinebooks.com

Designed for frontline mental health clinicians working with children with serious emotional disturbances; shows how to make childrens' worlds more supportive by changing the places, activities and people in their lives. *$15.95*

256 pages
ISBN 1-571290-57-5

2781 Edades y Etapas: Un Cuestionario Completad o por los Padres para Evaluar al los Ninos

Brookes Publishing
PO Box 10624
Baltimore, MD 21285
410-337-9580
800-638-3775
FAX: 410-337-8539
e-mail: custserv@brookespublishing.com
www.brookespublishing.com

This easy to use child-monitoring system is available in Spanish. Consists of a step-by-step User's Guide in English and a set of questionnaires for Spanish-speaking families to complete. Thirty questions covering five developmental domains: gross motor, fine motor, communication, personal-social, and problem solving. *$165.00*

ISBN 1-557663-69-6

2782 Educating Children with Multiple Disabilities: A Transdisciplinary Approach

Brookes Publishing
PO Box 10624
Baltimore, MD 21285
410-337-9580
800-638-3775
FAX: 410-337-8539
e-mail: custserv@brookespublishing.com
www.brookespublishing.com

Emphasizing transdisciplinary cooperation between teachers, therapists, nurses and parents, this book describes a general model and specific techniques for effectively educating children with multiple disabilities. *$29.00*

496 pages Paperback
ISBN 1-557662-46-0

2783 **Educating Students Who Have Visual Impairments with Other Disabilities**

Brookes Publishing
PO Box 10624
Baltimore, MD 21285 **410-337-9580**
800-638-3775
FAX: 410-337-8539
e-mail: custserv@brookespublishing.com
www.brookespublishing.com

This introductory text provides techniques for facilitating functional learning in students with a wide range of visual impairments and multiple disabilities. With a concentration on educational needs and learning styles, the authors of this multidisciplinary volume demonstrate functional assessment and teaching adaptations that will improve students' inclusive learning experiences. *$49.95*

552 pages Paperback
ISBN 1-557662-80-0

2784 **Educating all Students in the Mainstream**

Paul H Brookes Publishing Company
PO Box 10624
Baltimore, MD 21285
800-638-3775
FAX: 410-337-8539

Incorporating the research and viewpoints of both regular and special educators, this textbook provides an effective approach for modifying, expanding, and adjusting regular education to meet the needs of all students. *$34.00*

304 pages 1989
ISBN 1-557660-22-0

2785 **Education and Deafness**

Longman Publishing Group
10 Bank Street
9th Floor
White Plains, NY 10606 **914-993-5000**
FAX: 914-421-5598

Roth Wilkofsky, Systems Contact

Provides coverage of the interrelated issues that affect the teaching of deaf students. Concentrates on the severely to profoundly hearing impaired and includes an entire chapter devoted to students whose impairments are less severe (hard-of-hearing students).

320 pages Paperback 1990
ISBN 0-801300-26-6

2786 **Educational Audiology for the Limited Hearing Infant and Preschooler, 3rd Edition**

Charles C Thomas
2600 S First Street
Springfield, IL 62704 **217-789-8980**
800-258-8980
FAX: 217-789-9130
e-mail: books@ccthomas.com
www.ccthomas.com

Doreen Pollack, Author
Donald Goldberg, Author
Nancy Coleffe-Schenck, Author

Offers information on current concepts and practices in audio-logic screening and evaluation, development of the listening function, development of speech, development of language, the role of parents, parent education, mainstreaming of the limited-hearing child, and program modifications for the severely learning disabled child. Also includes information on auditory assessment, sensory aides, cochlear implants, acoupedics and auditory verbal programs. *$69.95*

430 pages paperback 1997
ISBN 0-39806 -28-1

2787 **Educational Dimensions of Acquired Brain Injury**

Pro-Ed Publications
8700 Shoal Creek Boulevard
Austin, TX 78757 **512-451-3246**
800-897-3202
FAX: 512-451-8542
e-mail: info@proedinc.com
www.proedinc.com

This book is a compilation of the working experiences of the professionals concerned about the educational dimensions of acquired brain injury. *$43.00*

574 pages Hardcover

2788 **Educational Intervention for the Student with Multiple Disabilities**

Charles C Thomas
2600 S First Street
Springfield, IL 62704 **217-789-8980**
800-258-8980
FAX: 217-789-9130
e-mail: books@ccthomas.com
www.ccthomas.com

Donna Irons-Reavis, Author

This text will assist those who want to teach severely, multiply disabled students by providing information on general principles of education and classroom organization and managing the behavior of students. Also available in cloth $34.95 (ISBN# 0-398-05793-1) *$24.95*

140 pages Softcover
ISBN 0-398061-73-4

2789 **Educational Prescriptions**

Educators Publishing Service
31 Smith Plaza
Cambridge, MA 02138 **617-367-2700**
800-225-5750
FAX: 617-547-0412
www.epsbooks.com

Lynne Meltzer, Author
Bethany Solomon, Author

This book provides specific recommendations for the classroom management of students who are experiencing subtle developmental and/or learning difficulties. Intended for regular classroom teachers, specific examples of accommodations teachers can make are provided for grades 1-3 and 4-6. *$13.50*

64 pages
ISBN 0-838819-90-7

2790 **Effective Instruction for Special Education, Second Edition**

Pro-Ed Publications
8700 Shoal Creek Boulevard
Austin, TX 78757 **512-451-3246**
800-897-3202
FAX: 512-451-8542
e-mail: info@proedinc.com
www.proedinc.com

This exciting and wide-ranging book provides special educators with effective methods for teaching students with mild and moderate learning and behavioral problems, as well as for teaching remedial students in general. *$37.00*

419 pages Paperback

2791 Effectively Educating Handicapped Students

Longman Publishing Group
10 Bank Street
9th Floor
White Plains, NY 10606 **914-993-5000**
FAX: 914-421-5598

For educators and other professionals who work with deaf and hearing impaired students in preschool and elementary programs. A developmental approach provides the foundation for several intervention methods including preparation for instruction, language, speech, audition and speechreading.

468 pages Paperback 1991
ISBN 0-801303-17-6

2792 Emotional Problems of Childhood and Adolescence

McGraw-Hill, School Publishing
220 E Danieldale Road
DeSoto, TX 75115 **972-224-1111**
800-442-9685
FAX: 972-228-1982
mhschool.com

For future special educators, psychologists and others who work with emotionally disturbed children and adolescents.

2793 Employment in the Mainstream

Mainstream
6930 Carroll Avenue
Suite 240
Takoma Park, MD 20912 **301-891-8777**
FAX: 301-891-8777
TTY:301-891-8777
e-mail: info@mainstreaminc.org
www.mainstreaminc.org

Reports on practical and legal issues affecting people with disabilities in the workplace. *$25.00*

32 pages Quarterly

2794 Enabling & Empowering Families: Principles & Guidelines for Practice

Brookline Books
PO Box 97
Newton Upper Falls, MA 02464 **617-558-8010**
800-666-2665
FAX: 617-558-8011
e-mail: milt@brooklinebooks.com
www.brooklinebooks.com

Carl Dunst PhD, Author
Carol Trivette MA, Author
Angela Deal MSW, Author

This book was written for practioners who must work with families but who have insufficient training in family systems assessment and intervention. The authors' system enables professionals to help the family identify its needs, locate the formal and informal resources to meet these needs and develop the abilities to effectively access these resources. *$24.95*

220 pages
ISBN 0-914797-59-X

2795 Enhancing Self-Concepts and Achievement of Mildly Handicapped Students

Charles C Thomas
2600 S First Street
Springfield, IL 62704 **217-789-8980**
800-258-8980
FAX: 217-789-9130
e-mail: books@ccthomas.com
www.ccthomas.com

Carroll J Jones, Author

This book is aimed towards students who are learning disabled, mildly mentally retarded, and who have behavior disorders. Individuals should be aware that unless they appreciate and understand themselves, it is difficult to relate to the world around them. This is no less true of exceptional than nonhandicapped learners. This book provides a wonderfully complete window of insight into the most tenuous of human aspects, the self-concept. Also available in cloth at $55.95 (ISBN# 0-398-05760-5) *$39.95*

294 pages Paperback
ISBN 0-398061-91-2

2796 Evaluation and Educational Programming of Deaf-Blind/Severly Multihandicapped Students:

Charles C Thomas
2600 S First Street
Springfield, IL 62704 **217-789-8980**
800-258-8980
FAX: 217-789-9130
e-mail: books@ccthomas.com
www.ccthomas.com

Offers information on the special education of deaf-blind students. *$41.95*

314 pages Softcover
ISBN 0-398055-15-7

2797 Evaluation and Treatment of the Psychogeriatric Patient

Haworth Press
10 Alice Street
Binghamton, NY 13904 **607-722-5857**
800-429-6784
FAX: 607-722-6362
e-mail: orders@haworthpress.com
www.haworthpress.com

Diane Gibson MS, OTR, Editor
S Harrington-Miller, Advertising

This pertinent book assists occupational therapists and other health care providers in developing up-to-date psychogeriatric programs and understands details of treating the cognitively impaired elderly. *$74.95*

111 pages Hardcover
ISBN 1-560240-52-0

2798 Exercise Activities for the Elderly

Springer Publishing Company
536 Broadway
New York, NY 10012 **212-431-4370**
877-687-7476
FAX: 212-941-7842
e-mail: marketing@springerpub.com
www.springerpub.com

Annette Imperati, Marketing/Sales Director

A variety of exercises geared to clients with such conditions as arthritis, diabetes and Parkinson's disease, and others which are designed to build up muscular strength and maintain flexibility. *$23.95*

240 pages Softcover
ISBN 0-82615 -10-9

2799 Facilitating Self Care Practices in the Elderly

Haworth Press
10 Alice Street
Binghamton, NY 13904 **607-722-5857**
800-429-6784
FAX: 607-722-6362
e-mail: orders@haworthpress.com
www.haworthpress.com

Barbara J Horn PhD, RN, Editor
S Harrington-Miller, Advertising

This up-to-date book is a synthesis of current knowledge from published sources and expert consultants relating to three commonly occurring problems in home health care practice: self-administration of medications, family caregiving issues, and teaching the elderly. *$ 74.95*

185 pages Hardcover

ISBN 1-560240-13-X

2800 Family Assessment in Early Intervention

Books on Special Children
PO Box 305
Congers, NY 10920 **845-638-1236**
FAX: 845-638-0847
e-mail: irene@boscbooks.com

Includes sources and measure used for assessment, strengths and weaknesses of families and comparisons between typical families and handicapped families. *$37.95*

280 pages Softcover

2801 Family-Centered Early Intervention with Infants and Toddlers

Paul H Brookes Publishing Company
PO Box 10624
Baltimore, MD 21285
800-638-3775
FAX: 410-337-8539

Karen G Radke, Marketing Director

This informative text provides professionals with insight and practical guidelines to help fulfill the federal requirements for provision of early intervention services. *$37.00*

368 pages Hardcover 1993

ISBN 1-557661-24-3

2802 Feeding Children with Special Needs

Arizona Department of Health Services
1740 W Adams
Office of Nutrition Services
Phoenix, AZ 85007 **602-542-1886**
FAX: 602-542-1890
www.hs.state.az.us/cfhs/ons/

Guide designed to help develop a greater awareness of the special challenges involved in the nutrition and feeding concerns for children with special health care needs, and ways to approach the issues. *$5.00*

2803 Focal Group Psychotherapy

New Harbinger Publications
5674 Shattuck Avenue
Oakland, CA 94609 **510-652-0215**
800-748-6273
FAX: 510-652-5472
e-mail: customerservice@newharbinger.com
www.newharbinger.com

Lauren Dockett, Publicity Director

Guide to leading brief, theme-based groups. This book offers an extensive week-by-week description of the basic concepts and interventions for 14 theme or focal groups for: codependency, rape victims, shyness, survivors of incest, agoraphobia, survivors of toxic parents, depression, child molesters, anger control, domestic violence offenders, assertiveness, alcohol and drug abuse, eating disorders, and parent training. *$59.95*

544 pages Cloth

ISBN 1-879237-18-0

2804 Free Hand: Enfranchising the Education of Deaf Children

TJ Publishers
817 Silver Spring Avenue
Suite 206
Silver Spring, MD 20910 **301-585-4440**
800-999-1168
FAX: 301-585-5930
e-mail: TJPubinc@aol.com

Angela K Thames, President
Jerald A Murphy, VP

A select group of nationally prominent educators, linguists and researchers met at Hofstra University to consider the most vital and controversial question in education of the deaf: What role should ASL play in the classroom? Become part of that discussion with A Free Hand. *$ 16.95*

204 pages Softcover 1990

ISBN 0-93266 -40-X

2805 Functional Assessment Inventory Manual

Stout Vocational Rehab Institute
University of Wisconsin-Stout
Menomonie, WI 54751 **715-232-1342**
FAX: 715-232-2356
e-mail: botterbuschd@uwstout.edu

Ronald R Fry, Manager
Darlene Botterbusch, Program Assistant

The Functional Assessment is a systematic enumeration of a client's vocationally relevant strengths and limitations. *$12.00*

96 pages Paperback

ISBN 0-916671-53-4

2806 Global Perspectives on Disability: A Curriculum

Mobility International USA
PO Box 10767
Eugene, OR 97440 **541-343-1284**
FAX: 541-343-6812
e-mail: info@miusa.org
www.miusa.org

Susan Sygall, Executive Director
Pamela Houston, Public Relations Coordinator
Tracy Scharn, Project Assistant

Designed for secondary and higher education instructors. Includes five lesson plans covering disability awareness, disability rights and international perspectives on disability. Available in alternative formats. *$40.00*

2807 Glossary of Terminology for Vocational Assessment/Evaluation/Work

Rehabilitation Resource University
University of Wisconsin-Stout
Menomonie, WI 54751 **715-232-1478**
FAX: 715-232-2356

Ronald R Fry, Manager
Darlene Botterbusch, Program Assistant

This glossary contains 254 terms and their definitions. Primary focus is on the terminology related to the practice and professionals of vocational assessment, vocational evaluation and work adjustment. *$9.50*

40 pages Softcover

2808 Graduate Technological Education and the Human Experience of Disability

Haworth Press
10 Alice Street
Binghamton, NY 13904
607-722-5857
800-429-6784
FAX: 607-722-6362
e-mail: orders@haworthpress.com
www.haworthpress.com

Robert C Anderson, Editor
S Harrington-Miller, Advertising

This book examines graduate schools of teology and their limited familiarity with the study of disability — and the presence of people with disabilities in particular — on their campuses. This text offers critical research and illuminates new pathways for theologia and practice in the community of faith. It offers suggestions for incorporating disability studies into theological education and religious life. *$34.95*

115 pages Hardcover
ISBN 0-789060-08-6

2809 HIV Infection and Developmental Disabilities

Paul H Brookes Pulishing Company
PO Box 10624
Baltimore, MD 21285
800-638-3775
FAX: 410-337-8539

Karen G Radke, Marketing Director

A resource for service providers pinpointing the most crucial medical, legal and educational issues to control HIV infection. *$47.00*

320 pages
ISBN 1-557660-83-2

2810 Handbook for Implementing Workshops for Siblings of Special Children

Special Needs Project
324 State Street
Suite H
Santa Barbara, CA 93101
800-333-6867
FAX: 805-962-5087
www.specialneeds.com

Based on three years of professional experience, this handbook provides guidelines and techniques for those who wish to start and conduct workshops for siblings. *$40.00*

2811 Handbook for Speech Therapy

Psychological & Educational Publications
1320 Sandy Prarie Road
PO Box 520
Hydesville, CA 95547
707-768-1807
800-523-5775

Morrison Gardner, President

Basic handbook for beginning speech teachers, shows how speech sounds are made, what thier individual characteristics are, how they relate to each other, what the most common errors are, and how to correct those errors.

143 pages paperback

2812 Handbook for the Special Education Administrator

Edwin Mellen Press
PO Box 450
Lewiston, NY 14092
716-754-2789
800-753-2788
FAX: 716-754-4056
e-mail: mellen@wzrd.com

Organization and procedures for special education. *$ 49.95*

96 pages Hardcover
ISBN 0-88946 -22-9

2813 Handbook of Developmental Education

Greenwood Publishing Group
88 Post Road W
Suite 5007
Westport, CT 06880
203-226-3571
FAX: 203-222-1502
www.greenwood.com

This comprehensive handbook has brought together the leading practitioners and researchers in the field of developmental education to focus on the developmental learning agenda. Hardcover.

400 pages $65 - $75
ISBN 0-275932-97-4

2814 Handbook on Supported Education for People with Mental Illness

Brookes Publishing
PO Box 10624
Baltimore, MD 21285
410-337-9580
800-638-3775
FAX: 410-337-8539
e-mail: custserv@brookespublishing.com
www.brookespublishing.com

Here you will find all necessary information that mental health professionals need in order to provide supported education services. There are specific suggestions on how to help people with mental illness return to or remain in college, trade school, or GED programs. Also addressed are funding and legal issues, accommodations, and specific interventions.

208 pages Paperback 1998
ISBN 1-55766 -52-1

2815 Head Injury Rehabilitation: Children

Taylor & Francis
47 Runway Drive
 # G
Levittown, PA 19057
FAX: 215-785-5515

Rehabilitation guide for the help of children or adolescents that have suffered brain injury.

460 pages Cloth
ISBN 0-85066 -67-1

2816 Health Care Management in Physical Therapy

Charles C Thomas
2600 S First Street
Springfield, IL 62704
217-789-8980
800-258-8980
FAX: 217-789-9130
e-mail: books@ccthomas.com
www.ccthomas.com

The focus of this book is on physical therapists as supervisors in health care settings of hospitals, nursing homes, home health agencies and in private practice. *$62.95*

328 pages Hardcover
ISBN 0-398056-42-0

2817 Health Care for Students with Disabilities

Paul H Brookes Publishing Company
PO Box 10624
Baltimore, MD 21285
800-638-3775
FAX: 410-337-8539

Karen G Radke, Marketing Director

This practical guidebook provides detailed descriptions of the 16 health-related procedures most likely to be needed in the classroom by students with disabilities. *$25.00*

304 pages Paperback 1990
ISBN 1-557660-37-9

2818 Helping Learning Disabled Gifted Children Learn Through Compensatory Play

Charles C Thomas
2600 S First Street
Springfield, IL 62704
217-789-8980
800-258-8980
FAX: 217-789-9130
e-mail: books@ccthomas.com
www.ccthomas.com

James H Humphrey, Author

About 3% of the school population is gifted and 5 to 8% of this number suffer from learning disabilities. These children experience a great deal more trauma than the normal child. *$24.95*

164 pages Softcover

ISBN 0-398061-62-9

2819 Helping Students Grow

American College Testing Program
2201 Dodge
168
Iowa City, IA 52243
319-337-1000
FAX: 319-351-2450

Designed to assist counselors in using the wealth of information generated by the ACT Assessment.

2820 How to Teach Spelling/How to Spell

Educators Publishing Service
31 Smith Place
Cambridge, MA 02138
617-367-2700
800-225-5750
FAX: 617-547-0412
www.epsbooks.com

Laura Toby Rudginsky, Author
Elizabeth Haskell, Author

This is a comprehensive resource manual based on the Orton-Gillingham approach to reading and spelling. It recommends what and how much to teach at each grade level at the beginning of each lesson or section. There are four student manuals that accompany this. *$22.50*

Teachers Manual

ISBN 0-838818-47-1

2821 Human Exceptionality: Society, School, and Family

Allyn & Bacon
75 Arlington Street
Suite 300
Boston, MA 02116
617-848-6000
800-852-8024
FAX: 617-848-7490
www.ablongman.com

Examination of the definitions, classification, prevalence and characteristics of each category of exceptionality in relation to the major topics and issues of the field of special education.

615 pages

ISBN 0-20528 -39-0

2822 I Heard That!

Alexander Graham Bell Association
3417 Volta Place NW
Washington, DC 20007
202-337-5220
FAX: 202-337-8314
e-mail: info@agbell.org
www.agbell.org

Provides a framework for teachers, clinicians and parents when writing objectives and designing activities to develop listening skills in children with hearing loss from newborn to 3 years. *$7.95*

36 pages

2823 I Heard That!2

Alexander Graham Bell Association
3417 Volta Place NW
Washington, DC 20007
202-337-5220
FAX: 202-337-8314
e-mail: info@agbell.org
www.agbell.org

Provides a framework for teachers, clinicians and parents when writing objectives and designing activities to develop listening skills in children who are deaf or hard of hearing. *$7.95*

36 pages

2824 Images of the Disabled, Disabling Images

Greenwood Publishing Group
88 Post Road W
Suite 5007
Westport, CT 06880
203-226-3571
FAX: 203-222-1502
www.greenwood.com

Combines an examination of the presentation of persons with disabilities in literature, film and the media with an analysis of the ways in which these images are expressed in public policy concerning the disabled. *$55.00*

227 pages Hardcover

ISBN 0-275921-78-6

2825 Implementing Family-Centered Services in Early Intervention

Brookline Books
PO Box 1047
Cambridge, MA 02238
617-868-0360
800-666-2665
FAX: 617-868-1772
e-mail: brooklinebks@delphi.com
www.brooklinebooks.com

This book describes a team-based decision-making workshop for implementing family-centered services in early interventions. Unlike a training curriculum, it focuses on the decisions that teams must make as they seek to become family-centered. *$19.95*

180 pages Paperback

ISBN 0-91479 -62-

2826 Including All of Us: An Early Childhood Curriculum About Disability

Educational Equity Concepts
114 E 32nd Street
New York, NY 10016
212-686-2531
FAX: 212-725-0947
TTY:212-725-1803
e-mail: information@equity.org
www.edequity.org

Barbara Sprung, Author

The first nonsexist, multicultural, mainstreamed curriculum. Step-by-step activities incorporate disability into three curriculum areas: Same/Different (hearing impairment), Body Parts (visual impairment), and Transportation (mobility impairment). *$14.95*

144 pages

ISBN 0-93162 -00-4

2827 **Including Students with Severe and Multiple Disabilites in Typical Classrooms**

Brookes Publishing
PO Box 10624
Baltimore, MD 21285 **410-337-9580**
800-638-3775
FAX: 410-337-8539
e-mail: custserv@brookespublishing.com
www.brookespublishing.com

This straightforward and jargon gree resource gives instructors the guidance needed to educate learners who have one or more sensory impairments in addition to cognitive and physical disabilities. *$32.95*

224 pages Paperback
ISBN 1-55766 -39-8

2828 **Including Students with Special Needs: A Practical Guide for Classroom Teachers**

Allyn & Bacon
75 Arlington Street
Suite 300
Boston, MA 02116 **617-848-6000**
800-852-8024
FAX: 617-848-7490
e-mail: ab_webmaster@abacon.com
vig.abacon.com

Focuses on educating students with special needs in inclusive settings based on substantive admisistrative backing, support for general education teachers, and an understanding that sometimes not all needs can be met in a single location.

544 pages
ISBN 0-20528 -85-4

2829 **Inclusive & Heterogeneous Schooling: Assessment, Curriculum, and Instruction**

Brookes Publishing
PO Box 10624
Baltimore, MD 21285 **410-337-9580**
800-638-3775
FAX: 410-337-8539
e-mail: custserv@brookespublishing.com
www.brookespublishing.com

Presents methods for successfully restructuring classrooms to enable all students, particularly those with disabilities, to flourish. Provides specific strategies for assessment, collaboration, classroom management, and age-specific instruction. *$34.95*

448 pages Paperback
ISBN 1-55766 -02-9

2830 **Independent Living Approach to Disability Policy Studies**

World Institute on Disability
510 16th Street
Suite 100
Oakland, CA 94612 **510-763-4100**
FAX: 510-763-4109
e-mail: wid@wid.org
www.wid.org

This collection of essays and bibliographies attempts to build a framework for understanding how the relationship between public policy, disability studies and disability policy studies will impact us in the future. *$17.50*

240 pages Paperback

2831 **Information & Referral Center**

Mississippi State University
PO Box 6189
Mississippi State, MS 39762 **662-325-2001**
800-675-7782
FAX: 662-325-8989
www.blind.msstate.edu

Kelly Schaefer, Publications Manager

A comprehensive website that includes information about client assistance programs, vocational rehabilitation agencies, low vision clinics and information about blindness and low vision. *$25.00*

150 pages

2832 **Instructional Methods for Students**

Allyn & Bacon
75 Arlington Street
Suite 300
Boston, MA 02116 **617-848-6000**
800-852-8024
FAX: 617-848-7490
e-mail: ab_webmaster@abacon.com
vig.abacon.com

Instructional methods for students with learning and behavior problems.

450 pages 1986
ISBN 0-205087-35-3

2833 **Interactions: Collaboration Skills for School Professionals**

Longman Education/Addison Wesley
95 Church Street
White Plains, NY 10601 **914-328-2090**
800-322-1377
FAX: 800-333-3328
www.longman.awl.com

Shows school professionals how to develop and use the skills necessary for effective collaboration among teachers, school support staff, and parents of children with special needs. *$35.00*

270 pages Paperback
ISBN 0-80131 -21-2

2834 **Interpreting Disability: A Qualitative Reader**

Teachers College Press
Columbia University
New York, NY 10027
800-575-6566
FAX: 212-678-4149

This book offers a collection of exemplary qualitative research affecting people with disabilities and their families. Instead of focusing upon methodological details, the chapters illustrate the variety of styles and formats that interpretive research can adopt in reporting its results. *$24.95*

328 pages Paperback
ISBN 0-807731-21-8

2835 **Intervention Research in Learning Disabilities**

Gallery Bookshop
PO Box 270
Mendocino, CA 95460 **707-937-2665**
FAX: 707-937-3737
e-mail: info@gallerybooks.com
www.gallerybooks.com

Bernice YL Wong, Editor

Based on the Symposium on Intervention Research, this volume presents 12 papers addressing issues in intervention research, academic interventions, social and behavioral interventions, and postsecondary interventions. *$30.00*

347 pages

2836 Introducing Students to Careers in Special Education and Related Services

Council for Exceptional Children
1110 N Glebe Road
Suite 300
Arlington, VA 22201
703-620-3660
FAX: 703-264-9494
www.cec.sped.org

Janice Burdick, President

Presents an array of activities appropriate for high school and college students to engage in to find out how it feels to be disabled. *$5.00*

25 pages

2837 Introduction to Learning Disabilities 2nd Edition

Allyn & Bacon
75 Arlington Street
Suite 300
Boston, MA 02116
617-848-6000
800-852-8024
FAX: 617-848-7490
e-mail: ab_webmaster@abacon.com
vig.abacon.com

Presents the current state of research in the area of learning disabilities, as well as intervention ideas and programs. Includes updated material on the 1997 re-authorization of IDEA (Individuals with Disabilities Education Act) and expanded coverage of ADHD and its relationship to learning disabilities. Presents the latest information on the characteristics of persons with learning disabilities, causes, and educational interventions.

608 pages
ISBN 0-20529 -43-4

2838 Introduction to Mental Retardation

Allyn & Bacon
75 Arlington Street
Suite 300
Boston, MA 02116
617-848-6000
800-852-8024
FAX: 617-848-7490
e-mail: ab_webmaster@abacon.com
vig.abacon.com

A thorough overview of mental retardation with a level of knowledge suitable for an undergraduate or beginning graduate student.

350 pages Casebound 1986
ISBN 0-134879-27-9

2839 Introduction to Special Education: Teaching in an Age of Challenge, 4th Edition

Allyn & Bacon
75 Arlington Street
Suite 300
Boston, MA 02116
617-848-6000
800-852-8024
FAX: 617-848-7490
e-mail: ab_webmaster@abacon.com
vig.abacon.com

Provides an applied approach to children with disabilities through the use of specific research and suggestions to focus on how the educational practices impact the lives of children, their families, and their teachers.

640 pages cloth
ISBN 0-20526 -94-4

2840 Introduction to the Nature and Needs of Students with Mild Disabilities

Charles C Thomas
2600 S First Street
Springfield, IL 62704
217-789-8980
800-258-8980
FAX: 217-789-9130
e-mail: books@ccthomas.com
www.ccthomas.com

Source of information for the special educator on the needs of students with mild disabilities. It has been designed as an introductory text for an undergraduate degree program in special education. The first chapter includes an overview of students who are at risk for academic failure. The remaining chapters are divided into three categorical units: students with mild mental retardation, behavior disorders, and learning disabilities.

300 pages Paperback
ISBN 0-398067-12-0

2841 Introduction to the Profession of Counseling

McGraw-Hill, School Publishing
220 E Danieldale Road
DeSoto, TX 75115
972-224-1111
800-442-9685
FAX: 972-228-1982
mhschool.com

Offers information, theories and techniques for counseling numerous cases from drug addiction to special populations.

464 pages

2842 Issues and Practices in Special Education

Longman Publishing Group
10 Bank Street
9th Floor
White Plains, NY 10606
914-993-5000
FAX: 914-421-5598

Roth Wilkofsky, Systems Contact

Utilizes current literature, classic articles and case histories to examine such topics as: withholding treatment from severely defective newborns, plastic surgery for Down Syndrome, handicapped offenders, and AIDS.

290 pages Paperback 1988
ISBN 0-582286-39-5

2843 Issues and Research in Special Education

Teachers College Press
Columbia University
New York, NY 10027
800-575-6566
FAX: 212-678-4149

Provides up-to-date research and discourse on a wide range of topics affecting professionals in the field of special education. *$38.00*

264 pages Hardcover
ISBN 0-807731-95-1

2844 Kendall Demonstration Elementary School Curriculum Guides

Gallaudet University Bookstore
800 Florida Avenue NE
Washington, DC 20002
202-651-5000
800-451-1073
FAX: 202-651-5489

These guides provide detailed information to help teachers organize curriculums and education programs. Pre-school: $15.95, Health: $8.95, Language Arts: $13.75, Social Studies: $14.95, Math: $11.95, Science: $17.95, Auditory & Speech: $10.95.

2845 Language Arts: Detecting Special Needs

Allyn & Bacon
75 Arlington Street
Suite 300
Boston, MA 02116
617-848-6000
800-852-8024
FAX: 617-848-7490
e-mail: ab_webmaster@abacon.com
vig.abacon.com

Describes special language arts needs of special learners.

180 pages paperback 1989

ISBN 0-205116-36-1

2846 Language Disabilities in Children and Adolescents

McGraw-Hill, School Publishing
220 E Danieldale Road
DeSoto, TX 75115
972-224-1111
800-442-9685
FAX: 972-228-1982
mhschool.com

A comprehensive review of research in language disabilities.

2847 Language Learning Practices with Deaf Children

Pro-Ed Publications
8700 Shoal Creek Boulevard
Austin, TX 78757
512-451-3246
800-897-3202
FAX: 512-451-8542
e-mail: info@proedinc.com
www.proedinc.com

This new edition describes the variety of language-development theories and practices used with deaf children without advocating anyone. *$38.00*

321 pages Hardcover

2848 Language and Communication Disorders in Children

McGraw-Hill, School Publishing
220 E Danieldale Road
DeSoto, TX 75115
972-224-1111
800-442-9685
FAX: 972-228-1982
mhschool.com

Comprehensive coverage encompassing all aspects of children's language disorders.

512 pages

2849 Learning Disabilities: Concepts and Characteristics

McGraw-Hill, School Publishing
220 E Danieldale Road
DeSoto, TX 75115
972-224-1111
800-442-9685
FAX: 972-228-1982
mhschool.com

Covers the conceptual basis of learning disabilities, identification, etiology and diagnosis.

448 pages

2850 Learning Disability: Social Class and the Cons. of Inequality In American Education

Greenwood Publishing Group
88 Post Road W
Suite 5007
Westport, CT 06880
203-226-3571
FAX: 203-222-1502
www.greenwood.com

Presents a detailed historical description of the social and educational assumptions integral to the idea of learning disability.

167 pages $43.95 - $47.95

ISBN 0-313253-96-X

2851 Learning and Individual Differences

National Association of School Psychologists
8455 Colesville Road
Suite 1000
Silver Spring, MD 20910
301-681-3223
FAX: 301-608-2514

A multidisciplinary journal in education.

2852 Learning to See: American Sign Language as a Second Language

Gallaudet University Press
11030 S Langley Avenue
Chicago, IL 60628
800-621-2736
FAX: 800-621-8476
TTY:800-621-9347
gupress.gallaudet.edu

Sherman Wilcox, Co-Author
Phyliss Wilcox, Co-Author

This important book has been updated to help teachers teach American Sign Language as a second language, including information on Deaf culture, the history and structure of ASL, teaching methods and issues facing educators. *$19.95*

160 pages Softcover

2853 Legal-Ethical Considerations, Restrictions and Obligations for Clinicians

Charles C Thomas
2600 S First Street
Springfield, IL 62704
217-789-8980
800-258-8980
FAX: 217-789-9130
e-mail: books@ccthomas.com
www.ccthomas.com

Legal-Ethical Considerations, Restrictions and Obligations for Clinicians who Treat Communicative Disorders is a clinical functioning of speech-language pathologists and audiologists is determined not only by their clinical skills but by their awareness of the legal-ethical restrictions and obligations they are required by law to consider in their relationships with their clients and their families *$51.95*

258 pages Softcover

ISBN 0-39806 -29-6

2854 Library Manager's Guide to Hiring and Serving Disabled Persons

McFarland & Company
PO Box 611
Jefferson, NC 28640
336-246-4460
800-253-2187
FAX: 336-246-5018

Information for library staff on hiring and serving disabled persons. *$35.00*

171 pages Illustrated

ISBN 0-89950 -16-3

2855 Life Beyond the Classroom: Transition Strategies for Young People

Brookes Publishing
PO Box 10624
Baltimore, MD 21285
410-337-9580
800-638-3775
FAX: 410-337-8539
e-mail: custserv@brookespublishing.com
www.brookespublishing.com

This textbook is an essential guide to planning, designing, and implementing successful transition programs for students with disabilities. *$44.00*

496 pages

ISBN 1-55766 -05-7

2856 Life-Span Approach to Nursing Care for Individuals with Developmental Disabilities

Brookes Publishing
PO Box 10624
Baltimore, MD 21285 **410-337-9580**
800-638-3775
FAX: 410-337-8539
e-mail: custserv@brookespublishing.com
www.brookespublishing.com

This reference book was written by and for nurses. This guide addresses fundamental nursing issues such as health promotion, infection control, seizure management, adaptive and assistive technology, and sexuality. Also offered are in-depth case studies, helpful charts and tables, and problem-solving strategies. *$49.95*

464 pages Hardcover
ISBN 1-557661-51-0

2857 Lipreading for Children

Health Publishing Company
PO Box 3805
San Francisco, CA 94119 **415-282-8585**
FAX: 415-750-6550

Collection of games, activities and stories has been used for many years by teachers, educational therapists and language audiologists working with hearing impaired children. *$19.25*

2858 Look, Now Hear This: Combined Auditory Training and Speech-Reading Instruction

Charles C Thomas
2600 S First Street
Springfield, IL 62704 **217-789-8980**
800-258-8980
FAX: 217-789-9130
e-mail: books@ccthomas.com
www.ccthomas.com

A manual on combined auditory training and speech reading instruction. Also available in cloth: $42.95 (ISBN# 0-398-03830-9) *$ 30.95*

230 pages Softcover
ISBN 0-398061-81-5

2859 MA Report

National Allergy and Asthma Network
3554 Chain Bridge Road
Suite 200
Fairfax, VA 22030 **703-385-4403**
FAX: 703-352-4354

Offers information on medical breakthroughs, patient care, public awareness, activities and events focusing on the allergy and asthma patient. This newsletter is the only Monthly Asthma Report that a patient will need to keep fully informed with medical articles written by experts in the field.

Monthly

2860 Mainstreaming Deaf and Hard of Hearing Students: Questions and Answers

Gallaudet University Bookstore
800 Florida Avenue NE
Washington, DC 20002 **202-651-5000**
800-451-1073
FAX: 202-651-5489

This booklet presents mainstreaming as one educational option and suggests some considerations for parents, teachers and administrators. *$6.00*

40 pages

2861 Mainstreaming Exceptional Students: A Guide for Classroom Teachers, 4th Edition

Allyn & Bacon
75 Arlington Street
Suite 300
Boston, MA 02116 **617-848-6000**
FAX: 617-848-7490
e-mail: ab_webmaster@abacon.com
vig.abacon.com

Covers the various categories of exceptional students and discusses educational strategies and classroom management.

464 pages paperback
ISBN 0-20515 -24-6

2862 Management of Autistic Behavior

Pro-Ed Publications
8700 Shoal Creek Boulevard
Austin, TX 78757 **512-451-3246**
800-897-3202
FAX: 512-451-8542
e-mail: info@proedinc.com
www.proedinc.com

This excellent reference is a comprehensive and practical book that tells what works best with specific problems. *$41.00*

450 pages

2863 Managing Diagnostic Tool of Visual Perception

Gallery Bookshop
PO Box 270
Mendocino, CA 95460 **707-937-2665**
FAX: 707-937-3737
e-mail: info@gallerybooks.com
www.gallerybooks.com

For diagnosing specific perceptual learning abilities and disabilities. *$14.00*

ISBN 0-80580 -83-4

2864 Medical Rehabilitation

Lippincott, Williams & Wilkins
227 E Washington Square
Philadelphia, PA 19106 **215-238-4200**
800-777-2295
FAX: 301-824-7390
www.lpub.com

Information for the professional on new techniques and treatments in the medical rehabilitation fields. *$80.50*

368 pages Illustrated
ISBN 0-88167 -85-5

2865 Mental Health Concepts and Techniques for the Occupational Therapy Assistant

Lippincott, Williams & Wilkins
227 E Washington Square
Philadelphia, PA 19106 **215-238-4200**
800-777-2295
FAX: 301-824-7390
www.lpub.com

This text offers clear and easily understood explanations of the various theoretical and practice health models. *$36.00*

344 pages
ISBN 0-88167 -53-X

2866 **Mental Health and Mental Illness**

Lippincott, Williams & Wilkins
227 E Washington Square
Philadelphia, PA 19106 **215-238-4200**
800-777-2295
FAX: 301-824-7390
www.lpub.com

Concise, comprehensive and completely up to date, this book presents the most current theory in mental health nursing for the student and the new practitioner. *$28.95*

480 pages
ISBN 0-39755 -73-7

2867 **Mentally Ill Individuals**

Mainstream
3 Bethesda Metro Center
Suite 830
Bethesda, MD 20814 **301-951-6122**
800-247-1380
FAX: 301-654-6714
e-mail: info@mainstreaminc.org

Mainstreaming mentally ill individuals into the workplace. *$2.50*

12 pages

2868 **Mentally Retarded Individuals**

Mainstream
3 Bethesda Metro Center
Suite 830
Bethesda, MD 20814 **301-951-6122**
800-247-1380
FAX: 301-654-6714
e-mail: info@mainstreaminc.org

Mainstreaming mentally retarded individuals into the workplace. *$2.50*

12 pages

2869 **Midland Treatment Furniture**

Sammons Preston Rolyan
4 Sammons Court
Bolingbrook, IL 60440 **630-226-1300**
800-323-5547
FAX: 630-226-1389
e-mail: spr@abilityone.com
www.sammonsprestonrolyan.com

This catalog has the biggest selection of OT/PT products anywhere. Whether you deal with larger or smaller caseloads, you need treatment furniture you can count on. Midland Treatment Furniture from SPR is designed and built to stand up to the heaviest use. From tilt tables and traction packages to mat platforms and parallel bars, you'll find the complete line of Midland Treatment Furniture inside this brochure. All products are assembled from premium materials and carefully crafted.

Free

2870 **Multidisciplinary Assessment of Children With Learning Disabilities and Mental Retardation**

Paul H Brookes Publishing Company
PO Box 270
Mendocino, CA 95460 **707-937-2665**
FAX: 707-937-3737
e-mail: info@gallerybooks.com
www.gallerybooks.com

James E Joy, Editor

Assessment of children with learning disabilities and mental retardation. *$24.00*

346 pages Illustrated
ISBN 0-93371 -62-1

2871 **Multisensory Teaching of Basic Language Skills: Theory and Practice**

Brookes Publishing
PO Box 10624
Baltimore, MD 21285 **410-337-9580**
800-638-3775
FAX: 410-337-8539
e-mail: custserv@brookespublishing.com
www.brookespublishing.com

This book presents specific multisensory methods for helping students who are having trouble learning to read due to dyslexia or other learning disabilities. Recommended techniques are offered for teaching alphabet skills, composition, comprehension, handwriting, math, organization and study skills, phonological awareness, reading and spelling. *$59.00*

608 pages Hardcover 1999
ISBN 1-557663-49-1

2872 **Negotiating the Special Education Maze: A Guide for Parents and Teachers**

Spina Bifida Association of America
4590 MacArthur Boulevard
Suite 250
Washington, DC 20007 **202-944-3285**
800-621-3141
FAX: 202-944-3295
e-mail: sbaa@sbaa.org
www.sbaa.org

An excellent aid for the development of an effective special education program. *$19.00*

2873 **No Longer Immune: A Counselor's Guide to AIDS**

American Counceling Association
PO Box 2513
Birmingham, AL 35201 **800-347-6647**
800-473-2329
FAX: 703-823-6862
www.counseling.org

Craig Kain, Editor

Covers a broad range of issues such as working with specific populations, handling pre and post testing situations, coping with fear, grief and survivor guilt, struggling with spiritual issues and dealing with counter transference. *$26.95*

295 pages
ISBN 1-55620 -64-1

2874 **Occupational Therapy Across Cultural Boundaries**

Haworth Press
10 Alice Street
Binghamton, NY 13904 **607-722-5857**
800-429-6784
FAX: 607-722-6362
e-mail: orders@haworthpress.com
www.haworthpress.com

S Harrington-Miller, Advertising

Examines the concept of culture from a unique perspective, that of individual occupational therapists who have worked in environments very different from those in which they were educated or had worked previously. *$74.95*

107 pages Hardcover
ISBN 1-560242-23-X

2875 Occupational Therapy Approaches to Traumatic Brain Injury

Haworth Press
10 Alice Street
Binghamton, NY 13904 **607-722-5857**
800-429-6784
FAX: 607-722-6362
e-mail: orders@haworthpress.com
www.haworthpress.com

Jerry Johnson EdD, OTR, Editor

Focuses on the disabled individual, the family, and the societal responses to the injured, this comprehensive book covers the spectrum of available services from intensive care to transitional and community living. *$74.95*

137 pages Hardcover
ISBN 1-560240-64-4

2876 Overcoming Dyslexia in Children, Adolescents and Adults

Pro-Ed Publications
8700 Shoal Creek Boulevard
Austin, TX 78757 **512-451-3246**
800-897-3202
FAX: 512-451-8542
e-mail: info@proedinc.com
www.proedinc.com

This book describes some forms of dyslexia in detail and then relates those problems to the social, emotional and personal development of dyslexic individuals. *$34.00*

350 pages Paperback

2877 Oxford Textbook of Geriatric Medicine

Oxford University Press
198 Madison Avenue
New York, NY 10016 **212-726-6000**
800-451-7556
FAX: 919-677-1303
www.oup-usa.org

This comprehensive text brings together extensive experience in clinical geriatrics with a strong scientific base in research. *$125.00*

784 pages

2878 PKU for Children: Learning to Measure

University of Washington, PKU Clinic
CHDD
Box 537920
Seattle, WA 98195 **206-685-1242**
FAX: 206-543-5771
e-mail: vam@u.washington.edu
www.depts.washington.edu/pku

Lesson format for parents and teachers.

2879 Pain Centers: A Revolution in Health Care

Lippincott, Williams & Wilkins
227 E Washington Square
Philadelphia, PA 19106 **215-238-4200**
800-777-2295
FAX: 301-824-7390
www.lpub.com

$103.00

280 pages

2880 Parental Concerns in College Student Mental Health

Haworth Press
10 Alice Street
Binghamton, NY 13904 **607-722-5857**
800-429-6784
FAX: 607-722-6362
e-mail: orders@haworthpress.com
www.haworthpress.com

Leighton C Whitaker PhD, Editor

An instructive guide for parents and mental health professionals regarding the most important issues about psychological development in college students. *$74.95*

204 pages Hardcover
ISBN 0-866567-20-8

2881 Parents and Teachers

Alexander Graham Bell Association
3417 Volta Place NW
Washington, DC 20007 **202-337-5220**
FAX: 202-337-8314
e-mail: info@agbell.org
www.agbell.org

This excellent book offers in-depth guidance to parents and teachers whose partnership can foster language in school-aged children with hearing impairments. The first section examines roles of parents, teachers, professionals and children in language acquisition, residual hearing and audiological management, language development stages and readying children for preschool. The second portion of the book presents specific objectives and teaching strategies to use at school and at home. *$27.95*

386 pages

2882 Patient and Family Education

Springer Publishing Company
536 Broadway
New York, NY 10012 **212-431-4370**
877-687-7476
FAX: 212-941-7842
e-mail: marketing@springerpub.com
www.springerpub.com

Annette Imperati, Marketing/Sales Director

This guide outlines the actual clinical content needed to develop, implement and maintain patient education programs. Conveniently arranged in one-hour long lesson plans, each disease or condition is organized in an easy-to-follow format. *$26.95*

272 pages Softcover
ISBN 0-82615 -41-7

2883 Peer Tutoring: A Guide for School Psychologists

National Association of School Psychologists
8455 Colesville Road
Suite 1000
Silver Spring, MD 20910 **301-681-3223**
FAX: 301-608-2514

In recent years the term peer tutoring has received more attention as an alternative to the traditional academic arrangements in the classroom for at-risk students. Remedial instruction is often needed by at-risk students and peer tutoring is an attractive alternative due to its use of available resources.

36 pages

2884 Person to Person: Guide for Professionals Working with the Disabled, 2nd Ed.

Paul H Brookes Publishing Company
PO Box 10624
Baltimore, MD 21285
800-638-3775
FAX: 410-337-8539

Karen G Radke, Marketing Director

This second edition of an already-popular book helps professionals approach interactions with a people-first, disability second attitude. *$29.00*

288 pages Paperback 1992
ISBN 1-557661-00-6

2885 Personality and Emotional Disturbance

Taylor & Francis
47 Runway Drive
 # G
Levittown, PA 19057
FAX: 215-785-5515

The brain injured person has unique needs. Recent findings have highlighted that it is the personality, behavioral and emotional problems which most prohibit a return to work, create the greatest burden for the long-term care and rehabilitation of physical and cognitive functions. *$72.00*

260 pages Cloth
ISBN 0-85066 -71-3

2886 Peterson's Guide to Colleges with Programs for Learning Disabled Students

Special Needs Project
324 State Street
Suite H
Santa Barbara, CA 93101
800-333-6867
FAX: 805-962-5087
www.specialneeds.com

The most complete and accurate guide to the more than 900 colleges with programs for the learning disabled. *$19.95*

406 pages

2887 Phenomenology of Depressive Illness

Human Sciences Press
233 Spring Street
New York, NY 10013
212-229-2859
800-221-9369
FAX: 212-463-0742

Provides the reader with a detailed knowledge of the clinical characteristics of depressive disorders that will permit judgement of the general ability of the various theoretical models of depressive disorders. *$42.95*

263 pages Cloth
ISBN 0-89885 -69-9

2888 Physical Disabilities and Health Impairments: An Introduction

McGraw-Hill, School Publishing
220 E Danieldale Road
DeSoto, TX 75115
972-224-1111
800-442-9685
FAX: 972-228-1982
mhschool.com

A comprehensive text which presents a wealth of up-to-date medical information for teachers.

2889 Physical Education and Sports for Exceptional Students

McGraw-Hill Company
2460 Kerper Boulevard
Dubuque, IA 52001
800-338-3987
FAX: 614-755-5654
www.mhhe.com/hper/physed

Physical education for exceptional students and teaching students with learning and behavior exceptionalities.

Cloth

2890 Physical Management of Multiple Handicaps: A Professional's Guide

Paul H Brookes Publishing Company
PO Box 10624
Baltimore, MD 21285
800-638-3775
FAX: 410-337-8539

Comprehensive guide, takes a transdisciplinary approach to therapeutic/technological management of persons with multiple handicaps. *$36.00*

352 pages Hardcover
ISBN 1-557660-47-6

2891 Physically Handicapped in Society

Ayer Company Publishers
RR 1 Box 85-1
N Stratford, NH 03590
603-669-9307
888-267-7323
FAX: 603-669-7945
e-mail: stg@ncia.net
bookfinder.com/dir/i/Physically_Handicapped_i

Kathy Train, Office Manager
Ellie Phipps, Customer Service

A group of 39 books. Biographies that offer studies on attitudes, sociological and psychological. Please write or call for catalog. *$965.00*

Hardcover
ISBN 0-40513 -00-3

2892 Practicing Rehabilitation with Geriatric Clients

Springer Publishing Company
536 Broadway
New York, NY 10012
212-431-4370
877-687-7476
FAX: 212-941-7842
e-mail: marketing@springerpub.com
www.springerpub.com

Annette Imperati, Marketing/Sales Director

Physical therapy in the geriatric client, psychological and psychiatric considerations in the rehabilitation of the elderly. *$ 32.95*

256 pages Hardcover
ISBN 0-82616 -80-5

2893 Pragmatic Approach

Educators Publishing Service
31 Smith Plaza
Cambridge, MA 02138
617-547-6706
800-225-5750
FAX: 617-547-0412
www.epsbooks.com

Monograph on evaluation of children's performances on Slingerland Pre-Reading Screening Procedures to Identify First Grade Academic Needs. *$6.00*

56 pages
ISBN 0-838816-85-1

2894 Preschoolers with Special Needs: Children At-Risk, Children with Disabilities, 2nd Edition

Allyn & Bacon
75 Arlington Street
Suite 300
Boston, MA 02116
617-848-6000
800-852-8024
FAX: 617-848-7490
e-mail: ab_webmaster@abacon.com
vig.abacon.com

Explores ways of providing preschool children with special needs and their families with a learning environment that will help them develop and learn. Emphasizes the needs of preschoolers age three to six and provides information to teachers and others who work with young children in all settings. Current models of curricula, which incorporate new features from research and practical expreiences with children who have special needs, are described and discussed. *$59.00*

336 pages cloth

ISBN 0-205358-79-9

2895 Preventing Academic Failure

Educators Publishing Service
31 Smith Place
Cambridge, MA 02138
617-367-2700
800-225-5750
FAX: 617-547-0412
www.epsbooks.com

Ungraded multisensory curriculum coordinating Orton-Gillingham and Merrill Linguistic reading techniques for language disabled students. Teaches phonics, spelling and reading to reinforce the development of language skills. A separate handwriting program is available. *$42.00*

284 pages Paperback

ISBN 0-838852-71-8

2896 Preventing School Dropouts

Pro-Ed Publications
8700 Shoal Creek Boulevard
Austin, TX 78757
512-451-3246
800-897-3202
FAX: 512-451-8542
e-mail: info@proedinc.com
www.proedinc.com

For secondary teachers, special education and regular, who have difficulty teaching youth in their classes. Presented are 120 tactics, specific instructional techniques, for helping adolescents to stay in school. Each tactic is written in a format that includes five sections. *$38.00*

509 pages

2897 Prevocational Assessment

Exceptional Education
PO Box 15308
Seattle, WA 98115
206-542-3971
FAX: 475-486-4510

JE Stewart, Owner

Use the PACG to assess your students in nine areas (attendance and endurance, learning and behavior, communication skills, social skills, grooming and eating and toileting) covering 46 specific workshop experiences. *$12.00*

16 pages Complete Set

ISBN 1-87786 -23-7

2898 Progress Without Punishment: Approaches for Learners with Behavior Problems

Teachers College Press
Columbia University
New York, NY 10027
800-575-6566
FAX: 212-678-4149

In this volume, the authors argue against the use of punishment, and instead advocate the use of alternative intervention procedures. *$17.95*

184 pages Paperback

ISBN 0-807729-11-6

2899 Promoting Postsecondary Education for Students with Learning Disabilities

Pro-Ed Publications
8700 Shoal Creek Boulevard
Austin, TX 78757
512-451-3246
800-897-3202
FAX: 512-451-8542
e-mail: info@proedinc.com
www.proedinc.com

Primarily designed for postsecondary service providers who are responsible for serving college students with learning disabilities. *$41.00*

440 pages

2900 Promoting Special Education Career Awareness

Council for Exceptional Children
1110 N Glebe Road
Suite 300
Arlington, VA 22201
703-620-3660
FAX: 703-264-9494
www.cec.sped.org

Janice Burdick, President

Written for use by individuals or groups interested in promoting careers in special education. *$10.00*

57 pages

2901 Psychiatric Mental Health Nursing

Lippincott, Williams & Wilkins
227 E Washington Square
Philadelphia, PA 19106
215-238-4200
800-777-2295
FAX: 301-824-7390
www.lpub.com

This text emphasizes and contrasts the roles of the generalist nurse and the psychiatric nurse specialist. *$52.00*

1120 pages Illustrated

2902 Psychoeducational Assessment of Hearing-Impaired Students

Pro-Ed Publications
8700 Shoal Creek Boulevard
Austin, TX 78757
512-451-3246
800-897-3202
FAX: 512-451-8542
e-mail: info@proedinc.com
www.proedinc.com

This book includes a comprehensive presentation of issues and procedures related to the assessment of hearing-impaired students. *$29.00*

251 pages Paperback

2903 Psychoeducational Assessment of Visually Impaired and Blind Students

Pro-Ed
8700 Shoal Creek Boulevard
Austin, TX 78757 **512-451-3246**
800-897-3202
FAX: 512-451-8542
e-mail: info@proedinc.com
www.proedinc.com

Professional reference book that addresses the problems specific to assessment of visually impaired and blind children. Of particular value to the practitioner are the extensive reviews of available tests, including ways to adapt those not designed for use with the visually handicapped. *$29.00*

140 pages Paperback
ISBN 0-890791-08-2

2904 Rational-Emotive Therapy with Alcoholics

Pergamon Press
655 Avenue of the Americas
New York, NY 10010 **212-213-8310**

Therapy text on alcoholism and substance abusers. *$15.95*

176 pages Softcover
ISBN 0-08033 -74-3

2905 Reading and Deafness

Pro-Ed Publications
8700 Shoal Creek Boulevard
Austin, TX 78757 **512-451-3246**
800-897-3202
FAX: 512-451-8542
e-mail: info@proedinc.com
www.proedinc.com

Three areas are looked at in this book: deaf children's prereading development of real-world knowledge, cognitive abilities and linguistic skills. *$39.00*

422 pages

2906 Reading and the Special Learner

Ablex Publishing Corporation
PO Box 811
Stamford, CT 06904
FAX: 203-661-0792

Explores the needs of the special learner: compensatory methods and adaptive means. *$73.25*

272 pages
ISBN 0-89391-95-9

2907 Readings on Research in Stuttering

Longman Publishing Group
10 Bank Street
9th Floor
White Plains, NY 10606 **914-993-5000**
FAX: 914-421-5598

Roth Wilkofsky, Systems Contact

Collection of the key journal articles published on stuttering over the past decade, addressing trends in recent research in the field.

231 pages Paperback 1991
ISBN 0-801304-10-5

2908 Recreation Activities for the Elderly

Springer Publishing Company
536 Broadway
New York, NY 10012 **212-431-4370**
877-687-7476
FAX: 212-941-7842
e-mail: marketing@springerpub.com
www.springerpub.com

Annette Imperati, Marketing/Sales Director

Included in this volume are simple crafts that utilize easily obtainable, inexpensive materials, hobbies focusing on collections, nature, and the arts' and games emphasizing both mental and physical activity. *$23.95*

240 pages Softcover
ISBN 0-82616 -30-1

2909 Reference Manual for Communicative Sciences and Disorders

Pro-Ed Publications
8700 Shoal Creek Boulevard
Austin, TX 78757 **512-451-3246**
800-897-3202
FAX: 512-451-8542
e-mail: info@proedinc.com
www.proedinc.com

An indispensable guide to standards and values essential in the assessment of communication disorders. *$54.00*

393 pages

2910 Rehabilitation Counseling and Services: Profession and Process

Charles C Thomas
2600 S First Street
Springfield, IL 62704 **217-789-8980**
800-258-8980
FAX: 217-789-9130
e-mail: books@ccthomas.com
www.ccthomas.com

Gives information on the rehabilitation and counseling process, work evaluation, work adjustment and more. *$52.95*

376 pages Cloth
ISBN 0-39052 -24-4

2911 Rehabilitation Interventions for the Institutionalized Elderly

Haworth Press
10 Alice Street
Binghamton, NY 13904 **607-722-5857**
800-429-6784
FAX: 607-722-6362
e-mail: orders@haworthpress.com
www.haworthpress.com

Ellen Dunleavy Taira Otr/L, Editor

Gerontology professionals offer suggestions to enrich the quality of rehabilitation services offered to the institutionalized elderly. This volume examines up to the minute ideas, some that would have been unlikely even a few years ago, that focus exclusively on rehabilitation services for the institutionalized elderly. *$44.95*

77 pages Hardcover
ISBN 0-866568-33-6

2912 Rehabilitation Nursing for the Neurological Patient

Springer Publishing Company
536 Broadway
New York, NY 10012 **212-431-4370**
877-687-7476
FAX: 212-941-7842
e-mail: marketing@springerpub.com
www.springerpub.com

Annette Imperati, Marketing/Sales Director

A practical new reference written especially for practicing nurses who work with neurologically disabled persons. *$32.95*

240 pages

2913 **Rehabilitation Resource Manual: VISION**

Resources for Rehabilitation
33 Bedford Street
Suite 19A
Lexington, MA 02420 **781-890-6371**
FAX: 781-867-7517

Susan Greenblatt

A desk reference that enables service providers, librarians and others to make effective referrals. Includes guidelines on establishing self-help groups, information on research and service organizations, and chapters on assistive technology, for special population groups and by eye condition. *$44.95*

Biennial

2914 **Rehabilitation Technology**

Haworth Press
10 Alice Street
Binghamton, NY 13904 **607-722-5857**
800-429-6784
FAX: 607-722-6362
e-mail: orders@haworthpress.com
www.haworthpress.com

Glenn Hedman MEME, Editor

Learn how the use of technological devices can enhance the lives of disabled children. Informs physical therapists, occupational therapists, and rehabilitation technologists about the devices that are available today and provides important background information on these devices. *$74.95*

173 pages Hardcover
ISBN 1-560240-33-4

2915 **Report Writing in Assessment and Evaluation**

Stout Vocational Rehab Institute
University of Wisconsin-Stout
Menomonie, WI 54751 **715-232-1478**
FAX: 715-232-2356

Ronald R Fry, Manager
Darlene Botterbusch, Program Assistant

This examines questions of who are you writing for and what does the referral source want. Defines characteristics of good reports, common problems, writing in different settings, types of reports, getting ready to write, and writing prescriptive recommendations. *$17.75*

188 pages Softcover

2916 **Resources for Rehabilitation**

33 Bedford Street
Suite 19A
Lexington, MA 02420 **781-862-6455**
FAX: 781-368-9096

R Frances Weisse, President

Provides training and information to professionals and the public about disabilities and resources available to help. Publishes resource guides, professional publications and patient/client educational materials. Conducts custom designed training programs and workshops.

2917 **Restructuring High Schools for All Students: Taking Inclusion to the Next Level**

Brookes Publishing
PO Box 10624
Baltimore, MD 21285 **410-337-9580**
800-638-3775
FAX: 410-337-8539
e-mail: custserv@brookespublishing.com
www.brookespublishing.com

Taking Inclusion to the Next Level. Details the process of creating an inclusive, collaborate community of learners and teachers at the secondary level. *$29.95*

304 pages Paperback 1998
ISBN 1-557663-13-0

2918 **Restructuring for Caring and Effective Education: Administrative Guide**

Brookes Publishing
PO Box 10624
Baltimore, MD 21285 **410-337-9580**
800-638-3775
FAX: 410-337-8539
e-mail: custserv@brookespublishing.com
www.brookespublishing.com

In this empowering book, leading general and special education schools reform experts synthesize the major school restructuring initiatives and describe the processes and rationale for changing the organizational structure and instructional practices of schools. *$ 29.00*

384 pages Paperback
ISBN 1-55766 -91-3

2919 **Screening in Chronic Disease**

Oxford University Press
2001 Evans Road
Cary, NC 27513 **212-726-6000**
800-451-7556
FAX: 919-677-1303
www.oup-usa.org

Early detection, or screening, is a common strategy for controlling chronic disease, but little information has been available to help determine which screening procedures are worthwhile. *$42.50*

256 pages

2920 **Selective Nontreatment of Handicapped**

Oxford University Press
2001 Evans Road
Cary, NC 27513 **212-726-6000**
800-451-7556
FAX: 919-677-1303
www.oup-usa.org

Information on selective nontreatment of handicapped newborns, moral dilemmas in neonatal medicine. *$17.95*

304 pages Paperback

2921 **Service Coordination for Early Intervention: Parents and Friends**

Brookline Books
PO Box 1047
Cambridge, MA 02238 **617-868-0360**
800-666-2665
FAX: 617-868-1772
e-mail: brooklinebks@delphi.com
www.brooklinebooks.com

This book helps administrators and professionals to structure early intervention and ongoing services so that professionals work collaboratively with parents to promote the health, well being and development of children with special needs. *$19.95*

110 pages Paperback
ISBN 0-91479 -91-3

2922 **Services for the Seriously Mentally Ill: A Survey of Mental Health Centers**

Nat'l Council for Community Behavioral Healthcare
12300 Twinbrook Parkway
Suite 320
Rockville, MD 20852 **301-984-6200**
FAX: 301-881-7159
www.nccbh.org

This ground-breaking report documents what administrators and practitioners have maintained for many years: community mental health organizations devote a significant percentage of the human and financial resources to serving the seriously mentally ill. *$30.00*

2923 **Shop Talk**

Research Press
PO Box 9177
Champaign, IL 61826 **217-352-3273**
800-519-2707
FAX: 217-352-1221
e-mail: rp@researchpress.com
www.researchpress.com

Russell Pence, VP Marketing

A well-structured group training program that covers five crucial communication areas: social communication routines, identification information, basic language skills, language-related concepts and cognitive components. The authors emphasize direct cooperation between educators and parents by providing over 100 interesting activities that focus on the student's affective impact on others, unique identify as a person, self-care, grooming, leisure and ability to work independently. *$25.95*

236 pages Paperback
ISBN 0-878222-29-4

2924 **Signed English Schoolbook**

Gallaudet University Press
11030 S Langley Avenue
Chicago, IL 60628
800-621-2736
FAX: 800-621-8476
TTY:800-621-9347
gupress.gallaudet.edu

Harry Bornstein, Co-Author
Karen L Saulnier, Co-Author

The Signed English Schoolbook provides vocabulary for teachers and others who serve school-age children and adolescents and covers the full range of school activities. *$13.95*

184 pages Softcover

2925 **Smart But Stuck: Emotional Aspects of Learning Disabilities and Imprisoned Intelligence**

Haworth Press
10 Alice Street
Binghamton, NY 13904 **607-722-5857**
800-429-6784
FAX: 607-722-6362
e-mail: orders@haworthpress.com
www.haworthpress.com

S Harrington-Miller, Advertising

Elaborates on new research about imprisoned intelligence and the emotional consequences of learning disabilities. It is also for psychoterapists, educators, school social workers, medical personnel, people dealing with prisons, etc. It helps those who struggle with learning disabilities (and people who help them) build self esteem, face LD obstacles, bypass weaknesses, and enhance strenghts. *$34.95*

228 pages Hardcover
ISBN 0-789014-66-1

2926 **Social Studies: Detecting and Correcting Special Needs**

Allyn & Bacon
75 Arlington Street
Suite 300
Boston, MA 02116 **617-848-6000**
800-852-8024
FAX: 617-848-7490
www.ablongman.com

Describes social studies and special needs for special learners.

180 pages 1990
ISBN 0-205121-51-9

2927 **Social and Emotional Development of Exceptional Students: Handicapped**

Charles C Thomas
2600 S First Street
Springfield, IL 62704 **217-789-8980**
800-258-8980
FAX: 217-789-9130
e-mail: books@ccthomas.com
www.ccthomas.com

Carroll J Jones, Author

Sixteen years after the passage of P.L. 94-142, the dream of special educators to educate the handicapped and nonhandicapped children and youth together resulting in increased academic gains and age-appropriate school skills for handicapped children and youth has not yet materialized. This book helps eliminate an existing void by providing teachers with understandable information regarding the social and emotional development of exceptional students. Also in cloth at $41.95 (ISBN# 0-398-05781-8) *$29.95*

218 pages Softcover
ISBN 0-398061-94-7

2928 **Special Education Today**

LifeWay Christian Resources Southern Baptist Conv.
127 9th Avenue N
Nashville, TN 37234 **615-251-2000**
800-458-2772
FAX: 651-251-5764
e-mail: specialed@lifeway.com
www.lifeway.com

Ellen Beene, Editor

This unique quarterly publications ministers to people with special education needs and to their families, the church, and other caregivers. It offers a variety of helps and encouragement, including: What's working in churches, Suggestions for adapting teaching techniques, inspirational stories about people who have disabilities, Parenting and family issues, Ideas for reaching, witnessing, worship, and recreation. *$4.25*

36 pages Quarterly

2929 **Special Education for Today**

Allyn & Bacon
75 Arlington Street
Suite 300
Boston, MA 02116 **617-848-6000**
800-852-8024
FAX: 617-848-7490
www.lifeway.com

An undergraduate introduction to special education covering all major areas of exceptionality. Contains pedagogical features designed to make the book accessible to the undergraduate.

576 pages hardcover 1984
ISBN 0-138264-53-8

2930 Speech and the Hearing-Impaired Child

Alexander Graham Bell Association
3417 Volta Place NW
Washington, DC 20007 **202-337-5220**
FAX: 202-337-8314
e-mail: info@agbell.org
www.agbell.org

This textbook for professionals deals with basic theoretical issues in the acquisition of speech and the form of language (phonetics and phonology) in children with hearing losses. It provides a systematic framework to develop and evaluate speech target behaviors and their underlying subskills. *$29.95*

402 pages Paperback

2931 Speech-Language Pathology and Audiology: An Introduction

McGraw-Hill, School Publishing
220 E Danieldale Road
DeSoto, TX 75115 **972-224-1111**
800-442-9685
FAX: 972-228-1982
mhschool.com

Offers classroom-tested coverage of clinical objectives and functioning.

301 pages

2932 Spinal Cord Dysfunction

Oxford University Press
2001 Evans Road
Cary, NC 27513 **212-726-6000**
800-451-7556
FAX: 919-677-1303
www.oup-usa.org

Offers information on restoration of function after spinal cord damage as seen from the point of view of identification of impaired or absent function in the nerve cells and processes which survive after the initial insult, intact but with impaired functions. *$95.00*

368 pages

2933 Spotting Language Problems

Los Amigos Research Associates
7035 Galewood Street
San Diego, CA 92120 **619-286-3162**
FAX: 619-286-3162

Donald R Omark, Partner

A screening tool for educators, clinicians, and paraprofessionals to help them identify students with language problems that may result in learing difficulties. Based on evaluating ordinary conversation. *$30.00*

2934 Strategies for Teaching Students with Learning and Behavior Problems

Allyn & Bacon
75 Arlington Street
Suite 300
Boston, MA 02116 **617-848-6000**
800-852-8024
FAX: 617-848-7490
www.ablongman.com

Provides descriptions of methods and strategies for teaching students with learning and behvior problems, managing professional roles, and collaborating with families, professionals, and paraprofessionals.

544 pages
ISBN 0-205113-89-3

2935 Students with Acquired Brain Injury: The School's Response

Brookes Publishing
PO Box 10624
Baltimore, MD 21285 **410-337-9580**
800-638-3775
FAX: 410-337-8539
e-mail: custserv@brookespublishing.com
www.brookespublishing.com

This book is designed for school professionals and describes a range of issues that this population faces and presents proven means of addressing them in ways that benefit all students. Included topics are hospital-to-school transitions, effective assessment strategies, model programs in public schools, interventions to assist classroom teachers, and ways to involve family members in the educational program. *$29.95*

424 pages Paperback 1997
ISBN 1-55766-85-1

2936 Students with Mild Disabilities in the Secondary School

Longman Group
1185 Avenue of the Americas
New York, NY 10036 **212-782-3300**
www.ablongman.com

Roth Wilkofsky, Systems Contact

Provides methods and strategies for curriculum delivery to students with mild disabilities at the secondary school level.

2313G pages Paperback 1991
ISBN 0-801301-66-1

2937 Support Groups for Practicing Special Education Professionals

Council for Exceptional Children
1110 N Glebe Road
Suite 300
Arlington, VA 22201 **703-620-3660**
FAX: 703-264-9494
www.cec.sped.org

Janice Burdick, President

The demands and logistics of teaching make it difficult for teachers to form and maintain professional support networks as part of their working day. *$10.00*

56 pages

2938 Supporting and Strengthening Families

Brookline Books
PO Box 1047
Cambridge, MA 02238 **617-868-0360**
800-666-2665
FAX: 617-868-1772
e-mail: brooklinebks@delphi.com
www.brooklinebooks.com

A collection of papers addressing the theory, methods, strategies, and practices involved in adopting an empowerment and family-centered resources approach to supporting families and strengthening individual and family functioning. *$30.00*

252 pages Paperback
ISBN 0-91479-94-8

2939 **Survival Guide for the First-Year Special Education Teacher**

Council for Exceptional Children
1110 N Glebe Road
Suite 300
Arlington, VA 22201
703-620-3660
FAX: 703-264-9494
www.cec.sped.org

Janice Burdick, President

Help for teachers. This survival guide was developed to help teachers be prepared for and enjoy the challenges of a new career. *$12.00*

47 pages

2940 **TESTS**

Slosson Educational Publications
PO Box 280
E Aurora, NY 14052
585-652-0930
800-828-4800
FAX: 800-665-3840
e-mail: slosson@slosson.com
www.slosson.com

Leslie Foote, Office Personnel
Peggy Meyer, Office Personnel

Slosson Educational Publications, Inc. offers educators an extensive selection of testing products, along with books on Autism. ADED and other Special needs materials. Our catalog includes 30 pages of Speech-Language Testing and language Rehabilitation Products. The behavioral conduct. Special needs section includes checklist and scales on aberrant/disruptive behavior, Tapes on ADD, as well as products for dyslexia and Remediation of reversals.

2941 **Teacher's Guide to Including Students with Disabilities in Regular Physical Education**

Brookes Publishing
PO Box 10624
Baltimore, MD 21285
410-337-9580
800-638-3775
FAX: 410-337-8539
e-mail: custserv@brookespublishing.com
www.brookespublishing.com

Provides simple and creative strategies for meaningfully including children with disabilities in regular physical education programs. *$39.00*

288 pages Paperback
ISBN 1-557661-56-1

2942 **Teachers Working Together**

Brookline Books
PO Box 1047
Cambridge, MA 02238
617-868-0360
800-666-2665
FAX: 617-868-1772
e-mail: brooklinebks@delphi.com
www.brooklinebooks.com

Hon Deshier, Author
Jean Schumaker, Author
Karen Harris, Author

This collection of papers describes collaboraborative efforts for such classroom settings as preschools, elementary, middle and high schools, for content area teaching and into the transition to work. Each chapter describes actual practice and analyzes what is required to accomplish this collaboration. *$19.95*

Paperback 1998
ISBN 1-57139 -66-4

2943 **Teaching Children with Autism: Strategies for Initiating Positive Interactions**

Brookes Publishing
PO Box 10624
Baltimore, MD 21285
410-337-9580
800-638-3775
FAX: 410-337-8539
e-mail: custserv@brookespublishing.com
www.brookespublishing.com

Stategies for initiating positive interactions and improving learning opportunities. This guide begins with an overview of characteristics and long-term strategies and proceeds through discussions that detail specific techniques for normalizing environments, reducing disruptive behavior, improving language and social skills, and enhancing generalization. *$32.95*

256 pages Paperback
ISBN 1-55766 -80-4

2944 **Teaching Disturbed and Disturbing Students: An Integrative Approach**

Pro-Ed Publications
8700 Shoal Creek Boulevard
Austin, TX 78757
512-451-3246
800-897-3202
FAX: 512-451-8542
e-mail: info@proedinc.com
www.proedinc.com

Using an integrative approach, this text provides teachers with step-by-step details of how to implement and use the methods and theories discussed in each chapter. *$37.00*

465 pages

2945 **Teaching Every Child Every Day: Integrated Learning in Diverse Classrooms**

Brookline Books
PO Box 1047
Cambridge, MA 02238
617-868-0360
800-666-2665
FAX: 617-868-1772
e-mail: brooklinebks@delphi.com
www.brooklinebooks.com

Collection of articles addressing various issues in teaching to diverse classrooms—varied in need for special educational services, English proficiency, and socioeconomic and racial backgrounds. *$19.95*

224 pages Paperback
ISBN 0-57129 -40-0

2946 **Teaching Infants and Preschoolers with Handicaps**

McGraw-Hill, School Publishing
220 E Danieldale Road
DeSoto, TX 75115
972-224-1111
800-442-9685
FAX: 972-228-1982
mhschool.com

Builds a solid background in early childhood special education.

380 pages

2947 **Teaching Language-Disabled Children: A Communication/Games Intervention**

Brookline Books
PO Box 1046
Cambridge, MA 02238
617-868-0360
800-666-2665
FAX: 617-868-1772
e-mail: brooklinebks@delphi.com
www.brooklinebooks.com

Susan Conant, Author
Milton Budoff, Author
Barbara Hecht, Author

Describes exactly how to play the communication games. It does not simply exhort practitioners to give topic-relevant responses and take advantage of opportunities. It provides specific teaching methods and not simply a new perspective on language remeditation. *$22.95*

Hardcover

ISBN 0-91479 -38-7

2948 Teaching Learners with Mild Disabilities: Integrating Research and Practice

Brooks/Cole Publishing Company
511 Forest Lodge Road
Pacific Grove, CA 93950 **831-373-0728**
FAX: 831-375-6414
e-mail: bc-info@brookscole.com

The authors illustrate interactions among regular teachers, special education teachers and students with mild disabilities through the use of hypothetical case studies of students and teachers.

496 pages Paperbound

ISBN 0-53421 -02-0

2949 Teaching Mathematics to Students with Learning Disabilities

Pro-Ed Publications
8700 Shoal Creek Boulevard
Austin, TX 78757 **512-451-3246**
800-897-3202
FAX: 512-451-8542
e-mail: info@proedinc.com
www.proedinc.com

Nancy S Bley, Author
Carl A Thornton, Author

New trends in school mathematics have surfaced in the teaching world. Problem-solving, estimation and the use of computers are receiving considerably greater emphasis than in the past and these areas are included in the new text. *$38.00*

486 pages Paperback

2950 Teaching Mildly and Moderately Handicapped Students

Allyn & Bacon
75 Arlington Street
Suite 300
Boston, MA 02116 **617-848-6000**
800-852-8024
FAX: 617-848-7490
www.ablongman.com

A cross-categorial text providing teaching ideas and techniques. Focuses on the theme of learning as a constructive process in which the learner interacts with the environment, constructing new systems of knowledge, Behavioral techniques and research are also presented.

hardcover 1986

ISBN 0-138939-00-4

2951 Teaching Reading to Children with Down Syndrome: A Guide for Parents and Teachers

Woodbine House
6510 Bells Mill Road
Bethesda, MD 20817 **301-843-7323**
800-843-7323
FAX: 301-897-5838
www.woodbinehouse.com

Alison Oelwein, Illustrator

Guide includes lessons customized to meet the unique interests and learning style of each child. *$16.95*

371 pages Paperback

ISBN 0-933149-55-7

2952 Teaching Reading to Disabled and Handicapped Learners

Charles C Thomas
2600 S First Street
Springfield, IL 62704 **217-789-8980**
800-258-8980
FAX: 217-789-9130
e-mail: books@ccthomas.com
www.ccthomas.com

Harold D Love, Author
Feddie W Litton, Author

Designed as a text for undergraduate and graduate students, it's aim is to help the many children, adolescents, and adults who encounter difficulty with reading. It guides prospective and present special education teachers in assisting and teaching handicapped learners to read. The text integrates traditional methods with newer perspectives to provide and effective reading program in special education. *$37.95*

260 pages Paperback

ISBN 0-398062-48-X

2953 Teaching Reading to Handicapped Children

Love Publishing Company
9101 E Kenyon Avenue
Denver, CO 80222 **303-221-7333**
FAX: 303-221-7444
e-mail: lovepublishing@compuserve.com

The author covers skills teaching through letter sound association, word identification, synthetic and analytic methods and others, plus testing and assessment. *$24.95*

ISBN 0-89108 -13-5

2954 Teaching Self-Determination to Students with Disabilities

Brookes Publishing
PO Box 10624
Baltimore, MD 21285 **410-337-9580**
800-638-3775
FAX: 410-337-8539
e-mail: custserv@brookespublishing.com
www.brookespublishing.com

Basic skills for successful transition. This teacher-friendly source will help educators prepare students with disabilities with the specific skills they need for a satisfactory, self-directed life once they leave school. *$34.95*

384 pages Paperback 1997

ISBN 1-55766 -02-5

2955 Teaching Students with Learning and Behavior Problems

Pro-Ed Publications
8700 Shoal Creek Boulevard
Austin, TX 78757 **512-451-3246**
800-897-3202
FAX: 512-451-8542
e-mail: info@proedinc.com
www.proedinc.com

Donald D Hammill, Author
Nettie Bartel, Author

Popular, classic text with a comprehensive overview of best practices in assessing and instructing students with mild-to-moderate learning and behavior problems. *$44.00*

520 pages Paperback

2956 Teaching Students with Mild and Moderate Learning Problems

Allyn & Bacon
75 Arlington Street
Suite 300
Boston, MA 02116
800-852-8024
FAX: 617-848-7490
www.ablongman.com

Provides teachers with skills for assisting students with mild to moderate handicaps in making successful transitions in school and community environments.

496 pages 1990
ISBN 0-205123-62-7

2957 Teaching Students with Moderate/Servere Disabilities, Including Autism

Charles C Thomas
2600 S First Street
Springfield, IL 62704
217-789-8980
800-258-8980
FAX: 217-789-9130
e-mail: books@ccthomas.com
www.ccthomas.com

This resource and guide was written to help teachers, parents, and other caregivers provide the best educational opportunities for their students with moderate and severe disabilities. The author addresses functional language and other language intervention strategies, vocational training, community based instruction, transition and postsecondary programming, the adolescent student with autism, students with multiple disabilities, parent and family issues, and legal concerns. *$58.95*

416 pages Paperback
ISBN 0-398067-01-5

2958 Teaching Students with Special Needs in Inclusive Settings

Allyn & Bacon
75 Arlington Street
Suite 300
Boston, MA 02116
617-848-6000
800-852-8024
FAX: 617-848-7490
www.ablongman.com

Tom Smith, Author
Ed Polloway, Author
James Patton, Author

This text is intended to be a survey text providing practical guidance to general education teachers. It will help them to meet the diverse needs of students with disabilities.

544 pages
ISBN 0-20527 -16-6

2959 Teaching Young Children to Read Brookline Books

PO Box 1047
Cambridge, MA 02238
617-868-0360
800-666-2665
FAX: 617-868-1772
e-mail: brooklinebks@delphi.com
www.brooklinebooks.com

Milt Budoff, Publisher

Detailed instructions on teaching reading to preschoolers. Gradually develops full fluency. *$16.95*

192 pages Paperback
ISBN 0-57129 -48-6

2960 Teaching and Mainstreaming Autistic Children

Love Publishing Company
9101 E Kenyon Avenue
Denver, CO 80222
303-221-7333
FAX: 303-221-7444
e-mail: lovepublishing@compuserve.com

Dr. Knoblock advocates a highly organized, structured environment for autistic children, with teachers and parents working together. His premise is that the learning and social needs of autistic children must be analyzed and a daily program designed with interventions that respond to this functional analysis of their behavior. *$24.95*

ISBN 0-89108 -11-9

2961 Teaching the Bilingual Special Education Student

Ablex Publishing Corporation
PO Box 811
Stamford, CT 06904
FAX: 201-767-6717

This book focuses on teaching those students who are bilingual, handicapped and in need of special instruction. It responds to the complex and practical issues of teaching these students in an effective way.

ISBN 0-89391 -23-4

2962 Teaching the Learning Disabled Adolescent

Love Publishing Company
9101 E Kenyon Avenue
Denver, CO 80222
303-221-7333
FAX: 303-221-7444
e-mail: lovepublishing@compuserve.com

This book gives expert strategies and methods for teaching learning disabled adolescents how, rather than what, to learn. *$34.95*

ISBN 0-89108 -94-5

2963 Teaching the Mentally Retarded Student: Curriculum, Methods, and Strategies

Allyn & Bacon
75 Arlington Street
Suite 300
Boston, MA 02116
617-848-6000
800-852-8024
FAX: 617-848-7490
www.ablongman.com

Represents a comprehensive approach to curriculum, methods and strategies for teaching the mildly mentally retarded student.

640 pages hardcover 1987
ISBN 0-205102-62-X

2964 Technology and Handicapped People

Springer Publishing Company
536 Broadway
New York, NY 10012
212-431-4370
877-687-7476
FAX: 212-941-7842
e-mail: marketing@springerpub.com
www.springerpub.com

Annette Imperati, Marketing/Sales Director

Important information for concerned professionals about new rehabilitation techniques and treatments for handicapped people. *$ 29.95*

224 pages Hardcover
ISBN 0-82614 -10-8

2965 **Textbooks and the Student Who Can't Read Them: A Guide for Teaching Content**

Brookline Books
PO Box 1046
Cambridge, MA 02238 **617-868-0360**
800-666-2665
FAX: 617-868-1772
e-mail: brooklinebks@delphi.com
www.brooklinebooks.com

Jean Ciborowski

Based on a careful analysis of 10 textbook programs, the author concisely and sensibly indicates the procedures that facilitate teachers' use of regular grade level textbooks with low-reading students. *$21.95*

Paperback
ISBN 0-91479 -57-3

2966 **There's a Hearing Impaired Child in My Class**

Gallaudet University Bookstore
800 Florida Avenue NE
Washington, DC 20002 **202-651-5000**
800-451-1073
FAX: 202-651-5489

This complete package provides basic facts about deafness, practical strategies for teaching hearing impaired children, and the question-and-answer information for all students. *$16.95*

44 pages

2967 **To Teach a Dyslexic**

AVKO Educational Research Foundation
3084 W Willard Road
Clio, MI 48420 **810-686-9283**
FAX: 810-686-1101

Don McCabe, Research Director

A dyslexic tells how luck enabled him to learn to read and how his blissful ignorance and stubbornness enabled him to discover how to teach other dyslexics to read and write. *$14.95*

288 pages Paperback

2968 **Toward Effective Public School Program for Deaf Students**

Teachers College Press
Columbia University
New York, NY 10027
800-575-6566
FAX: 212-678-4149

This book translates research and data into useable recommendations and possible courses of action for organizing effective public school programs for deaf students. *$22.95*

272 pages Paperback
ISBN 0-807731-59-5

2969 **Traumatic Brain Injury: Mechanisms of Damage, Assessment & Intervention**

Pro-Ed Publications
8700 Shoal Creek Boulevard
Austin, TX 78757 **512-451-3246**
800-897-3202
FAX: 512-451-8542
e-mail: info@proedinc.com
www.proedinc.com

Traumatic Brain Injury ranks as one of the most prevalent disorders with estimates ranging in hundreds of thousands of new cases each year. This book focuses on the mechanisms of acquired brain injury and the methods of assessment, along with treatment and outcome variables. *$41.00*

458 pages Hardcover

2970 **Treating Cerebral Palsy for Clinicians by Clinicians**

Pro-Ed Publications
8700 Shoal Creek Boulevard
Austin, TX 78757 **512-451-3246**
800-897-3202
FAX: 512-451-8542
e-mail: info@proedinc.com
www.proedinc.com

A clinical manual for professionals beginning to work with persons who have cerebral palsy. *$31.00*

312 pages

2971 **Treating Disordered Speech Motor Control**

Pro-Ed Publications
8700 Shoal Creek Boulevard
Austin, TX 78757 **512-451-3246**
800-897-3202
FAX: 512-451-8542
e-mail: info@proedinc.com
www.proedinc.com

This book about neuromotor disturbances of speech production is aimed at practicing professionals and advanced graduate students interested in the neuropathologies of communication. *$36.00*

410 pages

2972 **Treating Families of Brain Injury Survivors**

Springer Publishing Company
536 Broadway
New York, NY 10012 **212-431-4370**
877-687-7476
FAX: 212-941-7842
e-mail: marketing@springerpub.com
www.springerpub.com

Annette Imperati, Marketing/Sales Director

Provides the mental health practitioner with a comprehensive program for helping families of head injury survivors cope with the change in their lives. Includes background on medical aspects of head injury, family structure functioning and special needs of various family members.

220 pages
ISBN 0-82616 -20-1

2973 **Understanding and Teaching Emotionally Disturbed Children & Adolescents**

Pro-Ed Publications
8700 Shoal Creek Boulevard
Austin, TX 78757 **512-451-3246**
800-897-3202
FAX: 512-451-8542
e-mail: info@proedinc.com
www.proedinc.com

The teacher's handbook provides information that will change misconceptions about children who are frequently labeled as emotionally disturbed. It also gives information about a wide variety of intervention methods and approaches for use in educational settings. *$41.00*

620 pages Hardover

2974 **Using the Dictionary of Occupational Titles in Career Decision Making**

Stout Vocational Rehab Institute
University of Wisconsin-Stout
Menomonie, WI 5413G
FAX: 715-232-2356

Robert R Fry, Manager
Darlene Botterbusch, Program Assistant

This is a self-study manual for learning how to use the 1991 U.S. Department of Labor's Dictionary of Occupational Titles. It gives the DOT user a tool to understand the DOT and then put its information to work. Shows how to quickly obtain information about the work performed in 12,741 occupations listed and described in the DOT and the worker requirements for those occupations. *$24.00*

142 pages Softcover

2975 **VBS Special Education Teaching Guide**

LifeWay Christian Resources Southern Baptist Conv.
127 9th Avenue N
Nashville, TN 37234
615-251-2000
800-458-2772
FAX: 651-251-5764
e-mail: specialed@lifeway.com
www.lifeway.com

Ellen Beene, Editor

This book contains teaching plans for five bible study sessions with reproducible handouts for learners. The plans use multisensory, experiential-based learning activities designed for adults and older youth who have mental retardation. Suggestions for Bible learning, crafts, recreation, snacks and theme interpretation are included. Designed primarily for Vacation Bible School, but may be used in camp/retreat settings. *$9.95*

56 pages Yearly

2976 **Vocational Rehabilitation and Employment**

Books on Special Children
PO Box 305
Congers, NY 10920
845-638-1236
FAX: 845-638-0847
e-mail: irene@boscbooks.com

Defines kinds of work, expectations, goals and programs. Contributions in general issues of supported employment, training and management and community based programs. *$47.00*

372 pages Hardcover

2977 **We Can Speak for Ourselves: Self Advocacy by Mentally Handicapped People**

Brookline Books
PO Box 1046
Cambridge, MA 02238
617-495-3682
800-666-BOOK
FAX: 617-868-1772
e-mail: brooklinebks@delphi.com

The fundamental right of speaking for oneself has long been denied people with developmental disabilities. This book offers practical advice and support for parents, group home residence workers, day activity workers, citizens and professionals interested in developing self-advocacy for mentally handicapped people. *$17.95*

Paperback
ISBN 0-253363-65-9

2978 **Wintergreen Orchard House**

Wintergreen Orchard House
PO Box 15899
New Orleans, LA 70175
504-866-8658
800-321-9479
FAX: 504-866-8710

Allan B Corderman, Publisher
$25.95

320 pages Annual

2979 **Working Bibliography on Behavioral and Emotional Disorders**

Natl. Clearinghouse for Alcohol & Drug Information
PO Box 2345
Rockville, MD 20847
800-729-6686
FAX: 301-468-6433
e-mail: info@health.org
www.health.org

Lizabeth J Foster, Librarian/Info. Resource Mgr.

NCADI is a service of the U.S. Substance Abuse and Mental Health Services Administration. As the national focal point for information on alcohol and other drugs, NCADI collects, prepares, classifies, and distributes information about alcohol, tobacco and other drugs, prevention strategies and materials, research, treatment, etc.

40 pages

2980 **Working Together with Children and Families: Case Studies**

Paul H Brookes Publishing Company
PO Box 10624
Baltimore, MD 21285
800-638-3775
FAX: 410-337-8539

Karen G Radke, Marketing Director

Early interventionists will be able to bridge the gap between theory and practice with this edited collection of case studies. *$23.00*

336 pages 1993
ISBN 1-557661-23-5

2981 **Working with Visually Impaired Young Students: A Curriculum Guide**

Charles C Thomas
2600 S First Street
Springfield, IL 62704
217-789-8980
800-258-8980
FAX: 217-789-9130
e-mail: books@ccthomas.com
www.ccthomas.com

Ellen Trief, Author

The first step in the education process of a visually impaired child is the early identification and treatment by an eye care specialist. This book is geared to the age of birth through 3-years. Available in cloth, paperback and hardcover. *$36.95*

208 pages Paperback
ISBN 0-398068-75-5

Testing Resources

2982 **AEPS Child Progress Report: For Children Ages Birth to Three**

Brookes Publishing
PO Box 10624
Baltimore, MD 21285
410-337-9580
800-638-3775
FAX: 410-337-8539
e-mail: custserv@brookespublishing.com
www.brookespublishing.com

This chart helps monitor change by visually displaying current abilities, intervention targets, and child progress. In packages of 30. *$18.00*

6 pages Gate-fold
ISBN 1-55766 -65-0

2983 AEPS Data Recording Forms: For Children Ages Birth to Three

Brookes Publishing
PO Box 10624
Baltimore, MD 21285 **410-337-9580**
800-638-3775
FAX: 410-337-8539
e-mail: custserv@brookespublishing.com
www.brookespublishing.com

These forms can be used by child development professionals on four separate occasions to pinpoint and then monitor a child's strengths and needs in the six key areas of skill development measured by the AEPS Test. Packages of 10. *$23.00*

36 pages Saddle-stiched
ISBN 1-55766 -97-2

2984 AEPS Measurement for Birth to Three Years (Volume 1)

Brookes Publishing
PO Box 10624
Baltimore, MD 21285 **410-337-9580**
800-638-3775
FAX: 410-337-8539
e-mail: custserv@brookespublishing.com
www.brookespublishing.com

This dynamic volume explains the Assessment, Evaluation and Programming System, provides the complete AEPS Test and parallel assessment/evaluation tools for families and includes the forms and plans needed for implementation. *$39.00*

352 pages

2985 AEPS Measurement for Three to Six Years

Brookes Publishing
PO Box 10624
Baltimore, MD 21285 **410-337-9580**
800-638-3775
FAX: 410-337-8539
e-mail: custserv@brookespublishing.com
www.brookespublishing.com

$57.00

400 pages Spiral-bound
ISBN 1-55766 -87-1

2986 AIR: Assessment of Interpersonal Relations

Pro-Ed Publications
8700 Shoal Creek Boulevard
Austin, TX 78757 **512-451-3246**
800-897-3202
FAX: 512-451-8542
e-mail: info@proedinc.com
www.proedinc.com

A thoroughly researched and standardized clinical instrument assessing the quality of adolescents' interpersonal relationships in a hierarchical fashion, including global relationship quality and relationship quality with three domains: Family, Social and Academic. *$89.00*

2987 ALST: Adolescent Language Screening Test

Pro-Ed Publications
8700 Shoal Creek Boulevard
Austin, TX 78757 **512-451-3246**
800-897-3202
FAX: 512-451-8542
e-mail: info@proedinc.com
www.proedinc.com

Provides speech/language pathologists and other interested professionals with a rapid thorough method for screening adolescents (ages 11-17). *$119.00*

2988 Academic Skills Problems

National Association of School Psychologists
8455 Colesville Road
Suite 100
Silver Spring, MD 20910 **301-657-0270**
FAX: 301-657-0275

Offers direct assessment and intervention information for professionals.

232 pages

2989 Adaptive Mainstreaming: A Primer for Teachers and Principals, 3rd Edition

Longman Publishing Group
1185 Avenue of the Americas
New York, NY 10036 **212-782-3300**
www.ablongman.com

An introduction to education for handicapped and gifted students. Presents research-based rationales for teaching exceptional students in the least restrictive environment. Provides historical perspectives, offers realistic descriptions of prevailing practices in the field, and reviews trends and new directions.

366 pages Paperback 1988
ISBN 0-582285-04-6

2990 Ages & Stages Questionnaires

Brookes Publishing
PO Box 10624
Baltimore, MD 21285 **410-337-9580**
800-638-3775
FAX: 410-337-8539
e-mail: custserv@brookespublishing.com
www.brookespublishing.com

ASQ is an economical and field-tested system for identifying whether infants and young children may require further developmental evaluation and offers a screening and tracking program that helps early intervention professionals, service coordinators, and administrators maximize financial resources while promoting the health and growth of the children they serve. Set includes 11 color-coded, reproducible questionnaires, 11 reproducible, age appropriate scoring sheets. *$135.00*

2991 Assessing Students with Special Needs

Longman Publishing Group
10 Bank Street
9th Floor
White Plains, NY 10606 **914-993-5000**
FAX: 914-997-8115

Step-by-step guide to informal, classroom assessment of students with special needs.

174 pages Paperback 1990
ISBN 0-801301-77-7

2992 Assessing Young Children

National Association of School Psychologists
8455 Colesville Road
Suite 1000
Silver Spring, MD 20910 **301-681-3223**
FAX: 301-608-2514

Assessment is the key topic in this manual which discusses why and how assessment is unique for the early childhood population.

63 pages

2993 Assessing and Screening Preschoolers

National Association of School Psychologists
8455 Colesville Road
Suite 1000
Silver Spring, MD 20910
301-681-3223
FAX: 301-608-2514

A comprehensive and practical source to help professionals in counseling, school, and clinical psychology, special education, and human development become more competent in assessing preschoolers with special needs.

484 pages

2994 Assessment Log & Developmental Progress Charts for the CCPSN

Brookes Publishing
PO Box 10624
Baltimore, MD 21285
410-337-9580
800-638-3775
FAX: 410-337-8539
e-mail: custserv@brookespublishing.com
www.brookespublishing.com

This 28-page booklet allows readers to actually chart the on-going progress of each preschool child. Available in packages of 10. *$22.00*

28 pages Saddle-stiched
ISBN 1-55766-39-5

2995 Assessment of Learners with Special Needs

Allyn & Bacon
75 Arlington Street
Suite 300
Boston, MA 02116
617-848-6000
800-852-8024
FAX: 617-848-7490
www.ablongman.com

The central goal of this book is to help teachers become sophisticated, informed test consumers in terms of choosing, using and interpreting commercially prepared tests for their special needs students.

508 pages Casebound 1989
ISBN 0-205227-33-3

2996 Benchmark Measures

Educators Publishing Service
31 Smith Place
Cambridge, MA 02138
617-367-2700
800-225-5750
FAX: 617-547-0412
www.epsbooks.com

Ungraded test containing three sequential levels that assess alphabet and dictionary skills, reading, handwriting and spelling, and correspond to the first three schedules of the Alphabetic Phonics curriculum. The tests can be used at any level to measure a student's general knowledge of phonics. *$64.40*

Kit

2997 CREVT: Comprehensive Receptive and Expressive Vocabulary Test

Pro-Ed Publications
8700 Shoal Creek Boulevard
Austin, TX 78757
512-451-3246
800-897-3202
FAX: 512-451-8542
e-mail: info@proedinc.com
www.proedinc.com

A new, innovative, efficient measure of both receptive and expressive oral vocabulary. The CREVT has two subtests and is based on the most current theories of vocabulary development, suitable for ages 4 through 17. *$174.00*

Complete Kit

2998 DAYS: Depression and Anxiety in Youth Scale

Pro-Ed Publications
8700 Shoal Creek Boulevard
Austin, TX 78757
512-451-3246
800-897-3202
FAX: 512-451-8542
e-mail: info@proedinc.com
www.proedinc.com

A unique battery of three norm-references scales useful in identifying major depressive disorder and overanxious disorders in children and adolescents. *$129.00*

Complete Kit

2999 DOCS: Developmental Observation Checklist System

Pro-Ed Publications
8700 Shoal Creek Boulevard
Austin, TX 78757
512-451-3246
800-897-3202
FAX: 512-451-8542
e-mail: info@proedinc.com
www.proedinc.com

Wayne P Hresko, Author
Shirley A Miguel, Author

A three-part system for the assessment of very young children with respect to general development, adjustment behavior and parent stress and support. *$124.00*

3000 Daytime Development Center

Joseph Willard Health Center
3750 Old Lee Highway
Fairfax, VA 22030
703-246-7180
FAX: 703-246-7307

Susan Delauter CU-SLP, Director Health Services
Allan Phillips, Director Early Intervention

Offers assessments, evaluations and educational/therapeutic infant programs for parents and their children.

Sliding Scale

3001 Developmental Services Center

Therapeutic Nursery Program
4525 Lee Street NE
Washington, DC 20019
202-388-3216
FAX: 202-576-8799

Alice Anderson

Offers assessment information and evaluation for developmentally delayed students.

3002 K-BIT: Kaufman Brief Intelligence Test

AGS
Publishers Building
PO Box 99
Circle Pines, MN 55014
800-328-2560
FAX: 763-786-9007
www.agsnet.com

Robert Zaske, Market Manager

Quick and easy-to-use, KBIT assesses verbal and non-verbal abilities through two reliable subtests - vocabulary and matricies. *$ 124.95*

Ages 4-90

3003 **K-FAST: Kaufman Functional Academic Skills Test**

AGS
Publishers Building
PO Box 99
Circle Pines, MN 55014

800-328-2560
FAX: 763-786-9007
www.agsnet.com

Robert Zaske, Market Manager

Helps assess a person's capacity to function effectively in society regarding functional reading and math skills. *$99.95*

Ages 15-85+

3004 **K-SEALS: Kaufman Survey of Early Academic and Language Skills**

AGS
Publishers Building
PO Box 99
Circle Pines, MN 55014

800-328-2560
FAX: 763-786-9007
www.agsnet.com

Robert Zaske, Market Manager

An individually administered test of children's of both expressive and receptive skills, pre-academic skills and articulation. K-SEALS offers reliable scores usually in less than 25 minutes. *$ 179.95*

Ages 3-0; 6-11

3005 **KLST-2: Kindergarten Language Screening Test Edition, 2nd Edition**

Pro-Ed
8700 Shoal Creek Boulevard
Austin, TX 78757

512-451-3246
800-897-3202
FAX: 512-451-8542
e-mail: info@proedinc.com
www.proedinc.com

Identifies children who need further diagnostic testing to determine whether or not they have language deficits that will accelerate academic failure. *$94.00*

3006 **Kaufman Test of Educational Achievement (K-TEA)**

AGS
Publishers Building
PO Box 99
Circle Pines, MN 55014

800-328-2560
FAX: 763-786-9007
www.agsnet.com

Robert Zaske, Market Manager

K-TEA is an individually administered diagnostic battery that measures reading, mathematics, and spelling skills. Setting the standards in achievement testing today, K-TEA Comprehensive provides the complete diagnostic information you need for educational assessment and program planning. The Brief Forum is indispensable for school and clinical psychologists, special education teachers when a quick a measure of achievement is needed. *$249.95*

3007 **Life Centered Career Education: A Contemporary Based Approach 4th Edition**

Council for Exceptional Children
1110 N Glebe Road
Suite 300
Arlington, VA 22201

703-620-3660
FAX: 703-264-9494
www.cec.sped.org

Janice Burdick, President

Provides a framework for building 97 functional skill competencies appropriate for preparing for adult life and special education students. *$28.00*

175 pages

3008 **Managing Attention Disorders in Children**

National Association of School Psychologists
8455 Colesville Road
Suite 1000
Silver Spring, MD 20910

301-681-3223
FAX: 301-608-2514

A guide for practitioners offering information on treating Attention Deficit Disorders.

3009 **Measure of Cognitive-Linguistic Abilities (MCLA)**

Speech Bin
1965 25th Avenue
Vero Beach, FL 32960

772-770-0007
800-477-3324
FAX: 772-770-0006
www.speechbin.com

A diagnostic test of cognitive-linguistic abilities of adolescents and adults with traumatically induced brain injuries. High level. Normed. *$89.00*

100 pages
ISBN 0-93785 -72-

3010 **ONLINE**

West Virginia Research and Training Center
PO Box 1004
Institute, WV 25112

304-766-4602
800-624-8284
FAX: 304-766-2689
e-mail: online @rtc2.icdi.wvu.edu
www.icdi.wvu.edu

On Line Editor

A quarterly newsletter offering information about hardware technology, software (commercial and home grown); applications that work and bonuses such as an exchange program for copyright-free software. *$25.00*

Quarterly

3011 **OWLS: Oral and Written Language Scales LC/OE & WE**

AGS
Publishers Building
PO Box 99
Circle Pines, MN 55014

800-328-2560
FAX: 763-786-9007
www.agsnet.com

Robert Zaske, Market Manager

One kit provides an assessment of listening comprehension while the other assesses oral expression tasks: semantic, syntactic, pragmatic, and supralinguistic aspects of language. Written Expression may be administered individually or in small groups. *$249.95*

3012 **PAT-3: Photo Articulation Test**

Pro-Ed Publications
8700 Shoal Creek Boulevard
Austin, TX 78757

512-451-3246
800-897-3202
FAX: 512-451-8542
e-mail: info@proedinc.com
www.proedinc.com

Stanley Dickey, Author
Anton Soder, Author
Barbara Lippke, Author

This test consists of 72 color photographs. The first 69 photos test consonants and all but one vowel and one diphthong. The remaining pictures test connected speech and the remaining vowel and diphthong. *$144.00*

Complete Kit

3013 Peabody Early Experiences Kit (PEEK)

AGS
Publishers Building
PO Box 99
Circle Pines, MN 55014
800-328-2560
FAX: 763-786-9007
www.agsnet.com

Robert Zaske, Market Manager

1,000 activities and all the materials you need to build youngsters' cognitive, social and language skills. Manuals, puppets, manipulatives, picture card deck, picture mini decks and more to teach early development concepts. *$789.95*

3014 Peabody Individual Achievement Test-Revised Normative Update (PIAT-R-NU)

AGS
Publishers Building
PO Box 99
Circle Pines, MN 55014
800-328-2560
FAX: 763-786-9007
www.agsnet.com

Robert Zaske, Market Manager

PIAT-R-NU is an efficient individual measure of academic achievement. Reading, mathematics, and spelling are assessed in a simple, non-threatening format that requires only a pointing response for most items. This multiple choice format makes the PIAT-R ideal for assessing individuals who hesitate to give a spoken response, or have limited expressive abilities. *$289.98*

3015 Peabody Language Development Kits (PLDK)

AGS
Publishers Building
PO Box 99
Circle Pines, MN 55014
800-328-2560
FAX: 763-786-9007
www.agsnet.com

Robert Zaske, Market Manager

The main goals of the Peabody Kit language program are to stimulate overall language skills in Standard English and, for each level of the program, advance children's cognitive skills about a year. *$ 649.95*

Level P

ISBN 0-88671 -25-1

3016 Pediatric Early Elementary (PEEX II) Examination

Educators Publishing Service
31 Smith Place
Cambridge, MA 02138
617-367-2700
800-225-5750
FAX: 617-547-0412
www.epsbooks.com

Assesses the second-fourth grade child's performance on thirty-two tasks in six specific areas of development: fine-motor function, language, gross-motor function, memory, visual processing, and delayed recall. At three points during the exam, the child is rated on selective attention and behavior and effect.

$15.40 - $93

ISBN 0-83888 -80-6

3017 Pediatric Exam of Educational-PEERAMID Readiness at Middle Childhood

Educators Publishing Service
31 Smith Place
Cambridge, MA 02138
617-367-2700
800-225-5750
FAX: 617-547-0412
www.epsbooks.com

Assesses the 4th-10th grade child's performance on thirty-one tasks in six specific areas: minor neurological indicators, fine-motor function, language, gross-motor function, temporal-sequential organization, and visual processing. Complete set.

$15.40 - $109

ISBN 0-83888 -99-3

3018 Pediatric Examination of Educational Readiness

Educators Publishing Service
31 Smith Place
Cambridge, MA 02138
617-367-2700
800-225-5750
FAX: 617-547-0412
www.epsbooks.com

Assesses the Pre-1st grade child's performance on twenty-nine tasks in six specific areas of development: orientation, gross-motor, visual-fine motor, sequential, linguistic and preacademic learning. The child is rated on ten dimensions of selective attention/activity processing efficiency and adaptation. Complete set.

$12.85 - $86.40

ISBN 0-83888 -80-1

3019 Pediatric Extended Examination at-PEET Three

Educators Publishing Service
31 Smith Place
Cambridge, MA 02138
617-367-2700
800-225-5750
FAX: 617-547-0412
www.epsbooks.com

Assesses the preschool-age child's performance on twenty-eight tasks in five basic areas of development: gross-motor, language, visual-fine motor, memory, and intersensory integration. Complete set.

$13.75 - $126

ISBN 0-83888 -79-4

3020 Pre-Reading Screening Procedures

Educators Publishing Service
31 Smith Place
Cambridge, MA 02138
617-367-2700
800-225-5750
FAX: 617-547-0412
www.epsbooks.com

This revised group test, for grades K-1, evaluates auditory, visual and kinesthetic strengths in order to identify children who may have some form of dyslexia or specific language disability. *$ 18.00*

Grades K-1

ISBN 0-83885 -23-4

3021 Preparing for ACT Assessment

American College Testing Program
2201 Dodge
 # 168
Iowa City, IA 52243
319-337-1000
FAX: 319-339-3020

Designed to help high school students ready themselves for the ACT Assessment's subject area tests, explains the purposes of the four tests, describes their content and format, provides tips and exercises to improve student's test-taking skills and includes a complete sample text with scoring key.

3022 Psycho-Educational Assessment of Preschool Children

National Association of School Psychologists
8455 Colesville Road
Suite 1000
Silver Spring, MD 20910 **301-681-3223**
FAX: 301-608-2514

This is a contributed text on assessing specific skills of preschool children.

592 pages

3023 RULES: Revised

Speech Bin
1965 25th Avenue
Vero Beach, FL 32960 **772-770-0007**
800-477-3324
FAX: 772-770-0006
www.speechbin.com

Jane Webb, Author
Barbara Duckett, Author

Treatment program for young children who have phonological disorders. *$43.95*

280 pages
ISBN 0-93785 -51-3

3024 Receptive-Expressive Emergent-REEL-2 Language Test, Second Edition

Pro-Ed Publications
8700 Shoal Creek Boulevard
Austin, TX 78757 **512-451-3246**
800-897-3202
FAX: 512-451-8542
e-mail: info@proedinc.com
www.proedinc.com

Kenneth R Bzoch, Author
Richard League, Author

A revision of the popular scale used for the multidimensional analysis of emergent language. The REEL-2 is specifically designed for use with a broad range of at risk infants and toddlers in the new multidisciplinary programs developing under P.L. 99-457. *$79.00*

3025 Slingerland High School/College Screening

Educators Publishing Service
31 Smith Place
Cambridge, MA 02138 **617-367-2700**
800-225-5750
FAX: 617-547-0412
www.epsbooks.com

Assessments of high school and college level students to determine specific language disability and predict academic strengths as well as difficulties.

$17 - $23.95
ISBN 0-83882 -78-2

3026 Slingerland Screening Tests

Educators Publishing Service
31 Smith Place
Cambridge, MA 02138 **617-367-2700**
800-225-5750
FAX: 617-547-0412
www.epsbooks.com

These tests, by Beth Slingerland, for individuals or groups of children, grades 1-6, identify children who show indications of having specific language disability in reading, handwriting, spelling or speaking. Form D evaluates personal orientation in time and space as well as the ability to express ideas in writing.

$14.80 - $27.45
ISBN 0-83882 -02-2

3027 Special Orientation and Sequencing Development Remedial Activities

Psychological & Educational Publications
1320 Sandy Prarie Road
PO Box 520
Hydesville, CA 95547 **707-768-1807**
800-523-5775

Morrison Gardner, President

Designed to be used to remediate those children who perform poorly on any one or more activities of the Test of Pictures test. *$ 59.95*

3028 Specific Language Disability Test

Educators Publishing Service
31 Smith Place
Cambridge, MA 02138 **617-367-2700**
800-225-5750
FAX: 617-547-0412
www.epsbooks.com

Tests for individuals or groups to evaluate students in grades 6-8. Sub-tests I-V evaluate perception in visual discrimination, visual memory, visual motor-coordination. Sub-tests VI-X evaluate auditory discrimination, auditory-visual coordination, auditory-motor coordination and comprehension. Teacher's manual, test booklet, charts and cards are also available.

$2.85 - $21.15
ISSN 0838-84 0

3029 Speech Bin

1965 25th Avenue
Vero Beach, FL 32960 **772-770-0007**
800-477-3324
FAX: 772-770-0006
www.speechbin.com

Catalog offering test materials, assessment information, books and special education resources for speech-language pathologists, occupational and physical therapists, audiologists, and other rehabilitation professionals in schools, hospitals, clinics and private practices.

ISSN 4773-324

3030 Stocker Probe: Revised

Speech Bin
1965 25th Avenue
Vero Beach, FL 32960 **772-770-0007**
800-477-3324
FAX: 772-770-0006
www.speechbin.com

Diagnostic and treatment program for stuttering and language impairment in children and adults. *$75.00*

144 pages
ISBN 0-93785 -58-0

3031 Stuttering Severity Instrument for Children and Adults

Psychological & Educational Publications
1320 Sandy Prarie Road
PO Box 520
Hydesville, CA 95547 **707-768-1807**
800-523-5775

Morrison Gardner, President

With this tool teachers can determine whether to schedule a child for therapy or to evaluate the effects of treatment.

3032 Survey of Educational Skills and the Survey of Problem-Solving Skills

Educators Publishing Service
31 Smith Place
Cambridge, MA 02138
617-367-2700
800-225-5750
FAX: 617-547-0412
www.epsbooks.com

Both surveys are process measures designed to characterize the problem-solving and learning strategies of students in middle childhood. A detailed rating system enables educators and psychologists to observe each child's performance, to analyze error patterns and to guide the assessment procedure. *$10.00*

96 pages $10.65 - $37.90

ISBN 0-83881 -56-

3033 Taking Part: Introducing Social Skills to Young Children

AGS
Publishers Building
PO Box 99
Circle Pines, MN 55014
800-328-2560
FAX: 763-786-9007
www.agsnet.com

Robert Zaske, Market Manager

The first social skills curriculum to be linked directly to an assessment tool. More than 30 lessons correlate with the skills assessed by the Social Skills Rating System, a multirater approach to assessing prosocial and problem behaviors. *$149.95*

3034 Teaching Resources & Assessment of Critical Skills

Becoming Independant
1425 Corporate Center Parkway
Santa Rosa, CA 95407
707-527-5904
FAX: 707-527-1206
www.nbrc.net/DayProg/DayProg.htm

John McCue, Chief Executive Officer
Tom Richardson, Chief Operating Officer

An independent living assessment tool consisting of four booklets and master forms and a cassette tape. The tool was developed by Becoming Independent/TRACE, incorporating over 15 years of experience in providing independent living services. *$129.00*

3035 Test Accommodations for Students with Disabilities

Charles C Thomas
2600 S First Street
Springfield, IL 62704
217-789-8980
800-258-8980
FAX: 217-789-9130
e-mail: books@ccthomas.com
www.ccthomas.com

Considers legal questions, theoretical issues, and practical methods for meeting the assessment needs of students with diabilities. The book is comprised of ten chapters and includes test accommodations topics relating to federal and state regulations (including the IDEA Amendments Act of 1997), problems concerning reliability and validity, and practical strategies for planning test accomodations and adapting and modifying tests. *$51.95*

340 pages Paperback 1998

ISBN 0-398068-45-3

3036 Test Critiques: Volumes I-X

Pro-Ed Publications
8700 Shoal Creek Boulevard
Austin, TX 78757
512-451-3246
800-897-3202
FAX: 512-451-8542
e-mail: info@proedinc.com
www.proedinc.com

Provides the professional and nonprofessional with in-depth, evaluative studies of more than 800 of the most widely used of these assessment instruments. *$649.00*

3037 Test of Early Reading Ability Deaf or Hard of Hearing

Pro-Ed Publications
8700 Shoal Creek Boulevard
Austin, TX 78757
512-451-3246
800-897-3202
FAX: 512-451-8542
e-mail: info@proedinc.com
www.proedinc.com

D Kim Reid, Author
Wayne P Hresko, Author
Donald D Hammill, Author

This adaptation of the TERA-2 for simultaneous communication of American Sign Language is the ONLY individually administered test of reading designed for children with moderate to profound sensory hearing loss. *$169.00*

Complete Kit

3038 Test of Language Development: Primary

Pro-Ed
8700 Shoal Creek Boulevard
Austin, TX 78757
512-451-3246
800-897-3202
FAX: 512-451-8542
e-mail: info@proedinc.com
www.proedinc.com

TOLD P:2 and TOLD 1:2 are the most popular tests of spoken language used by clinicians today. They are used to identify children who have language disorders and to isolate the particular types of disorders they have. Primary Edition for ages 1-4 to 8-11: Intermediate Edition for ages 8-6 to 12-11.

3039 Test of Mathematical Abilities Second Edition

Pro-Ed Publications
8700 Shoal Creek Boulevard
Austin, TX 78757
512-451-3246
800-897-3202
FAX: 512-451-8542
e-mail: info@proedinc.com
www.proedinc.com

Virginia Brown, Author
Mary Cronin, Author
Elizabeth McEntire, Author

The latest version was developed for use in grades 3 through 12. It measures math performance on the two traditional major skill areas in math as well as attitude, vocabulary and general application of math concepts in real life. *$84.00*

3040 Test of Nonverbal Intelligence Third Edition

Pro-Ed Publications
8700 Shoal Creek Boulevard
Austin, TX 78757
512-451-3246
800-897-3202
FAX: 512-451-8542
e-mail: info@proedinc.com
www.proedinc.com

Linda Brown, Author
Rita J Sherbenou, Author
Susan K Johnson, Author

A language-free measure of intelligence, aptitude and reasoning. The administration of the test requires no reading, writing, speaking or listening on the part of the test subject. The items included in this test are problem-solving tasks that increase in difficulty. Each item presents a set of figures in which one or more components is missing. The test items include one or more of the characteristics of shape, position, direction, rotation, contiguity, shading, size, movement or pattern. *$229.00*

Complete Kit

3041 Test of Phonological Awareness

Pro-Ed Publications
8700 Shoal Creek Boulevard
Austin, TX 78757 **512-451-3246**
800-897-3202
FAX: 512-451-8542
e-mail: info@proedinc.com
www.proedinc.com

Measures young children's awareness of the individual sounds in words. Children who are sensitive to the phonological structure of words in oral language have a much easier time learning to read than children who are not. *$143.00*

3042 Test of Pictures/Forms/Letters/Numbers Spatial Orientation Skills

Psychological & Educational Publications
1320 Sandy Prarie Road
PO Box 520
Hydesville, CA 95547 **707-768-1807**
800-523-5775

Morrison Gardner, President

Developed to aid professionals in determining a child's ability to visually perceive forms and letters in the correct direction. *$35.00*

ISBN 0-93142 -09-8

3043 Test of Visual-Motor Skills: Upper Level

Psychological & Educational Publications
1320 Sandy Prarie Road
PO Box 520
Hydesville, CA 95547 **707-768-1807**
800-523-5775

Morrison Gardner, President

Measures eye-hand coordination. *$59.00*

ISBN 0-93142 -72-1

3044 Test of Written Spelling Third Edition

Pro-Ed Publications
8700 Shoal Creek Boulevard
Austin, TX 78757 **512-451-3246**
800-897-3202
FAX: 512-451-8542
e-mail: info@proedinc.com
www.proedinc.com

This revised edition assesses the student's ability to spell words whose spellings are readily predictable in sound-letter patterns, words whose spellings are less predictable and both types of words considered together. *$74.00*

3045 Welcoming Students who are Deaf-Blind into Typical Classrooms

Brookes Publishing
PO Box 10624
Baltimore, MD 21285 **410-337-9580**
800-638-3775
FAX: 410-337-8539
e-mail: custserv@brookespublishing.com
www.brookespublishing.com

Facilitating School Participation, Learning, and Friendships. Examines successful inclusive educational practices that encourage the participation of students who are deaf-blind. *$37.00*

480 pages Paperback
ISBN 1-55766 -44-8

3046 Woodcock Reading Mastery Tests

AGS
Publishers Building
PO Box 99
Circle Pines, MN 55014
800-328-2560
FAX: 763-786-9007
www.agsnet.com

Robert Zaske, Market Manager

The Woodcock Reading Mastery Tests - Revised provides an interpretive system and age range to help you assess reading skills of children and adults. Two forms, G and II, make it easy to test and retest, or you can combine the results of both forms for a more comprehensive assessment. Revised with recent updates. *$329.95*

3047 Young Children with Special Needs: A Developmentally Appropriate Approach

Allyn & Bacon
75 Arlington Street
Suite 300
Boston, MA 02116 **617-848-6000**
800-852-8024
FAX: 617-848-7490
www.ablongman.com

This book is designed to prepare students in making curriculum decisions in order to care for and foster the development of young children with special needs in normal early childhood settings.

270 pages
ISBN 0-20518 -94-X

General

3048 **American Institute for Foreign Study**

River Plaza
9 W Broad Street
Stamford, CT 06902

800-727-2437
FAX: 203-399-5598
e-mail: info@aifs.com
www.aifs.org

Anthony Cook, Executive Director

Provides summer travel programs overseas and in the US ranging from one week to a full academic year.

3049 **American Universities International Programs**

305 W Magnolia Street
Suite 221
Fort Collins, CO 80521

970-495-0869
FAX: 970-484-6997
e-mail: auip@fru.com

Linda Detling, Program Coordinator AUIP

Study abroad organization sending students to universities in Australia and New Zealand.

3050 **American-Scandinavian Foundation**

58 Park Avenue
New York, NY 10016

212-879-9779
FAX: 212-879-2301
e-mail: info@amscan.org
www.amscan.org

Jean Prahl, Director Training

Offers young US citizens the opportunity to live in Scandinavia and train in their professional field.

3051 **Antioch College**

795 Livermore Street
Yellow Springs, OH 45387

937-767-7331
FAX: 937-767-6429
e-mail: aea@antioch-college.edu
www.antioch-college.edu

Education abroad offers numerous programs which can be included in undergraduate and graduate study programs.

3052 **Army and Air Force Exchange Services**

PO Box 660202
Dallas, TX 75266

214-312-3333
FAX: 214-312-3429

Management Recruiter, Contact

A worldwide retail, food and service business. All careers include job training and education, on-the-job training and classroom instruction. The AAFES accepts responsibility for ensuring accessibility and making reasonable accommodations when needed. This program focuses on ability not disability.

3053 **Association for International Practical Training**

10400 Little Patuxent Parkway
Suite 250
Columbia, MD 21044

410-997-2200
FAX: 410-992-3924
e-mail: aipt@aipt.org
www.aipt.org

Molly Fritts, Communications Manager

Nonprofit organization dedicated to encouraging and facilitating the exchange of qualified individuals between the US and other countries so they may gain practical work experience and improve international understanding.

3054 **Basic Facts on Study Abroad**

International Education
809 United Nations Plaza
New York, NY 10017

212-949-1840
FAX: 212-963-3489
e-mail: publications@un.org

Information book including foreign study planning, educational choices, finances and study abroad programs. *$35.00*

30 pages

3055 **Beaver College**

450 S Easton Road
Glenside, PA 19038

215-572-2901
888-232-8379
FAX: 215-572-2174
e-mail: cea@beaver.edu
www.beaver.edu/cea

Lorna Stern, Deputy Director

One of the largest college-based study abroad programs in the country. Prices from $8000.00 semester to $22000.00 a year.

3056 **Davidson College, Office of Study Abroad**

PO Box 1719
Davidson, NC 28036

704-892-2351
FAX: 704-892-2120
e-mail: caortmayer@davidson.edu
www.davidson.edu/academic/sasian/application.

Carolyn Ortmayer, Coordinator of Study Abroad

Recognizes the value of study abroad for both the development of world understanding and the development of the student as a broadminded, objective and mature individual. 1. Junior year abroad in Wurzburg, Germany. 2. Fall, Spring or full year in tours, France.

3057 **High School Students Guide to Study, Travel, and Adventure Abroad**

205 E 42nd Street
New York, NY 10017

888-COU-NCIL
FAX: 212-822-2649
www.councilexchanges.org

Priscilla Tovey, Information Services
Cheryl Jeffries, Administrative Asst.

This guide provides high school students with all the information they need for a successful trip abroad. Included are sections to help students find out if they're ready for a trip abroad, make the necessary preparations and get the most from their experience. Over 200 programs are described including language study, summer camps, homestays, study tours and work camps. The program descriptions include information for people with disabilities. *$13.95*

308 pages Biennial
ISBN 0-31211-22-8

3058 **Higher Education Consortium for Urban Affairs (HECUA)**

2233 University Avenue W
Suite 210
St. Paul, MN 55114

651-646-8831
800-554-1089
FAX: 651-659-9421
e-mail: info@hecua.org
www.hecua.org

Michael Eaton, Director Student Services

HECUA offers college-level off-campus study programs in Latin America, Asia, Europe and the U.S. Internships, field projects and other forms of experimental learning are combined with academic study. Programs focus on issues of inequality and ways to bring about positive social change. HECUA has thirty years of experience and a national reputation for the best in teaching and learning that engages students in meaningful study and action. Students with disabilities welcome to apply.

3059 International Christian Youth Exchange

134 W 26th Street
New York, NY 10001 **212-206-7307**
FAX: 212-633-9085

Ed Gragert

Offers participants a unique experience to learn about another culture and make friends from different countries.

3060 International Partnership for Service-Learning

815 2nd Avenue
Suite 315
New York, NY 10017 **212-986-0989**
FAX: 212-986-5039
e-mail: info@ipsl.org
www.ipsl.org

Linda A Chisholm, President
Sarah Callahan, Coordinator of Special Projects

An organization of colleges, universites, service agencies, and related organizations united to foster and develop programs linking volunteer service and academic study for credit. Administers 13 undergraduate programs in 12 nations, and offers an MA Degree program in International Service.

1982

3061 International University Partnerships

University of Pennsylvania
1011 S Drive
Indiana, PA 15705 **724-357-2295**
FAX: 724-357-2514

Dr. Robert Morris

Offers a variety of international educational exchange programs to students who wish to study overseas.

3062 Lake Erie College

Academic Programs Abroad
Painesville, OH 44077 **440-942-3872**
FAX: 440-352-3533

Catherine Shaw

Sends students abroad for a term or longer to develop intellectual awareness and individual maturity.

3063 Lane Community College

4000 E 30th Avenue
Eugene, OR 97405 **541-747-4501**
FAX: 541-744-4171
www.lanecc.edu

Work Experience Program students work for credit and in some cases pay, in Europe, Asia, Mexico and Turkey.

3064 Lions Clubs International

300 22nd Street
Oak Brook, IL 60523 **630-571-5466**
FAX: 630-571-8890
e-mail: info@lionsclubs.org
www.lionsclubs.org

Deborah O'Malley, Health Research Coordinator

Over 44,500 individual clubs in over 186 countries and geographical areas which provide community service and promote better international relations. Clubs work with local communities to provide needed and useful programs for sight, diabetes and hearing.

3065 Lisle

900 County Road 269
Leander, TX 78641 **512-259-7621**
FAX: 512-259-0392
e-mail: mkinney@utnet.utoledo.edu
www.lisle.utoledo.edu

Barbara Bratton, Executive Director

Educational organization which works toward world peace and better quality of human life through increased understanding between persons of similar and different cultures.

$750 - $3,500

3066 National 4-H Council

7100 Connecticut Avenue
Chevy Chase, MD 20815 **301-961-2800**
FAX: 301-961-2894
www.fourhcouncil.edu

Edith Cowper

Offers two different types of international exchange programs.

3067 New Directions for People with Disabilities

135 S Mount Zion Road
Suite 207
Lebanon, IN 46052
FAX: 800-882-8583
e-mail: newdirec@sikom.com
www.newdirectionstravel/index.htm

Dee Duncan, Executive Director

Dedicated to providing local, national, and international travel and foreign exchange programs for people with disabilities. Promote understanding, acceptance, and appreciation of people with disabilties as important and contributing members of our society as well as to promote a sense of accomplishment, belinging, and self-worth.

3068 People to People International

501 E Armour Boulevard
Kansas City, MO 64109 **816-531-4701**
800-676-7874
FAX: 816-561-7502
e-mail: ptpi@ptpi.org
www.ptpi.org

Jill Sigler, Adult Programs Coordinator

Nonpolitical, nonprofit organization working outside the government to advance the cause of international undestanding through international contact. We offer overseas internships and volunteering opportunities.

3069 Rotary Youth Exchange

Rotary International
One Rotary Center
Evanston, IL 60201 **847-866-3000**
FAX: 847-866-6116
www.rotary.org

Exchanges for disabled youth are run by local Rotary clubs and districts. The exchanges can either be short term or long term exchanges. Contact your local Rotary Club for information.

3070 Scandinavian Seminar
24 Dickinson Street
Amherst, MA 01002
413-253-9736
800-828-3343
FAX: 413-253-5282
www.scandinavianseminar.com

Leslie Evans

Student exchange program founded in 1949.

3071 Sister Cities International
1301 Pennysylvania Avenue
Suite 830
Washington, DC 20004
202-347-8630
FAX: 202-393-6524
e-mail: info@sister-cities.org
www.sister-cities.org

Tim Honey, Executive Director
Cynthia M Makin, Assistant Executive Director

3072 Southern Illinois University at Carbondale
Room B220 NW Annex
Carbondale, IL 62901
618-453-7670
FAX: 618-453-7647
e-mail: studyabr@siu.edu
www.siu.edu/departments/study_abroad

Study Abroad Programs

Main emphasis in international programs abroad are school-to-school direct exchanges and exchanges through organizations such as the International Student Exchange Program.

3073 State University of NY College at Buffalo
1300 Elmwood Avenue
Cleveland Hall 416
Buffalo, NY 14222
716-878-4620
FAX: 716-878-3054
e-mail: intleduc@buffalostate.edu
www.buffalostate.edu/intnated

Dr Lee Ann Grace, Director, Intl Education

Provides international educational exchange opportunities for students of university age and older through its Office of International Education.

3074 State University of New York
1400 Washington Avenue
Albany, NY 12222
518-442-3300
FAX: 518-442-3235
www.albany.edu

Dr. Reynold Bloom

Offers over 150 international educational exchange programs in 37 different countries.

3075 University of Minnesota at Crookston
2900 University Avenue
Crookston, MN 56716
218-281-8508
800-UMC-MINN
FAX: 218-281-8050
e-mail: mprada@mail.crk.umn.edu
www.crk.umn.edu

Mario Prada, Program Director

A four-year college with innovative educational programs for the acquisition of technical skills and a liberal arts education.

3076 University of Oregon International Service
330 Oregon Hall
5209 University of Oregon
Eugene, OR 97403
541-346-3206
FAX: 541-346-1232
www.uoregon.edu

Paul Primak

International programs offered through the University of Oregon offer participants the opportunity to gain academic, cultural, and personal experience.

3077 University of Portland
5000 N Willamette Boulevard
Portland, OR 97203
503-943-7911
FAX: 503-943-7178

Thompson Faller

Study/cultural experience is available in Tokyo and other Japanese cities as part of the Japan Studies Program at the University.

3078 Western Washington University
International Programs & Exchanges
Old Main 530E
Bellingham, WA 98225
360-650-3910
FAX: 360-650-9046
e-mail: ipewwu@cc.wwu.edu
www.wwu.edu/~ipewwu

Liz Partolan-Fray, Director International Programs

Provides international educational exchange opportunities for students through various programs.

3079 World Experience
2440 S Hacienda Boulevard
Suite 116
Hacienda Heights, CA 91745
626-330-5719
800-633-6653
FAX: 626-333-4914
www.worldexperience.org

Nonprofit organization which sponsors, develops and carries out international student exchange programs for study and service abroad.

3080 Youth for Understanding International Exchange
3501 Newark Street NW
Washington, DC 20016
202-966-6800
800-TEE-NAGE
FAX: 202-895-1104
e-mail: info@yfu.org
www.youthforunderstanding.org

Youth for Understanding (YFU) International Exchange, an educational, nonprofit organization, prepares young people for the opportunities and responsabilities in a changing, independent world. With YFU, students can choose a year, semenster, or summer program in one or more than 35 countries worldwide. More than 200,000 young people from more than 50 nations in Asia, Europe, North and South America, Africa and the Pacific have participated in YFU exchanges.

Alabama

3081 **Alabama Power Foundation**

600 18th Street N
17th Floor
Birmingham, AL 35203 **205-257-1000**
FAX: 205-226-1441

Giving is limited to Alabama. No support is given for religious or political organizations, individuals or for operating funds that duplicate the United Way support.

3082 **Andalusia Health Services**

PO Box 667
Andalusia, AL 36420 **334-222-2030**
FAX: 334-222-7844
e-mail: chamber@alaweb.com

George Proctor Sr, President

Only offers grants to the residents of Covington County in Alabama who are pursuing a degree in a medical field.

3083 **Arc of Alabama**

300 S Hull Street
Montgomery, AL 36104 **334-262-7688**
FAX: 334-834-9737
e-mail: arcalabama@juno.com
www.arcalabama.org

Thomas B Holmes, Executive Director

The Arc of Alabama is committed to securing for all people with mental retardation the opportunity to choose and realize their goals in regard to where and how they learn, live, work and play.

3084 **Blount Foundation**

4520 Executive Park Drive
Montgomery, AL 36116 **334-244-4000**

D Joseph McInnes

Established in 1970, the Foundation was created to serve as the voice with which the Blount Companies address the need to provide financial assistance to a variety of activities and programs concerned with the general welfare of our country and its citizens. The Foundation has a strong commitment to corporate citizenship and endorses the concept that companies, as well as individuals, must contribute to the well-being of society.

Alaska

3085 **Arc of Alaska**

2211-A Arca Drive
Anchorage, AK 99508 **907-277-6677**

3086 **Rasmuson Foundation**

301 W Northern Lights Boulevard
Suite 400
Anchorage, AK 99503 **907-297-2700**
FAX: 907-297-2770
e-mail: rasmusonfdn@rasmuson.org
www.rasmuson.org

Grants for Alaska 501C3 nonprofits only.

Arizona

3087 **Arc of Arizona**

5610 S Central Avenue
Phoenix, AZ 85040 **602-243-1787**
800-252-9054
FAX: 602-268-7483
e-mail: Arcofarizona@aol.com
www.arcofarizona.org

Richard Young, Executive Director

The Arc, a national organization on mental retardaion, is committed to securing for all people with developmental disabilities the opportunity to choose and realize their goals in regard to where they live, learn, work and play.

3088 **Arizona Community Foundation**

2122 E Highland Avenue
Suite 4000
Phoenix, AZ 85016 **602-381-1400**
800-222-8221
FAX: 602-381-1575
e-mail: rmayberry@azfoundation.com
www.azfoundation.org

Bennett Dorrance, Chairperson

3089 **JW Kieckhefer Foundation**

116 E Gurley Street
PO Box 750
Prescott, AZ 86302 **928-445-4010**

John Kieckhefer, Trustee

3090 **Margaret T Morris Foundation**

PO Box 592
Prescott, AZ 86302 **928-445-6633**
FAX: 928-445-5368

Eugene P Polk

Arkansas

3091 **Arc of Arkansas**

2004 S Main Street
Little Rock, AR 72206 **501-375-7770**
FAX: 501-372-4621

3092 **Roy and Christine Sturgis Charitable Trust**

PO Box 92
Malvern, AR 72104 **501-337-5109**

Physically disabled, hospitals, child welfare and visually impaired are priorities of giving for this foundation.

3093 **Winthrop Rockefeller Foundation**

308 E 8th Street
Little Rock, AR 72202 **501-376-6854**
FAX: 501-374-4797

Mahlon Martin

Mission is to improve the quality of life in Arkansas. It focuses its grantmaking efforts in three areas: education, economic development and civic affairs. Education projects funded in the past have included grants to schools that are working to involve teachers and parents in making decisions about what happens at their schools, projects that work to remove prejudice from the educational process and more. Major grants are made to support the development of new programs.

California

3094 Ahmanson Foundation
9215 Wilshire Boulevard
Beverly Hills, CA 90210 **310-278-0770**

Lee Walcott, Managing Director
Robert Ahmanson, President

The Foundation primarily gives in Southern California with major emphasis in Los Angeles County. The Foundation focuses on the arts and humanities, education, mental health and support for a broad range of social welfare programs.

3095 Alice Tweed Touhy Foundation
205 E Carrillo Street
Suite 219
Santa Barbara, CA 93101 **805-962-6430**

Harris Seed, President
Eleanor Van Cott, Executive VP

Rehabilitation, recreation and building funds are given to organizations only within the Santa Barbara area.

3096 Alternating Hemiplegia of Childhood Foundation
239 Nevada Street
Redwood City, CA 94062 **650-365-5798**
800-225-3353
FAX: 650-365-5798
e-mail: laegan6@sbcglobal.net
www.ahckids.org

Lynn Egan, VP
Carol Presunka, Secretary

Voluntary not-for-profit organizations dedicated to promoting professional and public awareness of Alternating Hemiplegia of Childhood (AHC) and providing current information to affected individuals and their families. Supports ongoing medical research into the cause, treatment and potential cure of AHC. Disseminates information about this disorder to promote proper diagnosis and maintains a registry of families, affected chidren and physicians who are familiar with AHC.

3097 Amateur Athletic Foundation of Los Angeles
2141 W Adams Boulevard
Los Angeles, CA 90018 **323-730-4600**
FAX: 323-730-9637
e-mail: info@aafla.org
www.aafla.org

Enables AAF to serve as an educational and research center for sport— a leading forum for the advancement of coaching, the exchange of ideas and exploration of important issues in sport.

3098 Annuziata Sanguinetti Foundation
420 Montgomery Street
5th Floor
San Francisco, CA 94104 **415-477-1000**

Eugene Ranghiasci

Hard-of-hearing, speech impaired and recreation. Serves only the San Francisco Bay area.

3099 Apple Computer
Worldwide Disability Solutions Group
2851 Park Avenue
Santa Clara, CA 95050 **408-996-1010**
800-692-7753
TTY:800-755-0601

Offers grants in the areas of education, health and in areas of company operations.

3100 Arc of California
1225 8th Street
Suite 590
Sacramento, CA 95814 **916-552-6619**
FAX: 916-441-3494
e-mail: arcca@quiknet.com

3101 Atkinson Foundation
1720 S Amphlett Boulevard
#100
San Mateo, CA 94402 **650-357-1101**
FAX: 650-357-1101
e-mail: atkinfdn@aol.com

Elizabeth Curtis, Administrator

The Foundation focuses and awards grants to community service and civic organizations serving the residents of San Mateo County, California through programs that benefit children, youth, seniors, the disadvantaged and those in need of rehabilitation. Grants are also made to local churches and schools, and overseas for sustainable development, health education and family planning. No grants to individuals or for research, travel, special events, annual campaigns, media and publications.

3102 Baker Commodities Corporate Giving Program
4020 Bandini Boulevard
Los Angeles, CA 90023 **323-268-2801**
FAX: 323-268-5166

Maxine Taylor, Executive Secretary

3103 Bank of America Foundation
315 Montgomery Street
8th Floor
San Francisco, CA 94104 **415-622-3456**
888-488-9802
FAX: 704-386-6444
www.bankamerica.com/foundation

Caroline Boitano

The Foundation will consider grants in four categories including: Health & Human Services, which provides support to health & human service organizations primarily through grants to the United Way campaigns; Education, with the focus on preparing people to become productive employees and participating citizens; Conservation & Environment, the improvement of California communities for the benefit of their citizens; and Culture & The Arts, supporting the leading performing and visual arts groups.

3104 Bergen Brunswig Corporation Contributions Program
4000 Metropolitan Drive
Orange, CA 92686 **714-385-4000**
FAX: 714-385-6948

Valerie Calleros, Chairperson

3105 Blind Babies Foundation
1200 Gough Street
San Francisco, CA 94109 **415-922-9185**
FAX: 415-771-9026

Dennak Murphy, Executive Director

Founded in 1949, provides services and programs that enable and empower families, professionals and the broader community to meet the unique needs of infants and preschool children who are blind or visually impaired. *$5.00*

3106 Bothin Foundation

PO Box 29906
San Francisco, CA 94129 **415-771-4300**
FAX: 415-771-4064

Lyman J Casey, Executive Director

The broad purpose of this foundation is to support public charities located in the five counties of San Francisco, Marin, Sonoma, San Mateo and Santa Barbara. Bothin elects to support charitable organizations that promote youth, elderly, disabled, health care, minorities, community social services and the environment. Grants for the arts are made mainly to those groups predominantly serving youth or with heavy emphasis on youth participation.

3107 Briggs Foundation

6106 La Flecha, Number 250
PO Box 1510
Rancho Santa Fe, CA 92067 **858-756-4875**

Blaine A Briggs

3108 Burns-Dunphy Foundation

5 Third Street
Suite 1200
San Francisco, CA 94103 **415-421-6995**
FAX: 415-882-7774

Walter Gleason

Grants are given to promote wellness for the visually impaired, physically and mentally disabled and to promote research in these areas.

3109 CNF Transportation Corporate Giving Program

3240 Hillview Avenue
Palo Alto, CA 94304 **650-494-2900**
FAX: 650-493-0360

Henry A Schmitt, Assistant Vice President

3110 California Community Foundation

445 S Figueroa Street
Suite 3400
Los Angeles, CA 90071 **213-413-4130**
FAX: 213-622-2979
www.calfund.org

Jack Shakely

Areas of funding priority include grants for the disabled, child welfare, rehabilitation, developmentally disabled, employment projects, research and computer projects. Giving is limited to the greater Los Angeles area.

3111 California Endowment

21650 Oxnard Street
Suite 1200
Woodland Hills, CA 91367 **818-703-3311**
800-449-4149
FAX: 818-703-4193
e-mail: bmartin@calendow.org
www.calendow.org

Rebecca Martin, Grants Manager

3112 Carrie Estelle Doheny Foundation

911 Wilshire Boulevard
Suite 1750
Los Angeles, CA 90017 **213-488-1122**
FAX: 413-488-1544
e-mail: doheny@earthlink.net

Robert A Smith III, Presedent

3113 Clorox Company Foundation

PO Box 24305
Oakland, CA 94623 **510-271-2199**

e-mail: community.relations@clorox.com
www.clorox.com/company/foundation

Patricia Marino, President

Community Support Programs are offered to make the communities in which we live and work stronger, while providing measurable benefits to the Company and its shareholders. The Foundation's primary concern continues to be youth and K-12 education. The Foundation is helping our young people to improve their educational and job skills and develop their leadership potential.

3114 Community Foundation of Santa Clara County

111 W Saint John Street
Suite 230
San Jose, CA 95113 **408-264-2437**

Peter Hero

Visually impaired, mentally and physically disabled, hard-of-hearing, special education, mental health and employment projects are areas of priority. Giving is limited to Santa Clara and surrounding counties.

3115 Crescent Porter Hale Foundation

220 Bush Street
Suite 1069
San Francisco, CA 94104
FAX: 415-986-5197

Ulla Davis, Executive Director

Serves organizations in the San Francisco Bay Area who are involved in the following areas of concern: education in the fields of art and music; private elementary, high school and university education; capital funding; and other worthwhile programs which can be demonstrated as serving broad community purposes, leading toward the improvement of the quality of life.

3116 Darrow Foundation

1000 4th Street
Suite 375
San Rafael, CA 94901 **415-453-0534**
FAX: 415-453-0441

DeWitt K MacDonald, Director

Grants are given in the areas of child welfare, visually impaired, projects involving independence, mentally and physically disabled.

3117 David and Lucile Packard Foundation

300 2nd Street
Suite 200
Los Altos Hills, CA 94022 **650-948-7658**
FAX: 650-947-8616
www.packfound.org

Richard Schlesburg, President

This foundation provides grants to nonprofit organizations in the following areas Conservation; Population; sciance; children, familes, and communities; Arts anf Organizational Effectiveness and Philanthropy. It provides national and international grants and also has a special focus on the Northern California Counties.

3118 **Deutsch Foundation**
2444 Wilshire Boulevard
Suite 600
Santa Monica, CA 90403 **310-862-3000**
FAX: 310-862-3100

Learning disabled, visually impaired, mental health, eye research, child welfare, speech and hearing impaired, physically disabled and independence projects are funded through this Foundation. Giving is limited to California.

3119 **Donald R Barker Foundation**
PO Box 936
Rancho Mirage, CA 92270 **760-321-2345**
FAX: 760-321-8662

Coeta Barker, Owner

It is an independent organization that gives its attention to organizations that are charitable or nonprofit under the laws of the state of Oregon or California.

3120 **East Bay Community Foundation**
200 Frank H Ogawa Plaza
Oakland, CA 94612 **510-836-3223**
FAX: 510-836-3287
e-mail: admin@eastbaycp.org
www.eastbaycf.org

David Pontecorvo, Program Director

A collection of funds created by many people, organizations and businesses, the Foundation helps those people and groups to support effective nonprofit organizations to the East Bay and beyond.

3121 **Evelyn and Walter Hans Jr**
1 Lombard Street
Suite 305
San Francisco, CA 94111 **415-398-4474**
FAX: 415-986-4779

Ira Hirschfield, President

A private foundation interested in programs which assist people who are hungry, homeless, or at risk of homelessness; enable older adults to maintain independent lives in the community and support Hispanic community development in San Francisco's Mission District. The Foundation also encourages proposals for corporate social responsibility efforts within the business community.

3122 **Fireman's Fund Foundation**
777 San Marin Drive
Novato, CA 94998 **415-899-2757**
FAX: 415-899-2126

Barbara Friede, Director

Provides discretionary grants to the disabled only in Marin and Sonoma counties in the San Francisco Bay area.

3123 **Foundation for the Junior Blind**
5300 Angeles Vista Boulevard
Los Angeles, CA 90043 **323-295-4555**
FAX: 323-296-0424
e-mail: info@fjb.org
www.fjb.org

Robert B Ralls, President

The Foundation for the Junior Blind is a private nonprofit agency that provides a wide range of programs and services for the blind, visually impaired and multiply disabled-blind children, youths and adults and their families. Programs include: Infant-Family Program; Children's Special Education School; Children's Residential Program; Davidson Program for Independence (for adults); and a year-round recreation program that includes a summer residential camp— Camp Bloomfield.

3124 **Fred Gellert Foundation**
1 Embarcadero Center
Suite 2480
San Francisco, CA 94111 **415-433-6147**
FAX: 415-433-7952

Fred Gellert Jr, Chairman

Focuses on organizations and programs serving residents of San Mateo and San Francisco and Marin counties in California, with the exception of environmentally concerned organizations.

3125 **Gallo Foundation**
PO Box 1130
Modesto, CA 95353 **209-341-3111**
FAX: 209-341-3307

Physically and mentally disabled, child welfare, Special Olympics, United Cerebral Palsy and Easter Seal Society are among the grants provided by this foundation.

3126 **Glaucoma Research Foundation**
200 Pine Street
Suite 200
San Francisco, CA 94104 **415-986-3162**
800-826-6693
FAX: 415-986-3763
e-mail: info@glaucoma.org
www.glaucoma.org

Tara L Steele, Executive Director

A national organization dedicated to protecting the sight of people with glaucoma through research and education. The Foundation conducts and supports research that contributes to improved patient care and a better understanding of the disease process. Provides education, advocacy and emotional support to patients and their families.

3127 **Harden Foundation**
PO Box 779
Salinas, CA 93902 **831-442-3005**
FAX: 831-443-1429

Joseph C Grainger, Executive Director

3128 **Harry and Grace Steele Foundation**
441 N Newport Boulevard
Suite 30
Newport Beach, CA 92663 **949-631-0418**
FAX: 949-631-1255

Marie Kowert

Gives grants to qualified tax-exempt charitable organizations which are not private foundations. Tax-supported organizations of any kind, and applications from individuals are not accepted. Grants are made for altruistic purposes, charitable, benevolent or educational, primarily local giving.

3129 **Henry J Kaiser Family Foundation**
2400 Samd Hill Road
Menlo Park, CA 94025 **650-854-9400**
800-656-4533
FAX: 650-854-4800
e-mail: rwells@kff.org
www.kff.org

Renee Wells, Grants and Contracts Manager

3130 **Henry W Bull Foundation**

Santa Barbara Bank & Trust
PO Box 2340
Santa Barbara, CA 93120
805-879-8405
FAX: 805-884-1404

Janice Gibbons, VP/Senior Trust Officer
Sharon McGinness, Sr Trust Admin Assistant

Grant given to a wide range of organizations that include those which provide services for the hard-of-hearing, speech impaired, visually impaired and physically disabled; arts, education services for elderly and youth grants awarded three times a year. Grant size ranges from $500 to $5,000. Proposal deadlines Jan 1, May 1, Sept 1.

3131 **Irvine Health Foundation**

18301 Von Kraman Avenue
Irvine, CA 92612
949-253-2959
FAX: 949-253-2962
e-mail: ebk@ihf.org
www.ihf.org

Edward B Kacic, President

3132 **Joseph Drown Foundation**

1999 Avenue of the Stars
Suite 1930
Los Angeles, CA 90067
310-277-4488
FAX: 310-277-4573
www.jdrown.org

Giving is focused primarily in California. No support for religious purposes or to individuals.

3133 **Kenneth T and Eileen L Norris Foundation**

11 Golden Shore
Suite 450
Long Beach, CA 90802
562-435-8444
FAX: 562-436-0584
e-mail: bover@ktn.org
www.norrisfoundation.org

Ronald Barnes, Executive Director
Nancy Boyer, Grants Manager
Savannah Gerringer, Grants Assistant

The Foundation is primarily focused on medicine and education. To a lesser extent the foundation contributes to community programs including visually impaired, autism, mentally and physically disabled, deaf and mental health in the Southern California area. Average grant size in this area is $5,000-$10,000. Grants are also given in the area of culture and youth.

3134 **Koret Foundation**

33 New Montgomery Street
Suite 1090
San Francisco, CA 94105
415-882-7740
FAX: 415-882-7775
e-mail: info@koretfoundation.org
www.koretfoundation.org

Rosemary Peterson

3135 **LJ Skaggs and Mary C Skaggs Foundation**

1221 Broadway
21st Floor
Oakland, CA 94612
510-451-3300
FAX: 510-451-1527

David Knight, Program Director

The Foundation presently makes grants under four program categories: performing arts, social concerns, projects of historic interest and special projects.

3136 **LK Whittier Foundation**

625 Fair Oaks Avenue
Suite 360
S Pasadena, CA 91030
626-441-5188
FAX: 626-441-3672

Linda Blinkenberg, Foundations Director

Giving is primarily offered to preselected organizations. No grants are given to individuals.

3137 **Lawrence Welk Foundation**

2700 Pennsylvania Avenue
Santa Monica, CA 90404
310-451-9077
FAX: 310-451-4268

Lisa Parker, Executive Director

Awards grants in the range of $500 to $10,000. They are given to private, nonprofit organizations in Southern California whose focus is social services agencies working in inner cities with families to alleviate the effects of poverty. Fund is unable to allocate funds to individuals, pass-through organizations, arts or environmental organizations, or to those requesting planning grants and prefers to fund capital improvements and seed or special projects rather than operating budgets.

3138 **Legler Benbough Foundation**

2550 5th Avenue
Suite 132
San Diego, CA 92103
619-235-8099
FAX: 619-235-8077

Peter K Ellsworth, President

3139 **Levi Strauss Foundation**

1155 Battery Street
7th Floor
San Francisco, CA 94111
415-501-1361
FAX: 415-501-3939
www.levistrauss.com/responsibility/foundation

Judy Belk, Executive Director

Has a funding initiative to support organizations which provide services for people with AIDS, and/or educational programs which help prevent the further spread of the HIV virus. The Foundation will assist in the development and enhancement of such services only in those communities where Levi Strauss & Co. has plants and distribution centers.

3140 **Louis R Lurie Foundation**

555 California Street
Suite 5100
San Francisco, CA 94104
415-392-2470
FAX: 415-421-8669

Robert Lurie

Visually impaired, hard-of-hearing and physically disabled in the San Francisco Bay Area and Metropolitan Chicago areas only.

3141 **Luke B Hancock Foundation**

360 Bryant Street
Palo Alto, CA 94301
650-321-5536
FAX: 650-321-0697

Joan Wylie

Has concentrated its resources over the past year on programs which provide job training and employment for at-risk youth. Consortium funding with other foundations in areas where there is unmet need; emergency and transitional funding; and selected funding for music education.

3142 Marin Community Foundation
17 E Sir Francis Drake Boulevard
Suite 200
Larkspur, CA 94939 **415-461-3333**
FAX: 415-464-2555
e-mail: mcf@marincf.org
www.marincf.org

Mark Koenig, Contact

3143 Mary A Crocker Trust
233 Post Street
2nd Floor
San Francisco, CA 94108 **415-982-0138**
FAX: 415-982-0141
e-mail: mact@best.com
www.mactrust.org

Barbaree Jernigan, Administrator

Established in 1889, the Foundation is interested in Bay Area programs such as environment, education and community relations.

3144 National Foundation of Wheelchair Tennis
940 Calle Amanecer
Suite B
San Clemente, CA 92673 **949-366-2410**
FAX: 949-361-6822

Bradley Parks, President

Founded in January of 1980, the intention of this foundation is to assist the newly physically disabled individual to realize his full potential in society by enhancing his esteem, independence productivity and physical capabilities regardless of age, sex, creed or disability extent.

3145 Optometric Extension Program Foundation
1921 E Carnegie Avenue
Suite 3-L
Santa Ana, CA 92705 **949-250-8070**
FAX: 949-250-8157
e-mail: smcorngold@oep.org
www.healthy.net/oep/

Offers continuing education in behavioral optometry for consumers and optometrists.

3146 Parker Foundation
4365 Executive Drive
Suite 1600
San Diego, CA 92121 **858-677-1431**
FAX: 858-677-1477

Robbin Powell, Assistant Secretary

The assets are directed to projects which will contribute to the betterment of any aspect of the people of San Diego County, California and solely to entities which, among other things, are organized exclusively for charitable purposes and are operating in San Diego County, California.

3147 Pasadena Foundation
16 N Marengo Avenue
Suite 300
Pasadena, CA 91101 **626-796-2097**
FAX: 626-583-4738
e-mail: pfstaff@pasadenafoundation.org
www.pasadenafoundation.org

Jennifer DeVoll, Executive Director

The mission of the Pasadena Foundation is to improve the quality of life for citizens of the Pasadena area through support of nonprofit organizations that provide services beneficial to the community.

3148 Peninsula Community Foundation
1700 S El Camino Real
Suite 300
San Mateo, CA 94402 **650-348-2764**
FAX: 650-358-9817

Sterling Speirn, President
Ellen Clear, VP Community Programs

For more than 36 years, Peninsula Community Foundation has built involvement and investment in the community. Develops resources and imaginative programs that make it easy for Peninsula and Silicon Valley residents— from Daly City to San Jose, from the Pacific Ocean to the San Francisco Bay— to support the common good and connect with causes they care about.

3149 RC Baker Foundation
PO Box 6150
Orange, CA 92863 **714-750-8987**

Established in 1952, for general philanthropic purposes. The bulk of assistance and support has been to religious, scientific, educational institutions and youth organizations.

3150 Ralph M Parsons Foundation
1055 Wilshire Boulevard
Suite 1701
Los Angeles, CA 90017 **213-482-3185**
FAX: 213-482-8878

Joseph Hurley, President

The Foundation is concerned with the encouragement and support of projects and programs deemed beneficial to mankind in several major areas of interest such as: education; social impact; civic and cultural; health and special products. Only funds in Los Angeles County.

3151 Robert Ellis Simon Foundation
152 S Lasky Drive
Beverly Hills, CA 90212 **310-275-7335**

Dr. Joan Willens

Mental health and visually impaired grants are the main concerns of this organization.

3152 San Francisco Foundation
225 Bush Street
 # 500
San Francisco, CA 94104 **415-733-8500**
FAX: 415-477-2783
www.sff.org

Robert Fisher

The Foundation's purpose is to improve life, promote greater equality of opportunity and assist those in need or at risk in the San Francisco Bay Area. The Foundation strives to protect and enhance the unique resources of the Bay Area, committed to equality of opportunity for all and the elimination of any injustice, seeks to enhance human dignity and seeks to establish mutual trust, respect and communication among the Foundation.

3153 Santa Barbara Foundation
15 E Carrillo Street
Santa Barbara, CA 93101 **805-963-1873**
FAX: 805-966-2345

Charles Slosserng, President/CEO
Rebecca Stebbins, Director Development
Suzanne Farwell, Communications Associate

Giving is limited to Santa Barbara County, California with no support given to individuals (except sutdent aid) or religious organizations.

3154 Sidney Stern Memorial Trust

PO Box 893
Pacific Palisades, CA 90272 **310-459-2117**

Peter Hooffers, Chair
Marvin Hoffenberg, Advisor

A Southern California-based foundation providing grants to nonprofit organizations for various projects. The foundation gives priority to the following areas of interest: education, health and science, community service projects, youth, services to the mentally and emotionally disabled, the arts, organizations and activities serving California. The Board prefers to make contributions to organizations that use the funds directly in the furtherance of their charitable and public purposes.

3155 Sierra Health Foundation

2525 Natomas Park Drive
Suite 200
Sacramento, CA 95833 **916-922-4755**
FAX: 916-635-3362

Dorothy Beaumont, VP

The Foundation strives to establish a collaborative relationship with its grantees, and with other funders and foundations, through an open dialogue. The Foundation approaches each grant as a partnership, with opportunities for the grantee and grantor to work cooperatively to enhance the effectiveness of the grant project.

3156 Sonora Area Foundation

20100 Cedar Road #E
PO Box 577
Sonsora, CA 95370 **209-533-2596**
FAX: 209-533-2412
e-mail: acorn@sonora-area.org
www.sonora-area.org

Mick Grimes, Executive Director

3157 Stella B Gross Charitable Trust

Bank of the West
PO Box 1121
San Jose, CA 95108 **408-947-5203**
FAX: 408-971-0933
e-mail: gpadilla@bankofthewest.com

Lori C Stetzenmyer, Trust Officer
Gabe Padilla, Trust Associate

Organization must be federal and state tax-exempt and reside within the bounds of Santa Clara County, California to be eligible.

3158 Teichert Foundation

3500 American River Drive
Sacramento, CA 95864 **916-484-3255**
FAX: 916-480-5559
e-mail: info@teichertfoundation.org
www.teichert.com

Frederick A Teichert, Executive Director

3159 Times Mirror Foundation

202 W 1st Street
Los Angeles, CA 90012 **213-237-3945**
FAX: 213-237-2116
www.timesmirrorfoundation.org

Michelle Williams, Executive Director
Vanessa Briseno, Contributions Coordinator

3160 WM Keck Foundation

550 S Hope Street
Suite 2500
Los Angeles, CA 90071 **213-680-3833**
FAX: 213-614-0934
www.wmkeck.org

Dr. Dorothy Fleisher, Program Director

Created to support accredited colleges and universities with particular emphasis on the sciences, engineering and medical research. The Foundation also maintains a Southern California Grant Program that provides support for non-profit organizations in the field of civic and community services, health care, precollegiate education and the arts.

3161 Willam G Gilmore Foundation

120 Montgomery Street
San Francisco, CA 94101 **415-546-1400**
FAX: 415-391-8732

Faye Wilson, Secretary

Colorado

3162 Adolph Coors Foundation

4100 E Mississippi Avenue
Suite 1850
Denver, CO 80246 **303-388-1636**
FAX: 303-388-1684
www.coorsfoundation.org

Sally Rippey, Executive Director

Applicant organizations must be classified as 501 and must operate within the United States. The areas covered by the Foundation are health, education, youth, community services, civic and cultural and public affairs.

3163 Anschutz Family Foundation

2400 Anaconda Tower
555 17th Street
Denver, CO 80202
FAX: 303-298-8881

Sue Anschutz Rodgers, President

The Foundation's interests are to support efforts helping the elderly, the young and the economically disadvantaged. The Foundation has supported over 600 public and private charities sharing in the concern for neighborhood strengthening and community cooperation.

3164 Arc of Colorado

8000 E Prentice Avenue
Suite D-1
Greenwood Village, CO 80111 **303-864-9334**
800-333-7690
FAX: 303-864-9330
e-mail: bbaesman@thearcfco.org
www.thearcofco.org

Bill Baesman, Executive Director

3165 Bonfils-Stanton Foundation

1601 Arapahoe Street
Suite 5
Denver, CO 80202 **303-825-3774**
www.bonfils-stantonfoundation.org

Eileen Greenawalt, Executive Secretary

Grants limited to Colorado 501 (c) (3) organizations. Grants are for general, charitable philanthropic activities within the State. Major categories include education, scientific (including hospital and health services), civic and cultural, community and human services. Organizations should request foundation guidelines before submitting a proposal.

3166 **Comprecare Foundation**
1145 Bannock Street
Denver, CO 80204 **303-629-8661**

JR Gilsdorf, Executive Director

3167 **Denver Foundation**
950 S Cherry Street
Suite 200
Denver, CO 80246 **303-300-1790**
FAX: 303-300-6547
e-mail: info@denverfoundation.org
www.denverfoundation.org

Robert Lee, Director

Neighbors helping neighbors, that's what the foundation is for. As Denver's only community foundation we've been accepting charitable donations since 1925. Those funds have been given back to the community in ongoing grants to nonprofit organizations - organizations that touch nearly every meaningful artistic, cultural, civic, health and human services interest of metro Denver's citizens.

3168 **El Pomar Foundation**
10 Lake Circle
Colorado Springs, CO 80906 **719-633-7733**
800-554-7711
FAX: 719-577-5702
www.elpomar.org

William J Hybl, Chairperson

3169 **Gates Family Foundation**
3200 Cherry Creek S Drive
Suite 630
Denver, CO 80209 **303-722-1881**
FAX: 303-698-9031
e-mail: Gatesfdn@aol.com

Charles Cannon, Executive Director

Purpose is to aid, encourage, initiate or carry on activities that will promote the health, well-being, security and education of all people. Because of a deep concern for and confidence in the future of Colorado, the foundation will invest primarily in institutions, projects and programs that will enhance the quality of life of those who live and work in the state, especially the Denver metropolitan area. Also finds ways to encourage greater cooperation between public and private sectors.

3170 **Helen K and Arthur E Johnson Foundation**
1700 Broadway
Suite 1100
Denver, CO 80290 **303-861-4127**
800-232-9931
FAX: 303-861-0607
e-mail: johnsonfon@cs.com
www.johnsonfoundation.net

Stan Kamprath, Executive Director
Brigit Davis, VP Program Officer

A nonprofit, grantmaking private foundation incorporated under the laws of the State of Colorado in 1948. The Foundation is a general purpose foundation whose grant program consists of a wide variety of creative efforts to solve problems and to enrich the quality of life. The areas of interest are: education, youth, health, community services, civic and culture and senior citizens. Grants limited to the state of Colorado.

3171 **Herbert F Parker Foundation**
First Interstate Bank of Denver
PO Box 5825
Denver, CO 80217

Cancer research, care and education of mentally retarded children and promoting sporting programs for youths.

3172 **Hill Foundation**
First Interstate Bank of Denver
PO Box 5825
Denver, CO 80217

Robert Lorentz, VP

Offers grants primarily for higher education (private), health and human services, cultural projects.

3173 **JM McDonald Foundation**
PO Box 3219
Evergreen, CO 80437 **303-674-9300**
FAX: 303-674-9216

Donald R McJunkin, President

3174 **Kitzmiller-Bales Trust**
PO Box 96
Wray, CO 80758 **970-332-3484**

Robert U Hansen

3175 **V Hunter Trust**
650 S Cherry Street
Suite 535
Denver, CO 80246 **303-399-5450**
FAX: 303-399-5499

Sharon Siddons, Secretary

Connecticut

3176 **Aetna Foundation**
151 Framington Avenue
Hartford, CT 06156 **860-273-6382**
www.aetna.com/foundation

Diana Kinosh, Consultant

3177 **Arc of Connecticut**
1030 New Britain Avenue
Suite 102-B
W Hartford, CT 06110 **860-953-8335**
e-mail: arcct@aol.com

3178 **Clipper Ship Foundation**
Hartford Insurance Group
Hartford Plaza
Hartford, CT 06115 **860-547-4945**

Richard M Madden, Director

The purpose of this Foundation is to offer financial help to federally, nonprofit operating organizations serving the poor and the sick of the greater Boston area in order to assist them in fulfilling their goals and broadening the scope of their activities. Priority will be given to organizations devoted to helping the homeless, destitute, handicapped, children and the aged, or supplying the special needs of minority, low-income families and individuals.

3179 Community Foundation of Southeastern Connecticut

1 Union Plaza
PO Box 769
New London, CT 06320 **860-442-3572**
FAX: 860-442-0582
e-mail: jenno@cfsect.org
www.cfsect.org

Alice F Fitzpatrick, Executive Director

3180 Connecticut Mutual Life Foundation

140 Garden Street
Hartford, CT 06154 **860-727-3000**

Astrida Olds, Executive Director

Distinguished throughout its long history by unusual commitment to high principles of corporate purpose and business ethics. That commitment has been reflected not only in the firm belief that normal business functions must be carried out with a sense of responsibility beyond that required by the marketplace. Maintains an ongoing program of corporate contributions, a nationwide matching gifts plan for all employees on behalf of private and public education, skills training programs, and more.

3181 Cornelia de Lange Syndrome Foundation

302 W Main Street 100
Avon, CT 06001 **860-693-0159**
800-223-8355

Provides information about birth defects caused by Cornelia de Lange Syndrome.

3182 Fidelco Guide Dog Foundation

PO Box 142
Bloomfield, CT 06002 **860-243-5200**
FAX: 860-243-7215
www.fidelco.org

Roberta C Kaman, President

Purpose is to breed, train and place Fidelco German shepherd guide dogs with persons who are visually impaired throughout the Northeast. Provides in community training services to persons receiving guide dogs, reviews performance of the guide dog teams to see that satisfactory level of achievement is maintained, utilizes genetic processes and clinical methods to improve and refine the breed and maintains an ongoing program for development and improvement of training methods.

3183 GE Foundation

3135 Easton Turnpike
Fairfield, CT 06431 **203-373-2178**
FAX: 203-373-3029

Joyce Hergenhan, President

Believes that our greatest national resource is the work force. If we are to successfully compete in the global arena, then we become involved in improving the education of all of our citizens. The Foundation sets examples for others to emulate helping people with their international grant program to higher education and to health care for children in developing countries.

3184 General Electric Foundation

3135 Easton Turnpike
Fairfield, CT 06828 **203-373-3180**
FAX: 203-373-3029
www.ge.com

Marc Saperstein, President

Blind, physically and mentally disabled and rehabilitation grants are among the priorities of the company.

3185 Hartford Foundation for Public Giving

85 Gillett Street
Hartford, CT 06105 **860-246-5236**
e-mail: hfpg2@ursa.hartnet.org
www.hartnet.org

R Malcolm Salter

Developmentally disabled, housing, deaf, recreation and education grants.

3186 Hartford Insurance Group

Hartford Plaza
Hartford, CT 06115 **860-547-5000**
www.thehartford.com

Sandra Sharr

Giving is primarily in the Hartford, CT area and in communities where the company has a regional office. No support is available for political or religious purposes. Grants are given in the areas of education, health and United Way organizations.

3187 Henry Nias Foundation

2 Batterson Park Road
Milford, CT 06460 **203-874-2787**

Charles D Fleischman, VP

3188 Heublein Foundation

PO Box 778
Hartford, CT 06142 **860-702-4000**

Moira E Burke, Treasurer

The Foundation awards grants to class organizations in communities where there is a high concentration of employees, or in which the company has a major operating facility. The areas of interest are charitable, civic and health and social care.

3189 Jane Coffin Childs Memorial Fund for Medical Research

Jane Coffin Childs Memorial Fund
333 Cedar Street
New Haven, CT 06510 **203-785-4612**
FAX: 203-785-3301
e-mail: jccfund@yale.edu
www.jccfund.org

Elizabeth M Ford, Administrative Director

The Fund awards fellowships to suitably qualified individuals for full time postdoctoral studies in the medical and related sciences bearing on cancer.

3190 John H and Ethel G Nobel Charitable Trust: Bankers Trust Company, Limited

I Fawcett Place
Greenwich, CT 06830 **203-629-7120**
FAX: 203-629-7170

Paul J Bisset, VP

3191 Scheuer Associates Foundation

Robert Scheuer
960 Lake Avenue
Greenwich, CT 06831 **203-869-3644**
FAX: 203-622-5002

3192 Swindells Charitable Foundation Trust
Shawmut Bank
777 Main Street
 # 242
Hartford, CT 06115 **860-728-4900**
FAX: 860-240-1210

Maggie Willard, Assistant VP
Joseph Giangreco, Personal Trust Assoc

Grants made to charitable organizations or societies incorporated for the relief of sick and suffering poor children and/or the relief of sick suffering and indigent aged men and women and/or the support of public charitable hospitals. Geographic area includes Hartford, CT area primarily. Application is required, deadlines are Feb. 1 and Aug. 1.

Delaware

3193 Arc of Delaware
1016 Centre Road
Suite 1
Wilmington, DE 19805 **302-996-9400**

3194 Laffey-McHugh Foundation
1220 Market Boulevard
PO Box 2207
Wilmington, DE 19899 **302-658-9141**
FAX: 302-654-1681

Arthor G Connolly Jr, Junior President

3195 Longwood Foundation
100 W 10th Street
Suite 1109
Wilmington, DE 19801 **302-654-2477**
FAX: 302-654-2323

David D Wakefield, Executive Secretary

Offers grants to the mentally and physically disabled - capital, program, education and housing grants in the state of Delaware.

District of Columbia

3196 Albert L and Elizabeth T Tucker Foundation
1120 20th Street NW
Suite 300
Washington, DC 20036 **202-457-1600**
FAX: 202-457-1678

Nicholas S McConnell

3197 Alexander and Margaret Stewart Trust
888 17th Street NW
Suite 210
Washington, DC 20006 **202-785-9892**
FAX: 202-785-0918

Doris Lustine, Executive Secretary

Grants are given only to the Washington, DC area organizations providing care or treatment to cancer patients or those with childhood afflictions.

3198 Arc of the District of Columbia
900 Varnum Street NE
Washington, DC 20017 **202-636-2950**
FAX: 202-636-2996
e-mail: arcdc@juno.com
www.arcdc.net

Mary Durso, Social Worker
Tasha Kluseman, Manager Employment Services
Monita Short-Ellis, Manger Commerical Services

Advocating for and providing services to persons with mental retardation.

3199 Charles Delmar Foundation
1918 16th Street NW
Number 203
Washington, DC 20006 **202-293-2494**
FAX: 202-293-1788

Mareen D Hughes, President

3200 Eugene and Agnes E Meyer Foundation
1400 16th Street NW
Suite 360
Washington, DC 20036 **202-483-8294**
FAX: 202-328-6850
www.meyerfoundation.org

Julie Rogers, President

Awards grants to projects dealing with the learning disabled, blind, mental health and vocational training in the Washington metropolitan area.

3201 Federal Student Aid Information Center
US Department of Education
400 Maryland Avenue SW
Washington, DC 20202 **202-260-2226**
800-433-3243
FAX: 202-401-0689
www.ed.gov/prog_info/SFA/StudentGuide

William J Ryan, Acting Director

Answers questions about Federal student aid from students, parents and Members of Congress, as well as financial aid administrators.

3202 GEICO Philanthropic Foundation
One Geico Plaza
Washington, DC 20076 **301-986-2911**
TTY:800-833-8255
www.geico.com

Hospitals, physically disabled and Special Olympics.

1980

3203 Giant Food Foundation
PO Box 1804
Washington, DC 20013 **301-341-4100**
FAX: 301-618-4667

Israel Sohen, Chairman

Offers grants in the areas of mental health, recreation, community and cultural programs, art, and educational programs for the health and prosperity of the greater Washington area.

3204 Jacob and Charlotte Lehrman Foundation
1027 33rd Street NW
2nd Floor
Washington, DC 20007 **202-338-8400**

Samuel Lehrman, President

3205 **John Edward Fowler Memorial Foundation**
1725 K Street NW
Suite 1201
Washington, DC 20006 **202-728-9080**
FAX: 202-728-9082

Richard Lee

Although not a program priority, the foundation does offer grants to the physically disabled in the Washington, DC area only.

3206 **Joseph P Kennedy Jr Foundation**
1325 G Street NW
Suite 500
Washington, DC 20005 **202-393-1250**
FAX: 202-824-0351
e-mail: info@jpkf.org
www.jpkf.org

Eunice Shriver, Executive VP
Sue Swenson, Executive Director
Susan Coe Brown, Bussiness Manager

Has two firm objectives: to seek the prevention of mental retardation, and to improve the way society deals with its citizens who are already mentally retarded. The Foundation uses its funds in areas where a multiplier effect can be achieved through development of innovative models for the prevention and amelioration of mental retardation, through provision of seed money that encourages new researchers, and thorough use of the Foundation's influence to promote public awareness.

3207 **Kiplinger Foundation**
1729 H Street NW
Washington, DC 20006 **202-887-6400**
FAX: 202-778-8976

Andrea Wilkes, Secretary

Limited to the greater Washington, DC area, the grants focus primarily on education, social welfare, cultural activities and community programs. Matching grants to eligible secondary or higher education institutions are provided on behalf of employees and retirees of Kiplinger Washington Editors, Inc. The Foundation does not fund scholarships.

3208 **Morris and Gwendolyn Cafritz Foundation**
1825 K Street NW
14th Floor
Washington, DC 20006 **202-223-3100**
www.cafritzfoundation.org

Anne Allen, Executive Director

Grants are awarded to only 501(c)(3) organizations that are in the DC area. Grants are not awarded for capitol purposes, special events, endowments, or to individuals.

3209 **Paul and Annetta Himmelfarb Foundation**
4545 42nd Street NW
Suite 203
Washington, DC 20016 **202-966-3795**

Lilian N Khronstadt, Executive Director

3210 **Public Welfare Foundation**
1200 U Street NW
Washington, DC 20009 **202-965-1800**
800-275-7934
FAX: 202-265-8851
e-mail: reviewcommittee@publicwelfare.org
www.publicwelfare.org

The foundation's funding is specifically targeted to economically disadvantaged populations. Proposals must fall within one of the following categories: criminal justice, disadvantaged elderly, disadvantaged youth, environment, health and population and reproductive health, human rights and global security, and community economic developmental and participation. Proposals should be addressed to the Review Committee.

Florida

3211 **Able Trust**
Florida Endowment Foundation for Vocational Rehab.
106 E College Avenue
Suite 820
Tallahassee, FL 32301 **850-224-4493**
888-838-2253
FAX: 850-224-4496
e-mail: info@abletrust.org
www.abletrust.org

Sharon Griffith, President/CEO
Kristen Knapp, VP Public Relations
Guenevere Crum, Director Grants Program

Provides grant funds for purchasing equipment for current employment for people with disabilities and employment-related programs for non-profit agencies in Florida. Assists families, individuals and agencies through an information and referral helpline, educational conferences, and youth training programs. Provides businesses free resources for hiring people with disabilities.

3212 **Arc of Florida**
411 E College Avenue
Tallahassee, FL 32301 **850-921-0460**
e-mail: arcofflorida@comcast.net
arcflorida.org

Promotes, for all people with mental retardation and other developmental disablilities, through education, awareness, research, advocacy and the support of families, friends and community.

3213 **BCR Foundation**
PO Box 13307
Pensacola, FL 32591 **850-438-2509**

Betty Rainwater, Director

3214 **Baron de Hirschmeyer Foundation**
407 Lincon Road
Suite 6J
Miami Beach, FL 33139 **305-672-0934**

Polly Lux de Hirshmeyer, President

3215 **Barron Collier Jr Foundation**
2600 Golden Gate Parkway
Suite 200
Naples, FL 34105 **239-262-2600**
FAX: 239-262-1840

Giving to the Special Olympics is a top priority of the Foundation.

3216 Camiccia-Arnautou Charitable Foundation
Bill T Smith Jr
980 N Federal Highway
Suite 402
Boca Raton, FL 33432
561-368-5757
FAX: 561-368-8505

3217 Chatlos Foundation
PO Box 915048
Longwood, FL 32791
407-862-5077
www.chatlos.org

William J Chatlos, President
Joy D'Arata, VP

Funds nonprofit organizations in the USA and around the globe. Funding is provided in the following areas of giving: Bible Colleges/Seminaries, Religious Causes, Medical Concerns, Liberal Arts Colleges and Social Concerns. Category of placement is determined by the organizations overall mission rather than the project under consideration. The Foundation does not make scholarship grants directly to individuals but rather to educational institutions which in turn select recipients.

1953

3218 Dade Community Foundation
200 S Biscayne Boulevard
Suite 2780
Miami, FL 33131
305-371-2711
FAX: 305-371-5342
e-mail: dadecomfdn@aol.com

Ruth Shack, President

3219 Dr. Jack Widrich Foundation
400 W Rivo Alto Drive
Miami Beach, FL 33139
305-868-1918

3220 EIS Foundation
6931 Queenferry Circle
Boca Raton, FL 33496
561-852-6854
FAX: 561-852-6884

Maurice L Schwarz, President

3221 Edyth Bush Charitable Foundation
199 E Welbourne Avenue
PO Box 1967
Winter Park, FL 32790
407-647-4322
888-647-4322
FAX: 407-647-7716
e-mail: dhessler@edythbush.org
www.edythbush.org

Deborah J Hessler, Program Associtate

funding is resrticted to 501c3 nonprofit organizations located and operating in Orange, Osceola, Seminole and Lake Counties, Florida. Visit www.edythbush.org for a list of funding policies.

3222 FPL Group Foundation
700 Universe Boulevard
Juno Beach, FL 33408
561-694-4000
800-222-4511
FAX: 561-694-4620

John L Kitchens

3223 Florida Rock Industries Foundation
155 E 21st Street
Jacksonville, FL 32206
904-355-1781
FAX: 904-791-1810

HB Horner, Secretary

3224 Frank Stanley Beveridge Foundation
301 Yamato Road
Suite 1130
Boca Raton, FL 33431
800-600-3723
FAX: 561-241-8388
e-mail: administrator@beveridge.org
www.beveridge.org

Philip Caswell, President

3225 Jack Eckerd Corporation Foundation
PO Box 4689
Clearwater, FL 33758
727-395-6000
FAX: 727-395-7934
e-mail: serve@eckerd.com
www.eckard.com

Tamz Alderman, MCR, PR

The foundation limits its giving to nonprofit, tax-exempt organizations located in Eckerd Drug Company's 13-state marketing area. The majority of our funds are committed to national health organizations, the United Way campaigns, and scholarship funding at various colleges of pharmacy.

3226 Jefferson Lee Ford III Memorial Foundation
9600 Collins Avenue
546487
Bal Harbour, FL 33154
305-885-5447
FAX: 305-868-2646

Herbert Kurras, Trustee
Suzanne Kingsbury, Trustee

Disabled children, hearing and speech center. Grants are only given to tax exempt organizations, no individual grants are offered.

3227 Jessie Ball duPont Fund
One Independent Drive
Suite 1400
Jacksonville, FL 32202
904-353-0890
800-252-3452
FAX: 904-353-3870
e-mail: jessie@dupontfund.org
www.dupontfund.org

Sherry P McGill PhD, President
JoAnn P Bennett, Director Administration

Established under the terms of the will of the late Jessie Ball duPont. The fund is a national foundation having a special though not exclusive interest in issues affecting the South. The Fund works with the approximately 325 individual institutions to which Mrs. duPont personally contributed during the five-year period, 1960 through 1964.

3228 Joe and Emily Lowe Foundation
249 Royal Palm Way
Palm Beach, FL 33480
561-659-1203
FAX: 561-655-7130

Bernard Sterm, President

Emphasis is on Jewish welfare funds, the arts, museums, higher education including medical education, hospitals, medical research, aid to the handicapped, underprivileged children's organizations and women's projects. The funding is limited to the New York Metropolitan Area including New Jersey and Palm Beach County, Florida. No grants are made to individuals.

3229 John E & Nellie J Bastien Memorial Foundation
440 E Sample Road
Suite 209
Pompano Beach, FL 33064 954-942-3203

3230 Lost Tree Village Charitable Foundation
11555 Lost Tree Way
North Palm Beach, FL 33408 561-622-3780
FAX: 561-622-7558
e-mail: itvcfi@aol.com

Pamela M Rue, Executive Director

3231 NationsBank Community Foundation
1800 2nd Street
Suite 750
Sarasota, FL 34236 941-957-0442
FAX: 941-957-3135

Debra Jacobs, Administrator

3232 Publix Super Markets Charities
1936 George Jenkins Boulevard
PO Box 407
Lakeland, FL 33802 863-688-1188
www.publix.com

Barbara O Hart, President

3233 Richard W Higgins Charitable Foundation Trust
hall & Ilsley Trust of Florida
800 Laurel Oak Drive
Suite 101
Naples, FL 34108 239-597-2933
800-874-2427
FAX: 239-592-2454

Georgia

3234 Community Foundation for Greater Atlanta
Hurt Building
Suite 449
Atlanta, GA 30303 404-688-5525
FAX: 404-688-3060
www.atlcf.org

Vilma Weekes, Grants Administrator

3235 Florence C and Harry L English Memorial Fund
SunTrust Bank Atlanta
PO Box 4418
Atlanta, GA 30302 404-827-6902
FAX: 404-724-3082
e-mail: raymond.king@suntrust.com
www.suntrustatlantafoundation.org

Raymond B King, Senior VP
Renee P Barnett, Foundation Administrator

Grants only made to Metro Atlanta non-profit organizations; no grants to churches or individuals.

3236 Georgia Arc Network
1996 Cliff Valley Way
Suite 102
Atlanta, GA 30329 404-634-5512
e-mail: gaarcnetwork@earthlink.net
www.arcga.org

Provides unified advocacy so that individuals with mental retardation or developmental disabilities and their families achieve valued lives throuh full, productive and dignified participation in their communities.

3237 Georgia Power Company Contributions Program
241 Ralph McGill Boulevard NE
Bin 10230
Atlanta, GA 30308 404-506-6784
FAX: 404-506-1485

Linda Leathers, Manager

3238 Grayson Foundation
PO Box 515
Grayson, GA 30017 770-554-1000
FAX: 770-554-1003
e-mail: graysonfoundation@yahoo.com
www.graysonfoundation.org

Sam B Grayson, President

Grayson Foundation enhances the quality of public educationfor the students of the Grayson cluster of schools by providing funds which enrich and extend educational oppurtunities.

3239 Harriet McDaniel Marshall Trust in Memory of Sanders McDaniel
SunTrust Bank Atlanta
PO Box 4418
Atlanta, GA 30302 404-827-6902
FAX: 404-724-3082
e-mail: raymond.king@suntrust.com
www.suntrustatlantafoundation.org

Raymond B King, Senior VP
Renee P Barnett, Foundation Administrator

Grants only made to Metro Atlanta non-profit organizations, no grants to churches or individuals.

3240 IBM Corporation
4111 Northside Parkway NW
Atlanta, GA 30327
FAX: 404-238-3409

Manages disability programs (which leverage IBM resources through partnerships) designed to train persons with disabilities and assist them in gaining employment. Also, disseminates information regarding products and resources for persons with disabilities with those of other companies and organizations.

3241 John H and Wilhelmina D Harland Charitable Foundation
3565 Piedmont Road NE
Atlanta, GA 30305 404-264-9912
e-mail: harland@randomc.com

John A Conant, Secretary
Margeret Dixon, Manager

3242 **Lettie Pate Whitehead Foundation**
50 Hurt Plaza
Suite 1200
Atlanta, GA 30303 404-522-7026
FAX: 404-522-7026
www.lpwhitehead.org

Charles H McTier, President

3243 **Patterson-Barclay Memorial Foundation**
6487 Peachtree Industrial Boulevard
Suite A
Atlanta, GA 30360 770-458-9888
FAX: 770-452-7704

Hugh R Powell Jr, Secretary

3244 **Perkins-Ponder Foundation**
Bank of America
PO Box 4007
Macon, GA 31213 478-744-6454

3245 **Rich Foundation**
11 Piedmont Center
Suite 204
Atlanta, GA 30305 404-262-2266
FAX: 404-262-4123

Anne Poland-Berg, Grant Consultant

3246 **Savannah Widows Society**
3025 Bull Street
Savannah, GA 31405 912-232-6312

Martha Peeples

3247 **SunTrust Bank, Atlanta Foundation**
SunTrust Bank Atlanta
PO Box 4418
Atlanta, GA 30302 404-827-6902
FAX: 404-724-3082
e-mail: raymond.king@suntrust.com
www.suntrustatlantafoundation.org

Raymond B King, Senior VP
Renee P Barnett, Foundation Administrator

Hawaii

3248 **Arc of Hawaii**
3989 Diamond Head Road
Honolulu, HI 96816 808-737-7995
FAX: 808-732-9531
e-mail: arc-hi@aloha.net
www.thearcinhawaii.org/

3249 **Atherton Family Foundation**
222 Merchant Street
Honolulu, HI 96813 808-537-6333

Jane Smith

Supports educational projects, programs and institutions have the highest priority, with the enterprises of a religious nature and those concerned with health and social services given careful attention. The Foundation is one of the largest private resources in the State devoted exclusively to the support of activities of a charitable nature.

3250 **Clarence TC Ching Foundation**
PO Box 4107
Honolulu, HI 96812 808-521-8841
FAX: 808-521-8835

Lawrence SL Ching, Chairperson

3251 **GN Wilcox Trust**
Pacific Century Trust
PO Box 3170
Honolulu, HI 96802 808-538-4540

3252 **Hawaii Community Foundation**
900 Fort Street Mall, Pioneer Plaza
Suite 1300
Honolulu, HI 96813 808-537-6333
888-731-6286
FAX: 808-521-6286
e-mail: info@hcf-hawaii.org
www.hcf-hawaii.org

Kevin Taketa, President

3253 **McInerny Foundation**
Pacific Century Trust
130 Merchant Street
Honolulu, HI 96813 808-538-4944

Lois C Loomis, VP

3254 **Sophie Russell Testamentary Trust**
PO Box 2390
Honolulu, HI 96804 808-524-4488
FAX: 808-523-2195

Lois Loomis, Secretary

Supports qualified tax-exempt charitable organizations, in the State of Hawaii only. Offers grants to the Humane Society and institutions giving nursing care and serving the physically and mentally handicapped.

Illinois

3255 **Abbott Laboratories Fund**
Contributions Committee
100 Abbott Park Road
Abbott Park, IL 60064 847-937-6100
FAX: 847-938-6511

An Illinois, nonprofit, philanthropic organization that makes a significant contribution to human welfare through the development and worldwide distribution of technologically advanced health care products.

3256 **Alfred Bersted Foundation**
231 S Lasalle Street
Chicago, IL 60604 312-251-8850

M Catherine Ryan

Grants are given to programs serving the mentally and physically disabled, organizations included in the broader focus of the foundation. Grants are restricted to organizations in four Illinois counties: DuPage, Kane, McHenry and DeKalb.

3257 **Alzheimer's Association**
Medical and Scientific Affairs
919 N Michigan Avenue
Suite 1000
Chicago, IL 60611
800-272-3900
FAX: 312-335-4034
e-mail: nico.stanculescu@alz.org
www.alz.org

Timothy J Morgan, Director Financial Operations

3258 **American Foundation for the Blind-Midwest**
401 N Michigan Avenue
Suite 350
Chicago, IL 60611 **312-396-4420**
800-232-5463
FAX: 312-527-4660
e-mail: chicago@afb.net
www.afb.org

Jay Stiteley, Director

3259 **American National Bank and Trust Company**
33 N LaSalle Street
Chicago, IL 60690 **773-376-1400**
FAX: 815-961-7745

Joan M Klaus, Foundation Director

Supports the endeavors of organizations working to meet the critical needs of the city and its surrounding communities. Success is greatly affected by the well-being of the communities the company serves, thus the foundation seeks to fulfill the social obligations both through financial funding and human resources. The Foundation funding categories include organizations and programs involved in economic development, education, community and social services, healthcare and culture and the arts.

3260 **Ameritech Corporation Contributions Program**
30 S Wacker Drive
34th Floor
Chicago, IL 60606 **312-750-5205**
FAX: 312-727-1496
www.ameritech.com

Michael E Kuhlin, Senior Director

3261 **Amerock Corporation**
4000 Auburn Street
PO Box 7018
Rockford, IL 61125 **815-963-9631**
FAX: 815-969-6029

Lawrence Gloyd

Grants are given to organizations promoting wellness, health and rehabilitation of the visually impaired and physically disabled.

3262 **Arc of Illinois**
18207-A Dixie Highway
Homewood, IL 60430 **708-206-1930**
FAX: 708-206-1171
e-mail: tony@thearcofil.org
www.thearcofil.org

The Arc of Illinois is committed to empowering persons qith disabilities toachieve full participation in community life thru in formed choices.

3263 **Benjamin Benedict Green-Field Foundation**
8 S Michigan Avenue FL 2900
Chicago, IL 60603 **312-984-0001**

Harriet Brady, VP
Colin Fisher, President

3264 **Blowitz-Ridgeway Foundation**
One Northfield Plaza
Suite 528
Northfield, IL 60093 **847-446-1010**
FAX: 847-446-6318

Tina M Erickson, Administrator

Provides limited program, capital and research grants to organizations aiding the physically and mentally disabled, and agencies serving children and youth. Grants generally limited to Illinois.

3265 **Burlington Northern Santa Fe Foundation**
5601 W 26th Street
Cicero, IL 60804 **630-222-4815**
FAX: 630-222-4857

Dick Russack, President

3266 **Chicago Community Trust and Affiliates**
111 E Wacker Drive
Suite 1400
Chicago, IL 60601 **312-372-3356**
FAX: 312-580-7411
TTY:312-853-0394
e-mail: info@cct.org
www.cct.org

Sandy Chears, Grants Manager

3267 **Community Foundation of Champaign County**
404 W Church Street
Champaign, IL 61820 **217-359-0125**
FAX: 217-352-6494

Jill Niles, Executive Director

3268 **Dr. Scholl Foundation**
1033 Skokie Boulevard
Suite 230
Chicago, IL 60062 **312-559-7430**
www.drschollfoundation.com

Pamela Scholl, President

3269 **Duchossois Foundation**
845 N Larch Avenue
Elmhurst, IL 60126 **630-279-3600**
FAX: 630-993-6911

Kimberly Duchossois Lenczuk, President

Established in 1984, the foundation returns dollars to the communities supporting its facilities and employees. Within these following areas, organizations are carefully selected on the basis of community needs and the organization's value and performance. Areas aimed at include: medical research, children/youth programs and cultural institutions.

3270 **Evenston Community Foundation**
828 Davis Street
Suite 300
Evanston, IL 60201 **847-475-2402**
FAX: 847-475-2469

Thomas K Jager, Administrator

3271 **Field Foundation of Illinois**
200 S Wacker Drive
Suite 3860
Chicago, IL 60606 **312-831-0910**

Handy Lindsey Jr, Executive Director

The Foundation awards grants to institutions and agencies in the fields of health, welfare, education, cultural and conservation activities, and urban and community affairs, primarily serving the people of the Chicago metropolitan area.

3272 Francis Beidler Charitable Trust

53 W Jackson Boulevard
Suite 530
Chicago, IL 60604 **312-922-3792**

Thomas B Dorris

3273 Fred J Brunner Foundation

9300 King Street
Franklin Park, IL 60131 **847-678-3232**
FAX: 847-678-0642

General disability grants.

3274 George M Eisenberg Foundation for Charities

2340 S Arlington Heights Road
Suite 480
Arlington Heights, IL 60005 **847-981-0545**
FAX: 847-941-0548

3275 George Zoltan Lefton Family Foundation

George Zoltan Lefton Company
3622 S Morgan Street
Chicago, IL 60609 **773-254-4344**

Magda Lefton, Secretary

3276 Green Bay Foundation

Goldman, Sachs & Company
233 S Wacker Drive
Suite 4900
Chicago, IL 60606

General disability grants.

3277 Grover Hermann Foundation

Paul K Rhoads
233 S Wacker Drive
Suite 7200
Chicago, IL 60606 **312-876-1000**
FAX: 312-258-5700

Paul Rhoads

Provides funds for educational, health, public policy, community and religious organizations throughout the United States. Its major interests are in higher education and health.

3278 Harry F and Elaine Chaddick Foundation

123 W Maddison Street
Suite 200
Chicago, IL 60602 **312-704-4100**

Elaine M Chaddick

3279 Helen Brach Foundation

55 W Wacker Drive
Suite 701
Chicago, IL 60601 **312-372-4417**
FAX: 312-372-0290

Raymond F Simon, President

3280 John D and Catherine T MacArthur Foundation

140 Dearborn Street
Suite 100
Chicago, IL 60603 **312-726-8000**
FAX: 312-920-6258
e-mail: 4answers@macfnd.org
www.macfdn.org

Richard Kaplan, Director

3281 LaSalle Chicago Community Trust

222 N Lasalle Street
Suite 1400
Chicago, IL 60601 **312-372-3356**
FAX: 312-580-7411
www.cct.org

Sandy Chears, Grants Manager

A community foundation established in 1915, which receives gifts and bequests from individuals, families or organizations interested in providing through the community foundation, financial support for the charitable agencies or institutions which serve the residents of metropolitan Chicago.

3282 Les Turne Amyotrophic Laterial Sclerosis Foundation

3325 Main Street
Skokie, IL 60076 **847-679-3311**
FAX: 847-679-9103
e-mail: info@lturner-als.org

Harvey Gaffen, President
Wendy Abrams, Executive Director

Voluntary health organization dedicated to raising funds for ALS research, patient services and public awareness. Provides educational mateials for affected individuals and family members, health care professionals, and the general public. Program services include referrals and counseling; audio-visual aids and periodic newsletters. Offers support groups and patient networking to affected individuals, family members, and caregivers.

3283 Little City Foundation

1760 W Algonquin Road
Palatine, IL 60067 **847-358-5510**
FAX: 847-358-3291
www.littlecity.org

Rena Zaid, Executive Director
Char Rivette, Director Children Services
Mary Ann Scott, Director Adult Services

Provides progressive community-based services and service coordination for children and adults with mental retardation or other developmental, emotional and behavioral challenges. Services include direct care with up to 24-hour per day support for children and adults, Foster Care, Families One, adoption opportunities, respite care, supported employment, studio and multidisciplinary fine arts, public education, and advocacy.

3284 MAGIC Foundation for Children's Growth

6645 W N Avenue
Oak Park, IL 60302 **708-383-0808**
800-362-4423
FAX: 708-383-0899
e-mail: mary@magicfoundation.org
www.magicfoundation.org

Dianne Andrews, Executive Director

This is a national nonprofit organization providing support and education regarding growth disorders in children and related adult disorders, including adult GHD. Dedicated to helping children whose physical growth is affected be a medical problem by assiating families of afflicted children through local support groups, public education/awareness, newsletters, specialty divisions an d programs for the children.

3285 McDonald's Corporation Contributions Program

McDonalds Plaza
Oak Brook, IL 60521 **630-623-7048**

www.mcdonalds.com/countries/usa/community/ind

Jackie Meara, Supervisor Contributions

3286 Michael Reese Health Trust

20 N Wacker Drive
Suite 760
Chicago, IL 60606 **312-726-1008**
FAX: 312-726-2797
e-mail: info@healthtrust.net
www.gih.org/usr_doc/may21,%202001.pdf

Dorothy H Gardner, President

3287 Moen Foundation

First National Bank of Chicago
1 S NW Highway
Park Ridge, IL 60068 **815-729-1850**
FAX: 815-729-5047

3288 National Eye Research Foundation (NERF)

910 Skokie Boulevard
Suite 207A
Northbrook, IL 60062 **847-564-4652**
800-621-2258
FAX: 847-564-0807
e-mail: nerfl955@aol.com
www.eyemac.com/nerf

Dedicated to improving eye care for the public and meeting the professional nees of eye care practitioners; sponsors eye research projects on contact lens applications and eye care problems. Special study sections in such fields as orthokertology, primary eyecare, pediatrics, and through continuing education programs. Provides eye care information for the public and professionals. Educational materials including pamphlets. Program activities include education and referrals.

3289 National Headache Foundation

5252 N Western Avenue
Chicago, IL 60625
800-843-2256
FAX: 773-525-7357

Headache physicians.

3290 OMRON Foundation

OMRON Systems
1 E Commerce Drive
Schaumburg, IL 60173 **847-843-7900**
FAX: 847-240-5362

Nicholas Hahn, Director

3291 Oris B Hastings Charitable Foundation

230 8th Street
PO Box 186
Cairo, IL 62914 **618-734-2800**

John G Holland

3292 Parkinson's Disease Foundation

833 W Washington Boulevard
Chicago, IL 60607 **312-733-1893**
FAX: 312-733-1896
e-mail: pdfshgo@enteract.com
PDF@info.org

Lewis P Rowland MD, President
Robin Elliot, Executive Director

International voluntary not-for-profit organization dedicated to patient services; education of affected individuals, family members, and healthcare professionals; and promotion and support of research for Parkinson's Disease and related disorders. Offers an extensive referral service to guide affected individuals to proper diagnosis and clinical care. Provides referrals to genetic counseling and support groups; promotes patient advocacy; and offers a variety of educational and support materials

3293 Peoria Area Community Foundation

124 SW Adams Street
Suite 1
Peoria, IL 61602
FAX: 309-674-8754
e-mail: PACF@worldnet.att.net

George H Kreiss, Executive Director

3294 Polk Brothers Foundation

420 N Wabash Avenue
Number 204
Chicago, IL 60611 **312-527-4684**
FAX: 312-527-4681

Nikki W Stein, Executive Director

3295 Retirement Research Foundation

8765 W Higgins Road
Suite 430
Chicago, IL 60631 **773-714-8080**
FAX: 773-714-8089
e-mail: info@rrf.org
www.rrf.org

Marilyn Hennessey, President
Sharon Markham, Associate VP
Nancy Zweibel PhD, Snior Program Officer

A private philanthropy with primary interest in improving the quality of life of older persons in the United States.

3296 Rush Hayward Masonic Fund

14 Bel Air Court
Champaign, IL 61820 **217-352-7099**

3297 Sears-Roebuck Foundation

Sears Tower
Department 903
Chicago, IL 60684 **847-286-2500**

3298 Siragusa Foundation

919 N Michigan Avenue
Chicago, IL 60611 **312-280-0833**
FAX: 312-943-4489

Irene S Phelps, Executive Director

3299 Square D Foundation

1415 S Roselle Road
Palatine, IL 60067
FAX: 847-397-8814

Makes donations for operating support, capital development needs, and special projects to nonprofit organizations that have been granted exemption from the Federal Income Tax. The Foundation has a strong commitment to the following areas: health and welfare, education, civic and community affairs, and culture and the arts. Support of higher education is also made for scholarships, endowments for facility and acquisition or expansion of equipment or facilities, through Matching Gift Program.

3300 WP and HB White Foundation

540 W Frontage Road
Suite 332
Northfield, IL 60093 **847-446-1441**

Margaret Blandford, Executive Director

The Foundation's funds are allocated on a continuing basis within the metropolitan area of Chicago where our founder's business prospered. The Foundation helps organizations specializing in the visually impaired, mental health, youth and recreation.

3301 Washington Square Health Foundation

875 N Michigan Avenue
Suite 3516
Chicago, IL 60611 **312-664-6488**
FAX: 312-664-7787
e-mail: washington@wshf.org
www.wshf.org

Howard Nochumson, Executive Director
Angelo Creticos, President
Authur Wirtz, VP

3302 Wheat Ridge Ministries

1 Pierce Place
Suite 250E
Itasca, IL 60143 **630-766-9066**
800-762-6748
FAX: 630-766-9622
e-mail: wrmin@aol.com
www.wheatridge.org

Indiana

3303 Arc of Indiana

22 E Washington
Suite 210
Indianapolis, IN 46204 **317-977-2375**
800-382-9100
FAX: 317-977-2385
e-mail: arcin@in.net

John Dickerson, Executive Director
Kim Dodson, Director Government Relations
Melissa Justice, Bookeeper

Arc of Indiana is commited to people with mental retardation and othe developmental disabilities realizing their goals of learning, living, working, and playing in the community.

3304 Ball Brothers Foundation

222 S Mulberry Street
 # 1408
Muncie, IN 47305
FAX: 765-741-5518

Douglas Bakken, Executive Director

Mentally and physically disabled, only serving Indiana area.

3305 Central Indiana Community Foundation

615 N Alabama Street
Suite 119
Indianapolis, IN 46204 **317-634-2423**
FAX: 317-684-0943
e-mail: program@cicf.org
www.cicf.org

Kenneth L Gladish PhD, Executive Director

3306 Community Foundation of Boone County

60 E Cedar Street
PO Box 92
Zionsville, IN 46077 **317-873-0210**
FAX: 317-873-0219
e-mail: cfbc@in-motion.net
www.bccn.boone.in.us/cf/index.html

Lisa Latz John, Executive Director

3307 Crown Point Community Foundation

Courthouse Square, Suite 302
PO Box 522
Crown Point, IN 46308 **219-662-7252**
FAX: 219-662-9493
e-mail: cpcf@urisp.com

Linda Davis, Executive Director
John Barney, President
Steve Leurck, First VP

Crown Point Community Foundation is a not for profit organization . Foundation serves as a facilitataor fot the community good, builds endowments, allocates grants and awards scholarships to better serve Crown Point and South Lake county area of Indiana.

3308 Eli Lilly and Company Corporate Contributions Program

Lilly Corporate Center
Indianapolis, IN 46285 **317-276-2000**
www.lilly.com/about/overview/access/foundatio

Kendy S Smith, Secretary

3309 Indianapolis Foundation

615 N Alabama Street
Room 119
Indianapolis, IN 46204 **317-634-2423**
FAX: 317-684-0943
www.indyfund.org

Kenneth L Gladish PhD, Executive Director
Rexford Early, Secretary, President
David Kleiman, Trustee Attorney

3310 John W Anderson Foundation

402 Wall Street
Valparaiso, IN 46383 **219-462-4611**

William N Vinovich, Vice-Chairman

Physically and mentally disabled, recreation and youth agencies in Northwest Indiana area.

3311 Trabant North Knox

Bank One, Trust Group
111 Monument Circle
Suite 1501
Indianapolis, IN 46277 **317-321-8030**

3312 **William H Willennar Foundation**
Fort Wayne National Bank
PO Box 110
Fort Wayne, IN 46801 260-426-0555

MC Haggarty, Secretary

Iowa

3313 **Arc of Iowa**
715 E Locust
Des Moines, IA 50309 515-283-2358
800-362-2927
e-mail: arciowa@aol.com

3314 **Hall-Perrine Foundation**
115 3rd Street SE
Suite 803
Cedar Rapids, IA 52401 319-362-9079

Jack B Evans, President

This foundation is dedicated tio improving the quality of life for peole in Linn County, IA by responding to the changing social, economic, and cultural needs of the community.

3315 **Homer G Barr Trust**
PO Box 370
Webster City, IA 50595 515-832-1133

3316 **Kinney-Lindstrom Foundation**
RR One
PO Box 18
Hanlontown, IA 50444 641-896-3888

Lowell Hall, Secretary

Offers grants only to the area of Iowa for projects to help; Special Olympics, physically disabled and art and cultural affairs.

3317 **Mid-Iowa Health Foundation**
553 39th Street
Suite 104
Des Moines, IA 50312 515-277-6411
FAX: 515-271-7579

Kathryn Bradley, Director

3318 **Principal Financial Group Foundation**
711 High Street
Des Moines, IA 50392 515-247-5091
FAX: 515-246-5475
e-mail: bassett.kendra@principal.con
www.principal.com/about/giving

Kendra Bassett, Contributions Assistant

3319 **Siouxland Foundation**
PO Box 2014
Sioux County, IA 51104 712-239-3303
FAX: 712-239-3303
e-mail: sxlfdn@aol.com

Debbie Hubbard, Executive Director

Kansas

3320 **Arc of Kansas**
3601 SW 29th Street
S-105
Topeka, KS 66614 785-271-8783
FAX: 785-272-4645
e-mail: thearcks@thearcks.org
www.thearcks.org

3321 **Cessna Foundation**
PO Box 7706
Wichita, KS 67277 316-517-7810
FAX: 316-517-7812

Marilyn Richwine, Secretary Treasurer

Some grants are available to organizations which meet the guidelines for serving the physically disabled. Grants are restricted to communities where Cessna has manufacturing facilities.

3322 **Hutchinson Community Foundation**
PO Box 298
Hutchinson, KS 67601 620-663-5293
FAX: 620-663-9277

Joseph A Hess
Lynette Lacy, President

Kentucky

3323 **Arc of Kentucky**
833 E Main Street
Frankfort, KY 40601 502-875-5225
800-281-1272
FAX: 502-875-5226
e-mail: arcofky@aol.com
www.arcofky.org

Patty Dempsey, Executive Director

The Arc of Kentucky helps in securing a postive future for individuals with mental retardation. The Arc vaules services and supports that enhance the quality of life through interdependence, friendship, choice and respect for individuals with mental retardation.

3324 **Kentucky Social Welfare Foundation**
PNC Bank NA
500 W Jefferson Street
Citizens Plaza
Louisville, KY 40296 502-581-2157

W Michael Hanks, VP

3325 **Omnicare Foundation**
1717 Dixie Highway
Suite 800
Fort Wright, KY 41011 859-426-3000
FAX: 859-426-3118

Cheryl D Hodges, Secretary

Louisiana

3326 **Arc of Louisiana**
PO Box 65129
Baton Rouge, LA 70896 225-383-1033

3327 **Baton Rouge Area Foundation**
406 N 4th Street
Baton Rouge, LA 70802
225-387-6126
FAX: 225-387-6153

John G Davies, President

3328 **Booth-Bricker Fund**
826 Union Street
Suite 300
New Orleans, LA 70112
504-581-2430

Gray S Parker, President

3329 **Community Foundation of Shreveport-Bossier**
401 Edwards Street
Suite 1111
Shreveport, LA 71101
318-221-0582
FAX: 318-221-7463
e-mail: cfsb@comfoundsb.org
www.comfoundsb.org

Dorothy Gwin, Executive Director

Public Foundation that makes grants only to 501C3 organizations.

Maine

3330 **UNUM Charitable Foundation**
2211 Congress Street
Portland, ME 04122
207-770-2211
FAX: 800-447-2498

Janine Manning, Manager

The Foundation encourages projects that: stimulate others in the private or public sector to participate in problem solving; advance innovative and cost-effective approaches for addressing defined, recognized needs; and demonstrate ability to obtain future project funding, if needed. The foundation generally limits its consideration of capital campaign requests to the Greater Portland, Maine area.

Maryland

3331 **American Health Assistance Foundation**
15825 Shady Grove Road
Suite 140
Rockville, MD 20850
301-948-3244
800-437-2423
FAX: 301-258-9454
www.ahaf.org

Eugene Micheals, President
Clayton Raymond, VP
Peter Feliciano, Secretary

3332 **American Occupational Therapy Foundation**
4720 Montgomery Lane
PO Box 31220
Bethesda, MD 20824
301-656-3620
FAX: 301-652-7711
www.aotf.org

Martha Kirkland, Executive Director

3333 **Arc of Maryland**
49 Old Solomons Island Road
Suite 205
Annapolis, MD 21401
410-571-9320
FAX: 410-974-6021
e-mail: info@thearcmd.org
www.thearcmd.org

3334 **Baltimore Community Foundation**
2 E Read Street
Latrobe Building, 9th Floor
Baltimore, MD 21202
410-332-4171
FAX: 410-837-4701

Timothy D Armbruster, President

3335 **Candlelighters Childhood Cancer Foundation**
3910 Warner Street
Kensington, MD 20895
800-366-2223
e-mail: info@candlelighters.org
www.candlelighters.org

An international organization providing information and support, and advocacy to parents of children with cancer and survivors of childhood cancer.Health and Education professionals also welcome as members.Network of local support groups. Information on disabilities related to treatment of childhood cancer. Publications.

3336 **Children's Fresh Air Society Fund**
Baltimore Community Foundation
2 E Read Street
Baltimore, MD 21202
410-332-4171
FAX: 410-837-4701
e-mail: khoeller@bcf.org
www.bcf.org

Anne Khoeller, Grants Administrator

Makes grants to nonprofit camps to provide tuition for disadvantaged and disabled Maryland children to attend summer camp.

3337 **Clark-Winchcole Foundation**
3 Bethesda Metro Center
Suite 550
Bethesda, MD 20814
301-654-3607
FAX: 301-654-3140

Laura Phillips

Supported tax-exempt charitable organizations operating in the metropolitan area of Washington, DC in the following areas: deaf, higher education and physically disabled.

3338 **Columbia Foundation**
10221 Wincopin Circle
Columbia, MD 21044
410-730-7840
FAX: 410-715-3043

Barbara K Lawson, Executive Director

3339 **Cystic Fibrosis Foundation**
6931 Arlington Road
Bethesda, MD 20814
301-654-4055
800-FIG-HTCF
FAX: 301-951-6378
e-mail: info@cff.org
www.cff.org/research.htm

Robert Dressing, President

3340 Foundation Fighting Blindness

11435 Cronhill Drive
Owings Mills, MD 21117
410-568-0150
800-683-5555
888-394-3937
FAX: 410-363-2393
www.blindness.org

Randall Hove, Interim CEO

The urgent mission of The Foundation Blindness is to fund the research with will discover the causes, treatments, preventive methods and cures for Retinitis Pigmentosa, Macular Degeneration, Usher Syndrome, Stargart disease, and the entire spectrum of retinal degenerative diseases.

3341 George Wasserman Family Foundation

Grossberg Company
6707 Democracy Boulevard
Suite 300
Bethesda, MD 20817
301-571-1900
FAX: 301-571-1932

Janice W Goldsten, President

3342 Harry and Jeanette Weinberg Foundation

7 Park Center
Owings Mills, MD 21117
410-654-8500
FAX: 410-654-4900

Bernard Siegel, President

3343 Miracle-Ear Children's Foundation

PO Box 59261
Minneapolis, MD 55459
612-520-9550
800-234-5422
FAX: 612-520-9793
TTY:612-520-9791
www.miracle-ear.com

Jerry Krbec, President
Richard C Brandt, Executive Director

Nonprofit organization that provides hearing aids to children whose families to not qualify for public assistance. Provides hearing aid fittings and follow-up care and services free of charge through Miracle-Ear Hearing Centers. Provides information on alternative communication. Offers educational materials and brochures.

3344 National Federation of the Blind

1800 Johnson Street
Baltimore, MD 21230
410-659-9314
FAX: 410-685-5653
e-mail: nfb@access.digex.net
www.nfb.org

Marc Maurer, President

The largest consumer membership organization of the blind, founded in 1940, it has 50,000 members nationwide in 52 affiliates and over 700 local chapters. Provides public education about blindness, support services to the newly blinded, scholarships, publications about blindness, adaptive equipment for the blind, advocacy services, Newsline for the Blind, assistive technology information and Job Opportunities for the Blind.

3345 National Retinitis Pigmentosa Foundation Fighting Blindness

11350 McCormick Road
 # 800
Hunt Valley, MD 21031
800-683-5555
FAX: 410-659-4086

Robert Gray, Executive Director

The Foundation provides information and referral services, support networks. The main focus of the Foundation is to fund research on causes, cures and prevention of RP and related retinal degenerations. Volunteer affiliates throughout the United States are offered to promote public awareness, raise funds and provide opportunity for those who have RP to interact.

3346 Ryland Group Corporate Giving Program

11000 Broken Land Parkway
Columbia, MD 21044
800-267-0998
FAX: 443-367-3500

Maurice M Simpkins, VP

3347 Sjogren's Syndrome Foundation

8120 Woodmont Avenue
Suite 530
Bethesda, MD 20814
301-718-0300
800-475-6473
FAX: 301-718-0322
e-mail: ssf@sjorgrens.org
www.sjogrens.org

Edna Scott, Office Manager
Suzanne Stone, Executive Director

Provides patients practical information and coping strategies that minimize the effects of Sjogren's syndrome. In addition, the Foundation is the clearinghouse for medical information and is the recognized national advocate for Sjogren's syndrome. *$25.00*

Monthly

Massachusetts

3348 Abbot and Dorothy H Stevens Foundation

PO Box 111
North Andover, MA 01845
978-688-7211
FAX: 978-686-1620
e-mail: 74722.637@compuserve.com

3349 Arc Massachusetts

217 S Street
Waltham, MA 02453
781-891-6270
FAX: 781-891-6271
e-mail: arcmass@arcmass.org
www.arcmass.org

Leo Sarkissian, Executive Director

3350 Bank of Boston Corporation Charitable Foundation

100 Federal Street
Boston, MA 02110
617-434-2659

Giving primarily to New England.

3351 Boston Foundation

1 Boston Place
24th Floor
Boston, MA 02108
617-723-7415
FAX: 617-723-7415
e-mail: alk@tbf.ork
www.tbf.org

Ann Kurk, Director Public Relations

3352 **Boston Globe Foundation**
135 Morrissey Boulevard
PO Box 2378
Boston, MA 02107 **617-929-2895**
FAX: 617-929-2041
e-mail: foundation@globe.com
www.bostonglobe.com/foundation

Seeks to empower low income families and children in the Boston area plus youth frequently excluded from equal participation in our society. The Foundation hopes their funding will have a special impact on children in communities of color. Focus areas are on: community services; education; culture; health care and environment.

3353 **Bushrod H Campbell and Ada F Hall Charity Fund**
Palmer & Dodge
111 Huntington Avenue
Boston, MA 02199 **617-239-0556**
FAX: 617-227-4420

Brenda Taylor, Foundation Administrator

The fund's areas of interest include organizations and/or their projects supporting aid to the elderly, healthcare and population control. Medical research grants are administered through the Medical Foundation. No grants are awarded to individuals and the geographical area of support is limited to organizations located in Massachusetts within the area of Boston and Route 128.

3354 **Clipper Ship Foundation**
Grants Management Associates
77 Summer Street
8th Floor
Boston, MA 02110 **617-426-7172**
FAX: 617-426-5441
agmconnect.org/clipper1.html

Raymond C Woodring, Foundation Assistant

3355 **Community Foundation of Western Massachusetts**
1500 Main Street, Suite 622
PO Box 15769
Springfield, MA 01115 **413-733-8565**
FAX: 413-732-2858
e-mail: wmass@communityfoundation.org

Kent W Faerber, President

3356 **Frank R and Elizabeth Simoni Foundation**
434 Providence Highway
Norwood, MA 02062 **781-762-3449**
FAX: 781-769-6166

Victor F Coletti, VP

3357 **Friendly Ice Cream Corporation Contributions Program**
Public Affairs Department
1855 Boston Road
Wilbraham, MA 01095 **413-543-2400**
FAX: 413-543-9355

Barbara Miller

3358 **Greater Worcester Community Foundation**
44 Front Street
Suite 530
Worcester, MA 01608 **508-755-0980**
FAX: 508-755-3406
e-mail: atlis@greaterworcester.org
www.greaterworcester.org

Ann T Lisi, Executive Director

3359 **Hyams Foundation**
175 Federal Street
14th Floor
Boston, MA 02110 **617-426-5600**
FAX: 617-426-5696
e-mail: info@hyamsfoundation.org
www.hyamsfoundation.org

Elizabeth B Smith, Executive Director

3360 **Nathaniel and Elizabeth P Stevens Foundation**
PO Box 111
Norht Andover, MA 01845 **978-688-7211**
FAX: 978-686-1620
e-mail: 74722.2637@compuserve.com

Elizabeth A Beland, Administrator

3361 **Raytheon Company Contributions Program**
141 Spring Street
Lexington, MA 02173 **781-862-6600**
FAX: 781-860-2172

Janet C Taylor, Manager

3362 **Spero Charitable Foundation**
Shirley Spero
79 Florence
Suite 200
Chestnut Hill, MA 02167 **617-244-3174**
FAX: 617-244-3174

3363 **TJX Foundation**
TJX Companies
770 Cochiuate Road
Route 1E
Framingham, MA 01701 **508-390-3199**
FAX: 508-390-2091

Christine A Strickland, Foundation Manager

3364 **Vision Foundation**
818 Mount Auburn Street
Watertown, MA 02172 **781-926-4232**
800-852-3029
FAX: 781-926-1412

Barbara Kibler, Executive Director

Offers counseling, support groups, seminars and transportation for the blind providing 600 members.

Michigan

3365 **Ann Arbor Area Community Foundation**
201 Main Street
Suite 801
Ann Arbor, MI 48104 **734-663-0401**
FAX: 734-663-3514
www.aaacf.org

Terry Foster, President
Cheryl Elliott, Program Director

Interested in funding projects which will improve the quality of life for citizens of the Ann Arbor Area. Eligible projects generally fall within these categories: education, culture, social service, community development, environmental awareness and health and wellness. The Foundation aims to support creative approaches to community needs and problems by making grants which will benefit the widest possible range of people.

3366 Arc of Michigan
1325 S Washington Avenue
Lansing, MI 48910
517-487-5426
800-292-7851
FAX: 517-487-0303
e-mail: arcmi@voyager.net
www.arcmi.org

3367 Berrien Community Foundation
2900 S State Street
Suite 2E
St Joseph, MI 49085
269-983-3304
FAX: 269-983-4939
e-mail: bcf@gtm.net

3368 Blind Children's Fund
4740 Okemos Road
Okemos, MI 48864
517-347-1357
FAX: 517-347-1459
e-mail: blindchfnd@aol.com
www.blindchildrensfund.org

Karla B Storrer, Executive Director

Provides parents and profesionsals informaion materials and resousces that help them scuccesfullly teach and nurture blind, visually and multi-impanred infants and preschoolers.

3369 Clarence & Grace Chamberlin Foundation
600 Woodbridge Place
Detroit, MI 48226
313-567-1000
FAX: 313-567-1001
e-mail: jking@berrymoorman.com

John L King, President

3370 Community Foundation of Monroe County
111 E 1st Street
PO Box 627
Monroe, MI 48161
734-242-1976
FAX: 734-242-1234
www.cfmonroe.org

Kristyn Theisen, Executive Director
Susan Gruber, Administrator

3371 Cowan Slavin Foundation
7881 Dell Road
Saline, MI 48176
734-944-0469
FAX: 734-944-3529

Marjorie Bovee, Executive Director

3372 Daimler Chrysler
Automobility Program
PO Box 3124
Troy, MI 48302
800-255-9877
FAX: 248-925-3053
TTY:800-922-3826

Kim Halbeisen, Supervisor

Provides a cash reimbursement to assist in reducing the cost of adaptive driving equipment and conversion aids installed on new model Daimler Chrysler LLC vehicles. Up to a maximum of $1000 on full size ram vans and up to $750 on all other vehicles.

3373 Frank S and Mollie S VanDervoort Memorial Foundation
4646 Okemos Road
Okemos, MI 48864
517-349-7232

Ann L Gessert, Secretary

3374 Fremont Area Foundation
4424 W 48th Street
PO Box B
Fremont, MI 49412
231-924-5350
FAX: 231-924-5391
e-mail: gzerlaut@tfaf.org
www.tfaf.org

Elizabeth Cherin, President/CEO

3375 Grand Rapids Foundation
209-Cg Waters Building
161 Ottawa NW
Grand Rapids, MI 49503
616-454-1751
FAX: 616-454-6455
e-mail: grfound@grfoundation.org
www.grfoundation.org

Marcia Rapp, VP Programs

3376 Granger Foundation
PO Box 22187
Lansing, MI 48909
517-393-1670
FAX: 517-393-0901
e-mail: tfate@grangerconstruction.com
www.grangerfoundation.org

Alton L Granger, Treasurer

3377 Harvey Randall Wickes Foundation
4800 Fashion Square Boulevard
Plaza North, Suite 472
Saginaw, MI 48604
989-799-9850
FAX: 989-799-3327

James Finkbeiner

Grants for rehabilitation.

3378 Havirmill Foundation
3503 Greenleaf Boulevard
Suite 203
Kalamazoo, MI 49008
269-375-1800
FAX: 269-375-1346

Jerry L Miller, President

3379 Kelly Services Foundation
999 W Big Beaver Road
Troy, MI 48084
248-362-4444
FAX: 248-244-5518

Lori Beirne-Kennedy, Director Marketing

3380 Kresge Foundation
3215 W Big Beaver Road
Troy, MI 48084
248-643-9630
FAX: 248-643-0588
www.kresge.org

John E Marshall III, President

This foundation offers challenge grants for capital projects, most often for construction or renovation of buildings, but also for the purchase of major equipment and real estate. As challenge grants, they are intended to stimulate new, private gifts in the midst of an organized fund raising effort. Offers special opportunities to build capacity, both in providing enhanced facilities in which to present programs and in generating private support. Only charitable organizations may apply.

3381 **Lanting Foundation**
c/o Arlyn Lanting
1575 S Shore Drive
Holland, MI 49423 **616-355-2740**

Arlyn Lanting, Partner

3382 **Ransom Fidelity Company Foundation**
702 Michigan National Tower
Lansing, MI 48933 **517-482-1538**
FAX: 517-482-1539

Grants for the schools, Native Americans, minorities, environmnt, youth and physically disabled.

3383 **Rollin M Gerstacker Foundation**
PO Box 1945
Midland, MI 48641 **989-631-6097**

EN Brandt, VP

3384 **Steelcase Foundation**
PO Box 1967, CH-4E
Grand Rapids, MI 49501 **616-246-4695**
FAX: 616-475-2200
e-mail: sbroman@steelcase.com

Susan Broman, Executive Director

Minnesota

3385 **Arc Minnesota**
770 Transfer Road
Suite 26
Saint Paul, MN 55114 **651-523-0823**
800-582-5256
FAX: 651-523-0829
e-mail: mail@arcminnesota.com
www.arcminnesota.com

3386 **Bush Foundation**
E-900 First National Bank Building
332 Minnesota Street
Saint Paul, MN 55101 **651-227-0891**
FAX: 651-297-6485
e-mail: kkleppe@bushfoundation.org
www.bushfoundation.org

Kelly Kleppe, Grant Manager

A regional grantmaking foundation, with broad interests in education, human services, health, arts and culture and in the development of leadership. The foundation is interested in encouraging education at all levels, seeks to support projects which will help prevent or resolve social problems, seeks to encourage the delivery of good healthcare, supports the arts, develops leadership potential and promotes programs for minorities and programs of interest to women.

3387 **Deluxe Corporation Foundation**
PO Box 64235
St. Paul, MN 55164 **651-483-7842**
FAX: 651-481-4371

Jennifer A Anderson, Director Foundations

3388 **General Mills Foundation**
PO Box 113
Minneapolis, MN 55440 **612-540-7891**
FAX: 612-540-4114
e-mail: mills999@mail.genmills.com
www.generalmills.com/corporate/about

Reatha Clark King, President/Executive Director

3389 **Hugh J Andersen Foundation**
PO Box 204
Bayport, MN 55003 **651-439-1557**
888-439-9508
FAX: 681-439-9480
www.workinggroup.org/lgbtfunders/FD/dstate.ht

Sarah J Andersen, President
Christine E Andersen, VP
William H Rubenstein, Secretary

Established in 1962, this fund is a nonprofit charitable corporation classified as a private foundation. The Foundation was established as a general charitable fund, but now identifies projects that build individual and community capacity to be a priority. Giving is focused primarily in the counties of Washington, Minnesota, & St, Croix, Polk and Pierce of Wl. Grants are given in the areas of human services, health, education, arts and culture, community services and the environment.

3390 **James R Thorpe Foundation**
5201 Eden Circle
Suite 202
Minneapolis, MN 55436 **612-373-9484**
FAX: 651-291-0969

Edith D Thorpe, President

3391 **Jay and Rose Phillips Family Foundation**
10 2nd Street NE
Suite 200
Minneapolis, MN 55413 **612-623-1654**
FAX: 612-623-1653
e-mail: phillipsfnd@phillipsfnd.org

Patricia A Cummings, Secretary/Executive Director

3392 **Minneapolis Foundation**
A200 Foshay Tower
821 Marquette Avenue S
Minneapolis, MN 55402 **612-339-7343**
FAX: 612-672-3870
www.mplsfoundation.org

Emmett D Carson, President

3393 **Ordean Foundation**
424 W Superior Street
Duluth, MN 55802 **218-726-4785**
FAX: 218-726-4848

Stephen A Mangan, Executive Director

Grants are given for a variety of purposes including: treatment and rehabilitation for persons who are chronically or temporarily mentally ill, persons whose physical capacity is impaired by injury or illness, promotes mental and physical health of the elderly, provide for youth guidance programs designed to avoid delinquency, and provides relief, aid and charity to people with no or low incomes. Grants are only offered to certain cities and townships near and around St. Louis County/Duluth.

3394 **Otto Bremer Foundation**
445 Minnesota Street
Suite 2000
St. Paul, MN 55101 **651-227-8036**
FAX: 651-227-2522
e-mail: obf@bfsi.com
fdncenter.org/grantmaker/bremer/contacts.htm

John Kostishack, Executive Director

3395 **Rochester Area Foundation**
21 First Street SW
Suite 350
Rochester, MN 55902 **507-282-0203**
FAX: 507-282-4938
e-mail: rafmn@aol.com

Steve Thornton, Executive Director

Mississippi

3396 **Arc of Mississippi**
7 Lakeland Circle
Suite 600
Jackson, MS 39216 **601-982-1180**
800-717-1180
FAX: 601-982-5792
e-mail: arcms@arcms.org
www.arcms.org

Missouri

3397 **Allen P & Josephine B Green Foundation**
222 S Jefferson Street
PO Box 523
Mexico, MO 65265 **573-581-5568**
FAX: 573-581-1714
e-mail: wstaley@greenfdn.org
www.greenfdn.org

Walter G Staley Jr, Secretary/Treasurer

While the Foundation makes grants in a variety of fields, in the past its major support was in the field of medical research. During a 20-year period, 1951-71, it contributed over $900,000 to research in Parkinson's and related diseases of the nervous system; $600,000 for research in pediatric neurology and lesser amounts in other areas of medical research, but the board is now treading in other disabilities. Grants are limited to Missouri and none are offered to individuals.

3398 **Anheuser-Busch Foundation**
1 Busch Place
Saint Louis, MO 63118 **314-577-2453**
FAX: 314-577-3251

Giving in areas of company operation.

3399 **Greater Kansas City Community Foundation and Affiliated Trusts**
1055 Broadway
Suite130
Kansas City, MO 64105 **816-842-0944**
FAX: 816-842-8079
http://www.gkccf.org

Janice C Kreamer, President

3400 **H&R Block Foundation**
4410 Main Street
Kansas City, MO 64111 **816-932-8453**
FAX: 816-931-7486

Barbara Allmon, President

A charitable organization under the not-for-profit corporation law of the state of Missouri. Grants are made only to organizations which are tax exempt from Federal Income taxation and which are not classified as private foundations. Major emphasis is placed in the metropolitan areas of Kansas City, Missouri: and Columbus, Ohio. The goal is to provide proportionately significant support of relatively few activities, as opposed to minor support for a great many.

3401 **James S McDonnell Foundation**
1034 S Brentwood Boulevard
Suite 1850
St. Louis, MO 63117 **314-721-1532**
FAX: 314-721-7421
www.jsmf.org

Dr. John T Bruer, President

3402 **Lutheran Charities Foundation of St. Louis**
211 N Broadway
Suite 1290
St. Louis, MO 63102 **314-231-2244**
FAX: 314-231-0799
e-mail: lcfjan@tetranet.net

Fred A Bleeke, President/CEO

3403 **Mary's Call**
504 W U S Highway 24
Salisbury, MO 65281 **660-388-5308**
FAX: 660-388-5453

Ray Goffinet, President

3404 **Oppenstein Brothers Foundation**
PO Box 13095
Kansas City, MO 64199 **816-234-8671**

Sheila K Rice, Contact

3405 **RA Bloch Cancer Foundation**
4400 Main Street
Kansas City, MO 64111 **816-932-8453**
800-433-0464
FAX: 816-931-7486
e-mail: hotline@hrblock.com
www.blochcancer.org

Vangie Rich, Assistant to Richard Bloch
Ann Hron, Co-Director Bloch Cancer Hotline

Provides a hotline that matches newly diagnosed cancer patients with someone who has survived the same kind of cancer. Offers free infomration, resources and support groups, and distributes lists of multidisciplinary second opnion centers. Also supplies three books at no charge: Fighting Cancer; Cancer... There's Hope; and A Guide for Cancer Supporters. All services and books are free of charge.

3406 **St. Louis Community Foundation**
319 Noth 4th Street
Suite 501
St. Louis, MO 63102 **314-588-8088**
FAX: 314-588-8200
e-mail: foff@anet.stl.com

Tullia Hamilton, Executive Director

3407 **Victor E Speas Foundation**
14 W 10th Street
PO Box 419119
Kansas City, MO 64141 816-979-7481

David P Ross, Sr VP Bank of America

Nebraska

3408 **Arc of Nebraska**
1672 Van Dorn Street
Lincoln, NE 68502 402-475-4407
800-666-7907
FAX: 402-475-0214
e-mail: arcneb@inetnebr.com
www.arc-nebraska.org

Arc of Nebraska is commited to helping children and adults with disabilities secure the oppurtunity to choose and realize their goals of where and how they learn, live, work, and play.

3409 **Cooper Foundation**
304 Cooper Plaza
Lincoln, NE 68508 402-476-7571
FAX: 402-476-2356

Elwood Thompson, President

Serves only Nebraska with the primary interest in education, arts and humanities and the human services area.

3410 **Hazel R Keene Trust**
152 E Sixth Street
Fremont, NE 68025 402-753-2246
FAX: 402-753-2204

Joe Twidwell, Contact

3411 **Slosburg Family Charitable Trust**
10040 Regency Circle
Suite 200
Omaha, NE 68114 402-391-7900
FAX: 402-391-6615

D David Slosburg, Treasurer

3412 **Union Pacific Foundation**
1416 Dodge Street
Room 802
Omaha, NE 68179 402-271-5600
FAX: 402-271-5477
e-mail: union_pacific_foundation@notes.up.com
www.up.com

Darlynn Herweg, Director

Nevada

3413 **Conrad N Hilton Foundation**
100 W Liberty Street
Suite 840
Reno, NV 89501 775-323-4221
FAX: 775-323-4150

Steven M Hilton, President

Our grant-making style is to initiate and develop major long-term projects and then seek out the organizations to implement them. As a consequence of this proactive approach, the Foundation does not generally consider unsolicited proposals. Our major projects currently include: blindness prevention and treatment, support the work of the Catholic Sisters, drug abuse prevention among youth, support of the Conrad N. Hilton College of Hotel and Restaurant Management, and much more.

3414 **EL Wiegand Foundation**
165 W Liberty Street
Reno, NV 89501 775-333-0310
FAX: 775-333-0314

Kristen A Avansino, President/Executive Director

3415 **Mark B Wallner Foundation**
5386 Hidden Valley Center
Reno, NV 89502 775-856-1166

Kimberly England, President

3416 **Nell J Redfield Foundation**
PO Box 61
1755 E Plumb Lane, Suite 212
Reno, NV 89502 775-323-1373
FAX: 775-323-4476

Gerald C Smith, Director

3417 **William N and Myriam Pennington Foundation**
441 W Plumb Lane
Reno, NV 89509 775-333-9100
FAX: 775-333-9111

Kent Green, Comptroller

New Hampshire

3418 **Agnes M Lindsay Trust**
660 Chestnut Street
Manchester, NH 03104 603-669-1366
866-669-1366
FAX: 603-665-8114
e-mail: admin@lindsaytrust.org
www.lindsaytrust.org

Robert Chiesa, Managing Trustee
Susan Bouchard, Administrative Director
Ernest Dion, Trustee

Funding for health and wefare organizations, special needs, mental health, blind, deaf and cultural programs to organizations, specifically for capital needs, not operating funds, located in the New England states of Maine, Massachusetts, New Hampshire and Vermont. We highly recommend you visit our web site.

3419 **Foundation for Seacoast Health**
100 Campus Drive
Suite 1
Portsmouth, NH 03801 603-422-8200
FAX: 603-422-8207
e-mail: ffsh@communitycampus.org
www.ffsh.org

Susan R Bunting EdD, President/CEO

Giving limited to Portsmouth, Rye, New Castle, Greenland, Newington, North Hampton, NH; and Kittery, Eliot, and York, ME.

New Jersey

3420 **American Express Foundation**
American Expressway
90 Hudson Street
Jersey City, NJ 07302 **212-640-2000**
FAX: 201-209-4303

Giving primarily in Arizona, California, Colorado, Florida, Georgia, Illinois, Minnesota, North Carolina, Nebraska, New York, Texas, Utah, Massachusetts and Pennsylvania. Also include international committees.

3421 **Arc of New Jersey**
985 Livingston Avenue
N Brunswick, NJ 08902 **732-246-2525**
FAX: 732-214-1834
e-mail: info@arcnj.org
www.arcnj.org

3422 **Arnold A Schwartz Foundation**
Bivona, Cohen, Kunzman, et. al.
15 Mountain Boulevard
Warren, NJ 07059 **908-757-7800**
FAX: 908-757-8039

Edwin D Kunzman, President

3423 **Campbell Soup Foundation**
Campbell Place
Camden, NJ 08103 **856-342-4800**
FAX: 856-342-3878

John M Coleman, Chairman
James J Baldwin, Vice Chairman

Goal of this foundation is to match the company's assets with community needs in order to help forge solutions to community challenges. The Foundation believes that involvement at the community level can play a catalytic role in improving the quality of life. Giving is located in the areas of education, nutrition and health, cultural and youth related programs. The major focus of the foundation is on nutrition and health related matters, and places a high priority on Camden, New Jersey areas.

3424 **Children's Hopes & Dreams Wish Fulfillment Foundation**
280 Route 46
Dover, NJ 07801 **973-361-7366**
800-IDR-EAM2
FAX: 973-361-6627
e-mail: chdfdover@juno.com
www.childrenswishes.org

Victor Franklin Jr, President
Mariann Oswald, Program Director

Provides continual support for children and their families through the International Pen-Pal Program and the Kid's Kare Packages program. All services are free. Fulfills the last dreams of children with life threatening illnesses.

3425 **Community Foundation of New Jersey**
PO Box 317
Morristown, NJ 07963 **973-267-5533**
FAX: 973-257-2903
www.cfnj.org

Giving limited to the state of New Jersey.

3426 **Cowles Charitable Trust**
PO Box 219
Rumson, NJ 07760 **732-936-9826**

Gardner Cowles III, President

3427 **F Mason Perkins Trust**
Summit Bank, Trust Department
210 Main Street
Hackensack, NJ 07601 **201-646-5225**
FAX: 201-646-9881

3428 **FM Kirby Foundation**
17 DeHart Street
PO Box 151
Morristown, NJ 07963 **973-538-4800**
FAX: 973-538-4801
fdncenter.org/grantmaker/kirby/

FM Kirby, President

3429 **Fannie E Rippel Foundation**
180 Mount Airy Road
Suite 200
Basking Ridge, NJ 07920 **908-766-0404**

e-mail: rippel@gti.net
www.mharc.com/fundpri-rz.htm

Edward W Probert, CEO/ President

3430 **Fund for New Jersey**
94 Church Street
Suite 303
New Brunswick, NJ 08901 **732-220-8656**
FAX: 732-220-8654
e-mail: info@fundformj.org
www.fundfornj.org

3431 **Merck Company Foundation**
1 Merck Drive
PO Box 100
Whitehouse Station, NJ 08889 **908-423-2042**
FAX: 908-423-1987

John R Taylor, Executive VP

3432 **Merrill Lynch & Company Foundation**
100 Union Avenue
Cresskill, NJ 07626 **201-871-0350**

Eddy Bayardelle, Dir. Philanthropic Progs.

3433 **Milton Schamach Foundation**
810 Belmont Avenue
Noth Haledon, NJ 07508 **973-423-9494**
FAX: 973-423-2376

Andrew ER Frommel Jr, Secretary/Treasurer

3434 **Nabisco Foundation**
Nabisco Plaza
7 Campus Drive
Parsippany, NJ 07054 **973-682-5000**
FAX: 973-503-3018

3435 **Ostberg Foundation**
278 Fountain Road
Englewood, NJ 07631 **201-569-6800**
FAX: 201-569-6606

Charles Borhan

3436 **Prudential Foundation**
751 Broad Street
15th Floor
Newark, NJ 07102 **973-802-4791**
FAX: 973-802-3345
www.prudential.com

Donald Treloar

Gives priority to national programs that further our objectives and programs serving areas where The Prudential has a substantial employee presence. Places special emphasis on the home state of New Jersey and the headquarters city, Newark.

3437 **Robert Wood Johnson Foundation**

Route One & College Road E
PO Box 2316
Princeton, NJ 08543 **609-452-8701**
FAX: 609-627-6406
e-mail: mail@rwjf.org
www.rwjf.org

Richard J Toth, Director Office/Proposal

3438 **Victoria Foundation**

40 S Fullerton Avenue
Montclair, NJ 07042 **973-783-4450**
FAX: 973-783-6664
e-mail: CMCFFarvic@aol.com

Catherine M McFarland, Executive Officer

3439 **Walking Tomorrow**

Christopher Reeve Paralysis Foundation
500 Morris Avenue
Springfield, NJ 07081
800-225-0292
FAX: 973-912-9433
e-mail: info@crpf.org
www.paralysis.org

Pam Gold, Director Special Projects

New Mexico

3440 **Arc of New Mexico**

3655 Carlisle NE
Albuquerque, NM 87110 **505-883-4630**
800-358-6493
FAX: 505-883-5564
e-mail: arcnm@arcnm.com
www.arcnm.com

Karen Fricks, President
Rebecca Shuman, Executive Director

Our mission is to improve the quality of life for individuals with developmental disabilities of all ages by advocating for equal opportunities and choices in where and how they learn, live, work, play and socialize. The Arc of New Mexico promotes self-determination, healthy families, effective community support systems and partnerships.

3441 **Frost Foundation**

511 Armijo Street
Suite A
Santa Fe, NM 87501 **505-986-0208**
FAX: 505-986-0430

Mary Whited-Howell, President

3442 **McCune Charitable Foundation**

345 E Alameda Street
Santa Fe, NM 87501 **505-983-8300**
FAX: 505-983-7887
e-mail: fsowers@trail.com
www.nmmccune.org

Frances R Sowers, Associate Director

3443 **Santa Fe Community Foundation**

516 Alto Street
PO Box 1827
Santa Fe, NM 87504 **505-988-9715**
FAX: 505-988-1829
e-mail: foundation@santafecf.org
www.santafecf.org

Elizabeth Bremner, Executive Director

New York

3444 **AT&T Foundation**

32 Avenue of Americas
24th Floor
New York, NY 10013 **212-387-4801**
FAX: 212-387-5097
e-mail: rdabney@att.com
http://www.att.com/foundation/

Ronald Dabney, Communications Manager

3445 **Achelis Foundation**

Morris & McVeigh
767 3rd Avenue
4th Floor
New York, NY 10017 **212-644-0322**
FAX: 212-759-6510
e-mail: main@achelis-bodman-fnds.org
fdncenter.org/grantmaker/achelis-bodman/

John N Irwin III, President/Treasurer
Russell P Pennoyer, First VP
Mary S Phipps, Second VP

Follows donor intent with distribution of funds for charitable, benevolent, educational and religious uses and purposes. Primarily funds in the New York City area.

1940

3446 **Alavi Foundation of New York**

500 5th Avenue
Floor 34
New York, NY 10110 **212-944-8333**
FAX: 212-921-0325
www.alavifoundation.org/index.html

Purposes are charitable and philanthropic with an emphasis on education and civic concerns.

1973

3447 **Altman Foundation**

521 5th Avenue
35th Floor
New York, NY 10175 **212-682-0970**

fdncenter.org/grantmaker/altman

Jane B O'Connell, President
Karen L Rosa, VP/Executive Director
John W Townsend, VP

For the benefit of such charitable and educational institutions in the City of New York as said directors shall approve. Foundation grants support programs and institutions that enrich the quality of life in the city, with a particular focus on initiatives that help individuals, families and communities benefit from the services and opportunities that will enable them to achieve their full potential.

1913

3448 Ambrose Monell Foundation
c/o Fulton Rowe, Hart & Coon
1 Rockefeller Plaza, Suite 301
New York, NY 10020 **212-586-0700**
FAX: 212-245-1863
e-mail: mailto:mjmorello@fultonrowe.com
www.monellvetlesen.org/monell/default.htm

George Row Jr, President

Voluntary aiding and contributing to religious, charitable, scientific, literary, and educational uses and purposes, in New York, elsewhere in the US and throughout the world.

3449 American Chai Trust
c/o Perleman & Perleman
220 5th Avenue, 7th Floor
New York, NY 10001 **212-889-0575**
FAX: 212-889-5228

Clifford Perlman, Treasurer

3450 American Foundation for the Blind
11 Penn Plaza
Suite 300
New York, NY 10001 **212-502-7600**
FAX: 212-502-7777
e-mail: afbinfo@afb.org
www.afb.org

Regina Genwright, Director Information Center

Dedicated to addressing issues of literacy, independent living, employment, and access through technology for the ten million Americans who are blind or visually impaired.

3451 Arthur Ross Foundation
20 E 74th Street
Suite 4C
New York, NY 10021 **212-737-7311**
FAX: 212-650-0332

Arthur Ross, President

3452 Artists Fellowship
c/o Salmagundi Club
47 5th Avenue
New York, NY 10003 **646-230-9833**

Richard Pionk, Treasurer

3453 Beatrice & Samuel A Seaver Foundation
c/o Eisner & Lubin
444 Madison Avenue
New York, NY 10022 **212-350-7050**
FAX: 212-750-3262

Hirschel E Levine, Treasurer

Autism Research

3454 Bell Atlantic Foundation
1095 Avenue of the Americas
Room 3200
New York, NY 10036
800-360-7955
FAX: 212-398-0951
e-mail: suzanne_dubose@smtp.nynex.com
www.npcnys.org/Foundations/Foundationnys.html

Suzanne A Du Bose, President

3455 Bodman Foundation
767 3rd Avenue
4th Floor
New York, NY 10017 **212-644-0322**
FAX: 212-759-6510
www.fdncenter.org/grantmaker/bodman

3456 Booth Ferris Foundation
60 Wall Street
46th Floor
New York, NY 10260 **212-809-1630**

Giving limited to the New York metropolitan area.

3457 Brooklyn Home for Aged Men
9701 Shore Road
PO Box 280062
Brooklyn, NY 11228 **718-745-1638**

Nancy K Munson, President

3458 Cancer Care
1180 Avenue of the Americas
New York, NY 10036 **212-221-3300**
800-813-HOPE
FAX: 212-719-0263
e-mail: info@cancercareinc.org
celebratinglife.org/Organization_Support.htm

Diane Blum, Executive Director

3459 Charles A Dana Foundation
745 5th Avenue
Suite 700
New York, NY 10151 **212-223-4040**
FAX: 212-593-7623
e-mail: danainfo@danany.dana.org
www.dana.org

David Mahoney, Chair

3460 Clark Foundation
250 Park Avenue
Suite 900
New York, NY 10177 **212-551-1100**
FAX: 212-986-4558

Giving in New York and New York City.

3461 Commonwealth Fund
1 E 75th Street
New York, NY 10021 **212-606-3800**
FAX: 212-606-3500
e-mail: cmwf@cmwf.org
www.cmwf.org

Karen Davis, President

A private foundation with the broad charge to enhance the common good. Carries out this mandate by supporting efforts that help people live healthy and productive lives, and by assisting certain groups with serious and neglected problems. Supports independent research on health and social issues and makes grants to improve heathcare practice and policy.

1918

3462 Community Foundation for Greater Buffalo
712 Main Street
Buffalo, NY 14202 **716-852-2857**
FAX: 716-852-2861
e-mail: cfgb@buffnet.net
www.cfgb.org

Jean M Brun, Program Officer

3463 Community Foundation for the Capitol Region
Executive Park Drive
Albany, NY 12203
518-446-9638
FAX: 518-446-9638
e-mail: info@cfcr.org
www.cfcr.org

Judith Lyons, Executive Director

3464 Community Foundation of Herkimer & Oneida Counties
270 Genesse Street
Utica, NY 13502
315-735-8212
FAX: 315-735-9363
e-mail: commfdn@borg.com

Susan D Smith, Sr Program Officer

3465 Comsearch: Broad Topics
Foundation Center
79 Fifth Avenue
Department ZE
New York, NY 10003
212-421-0771
800-424-9836
FAX: 212-807-3677
www.fdncenter.org

Thomas Buckman, President

Subset publications of The Foundation Grants Index, are printouts of actual foundation grants, covering 26 key areas of grantmaking. This tool is designed for fundraisers who wish to examine grantmaking activities in a broad field of interest. *$55.00*

3466 DE French Foundation
120 Genesee Street
Room 503
Auburn, NY 13021
315-253-9321

J Douglas Pedley, President

3467 David J Green Foundation
599 Lexington Avenue
Suite 12
New York, NY 10022
212-371-4200
FAX: 212-371-5099

Barbara A McBride, Secretary

3468 Easter Seals New York
230 Washington Avenue Extension
Albany, NY 12203
518-456-4880
800-727-8785
ny.easter-seals.org

Christine McMahon, Chief Operating Officer

Offers resources and expertise that allow children and adults with disabilities to live with dignity and independence. A long standing commitment to serve those for whom no other resources exist. Statewide, provides innovative solutions that enhance the lives of people with disabilities, while heightening community awareness and acceptance.

3469 Edward John Noble Foundation
32 E 57th Street
Floor 19
New York, NY 10022
212-759-4212

Noble Smith, Executive Director

3470 Epilepsy Foundation of Long Island
506 Stewart Avenue
Garden City, NY 11530
516-739-7733
888-672-7154
e-mail: rdaly@epil.org
www.epilepsyfoundation.org/longisland

Richard E Daly, Executive Director
Henry Hertl, Associate Executive Director
Elaine Lubelsky, Controller

Provides education, counseling and residential care to Long Island residents with epilepsy and related conditions.

1953

3471 Epilepsy Society of New York
305 7th Avenue
12th Floor
New York, NY 10001
212-633-2930
FAX: 212-633-2991
e-mail: epsocny@aol.com

George H Smith, Executive Director

3472 Episcopal Charities
1047 Amsterdam Avenue
New York, NY 10025
212-316-7426
FAX: 212-316-7431
e-mail: EPCHARNY@aol.com

David P Shover, Executive Director

3473 Esther A & Joseph Klingenstein Fund
787 7th Avenue
6th Floor
New York, NY 10019
212-492-6181
FAX: 212-492-7007

John Klingenstein, President

3474 Fay J Lindner Foundation
1161 Meadowbrook Road
Merrick, NY 11566
516-292-1331

Ruth Torito, Director

3475 Florence V Burden Foundation
630 5th Avenue
Suite 2900
New York, NY 10111
212-332-1100

Edward P H Burden, President

Publishes an annual or periodic report.

3476 Ford Foundation
320 E 43rd Street
New York, NY 10017
212-573-5000
FAX: 212-351-3677
www.fordfound.org

Joan Dassin, Director
Ashok Gurung, Program Officer
Susan V Berresford, President

A resource for innovative people and institutions worldwide. Goals are to: strenghthen democratic values; reduce poverty and injustice; promote international cooperation; and advance human achievement.

3477 **Fortis Foundation**

1 World Trade Center
Suite 5001
New York, NY 10048
FAX: 212-859-7058

Jacqueline A Gentile, Director

Grants are offered in healthcare fields, especially in medical research ($500-$5,000). New York City social, educational organizations also receive funds ($250-$5,000).

3478 **Foundation Center Library Services**

Foundation Center
79 Fifth Avenue
Department ZE
New York, NY 10003
212-421-0771
800-424-9836
FAX: 212-807-3677
www.fdncenter.org

Thomas Buckman, President

The Center disseminates current information on foundation and corporate giving through our national collections in New York City and Washington D.C., our field offices in San Francisco and our network of over 180 cooperating libraries in all 50 states and abroad.

3479 **Foundation for Advancement in Cancer Therapy**

PO Box 1242
Old Chelsea Station
New York, NY 10113
212-741-2790
www.fact-ltd.org

A clearinghouse for information regarding alternative cancer therapies, emphasizing nutritional and metabolic approaches.

3480 **Foundation for the Advancement of Innovative Medicine**

2 Executive Boulevard
Suffern, NY 10601
877-634-3246
FAX: 518-758-7967
e-mail: faim@healthlobby.com
www.faim.org

Howard G Hindin DDS, President
Monica Miller, Member Services/Gov't Relations
Alan Lambert MD JD, Legal Counsel

A voice for innovative medicine's professionals, patients, and suppliers. Defines innovative medicine as a treatment or therapy of empirical clinical benefit that is yet outside the mainstream of conventional medicine. Complementary to conventional medicine, offering alternatives as an individual situation may warrant.

1989

3481 **Gebbie Foundation**

110 W 3rd Street
Suite 308
Jamestown, NY 14701
716-487-1062
FAX: 716-484-6401

Giving in Chautauqua County, and secondly, in neighboring areas of western New York. Giving is offered in other areas only when the project is consonant with program objectives that cannot be developed locally.

3482 **Gladys Brooks Foundation**

226 7th Street
Garden City, NY 11530
516-248-8660

Harman Hawkins, Chairman
James J Daly, Board of Governors

The purpose of this Foundation is to provide for the intellectual, moral and physical welfare of the people of this country by establishing and supporting nonprofit libraries, educational institutions, hospitals and clinics. The Foundation will make grants only to private, publicly supported, nonprofit, tax-exempt organizations.

3483 **Glickenhaus Foundation**

6 E 43rd Street
New York, NY 10017
212-953-7867

Maddy Wehle

3484 **Graphic Controls Corporate Giving Program**

189 Van Rensselaer Street
PO Box 1271
Buffalo, NY 14240
716-853-7500

Phyllis Rudz

3485 **Guide Dog Foundation for the Blind**

371 E Jericho Turnpike
Smithtown, NY 11787
631-265-2121
800-548-4337
FAX: 516-361-5192
e-mail: guidedog@guidedog.org
www.guidedog.org

Wells B Jones CAE CFRE, Executive Director
Catherine I McDougall, Office Manager

Established in 1946, the Foundation provides rehabilitation for the blind by breeding and training guide dogs. A fully trained guide dog is given to blind applicants from all over the United States and some foreign countries. They train together as a team for 25 days on campus. All of these programs, including the cost of transportation and after-care programs, are given without cost to the blind recipients. Quarterly newsletter, video cassette, audio cassette.

3486 **Hearst Foundation**

888 7th Avenue
45th Floor
New York, NY 10106
212-586-5404

Robert M Frehs Jr, VP/Executive Director

3487 **Henry and Lucy Moses Fund**

Moses and Singer
1301 Avenue of the Americas
New York, NY 10019
212-554-7800

3488 **Herman Goldman Foundation**

61 Broadway, 18th Floor
New York, NY 10006
212-797-9090

Richard K Baron, Executive Director

3489 **Horace W Goldsmith Foundation**

375 Park Avenue
Suite 1602
New York, NY 10152
212-319-8700

James C Slaughter, CEO

3490 **International Paper Company Foundation**

2 Manhattanville Road
Purchase, NY 10577
914-397-1500
FAX: 914-397-1500
www.internationalpaper.com

3491 **JM Foundation**
60 E 42nd Street
Room 1651
New York, NY 10165
212-687-7735
FAX: 212-697-5495

Carl O Helstrom, Assistant Executive Director

3492 **Jedra Charitable Foundation**
110-11 Queens Boulevard
Apartment 208
Forest Hills, NY 11375
718-263-4956

David Shechet, President

3493 **Joseph Alexander Foundation**
400 Madison Avenue
Room 906
New York, NY 10017
212-980-0600

3494 **Kenneth & Evelyn Lipper Foundation**
c/o Lipper & Company
101 Park Avenue, 6th Floor
New York, NY 10178
212-883-6333

Kenneth Lipper, Treasurer

3495 **Louis and Anne Abrons Foundation**
First Manhattan Company
437 Madison Avenue
New York, NY 10022
212-756-3100
FAX: 212-832-6698

3496 **Margaret L Wendt Foundation**
40 Fountain Plaza
Suite 277
Buffalo, NY 14202
716-855-2146
FAX: 716-855-2149

Robert J Kresse, Secretary/Treasurer

3497 **Marquis George MacDonald Foundation**
The Chase Manhattan Bank NA
270 Park Avenue
New York, NY 10017
212-270-6000

Donna M Bowers, Administrator

3498 **MetLife Foundation**
1 Madison Avenue
New York, NY 10010
212-578-6272
FAX: 212-685-1435
e-mail: sjacobson@metlife.com
www.metlife.org

Sibyl Jacobson, President/CEO

3499 **Metzger-Price Fund**
230 Park Avenue
Suite 2300
New York, NY 10169
212-867-9500
FAX: 212-599-1759

Isaac A Saufer, Secretary/Treasurer

3500 **Morgan Stanley Foundation**
1221 Avenue of the Americas
27th Floor
New York, NY 10020
212-762-7848
FAX: 212-762-7790

Joan Steinberg, Director Community Affairs

3501 **National Foundation for Facial Reconstruction**
317 E 34th Street
Room 901
New York, NY 10016
212-263-6656
FAX: 212-263-7534
www.nffr.org

A nonprofit organization whose major purposes are to provide facilities for the treatment and assistance of individuals who are unable to afford private reconstructive surgical care, to train and educate professionals in this surgery, to encourage research in the field and to carry on public education.

3502 **National Hemophilia Foundation**
Soho Building
110 Greene Street
Suite 406
New York, NY 10012

3503 **National Neurofibromatosis Foundation**
95 Pine Street
16th Floor
New York, NY 10005
212-344-6633
800-323-7938
FAX: 212-747-0004
e-mail: nnff@nf.org
www.nf.org

Peter Bellermann, President
Jacqueline Medina, Director Programs

A nonprofit 501 (c)(3) medical foundation, dedicated to improving the health and well-being of individuals and families affected by neurofibromatosis. The Foundation sponsors medical research, clinical services, public education programs and patient support services. It is the central source for up-to-date and accurate information about NF. It also assists patients and families with referrals to NF clinics and healthcare professionals specializing in NF. The goal is to find a cure for NF.

3504 **Neisloss Family Foundation**
1737-7 Veterans Highway
Central Islip, NY 11722
631-234-1600
FAX: 631-234-1066

Stanley Neisloss, President

3505 **New York Community Trust**
2 Park Avenue
24th Floor
New York, NY 10016
212-686-0010
FAX: 212-532-8528
www.nycommunitytrust.org

Lorie A Slutsky, President/Director

3506 **New York Foundation**
350 5th Avenue #2901
Room 2901
New York, NY 10118
212-594-8009
www.nyf.org

Madeline Lee, Executive Director

3507 **Northern New York Community Foundation**
120 Washington Street
Watertown, NY 13601
315-782-7110
FAX: 315-782-0047

Alex C Velto, Executive Director

3508 **Parkinson's Disease Foundation**

710 W 168th Street
New York, NY 10032
212-923-4700
800-457-6676
FAX: 212-923-4778
e-mail: info@pdf.org
www.pdf.org

Robin Elliott, Executive Director
Renay D Crooms, Assistant Director

National not-for-profit organization dedicated to funding scientific research to investigate the cause and cure of Parkinson's disease and related disorders. The Foundation has a post-doctoral training program, Interntional Research Grant Program, and makes referrals to physicians who treat PD. Other services include supporting advocacy efforts, making referrals to self-help groups, conducting educational symposiums for patients and professionals.

3509 **Reader's Digest Foundation**

Reader's Digest Road
Pleasantville, NY 10570
914-238-1000
FAX: 914-238-4559
www.readersdigest.com

3510 **Research to Prevent Blindness**

645 Madison Avenue
21st Floor
New York, NY 10022
212-752-4333
800-621-0026
FAX: 212-688-6231
e-mail: info@rpbusa.org
www.rpbusa.org

James V Romano PhD, COO
Thomas Furlong, Director Public Information

National voluntary health foundation supported by foundations, corporations and voluntary gifts and bequests from individuals. Established to stimulate basic and applied research into the causes, prevention and treatment of blinding eye diseases.

3511 **Rita J and Stanley H Kaplan Foundation**

866 United Nations Plaza
Suite 306
New York, NY 10017
212-688-1047
FAX: 212-688-6907

Rita J Kaplan, Director

3512 **Robert Sterling Clark Foundation**

135 E 64th Street
New York, NY 10021
212-288-8900
FAX: 212-288-1033

Margaret Ayers, Executive Director

Giving primarily in New York with emphasis on advocacy, research, and public education aimed at informing New York City of state policies.

3513 **Skadden Fellowship Foundation**

Four Times Sqaure
Room 40/228
New York, NY 10086
212-735-2956
FAX: 917-777-2956
www.skadden.com

Susan Plum, Director

3514 **St. George's Society of New York**

175 9th Avenue
New York, NY 10011
212-924-1434
FAX: 212-727-1566

John Shannon, Executive Director

3515 **Stanley W Metcalf Foundation**

120 Genesse Street
Room 503
Auburn, NY 13021
315-253-9321

J Douglas Pedley, President

3516 **Stonewall Community Foundation**

119 W 24th Street
9th Floor
New York, NY 10011
212-367-1155
FAX: 212-367-1157
e-mail: STNWLCMFD@aol.com

William P Epke, Executive Director

3517 **Surdna Foundation**

330 Madison Avenue
30th Floor
New York, NY 10017
212-557-0010
FAX: 212-557-0003
e-mail: request@surdna.org

3518 **Sydney & Helen Jacoff Foundation**

c/o Berlack, Israels & Liberman
120 W 45th Street
New York, NY 10036
212-704-0100
FAX: 212-704-0196

3519 **Tisch Foundation**

655 Madison Avenue
8th Floor
New York, NY 10021
212-521-2930
FAX: 212-521-2983

Mark J Krinsky, VP

3520 **Van Ameringen Foundation**

509 Madison Avenue
New York, NY 10022
212-758-6221
www.vanamfound.org/right.htm

Henry P van Amerigen, President

3521 **Western New York Foundation**

Main Seneca Building Suite 1402
237 Main Street
Buffalo, NY 14203
716-847-6440
FAX: 716-847-6440

Welles V Moo Jr, President

3522 **William T Grant Foundation**

570 Lexington Avenue
18th Floor
New York, NY 10022
212-752-0071
FAX: 212-752-1398
e-mail: info@wtgrantfdn.org
www.wtgrantfoundation.org

Karen Hein, President
Sharon Brewster, Grants Coordinator

North Carolina

3523 Arc of North Carolina
4200 Six Forks Road
Suite 100
Raleigh, NC 27609
919-782-4632
800-662-8706
FAX: 919-782-4634
e-mail: arcfnc@arcnc.org
www.arcnc.org

3524 Bob & Kay Timberlake Foundation
c/o Bob Timberlake
1660 E Center Street
Lexington, NC 27292
336-248-5092

3525 Broyhill Family Foundation
PO Box 500
Lenoir, NC 28645
828-758-5505
FAX: 828-754-7335

3526 Duke Endowment
100 N Tryon Street
Suite 3500
Charlotte, NC 28202
704-376-0291
FAX: 704-376-9336
e-mail: info@tde.org
www.dukeendowment.org

3527 First Union Foundation
c/o First Union Corporation
301 S College Street
Charlotte, NC 28288
704-374-4689
FAX: 704-374-2484

Judy Allison, Director

3528 Foundation for the Carolinas
1043 E Morehead Street
Suite 100
Charlotte, NC 28204
704-376-9541
FAX: 704-376-1243
www.fftc.org

Giving primarily to organizations serving the citizens of North and South Carolina.

3529 John H Wellons Foundation
PO Box 1254
Dunn, NC 28335
910-892-0436
FAX: 910-892-4888

John H Wellons, Sr President

3530 Kate B Reynolds Charitable Trust
128 Reynolda Village
Winston-Salem, NC 27106
620-723-1456
FAX: 336-723-7765
www.kbr.org

E Ray Cope, President

Grants resricted to the state of North Carolina only.

3531 Kathleen Price and Joseph M Bryan Family Foundation
220 S Eugene Street
Greensboro, NC 27401
336-273-0080
FAX: 336-288-5458

Nancy H Poteet, Interim Director
Joseph M Bryan Jr, President

Only organizations or projects demonstrating direct benefits to North Carolina are eligible for consideration with emphasis on Greensboro and Guilford County and rural communities in North Carolina with financial need. The Foundation does not consider support for annual campaigns, conferences, video production, individuals, research, travel for band and sports teams. There are no discretionary or emergency funds.

3532 Mary Reynolds Babcock Foundation
102 Reynolda Village
Winston Salem, NC 27106
FAX: 919-777-0095
e-mail: info@mrbf.org

Gayle W Dorman, Executive Director

For 1994, this foundation is committed to an extensive educational and planning process to better understand the Southeast and to articulate the role the foundation seeks to play in the region into the twenty-first century.

3533 Triangle Community Foundation
100 Park Offices, Suite 209
PO Box 12834
Research Triangle Park, NC 27709
919-549-9840
FAX: 919-990-9066
e-mail: polly@trianglecf.org
www.trianglecf.org

Polly Guthrie, Program Director

North Dakota

3534 Alex Stern Family Foundation
Bill Stern Building, Suite 205
609 1/2 1st Avenue N
Fargo, ND 58102
701-237-0170
FAX: 701-234-9724

EG Preston, Executive Director

3535 Arc of North Dakota
c/o Arc, Upper Valley
2500 DeMers Avenue, PO Box 12420
Grand Forks, ND 58208
701-772-6191
877-250-2022
FAX: 701-772-2195

3536 North Dakota Community Foundation
1025 N 3rd Street
PO Box 387
Bismarck, ND 58502
701-222-8349
www.ndcf.net

Kevin J Dvorak, President
Valerie Bren, Excutive Assistant

Ohio

3537 Akron Community Foundation
345 W Cedar Street
Akron, OH 44307
330-376-8522
FAX: 330-376-0202
e-mail: acf_fund@ix.netcom.com
www.akroncommunityfdn.org/financialadvisor/

Jody Bacon, Executive Director

3538 Albert G and Olive H Schlink Foundation

49 Benedict Avenue
Suite C
Norwalk, OH 44857
419-668-8211
FAX: 419-668-2813

Robert A Wiedemann, President

3539 American Foundation Corporation

720 National City Bank Building
Cleveland, OH 44114
216-241-6664

William Murphy, President

3540 Arc of Ohio

1335 Dublin Road
Suite 205-C
Columbus, OH 43215
614-487-4720
800-875-2723
FAX: 614-487-4725
e-mail: thearcohio@aol.com
www.thearcofohio.org

3541 Britton Fund

1422 Euclid Avenue
Suite 1010
Cleveland, OH 44115
216-363-6481

Nick Valentino, Treasurer

3542 Cleveland Foundation

1422 Euclid Avenue
Suite 1400
Cleveland, OH 44115
216-861-3810
FAX: 216-861-1729
www.clevelandfoundation.org

Steven A Minter, Executive Director

3543 Columbus Foundation and Affiliated Organizations

1234 E Broad Street
Columbus, OH 43206
614-251-4000
FAX: 614-251-4009
e-mail: info@columbusfoundation.com
www.columbusfoundation.org

James I Luck, President

3544 Eleanora CU Alms Trust

Fifth Third Bank
Dept 00864
9990 Montgomery Road
Cincinnati, OH 45263
513-793-2200

Giving limited to Cincinnati, OH.

3545 Emma Leah and Laura Bell Bahmann Foundation

8041 Hosbrook Road
Suite 210
Cincinnati, OH 45236
513-891-3799
FAX: 513-891-3722

John T Gatch, Executive Director

3546 Eva L and Joseph M Bruening Foundation

627 Hanna Building
1422 Euclid Avenue
Cleveland, OH 44115
216-621-2632
FAX: 216-621-8198
e-mail: fmscleveland.com/bruening

Janet E Narten, Executive Director

Charitable foundation providing grants to noprofit organizations located inCuyahoga county Ohio. No grant are awarded to inviduals.

3547 Fred & Lillian Deeks Memorial Foundation

Star Bank NA
PO Box 1118, ML 5145
Cincinnati, OH 45201
937-339-2329
FAX: 937-339-1861

3548 GAR Foundation

50 S Main Street
PO Box 1500
Akron, OH 44309
330-643-0201
FAX: 330-252-5584
e-mail: rob_briggs@akron.BDBLaw.com
www.garfdn.org

Robert W Briggs, Executive Director

3549 George Gund Foundation

1845 Guildhall Building
45 Prospect Avenue W
Cleveland, OH 44115
216-241-3114
FAX: 216-241-6560
www.gundfdn.org

David Bergholz, Executive Director

3550 Greater Cincinnati Foundation

300 W 4th Street
Suite 200
Cincinnati, OH 45202
513-241-2880
FAX: 513-852-6886
www.greatercincinnatifdn.org

3551 HCR Manor Care Foundation

PO Box 10086
333 N Summit Street
Toledo, OH 43699
FAX: 724-525-5521
e-mail: jsteiner@hcr-manorcare.com
www.hcr-manorcare.com

Jennifer Steiner, Executive Director

3552 Harry C Moores Foundation

100 S 3rd Street
Columbus, OH 43215
614-227-8884

Mary B Cummins

3553 Helen Steiner Rice Foundation

221 E 4th Street, Suite 2100
PO Box 58665
Cincinnati, OH 45258
513-451-9241
www.helensteinerrice.com

3554 Herbert W Hoover Foundation

220 Market Avenue S
United Bank Plaza, Suite 40
Canton, OH 44701
330-453-5555
FAX: 330-453-5622

3555 John P Murphy Foundation

Tower City Center
924 Terminal Tower, 50 Public Sq.
Cleveland, OH 44113
216-623-4770
FAX: 216-623-4773

Herbert E Strawbridge, President/Treasurer

3556 **Nationwide Foundation**
One Nationwide Plaza
Columbus, OH 43215 **614-249-4310**
www.nationwide.com

Stephan A Rish, President

3557 **Nordson Corporate Giving Program**
28601 Clemens Road
Westlake, OH 44145 **440-892-1580**
e-mail: kladiner@nordson.com
www.nordson.com

Constance T Haqq, Executive Director

3558 **Parker-Hannifin Foundation**
6035 Parkland Boulevard
Cleveland, OH 44124 **216-896-3000**
FAX: 216-896-4057

3559 **Reinberger Foundation**
27600 Chagrin Boulevard
Cleveland, OH 44122 **216-292-2790**
FAX: 216-292-4466

Robert N Reinberger, Director

3560 **Robert Campeau Family Foundation**
7 W 7th Street
Cincinnati, OH 45202 **513-579-7000**
FAX: 513-579-7555

3561 **Sisler McFawn Foundation**
PO Box 149
Akron, OH 44309 **330-849-8887**
FAX: 330-996-6215

Charlotte M Stanley, Grants Manager
Our character restricts our giving to certain programs and types of organizations. You can see what out recent giving has been by referring to the list of grants approved and paid during the past year.

3562 **Stark Community Foundation**
The Saxton House
331 Market Avenue S
Canton, OH 44702 **330-454-3426**
FAX: 330-454-5855
e-mail: starkcf@cannet.com

James A Bower, President

3563 **Stocker Foundation**
559 Broadway Avenue
2nd Floor
Lorain, OH 44052 **440-246-5719**
FAX: 440-246-5720
e-mail: pobrien@stockerfoundation.org
www.stockerfoundation.org

Patricia O'Brien, Executive Director

3564 **Toledo Community Foundation**
608 Madison Avenue
Suite1540
Toledo, OH 43604 **419-241-5049**
FAX: 419-242-5549

Pam Howell-Beach, Director

3565 **William J and Dorothy K O'Neill Foundation**
30195 Chagrin Boulevard
Suite 310
Cleveland, OH 44124 **216-831-9667**
FAX: 216-831-3779
e-mail: oneillfdn@aol.com
www.oneillfdn.org

Christine E Henry, Director

3566 **Youngstown Foundation**
Dollar Savings & Trust Company
PO Box 450
Youngstown, OH 44501 **330-744-0320**
FAX: 330-744-0344

Oklahoma

3567 **Anne and Henry Zarrow Foundation**
401 S Boston
Suite 900
Tulsa, OK 74103 **918-295-8000**
FAX: 918-295-8049
e-mail: ZFFound@aol.com

Jeanne Gillert, Grants Manager

3568 **International Bio-Oxidative Medicine Foundation (IBOM)**
1015 Waterwood Parkway
Suite G
Edmond, OK 73034 **405-478-4266**

Offers educational programs, referrals and a newsletter.

3569 **Sarkeys Foundation**
530 E Main
Suite 219
Norman, OK 73021 **405-364-3703**
FAX: 405-364-8191
sarkeys.org

Cheri D Cartwright, Executive Director
Susan C Frantz, Program Officer
Ann M Way, Program Officer
Improves the quality of life in Oklahoma. Offers contributions in the areas of social services, arts and cultural programs, educational funding and health care and medical research. Funding only in agencies in the state of Oklahoma.

3570 **William K Warren Foundation**
PO Box 470372
Tulsa, OK 74147 **918-481-7900**
FAX: 918-481-7935

Oregon

3571 **Arc of Oregon**
1745 State Street
Salem, OR 97301 **503-581-2726**
800-581-2726
877-581-2726
FAX: 503-363-7168
e-mail: arcofor@callatg.org
www.arcoregon.org

Linda Drummond, Excutive Director
Guardianship, Advocacy and Planning Services. Oregon special needs trust; information and referral.

3572 **Arc of Pennsylvania**
2001 N Front Street
Suite 221
Harrisburg, PA 17102 **717-234-2621**
800-692-7258
FAX: 717-234-7615
e-mail: lindadrummond@thearcpa.org
www.thearcpa.org

Linda Drummond, Excutive Director

3573 **Chiles Foundation**
111 SW 5th Avenue
Suite 4050
Portland, OR 97204 **503-222-2143**

Giving in Oregon, with emphasis on Portland, and the Pacific Northwest.

3574 **Jackson Foundation**
PO Box 3168
Portland, OR 97208 **503-275-6564**

Robert H Depew, VP US Bank, N.A.

3575 **Leslie G Ehmann Trust**
c/o US Bank Idaho, Trust Group
PO Box 3168
Portland, OR 97208 **503-275-5929**
FAX: 503-275-4117

Marilyn Norquist

3576 **Samuel S Johnson Foundation**
PO Box 356
Redmond, OR 97756 **541-548-8104**
FAX: 541-548-2014
e-mail: ssjohnson@empnet.com

Elizabeth H Johnson, President

Pennsylvania

3577 **Acorn Alcinda Foundation**
RR 4 Box 710
Mifflintown, PA 17059 **717-436-6597**

Robert J Kennedy, President/Treasurer

3578 **Air Products Foundation**
7201 Hamilton Boulevard
Allentown, PA 18195 **610-481-4911**
FAX: 610-481-5900

Giving primarily in areas of company operations throughout the US.

3579 **Arc of Pennsylvania**
2001 N Front Street
Building #2, Suite 221
Harrisburg, PA 17102 **717-234-2621**

3580 **Arcadia Foundation**
105 E Logan Street
Norristown, PA 19401 **610-275-8460**

Marilyn L Steinbright, President

3581 **Brachial Plexus Palsy Foundation**
210 Spring Haven Circle
Royersford, PA 19468 **610-792-0974**
FAX: 610-792-0974
e-mail: brachial@aol.com
www.membrane.com/bpp

Thomas J Cirino, President
Michael F Cirino, Executive Director

Nonprofit organization dedicated to raising funds for support of families who hae children with brachial plexus injuries. Supports medical facilities that research and treat such injuries, holds fund-raising events to support further research, has support groups, and produces educational materials including a newsletter, Outreach, and brochures.

3582 **Claude Washington Benedum Foundation**
1400 Benedum
Trees Building
Pittsburgh, PA 15222 **412-288-0360**
FAX: 412-288-0366

Giving limited to West Virginia and southwestern Pennsylvania.

3583 **Columbia Gas of Pennsylvania/Columbia Gas of Maryland - Corporate Giving**
650 Washington Road
Pittsburgh, PA 15228 **412-572-7104**
FAX: 412-572-7140
e-mail: mmarti@columbiaenergygroup.com
www.columbiagaspamd.com/html/

Rosemary Martinelli, Manager Corporation

3584 **Connelly Foundation**
1 Tower Bridge
Suite 1450
W Conshohocken, PA 19428 **610-834-3222**
FAX: 610-834-0866
e-mail: info@connellyfdn.org
www.connellyfdn.org

3585 **Dolfinger-McMahon Foundation**
c/o Duane, Morris & Heckscher
1 Liberty Plaza
Philadelphia, PA 19103 **215-979-1768**

Marlene Valcich, Executive Secretary

3586 **Harry C Trexler Trust**
33 S 7th Street
Suite 205
Allentown, PA 18101 **610-434-9645**
FAX: 610-437-5721

Thomas Christman, Secretary Trustees
Giving limited to Lehigh County, Pennsylvania.

3587 **Henry L Hillman Foundation**
2000 Grant Building
Pittsburg, PA 15219 **412-338-3466**
FAX: 412-338-3463
e-mail: foundation@hillmanfo.com

Ronald W Wertz, Secretary/Executive Director

3588 **Howard Heinz Endowment**
625 Liberty Avenue
Pittsburgh, PA 15222 **412-227-1599**

3589 **Hoxie Harrison Smith Foundation**

350 Pond View
Devon, PA 19333 **610-688-0143**
FAX: 610-688-0143

Bruce M Brown, Secretary/Treasurer

3590 **Jewish Healthcare Foundation of Pittsburgh**

Centre City Tower, Suite 2330
650 Smithfield Street
Pittsburgh, PA 15222 **412-594-2550**
FAX: 412-232-6240
e-mail: info@jhf.org
www.jhf.org

Karen W Feinstein, President

3591 **Juliet L Hillman Simonds Foundation**

2000 Grant Building
Pittsburgh, PA 15219 **412-338-3466**
FAX: 412-338-3463
e-mail: foundation@hillmanfo.com

Ronald W Wertz, Secretary

3592 **Oberkotter Foundation**

1600 Market Street
Suite 3600
Philadelphia, PA 19103 **215-751-2601**
FAX: 215-751-2678
e-mail: george_nofer@shsl.com

George H Nofer, Executive Director

3593 **PECO Energy Company Contributions Program**

2301 Market Street
7th Floor
Philadelphia, PA 19103 **215-841-4124**
FAX: 215-841-4040

Anne Baker, Manager

3594 **PNC Bank Foundation**

1 PNC Plaza
249 5th Avenue
Pittsburgh, PA 15222 **412-762-2000**
FAX: 412-768-3779
www.pncbank.com

3595 **Philadelphia Foundation**

1234 Market Street
Suite 1800
Philadelphia, PA 19107 **215-563-6417**
FAX: 215-563-6882
e-mail: parkow@philafound.org
www.philafound.org

R Andrew Swinney, President
Jeffery W Perkins, VP Finance/Administrator

3596 **Pittsburgh Foundation**

1 PPG Place, 30th Floor
Pittsburgh, PA 15222 **412-391-5122**
FAX: 421-391-7259
e-mail: email@pghfdn.org
www.pittsburghfoundation.org

Alfred W Wishart Jr, President/CEO

3597 **Shenango Valley Foundation**

41 Chestnut Street
Sharon, PA 16146 **724-981-5882**
FAX: 724-981-5480

Larry Haynes, Executive Director

3598 **Snee-Reinhardt Charitable Foundation**

2101 1 Mellon Bank Center
500 Grant Street
Pittsburgh, PA 15219 **412-390-2677**
FAX: 412-390-2686

Joan E Szymanski, Foundation Manager

3599 **Staunton Farm Foundation**

Center City Tower, Suite 210
650 Smithfield Street
Pittsburgh, PA 15222 **412-281-8020**
FAX: 412-232-3115
e-mail: info@stauntonfarm.org
www.stauntonfarm.org

Joni Schwager, Executive Director

3600 **Stewart Huston Charitable Trust**

76 S 1st Avenue
Coatesville, PA 19320 **610-384-2666**
FAX: 610-384-3396
e-mail: admin@stewarthuston.org

Scott G Huston, Program Director

3601 **Teleflex Foundation**

630 W Germantown Pike
Suite 461
Plymouth Meeting, PA 19462 **610-834-6378**
FAX: 610-834-0248

Thelma A Fretz, Executive Director

3602 **USX Foundation**

600 Grant Street
Suite 685
Pittsburgh, PA 15219 **412-433-5237**
FAX: 412-433-6847

CD Mallick, General Manager
Patricia Funaro, Program Manager

Giving primarily in areas of company operations located within the United States.

3603 **WW Smith Charitable Trust**

3515 W Chester Pike
Suite E
Newtown Square, PA 19073 **610-359-1811**
FAX: 610-359-9717

Frances R Pemberton, Trust Administrator

3604 **William B Dietrich Foundation**

PO Box 58177
Philadelphia, PA 19102 **215-979-1919**

William B Dietrich, President

3605 **William Talbott Hillman Foundation**

2000 Grant Building
Pittsburg, PA 15219 **412-338-3466**
FAX: 412-338-3463
e-mail: foundation@hillmanfo.com

Ronald W Wertz, Secretary

3606 **William V and Catherine A McKinney Charitable Foundation**

National City Center [25-154]
20 Stanwix Street
Pittsburgh, PA 15222 **412-644-8332**
FAX: 412-644-6058

William M Schmidt, VP National City Bank of PA

Rhode Island

3607 Arc South County Chapter
24 Salt Pond Road
Building G3
Wakefield, RI 02879
401-789-4386
FAX: 401-789-4394

3608 Arc of Northern Rhode Island
320 Main Street
Woonsocket, RI 02895
401-765-3700
FAX: 401-766-0910

3609 Arc-Down Syndrome Society of Rhode Island
99 Bald Hill Road
Cranston, RI 02920
401-463-5751

3610 Blackstone Valley Chapter RI Arc
115 Manton Street
Pawtucket, RI 02861
401-727-0150
FAX: 401-727-0153
e-mail: contact@bvcriarc.org
www.bvcriarc.org

Peter Holden, Executive Director
Barbara Lindsay, Development Director

Aprivate nonprofut organization providing residential developmental employment and recreational programs and services to more than 400 individuals with mental retardation and realted disabilities.

3611 Bristol County Chapter Arc
PO Box 711
Bristol, RI 02809
401-253-5900
FAX: 401-253-7880

3612 Champlin Foundations
300 Centerville Road
Suite 300S
Warwick, RI 02886
401-736-0370
FAX: 401-736-7248

David King, Director

Giving in the Rhode Island area.

3613 Cranston Arc
905 Pontiac Avenue
Cranston, RI 02920
401-941-1112
FAX: 401-941-2516
www.cranstonarc.org

3614 Greater Providence Arc
220 Woonasquatucket Avenue
North Providence, RI 02911
401-353-7000
FAX: 401-353-0320

3615 Horace A Kimball and S Ella Kimball Foundation
c/o The Washington Trust Company
23 Broad Street
Westerly, RI 02891
401-364-3565
FAX: 401-364-7799

Thomas F Black III, President

3616 Kent County Arc
3445 Post Road
Warwick, RI 02886
401-739-2700
FAX: 401-737-8907

3617 Newport County Arc
PO Box 4390
Middletown, RI 02842
401-846-4600
FAX: 401-849-4267

3618 Rhode Island Arc
99 Bald Hill Road
Cranston, RI 02920
401-463-9191
FAX: 401-463-9244
riarc@compuserve.com

3619 Rhode Island Foundation
1 Union Station
Providence, RI 02903
410-274-4564
FAX: 401-331-8085
www.rifoundation.org

Ronald D Thorpe, VP Programming

3620 Westerly Chariho Arc
Frank A Olean Cye
93 Airport Road
Westerly, RI 02891
401-596-2091
FAX: 401-596-3945

South Carolina

3621 Arc of South Carolina
PO Box 8707
Columbia, SC 29210
803-935-5266
FAX: 803-935-5250
e-mail: thearcssc@aol.com

3622 Center for Developmental Disabilities
University of South Carolina
8301 Farrow Road
School of Medicine, Education Bldg.
Columbia, SC 29208
803-935-5231
FAX: 803-935-5059
e-mail: scsis@dccisc.edu
www.scsis.org

Denise Rivers, Project Coordinator

A University Affiliated Program which develops model programs designed to serve persons with disabilities and to train students in fields related to disabilities.

3623 Colonial Life and Accident Insurance Company Contributions Program
1200 Colonial Life Boulevard
Columbia, SC 29202
803-798-7000
FAX: 803-213-7245

Edwina Carns, Public/Community Relations

3624 Pickens County Arc
PO Box 1308
Easley, SC 29641
864-859-5416

Tennessee

3625 Arc Putnam County
453 Gould Drive
Cookville, TN 38506
931-432-5981
FAX: 931-432-5987

3626 Arc of Anderson County
PO Box 4823
Oak Ridge, TN 37831
865-481-0550

3627 Arc of Davidson County
1207 17th Avenue S
Suite 100
Nashville, TN 37212
615-321-5699
FAX: 615-322-9184

3628 Arc of Hamilton County
4613 Brainerd Road
Chattanooga, TN 37411
423-624-6887
FAX: 423-624-3974

3629 Arc of Tennessee
44 Vantage Way
Suite 550
Nashville, TN 37228
615-248-5878
800-835-7077
FAX: 615-248-5879
e-mail: pcooper@thearctn.org
www.thearctn.org

Walter Rogers, Executive Director
Peggy Cooper, Office Manager

Advocacy, information and support for people with developmental disabilities and their families.

3630 Arc of Washington County
2700 S Roan Street
Suite 300B
Johnson City, TN 37601
423-928-9362
FAX: 423-928-7431

3631 Arc of Williamson County
129 W Fowlkes Street
Suite 151
Franklin, TN 37064
615-790-5815
FAX: 615-790-5891

3632 Benwood Foundation
736 Market Street
Suite 1600
Chattanooga, TN 37402
423-267-4311
FAX: 423-267-9049

Corinne A Allen, Executive Director

Giving primarily in the Chattanooga area.

3633 Community Foundation of Greater Chattanooga
1270 Market Street
Chattanooga, TN 37402
423-265-0586
FAX: 423-265-0586
e-mail: pcooper@cfgc.org
www.cfgc.org

Peter T Cooper, Executive Director

3634 Education and Auditory Research Foundation
1817 Patterson Street
Nashville, TN 37203
615-329-7807
800-545-4327
FAX: 615-329-7935
TTY:615-329-7849
e-mail: tef@earfoundation.org
www.earfoundation.org

Sam Hook, Executive Director

Not-for-profit organization dedicated to integrating persons with hearing impairments into the mainstream of society through public awarness and medical education. Sponsors a variety of programs including a medical educatin program that offers continuing medical education courses to physicians, the young ears program which focuses on raising the level of hearing loss prevention in grades K-3rd. Minnie Pearl scholorship program for hearing impaired high school seniors.

3635 Montgomery County Arc
PO Box 2145rive
Clarksville, TN 37042
931-905-0900
FAX: 931-905-0900

Texas

3636 Abell-Hangar Foundation
303 W Wall
Suite 615
Midland, TX 79701
423-684-6655
FAX: 423-684-4474
e-mail: AHF@abell-hanger.org

David L Smith, Executive Director

Giving limited to Texas, preferably within the Permian Basin.

3637 Albert & Bessie Mae Kronkosky Charitable Foundation
112 E Pecan
Suite 830
San Antonio, TX 78205
210-475-9000
FAX: 210-354-2204
e-mail: kronfdn@kronkosky.org
www.kronkosky.org

Palmer Moe, Executive Director

3638 American Foundation for the Blind: Southwest
260 Treadway Plaza
Exchange Park
Dallas, TX 75235
903-352-7222
FAX: 903-352-3214
e-mail: dallas@afb.net
www.afb.org

Mary Ann Siller, National Education Consultant

3639 Arc of Texas
1600 W 38th Street
Suite 200
Austin, TX 78731
512-454-6694
800-252-9729
FAX: 512-454-4956
e-mail: secretary@thearcoftexas.org
www.thearcoftexas.com

Mike Bright, Executive Director

3640 Arch and Stella Rowan Foundation
307 W 7th Street
Number 1900
Fort Worth, TX 76102
817-336-2679
FAX: 817-336-2679

Alice B Myatt, Secretary

3641 BA and Elinor Steinhagen Benevolent Trust
Chase Bank of Texas
PO Box 3928
Beaumont, TX 77704
FAX: 409-880-1437

Jean Monica, VP

3642 Brown Foundation
2217 Welch Street
PO Box 130646
Houston, TX 77019
713-523-6867
FAX: 713-523-2917
e-mail: bfi@brownfoundation.org
www.brownfoundation.org

Giving primarily in Texas, with emphasis on Houston.

3643 Burlington Northern Foundation
3800 Colonial Plaza
777 Main Street
Fort Worth, TX 76102
817-878-2000
FAX: 800-677-4816

Beverly Edwards, President
Becky Blankenship, Administrator

Giving primarily in the areas of company operations, included, but not limited to the areas of civic service, culture and the arts, education, federated, human service and youth.

3644 Burnett Foundation
801 Chrry Street
Suite 1585
Fort Worth, TX 76102
817-877-3344

Thomas F Beech, Executive VP

3645 CH Foundation
PO Box 16458
Lubbock, TX 79490
806-792-0448
FAX: 806-792-7824

Nelda Thompson, Secretary

3646 Cockrell Foundation
1600 Smith Street
Suite 3900
Houston, TX 77002
713-209-7300

Jennifer Delaney, Assistant to the Board
M Nancy Williams, Executive VP

Purpose is for giving for higher education at the University of Texas at Austin; support also for cultural programs, social services, youth services and health care. Limitations are giving in Houston, Texas and no grants are awarded to individuals.

3647 Communities Foundation of Texas
4605 Live Oak Street
Dallas, TX 75204
214-826-5231
FAX: 214-823-7737
e-mail: jsmith@cftexas.org
www.cftexas.org

Giving in the Dallas area.

3648 Community Foundation of the Metropolitan Tarrant County
306 W 7th Street, Suite 702
Fort Worth Club Building
Fort Worth, TX 76102
817-877-0702
FAX: 817-877-1215
e-mail: hdowd@cfmtc.com
www.cfmtx.org/history.asp

Homer M Dowd, President

3649 Cullen Foundation
601 Jefferson Street
40th Floor
Houston, TX 77002
713-659-7839
FAX: 713-651-2374

Alan M Stewart, Executive Director

Grants are restricted to Texas-based organizations for programs in Texas, primarily in the Houston area.

3650 Curtis & Doris K Hankamer Foundation
9039 Katy Freeway
Suite 530
Houston, TX 77024
713-461-8140

Gregory A Herbst

3651 Dallas Foundation
900 Jackson Street
Dallas, TX 75202
214-741-9848
FAX: 214-741-9848
e-mail: mjalonick@dallasfoundation.org
www.dallasfoundation.org

Mary M Jalonick, Executive Director

3652 David D & Nona S Payne Foundation
Hughes Building
Suite 436
Pampa, TX 79065
806-665-7281

Adelaide S Colwell, Secretary

3653 El Paso Natural Gas Foundation
PO Box 2511
Houston, TX 77252
713-420-3750

Karen King

3654 Epilepsy Foundation of Greater North Texas
2906 Swiss Avenue
Dallas, TX 75204
214-823-8809
800-447-7778
e-mail: postmaster@afgnt.org
www.efgnt.org

3655 Epilepsy Foundation of Southeast Texas
2650 Fountain View
Suite 316
Houston, TX 77057
713-789-6295
888-548-9716
e-mail: dstahlhut@efset.org
www.efset.org

Donna Stahlhut, Executive Director

3656 Epilepsy Foundation: Central and South Texas
10615 Perrin Beitel
Suite 602
San Antonio, TX 78217
210-653-5353
888-606-5353
e-mail: sindi@efcst.org
www.efcst.org

Sindy Rosales, Executive Director

3657 Gil and Dody Weaver Foundation
500 W 7th Street
Suite 1714
Fort Worth, TX 76102
817-877-1712

William R Weaver

3658 Harris and Eliza Kempner Fund
2201 Market Street
Suite 601
Galveston, TX 77550
409-762-1603
FAX: 409-762-5435

Elaine R Perachio, Executive Director

3659 Henry & Tommy Lehmann Charitable Foundation
PO Box 223
Giddings, TX 78942
979-542-3636

Jake Jacobson, Chairperson

3660 Hesta Stuart Christian Charitable Trust
Bank One, Texas NA
PO Box 2050
Fort Worth, TX 76113
817-884-4151

Robert Lansford, Trust Officer

3661 Hillcrest Foundation
Bank of America
PO Box 830214
Dallas, TX 75283
214-209-1965

Daniel Kelly, VP

3662 Hoblitzelle Foundation
5956 Sherry Lane
Suite 901
Dallas, TX 75225
214-373-0462
home.att.net/~hoblitzelle

Paul W Harris, Executive VP

3663 Houston Endowment
600 Travis Street
Suite 6400
Houston, TX 77002
713-238-8100
FAX: 713-238-8810
www.houstonendowment.org

H Joe Nelson III, President

3664 John G and Marie Stella Kennedy Memorial Foundation
1700 First City Tower II
Corpus Christi, TX 78478

3665 John S Dunn Research Foundation
3355 W Alabama
Suite 702
Houston, TX 77098
713-626-0368

Lloyd J Gregory Jr MD, Executive VP

3666 Kent Waldrep National Paralysis Foundation
16415 Addison Road
Suite 550
Addison, TX 75001
972-248-7100
877-724-2873
FAX: 972-248-7313
e-mail: lkoen@spinalvictory.org
www.spinalvictory.org

Lisa Koen, Office Manager/Media Coordinator

Not-for-profit organization dedicated to raising funds for research to find a cure for paralysis caused by brain injury, spinal cord injury, or stroke. Educational materials include brochures and a quarterly newsletter.

3667 Lola Wright Foundation
PO Box 1138
Georgetown, TX 78627
512-869-2574

Patrick H O'Donnell, President

3668 Marcia & Otto Koehler Foundation
Bank of America
PO Box 121
San Antonio, TX 78291
210-270-5371

Gregg Muenster, Senior VP

3669 Meadows Foundation
2922 Swiss Avenue
Dallas, TX 75204
214-821-3290
FAX: 214-827-7042
e-mail: grants@mfi.org
www.mfi.org

3670 Moody Foundation
704 Moody National Bank Building
Galveston, TX 7550
409-763-5333

Peter M Moore, Director Grants

3671 Pearle Vision Foundation
2534 Royal Lane
Dallas, TX 75229
972-277-5993

Trina Parasiliti, Secretary

3672 Rockwell Foundation
1360 Post Oak Road
Suite 780
Houston, TX 77056
713-629-9022
FAX: 713-629-7702

R Terry Bell, President

3673 San Antonio Area Foundation
PO Box 120366
San Antonio, TX 78212
210-225-2243
FAX: 210-225-1980
e-mail: saaf@dcci.com
www.saafdn.org

Marion T Lee, Executive Director

3674 **Shell Oil Company Foundation**
One Shell Plaza, Suite 4137
PO Box 2099
Houston, TX 77252 **713-241-3616**
FAX: 713-241-3329
e-mail: socfoundation@shellus.com
www.countonshell.com

AH Myresty, VP
BL McHam, Executive Director

A not-for-profit foundation funded by donations from Shell Oil Company and other participating Shell companies and subsidiaries.

3675 **South Texas Charitable Foundation**
PO Box 2459
Victoria, TX 77902 **512-573-4383**

Rayford L Keller, Secretary

3676 **Sterling-Turner Foundation**
811 Rusk
Suite 205
Houston, TX 77002 **713-237-1117**
FAX: 713-223-4638

Eyvonne Moser, Assistant Secretary

3677 **Swalm Foundation**
11511 Katy Freeway
Suite 430
Houston, TX 77079 **281-497-5280**
FAX: 281-497-7340

Miriam Minkoff, Secretary

3678 **TLL Temple Foundation**
109 Temple Boulevard
Lufkin, TX 75901 **936-639-5197**
e-mail: tlltf@lcc.com

A Wayne Corely, Executive Director

3679 **Vale-Asche Foundation**
1010 River Oaks Bank Building
2001 Kirby Drive
Houston, TX 77019 **713-520-7334**

Vale-Asche Russell, President

3680 **William Stamps Farish Fund**
1100 Louisiana Street
Suite 1250
Houston, TX 77002 **713-227-0408**

Primary giving in Texas.

Utah

3681 **Arc of Utah**
455 E 400 S
Suite 202
Salt Lake City, UT 94111 **801-364-5060**
e-mail: Arcutah@burgoyne.com

3682 **Ben B and Iris M Margolis Foundation**
First Security Bank of Utah
PO Box 628
Salt Lake City, UT 84110 **801-350-5583**

Julie Webster

3683 **Marriner S Eccles Foundation**
701 Deseret Building
79 South Main Street
Salt Lake City, UT 84111 **801-246-5157**

Shannon K Toronto

3684 **Questar Corporation Contributions Program**
180 E 1st S Street
PO Box 45433
Salt Lake City, UT 84145 **801-324-5435**
FAX: 801-324-5435

Janice Bates, Director Community Affairs

Vermont

3685 **Vermont Community Foundation**
3 Court Street
PO Box 30
Middlebury, VT 05753 **802-388-3355**
FAX: 802-388-3398
e-mail: vcf@vermontcf.org
www.vermontcf.org

Judy Dunning

Virginia

3686 **Arc of Virginia**
6 N 6th Street
Suite 403-A
Richmond, VA 23219 **804-649-8481**
e-mail: arcva@richmond.infi.net

3687 **Bell Atlantic Foundation**
1310 N Ct House Road
Arlington, VA 22201 **703-524-9761**
FAX: 703-974-0131
www.foundation.verizon.com/04014.shtml

James Cullen, President
Denise Bailey, Director

Concentrates efforts on programs that support its vision to produce more scientifically and technically literate population effecting measurable improvements in the way pre-collegiate science, math and technology education is delivered to and understood by students.

3688 **Camp Foundation**
PO Box 813
Franklin, VA 23851 **757-562-3439**

Bobby B Worrell, Executive Director

3689 **Community Foundation Serving Richmond & Central Virginia**
7325 Beaufont Springs Drive
Suite 210
Richmond, VA 23225
804-330-7400
FAX: 804-330-5992
www.tcfrichmond.org

Darcy S Oman, President

3690 **Gannett Foundation**
1100 Wilson Boulevard
30th Floor
Arlington, VA 22234
FAX: 703-558-3819
e-mail: isimpson@gcil.gannett.com
www.gannett.com

Irma Simpson, Manager

3691 **Greater Lynchburg Community Trust**
Federal Fidelity
National Bank Building, 19th Floor
PO Box 714
Lynchburg, VA 24505
434-845-6500
FAX: 434-845-6530
e-mail: glct@inmind.com

Stuart J Turille, Executive Director

3692 **John Randolph Foundation**
106 Norht Main Street, Suite B
PO Box 1606
Hopewell, VA 23860
804-458-2239
FAX: 804-458-3754
e-mail: jrf@new-quest.net

3693 **Norfolk Foundation**
1410 Nations Bank Court
Norfolk, VA 23510
757-622-7951

Lee C Kitchin, Executive Director

3694 **Robey W Estes Family Foundation**
Robey W Estes Jr
PO Box 25612
Richmond, VA 23260
804-353-1900

3695 **Virginia Beach Foundation**
PO Box 4329
Virginia Beach, VA 23454
757-422-5249
FAX: 757-422-1849
fdncenter.org/grantmaker/vbf

Ted Clarkson, Executive Director

3696 **W Alton Jones Foundation**
232 E High Street
Charlottesville, VA 22902
434-295-2134
FAX: 434-295-1648
www.whn.org

Washington

3697 **Arc of Washington State**
2600 Martin Way E
Suite D
Olympia, WA 98506
360-357-5596
888-754-8798
FAX: 360-357-3279
e-mail: thearc@nwrain.com
www.arcwa.org

Sue Elliott, Executive Director

3698 **Ben B Cheney Foundation**
1201 Pacific Avenue
Suite 1600
Tacoma, WA 98402
253-572-2442
FAX: 253-572-2902

William Rieke MD, Executive Director

3699 **Foundation Northwest**
555 Paulson Court
421 W Riverside Aveune
Spokane, WA 99201
509-624-2606
FAX: 509-624-2608

Peter A Jackson, President

3700 **Glaser Foundation**
2601 Elliott Avenue
Seattle, WA 98121
206-728-1050
FAX: 206-728-1123

Martin Collier, Executive Director

3701 **Greater Tacoma Community Foundation**
PO Box 1995
Tacoma, WA 98401
253-383-5622
FAX: 253-272-8099
e-mail: margy@gtcf.org

Margy McGroarty

3702 **Greater Wenatchee Community Foundation**
7 N Wenatchee Avenue, Suite 201
PO Box 3332
Wenatchee, WA 98807
868-663-7716
FAX: 509-664-9569

Raymond Taylor, President/CEO

3703 **Medina Foundation**
801 2nd Avenue
#1300
Seattle, WA 98104
206-652-8783
FAX: 206-652-8791
e-mail: info@medinafoundation.org
www.medinafoundation.org

Gregory P Barlow, Executive Director

3704 **Norcliffe Foundation**
999 3rd Avenue
Suite 1006
Seattle, WA 98104
206-682-4820
FAX: 206-682-4821
e-mail: arline@thenorcliffefoundation.com

Arline Hefferline, Principal

Geographic area of funding limited to the Puget Sound Region in and around Seattle, Washington.

3705 **Stewardship Foundation**
PO Box 1278
Tacoma, WA 98401 253-620-1340
FAX: 253-572-2721
e-mail: info@stewardshipfdn.org
www.stewardshipfdn.org

Christian, evangelical organizations - national or international impact.

3706 **Weyerhaeuser Company Foundation**
Box CH1L32
Tacoma, WA 98477 253-924-6731
FAX: 253-924-3658

Karen Veitenhans, Finance Manager

Although the foundation does fund programs for disabled persons from time to time, it is not a specific priority for the foundation. Since it was formed in 1948, the foundation has given more than $81.1 million to nonprofit organizations and is one of the oldest funds for corporate philanthropy in the country. Nearly all of its contributions have been made within the communities where Weyerhaeuser employees live and work and awards approximately 600 grants annually.

West Virginia

3707 **Bernard McDonough Foundation**
311 4th Street
Parkersburg, WV 26101 304-424-6280
FAX: 304-424-6281

James T Wakley, President

Wisconsin

3708 **Arc of Dane County**
1320 Mendota Street
Suite 111A
Madison, WI 53714 608-257-9738
FAX: 262-635-2640
e-mail: arcdane@chorus.net

3709 **Arc of Dunn County**
390 Red Cedar Street
Suite G
Menomonie, WI 54751 715-235-7373
FAX: 715-233-3565
e-mail: thearc@wwt.net

Advocating for the rights of citizens with disabilities.

3710 **Arc of Eau Claire**
513 S Barstow Street
Eau Claire, WI 54701 715-834-7204

3711 **Arc of Outagamie County**
633 W Wisconsin Avenue
Appleton, WI 54911 715-235-7373
FAX: 920-731-9850

3712 **Arc of Racine County**
818 Sixth Street
Racine, WI 53403 262-634-6303
FAX: 262-635-2640

3713 **Arc of Wisconsin Disability Association**
600 Williamson Street
Suite J
Madison, WI 53703 608-251-9272
FAX: 608-251-1403
e-mail: arcw@itis.com
www.wfv.org

The Arc-Wisconsin strives to be a majornforce in advocating and promoting self-determined quality of life opportunities for poeple with developmental and related disabilities and their families.

3714 **Faye McBeath Foundation**
1020 N Broadway
Milwaukee, WI 53202 414-272-2626
FAX: 414-272-6235
e-mail: mcbeath@execpc.com

Sarah M Dean, Executive Director

3715 **Helen Bader Foundation**
233 N Water Street
Milwaukee, WI 53202 414-244-6464
FAX: 414-244-1441
e-mail: info@hbf.org
www.hbf.org

Daniel J Badger, President

3716 **Johnson Controls Foundation**
PO Box 591
Milwaukee, WI 53201 414-228-1200
800-333-2222
FAX: 414-228-3200

Denise Zutz, Secretary Advisory
Valerie Adisek, Administrative Secretary

Organized and directed to be operated for charitable purposes which include the distribution and application of financial support to soundly managed and operated organizations or causes which are fundamentally philanthropic.

3717 **Lynde and Harry Bradley Foundation**
PO Box 92848
Milwaukee, WI 53202
FAX: 414-291-9991
www.townhall.com

Dr. Hillel Fradkin, VP

The Foundation recognizes that responsible self-government depends on enlightened citizens and informed public opinion. The Foundation offers grants to areas of concern such as educational activities of Wisconsin's universities. Supports initiatives to improve the cultural and economic areas of the Metropolitan area.

3718 **Milwaukee Foundation**
1020 N Broadway
Milwaukee, WI 53202 414-272-5805
FAX: 414-272-6235
e-mail: milwfdn@execpc.com
www.greatermilwaukeefoundation.org

Douglas M Jansson, Executive Director

3719 **Northwestern Mutual Life Foundation**
720 E Wisconsin Avenue
Milwaukee, WI 53202 414-271-1444
FAX: 414-665-2199
www.northwesternmutual.com

Fredric H Sweet, Executive Vice President

3720 **Patrick and Anna M Cudahy Fund**

PO Box 11978
Milwaukee, WI 53211 **414-271-6020**
FAX: 847-475-0679
e-mail: jborcher@ix.netcom.com
www.cudahyfund.org

Judith L Borchers, Executive Director

3721 **SB Waterman & E Blade Charitable Foundation**

Marshall & Ilsley Trust Company
PO Box 2980
Milwaukee, WI 53201 **414-287-7228**
FAX: 414-298-8097

Thomas C Boettcher

Wyoming

3722 **Arc of Wyoming**

PO Box 2161
Casper, WY 82602 **307-237-9110**
800-801-0569
FAX: 307-577-4014
www.arcofwyoming.org

Victor Orr, President

Funding Directories

3723 **AIDS Funding**

Foundation Center
79 Fifth Avenue
Department ZE
New York, NY 10003 **212-421-0771**
800-424-9836
FAX: 212-807-3677
www.fdncenter.org

Thomas Buckman, President

Gives vital information on over 450 foundations, corporate giving programs, and public charities; more than twice the number of grantmakers appeared in the last edition. All the grantmakers listed have proven their commitment by funding projects such as direct relief, medical research, legal aid and other programs to empower AIDS victims and combat the disease. *$60.00*

ISBN 0-87954 -82-5

3724 **Chronicle Guide to Grants**

Chronicle Guide to Grants
1255 23rd Street NW
Washington, DC 20037 **202-331-4267**
800-287-6072
FAX: 202-659-2236

Edward R Weidlein, Publisher

A computerized research tool, on floppy disks or a CD-ROM, for immediate use on any IBM compatible personal computer. Offers electronic listings of 10,000 grants from hundreds of foundations, with a subscription that offers 1,000 plus new listings every two months. Each listing offers grant information as well as names, addresses and phone numbers of the grant-making organizations. *$295.00*

3725 **Community Health Funding Report**

CD Publications
8204 Fenton Street
Silver Spring, MD 20910 **301-588-6380**
800-666-6380
FAX: 301-588-6385
e-mail: chf@cdpublications.com
www.cdpublications.com

Mike Gerecht, Publisher

Gives the widest range of funding information available anywhere, including public and private grant announcements, reports on successful health programs nationwide, interviews with grant officials, plus national news on health policy topics affecting various organizations. *$339.00*

18 pages BiWeekly

3726 **Corporate Foundation Files**

Foundation Center
79 Fifth Avenue
Department ZE
New York, NY 10003 **212-421-0771**
800-424-9836
FAX: 212-807-3677
www.fdncenter.org

Thomas Buckman, President

Provides an even more updated in-depth examination of over 250 of America's top corporate foundations, grantmakers with assets of $1 million plus or annual giving of $100,000 or more. This book supplements information presented on leading corporate foundations and provides 4-6 page reports with full background data on each Corporation and foundation structure plus a complete grants analysis and listing of sample grants awarded to nonprofit organizations. *$125.00*

ISBN 0-87954 -36-1

3727 **Corporate Foundation Profiles**

Foundation Center
79 Fifth Avenue
Department ZE
New York, NY 10003 **212-421-0771**
800-424-9836
FAX: 212-807-3677
www.fdncenter.org

Offers foundation portraits, grants analysis and grants list. *$135.00*

3728 **Crime and Justice**

Foundation Center
79 Fifth Avenue
Department ZE
New York, NY 10003 **212-421-0771**
800-424-9836
FAX: 212-807-3677
www.fdncenter.org

Thomas Buckman, President

This comprehensive work examines foundation funding for programs involved with crime prevention, juvenile justice, law enforcement, correction facilities, rehabilitation and victim assistance. This book looks at significant developments in the criminal justice field, changing public perceptions of crime and cuts in governmental expenditures. *$35.00*

ISBN 0-87954 -90-6

3729 **Directory of Japanese Giving**

Foundation Center
79 Fifth Avenue
Department ZE
New York, NY 10003 **212-421-0771**
800-424-9836
FAX: 212-807-3677
www.fdncenter.org

Offers crucial information on the fastest growing sector of corporate philanthropy. *$190.00*

3730 **Directory of New and Emerging Foundations**

Foundation Center
79 Fifth Avenue
Department ZE
New York, NY 10003 **212-421-0771**
800-424-9836
FAX: 212-807-3677
www.fdncenter.org

Provides information on over 3,000 foundations that have incorporated as grantmaking institutions in the United States. *$95.00*

3731 **Directory of Venture Capital Firms**

Grey House Publishing
185 Millerton Road
PO Box 860
Millerton, NY 12546 **518-789-8700**
800-562-2139
FAX: 518-789-0545
e-mail: books@greyhouse.com
www.greyhouse.com

Leslie Mackenzie, Publisher

Annual

3732 **Disability Funding News**

CD Publications
8204 Fenton Street
Silver Spring, MD 20910 **301-588-6380**
800-666-6380
FAX: 301-588-6385
e-mail: cdpubs@clark.net
www.cdpublications.com

Wayne Welch, Editor
Leonard Curry, Associate Publisher

Offers comprehensive listings on federal grants, detailed listings of foundations, legal news, grant-seeking techniques and more. *$249.00*

18 pages SemiWeekly
ISSN 1069-13 9

3733 **Federal Funding to Fight AIDS**

Government Information Services
4301 Fairfax Drive
Suite 875
Arlington, VA 22203 **703-465-9100**
800-876-0226
FAX: 800-926-2012

Describes all the federal government grants and financial aid programs to fight the AIDS epidemic. Includes agency-by-agency description of $1.9 billion in available grants, including the name, address and telephone number of the federal official responsible for each program. *$57.00*

74 pages Special Report

3734 **Federal Grants & Contracts Weekly**

Capitol Publications
1101 King Street
Suite 444
Alexandria, VA 22314 **703-683-4100**
800-655-5597
FAX: 703-736-6501

Pam Moore, Editor
Claudia Moran, Marketing Manager

The latest funding announcements of federal grants for project opportunities in research, training and services. Provides profiles of key programs, tips on seeking grants, updates on legislation and regulations, budget developments and early alerts to upcoming funding opportunities. *$369.00*

Weekly

3735 **Financial Aid for Asian Americans**

Reference Service Press
5000 Windplay Drive
Suite 4
El Dorado Hills, CA 95762 **916-939-9620**
FAX: 916-939-9626
e-mail: findaid@aol.com
www.rspfunding.com

Gail Ann Schlachter, Author
R David Weber, Author

This is the source to use if you are looking for financial aid for Asian Americans; nearly 1,000 funding opportunities are described. *$35.00*

336 pages 1999
ISBN 1-588410-02-1

3736 **Financial Aid for Hispanic Americans**

Reference Service Press
5000 Windplay Drive
Suite 4
El Dorado Hills, CA 95762 **916-939-9620**
FAX: 916-939-9626
e-mail: findaid@aol.com
www.rspfunding.com

Gail Ann Schlachter, Author
R David Weber, Author

Nearly 1,300 funding programs open to Americans of Mexican, Puerto Rican, Central American, or other Latin American heritage are described here. *$37.50*

472 pages 1999
ISBN 1-588410-03-X

3737 **Financial Aid for Native Americans**

Reference Service Press
5000 Windplay Drive
Suite 4
El Dorado Hills, CA 95762 **916-939-9620**
FAX: 916-939-9626
e-mail: findaid@aol.com
www.rspfunding.com

Gail Ann Schlachter, Author
R David Weber, Author

Detailed information is provided on 1,500 funding opportunities open to American Indians, Native Alaskans, and Native Pacific Islanders. *$37.50*

546 pages
ISBN 1-588410-04-8

3738 Financial Aid for Veterans, Military Personnel and Their Dependents

Reference Service Press
1100 Industrial Road
Suite 9
San Carlos, CA 94070 **510-841-2636**
FAX: 650-594-0411
e-mail: findaid@aol.com
www.rspfunding.com

According to Reference Book Review, this directory (with its 1,100 entries) is the most comprehensive guide available on the subject. *$40.00*

392 pages
ISBN 1-588410-43-9

3739 Financial Aid for the Disabled and their Families

Reference Service Press
5000 Windplay Drive
Suite 4
El Dorado Hills, CA 95762 **916-939-9620**
FAX: 916-939-9626
e-mail: info@rspfunding.com
www.rspfunding.com

Gail Ann Schlachter, Author
R David Weber, Author

Organized to easily identify funding opportunities not only by type, but by specific subject coverage, sponsoring organization, program title, residency requirements, where the money can be spent, and even deadline date; includes detailed program descriptions. Program profiles indicate purpose, eligibility, financial data, duration, special features, limitations, number awarded, and application. Complete contact information is also provided including fax numbers, toll-free, and email/website. *$37.50*

508 pages Every other yr. 1999
ISBN 1-588410-01-3

3740 Foundation & Corporate Grants Alert

Capitol Publications
1101 King Street
Suite 444
Alexandria, VA 22314 **703-683-4100**
800-655-5597
FAX: 703-736-6501

Patricia Hagmann, Editor
Claudia Moran, Marketing Manager

A complete guide to foundation and corporate grant opportunities for nonprofit organizations. Tracks developments and trends in funding and provides notification of changes in foundations' funding priorities. *$245.00*

Monthly
ISSN 1062-46 6

3741 Foundation 1000

Foundation Center
79 Fifth Avenue
Department ZE
New York, NY 10003 **212-421-0771**
800-424-9836
FAX: 212-807-3677
www.fdncenter.org

Full profiles of all 1,000 grantmakers across the United States. *$195.00*

3742 Foundation Center's User-Friendly Guide

Foundation Center
79 Fifth Avenue
Department ZE
New York, NY 10003 **212-421-0771**
800-424-9836
FAX: 212-807-3677
www.fdncenter.org

Thomas Buckman, President

This helpful book answers the most commonly asked questions about fundraising in an upbeat, easy-to-read style. Specifically designed for novice grantseekers, this publication will lead you through the maze of unfamiliar jargon and the wide range of research guides used successfully by professional grantseekers everyday. *$9.95*

ISBN 0-87954 -42-6

3743 Foundation Directory

Foundation Center
79 Fifth Avenue
Department ZE
New York, NY 10003 **212-421-0771**
800-424-9836
FAX: 212-807-3677
www.fdncenter.org

Thomas Buckman, President

An expanded, updated version of the fundraising research classic, offers a chance to bolster your prospect files with newly gathered data on these influential funders: over 7,500 foundation entries and over 1,100 foundations covered for the very first time in a Foundation Directory. *$140.00*

ISBN 0-87954 -45-0

3744 Foundation Grants to Individuals

Foundation Center
79 Fifth Avenue
Department ZE
New York, NY 10003 **212-421-0771**
800-424-9836
FAX: 212-807-3677
www.fdncenter.org

The only publication that provides extensive coverage of foundation funding prospects for individual grantseekers. *$40.00*

Biennially

3745 From the State Capitals: Public Health

Wakeman/Walworth
300 N Washington Street
Alexandria, VA 22314 **703-768-9600**
800-876-2545
FAX: 703-768-9690
e-mail: newsletters@statecapitals.com
www.statecapitals.com

Keyes Walworth, Publisher
Christine Ryan, Circulation

Digest of state and municipal health care financing and cost containment measures, includes medical legislation, disease control, etc. *$245.00*

6 pages

3746 Guide to Federal Funding for Child Care and Early Childhood Development

Government Information Services
4301 Fairfax Drive
Suite 875
Arlington, VA 22203 **703-465-9100**
800-225-5750
FAX: 703-528-6060

James J Marshall, Publisher
Joel M Drucker, Associate Publisher

Describes more than 60 federal grant, loan and tax credit programs to assist child care and early childhood development programs. The guide describes more than $25 billion in federal aid for traditional day care, developmental programs such as Head Start and school-based early childhood education programs such as Even Start. *$169.00*

372 pages 3-Ring Binder

3747 Guide to Federal Funding for Hospitals and Health Centers

Government Information Services
4301 Fairfax Drive
Suite 875
Arlington, VA 22203 **703-465-9100**
800-225-5750
FAX: 703-528-6060

James J Marshall, Publisher
Joel M Drucker, Associate Publisher

Describes approximately 150 federal grant and loan programs for hospitals, health centers, and other agencies involved in administering health services. *$297.00*

958 pages 3-Ring Binder

3748 Guide to Federal Funding for Volunteer Programs & Community Service

Government Information Services
4301 Fairfax Drive
Suite 875
Arlington, VA 22203 **703-465-9100**
800-225-5750
FAX: 703-528-6060

James J Marshall, Publisher
Joel M Drucker, Associate Publisher

Guide describes in detail roughly 60 federal programs that provide aid to establish and operate volunteer programs. *$85.00*

3-Ring Binder

3749 International Encyclopedia of Foundations

Foundation Center
79 Fifth Avenue
Department ZE
New York, NY 10003 **212-421-0771**
800-424-9836
FAX: 212-807-3677
www.fdncenter.org

Thomas Buckman, President

Compiled volume of useful and often hard-to-find information on the history and operation of major foundations located outside the U.S. One of the very few book-length accounts of international foundations in English, the book is made up of 146 historical sketches of the most significant foundations in 31 countries. *$75.00*

ISBN 0-31325 -83-6

3750 Japanese Corporate Connection: A Guide for Fundraisers

Foundation Center
79 Fifth Avenue
Department ZE
New York, NY 10003 **212-421-0771**
800-424-9836
FAX: 212-807-3677
www.fdncenter.org

Shows how certain U.S. nonprofits have successfully approached major Japanese philanthropics. *$90.00*

3751 National Data Book of Foundations

Foundation Center
79 Fifth Avenue
Department ZE
New York, NY 10003 **212-421-0771**
800-424-9836
FAX: 212-807-3677
www.fdncenter.org

Thomas Buckman, President

Gives fast access to vital information on 32,000 U.S. foundations, the most complete listing of grantmakers ever published. It reflects the broad scope of this important foundation locator. It can help you quickly develop a list of initial funding prospects from the largest national to the smallest local foundations. *$125.00*

ISBN 0-87954 -85-0

3752 National Directory of Corporate Giving

Foundation Center
79 Fifth Avenue
Department ZE
New York, NY 10003 **212-421-0771**
800-424-9836
FAX: 212-807-3677
www.fdncenter.org

Offers over 2,000 corporate funders, current giving reviews and profiles of sponsoring companies. *$195.00*

3753 National Guide to Funding Religion

Foundation Center
79 Fifth Avenue
Department ZE
New York, NY 10003 **212-421-0771**
800-424-9836
FAX: 212-807-3677
www.fdncenter.org

Thomas Buckman, President

This book gives access to a fundraising guide designed specifically for them. This new subject directory brings together a group of 2,800 foundations and corporate direct giving programs, all of which have a history of funding churches, religious welfare and religious education programs. *$125.00*

ISBN 0-87954 -80-9

3754 National Guide to Funding for Children, Youth & Families

Foundation Center
79 Fifth Avenue
Department ZE
New York, NY 10003 **212-421-0771**
800-424-9836
FAX: 212-807-3677
www.fdncenter.org

Thomas Buckman, President

Caters specifically to development professionals for organizations serving the needs of children, youth and families. With over 2,400 listings of funding sources, both foundations and direct giving programs and over 8,000 sample grants. *$125.00*

ISBN 0-87954 -91-5

3755 National Guide to Funding for Elementary & Secondary Education

Foundation Center
79 Fifth Avenue
Department ZE
New York, NY 10003
212-421-0771
800-424-9836
FAX: 212-807-3677
www.fdncenter.org

Thomas Buckman, President

This guide gathers together, in one convenient source, a list of grantmakers committed to improving pre-college education. This book provides full profiles for over 1,400 foundations and corporate direct giving programs. *$125.00*

ISBN 0-87954 -94-9

3756 National Guide to Funding for Libraries and Information Services

Foundation Center
79 Fifth Avenue
Department ZE
New York, NY 10003
212-421-0771
800-424-9836
FAX: 212-807-3677
www.fdncenter.org

Thomas Buckman, President

This guide features a long list of grantmakers that support facilities. This directory provides essential data on over 400 foundations and corporate direct giving programs. In addition, many of these grantmaker entries include grant lists. *$75.00*

ISBN 0-87954 -95-7

3757 National Guide to Funding for Women and Girls

Foundation Center
79 Fifth Avenue
Department ZE
New York, NY 10003
212-421-0771
800-424-9836
FAX: 212-807-3677
www.fdncenter.org

Thomas Buckman, President

Fundraisers who seek support for nonprofits that provide services and advocate women and girls can now turn to this new subject directory. This book offers grantseekers the benefit of over 700 foundations and corporate direct giving program entries. *$95.00*

ISBN 0-87954 -93-0

3758 National Guide to Funding in Aging

Foundation Center
79 Fifth Avenue
Department ZE
New York, NY 10003
212-421-0771
800-424-9836
FAX: 212-807-3677
www.fdncenter.org

Thomas Buckman, President

Professional fundraisers recognize this book as the premier source of information on the agencies and foundations that support aging projects. This volume covers federal and state programs as well as foundations and other voluntary organizations. *$75.00*

ISBN 0-87954 -33-7

3759 National Guide to Funding in Arts and Culture

Foundation Center
79 Fifth Avenue
Department ZE
New York, NY 10003
212-421-0771
800-424-9836
FAX: 212-807-3677
www.fdncenter.org

Thomas Buckman, President

Designed specifically to meet the needs of development professionals in the field of arts and culture, this guide thoroughly prepares you for an informed grant search. With over 3,300 listings of foundations and corporate direct giving programs, the volume offers fundraisers in the field an excellent opportunity to increase their funding base. *$125.00*

ISBN 0-87954 -48-9

3760 National Guide to Funding in Health

Foundation Center
79 Fifth Avenue
Department ZE
New York, NY 10003
212-421-0771
800-424-9836
FAX: 212-807-3677
www.fdncenter.org

Thomas Buckman, President

Contains essential facts on more than 2,500 foundations and corporate direct giving programs, each with a history of awarding grant dollars to hospitals, universities, research centers, community-based facilities, rural health-care projects and a range of other health-related programs and projects. *$125.00*

ISBN 0-87954 -79-5

3761 National Guide to Funding in Higher Education

Foundation Center
79 Fifth Avenue
Department ZE
New York, NY 10003
212-421-0771
800-424-9836
FAX: 212-807-3677
www.fdncenter.org

Thomas Buckman, President

Designed for those seeking foundation support for higher education, this National Guide allows researchers to immediately find information on top funders in the field. This directory covers nearly 3,000 foundations, all with a history of awarding grants to colleges, universities, graduate programs and research institutes. *$125.00*

ISBN 0-87954 -90-1

3762 New York State Foundations

Foundation Center
79 Fifth Avenue
Department ZE
New York, NY 10003
212-421-0771
800-424-9836
FAX: 212-807-3677
www.fdncenter.org

Provides a complete list of every grantmaking foundation in the state. *$150.00*

3763 Report on Disability Programs

Business Publishers
8737 Colesville Road
Suite 1100
Silver Spring, MD 20910
800-274-6737
FAX: 301-587-4530
e-mail: bpinews@bpinews.com
www.bpinews.com

Leonard A Eiserer, Publisher
Bob Grupe, Editor
Melissa Reid, Marketing Manager

Follows all programs and funding sources in education, housing, job training, therapy, Social Security Supplemental Security Income, Medicare, Medicaid and more of importance to persons with disabilities. Also covers the latest on the Americans with Disabilities Act. Publishes a newsletter. *$327.00*

25x Year

3764 Source Book Profiles

Foundation Center
79 Fifth Avenue
Department ZE
New York, NY 10003
212-421-0771
800-424-9836
FAX: 212-807-3677
www.fdncenter.org

Thomas Buckman, President

Now the fundraising resource that publishes comprehensive portraits of the country's most influential foundations over a two-year cycle offers even more for your research dollars. A database publication which means that it is now more flexible and efficient than ever before, an even more essential part of your philanthropic library. *$350.00*

ISBN 0-87954 -83-3

3765 Student Guide

US Department of Education
400 Maryland Avenue SW
Washington, DC 20202
202-260-2226
800-872-5376
FAX: 202-401-0689
TTY:800-437-0833
e-mail: customerservice@inet.ed.gov
www.ed.gov/prog_info/SFA/studentguide

William J Ryan, Acting Director

Describes the major student aid programs the US Department of Education administers and gives detailed information about program procedures.

74 pages Annual

3766 Substance Abuse Funding News

CD Publications
8204 Fenton Street
Silver Spring, MD 20910
301-588-6380
800-666-6380
FAX: 301-588-6385
e-mail: cdpubs@clark.net
www.cdpublications.com

Carol Solomon, List Manager
Mike Blankenheim, Editor
Mike Gerecht, Publisher

Newsletter covers private and federal funding opportunities for alcohol, tobacco and drug abuse programs. Plus advice on grantseeking and proposal writing, tips from funding officials and reports on the latest federal and state initives to address substance abuse and related concerns.

18 pages 2x Month

Federal

3767 ADA Regulation for Title II

US Department of Justice
950 Pennsylvania Avenue NW DRS-NYAV
Washington, DC 20530
202-307-0663
800-574-0301
FAX: 202-307-1197
www.ada.gov

The Department of Justice's regulation implementing title II, subtitle A, of the ADA which prohibits descrimination on the basis of disability in the services, programs, and activities provided by state and local governments.

3768 ADA Regulation for Title III

US Department of Justice
950 Pennsylvania Avenue NW DRS-NYAV
Washington, DC 20530
202-307-0663
800-574-0301
FAX: 202-307-1197
www.ada.gov

The Department of Justice's regulation implementing title III of the ADA which prohibits discrimination on the basis of disability by businesses and non-profit service agencies.

3769 Administration on Developmental Disabilities

US Department of Health and Human Services
370 L'Enfant Promenade SW
Washington, DC 20447
202-690-6590
877-696-6775
FAX: 202-690-6904
www.acf.dhhs.gov/programs/add/

Patricia Morrissey PhD, Commissioner
Faith McCormick, Executive Assistant

Ensures that individuals with developmental disabilities and their families participate in the design of and have access to culturally competent services, supports, and other assistance and opportunities that promote indepdnence, productivity, and integration and inclusion into the community.

3770 Administration on the Aging

US Department of Health and Human Services
3330 Independence Avenue SW
Washington, DC 20201
202-401-4541
800-677-1116
FAX: 202-260-1012
e-mail: AoAInfo@aoa.gov
www.aoa.gov

Carol Fish, Commissioner

Administers the Older Americans Act of 1965 to assist states and local communities to develop programs for older persons.

3771 Clearinghouse on Disability Information: Office of Special Education & Rehab

US Department of Education
330 C Street SW
Room 3132
Washington, DC 20202
202-205-8241
FAX: 202-401-2608
www.ed.gov/OFFICE/OSERS

Carolyn Corlett, Director

Provides information to people with disabilities or anyone requesting information, by doing research and providing documents in response to inquiries. The information provided includes areas of federal funding for disability-related programs. Information provided may be useful to disabled individuals and their families, schools and universities, teacher's and/or school administrators, and organizations who have persons with disabilities as clients.

3772 Committee for Purchase from People Who Are Blind or Severely Disabled

1421 Jefferson Davis Highway
Suite 10800
Arlington, VA 22202
703-603-7740
FAX: 703-603-0655
e-mail: info@jwod.gov
www.jwod.gov

Leon A Wilson Jr, Executive Director
Annmarie Hart-Bookbinder, Manager, Communications
Robert M Hartt, Manager, Legislative Affairs

A federal agency that administers the Javits-Wagner-O'Day Program, directing federal agencies to purchase products and services from nonprofit agencies that employ people who are blind or have other severe disabilities. Provides a wide range of vocational options to individuals with severe disabilities.

3773 Enforcing the ADA: Looking Back on a Decade of Progress

US Department of Justice
950 Pennsylvania Avenue NW DRS-NYAV
Washington, DC 20530
202-307-0663
800-574-0301
FAX: 202-307-1197
www.ada.gov

A 41-page special edition of the Department of Justice's quarterly status report highlighting accomplishments and activities over the decade 1990 through 2000.

3774 Equal Opportunity Employment Commission

1801 L Street NW
Washington, DC 20036
202-663-4900
800-669-4000

This agency is responsible for drafting and implementing the regulations of Title I of the ADA.

3775 Eric Clearinghouse on Disabilities and Gifted Education

1110 N Glebe Road
Suite 300
Arlington, VA 22201
703-620-3660
FAX: 703-264-9494
www.cec.sped.org

Janice Burdick, President

Provides information on special and gifted education. Provides referrals, offers patient networking services and provides information on current research programs. Focuses its efforts on prevention, identification, assessment, intervention and enrichment both in special settings and within mainstream communities. Offers a variety of materials including brochures and Spanish language matereials.

3776 Federal Communications Commission

445 12th Street SW
Washington, DC 20554
202-418-0008
888-225-5322
FAX: 866-418-0232
e-mail: fccinfo@fcc.gov
www.fcc.gov

Jennifer Simpson, Specialist

Enforces ADA telecommunications provisions which require that companies offering telephone service to the general public must offer telephone relay services to individuals who use text telephones or similar devices. Also enforces closed captioning rules, hearing compatibility and access to equipment and services for people with disabilities.

3777 **Health Care Financing Administration**

200 Independence Avenue SW
Washington, DC 20201 **202-690-6726**
FAX: 202-690-6262

William Roper, Administrator

Through the Social Security administration, it administers the Medicare program under Title XVIII of the Social Security Act. Administers grants to the states for Medicaid under Title XIX of the Social Security Act for individuals who are medically indigent.

3778 **National Coalition of Federal Aviation Employees with Disabilities**

Federal Aviation Administration
6500 S Mac Authur Street
AMP-400
Oklahoma City, OK 73169 **405-954-7398**
FAX: 405-954-4490
TTY:405-954-4587
www.faa.gov/acr/ncfaed.htm

Becky Pritchett, Tres., Special Advisor on ADA
Alan Jones, Aeronautical Ctr Chapter, Pres.

NCFAED is working on: 1) Improvement of work conditions for employees; 2) Expansion on National Coalition to serve all FAA employees; 3) Promote equal opportunity for people with disabilities in the FAA workplace; 4) Assist the FAA in its commitment to remove physical and attudinal barriers which inhibit opportunities for people with disabilities; 5) Align with internal and external organizations to attract future generations of people with disabilities to the FAA as employees.

3779 **National Council on Disability**

1331 F Street NW
Suite 850
Washington, DC 20004 **202-272-2004**
FAX: 202-272-2022
www.ncd.gov

Mark Quigley, Communications Director

Federal agency led by 15 members appointed by the President of the United States and confirmed by the United States Senate. The overall purpose of the National Council is to promote policies, programs, practices and procedures that guarantee equal opportunity for all people with disabilities, regardless of the nature of severity of the disability; and to empower people with disabilities to achieve economic self-sufficiency, independent living and integration into all aspects of society.

3780 **National Division of the Blind and Visually Impaired**

330 C Street NW
Washington, DC 20001 **202-205-8520**

Chester Avery, Director

Develops methods, standards and procedures to assist state agencies in the rehabilitation of blind persons. Administers the Randolph-Sheppard Act, which assures priority for blind persons in the operation of vending facilities on federal property and serves as a program manager for the Helen Keller National Center for Youth who are deaf-blind.

3781 **National Institutes of Health: National Eye Institute**

10 Center Drive, MSC 1860
Building 10/10N226
Bethesda, MD 20892 **301-402-8714**
FAX: 301-496-9970
e-mail: abg@b31.9ei.nih.gov
www.nei.nih.gov

Carl Kupfer, Director

Finances intramural and extramural research on eye diseases and vision disorders. Supports training of eye researchers.

3782 **Office of Policy**

Social Security Administration
2100 M Street NW
Washington, DC 20037 **202-523-0412**
800-772-1213
TTY:800-325-0778
www.ssa.gov/policy

Administers grants to the states for social services under Title XX of the Social Security Act to welfare recipients and others likely to become them.

3783 **Office of Special Education Programs: Department of Education**

370 L'Enfant Promenade SW
Washington, DC 20447 **202-619-0364**
FAX: 202-205-9519
e-mail: gblumenthal@acs.dhhs.gov

Gary Baumantha, Director
Madeline Will, Assistant Secretary

Administers the Education of the Handicapped Act and related programs for the education of handicapped children, including grants to institutions of higher learning and fellowships to train educational personnel. Grants to states for the education of handicapped children, research and demonstration.

3784 **President's Committee on Mental Retardation Administration for Children & Families**

369 K'Enfant Promenade SW
Washington, DC 20447 **202-619-0364**
FAX: 202-205-9519
e-mail: gblumenthal@acf.dhhs.gov
www.acf.dhhs.gov/programs/pcmr

Gary Blumenthal, Executive Director
Olivia Golden, Asst. Sec. for Children/Families

Administers the Education of the Handicapped Act and related programs for the education of handicapped children, including grants to institutions of higher learning and fellowships to train educational personnel. Grants to states for the education of handicapped children, research and demonstration.

3785 **Rehabilitative Services Administration**

330 C Street
Room 3028
Washington, DC 20202 **202-205-5482**
FAX: 202-205-9874

3786 **Social Security Administration**

6401 Security Boulevard
Baltimore, MD 21235
800-772-1213
www.ssa.gov

Martha McSteen, Acting Commissioner

Administers old age, survivors, and disability insurance programs under Title II of the Social Security Act. Also administers the federal income maintenance program under Title XVI of the Social Security Act. Maintains network of local/regional offices nationwide.

3787 US Department of Education Office of Civil Rights

300 C Street NW
Room 5414
Washington, DC 20202 **202-205-5413**
800-421-3481

Prohibits discrimination on the basis of disability in programs and activities funded by the Department of Education. Investigates complaints and provides technical assistance to individuals and entities with rights and responsibilities under Section 504.

3788 US Department of Education: Office of Civil Rights

400 Maryland Avenue SW
Washington, DC 20202 **202-260-2226**
FAX: 202-401-0689

Prohibits discrimination on the basis of disability in programs and activities funded by the Department of Education. Investigates complaints and provides technical assistance to individuals and entities with rights and responsibilities under Section 504.

3789 US Department of Justice

Civil Rights Division/Disability Rights Section
950 Pennsylvania Avenue NW DRS-NYAV
Washington, DC 20530 **202-307-0663**
800-574-0301
FAX: 202-307-1197
www.ada.gov

The US Department of Justice answers questions about the American Disabilities Act (ADA) and provides free publications by mail and fax through its ADA Information Line.

3790 US Department of Labor: Office of Federal Contract Programs

200 Constitution Avenue NW
Washington, DC 20210
888-376-3227
FAX: 202-693-1304

Prohibits discrimination on the basis of disability and requires federal contractors and sub-contractors with contracts of $2,500 or more to take affirmative action to employ and advance individuals with disabilities.

3791 US Department of Transportation

400 7th Street SW
Washington, DC 20590 **202-366-2680**
FAX: 202-366-9313
www.dot.gov

Rodney Slater, Director

Enforces ADA provisions that require nondiscrimination in public and private mass transportation systems and services.

3792 US Office of Personnel Management

1900 E Street NW
Washington, DC 20415 **202-606-8160**
FAX: 202-606-1637
www.opm.gov

Constance Horner, Director

Establishes policies for employment of the handicapped within the federal service. Administers a merit system for the federal employment that includes recruiting, examining, training, and promoting people on the basis of knowledge and skills, regardless of sex, race, religion or other factors.

Alabama

3793 Alabama Department of Public Health

20 Monroe Street, Suite 1552
PO Box 303017
Montgomery, AL 36104 **334-206-5200**
FAX: 334-206-5520
www.adph.org

Claude Fox, State Health Officer
Donald Williamson, Administrator

Provides professional services for the improvement and protection of the public's health through disease prevention and the assruance of public health services to resident and transient populations of the state regardless of social circumstances or the ability to pay.

3794 Alabama Department of Rehabilitation Services

2129 E S Boulevrad
Montgomery, AL 36116 **334-281-8780**
800-441-7607
FAX: 334-281-1973
e-mail: sshiver@rehab.state.al.us
www.rehab.state.al.us

Steve Shivers, Commissioner
Jim Harris III, Assistant Commissioner

3795 Alabama Department of Senior Services

770 Washington Street
RSA Plaza, Suite 470
Montgomery, AL 36131 **334-242-5743**
877-425-2243
FAX: 334-242-5594
e-mail: ageline@adss.state.al.us
www.adss.state.al.us

Melissa Mauser Galvin PhD, Executive Director

3796 Alabama Developmental Disability Planning Council

RSA Union Building
PO Box 310410
Montgomery, AL 36130 **334-242-3973**
800-232-2158
FAX: 334-242-0797

Sheryl R Matney, Executive Director
Elizabeth Prince, Council Chairperson

Made up of adults with disabilities, parents of children with disabilities, and representatives of all service provider agencies that serve people with disabilities. The Council generates a state plan and identifies priority areas for service planning.

3797 Alabama Disabilities Advocacy Program

University of Alabama
Box 870395
Tuscaloosa, AL 35487 **205-348-4928**
800-826-1675
FAX: 205-348-3909
e-mail: adap@ban.ua.edu
www.adap.net

Reuben W Cook, Director
Ann Marshall, Outreach/Training
Ellen Gillespie, Associate Director

The federally mandated statewide protection and advocacy system serving eligible individuals with disabilities in Alabama. ADAP has five program components: Protection and Advocacy for persons with developmental disabilities (PADD), protection and advocacy for individuals with mental illness (PAIMT), Protection and Advocacy of individual rights (PAIR), Protection and Advocacy for Assistive Technology (PAAT) and Protection & Advocacy For Beneficiaries of Social Security (PABSS).

3798 **Alabama Division of Rehabilitation and Crippled Children**
2129 E S Boulevard
Montgomery, AL 36116 **334-281-8780**
800-441-7607
FAX: 334-281-1973
e-mail: sshiver@rehab.state.al.us
www.rehab.state.al.us

Lamona Lucas, Director

3799 **Alabama State Department of Human Resources**
3030 Mobile Highway
PO Box 250380
Montgomery, AL 36125 **334-293-3100**
FAX: 334-293-3453
e-mail: ogapi@dhr.state.al.us
www.dhr.state.al.us/fsd/Child_Care.asp

Tarilton Benton, Director

Partners with communities to promtoe family stability and provide for the safety and self-sufficiency of vulnerable Alabamians.

3800 **Client Assistance Program: Alabama**
2129 E S Boulevard
Montgomery, AL 36111 **334-281-8780**
FAX: 334-281-1973
www.rehab.state.al.us

Lamona Lucas, Director

3801 **Disability Determination Service: Birmingham**
PO Box 830300
Birmingham, AL 35283 **205-870-1205**
FAX: 256-773-2296

Tammy Warren, Director

3802 **Governor's Committee on Employment of Persons with Disabilities**
Division of Rehabilitation Service
PO Box 11586
Montgomery, AL 36111 **334-242-9102**
FAX: 334-613-3893

Lamona Lucas, Director

3803 **Protection & Advocacy for Persons with Disabilities: Alabama**
Box 870395
Tuscaloosa, AL 35487 **205-348-4920**
800-826-1675
FAX: 205-348-3909
e-mail: adap@ban.ua.edu
www.adap.net

Reuben W Cook, Director
Ann Marshall, Outreach/Training
Ellen Gillespie, Associate Director

3804 **Social Security: Mobile Disability Determination Services**
PO Box 2371
Mobile, AL 36652 **251-433-2820**
800-772-1213
FAX: 251-436-0599
www.ssa.gov

3805 **Workers Compensation Board Alabama**
Department of Industrial Relations
Industrial Relations Building
Montgomery, AL 35131 **205-362-9040**
FAX: 334-261-3143

Alaska

3806 **ATLA**
2217 Tudor Road
Suite 4
Anchorage, AK 99501 **907-563-2599**
FAX: 907-563-0699
e-mail: atla@atlaak.com
www.atlaak.com

Assistive Technology sales and services.

3807 **Alaska Commission on Aging**
Pouch C Mail Station 0209
Juneau, AK 99811 **907-465-3250**
FAX: 970-465-4716
TTY:970-465-2205

Connie Sipe, Director

3808 **Alaska Department of Handicapped Children**
1231 Gambell Street
Room 314
Anchorage, AK 99501 **907-269-3400**

Rita Schmidt, Chief

3809 **Alaska Division of Mental Health and Developmental Disabilities**
350 Main Street
 # 110620
Juneau, AK 99801 **907-465-3562**
FAX: 907-465-2668
www.state.ak.us

Julie Neyhart, Director
Mike Renfro, Program Director

The Division plans for and provides appropriate prevention, treatment and support for families impacted by mental disorders or developmental disabilities while maximizing self-determination. Community based services are provided by grantees. Inpatient services are provided in two division operated facilities.

3810 **Alaska Division of Vocational Rehabilitation**
801 W 10th Street
Suite A
Juneau, AK 99801 **907-465-2814**
FAX: 907-465-2856

Duane French, Director
David Quisenberry, Rehab. Services Chief

Provides comprehensive services to people with disabilities to assist in achieving an employment outcome.

3811 **Alaska Welcomes You**
PO Box 91333
Anchorage, AK 99509 **907-349-6301**
800-349-6301
FAX: 907-344-3259
e-mail: akwy@customcpu.com
www.accessiblealaska.com

Paul Sandhofer, President

Corporation that researches, inspects and assesses accommodations, restauraunts, parks, fishing, cruises, trails, trains, tours and other Alaskan activities for travelers with disabilities. Additionally, they assess trails and design map for hikers with special needs.

3812 Client Assistance Program: Alaska

ASIST
2900 Boniface Parkway
Suite 100
Anchorage, AK 99504
907-333-2211
800-478-0047
FAX: 907-333-1186
e-mail: akcap@alaska.com
www.home.gci.net/~alaskacap

Pam Stratton, Director

We provide Informatory Referral to other programs in Alaska that are funded under the rehabilitation Act of 1973 as a amended; Individual Assistance or Advocacy, if an individual with disability has applied for or received services from an agency funded under the rehabilitation act and has concerns or questions we will work with them to help resolve their concerns with the agency.

3813 Governor's Committee on Employment and Rehab. of People with Disabilities: Alaska

801 W 10th Avenue
Suite A
Juneau, AK 99801
907-465-2814
FAX: 907-465-2856
e-mail: Velja_Elstad@labor.state.ak.us
www.afscme.org/wrkplace/disab_14.htm

Velja Elstad, Staff Liaison

Carries on a continuing program to promote the employment and rehabilitation of citizens with disabilities in the State of Alaska. Advocates for a comprehensive statewide system for access to assistive technology. Obtains and maintains co-operation with public and private groups and individuals in this field.

3814 Governor's Council on Disability and Special Education

3601 C Street
Suite 740
Anchorage, AK 99524
907-269-8990
FAX: 907-269-8995

3815 Protection & Advocacy System: Alaska

Disability Law Center of Alaska
3330 Arctic Boulevard
Suite 103
Anchorage, AK 99503
800-478-1234
e-mail: akpa@dlcak.org
www.dlcak.org

Deals with rights of the disabled. Works in conjunction with agencies, law offices and family members.

3816 Protection & Advocacy for Persons with Developmental Disabilities: Alaska

Advocacy Services of Alaska
615 E 82nd Avenue
Suite 101
Anchorage, AK 99518
FAX: 907-349-1002
e-mail: rtessardore@dlcakelcak.org

Rick Tessardore, Director

3817 Workers Compensation Board Alaska

Department of Labor
PO Box 25512
Juneau, AK 99802
907-465-2790
FAX: 907-465-2797
www.labor.state.ak.us

Paul Grossi, Director

Arizona

3818 Arizona Department of Aging

1789 W Jefferson
Phoenix, AZ 85007
602-542-4446
FAX: 602-542-6575
www.de.state.az.us/aaa/aaa_links/default.asp

Henry Blanco, Program Administrator

3819 Arizona Department of Children's Rehabilitative Services

1740 W Adams Street
Room 205
Phoenix, AZ 85007
520-604-1801

W Sundin Applegate

3820 Arizona Department of Economic Security

1717 W Jefferson Street
Phoenix, AZ 85007
520-604-1801

Linda J Blessing, Director

The Department of Economic Security is a human service agency providing services in six areas: Aging and Community Services, Benefits and Medical Eligibility, Child Support Enforcement, Children and Family Services, Developmental Disabilities and Employment and Rehabilitation Services.

3821 Arizona Department of Family Health Services

1740 W Adams Street
Room 202
Phoenix, AZ 85007
520-604-1801

Rosilyn Ryals

3822 Arizona Department of Handicapped Children

1740 W Adams Street
Room 205
Phoenix, AZ 85007
520-604-1801
FAX: 602-542-2589

W Sundin Applegate, Chief

3823 Arizona Rehabilitation State Services for the Blind and Visually Impaired

4620 N 16th Street
Suite 100
Phoenix, AZ 85016
602-439-4200

Kenneth House, State Manager

Offers clients a conservation program, eye examinations, treatments, counseling, social work, psychological testing and evaluation, professional training, computer training and more for the visually impaired. The staff includes 56 full time employees.

3824 Developmental Disability Council: Arizona

1717 W Jefferson Street
Phoenix, AZ 85007
602-542-4791
FAX: 602-547-5320

Bill Hixon, Director

3825 **Governor's Council on Developmental Disabilities**

1717 W Jefferson Street
Site Code 0742
Phoenix, AZ 85007
602-542-4049
800-889-5893
FAX: 602-542-5320
e-mail: mward@mail.dc.state.us

Michael Ward, Executive Director

The purpose of the Council is to advocate for and assure that individuals with developmental disabilities and their families participate in the design of and have access to culturally competent services, supports and provides opportunities to become integrated and included in the community.

3826 **International Dyslexia Association: Arizona Branch**

PO Box 6284
Scottsdale, AZ 85261
480-941-0308
800-222-3123
e-mail: info@interdys.org
www.interdys.org

Judy Zola, President

Provides free information and referral services for diagnosis and tutoring for parents, educators, physicians, and individuals with dyslexia. The voice of our membership is heard in 48 countries. Membership includes yearly journal and quarterly newsletter. Call for conference dates.

3827 **Protection & Advocacy for Persons with with Disabilities: Arizona**

Arizona Center for Disability Law
3839 N 3rd Street
Suite 209
Phoenix, AZ 85012
602-274-6287
800-927-2260
FAX: 602-274-6779
e-mail: center@acdl.com

Jami Snyder, Information/Outreach Director

3828 **Social Security: Phoenix Disability Determination Services**

PO Box 6123
Phoenix, AZ 85005
800-772-1213
www.ssa.gov

3829 **Social Security: Tucson Disability Determination Services**

PO Box 40060
Tucson, AZ 85717
800-772-1213
www.ssa.gov

3830 **Workers Compensation Board Arizona**

Industrial Commission
800 W Washington Street
Phoenix, AZ 85007
602-542-5141

Arkansas

3831 **Arkansas Assistive Technology Projects**

Increasing Capabilities Access
2201 Brookwood Drive
Suite 117
Little Rock, AR 72202
501-666-8868
800-828-2799
FAX: 501-666-5319
e-mail: aehurst@ars.state.ar.us
www.arkansas-ican.org

Barbara Gullett, Project Director
Lou Kirkpatrick, Supervisor
Linda Morgan, Occupational Therapist

A consumer responsive statewide program promoting assistive technology devices and sources for persons of all ages with all disabilities. Referral and information services provide information about devices, where to obtain them and their cost.

3832 **Arkansas Division of Aging & Adult Services**

Department of Human Services
PO Box 1437, Slot 1412
Little Rock, AR 72203
501-682-2441
FAX: 501-682-8155
e-mail: ron.tatus@mail.state.ar.us
www.state.ar.us/dhs/aging

Herb Sanderson, Director
Suzanne Crisp, Assistant Director
Sandra Barrett, Assistant Director

The division provides services geared for adults and the elderly including supervised living, home delivered meals, adult day care, senior centers, personal care, household chores, and adult protective services.

3833 **Arkansas Division of Developmental Disabilities Services**

PO Box 1437
Little Rock, AR 72203
501-682-8654
FAX: 501-682-8380

Mike McCreight, Director

State agency to assist persons with developmental disabilities and their family in obtaining appropriate assistance and services.

3834 **Arkansas Division of Services for the Blind**

411 S Victory Street
 # 3237
Little Rock, AR 72201
501-682-8654

James Hudson, Commissioner

State program which offers services in the areas of health, counseling, social work, self help and education for the visually and multihandicapped. The staff includes 4 full time and 13 part time members including mobility specialists and rehabilitation teachers.

3835 **Baptist Health Rehabilitation Institute**

9601 Interstate 630 Ext 7
Little Rock, AR 72205
501-202-7011
FAX: 501-202-7259
www.baptist-health.com

Doug Weeks, Senior VP/Administrator

Acute rehab facility serving patients with ortho, spinal cord injury, brain injury, CVA, arthritis, cardiac and generalized weakness; JCAHO and CARF accredited; 17 outpatient therapy centers throughout central Arkansas.

3836 Children's Medical Services
PO Box 1437, Slot S-380
Little Rock, AR 72203
501-682-8224
800-482-5850
FAX: 501-682-8247

Gilbert Buchanan, Medical Director
Nancy Holder, Program Director
Iris Fehr, Nursing Director

3837 Developmental Disability Council: Arkansas
4815 W Markham Street
Little Rock, AR 72205
501-661-2262
FAX: 501-661-2399

Wilma Stewart, Director

3838 President's Committee on People with Disabilities: Arkansas
7th & Main Street
Little Rock, AR 72203

3839 Social Security: Arkansas Disability Determination Services
701 S Pulaski Street
Little Rock, AR 72201
800-772-1213
FAX: 501-682-7553
www.ssa.gov

California

3840 California Department of Aging
1600 K Street
Sacramento, CA 95814
916-445-2417

Chris Arnold, Director

3841 California Department of Handicapped Children
714 P Street
Room 323
Sacramento, CA 95814
916-657-0582

Maridee Gregory

3842 California Department of Rehabilitation
830 K Street Mall
Sacramento, CA 95814
916-654-5326
TTY:916-445-3971
e-mail: doroa.bpremo@hwl.cahwnet.gov

Brenda Premo, Director

Assists people with disabilities, particularly those with severe disabilities, in obtaining and retaining meaningful employment and living independently in their communities. The Department develops, purchases, provides and advocates for programs and services in vocational rehabilitation, habilitation and independent living with a priority on serving persons with all disabilities, especially those with the most severe disabilities.

3843 California Governor's Committee on Employment of People with Disabilities
PO Box 826880
MIC 41
Sacramento, CA 94280
916-654-8055
800-695-0350
FAX: 916-654-9821
www.disabilityemployment.org

Provides sensitivity training kits designed to help participants examine their own attitudes, fears, and biases towards people with disabilities in the workplace.

3844 California Protection & Advocacy (PAI) A Nonprofit Organization
Protection and Advocacy (PAI)
100 Howe Avenue
Suite 235 N
Sacramento, CA 95825
916-488-9955
800-776-5746
FAX: 916-488-2365
e-mail: ruth.ordas@pai-ca.org
www.pai-ca.org

Catherine Blakemore, Executive Director
Virginia Knowlton, Director of Public Policy

Advancing the human and legal rights of people with disabilities.

3845 California State Council on Developmental Disabilities
2000 O Street
Suite 100
Sacramento, CA 95814
916-322-8481
FAX: 916-443-4957
e-mail: scdd@dss.ca.gov
www.scdd.ca.gov

Judy McDonald, Executive Director

3846 Client Assistance Program: California
2000 Evergreen Street
Sacramento, CA 95815
916-263-7367
800-952-5544
FAX: 916-263-7464
e-mail: smentkow@dor.ca.gov
www.dor.ca.gov

Sheila Conlon Mentkowski, Chief

3847 Governor's Committee for Employment of the Disabled: California
PO Box 826880
Sacramento, CA 94280
916-654-9072

3848 International Dyslexia Association: Central California Branch
4594 Michigan Avenue
Fresno, CA 93703
559-251-9385
800-222-3123
FAX: 599-252-1216
e-mail: dyslexias@attbi.com
www.interdys.org

Joy Moody, President

Provides free information and referral services for diagnosis and tutoring for parents, educators, physicians, and individuals with dyslexia. The voice of our membership is heard in 48 countries. Membership includes yearly journal and quarterly newsletter. Call for conference dates. Other locations also available in California.

3849 **Long Beach Department of Health and Human Services**
2525 Grand Avenue
Long Beach, CA 90815
562-570-4000
FAX: 562-570-4049
e-mail: info@ci.long-beach.ca.us/health
www.ci.long-beach.ca.us/health

3850 **Los Angeles County Department of Health Services**
313 N Figueroa Street
Los Angeles, CA 90012
213-250-8055

e-mail: webmaster@dhs.co.la.ca.us
www.ladhs.org

3851 **Social Security: California Disability Determination Services**
2600 Wilshire Road
Suite 102
Los Angeles, CA 90060
213-736-7006
800-772-1213
FAX: 213-736-7027
www.ssa.gov

3852 **Social Security: Fresno Disability Determination Services**
1052 C Street
Fresno, CA 93706
599-440-5371
800-772-1213
FAX: 800-869-0195
www.ssa.gov

3853 **Social Security: Oakland Disability Determination Services**
1111 Jackson Street
Oakland, CA 94623
800-325-0778
800-772-1213
www.ssa.gov

3854 **Social Security: Sacramento Disability Determination Services**
8351 Fulton Boulevard
Sacramento, CA 95826
916-263-5251
800-772-1213
FAX: 916-263-5310
TTY:800-325-0778
www.ssa.gov

3855 **Social Security: San Diego Disability Determination Services**
880 Front Street
Suite 1265
San Diego, CA 92101
619-278-4542
800-772-1213
FAX: 619-278-4303
TTY:800-325-0778
e-mail: josesanbria@ssa.gov
www.ssa.gov

Colorado

3856 **Colorado Department of Aging**
1575 Sherman Street
10th Floor
Denver, CO 80203
303-866-5994
FAX: 303-620-4191

Rita Barreras, Manager

3857 **Colorado Developmental Disabilities Planning Council**
777 Grant Street
Suite 304, CO 80203
303-894-2345
FAX: 303-894-2880
e-mail: cddpc@aol.com

3858 **Colorado Division of Mental Health**
3520 W Oxford Avenue
Denver, CO 80236
303-866-7253
FAX: 303-762-4373

George Kawamura, Director

3859 **Colorado Health Care Program for Children with Special Needs**
4300 Cherry Creek Drive S
Denver, CO 80246
303-692-2370
FAX: 303-782-5576

Sue Dunn

Provides information and state aid to children with disabilities.

3860 **Eastern Colorado Services for the Disabled**
211 W Main Street
Sterling, CO 80751
970-842-2413
FAX: 970-522-7121

Charles W Hayes, Executive Director
MaryLu Walton, Administrative Assistant

Case coordination, infant stimulation, family support, residential and vocational programs.

3861 **International Dyslexia Association: Rocky Mountain Branch (CO, UT, WY)**
PO Box 3598
Boulden, CO 80307
303-721-9425
800-222-3123
e-mail: info@interdys.org
www.interdys.org

Holly Graves, VP

Provides free information and referral services for diagnosis and tutoring for parents, educators, physicians, and individuals with dyslexia. The voice of our membership is heard in 48 countries. Membership includes yearly journal and quarterly newsletter. Call for conference dates.

3862 **Legal Center for People with Disabilities & Older People**
455 Sherman Street
Suite 130
Denver, CO 80203
303-722-0300
800-288-1376
FAX: 303-722-0720
e-mail: tlcmail@thelegalcenter.org
www.thelegalcenter.org

Mary Anne Harvey, Executive Director

Uses the legal system to protect and promote the rights of people with disabilities and older people in Colorado through direct legal representation, advocacy, education and legislative analysis. The Legal Center is Colorado's Protection and Advocacy System. We are also the State Ombudsman for nursing homes and assisted living facilities. Call for a free publications and products list.

3863 **Workers Compensation Board Colorado**

Division of Labor
1515 Arapahoe
14th Floor
Denver, CO 80202

318-870-0666
888-390-7936
FAX: 303-318-8710
www.coworkforce.com/dwc/

Connecticut

3864 **Bureau of Rehabilitation Services Disability Determination Services**

10 Griffin Road N
Windsor, CT 06095

860-298-2014
800-537-2549
FAX: 860-298-9590
TTY:860-298-2018
e-mail: cttap@aol.com

John Ficarro, Project Director

Provides vocational rehabilitation, independent living and social security disability determination services to persons with disabilities.

3865 **Connecticut Board of Education and Service for the Blind**

184 Windsor Avenue
Windsor, CT 06095

860-602-4000
FAX: 860-602-4020
TTY:860-602-4002
www.besb.state.ct.us

Donna Balaski, Executive Director

Offers rehabilitative services and information for persons with legal blindness and childrenwhonare visually impaired that are residents of Connecticut.

3866 **Connecticut Commission on Aging**

25 Sigourney Street
Hartford, CT 06106

860-424-5360
FAX: 860-424-4985
e-mail: commission.aging@po.state.ct.us
www.coa.state.ct.us

Mary Ellen Klinick, Commissioner

An Advocacy organiztion which advocates on behalf of elderly persons in CT by monitoring their status, assessing the impact of current and proposed iniatives and conducting activities which promote the interest of these individuals and to report to Govenor and the Legislative.

3867 **Connecticut Department of Children and Youth Services**

505 Hudson Street
Hartford, CT 06106

860-270-8131
FAX: 860-566-7947

Linda D'Amario Rossi, Commissioner

3868 **Connecticut Developmental Disabilities Council**

460 Capitol Avenue
Hartford, CT 06106

860-418-6160
FAX: 800-653-1134
TTY:860-418-6172
www.state.ct.us/ctcdd/

3869 **Connecticut Office of Protection and Advocacy for Persons with Disabilities**

60 B Weston Street
Hartford, CT 06120

860-297-4300
800-842-7303
FAX: 860-566-8714
TTY:860-566-2102
e-mail: OPA-Information@po.state.ct.us
www.state.ct.us/opapd

Stan Kosloski, Assistant Director

Seeks to protect the rights of and to advocate for people with disabilities. The Consumer Information Section provides information, referral services and short-term advocacy assistance. The Case Services unit staff advocates and attorney's for individuals who have been discriminated against based on disability or who have been denied needed services to which they are entitled to under state or federal law. Offers training & technical assistance to individuals and groups to promote self-advocacy.

3870 **Social Security: Hartford Area Office**

309 Wawarme Avenue
Hartford, CT 06114

860-466-6105
800-772-1213
FAX: 860-566-1795
www.ssa.gov

Jan Gilbert, Professional Relations Coord.

Delaware

3871 **Delaware Assistive Technology Initiative**

Univ. of Delaware/DuPont Hospital for Children
1600 Rockland Road
200 Research & Administration Bldg.
Wilmington, DE 19803

800-870-DATI
FAX: 302-651-6793
TTY:302-651-6794
e-mail: dati@asel.udel.edu
www.asel.udel.edu/dati

Beth Mineo Mollica, Project Director

As one of the projects funded under the Assistive Technology Act of 1998, the DATI focuses on improving public awareness, public access to information, training, technical assistance, and funding for assistive technology devices and services. The project maintains three resource centers that house assistive technology devices and materials that are available for demonstration and short-term loan.

3872 **Delaware Client Assistance Program**

United Cerebral Palsy Association
254 E Camden-Wyoming Avenue
Camden, DE 19934

302-698-9336
800-640-9336
FAX: 302-698-9338
e-mail: capdir@magpage.com

Melissa Shahan, Director

Provides advocacy services for persons involved with programs covered under the Rehabilitation Act of 1973 as amended, information and referrals on ADA, Title I.

3873 **Delaware Department of Health and Social Services**

Administration Building DHSS Campus
1901 N Dupont Highway
New Castle, DE 19720

302-577-4500
800-464-HELP
FAX: 302-577-4510
e-mail: dhssinfo@state.de.us

Vincent Meconi, Secretary

3874 **Delaware Department of Public Instructing**
PO Box 1402
Dover, DE 19903
302-739-4686
800-433-5292
FAX: 302-739-3092

Dr. Pascal D Forgione Jr, Superintendent

A publicly funded state agency that gives information about local facilities and administers supplemental funds for visually handicapped students in local schools. It also maintains special teachers of sight conservation and braille programs for both children and adults.

3875 **Delaware Developmental Disability Council**
410 Federal Street
Suite 2
Dover, DE 19901
302-739-3623
FAX: 302-739-2015
e-mail: arose@state.de.us

Alexander Rose, Social Services

3876 **Delaware Division for the Visually Impaired**
1901 N DuPont Highway
New Castle, DE 19720
302-255-9800
FAX: 302-255-4441
e-mail: dhssinfo@state.de.us
www.state.de.us

Harry Hill, Director
Ken Sutton, Program Spec/Staff Dev Officer

State agency serving the visually impaired persons from birth, with or without other handicaps. Services offered include educational, computer training, employment and pre-vocational training.

3877 **Delaware Division of Child Mental Health Services**
Excelsior Building
Wilmington, DE 19801
302-652-7441
FAX: 302-633-2614

Julian Taplin, Executive Director

3878 **Delaware Industries for the Blind**
1901 N Dupont Highway
New Castle, DE 19720
302-577-4760
FAX: 302-577-4763
e-mail: awingrove@state.de.us
www.promoplace.com/dib

Alan B Wingrove, General Manager

Industry for the blind, provides jobs for blind and visually impaired via sales of products and services.

3879 **Delaware Protection & Advocacy for Persons with Disabilities**
144 E Market Street
Georgetown, DE 19947
302-856-6019
FAX: 305-856-6133

3880 **Delaware Workers Compensation Board**
Industrial Accident Board
4425 N Market Street
Wilmington, DE 19802
302-422-1392
www.delawareworks.com

3881 **Social Security: Wilmington Disability Determination**
PO Box 8862
Wilmington, DE 19899
800-772-1213
www.ssa.gov

District of Columbia

3882 **District of Columbia Department of Handicapped Children**
DC General Hospital
1900 Massachusetts Avenue SE
Building #10
Washington, DC 20003
202-675-5214
FAX: 202-675-7694

Jacqueline McMorris, Acting Chief

3883 **District of Columbia Office on Aging**
441 4th Street NW
9th Floor
Washington, DC 20001
202-638-5448
FAX: 202-724-4979

E Veronica Pace, Executive Director

Serves the District of Columbia residents 60 years of age and older. Contact the Information and Assistance Unit for more information about innovative programs and services offered by the Office.

3884 **Information, Protection & Advocacy for Persons with Disabilities**
IPACHI
4455 Connecticut Avenue NW
Suite B
Washington, DC 20008
FAX: 202-966-6313

Vivianne Hardy-Townes, Executive Director
Ronald Tyson, Information/Referral

Offers services and support for persons with disabilities in the Washington, DC area.

3885 **Information, Protection and Advocacy Center for Handicapped Individuals**
4455 Connecticut Avenue NW
Suite B100
Washington, DC 20008
202-775-6932
FAX: 202-966-6313

Vivianne Hardy-Townes, Executive Director

Serves all persons with disabilities in the DC, Maryland and Virginia areas offering them legal representation and advocacy, information and referrals and several publications.

3886 **International Dyslexia Association of DC**
5914 Reservoir Heights Avenue
Alexandria, VA 22311
703-827-9019
800-222-3123
e-mail: info@interdys.org
www.interdys.org

Ruth Tifford, VP

Provides free information and referral services for diagnosis and tutoring for parents, educators, physicians and individuals with dyslexia. The voice of our membership is heard in 48 countries. Membership includes yearly journal and quarterly newsletter. Call for conference dates.

3887 **Wage and Hour Division of the Employment Standards Administration**
US Department of Labor
200 Constitution Avenue NW
Washington, DC 20210
202-693-0519
FAX: 202-693-1406
www.dol.gov

Administers regulations governing the employment of individuals with disabilities in sheltered workshops and the disabled workers industries.

3888 **Washington Hearing and Speech Society**

1934 Calvert Street NW
Washington, DC 20009 **202-265-7335**
e-mail: support@dcsha.org

Judyth Tinsley

Offers individuals with hearing or speech impairments, in the DC area, speech reading classes, audiological services and new aids.

3889 **Well Mind Association of Greater Washington**

18606 New Hampshire
Ashton, MD 20861 **301-774-6617**
FAX: 301-946-1402

Holistic mental health information and publications, public lectures in the Washington D.C. area, and nationwide referrals.

3890 **Workers Compensation Board: District of Columbia**

1200 Upshur Street NW
Washington, DC 20011

Florida

3891 **ARC Gateway**

3916 N 10th Avenue
Pensacola, FL 32503 **850-434-2638**
FAX: 850-438-2180
e-mail: aresc@aol.com
www.arc-gateway.org

Donna Fassett, Executive Director

To secure for all people with developmental disabilities the opportunity to choose and realize their goals of where and how they learn, live, work and play. ARC Gateway is committed to increasing the opportunities for all persons with, or at risk of, development disabilities the opportunity to choose where, how and with whom they live, learn, work and play.

3892 **Advocacy Center for Persons with Disabilities**

2671 W Executive Center
Suite 100
Tallahassee, FL 32301 **850-488-9071**
800-342-0823
FAX: 850-488-8640
e-mail: info@advocacy.org
www.advocacycenter.org

Marjorie Menzel, Communications Director

3893 **Assistive Technology Educational Network of Florida**

1207 Mellonville Avenue
Sanford, FL 32771
800-328-3678
FAX: 407-688-4593

Phyllis Neal-Wilson, Administrator

Provides state-wide information, awareness and training for students, family members, teachers and other professionals in the area of assisted technology; a quarterly newsletter and a network of specialists (Local Assistive Technology Specialists) trained by ATEN to provide support at the district level.

3894 **Bureau of Education for Exceptional Children**

Turlington Building
Tallahassee, FL 32399 **850-245-0477**
FAX: 850-245-0987

Shan Goff, Bureau Chief

Provides consultative services for the establishment and operation of school programs for visually impaired students. Provides assistance for in-service teacher training through state or regional workshops or technical assistance to individual programs.

3895 **Department of Health & Rehabilitative Services**

1317 Winewood Boulevard
Tallahassee, FL 32399 **850-488-8304**

Offers counseling and referrals on rehabilitation facilities.

3896 **Division of Workers Compensation**

310 Hartman Building
2012 Capital Circle SE
Tallahassee, FL 32399 **850-488-2514**
FAX: 850-922-6779
www2.myflorida.com/les/wc/

3897 **Florida Adult Services**

1317 Winewood Boulevard
Suite 2
Tallahassee, FL 32399 **850-488-2881**
FAX: 850-922-4193

Nancy J Fulton, Director

3898 **Florida Client Assistance Program**

2671 Executive Center W
Suite 100
Tallahassee, FL 32301

3899 **Florida Department of Handicapped Children**

1317 Winewood Boulevard
Building 5
Tallahassee, FL 32399 **850-488-8304**
FAX: 850-488-3813

WW Ausbon, Director

3900 **Florida Department of Mental Health and Rehabilitative Services**

1317 Winewood Boulevard
Tallahassee, FL 32399 **850-488-8304**
FAX: 850-487-2239

Dr. Ira Rose, Director

3901 **Florida Developmental Disabilities Council**

124 Marriott Drive
Suite 203
Tallahassee, FL 32301 **850-488-4180**
850-580-7801
FAX: 850-922-6702
e-mail: fddc@netally.com
www.fddc.org

K Joseph Krieger, Director

3902 **Florida Division of Vocational Rehabilitation**

2002 Old St. Augustine Road
Building A
Tallahassee, FL 32301 **850-488-6210**
FAX: 850-921-7215
TTY:850-488-2867
e-mail: costin@vr.doe.state.fl.us

Loretta Costin, Director
Sheree Keeler, Assistant Director

State agency serving individuals with physical or mental disabilities that interfere with them keeping or maintaining employment.

3903 **International Dyslexia Association: Florida Branch (FL, Puerto Rico)**

5005 Laurel
Suite 100
Tampa, FL 33607
813-281-2859
800-222-3123
e-mail: info@interdys.org
www.interdys.org

Barbara King, President

Provides free information and referral services for diagnosis and tutoring for parents, educators, physicians, and individuals with dyslexia. The voice of our membership is heard in 48 countries. Membership includes yearly journal and quarterly newsletter. Call for conference dates.

3904 **Social Security Administration**

227 N Bronough Street
Suite 2070
Tallahassee, FL 32301
800-772-1213
FAX: 850-942-8980
www.ssa.gov

Mary Ann Phillips, Operations Supervisor
Verdine Spicer, Staff Assistant

Administers the Title II and Title XVII disability programs. To be insured for Title II benefits, applicants must have worked in covered employment for at least five of the last ten years prior to becoming disabled. To be eligible for Title XVII disability benefits, applicants must meet an income and resource test.

3905 **Social Security: Miami Disability Determination**

9495 Sunset Drive
Suite B100
Miami, FL 33173
800-772-1213
www.ssa.gov

3906 **Social Security: Orlando Disability Determination**

PO Box 144040
Orlando, FL 32814
800-772-1213
www.ssa.gov

3907 **Social Security: Tampa Disability Determination**

PO Box 15550
Tampa, FL 33684
800-772-1213
www.ssa.gov

Georgia

3908 **ADA Technical Assistance Program**

Southeast Disability and Business Technical Center
490 Tenth Street
Atlanta, GA 30318
404-385-0636
800-949-4232
FAX: 404-385-0641
e-mail: sedbtac@catea.org
www.sedbtac.org

Amy Oliveras, Administrative Assistant
Shelley Kaplan, Director
Pam Williamson, Assistant Director

One of ten regional centers funded by NIDRR, to provide information and technical assistance to assist in voluntary compliance with the Americans with Disabilities Act accessible education-based information technology.

3909 **Division of Birth Defects and Developmental Disabilities**

4740 Buford Highway NE
Mailstop F-34
Atlanta, GA 30341
770-488-7150
FAX: 770-488-7156

3910 **Georgia Advocacy Office**

100 Crescent Centre Parkway
Suite 520
Tucker, GA 30084
770-493-4998
800-537-2329
FAX: 770-414-2948
e-mail: info@thegao.org
www.thegao.org

Protection and advocacy services for Georgians with disabilities.

3911 **Georgia Client Assistance Program**

Division of Rehabilitation Services
2 Peachtree Street
Room 23-307
Atlanta, GA 30303
404-657-2410
800-822-9727

Helps eligible persons with complaints, appeals and understanding available benefits under the 1992 Rehabilitation Act Amendments and Title I of the Americans with Disabilities Act. CAP investigates complaints, mediates conflict, represents complainants in appeals, provides legal services if warranted, advocates for due process, identifies and recommends solutions to system problems, advises of benefits available under the 1992 Rehab Act Amendments and Americans with Disabilities Act.

3912 **Georgia Department of Aging**

878 Peachtree Street NE
Apartment 318
Atlanta, GA 30309
404-657-2410
FAX: 404-730-7950

Fred McGinnis, Director

3913 **Georgia Department of Handicapped Children**

2600 Skyland Drive NE
Atlanta, GA 30319
404-679-4700

Linnette Jackson-Hunt, Manager

3914 **Georgia Division of Mental Health, Developmental Disabilities & Addictive Diseases**

2 Peachtree Street
Suite 22-224
Atlanta, GA 30303
404-657-2252
FAX: 404-657-1137

Kari H Schwarxkopf PhD, Director

3915 **Georgia State Board of Workers' Compensation**

270 Peachtree Street NW
Atlanta, GA 30303
404-656-3875
800-533-0682
FAX: 404-657-1767
www.ganet.org/sbwc

Stan Carter, Executive Director

3916 Governor's Council on Developmental Disabilities
Two Peachtree Street
Suite 8-210
Atlanta, GA 30303 **404-657-2126**
888-275-4233
FAX: 404-657-2132
TTY:404-657-3000
e-mail: eejacobson@dhr.state.ga.us
www.gcdd.org

Eric E Jacobson, Executive Director
Beth Spinning, Program Director
Yau Seidu, Public Information Officer

Advocacy and support organization focusd on improving the lives of people with disabilities and their families.

3917 International Dyslexia Association: Georgia Branch
1951 Greystone Road
Atlanta, GA 30318 **404-256-1232**
800-222-3123
e-mail: info@interdys.org
www.interdys.org

Laurie Spegener, President

Provides free information and referral services for diagnosis and tutoring for parents, educators, physicians, and individuals with dyslexia. The voice of our membership is heard in 48 countries. Membership includes yearly journal and quarterly newsletter. Call for conference dates.

3918 Social Security: Atlanta Disability Determination
878 Peachtree Street NE
Apartment 706
Atlanta, GA 30309
800-772-1213
www.ssa.gov

3919 Social Security: Decatur Disability Determination
PO Box 1187
Decatur, GA 30031
800-772-1213
www.ssa.gov

Hawaii

3920 Diabetes Network of East Hawaii
1221 Kilauea Avenue
Suite 70
Hilo, HI 96720 **808-933-9718**

Mary Glass, Executive Director

3921 Disability and Communication Access Board
919 Ala Moana Boulevard
Suite 101
Honolulu, HI 96814 **808-586-8121**
FAX: 808-586-8129
e-mail: accesshi@aloha.net
www.hawaii.gov/health/dcab

Francine Wai, Executive Director
Charlotte Townsend, Assistant Director
Debbra Jackson, Program Specialist

Clearinghouse of information related to disability issues, lead agency in the community for dissemination of ADA information, systems advocacy provided through the introduction and lobbying of bills at the State Legislation, review of blueprints for State and county renovation and new construction to make recommendations for physical accessibility; establishment of guidelines for communication access, including sign language interpreters and conducts state test to credential interpreters.

3922 Hawaii Assistive Technology Training and Services
414 Kuwili Street
 # 104
Honolulu, HI 96822 **800-532-7110**
800-645-3007
FAX: 808-532-7120
e-mail: bflapixi.com
www.icdri.org/legal/hawaii.htm

Barbara Fischlowitz-Leong, Executive Director

Provides information and referral to anyone interested in assistive technology devices and services. Operates eight equipment loan banks. Provides training to consumer and professional groups including self-advocacy skills for consumers and family members. Works to ensure that schools, vocational rehabilitation agencies and health insurers provide assessments, funding and training in the use of assistive technology devices and services for their clients. Low-interest loan programs available.

3923 Hawaii Department for Handicapped Children
741A Sunset Avenue
Honolulu, HI 96816 **808-733-9030**

Alan Taniguchi, Chief

3924 Hawaii Department of Health, Adult Mental Health Division
PO Box 3378
Honolulu, HI 96801 **808-586-4688**
FAX: 808-586-4745

Thomas W Hester MD, Chief

3925 Hawaii Department of Human Services
Services for the Blind Branch
1901 Bachelot Street
Honolulu, HI 96817 **808-586-5282**

Provides services to blind and visually impaired persons in Adjustment to Blindness, Vocational Rehabilitation, Low Vision evaluation and assistance. Work Evaluation, Work Activities Center, Vending training and operates the Ho'opono Workshop, a sheltered workshop program for the blind and visually impaired persons.

3926 Hawaii Disability Compensation Division Dept. Labor and Ind. Relations
830 Punchbowl Street
Room 211
Honolulu, HI 96813 **808-586-9151**
FAX: 808-586-9219

Gary Hamada, Administrator
Clyde Imada, Workers Comp Chief

Administers Hawaii's Workers' Compensation Program.

3927 Hawaii Disability Rights Center
900 Fort Street Mall
Suite 1040
Honolulu, HI 96813 **808-949-2922**
800-882-1052
FAX: 808-949-2928
e-mail: pahi@pixi.com
www.pixi.com/~pahi

Gary L Smith, President

3928 **Hawaii Executive Office on Aging**
250 S Hotel Street
Suite 406
Honolulu, HI 96813
808-586-0100
800-468-4644
FAX: 808-586-0185
e-mail: pasasaki@health.state.hi.us
www2.state.hi.us/eoa/

Pat Sasaki, Executive Director

State unit on aging responsible for policy formulation, program development, planning, information dissemination, advocacy and other activities, for persons age 60 and over.

3929 **Hawaii State Council on Developmental Disabilities**
919 Ala Moana Boulevard
Honolulu, HI 96814
808-586-8100
FAX: 808-586-7543
e-mail: hiddc@pixi.com

Waynette K Y Cabral, Administrator

The mission of the Council is to support people with developmental disabilities to control their own destiny and determine the quality of life they desire.

3930 **International Dyslexia Association: Hawaii Branch**
PO Box 51510
Honolulu, HI 96839
808-538-7007
800-222-3123
FAX: 808-538-7007
e-mail: info@interdys.org
www.interdys.org

Sandra Keawe, Co-President
Ron Yashimoto, Co-President

Provides free information and referral services for diagnosis and tutoring for parents, educators, physicians, and individuals with dyslexia. The voice of our membership is heard in 48 countries. Membership includes yearly journal and quarterly newsletter. Call for conference dates.

3931 **Social Security: Honolulu Disability Determination**
PO Box 339
Honolulu, HI 96809
808-586-5355
800-772-1213
e-mail: hivrsbd@kestrok.com
www.ssa.gov

Neil Shim, Administrator

3932 **State Planning Council on Developmental Disabilities**
919 Ala Moana Boulevard
Suite 113
Honolulu, HI 96814
808-586-8121
FAX: 808-586-8129
e-mail: tiza100w@wonder.cm.cdc.gov

Diana Tizard, Executive Director

Consists of 25 Hawaii residents appointed by the Governor. The council addresses the needs of the people with developmental disabilities: specifically, develops a state plan that sets the priorities for persons with developmental disabilities.

Idaho

3933 **Idaho Commission on Aging**
3380 Americana Terrace
Suite 120
Boise, ID 83706
208-334-3833
877-471-2777
FAX: 208-334-3033
e-mail: senglesb@icoa.state.id.us
www.idahoaging.com

Richard Juenglinge, Director
Gioia M Frahm, Planner/Statistician
Cathy Hart, State Ombudsman

3934 **Idaho Council on Developmental Disabilities**
802 W Bannock Street
#308
Boise, ID 83702
800-544-2433
FAX: 208-334-3417
e-mail: msword@icdd.state.id.us
www.state.id.us/icdd

Marilyn B Sword, Executive Director

3935 **Idaho Department of Handicapped Children**
Statehouse
Boise, ID 83720
208-334-4200

Thomas Bruck, Chief

3936 **Idaho Disability Determinations Service**
1505 McKinney Street
PO Box 21
Boise, ID 83707
208-327-7333
800-626-2681
FAX: 208-373-7287
www.accessidaho.org/dds.html

Barbara Bauer, Director

Under contract with the Social Security Administration, makes determinations of medical eligibility for disability benefits.

3937 **Idaho Industrial Commission**
317 Main Street
PO Box 83720
Boise, ID 83720
208-334-6000
800-950-2110
FAX: 208-334-2321
www2.state.id.us/iic

Free rehabilitation services to workers' who have suffered on the job injuries in Idaho. Field offices throughout the state.

3938 **Idaho Mental Health Center**
1720 Westgate Drive
Boise, ID 83704
208-334-0800
FAX: 208-334-0828

Dr. Gary Payne, Director

Illinois

3939 **Attorney General's Office: Disability Rights Bureau & Health Care Bureau**

100 W Randolph Street
Chicago, IL 60601 **312-814-5684**
FAX: 312-814-3212
www.ag.state.il.us/disabilities/

Lisa Danna, Chief, Disability Rights Bureau
Raymond Throlkeld, Chief, Health Care Bureau

Information on Illinois' Comprehensive Health Insurance Plan and architectural accessibility. Enforcement of Illinois' access law and standards and other disability rights laws. Information on initiatives such as: Opening the Courthouse Doors to People with Disabilities; the abuse, neglect or financial exploitation of people with disabilities and voter accessibility. Other information and referrals.

3940 **Client Assistance Program (CAP)**

Illinois State Board of Education
100 N 1st Street
1st Floor
Springfield, IL 62777 **217-782-4321**
800-641-3929
FAX: 217-524-1790
TTY:217-782-1900
www.isbe.state.il.us/

3941 **Equip for Equality**

11 E Adams Street
Suite 1200
Chicago, IL 60603 **312-341-0022**
800-537-2632
FAX: 312-341-0295
e-mail: contactus@equipforequality.org

Joanne Schwartz

Their mission is to advance the human and civil rights of individuals with physical and mental disabilities or who have a disability as defined by the American with Disabilities Act.

3942 **Illinois Assistive Technology Project**

1 W Old State Capitol Plaza
Springfield, IL 62701 **217-522-7985**
800-852-5110
FAX: 217-522-8067
TTY:217-522-9966
www.iltech.org

Sherry Edwards, Information/Assistance
Sue Castles, Info./Assistance Funding Advoc.

Directed by and for people with disabilities and their family members. As a federally mandated program, IATP strives to break down barriers and change policies that make getting and using technology difficult. IATP offers solutions to help people find what is available in products and services that will best meet their needs, where to find it, and how to get it.

3943 **Illinois Council on Developmental Disability**

State of Illinois Center
100 W Randolph Street
Chicago, IL 60601 **312-814-2700**
FAX: 312-814-7441

Rene Leininger, Director

3944 **Illinois Department of Mental Health and Developmental Disabilities**

401 Stratton Office
Springfield, IL 62765 **217-782-7820**
FAX: 217-524-0835

Jess McDonald, Director

3945 **Illinois Department of Rehabilitation**

622 E Washington Street
Springfield, IL 62701 **217-782-7820**
FAX: 217-557-0142

Susan Suter, Director

3946 **Illinois Department on Aging**

421 E Capitol Avenue
 # 100
Springfield, IL 62701 **217-785-3356**
800-252-8966
FAX: 217-785-4477
e-mail: ilsenior@age084r1.state.il.us
www.state.il.us/aging

Charles D Johnson, Director
Nikki Smith, Communications Director

3947 **International Dyslexia Association: Illinois Branch (IL, E/MO)**

751 Roosevelt Road
Building 7, Suite 301
Glen Ellyn, IL 60137 **630-469-6900**
800-222-3123
FAX: 808-538-7007
e-mail: slonghall@aol.com
www.interdys.org

Susan Hall, President
Maria Leibold, Executive Director

Provides free information and referral services for diagnosis and tutoring for parents, educators, physicians, and individuals with dyslexia. The voice of our membership is heard in 48 countries. Membership includes yearly journal and quarterly newsletter. Call for conference dates.

3948 **Social Security: Springfield Disability Determination**

PO Box 19429
Springfield, IL 62794
800-772-1213
www.ssa.gov

3949 **Workers Compensation Board Illinois**

100 W Randolph Street
Suite 8-200
Chicago, IL 60601
FAX: 312-814-6523

John Hallock Jr, Director

Indiana

3950 **Indiana Client Assistance Program**

850 N Meridian Street
Suite 2C
Indianapolis, IN 46204 **317-888-8366**
800-622-4845

3951 **Indiana Developmental Disability Council**

143 W Market Street
Suite 404
Indianapolis, IN 46204 **317-231-7100**

3952 Indiana Protection & Advocacy Services

4701 N Keystone Avenue
222
Indianapolis, IN 46205
317-722-5555
800-622-4845
FAX: 317-722-5564
www.state.in.us/ipas

Thomas Gallagher, Executive Director
Milo Gray, Client & Legal Services Director
Gary Richter, Support Services Director

An independent state agency established to protect and promote the rights of individuals with disabilities through empowerment and advocacy.

3953 Indiana State Commission for the Handicapped

PO Box 1964
Indianapolis, IN 46206
317-233-1292

3954 International Dyslexia Association: Indiana Branch

1100 W 42nd Street
Suite 385
Indianapolis, IN 46208
317-926-1450
800-222-3123
FAX: 317-573-0146
e-mail: info@interdys.org
www.interdys.org

Wayne L Lamade, President

Provides free information and referral services for diagnosis and tutoring for parents, educators, physicians, and individuals with dyslexia. The voice of our membership is heard in 48 countries. Membership includes yearly journal and quarterly newsletter. Call for conference dates.

Iowa

3955 International Dyslexia Association: Iowa Branch

1155 330th Street
Box 50A
Gowrie, IA 50543
515-352-3548
800-222-3123
e-mail: info@interdys.org
www.interdys.org

Marlin Geisler, President

Provides free information and referral services for diagnosis and tutoring for parents, educators, physicians, and individuals with dyslexia. The voice of our membership is heard in 48 countries. Membership includes yearly journal and quarterly newsletter. Call for conference dates.

3956 Iowa Child Health Specialty Clinics

100 Hawkins Drive
Room 247
Iowa City, IA 52242
319-356-1469
FAX: 319-356-3715

Jeffrey Lobas, Director
Lucia Dhooge, Associate Director
Brian Wilkes, Health/Disease Manager

Child Health Specialty Clinics has a mission to improve the health, development, and well-being of Iowa's children and youth with special health care needs in partnership with families, service providers, and communities.

3957 Iowa Commission of Persons with Disabilities

Locust Street
Des Moines, IA 50309
515-242-6172
FAX: 515-242-6119
e-mail: dhr.disabilities@dhr.state.ia.us
www.state.ia.us/government

3958 Iowa Compass

Center for Disabilities and Development
100 Hawkins Drive
Iowa City, IA 52242
800-779-2001
FAX: 319-356-1343
TTY:877-686-0032
e-mail: iowacompass@uiowa.edu
www.medicine.uiowa.edu/uhs/infomall.cfm

Jane Gay, Project Director

A statewide program provides free information and referral about disability related services and resources: advocacy, assistive technology, community services, early intervention, education, financial support, healthcare, legal aid, residential services and transportation.

BiMonthly

3959 Iowa Department for the Blind

524 4th Street
Des Moines, IA 50309
515-281-1333
800-362-2587
FAX: 515-281-1263
TTY:515-281-1355
e-mail: harrisallen.craig@blind.state.ia.us
www.blind.state.ia.us

Allen C Harris, Director

Offers services to blind, and visually impaired persons. Provides counseling, educational, recreational, library rehabilitation, computer training and professional training services.

3960 Iowa Department of Elder Affairs

200 10th Streete
Des Moines, IA 50319
515-242-3333
800-532-3213
FAX: 515-242-3300
www.state.ia.us/elderaffairs

Mark Haverland, Director
Sherry James, Administrative Assistant

3961 Iowa Department of Human Services

1305 E Walnut Street
Hoover State Office Building
Des Moines, IA 50319
515-281-5521
800-972-2017
FAX: 515-242-6036
e-mail: mnelson1@dhs.state.ia.us
www.dhs.state.ia.us

Mary Nelson, Administrator

3962 Iowa Developmental Disability Council

Hoover
1st Floor
Des Moines, IA 50319
515-242-6892

3963 Iowa Protection & Advocacy for the Disabled

3015 Merle Hay Road
Suite 6
Des Moines, IA 50310
515-278-2502
FAX: 515-278-0539
e-mail: hn5317@handsnet.org

Marvin Roth, Director

3964 Social Security: Des Moines Disability Determination
510 E 12th Street
Des Moines, IA 50309
800-532-1486
FAX: 515-281-3507
TTY:515-281-1333
e-mail: dmrb@edu.gte.net
www.ssa.gov

Marge Knudsen, Administrator

3965 Workers Compensation Board Iowa
1000 E Grand Avenue
Des Moines, IA 50319
515-281-6647

Kansas

3966 Beach Center on Families and Disability
University of Kansas
3111 Haworth Hall
Lawrence, KS 66044
785-864-7600
FAX: 785-864-7605
e-mail: beach@dole.lsi.ukans.edu
www.beachcenter.org

A federally funded center that conducts research and training in the factors that contribute to the successful functioning of families with members who have disabilities.

3967 International Dyslexia Association: Kansas/West Missouri Branch
2812 SW Osborn Road
Topeka, KS 66614
785-228-1717
FAX: 785-271-6453
e-mail: cwajr@compuserve.com
www.interdys.org

Wilson Anderson, President
Michele Bay PhD, VP

Provides free information and referral services for diagnosis and tutoring for parents, educators, physicians, and individuals with dyslexia. The voice of our membership is heard in 48 countries. Membership includes yearly journal and quarterly newsletter. Call for conference dates.

3968 Kansas Advocacy and Protective Services
3745 SW Wanamaker
Topeka, KS 66610
785-776-1541
877-776-1541
FAX: 785-776-5783
e-mail: michelle@ksadv.org
www.ksadv.org

James Germer, Executive Director
Tim Voth, Attorney
Michelle Rola, Director Operations

Protection and advocacy for persons with disabilities.

3969 Kansas Client Assistance Program
300 SW Oakley Avenue
Topeka, KS 66606
785-296-4454

3970 Kansas Commission on Disability Concerns
1430 SW Topeka Boulevard
Topeka, KS 66612
785-296-1722
800-295-5232
FAX: 785-296-0466
e-mail: mkgabeha@hr.state.ks.us
www.hr.state.ks.us/dc

Martha Gabehart, Executive Director
Randy Fisher, Employment/Training Liaison
Kerrie Bacon, Legislative Liasion

KCDC believes that all people with disabilities are entitled to be equal citizens and partners in Kansas society. The purpose is to involve all segments of the Kansas Community through legislative advocacy, education and resource networking to ensure full and equal citizenship for all Kansans with disabilities.

3971 Kansas Department on Aging
New England Building
503 S Kansas
Topeka, KS 66603
785-296-4986
800-432-3535
FAX: 785-296-0256
www.agingKansas.org

Wilda Davison, Customer Relations Director
Doug Farmer, Public Information Officer

Services and information for Kansas seniors.

3972 Kansas Developmental Disability Council
Docking State Office
Building # 141
Topeka, KS 66612

Kentucky

3973 Kentucky Council on Developmental Disability
100 Fair Oakes Lane
Suite 4 EF
Frankfort, KY 40621
502-564-7841
877-367-5332
FAX: 502-564-9826
e-mail: pat.seybold@mail.state.ky.us
www.kddc.org

Patricia Seybold, Executive Director

Implementation of Developmental Disabilities Planning Council responsible under P.L. 101-496.

3974 Kentucky Department for Mental Health: Mental Retardation Services
100 Fair Oaks Lane
Suite 4E-B
Frankfort, KY 40621
502-564-4527
FAX: 502-564-5478
dmhmrs.chr.state.ky.us

Margaret Pennington, Commissioner

The Department for Mental Health and Mental Retardation Services contracts with fourteen regional community mental health and mental broads to provide an array of community based mental health services; operates three psychiatric hospitals and contracts with two additional hospitals; operates or contracts for 10 ICFs/MR; also operates two nursing facilities.

3975 Kentucky Department for the Blind
209 St Clair Street
PO Box 757
Frankfort, KY 40601
502-695-6350
800-321-6661
TTY:502-564-2929
e-mail: dbohannon@state.ky.us.dfblind
www.state.ky.us/agencies/wforce

Denise Placido, Commissioner (Acting)

Provides career services and assistance to adults with severe visual handicaps who want to become productive in the home or work force. Also provides the Client Assistance Program established to provide advice, assistance and information available from rehabilitation programs to persons with handicaps.

3976 Kentucky Office of Aging Services
Cabinet for Health Services
275 E Main Street
 # 5W-A
Frankfort, KY 40621
502-564-6663
FAX: 502-564-4595
e-mail: sarah.watson@mail.state.ky.us

Sarah Watson, Human Services Manager

The Kentucky Office of Aging Services is the state agency directly responsible for programs and services for people with disabilities. Efforts are made to fully integrate the service response info and klutheric model that considers broad farmiliar implications.

3977 Kentucky Protection & Advocacy Division
100 Fair Oaks Lane
3rd Floor
Frankfort, KY 40601
502-564-2967
800-372-2988
FAX: 502-564-0848
e-mail: info@mail.pa.state.ky.us
www.kypa.net

Protecting the rights of persons with disabilities in Kentucky with a disability-related rights violation, providing information and referral, training and technical assistance.

3978 Social Security: Frankfort Disability Determination
330 W Broadway
2nd Floor
Frankfort, KY 40601
502-875-2232
800-772-1213
TTY:502-226-4519
www.ssa.gov

3979 Social Security: Louisville Disability Determination
601 W Broadway
Room 101
Louisville, KY 40202
502-582-6690
800-772-1213
www.ssa.gov

Louisiana

3980 Louisiana Assistive Technology Access Network
PO Box 3455
Baton Rouge, LA 70821
225-342-6804
800-922-3452
FAX: 225-342-8823

Jill Revers, Project Director

An information and training resource on Assistive Technology for the State of Louisiana. LATAN operates three regional centers to provide better access for consumers.

3981 Louisiana Center for Dyslexia and Related Learning Disorders
Nicholls State University
PO Box 2050
Thibodaux, LA 70310
985-448-4214
FAX: 985-448-4423
e-mail: dc-csr@nicholls.edu
www.nicholls.edu/dyslexia

Carol Ronka, Director

Provides free information and referral services for diagnosis and tutoring for parents, educators, physicians and individuals with dyslexia. The voice of our membership is heard in 48 countries. Membership includes yearly journal and quarterly newsletter. Call for conference dates.

3982 Louisiana Client Assistance Program
225 Baronne Street
Suite 2112
New Orleans, LA 70112
504-522-2387
800-960-7705
FAX: 504-522-5507
e-mail: advocacycenter@advocacyla.org
www.advocacyla.org

Diane Mirvis, CAP Director

Assistance to persons seeking, receiving or who have been denied rehabilitation services from Louisiana Rehabilitaton Services (LRS) or other projects, programs or facilities funded under the Rehabilitation Act (such as Vocational Rehabilitation, Independent Living or Supported Living). Must be a Louisiana resident and have a physical or mental disability.

3983 Louisiana Department of Aging
Office of Elderly Affairs
4550 N Boulevard
2nd Floor
Baton Rouge, LA 70806
225-927-4583
FAX: 225-342-7100

Richard Collins, Director

3984 Louisiana Developmental Disability Council
PO Box 3455
Baton Rouge, LA 70821
225-342-6804
800-922-DIAL
FAX: 225-342-1970

Clarice Eichelberger, Executive Officer

3985 Louisiana Division of Mental Health
PO Box 4049
Baton Rouge, LA 70821
225-342-2540
FAX: 504-342-5066

Jerry Vincent, Director

3986 Louisiana Learning Resources System
2525 Wyandotte Street
Baton Rouge, LA 70805
225-355-6197
FAX: 225-357-3508

Dr. Charlene Bishop, Director

Provides consultation on educational services for local schools, offers psychological testing and evaluation, maintains resource rooms in district schools and more for the blind and handicapped throughout the state.

3987 Louisiana Protection & Advocacy for Persons with Developmental Disabilities

225 Baronne Street
Suite 2112
New Orleans, LA 70112
504-566-1600
800-960-7705
FAX: 504-522-5507
e-mail: adce@advocacyla.org

Lois Simpson, Executive Director

Legal and advocacy services and training to persons whose legal issue is directly related to their disablity and has been designated an AC priority issue. Provides legal representation, counseling, information and referral, outreach, technical assistance, special subject speakers, and staff/professional training.

3988 Protection & Advocacy of Individual Rights

Advocacy Center
225 Baronne Street
Suite 2112
New Orleans, LA 70112
504-522-2337
800-960-7705
FAX: 504-522-5507
e-mail: adce@advocacyla.org

Lois Simpson, Executive Director

Legal services and training to people whose legal issue is directly related to their disability and has been designated an AC priority issue. Provides legal representation, counseling, information and referral, outreach, technical assistance, special subject speakers, and staff/professional training.

3989 Social Security: Baton Rouge Disability Determination

PO Box 94065
Baton Rouge, LA 70804
800-772-1213
FAX: 225-342-4252
www.ssa.gov

3990 Workers Compensation Board Louisiana

PO Box 94040
Baton Rouge, LA 70804
225-342-7555
FAX: 504-342-655

Maine

3991 Maine Assistive Technology Projects

University of Maine at Augusta
University Heights
Augusta, ME 04330
207-621-3000
FAX: 207-772-1302

Kathleen Powers, Project Director

A statewide program promoting assistive technology devices and services for persons of all ages with all disabilities.

3992 Maine Bureau of Elder and Adult Services

11 State House Station
Augusta, ME 04333
207-287-2826
FAX: 207-624-5361
www.state.me.us/dhs/beas

Christine Gianopoulos, Director

3993 Maine Department of Mental Health, Mental Retardation & Substance Abuse Services

State House Station
 # 40
Augusta, ME 04333
207-287-4223
FAX: 207-287-4268
e-mail: lynn.f.duby@state.me.us.web
www.state.me.us/dmhmrsa

Lynn F Duby, Commissioner

Provision of services to people with Mental Illness, Mental Retardation, Substance Abuse issues, Children with Special needs and people with developmental disabilities.

3994 Maine Developmental Disability Council

45 Memorial Circle
Suite 3
Augusta, ME 04330
207-622-6345
FAX: 207-622-6346
www.mdf.org

3995 Maine Division for the Blind and Visually Impaired

2 Anthony Avenue
Augusta, ME 04333
207-624-5120
800-760-1573
FAX: 207-624-5133
TTY:800-698-4440
e-mail: harold.j.lewis@state.me.us
www.state.me.us/rehab

Harold Lewis, Director

Works to bring about full access to employment, independence and community integration for people with disabilities in Maine.

3996 Maine Workers' Compensation Board

27 State House Station
AMHI Complex-Deering Building
Augusta, ME 04333
207-287-3751
888-801-9087
FAX: 207-287-7198
www.state.me.us/wcb

3997 Social Security: Maine Disability Determination

40 Western Avenue
Room G20 Federal Building
Augusta, ME 04330
207-622-1451
800-772-1213
TTY:207-623-4190
www.ssa.gov

Maryland

3998 Health Resources & Services Administration : State Bureau of Health

5600 Fishers Lane
Rockville, MD 20857
301-443-2216
FAX: 301-443-2111

Thomas Hatch, Director

Through appropriated funds, supports education programs, credentialing analysis, and development of human resources needed to staff the U.S. health care system.

3999 International Dyslexia Association: Maryland Branch

8600 La Salle Road
Suite 382
Baltimore, MD 21286
410-296-0232
800-222-3123
FAX: 410-321-5069
e-mail: info@interdys.org
www.interdys.org

Jean-Fryer Schedler, President

Nonprofit organization providing free information and referral services for diagnosis and tutoring for parents, educators, physicians, and individuals with dyslexia. The voice of our membership is heard in 48 countries. Membership includes yearly journal and quarterly newsletter. Call for conference dates.

4000 Maryland Client Assistance Program Division of Rehabilitation Services

2301 Argonne Drive
Baltimore, MD 21218
410-554-9385
800-638-6243
FAX: 410-554-9362
TTY:800-735-2258
e-mail: dors@msde.state.md.us

Beth Lash, Program Director

Helps individuals with disabilities understand the rehabilitation process and receives appropriate and quality services from the Division of Rehabilitation Services and other programs and facilities providing services under the Rehabilitation Act of 1973.

4001 Maryland Department of Aging

State Office Building
301 W Preston Street
Suite 1007
Baltimore, MD 21201
410-767-1100
800-243-3425
FAX: 410-333-7943
e-mail: drb@mail.ooa.state.md.us
www.mdoa.state.md.us/

Dakota Burgess, Sr Information Program Manager

4002 Maryland Department of Handicapped Children

201 W Preston Street
Unit 50
Baltimore, MD 21201
410-396-4476

Judson Force, Director

Children's Medical Services is a joint federal/state/local program which assists in obtaining specialized medical, surgical and related habilitative/rehabilitative evaluation and treatment services for children with special health care needs and their families. To be eligible for the program's services, an individual must be a resident of Maryland, younger than 22 years, have or be suspected of having an eligible medical condition and meet both medical and financial criteria.

4003 Maryland Developmental Disabilities Council

300 W Lexington Street
Box 10
Baltimore, MD 21201
410-333-3688
800-305-6441
FAX: 410-333-3686
e-mail: info@md-counicl.org
www.md-council.org

4004 Maryland Division of Mental Health

2301 Argonne Drive
Baltimore, MD 21218
410-243-7495
FAX: 410-333-7482

4005 Maryland's Protection & Advocacy System for Persons with Disabilities

Maryland Disability Law Center
1800 N Charles Street
Suite 400
Baltimore, MD 21201
410-727-6352
800-233-7201
FAX: 410-727-6389
TTY:410-727-6387
e-mail: MDLCBalto.org

Philip Fornaci, Executive Director

Legal assistance provided to Maryland residents with any mental and or physical disability and to their families for disability related problems. Due to limited resources, not all cases are accepted, no criminal, domestic or employment cases.

4006 Social Security: Baltimore Disability Determination

711 W 40th Streete
Room 212
Baltimore, MD 21211
800-772-1213
TTY:800-325-0778
www.ssa.gov

4007 Workers Compensation Board Maryland

10 E Baltimore Street
Baltimore, MD 21202
410-864-5100
800-492-0479
FAX: 410-864-5101
e-mail: wcc@charm.net
www.whitelung.org

Sheldon Press, Vice Chairman

Massachusetts

4008 Center for Public Representation PAIMI Program for MA

22 Green Street
Northampton, MA 01060
413-587-6265
FAX: 413-586-5711
e-mail: info@cpr-ma.org
www.centerforpublicrep.org

Robert Fleischner, PAIMI Director

4009 International Dyslexia Association of New England (CT, ME, NH, RI, VT)

PO Box 662
Lincon, MA 01773
800-222-3123
e-mail: info@interdys.org
www.interdys.org

Mary Ann Bonneau, President
Isabel Wesley, Regional Representative

Provides free information and referral services for diagnosis and tutoring for parents, educators, physicians, and individuals with dyslexia. The voice of our membership is heard in 48 countries. Membership includes yearly journal and quarterly newsletter. Call for conference dates.

4010 Massachusetts Assistive Technology Partnership

MATP Center
1295 Boylston Street
Suite 310
Boston, MA 02215
800-848-8867
FAX: 617-345-6345

Judy Brewer, Project Director

A statewide program promoting assistive technology devices and services for persons with all disabilities.

4011 Massachusetts Client Assistance Program

Massachusetts Office on Disability
1 Ashburton Place
Room 1305
Boston, MA 02108
617-727-7440
800-322-2020
FAX: 617-727-0965
e-mail: barbara.lybarger@state.ma.us
www.state.ma.us/mod/MSCAPBRO.html

Barbara Lybarger, Assistant Director

Provides advocacy and information services.

4012 Massachusetts Department of Mental Health

25 Staniford Street
Boston, MA 02114
617-367-0944
FAX: 617-727-4350

Eileen Elias, Commissioner

4013 Massachusetts Developmental Disabilities Council

1150 Hancock Street
Quincy, MA 02169
617-770-7676
FAX: 617-770-1987
e-mail: adelia.deltrecco@state.ma.us
www.state.ma.us/mddc/

Adelia DelTrecco, Executive Assistant
Harold Lieberman, Administrative Assistant
Dan Shannon, Executive Director

Group of citizens which analyzes needs of people with severe, lifelong disabilities and works to improve public policy. MDDC produces several publications and has committees and a grants program to study and advocate for changes in the service system.

4014 Social Security: Boston Disability Determination

27 Wormwood Street
 # 43
Boston, MA 02210
800-772-1213
FAX: 617-727-1354
www.ssa.gov

4015 Workers Compensation Board Massachusetts

1 Ashburton Place
Room 211
Boston, MA 02108
617-727-2720
FAX: 617-727-3285
www.state.ma.us/dia

James J Campbell, Director

Michigan

4016 Bureau of Workers' & Unemployment Compensation

PO Box 30016
Lansing, MI 48909
888-396-5041
FAX: 517-322-1808
e-mail: bwdcinfo@cis.state.mi.us
www.michigan.gov

4017 Department of Blind Rehabilitation

Western Michigan University
3404 Sangren Hall
Kalamazoo, MI 49008
269-657-2223
FAX: 617-387-3567

Dr. William Wiener, Chairperson

4018 Michigan Association for Deaf, Hearing and Speech Services

2929 Covington Court
Suite 200
Lansing, MI 48912
517-487-0066
800-968-7327
FAX: 517-487-2586
e-mail: yourear@msu.edu
www.madhs.org

Jennifer Mora, Associate Director

Substance abuse prevention for deaf and hard of hearing students (alcohol, marijuana, inhalants) acted in sign language, voicing and captioning. HIV/AIDS prevention and information for the deaf and hard of hearing. Lending library books, videos and audio tapes. Accessibility in Courts video and information. TTY distribution Program.

4019 Michigan Client Assistance Program

Michigan Protection and Advocacy Service
PO Box 30008
Lansing, MI 48909
517-487-1755
800-288-5923
FAX: 517-487-0827
e-mail: molsen@mpas.org
www.mpas.org

Amy Maes, CAP Manager

4020 Michigan Coalition for Staff Development and School Improvement

530 W Ionia
Suite C
Lancing, MI 48933
734-513-9080
800-444-2014
FAX: 517-371-1170

4021 Michigan Commission for the Blind: Lansing

201 N Washington
2nd Floor
Lansing, MI 48909
517-373-6425
FAX: 517-335-5140
www.mfia.state.mi.us

4022 Michigan Commission for the Blind - Gaylord

209 W First Street
Suite 102
Gaylord, MI 49735
989-732-2448
FAX: 989-731-3587
www.mfia.state.mi.us

4023 Michigan Commission for the Blind

201 N Washington Square
PO Box 30652
Lansing, MI 48933
517-373-2062
800-292-4200
FAX: 517-335-5140
TTY:517-373-4025
e-mail: cannonp@mi.gov

Patrick Cannon, Director

The Commission for the Blind serves as the vocational rehabilitation agency for the blind. The Commission also operates a residential training center in Kalamazoo, provides independent living services for Michigan's older blind population, low-vision services for the state's youth, a deaf/blind program, and entrepreneurial opportunities for blind persons through its Business Enterprise Program.

4024 Michigan Commission for the Blind Training Center
1541 Oakland Drive
Kalamazoo, MI 49008
269-337-3848
800-292-4200
FAX: 269-337-3872
www.mcb1.gov

Melody Lindsey, Director

Residential facility that provides instruction to legally blind adults in Braille, computers, handwriting, keyboarding, cane travel, adaptive kitchen skills, daily living, industrial arts and also crafts. Clients may also learn to use a variety of adaptive devices such as raised dot timers and watches, hand tools, talking calculators, tape recorders, reading machines and computers. Special training is also offered in vending stand operation, college preparation and job seeking skills.

4025 Michigan Commission for the Blind: Escanaba
State Office Building
305 Ludington
Escanaba, MI 49829
906-786-8602
800-323-2535
FAX: 906-786-4638
www.mfia.state.mi.us

4026 Michigan Commission for the Blind: Flint
125 E Union
7th Floor
Flint, MI 48502
810-760-2030
FAX: 810-760-2032
www.mfia.state.mi.us

4027 Michigan Commission for the Blind: Grand Rapids
State Office Building, 2nd Floor
350 Ottawa NW
Grand Rapids, MI 49503
616-356-0180
FAX: 616-356-0199
www.mfia.state.mi.us

4028 Michigan Council of the Blind and Visually Impaired (MCBVI)
Neal Freeling
1037 Winchester Avenue
Lincoln Park, MI 48146
313-381-7844
888-956-2284
e-mail: freeling@concentric.net

Neal Freeling, Information & Refferal

Advocate for blind and visually impaired people throughout the state of Michigan.

4029 Michigan Department of Community Health
Lewis Cass Building
320 S Walnut
Lansing, MI 48913
517-373-3740
FAX: 517-335-3090
www.michigan.gov/mdch

Janet Olszewski, Director

4030 Michigan Department of Handicapped Children
3423 N Logan Street
Lansing, MI 48906
517-335-8873
FAX: 517-335-9222

Karen Schrock, Chief

4031 Michigan Developmental Disability Council
Cass Building
320 S Walnut
Lansing, MI 48913
517-334-6123
FAX: 517-334-7353
TTY:517-334-7354
e-mail: collinsve@michigan.gov

Venoella Collins, Executive Director
Karla L Kirkland, Council Chair
Mitzi Allen, Administrative

4032 Michigan Office of Services to the Aging
PO Box 30026
Lansing, MI 48909
517-373-0219
FAX: 517-373-4092

Diane K Braunstein, Director

State unit on aging; allocates and monitors state and federal funds for the Older American Act services: nutrition, community services, administers home and community based waiver, develops programs through Area Agencies on Aging, advocates on behalf of seniors with legislature, governor, state departments, federal government, responsible for state planning of aging services, develops formula for distribution of state and federal funds.

4033 Michigan Rehabilitation Services
PO Box 30010
Lansing, MI 48909
517-373-3390
800-605-6722
FAX: 517-373-0565
TTY:517-373-4035
www.mrs.state.mi.us

A state and federally funded program that helps persons with disabilities prepare for and fund a job that matches their interests and abilities. Assistance is also available to workers with disabilities who are having difficulty keeping a job. A person is eligible for MRS services if he or she has a disability, is unemployed and needs vocational rehabilitation services to prepare for and find a job or independent living services.

4034 Social Security: Lansing Disability Determination
5210 Perry Robinson Circle
Lansing, MI 48911
517-393-3876
800-772-1213
FAX: 517-393-4686
TTY:800-366-3404
e-mail: mi.fo.lansing@ssa.gov
www.ssa.gov

Linda Dorn, State Director

4035 State of Michigan/Bureau of Workers' Disability Compensation
PO Box 30016
Lansing, MI 48909
888-396-5014
FAX: 517-322-1808
www.cis.state.mi.us/wkrcomp

Minnesota

4036 International Dyslexia Association: Minnesota Branch
5021 Vernon Avenue
Minneapolis, MN 55436
651-450-7589
800-222-3123
e-mail: info@interdys.org
www.interdys.org

Hannah Toiles, President

Provides free information and referral services for diagnosis and tutoring for parents, educators, physicians, and individuals with dyslexia. The voice of our membership is heard in 48 countries. Membership includes yearly journal and quarterly newsletter. Call for conference dates.

4037 Minnesota Assistive Technology Project

STAR
50 Sherburne Avenue
Suite 309
St Paul, MN 55155
651-296-2771
800-657-3862
FAX: 651-282-6671
e-mail: star.program@state.mn.us
www.admin.state.mn.us/assistivetechnology

Chuck Rassbach, Executive Director

A statewide program promoting assistive technology devices and services for persons of all ages with all disabilities.

4038 Minnesota Board on Aging

444 Lafayette Road N
Saint Paul, MN 55155
551-296-2770
800-882-6262
FAX: 651-297-7855
e-mail: mba.dhs@state.mn.us
www.mnaging.org

Jim Varpness, Director

A state unit on aging for the state of Minnesota. Funds 14 area agencies on aging throughout the state that provide services at the local level. The mission is to keep older people in the homes or places of residence for as long as possible.

4039 Minnesota Children with Special Needs, Minnesota Department of Health

PO Box 64882
St Paul, MN 55164
651-215-8956
800-728-5420
FAX: 651-281-9988

Guidelines of care for children with special health needs: Down Syndrome, Cerebral Palsy, Cystic Fibrosis, Asthma, Diabetes, Hemophilia, Seizure Disorders, Congenital Heart Disease and Spina Bifida, neurofibromatosis, Deaf & Hard of Hearing, Juvenile Rheumatoid Arthritis, Sickle Cell Disease, Muscular Dystrophy, Pheneylketoneurea, Cleft Lip and Palate.

4040 Minnesota Department of Labor & Industry Workers Compensation Division

443 Lafayette Road N
Saint Paul, MN 55155
651-296-2464
800-342-5354
FAX: 651-296-9634
e-mail: dli.workcomp@state.mn.us
www.doli.state.mn.us

To reduce the impact of work related injuries for employees and employers. Advice is given and questions answered on the toll-free number.

4041 Minnesota Disability Law Center

430 1st Avenue N
Suite 300
Minneapolis, MN 55401
612-332-1441
FAX: 612-334-5755
www.mnlegalservices.org/mdlc

Lisa Cohen, Administrator
Pamela Hoopes, Legal Director

Provides free civil legal assistance to Minnesotans with disabilities on issues related to their disability.

4042 Minnesota Governor's Council on Developmental Disabilities GCDD

370 Centennial Office Building
658 Cedar Street
St. Paul, MN 55155
651-296-4018
877-348-0505
FAX: 651-297-7200
e-mail: admin.dd@state.mn.us
www.mncdd.org

Colleen Wieck PhD, Executive Director

The GCDD works to assure that people with developmental disabilities and their families receive the necessary services and support to increase independence, productivity, self determination, and intergration with the community. Publications could be ordered, and text and pdf versions could be downloaded directly ordered on the website.

4043 Minnesota Mental Health Division

Human Services Building
444 Lafayette Road N
Saint Paul, MN 55155
651-582-1990
e-mail: dhs.info@state.mn.us
www.dhs.state.mn.us/Provider/faqs/mental_heal

Edwin Swenson, Director

Oversees the provision of services to people with mental illness in the state of Minnesota. Services are provided on the local level through a network of 87 county social service departments.

4044 Minnesota Protection & Advocacy for Persons with Disabilities

Minnesota Disability Law Center
430 1st Avenue N
Suite 300
Minneapolis, MN 55401
612-332-1441
800-292-4150
FAX: 612-334-5755
www.mnlegalservices.org/mdlc

Lisa Cohen, Administrator
Pamela Hoopes, Legal Director

4045 Minnesota State Council on Disability (MSCOD)

121 7th Place E
Suite 107
St Paul, MN 55101
651-296-6785
800-945-5913
FAX: 651-296-5935
e-mail: margot.imdieke@state.mn.us
www.disability.state.mn.us

Margot Imdieke Cross, Information Officer

The MSCOD collaborates, advocates, advises and provides information to expant opportunities, increase the quality of life and empower all persons with disabilities. This mission is accomplished by: providing information, referral and technical assistance to thousands of individuals every year via email, letter or telephone; through trainings on a variety of disability related topics; through publications and its web site; and through its advocacy and advisory work.

4046 Minnesota State Services for the Blind

2200 University Avenue W
Suite 240
St Paul, MN 55114
651-642-0500
800-652-9000
FAX: 651-649-5927
www.mnssb.org

Lyle Lundquist, Self-Sufficiency Supervisor
Chuk Hamilton, Acting Director
Pam Brown, Workforce Development Director

State agency serving blind and visually impaired persons with rehabilitation, information access, assistive technology, training and job placement services. Extensive older blind program.

4047 Social Security: St. Paul Disability Determination

Metro Square Building
Suite 300
St. Paul, MN 55101

800-772-1213
FAX: 651-297-5167
www.ssa.gov

Noreen Hale, Director

Mississippi

4048 International Dyslexia Association: Mississippi Branch

PO Box 2485
Laurel, MS 39442 **601-428-0857**
800-222-3123
e-mail: info@interdys.org
www.interdys.org

Judy Robinson, President

Provides free information and referral services for diagnosis and tutoring for parents, educators, physicians, and individuals with dyslexia. The voice of our membership is heard in 48 countries. Membership includes yearly journal and quarterly newsletter. Call for conference dates.

4049 Mississippi Assistive Technology Division

PO Box 1698
Jackson, MS 39215 **601-853-5100**
FAX: 601-853-5158
www.mdrs.state.ms.us

Kim Read

A statewide program promoting assistive technology devices and services for persons of all ages with all disabilities.

4050 Mississippi Bureau of Mental Retardation

1101 Robert E Lee Building
Jackson, MS 39201 **601-359-1288**
FAX: 601-359-6295

Ed LeGrand, Chief

4051 Mississippi Client Assistance Program

3226 N State Street
Jackson, MS 39216 **601-362-2585**
FAX: 601-982-1951

Presley Posey, Director

Advocacy program for clients/client applicants for state of MS vocational services.

4052 Mississippi Department of Mental Health

1101 Robert E Lee Building
Jackson, MS 39201 **601-359-1288**
FAX: 601-359-6295

Albert Hendrix PhD, Executive Director

Administers Mississippi's public programs of serving persons with mental illness, mental retardation, alcohol and substance abuse problems, and Alzheimer's Disease and related dementia.

4053 Mississippi Division of Aging and Adult Services

Mississippi Department Of Human Services
750 N State Street
Jackson, MS 39202 **601-359-4929**
800-948-3090
FAX: 601-359-3664
e-mail: webspinner@mdhs.state.ms.us
www.mdhs.state.ms.us/

Edna Caston, Director

Protects the rights of older citizens while expanding their opportunities and access to quality services.

4054 Mississippi State Department of Health

Children's Medical Program
PO Box 1700
Jackson, MS 39215 **601-987-3965**
800-844-0898
FAX: 601-987-5560

Mike Gallarno MSSW LCSW, Director
Mary Marbury RN, State Nursing Coord.
Marilyn Graves MD, Medical Director

Financial assistance to families of children with physical handicaps. Rehabilitative in nature and has as its goal the correction or reduction of physical handicaps. Eligibility determined by diagnosis and provided to children from birth to age twenty-one. Financial eligibility is determined by factors of family income, family size, estimated cost of treatment and family liabilities. Categories include, but are not limited to: orthopedic, congenital heart defects, cerebral palsy, etc.

4055 Mississippi: Workers Compensation Commission

1428 Lakeland Drive
Jackson, MS 39216 **601-987-4200**
FAX: 601-987-4233
www.mwcc.state.ms.us

Ray Minor, Director

Missouri

4056 Institute for Human Development

University of Missouri-Kansas City
2220 Holmes Street
Health Sciences Building, 3rd Floor
Kansas City, MO 64108 **816-235-1770**
800-444-0821
FAX: 816-235-1762
e-mail: ellerbuschk@umkc.edu
www.ihd.umkc.edu

Carl Calkins, Director

A statewide program promoting person-centered planning and services for persons of all ages with all disabilities.

4057 Missouri Division of Mental Retardation & Developmental Disabilities

Department of Mental Health
PO Box 687
Jefferson City, MO 65102 **573-751-4054**
FAX: 573-751-9207
e-mail: mzdeata@mail.amh.state.mo.us

Anne Deaton, Division Director

4058 **Missouri Protection & Advocacy Services**

925 S Country Club Drive
Jefferson City, MO 65109
573-893-3333
800-392-8667
FAX: 573-893-4231
e-mail: mopasjc@earthlink.net
www.moadvocacy.org

Shawn T de Loyola, Executive Director
Linda Snider, Information Specialist
Connie Wright, Information Specialist

MO P&A provides protection of the rights of persons with disabilities in Missouri and assistance to clients who have disabilities through information, referral, advocacy or legal counsel. Informational brochures, Alliance newsletter, Client Assistance Program (CAP) Manual available upon request.

4059 **Missouri Rehabilitation Services for the Blind**

3418 Knipp Drive
PO Box 88
Jefferson City, MO 65103
573-751-4249
800-592-6004
FAX: 573-751-4984
e-mail: mmerrick@mail.state.mo.us
www.dss.state.mo.us/dfs/rehab/rehab.htm

Sally Howard, Director

Offers services for the totally blind, legally blind, visually impaired, including counseling, educational, recreational, rehabilitation, computer training and professional training services.

4060 **Social Security: Jefferson City Disability Determination**

2401 E McCarty Street
Jefferson City, MO 65101
800-772-1213
FAX: 573-751-1441
www.ssa.gov

Dr. Don Gann, Director

4061 **Workers Compensation Board Missouri**

PO Box 58
Jefferson City, MO 65102
573-751-4231
FAX: 573-751-2012
www.dolir.state.mo.us

Montana

4062 **Addictive & Mental Disorders Division**

555 Fuller Avenue
PO Box 202905
Helena, MT 59620
406-444-3964
FAX: 406-444-4435
www.dphhs.state.mt.us

Dan Anderson, Administrator
Roland Mena, CD Bureau Chief
Lou Thompson, MH Bureau Chief

4063 **Montana Advocacy Program**

PO Box 1680
Helena, MT 59624
406-449-3266
800-245-4743
FAX: 406-449-2418
TTY:800-245-4743
e-mail: advocate@mt.net
www.mtadv.org

Bernadette Franks-Ongoy, Executive Director

Protects and advocates the human and legal rights of Montanans with mental and physical disabilities while advancing dignity, equality, and self-determination. Designated federal P&A, with AT, CAP, PADD, PAIMI and PAIR programs. Advocacy and legal services for abuse, neglect, rights violations, access, discrimination in employment, accommodations and housing, and assistance with vocational rehabilitation/visual services.

4064 **Montana Blind & Low Vision Services**

111 Sanders Street
PO Box 4210
Helena, MT 59604
406-444-2590
FAX: 406-444-0230
www.dphhs.state.mt.us/dsd

Janice Frisch, Chief Management Operations

Mission: Promoting work and independence for Montanans with disabilities.

4065 **Montana Department of Aging**

Capitol Station
Room 219
Helena, MT 59620
406-225-4411
FAX: 406-444-5529

Hank Hudson, Aging Coordinator

4066 **Montana Department of Handicapped Children**

Cogswell Building
Helena, MT 59620
406-225-4411
FAX: 406-444-2606

Sidney Pratt, Bureau Chief

4067 **Montana Developmental Disability Council**

PO Box 526
Helena, MT 59624
406-444-1334
FAX: 406-444-5999
e-mail: dswingley@state.mt.us
www.ddpac.org

Deborah Swingley, Executive Director

4068 **Montana Protection & Advocacy for Persons with Disabilities**

400 N Park
Second Floor
Helena, MT 59624
406-449-2344
800-245-4743
FAX: 406-449-2418
e-mail: advocate@mtav.org
www.mtadv.org

Bernadette Franks, Executive Director

4069 **Montana State Fund**

5 S Last Chance Gulch Street
Helena, MT 59601
800-332-6102
FAX: 406-444-5963

Laurence Hubbard, President/CEO

4070 **Montech Rural Institute on Disabilities**

634 Eddy Avenue
Missoula, MT 59812
406-243-5676
800-732-0323
e-mail: montech@selway.utm.edu
ruralinstitute.umt.edu

Gail McGregor, Program Officer
Peter Leech, Director

A statewide program promoting assistive devices and services for persons of all ages with all disabilities.

4071 **Social Security: Helena Disability Determination**
10 W 15th Street
Suite 1600
Helena, MT 59604
140-644-1127
800-772-1213
TTY:406-441-1278
www.ssa.gov

Nebraska

4072 **International Dyslexia Association: Nebraska Branch**
611 S 32nd Street
Lincoln, NE 68516
402-434-6432
800-222-3123
e-mail: gcrlson@lps.org
www.interdys.org

Gwelda Carlson, President

Provides free information and referral services for diagnosis and tutoring for parents, educators, physicians, and individuals with dyslexia. The voice of our membership is heard in 48 countries. Membership includes yearly journal and quarterly newsletter. Call for conference dates.

4073 **Nebraska Advocacy Services**
134 S 13th Street
Suite 600
Lincoln, NE 68508
402-474-3183
800-422-6691
FAX: 402-474-3274
e-mail: nas@nas-pa.org

Timothy Shaw, Director

Offers protection and advocacy services to people with developmental disabilities or mental illness. Direct assistance provided if issue within broad case priorities. Sliding scale fee. Information and referral at no cost.

4074 **Nebraska Client Assistance Program**
301 Centennial Mall S
Box 94987
Lincoln, NE 68509
402-471-3656
800-742-7594
FAX: 402-471-0117
e-mail: victoria@cap.state.ne.us
www.cap.state.ne.us/

Victoria Rasmussen, Director

4075 **Nebraska Commission for the Blind & Visually Impaired**
4600 Valley Road
Suite 100
Lincoln, NE 68510
402-471-2891
FAX: 402-471-3009
e-mail: pvanz@ncbvi.state.ne.us
www.ncbvi.state.ne.us

Pearl Van Zandt PhD, Executive Director

Offers services for the totally blind, legally blind, visually impaired, mentally retarded blind and more with health, counseling, educational, recreational, rehabilitation, computer training and professional training services.

4076 **Nebraska Department of Health & Human Resources of Medically Handicapped Children's Prgm**
301 Centennial Mall Square
5th Floor
Lincoln, NE 68509
402-471-9310
FAX: 402-471-6352
e-mail: roger.hillman@hhss.ne.us

Jeanne Garvin MD, Medical Director
Roger Hillman, Program Specialist
Roland Snuttjer, Program Manager

Maternal and child health, Title V, children with special health care needs. Community based, statewide programs to facilitate diagnoses and care of children with disabilities and chronic medical conditions.

4077 **Nebraska Department of Health and Human Services, Division of Aging Services**
PO Box 95044
Lincoln, NE 68509
402-471-2307
FAX: 402-471-4619
e-mail: pattie.flury@hhss.state.ne.us

Pattie Flury, Long Term Care Liason

4078 **Nebraska Department of Mental Health**
301 Centennial Mall S
Lincoln, NE 68508
402-471-4997
FAX: 402-423-7045
www.nmhc-clinics.com

4079 **Nebraska Developmental Disability Council**
PO Box 95007
Lincoln, NE 68509
402-471-2871
FAX: 402-471-0180

Mary Gorden, Director

4080 **Nebraska Workers' Compensation Court**
PO Box 98908
Lincoln, NE 68509
402-471-6468
800-599-5155
FAX: 402-471-2700

Glen Morton, Administrator
Su Davis, Public Information Manager

4081 **Social Security: Lincoln Disability Determination**
PO Box 94987
Lincoln, NE 68509
402-471-3649
800-772-1213
FAX: 471-362-6
TTY:402-471-3659
e-mail: flloyd@nde4.nde.state.ne.us
www.ssa.gov

Frank Lloyd, Assistant Commissioner

Nevada

4082 **Assistive Technology Center at NCEP: Nevada Community Enrichment Program**
2820 W Charleston Boulevard
D-37
Las Vegas, NV 89102
702-259-1903
FAX: 702-259-1907

Terry Sjoberg OTR/L, Manager
Robert Hogan, Executive Director
Reggie Bennett, Independent Living Coordinator

Provides information, demonstration and training to adults and children with disabilities in the use of microcomputers and other assistive technology product systems and devices. ATC offers peer screening, pre-service financial and resource planning, low interest loan program, technology matching, rehabilitation engineering, outreach training, and maintains a product information database.

4083 **Nevada Assistive Technology Project**

3656 Research Way
Suite 32
Carson City, NV 89706 **775-687-4452**
888-337-3839
FAX: 775-687-3292

Kelleen Preston, Project Manager

Serves all ages and all disabilities through partnerships with community organizations. The NATP provides training, advocacy, funding, information and referral services, a newsletter and weekly television show.

4084 **Nevada Bureau of Services to the Blind and Visually Impaired**

505 E King Street
Room 501
Carson City, NV 89701 **775-684-4244**
FAX: 775-687-5980
e-mail: detradmn@nvdetr.org
http://detr.state.nv.us/rehab/reh_bvi.htm

Offers services for the totally blind, legally blind, visually impaired, mentally retarded blind and more with health, counseling, educational, recreational, rehabilitation, computer training and professional training services.

4085 **Nevada Department of Mental Health: Neuro Clinic**

505 E King Street
Room 602
Carson City, NV 89701 **775-684-5943**
FAX: 775-684-5966
e-mail: mhds@govmail.state.nv.us
http://mdhs.state.nv.us

Pat Hardy, Director

Offers treatment, prevention, education, habitation and rehabilitation for mental disorders. Works with advocacy groups, families, agencies and the community.

4086 **Nevada Developmental Disability Council**

505 E King Street
Suite 502
Carson City, NV 89701 **775-687-4440**
FAX: 687-329-2

4087 **Nevada Disability Advocacy and Law Center NDALC**

1311 N McCarran
Suite 106
Sparks, NV 89431 **775-333-7878**
800-992-5715
FAX: 775-788-7825
TTY:702-788-7824
e-mail: reno@ndalc.org
www.ndalc.org

Nevada's protection and advocacy system for the human legal and service rights of individuals with disabilities. NDALC has offices in Reno/Sparks and Las Vegas, with services provided statewide.

4088 **Nevada Division for Aging: Carson City**

3416 Goni Road, Building D
Suite 132
Carson City, NV 89706 **775-687-4210**
FAX: 775-687-4264
e-mail: dascc@govmail.state.nv.us
www.nvaging.net

Carol Sala, Administrator

Provides services for seniors in Nevada including community based care. advocacy and volunteer programs. Call write or e-mail for more information.

4089 **Nevada Division for Aging: Las Vegas**

3100 W Sahara Avenue
Suite 103
Las Vegas, NV 89102 **702-486-3545**
FAX: 702-486-3572

Develops, coordinates and delivers a comprehensive support service system in order for Nevada' senior citizens to lead independent, meaningful and dignified lives.

4090 **Social Security: Carson City Disability Determination**

505 E King Street
Carson City, NV 89701
800-772-1213
FAX: 775-684-4010
www.ssa.gov

Dan Mooney, Director

4091 **State of Nevada Client Assistance Program**

2450 Wrondel Street
Suite E
Reno, NV 89502 **775-688-1440**
800-633-9879
FAX: 775-688-1627

4092 **Workers Compensation Board Nevada**

6515 E Musser Street
Carson City, NV 89714 **775-687-6492**
FAX: 775-687-5786

New Hampshire

4093 **New Hampshire Workers Compensation Board**

46 Donovan Street
Concord, NH 03301 **603-225-2841**
FAX: 603-226-6903

4094 **New Hampshire Assistive Technology Projects**

Department of Education
State of New Hampshire
Concord, NH 03824 **603-862-2260**
FAX: 603-228-2468

Jan Nisbet

A statewide program promoting assistive technology devices and services for persons of all ages with all disabilities.

4095 **New Hampshire Client Assistance Program**

57 Regional Drive
Concord, NH 03301 **603-271-4175**
FAX: 603-271-2837
www.state.nh.us/disability/caphomepage.html

4096 New Hampshire Commission for Human Rights

2 Chenell Drive
Concord, NH 03301
603-271-2767
FAX: 603-271-6339
e-mail: humanrights@state.nh.us
www.state.nh.us

Katharine A Daly, Executive Director

Enforces NH law against discrimination in housing, employment or public accomodations. Disability discrimination is prohibited under NH law. Takes formal charges and investigates them.

4097 New Hampshire Department of Mental Health

State Office Park S
Concord, NH 03301
603-226-0111
FAX: 603-271-5058

Donald Shumway, Director
Paul Garmon

4098 New Hampshire Developmental Disabilities Council

10 Ferry Street
Concord, NH 03301
603-271-3236
FAX: 271-115-6
e-mail: NHDDCNCL@aol.com
www.nhddc.org

Gordon Allen, Executive Director
Leslie Nelson, Director Of Policy And Planning
Jennifer Daniels, Administrative Assistant

Offers information, referral and support services to disabled persons. A federally funded state agency.

4099 New Hampshire Division of Developmental Services

105 Pleasant Street
Concord, NH 03301
603-271-5034
FAX: 603-271-5166
e-mail: dpowers@dhhs.state.nh.us
www.nhdds.org

Dennis Powers, Director
Michelle Rosado, Administrative Assistant

Developmental Services promotes opportunities for normal life experiences for persons with developmental disabilities and aquired brain disorders in all areas of community life: employment, housing, recreation, social relationships and community association. Services and supports are organized throught a central state office and twelve private nonprofit community area agencies. Family support is provided to families of children with chronic health conditions or are developmentally disabled.

4100 New Hampshire Division of Elderly and Adult Services

DEAS Office Park South
129 Pleasant Street
Concord, NH 03301
603-271-4394
800-351-1888
FAX: 603-271-4643

Catherine Keane, Director
Mary Maggioncaida, Manager Program Development

State agency on aging services; limited services to incapacitated adults, age 18 and older.

4101 New Hampshire Governor's Commission on Disability

57 Regional Drive
Concord, NH 03301
603-271-4175
FAX: 603-271-2837

4102 New Hampshire Protection & Advocacy for Persons with Disabilities

PO Box 3660
Concord, NH 03302
603-225-0432
800-834-1721
FAX: 603-225-2077
e-mail: advocacy@drcnh.org

Richard Coluor, Executive Director
Ron Lospennato, Legal Director

Legal services for individuals with disabilities; I & R.

4103 Social Security: Concord Disability Determination

70 Commercial Street
Suite 100
Concord, NH 03301
603-224-1939
800-772-1213
TTY:603-225-8475
www.ssa.gov

4104 Workers Compensation Board New Hampshire

95 Pleasant Street
Concord, NH 03301
603-271-3483
800-272-4353
FAX: 603-271-6149
e-mail: workerscomp@labor.state.nh.us
www.labor.state.nh.us

New Jersey

4105 Division of Developmental Disabilities

PO Box 726
Trenton, NJ 08625
609-292-3742
800-932-9173
FAX: 609-292-6610
e-mail: advoca@njpanda.org
www.njpanda.org

James W Smith, Jr, Extecutive Director

New Jersey's designated protection and advocacy system for poeple with disabilities and provides legal, nonlegal individual and systems advocacy.

4106 International Dyslexia Association: New Jersey Branch

Box 32
Long Valley, NJ 07853
908-879-0466
FAX: 908-879-0466
e-mail: info@interdys.org
www.interdys.org

David Katz, President

Provides free information and referral services for diagnosis and tutoring for parents, educators, physicians, and individuals with dyslexia. The voice of our membership is heard in 48 countries. Membership includes yearly journal and quarterly newsletter. Call for conference dates.

Quarterly

4107 New Jersey Commission for the Blind and Visually Impaired

153 Halsey Street, 6th Floor
PO Box 47017
Newark, NJ 07102
973-648-2324
877-685-8878
FAX: 973-648-7364
e-mail: Vito.DeSantis@dhs.state.nj.us
www.state.nj.us/humanservices/cbvi

Vito J DeSantis, Executive Director
Pamela Gaston, Executive Assistant
Khmbrly Howard PhD, Deputy Executive Director

Offers services for the totally blind, legally blind, visually impaired, deaf blind and more with eye health, counseling, educational, recreational, rehabilitation, computer training and vocational services.

4108 New Jersey Department of Aging

S Broad and Front Street
Trenton, NJ 08608 **609-292-3766**

Ruth Leader, Director

4109 New Jersey Department of Health/Special Child Health Services

PO Box 364
Trenton, NJ 08625 **609-777-7778**
FAX: 609-292-3580
e-mail: plisciotto@doh.state.nj.us
www.state.nj.us/health/fhs/scservic.htm

Pauline Lisciotto, Administrator

Provides services for New Jersey children that will prevent or reduce the effects of a developmental delay, chronic illness or behavioral disorder.

4110 New Jersey Division of Mental Health Services

50 E State Street
Capitol Center
Trenton, NJ 08625 **609-341-3330**
800-382-6717
FAX: 609-341-3333
e-mail: lgates@dhs.state.nj.us
www.state.nj.us/humanservices/dmhs/index.html

Lyn Gates, Bureau Chief

Oversees the public mental health system for the state of New Jersey. Operates six regional and specialty psychiatric hospitals, and contracts with over 125 not-for-profit agencies to provide a comprehensive system of community mental health services throughout all counties in the state.

4111 New Jersey Governor's Liaison to the Office of Disability Employment Policy

New Jersey Dept of Labor
P.O. Box 052
Trenton, NJ 08625 **609-292-2323**
FAX: 609-633-9271
e-mail: cmycoff@dol.state.nj.us
www.state.nj.us/labor

Mark B Boyd, Commisioner
Al Kirk, Assistant Director
Rick Shanberg, Program Assistant

The Division of Vocational Rehabilitation Services providesa vocational rehabilitation services to prepare and place in employment eligilbe individuals with disabilities who, because of their disabling conditions, would otherwise be unable to secure and/or mantain employment

4112 New Jersey Protection & Advocacy for Persons with Disabilities

Trenton, NJ 08625 **609-530-5200**
FAX: 609-292-6610

Robert Nickolas, Director

4113 Regional ADA Technical Assistance Center

354 S Broad Street
Trenton, NJ 08608 **609-392-4004**
800-949-4232
FAX: 609-362-3505
TTY:609-392-7044
e-mail: BTACUPNJ@aol.com
home.earthlink.net/~dawwn/dbtac.htm

Richard Dodds, Contacts

4114 Social Security Administration

50 E State Street
Second Floor
Trenton, NJ 08608
800-772-1213
TTY:800-325-0778
www.ssa.gov

Social Security disability is a social insurance program that workers and employers pay for with their Social Security taxes. Eligibility is based on your work history, and the amount of your benefit is based on your earnings. Social Security also has a disability program for people with limited income and resources- the Supplemental Security Income (SSI) program. For more information on these federal programs, please call our nationwide toll-free number.

New Mexico

4115 New Mexico Aging and Long-Term Care Dept

228 E Palace Avenue
La Villa Rivera Bldg, Ground Floor
Santa Fe, NM 87501 **505-827-7640**
800-432-2080
FAX: 505-827-7649
e-mail: nmaoa@state.nm.us
www.nmaging.state.nm.us

Michelle Lujan Grisham, Director
Patsy Trujillo-Knaver, Deputy Director
Kay Bird, Public Information Officer

Information and services for seniors, people with disabilities and their families.

4116 New Mexico Client Assistance Program

1720 Louisiana Boulevard NE
Suite 204
Albuquerque, NM 87110 **505-256-3100**
800-342-4682
FAX: 505-256-3184
e-mail: nmpanda@nmprotection-advocacy.com
www.nmpanda.org

James Jackson, Director

4117 New Mexico Commission for the Blind

2905 Rodeo Park Drive E
Building 4, Suite 100
Santa Fe, NM 87505 **505-476-4479**
FAX: 505-476-4475
e-mail: greg.trapp@state.nm.us
www.state.nm.us/cftb

Greg Trapp, Executive Director

Offers services for the totally blind, legally blind, visually impaired, mentally retarded blind and more with health, counseling, educational, recreational, rehabilitation, computer training and professional training services.

4118 New Mexico Department of Health: Children's Medical Services

1190 S Saint Francis Drive
Santa Fe, NM 87505 **505-827-2548**
FAX: 505-827-1697
e-mail: lchristiansen@doh.state.nm

Lynn Christiansen, Program Manager

Title V MCH Program for children with special health care needs from birth to age 21 years. Services provided include: diagnosis, medical intervention, clinics and service coordination.

4119 New Mexico Governor's Committee on Concerns of the Handicapped

491 Old Santa Fe Trail
Santa Fe, NM 87501
505-471-5242
FAX: 505-827-6328

4120 New Mexico Protection & Advocacy for Persons with Disabilities

1720 Louisiana Boulevard NE
Suite 204
Albuquerque, NM 87110
505-256-3100
800-432-4687
FAX: 505-256-3184
e-mail: nmpanda@inmprotection-advocacy.com
www.nmprotection-advocacy.com

James Jackson, Director

4121 New Mexico Technology Assistance Program

New Mexico State Department of Education
Division /Vocational Rehabilitation
435 Saint Michaels Drive, Bldg D
Santa Fe, NM 87505
505-954-8533
800-866-2253
FAX: 505-954-8562
TTY:800-659-4915
e-mail: aklaus@state.nm.us
www.nmtap.com

Alan Klaus, Project Director
Caroll Cadena, Public Contact

Examines and works to eliminate barriers to obtaining assistive technology in New Mexico. Has established a statewide program for coordinating assistive technology services; is designed to assist people with disabilities to locate, secure, and maintain assistive technology.

4122 New Mexico Workers Compensation Administration

PO Box 27198
Albuquerque, NM 87125
505-841-6000
866-WOR-KOMP
FAX: 505-841-6866
www.state.nm.us/wca

Alan Varela, Director

Regulates workers' compensation in New Mexico.

4123 Social Security: Santa Fe Disability Determination

604 W San Mateo Road
Santa Fe, NM 87505
FAX: 505-827-3512
e-mail: terryb@oscar.state.nm.us

Terry Brigance, Director

4124 Southwest Branch of the International Dyslexia Association

PO Box 25891
Albuquerque, NM 87125
505-255-8234
FAX: 505-262-8547
e-mail: swida84@hotmail.com
www.interdys.org

Mary Gilroy, President

Provides free information and referral services for diagnosis and tutoring for parents, educators, physicians, and individuals with dyslexia. The voice of our membership is heard in 48 countries. Membership includes yearly journal and quarterly newsletter. Call for conference dates.

4125 Workers Compensation Board New Mexico

PO Box 27198
Albuquerque, NM 87125
505-841-6039
FAX: 841-606-0

Steven Kennedy, Director

New York

4126 Albany County Department for Aging

112 State Street
Room 710
Albany, NY 12207
518-447-7198
FAX: 518-447-7188
e-mail: aging@albanycounty.com
www.albanycounty.com

Vincent Colonno, Commisioner

4127 International Dyslexia Association of NY: Buffalo Branch

40 Gow School Emery Road
S Wales, NY 14139
585-687-2030
800-222-3123
e-mail: bufida@gow.org
www.interdys.org

Denise Lawton, Contact
Kathy Rose, President

Provides free information and referral services for diagnosis and tutoring for parents, educators, physicians, and individuals with dyslexia. The voice of our membership is heard in 48 countries. Membership includes yearly journal and quarterly newsletter. Call for conference dates. Other locations available in New York State.

4128 Jawonio Vocational Center

Jawonio Vocational Center
260 N Littletor Road
New City, NY 10956
845-634-4648
FAX: 845-634-7731

Esther White, Associate Dir of Employment Svcs

Offers vocational evaluation, training, counseling and job placement services.

4129 NYS Commission on Quality of Care for the Mentally Disabled

401 State Street
Schenectady, NY 12305
518-381-7000
FAX: 518-381-7079
www.cqc.state.ny.us

4130 NYS Office of Advocacy for Persons with Disabilities

1 Empire State Plaza
Suite 1001
Albany, NY 12223
518-474-5567
800-522-4369
FAX: 518-473-6005
e-mail: oapwdinfo@advoc4diabled.state.ny.us
www.advoc4disabled.state.ny.us/

Richard Warrender, State Advocate
Yvonne Williams, Assistant Advocate

4131 NYSARC

393 Delaware Avenue
Delmar, NY 12054
518-439-8311
800-724-2094
FAX: 518-436-1893
e-mail: brandtm@nysarc.org
www.nysarc.org

Marc Brandt, Executive Director

4132 **National Alliance for the Mentally Ill of NY State**
260 Washington Avenue
Albany, NY 12210 518-462-2000
800-950-3228
e-mail: info@naminys.org
www.naminys.org

Michael Silverberg, President
David Seay, Executive Director

4133 **New York Client Assistance Program**
99 Washington Avenue
Suite 1002
Albany, NY 12210 518-869-1543
FAX: 518-474-2652
www.nls.org/caplist.htm

4134 **New York Department of Handicapped Children**
Department of Health
175 Green Street
PO Box 678
Albany, NY 12201 518-447-4691
FAX: 518-447-4573
e-mail: jcrucetti@albanycounty.com
www.health.state.ny.us

Thomas Blake, Acting Bureau Chief
James Crucetti, Commisioner

4135 **New York State Commission for the Blind**
52 Washington Street
South Building, Room 201
Rensselaer, NY 12144 518-474-6812
FAX: 518-486-5819

Thomas Robertson, Associate Commissioner

Offers services for the totally blind, legally blind, visually impaired, mentally retarded blind and more with health, counseling, educational, recreational, rehabilitation, computer training and professional training services.

4136 **New York State Commission on Quality of Care**
401 State Street
Schenectady, NY 12305 518-388-2892
FAX: 518-388-2890
e-mail: marcelc@cqc.state.ny.us
www.cqc.state.ny.us

Marcel Chaine, Director Advocacy Services

4137 **New York State Congress of Parents and Teachers**
One Wembley Square
Albany, NY 12205 518-452-8808
FAX: 518-452-8105
e-mail: office@nypta.com
www.nypta.com

Penny Leask, President
Maria DeWald, First VP

4138 **New York State Office of Advocate for Persons with Disabilities**
1 Empire State Plaza
Suite 1001
Albany, NY 12223 518-474-5567
800-522-4369
FAX: 518-473-6005
e-mail: oapwdinfo@advoc4disabled.state.ny.us
www.advoc4disabled.state.ny.us

Richard Warrender, State Advocate

Provides information and referral services; administers NYS Tech Art Project; promotes implementation of disability-related laws.

4139 **New York State Office of Mental Health**
44 Holland Avenue
Albany, NY 12229
800-597-8481
FAX: 518-474-1846
www.omh.state.ny.us

James L Stone MSW CSW, Commissioner

4140 **New York State TRAID Project**
1 Empire State Plaza
Suite 1001
Albany, NY 12223 518-474-2825
800-522-4369
FAX: 518-473-6005
e-mail: traid@emi.com
www.advoc4disabled.state.ny.us

Deborah Buck, Project Director

4141 **Parent to Parent of New York State**
500 Balltown Road
Schenectady, NY 12304 518-381-4350
800-305-8817
e-mail: info@parenttoparentnys.org
www.parenttoparentnys.org

Carolyn Schimanski, Director

4142 **Protection and Advocacy Agency of NY**
401 State Street
Schenectady, NY 12305 518-388-2892
FAX: 518-388-2890
e-mail: marcelc@cqc.state.ny.us
www.cqc.state.ny.us

Marcel Chaine, Director Advocacy Services

4143 **Regional Early Childhood Director Center**
Box 671
601 Elmwood Avenue
Rochester, NY 14642 585-275-2263
800-462-4344
FAX: 585-275-3366
e-mail: mike_reif@boces.monroe.edu
www.vesid.nysed.gov

Michael Reif, Director

4144 **Resources for Children with Special Needs**
116 E 16th Street
5th Floor
New York, NY 10003 212-667-4650
FAX: 212-254-4070
e-mail: info@resourcesnyc.org
www.resourcesnyc.org

Karen Schlesinger, Executive Director
Dianne Littwin, Director Publications

An independent nonprofit organization that provides information, referral, advocacy, training and support for parents and professionals in the New York City metropolitan area who are looking for programs and services for children from birth to 21 with learning, developmental, emotional or physical disabilities.

4145 **Singeria/Metropolitan Parent Center**
15 W 65th Street
6th Floor
New York, NY 10023 212-496-1300

e-mail: Sinergia@panix.com
www.sinergiany.org

Donald Lash, Acting Executive Director

4146 **Social Security: Albany Disability Determination**
40 N Pearl Street
Albany, NY 12243
518-474-6812
800-772-1213
FAX: 518-473-9286
TTY:518-474-7501
www.ssa.gov

Thomas A Robertson, Assistant Commissioner

4147 **State Agency for the Blind and Visually Impaired**
52 Washington Street
South Building, Room 201
Rensselaer, NY 12144
518-474-6812
FAX: 518-486-5819

Thomas Robertson, Associate Commissioner

4148 **State Education Agency Rural Representative**
Education Building Annex
Room 876
Albany, NY 12234
518-474-3936
FAX: 518-473-2860
e-mail: sspear@mail.nysed.gov
www.nysed.gov

Suzanne Spear, Supervisor

4149 **State Mental Health Agency**
44 Holland Avenue
Albany, NY 12229
518-474-4403
FAX: 518-474-2149
e-mail: cocojls@omh.state.ny.us

James Stone, Commissioner

4150 **State Mental Health Representative for Children and Youth**
44 Holland Avenue
Albany, NY 12229
518-473-6902
e-mail: cocompz@omh.state.ny.us

Michale Zuber, Associate Commissioner

4151 **State Mental Retardation Program**
44 Holland Avenue
Albany, NY 12229
518-473-1997
FAX: 518-473-1271
www.omr.state.ny.us

Thomas Maul, Commissioner

4152 **State Vocational Rehabilitation Agency**
1606 One Commerce Plaza
Albany, NY 12234
518-474-2714
FAX: 518-416-4182
www.nysed.gov

Lawrence Gloeckler, Deputy Commissioner
Richard Mills, Comissioner

4153 **United We Stand of New York**
202 Union Street
Suite L
Brooklyn, NY 11211
718-302-4313
FAX: 718-302-4315
e-mail: uwsofny@aol.com
www.taalliance.org/ptis/uws/

Lourdes Rivera-Putz, Program Director

4154 **University Afiliated Program/Rose F Kennedy Center**
1300 Morris Parkway S
Bronx, NY 10461
718-430-8518
bxcb11biz.com/comhospitals.html

Hebert J Cohen, Director

4155 **University of Rochester Medical Center**
601 Elmwood Avenue
Box 671
Rochester, NY 14642
585-275-0355
FAX: 585-275-3366
e-mail: phil_davidson@urmc.rochester.edu
www.urmc.rochester.edu/strong/scdd

Philp W Davidson, Director

4156 **VSA Arts of New York City**
18-05 215 Street Bayside
Suite 15N
Bayside, NY 11360
718-225-6305
FAX: 717-225-6305
TTY:718-229-5590
e-mail: Bbvsanyc@msn.com

Dr. Bebe Berenstein, Director

4157 **WIHD/ University Affiliated Program**
Weschester Medical Center
Valhalla, NY 10595
914-493-8204
FAX: 914-493-1973
e-mail: Ansley_Bacon@NYMC.edu
www.nymc.edu/wihd

Ansley Bacon, Director

4158 **Workers Compensation Board New York**
111 Livingston Street
Brooklyn, NY 11201
800-877-1373

Joesph McHugh, Administrator
Tom Agostino, Manager

North Carolina

4159 **Developmental Disability Services Section**
Albemarle Bldg, 325 N Salisbury St.
Mail Service Center 3001
Raleigh, NC 27699
919-733-7011
FAX: 919-733-9455
e-mail: rich.visingardi@ncmail.net
www.dhhs.state.nc.us/mhddsas/

Rich Visingardi, Director
Phillip Bickham, Human Resource Manager

Makes policies and monitors public services and supports to people with mental illness, developmental disabilities and substance abuse throughout North Carolina.

4160 **International Dyslexia Association: North Carolina Branch**
184-D2 Mountain Club
Vilason, NC 28692
252-243-8843
800-222-3123
e-mail: tommcd@boone.netg
www.interdys.org

Tom McDonocgh, President

Provides free information and referral services for diagnosis and tutoring for parents, educators, physicians, and individuals with dyslexia. The voice of our membership is heard in 48 countries. Membership includes yearly journal and quarterly newsletter. Call for conference dates.

4161 North Carolina Workers Compensation Board
430 N Salisbury Street
Raleigh, NC 27611
919-676-2288
FAX: 919-715-0282
www.comp.state.nc.us/

J Bunn Jr, Director

4162 North Carolina Assistive Technology Project
1110 Navaho Drive
Suite 101
Raleigh, NC 27609
919-676-2288
FAX: 919-850-2792
e-mail: ncatp@minespring.com
www.ncatp.org

Ricki Cook, Project Director
Annette Lauber, Funding Specialist
Jacquelyne Gordon, Consumer Resource Specialist

The North Carolina Assistive Technology Project exists to create a statewide, consumer-responsive system of assistive technology services for all North Carolinians with disabilities. The project's activities impact children and adults with disabilities across all aspects of their lives.

4163 North Carolina Children & Youth Branch
1928 Mail Service Center
Raleigh, NC 27699
919-733-7437
800-737-3028
FAX: 919-715-3187

Carol Tant, Head Children/Youth Branch
Cheryl Walker, Unit Manager Spec. Service
Dianne Tyson, Help Line Manager

4164 North Carolina Client Assistance Program
2801 Mail Service Center
Raleigh, NC 27699
919-855-3600
FAX: 919-715-2456
e-mail: kathy.brack@ncmail.net

Kathy Brack, Director

4165 North Carolina Developmental Disabilities
1001 Navaho Drive
Suite GL-103
Raleigh, NC 27609
919-850-2833
800-357-6916
FAX: 919-850-2895
e-mail: Holly.Riddle@ncmail.net
www.nc-ddc.org

Holly Riddle

A planning council established to assure that individuals with developmental disabilities and their families participate in the planning of and have access to culturally competent services, supports, and other assistance and opportunities that promote independence, productivity, and integration and inclusion into the community; and to promote, through systemic change, capacity building and advocacy activities, a consumer and family-centered comprehensive system.

4166 North Carolina Division of Aging
2101 Mail Service Center
Raleigh, NC 27699
919-733-3983
FAX: 919-733-0443
www.dhhs.state.nc.us/aging/home.htm

Karen Gottovi, Director

4167 North Carolina Industrial Commission
430 N Salisbury Street
Raleigh, NC 27603
919-733-3484
FAX: 919-715-0282
www.comp.state.nc.us

J Howard Bunn Jr, Chairman

4168 Social Security: Raleigh Disability Determination
4405 Bland Road
Suite 150
Raleigh, NC 27603
919-790-2782
800-772-1213
TTY:919-790-2773
www.ssa.gov

North Dakota

4169 Division of Mental Health and Substance Abuse
600 S 2nd Street
Suite 1D & 1E
Bismark, ND 58504
701-328-8924
800-755-2745
FAX: 701-328-8969
TTY:701-328-8968
e-mail: solark@state.nd.us
www.discovernd.com/healthsafety

Karen Romiglarson, Director
Bonnie Selzler, Assistant Director Mental Health
Don Wright, Ass't. Director Substance Abuse

4170 North Dakota Workers Compensation Board
50 E Front Avenueet
Bismarck, ND 58504
701-328-3800
800-777-5033
FAX: 701-329-9911
TTY:701-328-3786
www.ndworkerscomp.com

Brent Edison, Director

4171 North Dakota Client Assistance Program
600 S 2nd Street
Suite 1B
Bismarck, ND 58504
701-328-8947
800-207-6122
FAX: 701-328-8969

4172 North Dakota Department of Aging
600 S Second Street
Suite 1C
Bismarck, ND 58504
701-328-8910
800-451-8693
FAX: 701-328-8989

Linda Wright, Director

4173 North Dakota Department of Human Services
Children's Special Health Services
600 E Boulevard Avenue
Department 325
Bismarck, ND 58505
701-328-2436
800-755-2714
FAX: 701-328-2359
e-mail: dhscshs@state.nd.us
www.state.nd.us/humanservices/

Tamara Gallud-Millner, Deputy Director

Provides services for children special health care needs and their families. Provides services and diagnosis, treatment, clinics, information, referral and care coordinators.

4174 North Dakota State Council On Developmenta l Disabilities

600 S 2nd Street
Suite 1B
Bismarck, ND 58504
701-328-8953
FAX: 701-328-8969
e-mail: sowalt@state.nd.us
www.ndcd.org

Tom Wallner, Executive Director

The SCDD advocates for policy changes and non profits that promote choice, independence, productivity and inclusion for persons with developmental disabilites and their families.

4175 Protection & Advocacy Project

400 E Broadway Avenue
Suite 409
Bismarck, ND 58501
701-328-2950
800-472-2670
FAX: 701-328-3934
e-mail: panda@state.nd.us
www.ndpanda.org

Teresa Larsen, Executive Director

The Protection and Advocacy is a state agency whose purpose is to advocate for and protect the rights of people with disabilities. The Protection and Advocacy Project has programs to serve people with developmental disabilities, mental illnesses and other types of disabilities. The projects programs and services are free to eligible individuals.

4176 Social Security: Bismarck Disability Determination

1680 E Capitol Avenue
Bismarck, ND 58501
701-250-4200
800-772-1213
TTY:701-250-4620
www.ssa.gov

4177 Workers Compensation Board North Dakota

4007 State Street
Bismarck, ND 58501
701-224-3800

Ohio

4178 Bureau for Children with Medical Handicaps - Ohio Department of Health

PO Box 1603
Columbus, OH 43216
614-466-1700
800-755-4769
FAX: 614-728-3616
e-mail: bcmb@gw.odh.state.oh.us
www.odh.state.oh.us

James Bryant MD, Bureau Chief

Provides funding for the diagnosis, treatment and coordination of services for eligible Ohio children, under age 21, with medical handicaps; conducts quality assurance activities to establish standards of care and determine unmet needs of children with handicaps and their families; collaborates with public health nurses to increase access to care; and assists families to access and use third party resources. Conducts a separate program for adults with cystic fibrosis.

4179 Epilepsy Council of Greater Cincinnati

895 Central Avenue
Suite 550
Cincinnati, OH 45202
513-721-2905
877-804-2241
FAX: 531-721-0799
e-mail: ecgc@fuse.net
www.epilespsyfoudation.org

Marge Frommeyer, Executive Director

4180 International Dyslexia Association: Central Ohio Branch

PO Box 16216
Columbus, OH 43216
614-899-5711
800-222-3123
e-mail: info@interdys.org
www.interdys.org

Anita Gardner, Co-President
Karen Bradford, Co-President
Cameron Jones, President

Provides free information and referral services for diagnosis and tutoring for parents, educators, physicians, and individuals with dyslexia. The voice of our membership is heard in 48 countries. Membership includes yearly journal and quarterly newsletter. Call for conference dates. Other locations available in Ohio state.

4181 Ohio Bureau of Worker's Compensation

30 W Spring Street
Columbus, OH 43215
800-644-6292
FAX: 877-520-6446
e-mail: ombudsperson@bwc.state.oh.us
www.ohiobwc.com

James Conrad, Chief Excutive Officer

4182 Ohio Client Assistance Program

30 E Broad Street
Room 120
Columbus, OH 43215
614-466-6920
FAX: 614-752-4197

4183 Ohio Department of Aging

50 W Broad Street
9th Floor
Columbus, OH 43215
614-466-5500
866-243-5678
888-243-5678
FAX: 614-466-5741
www.state.oh.us/age

Joan W Lawrence, Director
Steve Proctor, Communications Chief

The department serves & represents about 2 million Ohioans age 60 & older. They advocate for the needs of all older citizens with emphasis on improving the quality of life, helping senior citizens live active, healthy, & independent lives, & promoting positive attitudes toward aging & older people. Committed to helping the frail elderly who choose to remain at home by providing home & community based services, their goal is to promote the level of choice, independence & self-care.

4184 Ohio Department of Mental Health

30 E Broad Street
8th Floor
Columbus, OH 43215
614-466-2596
FAX: 614-466-1571
www.mh.state.oh.us

Mike Hogan, Director

4185 **Ohio Developmental Disability Council**

8 E Long Street
12th Floor
Columbus, OH 43215
614-466-5205
800-766-7426
FAX: 614-466-0298
e-mail: david.zwyer@dmr.state.oh.us
www.state.oh.us/ddc

David Zwyer, Director

The Ohio Developmental Disabilities Council is one of 55 Councils found in all states and territories which provides funding for grant projects. The DD Council is a planning and advocacy agency that seeks to improve the lives of Ohioans with disabilities.

4186 **Ohio Governor's Council on People with Disabilities**

400 E Campus View Boulevard
Columbus, OH 43235
614-438-1391
FAX: 614-438-1274
e-mail: lucille.walls@rsc.state.oh.us
www.state.oh.us/gcpd

Lucille Walls, Executive Director
Leslie Alloway, Program Specialist
Marcella Eblin, Secretary

Advisory body to the governor and the legislature on issues that concern Ohioans with disabilities. State liaison to US Department of Labor, Office of Disability Employment policy and National Organization on Disability.

4187 **Ohio Legal Rights Service**

8 E Long Street
5th Floor
Columbus, OH 43215
614-466-7264
800-282-9181
FAX: 614-644-1888
www.state.oh.us/OLRS/

4188 **Ohio Rehabilitation Services Commission**

400 E Campus View Boulevard-SW5F
Columbus, OH 43235
614-438-1200
FAX: 614-438-1257
www.state.oh.us/rsc

John M Connelly, Executive Director

Is a state/federal program working in partnership with people with disabilities to assist them in achieving greater community participation through opportunities for employment and independence.

4189 **Social Security: Columbus Disability Determination**

400 E Campus View Boulevard
Columbus, OH 43235
800-772-1213
FAX: 614-438-1251
www.ssa.gov

Robert Rabbe, Director

4190 **Workers Compensation Board Ohio**

246 N High Street
Columbus, OH 43215
614-466-4110

Oklahoma

4191 **Oklahoma Workers Compensation Board**

400 N Lincon Boulevard
Oklahoma City, OK 73105
405-528-1500
888-269-5353
FAX: 405-528-5751
www.okdol.state.ok.us/workcomp/index.htm

4192 **Oklahoma Client Assistance Program**

2712 Villa Prom
Oklahoma City, OK 73107
405-521-3756
FAX: 405-522-6695

James Sirmans, Director

4193 **Oklahoma Department of Children with Disabilities**

4001 N Lincoln Boulevard
4th Floor
Oklahoma City, OK 73105
405-528-1500

Charles Brodt, Assistant Director

4194 **Oklahoma Department of Human Services Aging Services Division**

PO Box 25352
Oklahoma City, OK 73125
405-521-2281
FAX: 405-521-2086
www.okdhs.org

Roy Keen, Director

4195 **Oklahoma Department of Mental Health & Substance Abuse Services**

1200 NE 13th Street
PO Box 53277
Oklahoma City, OK 73152
405-522-3908
800-522-9054
FAX: 405-522-3650
www.odmhsas.org

Terry Cline PhD, Commissioner

State agency providing mental helath , substance abuse and domestic violence services.

4196 **Oklahoma Department of Rehabilitation Services - Division of Visual Services**

3535 NW 58th Street
Suite 500
Oklahoma City, OK 73112
405-951-3400
800-845-8476
FAX: 405-951-3529
e-mail: jprice@drs.state.ok.us
www.okrehab.org

Jody Harlem, Public Information Administrator

Offers services for the totally blind, legally blind, visually impaired, mentally retarded blind and more with health, counseling, educational, recreational, rehabilitation, computer training and professional training services.

4197 **Workers Compensation Board Oklahoma**

1915 N Stiles Avenue
Oklahoma City, OK 73105

Oregon

4198 **International Dyslexia Association: Oregon Branch**

PO Box 3677
Portland, OR 97208
503-228-4455
800-530-2234
FAX: 503-228-3152
e-mail: orbida@aracnet.com
www.aracnet.com

Betsy Ramsey, President
Charlie Weswig, VP

Provides free information and referral services for diagnosis and tutoring for parents, educators, physicians, and individuals with dyslexia. The voice of our membership is heard in 48 countries. Membership includes yearly journal and quarterly newsletter. Call for conference dates.

4199 Oregon Advocacy Center

620 SW 5th Avenue
5th Floor
Portland, OR 97204
503-243-2081
FAX: 503-243-1738
e-mail: oradvocacy@aol.com

The protection and advocacy system for Oregon.

4200 Oregon Client Assistance Program

620 SW 5th Avenue
Suite 500
Portland, OR 97204
503-243-2081
FAX: 503-243-1738
www.oradvocacy.org

4201 Oregon Commission for the Blind

535 SE 12th Avenue
Portland, OR 97214
503-731-3221
FAX: 503-731-3230
e-mail: linda.mock@state.or.us
www.cfb.state.or.us

Linda Mock, Administrator

4202 Oregon Department of Mental Health

2600 Center Street NE
Salem, OR 97310
503-945-9499
FAX: 503-945-2807

Stan Mazurhart, Director

4203 Oregon Technology Access for Life

3070 Lancaster Drive NE
Salem, OR 97310
503-361-1201
FAX: 503-370-4530
e-mail: ati@orednet.org
www.tal.org

Laurie Brooks, Project Director

A statewide program promoting assistive technology devices and services for persons of all ages with all disabilities.

4204 Social Security: Salem Disability Determination

530 Center NE Street
Suite 530
Salem, OR 97310
800-722-1213
TTY:800-325-0778
www.ssa.gov

4205 Vocational Rehabilitation Division

500 Summer Street NE
Salem, OR 97310
503-945-5880
FAX: 503-947-5025
TTY:503-378-3933

Joil A Southwell, Administrator
Lynnae Ruttledge, Assistant Administrator

The mission of the Division is to assist Oregonians with disabilities to achieve and maintain employment and independence.

4206 Washington County Disability, Aging and Veteran Services

133 SE Second Avenue
Hillsboro, OR 97123
503-640-3489
FAX: 503-640-6167

Pennsylvania

4207 International Dyslexia Association: Pennsylvania Branch

PO Box 251
Bryn Mawr, PA 19010
610-527-1548
800-ABC-D123
FAX: 610-527-5011
e-mail: dyslexia@pbida.org
www.GPBIDA.org

Marianne Cook, President
Amy Ress, Office Manager

Provides free information and referral services for diagnosis and tutoring for parents, educators, physicians, and individuals with dyslexia. The voice of membership is heard in 48 countries. Membership includes yearly journal and quarterly newsletter. Call for conference dates.

4208 Mental Health Association in Pennysylvania

1414 N Cameron Street
Second Floor
Harrisburg, PA 17103
717-236-8110
e-mail: swalther@paonline.com

Susan Walther, Executive Director

4209 Pennsylvania Workers Compensation Board

1171 S Cameron Street
Room 103
Harrisburg, PA 17104
717-939-9551
FAX: 717-772-0342

4210 Pennsylvania Bureau of Blindness

PO Box 2675
Harrisburg, PA 17105
717-787-6176
FAX: 717-787-3210
e-mail: jbirt@dpw.state.pa.us

Jay Birt, Interim Director

Offers services for the totally blind, legally blind, visually impaired, mentally retarded blind and more with health, counseling, educational, recreational, rehabilitation, computer training and professional training services.

4211 Pennsylvania Client Assistance Program

1650 Arch Street
Suite 2310
Philadelphia, PA 19103
215-988-4750
FAX: 610-555-7602

4212 Pennsylvania Department of Aging

555 Walnut Street
5th Floor
Harrisburg, PA 17101
717-783-1550
FAX: 717-783-6842
www.aging.state.pa.us

Nora Dowd Eisenhower, Secretary

4213 Pennsylvania Department of Children with Disabilities

PO Box 90
Harrisburg, PA 17108
717-783-1289
FAX: 717-772-0323

Donna Wenger, Acting Director

4214 Pennsylvania Developmental Disabilities Council
569 Forum Building
Harrisburg, PA 17120 **717-939-9551**
FAX: 717-772-0738
e-mail: paddpc@aol.com

Graham Mulholland, Executive Director

4215 Pennsylvania Protection & Advocacy for Persons with Disabilities
1414 N Cameron Street
Second Floor
Harrisburg, PA 17103 **717-236-8110**
800-692-7443
FAX: 717-236-0192
e-mail: ppa@ppaninc.org
www.ppainc.org

Provide advocacy, information and referral for persons with disabilities and mental illness issues.

4216 Public Interest Law Center of Philadelphia
125 S 9th Street
Suite 700
Philadelphia, PA 19107 **215-985-1113**
FAX: 215-627-3183
e-mail: pobint@aol.com

Mike Churchill, Chief Counsel
Judith Gramd, Director

A non-profit, public interest law firm with a Disabilities Project specializing in class action suits brought by individuals and organizations.

4217 Social Security: Harrisburg Disability Determination
555 Walnut Street
Harrisburg, PA 17101 **717-782-3400**
800-722-1213
TTY:717-783-8917
e-mail: ovr@dli.state.pa.us
www.ssa.gov

Susan Aldrete, Executive Director

4218 Workers Compensation Board Pennsylvania
1171 S Cameron Street
Suite 103
Harrisburg, PA 17104 **717-783-5421**
FAX: 717-772-0342

Rhode Island

4219 Department of Mental Health, Retardation and Hospitals of Rhode Island
14 Harrington Road
Cranston, RI 02920 **401-462-3201**
FAX: 401-462-3204

A Kathryn Power, Director

State department responsible for creating and administering systems of care for individuals with disabilities, specifically focused on mental health and mental illness; developmental disabilities, substance abuse and long term hospital care.

4220 Rhode Island Department Health
3 Capitol Hill
Providence, RI 02908 **401-222-5981**
FAX: 401-222-1442

Michael Spoerri, Disability & Health Program
Colleen Polselli, Pediatric Specialty Services
Sue Curley, Early Intervention Program

4221 Rhode Island Department of Elderly Affairs
160 Pine Street
Providence, RI 02903 **401-222-2858**
FAX: 401-222-3389
www.dea.state.ri.us

Barbara Rayner, Director

4222 Rhode Island Department of Mental Health
Cottage 405 Ct B
Cranston, RI 02920 **401-467-9200**
FAX: 401-464-2005

Reed Cosper, Director

4223 Rhode Island Developmental Disabilities Council
600 New London Avenue
Cranston, RI 02920 **401-462-3588**
FAX: 401-462-3570
e-mail: ac808.osfn.rhilinet@gov
www.riddc.org

Marie Citrone, Executive Director

The Rhode Island Developmental Disabilities Council works to make Rhode Island a better place for people with developmental disabilities to live, work, go to school, and be part of their community.

4224 Rhode Island Governor's Commission on Disabilities
John O Pastore Center
41 Cherry Dale Court
Cranston, RI 02920 **401-462-0100**
FAX: 401-462-0106
e-mail: disabilities@gcd.state.ri.us
www.gcd.state.ri.us

Doreen McConaghy, Chairperson
Bob Cooper, Executive Secretary

Assures the rights of persons with disabilities, deals with State and Federal regulations, building codes. Assists in the employment and education of disabled persons.

4225 Rhode Island Parent Information Network
175 Main Street
1st Floor
Pawtucket, RI 02860 **401-727-4144**
800-464-3399
FAX: 401-727-4040
e-mail: ripin@ripin.org
www.ripin.org

Vivian Weisman, Executive Director
Debra Spaziano, Intake Coordinator

A nonprofit organization established by parents and concerned professionals providing culturally appropriate information, training and support for families and professionals designed to improve educational and life outcomes for all children. Serving the state of Rhode Island.

4226 Rhode Island Protection & Advocacy for Persons with Disabilities
Rhode Island Disability Law Center
349 Eddy Street
Providence, RI 02903 **401-831-3150**
FAX: 401-274-5568

Raymond Bandusky, Executive Director

4227 Rhode Island Services for the Blind and Visually Impaired

40 Fountain Street
Providence, RI 02903
401-277-2300
800-752-0888
FAX: 401-222-1328
TTY:401-277-3010
e-mail: thompson@ors.state.ri.us

Jack Thompson, Deputy Administrator

Offers services for the totally blind, legally blind, visually impaired, mentally retarded blind and more with health, counseling, educational, recreational, rehabilitation, computer training and professional training services.

4228 Services for the Blind and Visually Impaired

40 Fountain Street
Providence, RI 02903
401-222-2300
FAX: 401-222-1322
e-mail: thompson@ors.state.ri.us
www.ors.state.ri.us

Jack Thompson, Deputy Administrator

Offers services for the blind and visually impaired.

4229 Social Security: Providence Disability Determination

380 Westminister Street
3rd Floor
Providence, RI 02903
401-528-4501
800-772-1213
TTY:401-273-6648
www.ssa.gov

4230 Workers Compensation Board Rhode Island

1 Darrance Plaza
Providence, RI 02903
401-458-5000
FAX: 401-421-3123

South Carolina

4231 Protection & Advocacy for People with Disabilities

3710 Landmark Drive
Suite 208
Columbia, SC 29204
803-782-0639
866-275-7273
FAX: 803-790-1946
e-mail: info@protectionandadvocacy-sc.org

Anne Trice, Director Administration

An Independent, non-profit organization responsible for safe guarding rights of South Carolinians with disabilities and other handicapped individuals without regard to age, income, severity of disability, sex, race, or religion.

4232 Social Security: West Columbia Disability Determination

1835 Assembly Street
Columbia, SC 29201
803-929-7635
800-772-1213
TTY:800-325-0078
www.ssa.gov

4233 South Carolina Assistive Technology Project

School of Medicine, CDR
University of South Carolina
Columbia, SC 29208
803-935-5263
FAX: 803-935-5342
TTY:803-935-5263
e-mail: jjendron@usit.net
www.sc.edu/scatp/

Evelyn Evans, Project Director
Janet Jendron, Program Coordinator
Mary Alice Bechtler, Program Coordinator

A statewide program promoting assistive technology devices and services for persons of all ages with all disabilities. Recently a statewide AT resource, demonstrations and equipment loan center and lab annual expo and training and workshops on a variety of disabilities and technology topics.

4234 South Carolina Client Assistance Program

Office of the Governor of South Carolina
1205 Pendleton Street
Room 306
Columbia, SC 29201
803-734-0285
800-868-0040
FAX: 803-734-0546
e-mail: lbarker@govpoepp.state.ce.us
www.govoepp.stat.sc.us/cap

Larry Barker PhD, Director

Provides information and advocacy to and for persons with disabilities in regards to vocational rehabilitation and independent living issues.

4235 South Carolina Commission for the Blind

1430 Confederate Avenue
PO Box 79
Columbia, SC 29201
803-898-8731
800-922-2222
FAX: 803-898-8852

Dr Nell Carney, Commissioner
Linda Johnston, Secretary

Offers services for the totally blind, legally blind, visually impaired, mentally retarded blind and more with health, counseling, educational, recreational, rehabilitation, computer training and professional training services.

4236 South Carolina Department of Children with Disabilities

2600 Bull Street
Columbia, SC 29201
803-734-5000

Ann Lee, Director

4237 South Carolina Department of Mental Health and Mental Retardation

PO Box 485
Columbia, SC 29202
803-898-8581
FAX: 803-898-8316
www.state.sc.us/dmh

Maureen Donnelly, Director

4238 South Carolina Developmental Disability Council

1205 Pendleton Street
Columbia, SC 29201
803-734-0465
FAX: 803-734-0465

Charles Lang, Director

4239 **South Carolina Services Information System**

University of South Carolina
School of Medicine
Columbia, SC 29208
803-935-5300
FAX: 803-935-5342
e-mail: scsis@cdd.sc.edu
www.scsis.org

Denise Rivers, Program Director

SCSIS provides information on aging and disability services in the state of South Carolina. Also, has a used equipment referral exchange where buyers and sellers are matched.

4240 **Workers Compensation Board South Carolina**

1612 Marien Street
PO Box 1715
Columbia, SC 29202
803-737-5744
FAX: 803-737-5764
www.state.sc.us/wcc

South Dakota

4241 **South Dakota Advocacy Services**

221 S Central Avenue
Pierre, SD 57501
605-224-8294
FAX: 605-224-5125
e-mail: sdas@sdadvocacy.com

Robert J Kean, Executive Director

Designated protection and advocacy progam for South Dakota providing legal, administrative, mediation and other services to elgible persons with disabilities in the state.

4242 **South Dakota Client Assistance Program**

221 S Central Avenue
Pierre, SD 57501
605-224-8641
FAX: 605-224-5125
e-mail: sdas@iw.net

Nancy Schade, Program Director

4243 **South Dakota Department of Aging**

700 Governors Drive
Pierre, SD 57501
605-773-3656
866-854-5465
FAX: 605-773-6834

Gail Ferris, Administrative

4244 **South Dakota Department of Children's Special Health Services**

615 E 4th Street
Pierre, SD 57501
605-773-3737
FAX: 605-773-5942

Nancy Hoyme, Program Director

4245 **South Dakota Department of Human Services Division of Mental Health**

E Highway 34, Hillsview Plaza
500 E Capitol
Pierre, SD 57501
605-773-5991
FAX: 605-773-7076
e-mail: infomh@dhs.state.sd.us
www.state.sd.us/dhs/dmh

Kim Malsam-Rysdon, Division Director
Amy Iversen-Pollreisz, Community Based Program Manager
Jennifer Fahey-Seale, Adult Svcs Program Specialist

4246 **South Dakota Developmental Disability Council**

700 Governors Drive
Pierre, SD 57501
605-773-3423
FAX: 605-773-5483

4247 **South Dakota Division of Rehabilitation**

700 Governors Drive
Pierre, SD 57501
605-773-3423
FAX: 605-773-5483

David Miller, Director

Offers diagnosis, evaluation and physical restoration services, counseling, social work, educational and professional training, employment and rehabilitation services for the disabled.

4248 **Workers Compensation Board South Dakota**

700 Governors Drive
Pierre, SD 57501
605-773-3423
FAX: 605-773-4211
e-mail: jamesmarsh@state.sd.us

James Marsh, Director

Tennessee

4249 **International Dyslexia Association: Tennessee Branch**

190 Woodcliff Circle
Signal Mountain, TN 37377
877-836-6432
800-222-3123
e-mail: info@interdys.org
www.interdys.org

Margaret Smith, President

Provides free information and referral services for diagnosis and tutoring for parents, educators, physicians, and individuals with dyslexia. The voice of our membership is heard in 48 countries. Membership includes yearly journal and quarterly newsletter. Call for conference dates.

4250 **Social Security: Nashville Disability Determination**

400 Deaderick Street
Nashville, TN 37243
800-772-1213
www.ssa.gov

4251 **Tennessee Assistive Technology Projects**

Doctor's Building
 # 300
Nashville, TN 37243
615-322-1210

EH Buddy White

A statewide program promoting assistive technology devices and services for persons of all ages with all disabilities.

4252 **Tennessee Client Assistance Program**

PO Box 121257
Nashville, TN 37212
615-298-1080
FAX: 615-298-2046

4253 **Tennessee Commission on Aging and Disability**

500 Deaderick Street
9th Floor
Nashville, TN 37243
615-741-2056
FAX: 615-741-3309
e-mail: tnaging.tnaging@state.tn.us

James Whaley, Executive Director

4254 Tennessee Council on Developmental Disabilities

500 Deaderick Street
Andrew Jackson Building 13th Floor
Nashville, TN 37243 **615-532-6615**
FAX: 615-532-6964
e-mail: tnddc@state.tn.us
www.state.tn.us/cdd

Wanda Willis, Executive Director

Provides leadership to ensure independence, productivity, integration and inclusion of individuals with disabilities in the community through promotion of systems change. The council works with members of the community, including public and private aencies, business, legislators and policymakers, to create a future in which: People with disabilities are full included in the community and experience no barriers related to attitudes about their disabilities as they persue their goals.

4255 Tennessee Department of Children with Disabilities

436 6th Avenue N
Room 525
Nashville, TN 37243 **615-532-5571**

Judy Womack, Director

4256 Tennessee Department of Mental Health and Developmental Disabilities

425 5th Avenue N
Cordell Hull Building 3rd Floor
Nashville, TN 37243 **615-532-6500**
FAX: 615-532-6514
e-mail: lola.potter@state.tn.us
www.state.tn.us/mental

Virginia Trotter Betts, Commissioner

4257 Tennessee Division of Rehabilitation

400 Deaderick Street
Nashville, TN 37243 **615-248-4996**

Patsy Matthews, Commissioner

Offers rehabilitation, medical and therapeutic information and referrals to the disabled.

4258 Workers Compensation Board Tennessee

710 James Robertson Parkway
Andrew Johnson Tower, Floor 2
Nashville, TN 37243 **615-741-2395**
FAX: 615-532-5929
www.state.tn.us/labor-wfd/wcomp.html

Texas

4259 Disability Policy Cosortium

7800 Shoal Creek Bolevard
Suite 171-E
Austin, TX 78757 **512-454-4816**

e-mail: klandrum@advodcacyinc.org
www.dpctexas.org

4260 Division of Special Education

1701 N Congress Avenue
Austin, TX 78701 **512-463-9414**

e-mail: glenz@tmail.tea.state.tx.us
www.tea.state.tx.us/special.ed

Gene Lenz, Senior Director

4261 Easter Seal of Greater Dallas, TX

4443 N Josey Lane
Carrollton, TX 75010 **972-394-8900**
800-580-4718
e-mail: rrabinowitz@easterseals.com
www.easterseals.com

Rebecca Rabinowitz, President/CEO

4262 Easter Seals Greater NW Texas

2100 Circle Drive
Fort Worth, TX 76119 **817-536-8693**
888-288-8324
e-mail: info@easterseals.fw.org

4263 El Valle Community Parent Resource Center

530 S Texas
Suite J
Weslaco, TX 78596 **956-969-3611**
800-680-0255
e-mail: texasfiestaedu.org
www.tfepodder.org

Laura Reagan, Project Coordinator

4264 Grassroots Consortium

6202 Belmark
Houston, TX 77087 **713-643-9576**

Speckids@aol.com

Agnes A Johnson, Director

4265 International Dyslexia Association: Austin Branch

5500 Ross Street
Del Valle, TX 78617 **512-452-7658**
800-222-3123
e-mail: info@interdys.org
home.austin.rr.com/aabida/resource.html

Sharon Roberts, President

Provides free information and referral services for diagnosis and tutoring for parents, educators, physicians, and individuals with dyslexia. The voice of our membership is heard in 48 countries. Membership includes yearly journal and quarterly newsletter. Call for conference dates. Other locations available in Texas state.

4266 NAMI Texas

611 S Congress Avenue
Suite 430
Austin, TX 78704 **512-693-2000**
800-633-3760
FAX: 512-693-8000
e-mail: namitexas@texami.org
tx.nami.org

NAMI Texas has a variety of programs directed to mental health consumers, family members, friends, professionals, other stake holders and the community at large to address the mental health needs of Texans. NAMI Texas works to inform the public about mental illness by distributing information about mental illness through every means of communication. Interviews are produced on television, stories are featured in newspapers, brochures are distributed, referrals are provided and more.

4267 Parent Connection

1020 Reverwood Court
Conroe, TX 77304 **936-756-8321**
800-839-8876
ParentCNCT@aol.com

4268 **Parents Supporting Parents Network**
601 N Texas Boulevard
Suite C
Weslaco, TX 78596 **956-447-8408**
888-857-8668
FAX: 512-454-4956
e-mail: CBTJr1@aol.com
www.thearcoftexas.org

Calvin Thomas, Program Director

4269 **Partners Resource Network**
1090 Longfellow Drive
Suite B
Beaumont, TX 77706 **409-898-4684**
800-866-4726
e-mail: path@partnerstx.org
www.partnerstx.org

Janice Meyer, Executive Director
Micheal Meyer, Director

4270 **Social Security: Austin Disability Determination**
903 San Jacinto Boulevard
Austin, TX 78704 **512-916-5404**
800-772-1213
TTY:512-916-5958
www.ssa.gov

4271 **Statewide Information at Texas School for the Deaf**
1102 S Congress Avenue
PO Box 3538
Austin, TX 78764 **512-462-5329**
e-mail: ercod@tsd.state.tx.us
www.tsd.state.tx.us

4272 **Texas Advocates Supporting Kids with Disabilities**
PO Box 162685
Austin, TX 78716 **512-310-2102**
FAX: 512-310-2102
e-mail: ASKTASK@aol.com
www.main.org/task/

4273 **Texas Commission for the Blind**
PO Box 12866
Austin, TX 78711 **512-459-2500**
800-252-5204
FAX: 512-459-2685

Terrell I Murphy, Executive Director

Offers services for the totally blind, legally blind, and visually impaired, with counseling, educational, recreational, rehabilitation, computer training and professional training services.

4274 **Texas Commission for the Deaf and Hard of Hearing**
PO Box 12904
Austin, TX 78711 **512-407-3250**
FAX: 512-451-9316
TTY:512-407-3251
e-mail: david.meyers@tcdhh.state.tx.us
www.tcdhh.state.tx.us

Bill Collins, Director Programs

4275 **Texas Council for Developmental Disabilities**
6201 E Oltorf
Suite 600
Austin, TX 78741 **512-437-5432**
800-262-0334
FAX: 512-437-5434
e-mail: TXDDC@txddc.state.tx.us
www.txddc.state.tx.us

4276 **Texas Department of Human Services**
701 W 51st Street
Austin, TX 78751 **512-438-3011**
888-834-7406
TTY:888-425-6889
e-mail: mail@dhs.state.tx.us
www.dhs.state.tx.us

Eric M McCain, Division Director
David Herndon, Chair
Carlela Vogel, Vice Chair

4277 **Texas Department of Mental Health & Mental Retardation**
PO Box 12668
Austin, TX 78711 **512-454-3761**
FAX: 512-206-4560
e-mail: karen.hale@mhmr.state.tx.us
www.mhmr.state.tx.us

Karen F Hale, Commissioner

Offers information and referrals.

4278 **Texas Department on Aging**
4900 N Lamar
Suite 4301
Austin, TX 78751 **512-424-6840**
800-252-9240
FAX: 512-424-6890
e-mail: mail@tdoa.state.tx.us
www.tdoa.state.tx.us

Mary Sapp, Executive Director
John Willis, Director Ombudsman

The state's visible advocate and steward for a full range of services and opportunities that allow older Texans to live healthy, dignified and independent lives.

4279 **Texas Federation of Families for Children's Mental Health**
7701 N Lamar Boulevard
Suite 505
Austin, TX 78752 **512-407-8844**
866-893-3264
FAX: 512-407-8266
e-mail: info@txffcmh.org
www.txffcmh.org

Patti Derr, Executive Director
Pat Calley, Board Chair
SG Barron, Director of Operations

Texas Federation of Families for Children's Mental Health is an organization comprised of family members of with emotional, behavioral and mental health needs; supporting families and youth through advocacy, links to resources and training.

4280 **Texas Governor's Committee on People with Disabilities**
1100 San Jacinto
Austin, TX 78701 **512-463-5739**
FAX: 513-463-5745
e-mail: ppound@governor.state.tx.us
www.governor.state.tx.us/disabilities

Pat Pound, Executive Director

4281 **Texas PTA**
408 W 11th Street
Austin, TX 78701 **512-476-6769**
800-825-5782
e-mail: txpta@txpat.org
www.txpta.org

Sylvia Ostos, President
Lynda Coleman, Chair

4282 **Texas Protection & Advocacy Services for Disabled Persons**

Advocacy
7800 Shoal Creek Boulevard
Suite 171-E
Austin, TX 78757
512-454-4816
800-252-9108
FAX: 512-323-0902
e-mail: infoai@advocacyinc.org
www.advocacyinc.org

Mary Faithfull, Executive Director
Shirley R DeBerry, Executive Assistant

A federally funded independent nonprofit agency that advocates for the legal, human and service rights of persons with disabilities. Publishes "Special Edition" newsletter, at a small fee and "It's a Good Idea!" a parent manual for $10, plus many other handouts free of charge.

4283 **Texas Respite Resource Network**

519 W Houston Street
San Antonio, TX 78207
FAX: 210-704-2797
e-mail: elizabethnewhouse@srhcc.org

Jennifer Cernoch, Director
Liz Newhouse, Assistant Director

A state clearinghouse and technical assistance network for respite in Texas. TRRN identifies, initiates and improves respite options for families caring for individuals with disabilities on the local, state and national levels. TRRN provides training/technical assistance to programs/groups wanting to establish respite services.

4284 **Texas Technology Access Project**

4030 W Braker Lane
Building 1, Suite 180
Austin, TX 78759
512-232-0740
800-828-7839
FAX: 512-232-0761
TTY:512-232-0762
e-mail: s.elrod@mail.utexas.edu
tatp.edb.utexas.edu/

Susanne Elrod, Project Director

Provides information, conducts training and technical assistance and works with policy makers to support children and adults with disabilities.

4285 **Texas UAP for Developmental Disabilities**

430 W Braker Lane
Building 1 Suite 180
Austin, TX 78712
512-232-0740
800-828-7839
FAX: 512-232-0761
e-mail: pseay@mail.utexas.edu
tcds.edu.utexas.edu/current.htm

Penny Seay, Executive Director

4286 **Texas Workers Compensation Commission**

4000 S IH 35
Austin, TX 78704
512-448-7900
FAX: 512-440-3547

4287 **United Cerebral Palsy of Texas**

5555 N Lamar Street
Suite L139
Austin, TX 78751
512-472-8696
800-798-1492
FAX: 512-472-8026
e-mail: ucptx@onr.com
www.ucpa.org

Jean Langendorf, Executive Director

Utah

4288 **Social Security: Salt Lake City Disability Determination**

555 E 300 S
Box 144032
Salt Lake City, UT 84114
801-321-6500
800-772-1213
FAX: 801-321-6599
www.ssa.gov

Dan Hooper, Director

4289 **Utah Assistive Technology Projects**

Utah State University
6855 Old Main Hill
Logan, UT 84322
435-797-3824
e-mail: garthe@coe.usu.edu

Marvin Fifield, Director

A statewide program promoting assistive technology devices and services for persons of all ages with all disabilities.

4290 **Utah Client Assistance Program**

455 E 400 S
Suite 410
Salt Lake City, UT 84111
801-363-1347
800-662-9080
FAX: 801-363-1437
www.disabilitylawcenter.org

Nancy Friel, Director

4291 **Utah Department of Aging**

120 N 200 W
Salt Lake City, UT 84103
801-538-3910
FAX: 801-538-4395
www.slcoagingservices.org/html/links.html

Helan Geddard, Director

4292 **Utah Department of Human Services: Division of Services for People with Disabilities**

120 N 200 W
Room 411
Salt Lake City, UT 84103
801-538-4200
800-837-6811
FAX: 801-538-4279
e-mail: dirdhs@utah.gov
www.hsdspd.utah.gov

Fran Morse PhD, Director
Krissie Summerhays, Constituent Services Rep

Information and referral services for people with disabilities, including DD/MR, Brain Injury and physical disabilities throughout the state of Utah.

4293 **Utah Department of Mental Health**

2001 S State Street
Suite 2600
Salt Lake City, UT 84190
801-530-6628
FAX: 801-530-6511

Dave Dangerfield, Director

4294 **Utah Division of Services for the Disabled**

660 S 200 E
Suite 400
Salt Lake City, UT 84111
801-238-4560
800-284-1823
FAX: 801-359-5627

William G Gibson, Director

Offers services for the totally blind, legally blind, visually impaired, mentally retarded blind and more with health, counseling, educational, recreational, rehabilitation, computer training and professional training services.

4295 **Utah Governor's Council for People with Disabilities**

155 S 300 W
Suite 100
Salt Lake City, UT 84101 **801-533-3965**
FAX: 801-533-3968
e-mail: alozano@hs.state.ut.us
http://www.gcpd.org/

4296 **Utah Labor Commission**

PO Box 146630
Salt Lake City, UT 84114 **801-530-6801**
800-222-1238
FAX: 801-530-7609
e-mail: sdanielson@utah.gov
www.laborcommission.utah.gov

R Lee Ellerston, Labor Commissioner
Alan Hennebold, Deputy Commisioner
Sherrie Hayashi, Director, Anti-Discrimination

4297 **Utah Protection & Advocacy Services for Persons with Disabilities**

Disability Law Center
455 E 400 S
Suite 410
Salt Lake City, UT 84111 **801-363-1347**
800-662-9080
FAX: 801-363-1437
e-mail: jstuart@disabilitylawcenter.org
www.disabilitylawcenter.org

Fraser Nelson, Executive Director
Ron Gardner Esq, Senior Counsel
Eric Dmitchell, Advocacy Director

Vermont

4298 **Disability Law Project**

57 N Main Street
Rutland, VT 05701 **852-775-0021**
800-769-7459
FAX: 802-775-0022
e-mail: nbreiden@vtlegalaid.org
vtlegalaid.org

Nancy Breiden, Director

Legal services (protection and advocacy) for people with disabilities on legal issues arising from disability. Statewide. Adults and children. Employment, education, discrimination, housing, public benefits, health care.

4299 **Social Security: Waterbury Disability Determination**

Two Pilgrim Park Road
Second Floor
Waterbury, VT 05676 **802-241-2463**
800-772-1213
FAX: 802-241-2492
www.ssa.gov

4300 **Vermont Assistive Technology Projects**

103 S Main Street
Weeks Building
Waterbury, VT 05671 **802-241-2620**
800-750-6355
FAX: 802-241-2174
TTY:802-241-1464
e-mail: jtucker@dad.state.vt.us
www.dad.state.vt.us

Julie Tucker, Project Director
Betsy Ross, Administrative Assistant

A statewide program promoting assistive technology devices and services for persons of all ages with all disabilities.

4301 **Vermont Client Assistance Program**

264 N Winoski Avenue
Burlington, VT 05401 **802-863-2881**
800-747-5022

Patrick Flood, Commissioner

4302 **Vermont Department of Aging and Disabilities**

Aging and Disabilities
103 S Main Street
Waterbury, VT 05671 **802-241-2400**
FAX: 802-241-2325
www.dad.state.vt.us

Patrick Flood, Commissioner

4303 **Vermont Department of Developmental and Mental Health Services**

103 S Main Street
Waterbury, VT 05671 **802-241-2614**
FAX: 802-241-1129
www.state.vt.us/dmh

Susan Besio, Commissioner
Theresa Wood, Director Development Services
Paul Blake, Director Division Mental Healths

4304 **Vermont Department of Health: Children with Special Health Needs**

108 Cherry Street
PO Box 70
Burlington, VT 05402 **802-863-7338**
FAX: 802-863-7635

Carol Hassler MD, Director

Multidisciplinary clinics and family support for children with chronic conditions, birth to age 21 years.

4305 **Vermont Developmental Disabilities Council**

103 S Main Street
Waterbury, VT 05671 **802-241-2612**
FAX: 802-241-2989
e-mail: vtddc@upgate1.ahs.state.vt.us

Phil Smith, Executive Director

The mission of the Vermont Developmental Disabilities Council is to assure that all people with developmental disabilities receive the opportunitites, assiatnce and services necessary to live independently and productivly in intergrated an inclusive community settings.

4306 **Vermont Division for the Blind and Visually Impaired**

103 S Main Street
Waterbury, VT 05671 **802-241-2210**
888-405-5005
FAX: 802-241-2128
e-mail: fredj@dad.state.vt.us
www.dad.state.vt.us/dbvi

Fred Jones, Director

Offers services for the totally blind, legally blind, visually impaired, mentally retarded blind and more with health, counseling, educational, recreational, rehabilitation, computer training and professional training services.

4307 **Vermont Protection and Advocacy**

141 Main Street
Suite 7
Montpelier, VT 05602
802-229-1355
800-834-7890
FAX: 802-229-1359
TTY:800-889-2047
e-mail: info@vtpa.org
www.vtpa.org

Ed Paquin, Executive Director
AJ Ruben, Supervising Attorney

Advocacy and legal services for people with mental illness on legal issues arising, out of disabilities. Children and adults.

4308 **Workers Compensation Board Vermont**

National Life Building
Drawer 20
Montpelier, VT 05602
802-828-2286
FAX: 802-828-2195

Virginia

4309 **Department for Rights of Virginians with Disabilities**

202 N Ninth Street
9th Floor
Richmond, VA 23219
804-225-2042
800-522-3962
FAX: 804-225-3221
www.vopa.state.va.us

Sandy Ferguson, Director

4310 **International Dyslexia Association: Virginia Branch**

13637 Prince William Drive
Midlothian, VA 23113
800-998-8336
800-222-3123
e-mail: info@interdys.org
www.interdys.org

Sherrell Sherron, President

Provides free information and referral services for diagnosis and tutoring for parents, educators, physicians, and individuals with dyslexia. The voice of our membership is heard in 48 countries. Membership includes yearly journal and quarterly newsletter. Call for conference dates.

4311 **Virginia Board for People with Disabilities**

202 N 9th Street
9th Floor
Richmond, VA 23219
804-786-0016
800-846-4464
FAX: 804-786-1118
e-mail: lindlekv@vbpd.state.va.us
www.vaboard.org

Barbara Ettner, Director Policy & Program
Heidi Lawyer, Director

4312 **Virginia Department for the Blind and Vision Impaired**

397 Azalea Avenue
Richmond, VA 23227
804-371-3140
FAX: 804-371-3351
e-mail: bowmanja@dbvi.state.va.us
www.vdbvi.org

Joseph A Bowman, Commissioner

Offers services for the totally blind, legally blind, visually impaired, mentally retarded blind and more with health, counseling, educational, recreational, rehabilitation, computer training and professional training services.

4313 **Virginia Department of Mental Health**

1220 Bank Street
PO Box 1797
Richmond, VA 23218
804-692-1849
FAX: 804-786-3827

Joe Damico, Director Administrative Services

4314 **Virginia Department of Veterans Services**

270 Franklin Road
SW Room 503
Roanoke, VA 24011
540-857-7104
FAX: 540-857-7573
e-mail: bboyd131@worldnet.att.net
www.vdva.vipnet.org

Colbert Boyd, Director

4315 **Virginia Developmental Disability Council**

101 N 14th Street
17th Floor
Richmond, VA 23219
804-225-3144
FAX: 804-225-3221

Sandra Reen, Director

4316 **Virginia Office Protection and Advocacy for People with Disabilities**

101 N 14th Street
17th Floor
Richmond, VA 23219
804-225-3144
FAX: 804-225-3221

4317 **Virginia Office for Protection & Advocacy**

202 N 9th Street
9th Floor
Richmond, VA 23219
804-225-2042
800-552-3962
FAX: 804-225-3221
www.vopa.state.va.us

Heidi Lawyer, Acting Director

An independent state agency that helps ensure that the rights of persons with disabiltiies in the Commonwealth are protected. The mission of DRVD is to provide zealous and effective advocacy and legal representation to protect and advance legal, human and civil rights of persons with disabilities, combat and prevent abuse, neglect and discrimination, and promote independence, choice and self-determination by persons with disabilities.

4318 **Virginia Office for Protection and Advocacy**

202 N 9th Street
9th Floor
Richmond, VA 23219
804-225-2042
800-532-3962
FAX: 804-225-3221

V Colleen Miller, Director

Washington

4319 DSHS/Aging & Adult Disability Services Administration

PO Box 45600
Woodland Square, Loop SE
Olympia, WA 98504
360-725-2300
800-422-3263
FAX: 360-407-0369
www.adsa.dshs.wa.gov

Kathy Leitch, Assistant Secretary

State agency providing services to eligible adults, children and their families. See our website for our publications list.

4320 International Dyslexia Association: Washington State Branch (AK, ID, MT, WA)

PO Box 7192
Seattle, WA 23113
206-382-1020
800-222-3123
e-mail: info@interdys.org
www.interdys.org

Stacy Turner, President

Provides free information and referral services for diagnosis and tutoring for parents, educators, physicians, and individuals with dyslexia. The voice of our membership is heard in 48 countries. Membership includes yearly journal and quarterly newsletter. Call for conference dates.

4321 Social Security: Olympia Disability Determination

402 Yauger Way SW
Olympia, WA 98504
800-772-1213
TTY:800-325-0778
www.ssa.gov

4322 WA Department of Services for the Blind

402 Legion Way
Suite 100
Olympia, WA 98504
360-586-1224
800-552-7103
FAX: 360-586-7627
www.wa.gov/dsb

Vocational rehabilitation for the blind.

4323 Washington Client Assistance Program

2531 Rainier Avenue S
Seattle, WA 98144
206-721-5999
800-544-2121
FAX: 206-721-5980
e-mail: capseattle@att.net

Jerry Johnsen, Director

Advocacy and information assistance for persons of disability seeking services through Vocational Rehabilitation or other program under the 1973 rehabilitation Act as commented. We provide counseling.

4324 Washington Department of Mental Health

PO Box 592
Olympia, WA 98507
888-713-6010
FAX: 360-902-7691

Dave Novseri, Director

4325 Washington Developmental Disability Council

2600 Martin Way E
Suite F
Olympia, WA 98504
360-586-3560
800-634-4473
FAX: 360-586-2424
e-mail: edh@cted.wa.gov
www.ddc.wa.gov

Ed Holen, Executive Director

4326 Washington Governor's Committee on Disability Issues & Employment

PO Box 9046
Olympia, WA 98507
360-753-6780
FAX: 360-438-3208

4327 Washington Office of Public Instruction

Old Capitol Building
Olympia, WA 98504
360-753-6738
FAX: 360-753-6712

Judy Schrag, Assistant Superintendent

Provides consultation on educational services for local schools, offers psychological testing and evaluation, maintains resource rooms in district schools and more for the blind and handicapped throughout the state.

4328 Washington Protection & Advocacy System

180 W Dayton
Suite 102
Edmonds, WA 98020
425-776-1199
800-562-2702
FAX: 425-776-0601
e-mail: wpas@wpas-rights.org

WPAS is a private, non-profit right protection agency for persons with disabilities residin in Washington state. Our advocacy services include information referral, technical assistance, training, publications and systemic advocacy.

4329 Workers Compensation Board Washington

7273 Linderson Way SW
Tumwater, WA 98501
360-902-4213
800-547-8367
www.lni.wa.gov

West Virginia

4330 Bureau of Employment Programs Division of Workers' Compensation

4700 MacCorkle Avenue
Charleston, WV 25304
304-926-5048
800-628-4265
e-mail: pgrinste@wvbep.org
www.state.wv.us

4331 Disability Determination Section

500 Quainier Street
Suite 500
Charleston, WV 25301
304-343-5055
FAX: 304-353-4212

4332 Social Security: Charleston Disability Determination

1800 Washington Street E
Charleston, WV 25305
800-772-1213
FAX: 304-353-4212
www.ssa.gov

4333 **West Virginia Advocates**

1207 Quarrier Street
4th Floor
Charleston, WV 25301
304-346-0847
800-950-5250
FAX: 304-346-0867
e-mail: wvadvocates@newwave.com

Intake Advocate

4334 **West Virginia Client Assistance Program**

West Virginia Advocates
1900 Kanawha Boulevard E
Building 6, Room 304
Charleston, WV 25305
304-558-2696
FAX: 304-346-0867
e-mail: vhuffman@access.k12.wv.us
http://wvde.state.wv.us/

4335 **West Virginia Department of Aging**

Holly Grove State Capitol
Charleston, WV 25305
304-755-5700
FAX: 304-558-0004
e-mail: hollygrove@juno.com

Patricia Bedford, Director

4336 **West Virginia Department of Children with Disabilities**

1116 Quarrier Street
Charleston, WV 25301
304-755-5700

Pat Kent, Administrative Director

4337 **West Virginia Department of Health**

1900 Capital Complex
Building 3
Charleston, WV 25305
304-755-5700
FAX: 304-558-1008

Taunja Willis-Miller, Secretary

4338 **West Virginia Developmental Disabilities Council**

110 Stockton Street
Charleston, WV 25312
304-558-0416
FAX: 304-558-0941
e-mail: jchankins@wvdhhr.org
www.state.wv.us/ddc

Jonathan Hankins, Office Manager

6-8 pages Quarterly Newsl

4339 **West Virginia Division of Rehabilitation Services**

1900 Washington Street E
Charleston, WV 25305
304-558-3428
e-mail: penneyh@mail.drs.state.wv.us

Penney Hal, Contact

Wisconsin

4340 **International Dyslexia Association: Wisconsin Branch**

2002 N Cambridge Avenue
Milwaukee, WI 53202
414-299-0551
800-222-3123
e-mail: lorej@nconnect.net
www.wis-dys.org

Nira Scherz-Busch, Co-President
William Kitz, Co-President

Provides free information and referral services for diagnosis and tutoring for parents, educators, physicians, and individuals with dyslexia. The voice of our membership is heard in 48 countries. Membership includes yearly journal and quarterly newsletter. Call for conference dates.

4341 **Social Security: Madison Disability Determination**

1 W Wilson Street
Madison, WI 53702
800-772-1213
www.ssa.gov

4342 **Wisconsin Assistive Technology Projects**

State Grants Program
1 W Wilson Street
8th Floor
Madison, WI 53702
608-266-6463
FAX: 608-243-5680

Sue Kidder, Director

A statewide program promoting assistive technology devices and services for persons of all ages with all disabilities.

4343 **Wisconsin Bureau of Aging**

1 W Wilson, Room 450
PO Box 7851
Madison, WI 53707
608-266-2536
FAX: 608-267-3203
e-mail: mcdowdb@dhfs.state.wi.us
www.dhfs.state.wi.us/aging

Donna McDowell, Director
Gail Schwersenska, Section Chief

Keeps and updates information and printed materials on senior housing directories, nursing home listings, and home care agencies.

4344 **Wisconsin Coalition for Advocacy: Milwaukee Office**

2040 W Wisconsin Avenue
Suite 678
Milwaukee, WI 53233
414-342-8700
800-708-3034
TTY:414-342-8700

The protection and advocacy agency for people with disabilities in Wisconsin. WCA provides guidance, advice, investigation, negotiation and in some cases legal representation to people with disabilities and their families. Local and state level systems advocacy and training are also provided.

4345 **Wisconsin Coalition for Advocacy: Madison Office**

16 N Carroll Street
Suite 400
Madison, WI 53703
608-250-3442
800-928-8778
FAX: 608-267-0368

Kim Hogan, Intake Specialist
Mr Lynn Breedolve, Director

The protection and advocacy agency for people with disabilities in Wisconsin. WCA provides guidance, advice, investigation, negotiation and in some cases legal representation to people with disabilities and their families. Local and state level systems advocacy and training are also provided.

4346 **Wisconsin Council on Developmental Disabilities (WCDD)**

600 Williamson Street
PO Box 7851
Madison, WI 53707
608-266-7826
FAX: 608-267-3906
TTY:608-266-6660
e-mail: wiswcdd@dhfs.state.wi.us
www.wcdd.org

Jennifer Ondrejka, Executive Director
Helen Hartman, WCDD Office Manager

Statewide systems advocacy group for people with developmental disabilities in Wisconsin.

4347 Wisconsin Department of Health and Family Services

Program for Children w/Special Health Care Needs
1 W Wilson, Room 351
PO Box 2659
Madison, WI 53701 **608-267-2945**
800-441-4576
FAX: 608-267-3824
e-mail: helmqp@dhfs.state.wi.us
www.dhfs.state.wi.us

Peggy Helm-Quest, Supervisor

The Department of Health and Family Services operates the federal Title V Maternal and Child Health Block Grant Program for Children with Special Health Care Needs. The program provides program monitoring, consultation and technical assistance to five regional CSHCN centers throughout Wisconsin; a Birth Defects Monitoring and Surveillance Program and a Universal Newborn Hearing Screening Program.

4348 Wisconsin Governor's Committee for People with Disabilities

PO Box 7852
Madison, WI 53707 **608-250-3442**
FAX: 608-267-0949

4349 Workers Compensation Board Wisconsin

PO Box 7901
Madison, WI 53707
FAX: 608-267-0394

Wyoming

4350 Social Security: Cheyenne Disability Determination

1100 Herschler
Cheyenne, WY 82002
800-772-1213
FAX: 800-972-2372
www.ssa.gov

Vicky Johnson, Director

4351 WY Department of Health: Mental Health Division

6101 Yellowstone Road
Room 259 B
Cheyenne, WY 82002 **307-777-7094**
FAX: 307-777-5580
TTY:307-777-5581
mentalhealth.state.wy.us

Dr Pablo Hernandez, Administrator
Marilyn J Patton, MSW, Deputy Administrator

State office responsible for purchase of service and program development policy.

4352 Workers Compensation Board Wyoming

122 W 25th Street
2nd Floor
Cheyenne, WY 82001 **307-777-7159**
FAX: 307-777-5946

4353 Wyoming Client Assistance Program

2424 Pioneer Avenue
Suite 101
Cheyenne, WY 82001 **307-638-7668**
FAX: 307-638-0815

Kristen Smith, Director

4354 Wyoming Department of Aging

6101 Yellowstone Road
Room 259 B
Cheyenne, WY 82002 **307-777-7986**
800-442-2766

Dan Stackis, Administrator
Ruth Davis, Excutive Secretary

4355 Wyoming Developmental Disability Council

122 W 25th Street
Cheyenne, WY 82001 **307-777-7230**
FAX: 307-777-5690

Lynn Achter, Director

4356 Wyoming Protection & Advocacy for Persons with Disabilities

320 W 25th Street
2nd Floor
Cheyenne, WY 82001 **307-638-7668**
FAX: 307-638-0815

Alabama

4357 **Birdie Thornton Center**
2309 Hine Street S
Athens, AL 35611
256-232-0366
FAX: 256-216-5681

Sharon Travis, Program Manager

4358 **Birmingham Independent Living Center**
PO Box 434
Jasper, AL 35502
205-387-0159
FAX: 205-387-0162
e-mail: pj,agik@bellsouth.net

4359 **Independent Living Center**
206 13th Street S
Birmingham, AL 35233
205-251-2223
FAX: 205-251-0605
www.birminghamilc.org

Linda Taylor, Director

Independent living center.

4360 **Independent Living Center of Mobile**
5304 Overlook Road
Mobile, AL 36618
251-460-0301
FAX: 251-341-1267
TTY:205-4602872
e-mail: ilc@zebra.net
www.ilcmobile.org

Michael Davis, Contact

Alaska

4361 **Access Alaska: ADA Partners Project**
121 W Fireweed
Suite 105
Anchorage, AK 99503
907-222-6166
888-462-1444
FAX: 907-222-6166
e-mail: adaalaska@netscape.net
www.adapartners.org

Mona McAleese, Coordinator

Since the passage of the Americans with Disabilities Act (ADA), Access Alaska developed the ADA Partners Project as a means of providing information, training and technical assistance, statewide to businesses and surrounding communities in better understanding and complying with this very important civil rights legislation.

4362 **Access Alaska: Anchorage**
3901 Taft Drive
Suites A and B
Anchorage, AK 99517
907-248-4777
800-770-4488
FAX: 907-248-0639
e-mail: access@alaska.net

Serena Dowling, Information/Referral Coordinator

Provides independent living services to persons with significant disabilities. Mission is to encourage and promote the total integration of persons with disabilities into the community of their choice. Services include independent living skills training, information and referral, advocacy, peer support, case management services, care coordination, interim accessible transportation and at home modifications.

4363 **Access Alaska: Fairbanks**
3550 Airport Way
Suite 3
Fairbanks, AK 99709
907-479-7940
800-770-7940
FAX: 907-474-4052
TTY:907-474-8619
e-mail: accessaccessalaska.net
www.accessalaska.net

David Jacobson, Statewide Director
Pat Bushman, Office Administrator

4364 **Access Alaska: Mat-Suvalley**
901 Commercial Drive
Wasilla, AK 99687
907-357-2588
800-770-0228
FAX: 907-352-2547

Provides independent living services to persons with significant disabilities. Mission is to encourage and promote the total integration of persons with disabilities into the community of their choice. Services include independent living skills training, information and referral, advocacy, peer support, case management services, care coordination, interim accessible transportation and at home modifications.

4365 **Alaska SILC**
1016 W Sixth Avenue
Suite 205
Anchorage, AK 99501
907-269-3571
FAX: 907-269-3636
TTY:907-269-3635

4366 **Arctic Access**
PO Box 903
Kotzebue, AK 99752
907-442-2393
FAX: 907-442-2393
e-mail: arcticac@ptialaska.net

Roger Wright

4367 **Hope Community Resources**
540 W International Airport Road
Anchorage, AK 99518
907-561-5335
FAX: 907-564-7429
www.hopealaska.org

Stephen Lesko, Director
Roy Scheller, Executive Deputy Director

Independent living centers offer peer counseling, disability education and awareness, attendant care registry and other services to the community.

4368 **Kenai Peninsula IL Center**
PO Box 2474
Homer, AK 99603
907-235-7911
FAX: 907-235-6236
e-mail: llc@xyz.net

Joyanna Geisler, Director

Offers peer counseling, disability education and awareness, attendant care registry and information on accessible housing.

4369 **Kenai Peninsula IL Center: Seward**
PO Box 3523
Seward, AK 99664
907-224-8711
FAX: 907-224-7793
e-mail: ilc@seward.net
www.peninsulailc.org

Joyanna Geisler, Executive Director

4370 **Kenai Peninsula IL Center: Soldotna**
47255 Princeton Avenue
Suite 1
Soldotna, AK 99669
907-262-6333
FAX: 907-260-4495
e-mail: solic@worldnet.att.net
peninsulaailc.org

Joyanna Geisler, Executive Director

4371 **SE Alaska ILC: Ketchikan**
1621 Tongass Avenue
Suite 205
Ketchikan, AK 99901
907-225-4735
FAX: 907-225-4753
TTY:907-225-4735
e-mail: sailktn@ptialaska.net
peninsulaailc.org

Joyanna Geisler, Executive Director

4372 **SE Alaska Independent Living Center (SAIL)**
3225 Hospital Drive
Suite 300
Juneau, AK 99801
907-586-4920
800-478-7245
FAX: 907-586-4980
e-mail: jokeefe@gci.net
www.sailinc.org

Joan Herbage-O'Keefe, Executive Director
Jerry Kainvlainen, Independent Livivng Coordinator
Sierra Kuden, ORCA Director

Offering a wide array of services for people with disabilities: Advocacy Information and Referral, Peer Support, IL Skills trainig Recreation, Benefits Counseling and more.

4373 **SE Alaska Independent Living: Sitka**
210 Lake Street
Suite A
Sitka, AK 99835
907-747-6859
FAX: 907-747-6783
TTY:907-747-6859
e-mail: sitka@sailinc.org

Jerry Kinulainem, IL Coordinator

4374 **Seward Independent Learning Center**
201 Third Avenue
Suite 102
Seward, AK 99664
907-224-7793
FAX: 907-224-8711
e-mail: ilc@mtaonline.com
www.peninsulailc.org

Jean Sether, Contact

Arizona

4375 **ASSIST! to Independence**
E Cedar Avenue & TCRHCC Parking Lot
Tuba City, AZ 86045
928-283-6261
888-848-1449
FAX: 928-283-6284
e-mail: assist@cybertrails.com
www.ASSISTtoIndependence.org

Michael Blatchford, Executive Director
ElizaBeth Pifer, Director Rehab Technology Svcs.
Elizabeth Fowler, Administrative Assistant

4376 **Arizona Bridge to Independent Living**
1229 E Washington Street
Phoenix, AZ 85034
602-256-2245
800-280-2245
FAX: 602-254-6407
e-mail: azbridge@abil.org
www.abil.org

Phil Pangnacio, Executive Director

Services include personal assistant training and referral, independent living skills instruction, home modification, information and referral, social/recreation activities, advocacy, peer support, Americans with Disabilities Act training and consulting.

4377 **Casa Del Rey**
PO Box W
Parker, AZ 85344
928-669-9695
FAX: 928-669-5280

4378 **Community Outreach Program for the Deaf**
268 W Adams Street
Tucson, AZ 85705
520-792-1906
FAX: 520-770-8514

Gail Lanham, Executive Director

Independent living centers offering peer counseling, disability education and awareness, advocacy and other services to the community.

4379 **Direct Center for Independence**
1023 N Tyndall Avenue
Tucson, AZ 85719
520-624-6452
800-342-1853
FAX: 520-792-1438
e-mail: directilc@earthlink.net
www.directilc.org

Ann Meyer, Executive Director

Offers peer counseling, disability education, information and referral services.

4380 **New Horizons Independent Living Center**
8085 E Manly Drive
Suite 1
Prescott Valley, AZ 86314
928-772-1266
800-406-2377
FAX: 928-772-3808
e-mail: nhilc@northlink.com
www.myweb.cableone.net/nhilc

Ken Edwards, Executive Director
Mary Hesselschwerdt, Outreach Coordinator
Jean Lasherc, Community Info Coordinator

4381 **Services Maximizing Independent Living and Empowerment (SMILE)**
1929 S Arizona Avenue
Suite 12
Yuma, AZ 85364
928-329-6681
FAX: 928-329-6715
e-mail: smile1929@adelphia.net
www.neiaw.com/smile/smileindex.htm

Kathryn N Robins, Executive Director

Independent Living Center.

4382 **Sterling Ranch: Residence for Special Women**
Sterling Ranch
PO Box 36
Skull Valley, AZ 86338
928-442-3289
FAX: 928-442-9272
e-mail: sterling.ranch@juno.com

Russell S Dryer, Executive Director

A nonprofit residence for mentally handicapped women which has been in operation since 1947. As a small facility (19 residents) the orientation is personal and family-like. Offers activities that range from gardening, quilting, academics, sign-language, crafts and a myriad of field trips and excursions. Private rooms and spacious living on 3 1/2 acres.

Arkansas

4383 Arkansas SILC
209 W Capitol
Suite 331
Little Rock, AR 72201
501-372-0607
FAX: 501-372-0598
TTY:501-372-0607
e-mail: 105344.1767@kcompuserve.com

4384 Delta Resource Center for Independent Living
400 S Main Street
Suite 118
Pine Bluff, AR 71601
870-535-2222
FAX: 870-536-7713
e-mail: deltar@seark.net

Billy Altom, Executive Director

Independent living center providing information and referrals, advocacy, peer counseling and independent living skills training to the Southeast region of Arkansas.

4385 Mainstream
1818 S University Avenue
Little Rock, AR 72204
501-280-0012
FAX: 501-280-9267
TTY:501-280-9262
e-mail: mainstreamlr@earthlink.net
www.mainstreamilrc.com

Rita Byers, Director

Peer counseling, disability education and awareness, and advocacy services, information and referrals, independent living skills training and more.

4386 Our Way
10434 W 36th Street
Little Rock, AR 72204
501-225-5030
FAX: 501-225-5190

Greg Goodwin, Project Manager

Advocacy and information services. One bedroom apartments for mobility impaired and elderly 62 years or older persons.

Based on income

4387 SE Alaska Independent Living Center
PO Box 35097
Juneau, AK 99803
907-789-9665
FAX: 907-789-9747

4388 Sources for Community IL Services
1918 N Birch Avenue
Fayetteville, AR 72703
479-442-5600
888-284-7521
888-284-7521
FAX: 479-442-5192
e-mail: sources@ursources.org
www.arsources.org

William Knight, Executive Director
Donna Henry, Administratove Assistant

Sources provides services, supports, and advocacy for persons with disabilities, their families, and the communities at large. We serve persons with all types of disabilities.

4389 Spa Area Independent Living Services
600 Main Street
Suite O
Hot Springs, AR 71913
501-624-7710
FAX: 501-624-7510
e-mail: sails@direclynx.net

Brenda Stinebuck, Contact

California

4390 Access Center of San Diego
1295 University Avenue
Suite 10
San Diego, CA 92103
619-293-3500
FAX: 619-293-3508
TTY:619-293-7757
e-mail: accesscentersd.org
www.accesscentersd.org

Louis Frick, Director

Offers peer counseling, disability awareness, advocacy services, client assistance programs, employment counseling, information and referral, personal assistant services, housing referral, financial benefits advocacy, durable medical equipment sales and repair, and assistance in compliance with the ADA (Americans with Disabilities Act).

4391 Access Center of San Diego N Branch
3355 Mission Avenue
Suite 131
Oceanside, CA 92054
760-435-9205
FAX: 760-435-9206
TTY:760-435-9213
www.accesscentersd.org

4392 CAPH Independent Living Center
3475 W Shaw AvenueWay
Suite 101
Fresno, CA 93711
209-927-6777
FAX: 209-927-6778
TTY:209-927-6779
e-mail: programdir@earthlink.net
www.cil-frenso.org

4393 CIL: Fresno
3475 W Shaw
Suite 101
Fresno, CA 93711
559-276-6777
FAX: 559-276-6778
TTY:209-276-6779
e-mail:
CILFMAILI@EATHLINK.NETprogram_dir@eathlin k.ne

4394 California Foundation for Independent Living Centers
910 K Street
Suite 350
Sacramento, CA 95814
916-325-1690
FAX: 916-325-1699
TTY:916-325-1695
e-mail: cfile@cfilc.org

4395 California State Independent Living Council (SILC)
1600 K Street
Suite 100
Sacramento, CA 95814
916-445-0142
FAX: 916-445-5973
TTY:916-445-5627
e-mail: casilc@calsilc.org.Michael C. Collins

4396 Center for IL
375 15th Street
Oakland, CA 94612
510-763-9999
FAX: 510-763-4910
TTY:510-444-1837
e-mail: ddaviscil@yahoo.com

4397 Center for Independence of the Disabled
875 Oneill Street
Belmont, CA 94002
408-733-5778
FAX: 407-895-5255

Kent Mickelson, Director

Counseling, disability education and awareness, attendant care registry, information on accessible housing and other services to the community.

4398 Center for Independent Living
2539 Telegraph Avenue
Berkeley, CA 94704
510-841-4776
FAX: 510-841-6168
e-mail: webmaster@cilberkeley.org
www.cilberkeley.org

Jan Garrett, Executive Director

The Center for Independent Living, Inc (CIL) is a national leader in helping people with disabilities live independently and become productive members of society. Founded in 1972, CIL is a pioneer advocating for greater accessibility in communities, designing techniques in independent living and providing direct services to people with disabilities. A partial list of services includes Information and Referral, Personal Assistance Services, Independent Living Skills Training and Peer Counseling.

4399 Center for Independent Living in Fresno
3475 W Shaw Avenue
Suite 101
Fresno, CA 93711
559-276-6779
FAX: 559-276-6778
e-mail: p_phillips@cil-frenso.org
www.cil-fresno.org

Fran Phillips, Executive Director

4400 Center for the Independence of the Disabled
875 Oneill Avenue
Belmont, CA 94002
650-595-0783
FAX: 650-595-0261
e-mail: rayp@cidbelmont.org
www.cidbelmont.org

Kent Mickelson, Contact
Ray Pittsinger, Program Manager
Arsie Tuquero-Zacarigs, Administrative Assistant

4401 Center of Independent Living: S Valley
204 E Main Street
Suite N
Visalia, CA 93291
559-622-9276
FAX: 559-622-9638

Robin Libbee, S Valley Office Manager

4402 Central Coast Center for IL: San Benito
San Benito Office
300 W Street
Hollister, CA 95023
831-638-1271
FAX: 831-638-1728

4403 Central Coast Center for Independent Living
234 Capitol Street
Suite A
Salinas, CA 93901
408-752-2968
FAX: 408-757-5549
TTY:408-752-2968
e-mail: info@progway.org

4404 Central Coast Center: Independent Living - Santa Cruz Office
1395 41st Avenue
Suite B
Capitola, CA 95010
831-462-8720
FAX: 831-462-8727

4405 Community Access Center
4960 Arlington Avenue
Suite C
Riverside, CA 92504
909-637-6900
FAX: 909-637-6906
TTY:909-637-6908
e-mail: lgwalls@flashcom.net

Lucille Walls, Contact
Paul Van Doren, Contact

4406 Community Access Center: Indio Branch
81-730 Highway 111
Suite 2
Indio, CA 92201
760-347-4888
FAX: 760-347-0722
e-mail: indiocac@aol.com
www.communityaccesscenter.org

Laurie Hoirup, Program Manager

4407 Community Rehabilitation Services
844 E Mission Road
Suite A
San Gabriel, CA 91775
626-307-2900
FAX: 626-307-1635
TTY:626-307-4188

4408 Community Rehabilitation Services
4716 Cesar E Chavez Avenue
Los Angeles, CA 90022
323-266-0453
FAX: 323-266-7992
TTY:213-266-3016

Juan Orantez, Info. And Ref./Stat. Coordinator
Yelanda Raminez, Care Services Program Director
Al Rivera, Executive Director

Community Rehabilitation Services, Inc. (CRS) is a private, non-profit agency established in 1974 to assist persons with disabilities within the East/North East areas of Los Angeles County to enhance their options for living independently. Any person who is 18 yrs of age or more with physical, sensory, mental/emotional or developmental disabilities can work with us to become more self-sufficient. Our intake procedures provide an orientation to the staff, facilities and services at CRS.

4409 Community Rehabilitation Services (CRS) Pasadena Office
980 N Fair Oaks Avenue
Room 16 & 17
Pasadena, CA 91103
626-794-9860
FAX: 626-794-9884

4410 Community Rehabilitation Services for Independent Living
4716 Brooklyn Avenue
Los Angeles, CA 90022
323-266-0453
FAX: 323-266-7992
e-mail: crsela@pacbell.net

Al Rivera, Director

Offer people with disabilities transportation, housing assistance, advocacy, attendant referral, peer counseling and information services. New programs include job club and independent living skills training and deaf services.

4411 Community Rehabilitation Services: Downtown Office

3325 Wilshire Boulevard
Suite 850
Los Angeles, CA 90010
323-427-9090
FAX: 323-427-0172
TTY:213-427-0173
e-mail: watu@pacbell.net

4412 Community Resources for Independence

980 Hopper Avenue
Santa Rosa, CA 95403
707-528-2745
800-528-7703
FAX: 707-528-9477
TTY:707-528-2151
e-mail: cri@cri-dove.org
www.cri-dove.org

Sandy Hobart, Executive Director

Offers peer counseling, disability education and awareness, attendant care, advocacy, housing access modification, disability law clinic, housing I&R. Serves Sonoma, Mendocino, Lake, Ukiah and Napa counties.

4413 Community Resources for Independence: Ukiah Office

1040 N State Street
Ukiah, CA 95482
707-463-8875

e-mail: cri_4@hotmail.com

4414 Community Resources for Independence: Fort Bragg Office

310 E Redwood Lane
Fort Bragg, CA 95437
707-964-6714
FAX: 707-961-1761
e-mail: Crifortbragg@excite.com

4415 Community Resources for Independence: Napa Office

1040 Main Street
Suite 301
Napa, CA 94559
707-528-0271
FAX: 707-528-0275
TTY:707-258-0274

4416 Community Resources for Independent Living Hayward

439 A Street
Hayward, CA 94541
510-881-5743
FAX: 510-881-1593
TTY:510-881-0218
e-mail: crilsvc4u@aol.com
www.cril-online.org

A resource center assisting persons with disabilities in becoming more independent

4417 DRAIL (Disability Resource Agency for Independent Living)

4555 Precissi Lane
Suite 2
Stockton, CA 95207
209-477-8143
FAX: 209-477-7730
e-mail: richard@drail.org
www.drail.org

Richard Gross, Coordinator

Provides services to meet the diverse needs of people who have a variety of disabilities in all age groups.

4418 Dayle McIntosh Center for the Disabled

150 W Cerritos Avenue
Building 4
Anaheim, CA 92805
714-772-8285
FAX: 714-772-8292
e-mail: rdevylde@pacbell.net
www.daylemcintoshcenter.org

Liz Gonzalez, Information & Referrals
Margaret Drda, Assistant Director
Anita Adams, Community Events Coordinator

Offers advocacy, counseling, attendant registry, information and referral, independent living skills training, communications, commend (medical emergency network for the deaf and children's services), housing, assistive technology, and emergency services.

4419 Dayle McIntosh Center/South County

27782 El Lazo Road
Suite 100
Laguna Niguel, CA 92677
949-643-7275
FAX: 949-643-7284
TTY:714-643-7282

Norma Vescovo, Contact
Kyle Minnis, Field Coordinator
Myvan Mguyen, Office Manager

4420 Disability Resource Agency for Independent Living: Modesto

221 McHenry Avenue
Modesto, CA 95354
209-521-7260
FAX: 209-521-4763
TTY:209-521-1425
e-mail: dwight@netfeed.com
www.drail.org

DRAIL provides services to persons with disabilities that lead to increased self-sufficiency and independent living. DRAIL's mission is to empower persons with disabilities to achieve their goals and dreams. Supports persons with disabilities that want to seek employment, live independently and feel good about themselves.

4421 Disabled Resources Center

2750 E Spring Street
Suite 100
Long Beach, CA 90806
562-427-1000
FAX: 562-427-2027
e-mail: info@drcinc.org
www.drcinc.org

Jeanette Nishikawa, Director
Dolores Nason, Associate Director

Offers peer support services, disability awareness, information on accessible housing, personal assistance services, benefits advocacy, assistive technology, socail security ticket to work and other services.

4422 FREED

508 J Street
Marysville, CA 95901
530-742-4474
FAX: 530-742-4476
TTY:530-742-4474
e-mail: tonyaar@ips.net
www.freed.org

4423 FREED Center for Independent Living

154 Hughes Road
Suite 1
Grass Valley, CA 95945
530-272-1732
FAX: 530-272-7793
e-mail: tony@freed.org
www.freed.org

Ann Guerra, Executive Director

Offers peer counseling, disability education and awareness, personal assistant care registry and information on accessible housing and assistive technology.

4424 First Step Independent Living
1174 Nevada Street
Redlands, CA 92374
800-362-0312
e-mail: cvsfs@deltanet.com

4425 IL Resource Center Fairfield
1545 Webster Street
Suite C
Fairfield, CA 94533
707-435-8174
FAX: 707-435-8177
TTY:707-435-8174
e-mail: wendy291@juno.com

4426 IL Resource of Contra Costa County
3200 Clayton Road
Concord, CA 94519
925-363-7293
FAX: 925-363-7296
e-mail: Robert@ilrccc.org

Robert LeGresley, Executive Director
Paul DeMange, Program Director
Rich Broaddus, Branch Manager

To empower people with disabilities to: control their own lives, provide advocacy and support for individuals with disabilities to live independently, create an accessible community free of physical and attitudinized barriers.

4427 IL Resource of Fairfield
1545 Webster Sat C
Fairfield, CA 94533
707-435-8174
FAX: 707-435-8177
e-mail: joanne@ilrccc.org

Joanne Bell, Executive Director
Paul DeMange, Program Director
Rich Broaddus, Branch Manager

To empower people with disabilities to: control their own lives, provide advocacy and support for individuals with disabilities to live independently, create an accessible community free of physical and attitudinal barriers.

4428 ILC Southern CA
23560 Lyons Avenue
Suite 201
Newhall, CA 91321
661-290-2569
FAX: 661-290-2569
TTY:661-290-2420

4429 Imperial Valley ILC
1450 Broadway
Suite 4
El Centro, CA 92243
760-353-4191
FAX: 760-353-4474
TTY:760-353-2802

4430 Independence Center
3640 S Sepulveda Boulevard
Suite 102
Los Angeles, CA 90034
310-202-7102
FAX: 310-202-7180
e-mail: judym@independencecenter.com
www.independencecenter.com

Judy Maizlish, Executive Director

A mainstreamed residential program teaching independent living to young adults (18-30+) with learning disabilities.

4431 Independent Living Center of Southern California
43805 Division
Suite A
Lancaster, CA 93535
661-945-6602
FAX: 661-945-5690
TTY:661-945-6604
e-mail: ilcsclanc@aol.com

Norma Vescovo, Contact

4432 Independent Living Center of Kern County
1631 30th Street
Bakersfield, CA 93301
661-325-1063
800-529-9541
FAX: 661-325-6702
e-mail: bonita.clyle@hotmail.com
www.ilcofkerncounty.org

Bonita Coyle, Contact

4433 Independent Living Center of Southern California
14354 Haynes Street
 # 103
Van Nuys, CA 91401
818-981-5000
FAX: 818-785-0330
TTY:818-988-3533
e-mail: ilcscserv1@aol.com

Cynthia Tovar, Supervisor of Services

Housing, advocacy, benefits counseling and independent living skills.

4434 Independent Living Resource Center
423 W Victoria Street
Santa Barbara, CA 93101
805-963-0595
FAX: 805-963-1350
e-mail: jblack3910@aol.com

Josephine Black, Executive Director
Kathleen Riel, Human Resources Director
Steven Wall, Peer Support

A private, nonprofit organization founded by and for persons with disabilities to assist individuals to achieve optimal levels of self-sufficiency. Services include personal assistant referrals, peer and benefits counseling, advocacy, sign language interpreter/communication services, independent living skills training, information and referrals, community education and systems advocacy, housing and employment assistance.

4435 Independent Living Resource Center: Ventura Office
1802 Eastman Avenue
Suite 112
Ventura, CA 93003
805-650-5993
FAX: 805-650-9278
e-mail: jblack@ilrc-trico.org
www.ilrc-trico.org

The ILRC Enables persons with persons with diabilites to take resposiblity for and control of their own lives to make decisions to reduce their dependence on people around them the ILRC Provides persons with disabilities the oppurtunties to develop the skills necessary to live their own lives. The ILRC Facilities independent living by making available on going support services thereby empowering persons with physical visual and or hearing disabilities to acheive self sufficiency.

4436 Independent Living Resource Center: San Francisco

649 Mission Street
3rd Floor
San Francisco, CA 94105
415-543-6222
FAX: 415-543-6318
e-mail: ilrcsf@earthlink.net
www.ilrcsf.org

Carol J Bradley, Executive Director
Herb Levine, Policy Director

ILRCSF provides a variety of services designed to assist disabled individuals to live independently. Offers independent living skills training; community living options planning, benefits counseling/advocacy for Social Security, SSI, and other government programs; peer counseling training and support groups; and self-advocacy workshops. Offers housing options counseling and housing referrals and placements.

4437 Independent Living Resource Center: Santa Maria Office

327 E Plaza Drive
Suite 3A
Santa Maria, CA 93454
805-925-0015
FAX: 805-349-2416
TTY:805-925-0015
e-mail: jblack@ilrc-trico.org
www.ilrc-trico.org

Madelena Nieto, Coordinator
Tina Horr, Benefits
Leeman Burke, Information/Referral

Peern and Benefit counseling, Independent living skills, Attendentr Recruitment/referral, American Sign language interpreting, Advocacy, housing and employment assistance information and referrals, Social Security benefit planning.

4438 Independent Living Resource Coast Country: Branch Office

1545 Webster Street
Suite Dc
Fairfield, CA 94553
707-743-8174
FAX: 707-743-8177
e-mail: joanne@ilrccc.org

JoAnne Bell, Executive Director
Paul Demange, Program Director
Rich Broaddus, Branch Manager

4439 Independent Living Resource of Contra Costa County - Antioch Office

310 W 10th Street
Antioch, CA 94509
925-754-0539

4440 Independent Living Service Northern California: Redding Office

1411 Yuba Street
Redding, CA 95001
530-242-8550
FAX: 530-241-1454
e-mail: ilsncrdg@maxinet.com

4441 Independent Living Services of Northern California

1161 E Avenue
Chico, CA 95926
530-893-8527
FAX: 530-893-8574

Jay Harris, Director of Services

Independent Living Services of Northern California is a consumer-run agency providing support services to help persons with disabilities maintain their optimal level of self-reliance and independence.

4442 Marin Center for Independent Living

1562 Cherokee Street
PO Box 151268
San Rafael, CA 94915
415-461-1440
FAX: 415-459-7047
e-mail: mcilbob@marincil.org
www.marincil.org

Bob Roberts, Executive Director

Offers peer counseling, disability education and awareness, attendant care registry and information on accessible housing.

4443 Placer Independent Resource Services

11768 Atwood Road
Suite 29
Auburn, CA 95603
530-885-6100
FAX: 530-885-3032
e-mail: tmiller@pirs.org
www.pirs.org

Independent Living Center providing advocacy and independent living services for people with disabilities in Placer, El Dorado and Alpine Counties, California.

4444 Resources for Independent Living

1211 H Street
Suite B
Sacramento, CA 95814
916-446-3074
FAX: 916-446-2443
e-mail: rIL@sna.com
www.ril-sacramento.org

Frances Gracechild, Contact

Independent living center serving Sacramento and Yolo counties.

4445 Rolling Start

570 W 4th Street
Suite 103
San Bernardino, CA 92401
909-884-2129
FAX: 909-386-7446
TTY:909-884-7396
e-mail: Fran Bates@yahoo.com
www.RollingStart.com

Claudia Hidek, Services Manager

Quarterly

4446 San Gabriel/Pomona Valley Center for Independent Living

963 W Bardille Avenue
Covina, CA 91722
626-967-0995
800-621-6722
FAX: 626-967-3132
TTY:626-967-4401
e-mail: scilcovn@tstonramp.com

Carol Lane, President/CEO
Anne Lamsden, Office Systems Manager
Rhonda Slattery, Project Manager

Cross-disability, non-profit agency providing advocacy services, housing listings, deaf services, assistive technology, peer counsiling and personal assists.

4447 Service Center for Independent Living: Covina Office

963 W Badillo Street
Covina, CA
626-967-0995
FAX: 626-967-3132
TTY:626-967-4401
e-mail: scilcovn@stonramp.com

4448 **Service Center for Independent Living**

PO Box 549
109 S Spring Street
Claremont, CA 91711
909-621-6722
FAX: 909-445-0727
TTY:909-621-0727
e-mail: scilclmt@tstonramp.com

4449 **Silicon Valley Independent Living Center: Gilroy Office**

7415 Eigleberry Street
Suite C
Gilroy, CA 95020
408-847-1805
FAX: 408-847-5595
e-mail: francesm@svilc.org
www.svilc.org

The mission of the Silicon Valley Independent Living Center is to empower prople with disabilities by providing the advocacy, training, skill development and services which enhance every individuals capabilities.

4450 **Silicon Valley Independent Living Center**

1601 Civic Center Drive
Suite 100
Santa Clara, CA 95050
408-985-1243
FAX: 408-985-067
TTY:408-985-9243
e-mail: vandanam@svilc.org

4451 **Southeast Center for Independent Living**

7830 Quill Drive
Suite D
Downey, CA 90242
562-862-6531
800-844-3089
FAX: 562-923-5274
TTY:562-869-0931
www.scrspwi.org/secil.html

Mary Rios, Executive Director
Steve Bramdt, Program Director

Offers peer counseling, disability awareness, information on accessible housing and other services to the community.

4452 **Southern California Rehabilitation Services**

7830 Quill Drive
Suite D
Downey, CA 90242
562-862-6531
FAX: 562-923-5274
TTY:562-869-0931
e-mail: scrsenid@aol.com

4453 **Through the Looking Glass**

2198 Sixth Street
Suite 100
Berkeley, CA 94710
510-848-1112
800-644-2666
FAX: 510-848-4445
e-mail: TLG@lookingglass.org
www.lookingglass.org

4454 **Tri-County Independent Living Center**

955 Myrtle Avenue
Eureka, CA 95501
707-445-8404
877-576-5000
FAX: 707-445-9751

Gay Larsen, Executive Director

Serving Humboldt, Del Norte and Trinity Counties in northern California.

4455 **Westside Center for Independent Living**

11201 S La Cienega Boulevard
Los Angeles, CA 90045
310-568-0107
FAX: 310-568-1015
TTY:310-568-0756
e-mail: wcil@aol.com
www.wcil.org

Colorado

4456 **Atlantis Community**

201 S Cherokee Street
Denver, CO 80223
303-733-9324
FAX: 303-733-6211
e-mail: terranceturner@hotmail.com
www.atlantiscommunity.net

Tim Thornton, Executive Co-Director
Terrance Turner, Executive Co-Director

Services offered Home Health Services, Support Services, Apartment Rental, and Apartment Modification.

4457 **Center for Disabilities**

1304 Berkley Avenue
Pueblo, CO 81004
719-546-1271
FAX: 719-546-1374
e-mail: ilcpueblo@yahoo.com

Larry Williams, Executive Director

4458 **Center for Independent Living**

16090 Ute Avenue
Suite 100
Grand Junction, CO 81501
970-241-0315
FAX: 970-245-3341
e-mail: cfi@gj.net
www.rmpbs.org/onourownterms/resource4.html

Mary Lynn McNutt, Contact

4459 **Center for People with Disabilities (CPWD)**

1675 Range Street
Boulder, CO 80301
303-442-8662
FAX: 303-442-0502
e-mail: info@cpwd-ilc.org
www.cpwd-ilc.org

Robert Trujillo, Deputy Director
David Bolin, Executive Director

Serving Boulder and Broomfield Counties since 1977, CPWD provides independent living services to people with disabilities.

4460 **Center on Deafness**

1490 Lafayette Street
Suite 408
Denver, CO 80203
303-839-8022
FAX: 303-839-8027
TTY:3038398022
e-mail: cod@pcisys.net
www.centerondeafness.org

Danielle Jansen

Offers sign language and oral interpreting services, sign language classes (both public and private), client services, ADA technical assistance, community education and advocacy.

4461 **Colorado Springs Independence Center**

21 E Las Animas
Colorado Springs, CO 80903 **719-471-8181**
FAX: 719-471-7829
e-mail: vickicsic@aol.com

Vicki Skoog, Director

Offers peer support, disability education and awareness, information on accessible housing, and classes on independent living.

4462 **Connections for Independent Living**

1024 - 9th Avenue
Suite E
Greeley, CO 80631 **970-330-2840**
FAX: 970-353-8058
e-mail: connectionsil!viawest.net

Beth Danielson, Executive Director

Certified IL Center, I and R advocacy, peer support, skills training, sign language interpretations, reader services, housing. Cross-disability, all ages.

4463 **Deaf Counseling Services at Mental Health Corporation of Denver**

4353 E Colfax Avenue
Denver, CO 80220 **303-504-1200**
FAX: 303-320-4830
e-mail: kmallah@mhcd.com
www.mhcd.com

Kara Mallah PhD, Program Manager

Provides conseling to deaf and hard of hearing persons who reside in Metro Denver. Our goal is to provide therapeutic service that respects the dignity, privacy, and unique needs of the person.

4464 **Denver CIL**

455 Sherman Street
Suite 140
Denver, CO 80203 **303-698-1900**

4465 **Disability Center for Independent Living**

5900 E 39th Avenue
Suite 4
Denver, CO 80207 **303-320-1345**
FAX: 303-320-1355
TTY:303-320-2330

John Pipe, Executive Director
Carol Reynolds, Deputy Director

4466 **Disabled Resource Services**

424 Pine Street
Suite 101
Fort Collins, CO 80524 **970-482-2700**
FAX: 970-407-7072
e-mail: drs@jymis.com
www.drs@fortnet.org

Nancy Jackson, Executive Director
Don Maroney, Branch Manager
Karen Hutchinson, Blind Program Administrator

Offers peer counseling, loan closet, employment assistance, information and referral, case management, volunteer coordination, equipment loan closet, advocacy, financial assistance, housing assistance, newsletter publication, and independent living skills, training to persons with disabilities to help increase their independence and quality of life.

4467 **Greeley Center for Independence**

2780 28th Avenue
Greeley, CO 80634 **970-339-2444**
800-748-1012
FAX: 970-339-0033
e-mail: gciinc.gci.org
www.gci.org

Hope Cassidy, Executive Director
Rob Rabe, Director Outpatient Services

Accessible apartments with home health care satff on site.

4468 **Martin Luther Homes: Denver**

2480 W 26th Avenue
Suite 120B
Denver, CO 80211 **303-455-8006**
FAX: 303-455-8106

Cecelia Camp, Administrator
Fred Naumann III, Communications

Providing a wide array of services to assist individuals and families in achieving positive life goals. Services to persons with disabilities and other special needs include community living options, training and employment options, spiritual growth and development options, training and counseling support.

4469 **Martin Luther Homes: Fort Collins**

109 Cameron Drive
Unit A
Fort Collins, CO 80525 **970-223-1751**
FAX: 970-223-1781
www.mlhs.com

Molly Kennis, Director

Providing a wide array of services to assist individuals and families in achieving positive life goals. Services to persons with disabilities and other special needs include community living options, training and employment options, spiritual growth and development options, training and counseling support.

4470 **Pueblo Goodwill Center for Independent Living**

250 S Santa Fe Avenue
Pueblo, CO 81003 **719-543-4483**
FAX: 719-545-5134

Bill Bolt, Director

Must be a client of DVR to be eligible for their program of independent living skills and work training skills.

4471 **Southwest Center for Independence**

801 Florida Road
Unit 3
Durango, CO 81301 **970-259-1672**
FAX: 970-259-0947
TTY:970-259-1672
e-mail: swcidur@frontier.net

Larry Wales, Executive Director

Offers peer counseling and disability education.

Connecticut

4472 **Center for Disability Rights**

764 A Campbell Avenue
W Haven, CT 06516 **203-934-7077**
FAX: 203-934-7078
TTY:203-934-7079
e-mail: CDR7077@aol.com

Marc K Gallurri, Executive Director
Carmen Conea, Information/Referral Specialist

4473 **Chapel Haven**

1040 Whalley Avenue
Westville, CT 06515
203-397-1714
FAX: 203-397-3692
www.chapelhaven.org

Judith Lefkowitz, Director Admissions

Independent living skills program that provides residential and community support services to adults with cognitive disabilities in life skills, employment, education, and recreation.

4474 **Co-Op Initiatives**

20-28 Sargeant Street
Suite 102
Hartford, CT 06105
860-724-4940
FAX: 860-724-7102
www.coopinit.org

Nichole Scappaticci, Administrative Assistant

Provides community based housing opppurtunities for people with disabilities in Connecticut.

4475 **Disabilities Network of Eastern Connecticut**

107 Route 32
North Franklin, CT 06254
860-823-1898
FAX: 860-886-2316
e-mail: dnec@snet.net

Carolyn Newcombe, Contact

4476 **Disability Resource Center of Fairfield County: Stratford Office**

80 Ferry Boulevard
Suite 210
Stratford, CT 06497
203-378-6977
FAX: 203-375-2748
TTY:203-378-3248
e-mail: info@drcfc.org
www.drcfc.org

DRCFC can assist individuals in identifying and accessing services and supports, benefits, assistive technology, housing, personal assistance serives, and other resources. DRCFC provides trianing in activities of daily living and the skills necessary for integration and full parcipation in the community for people with disabilities.

4477 **Independence Northwest Center for Independent Living**

1183 New Haven Road
Suite 200
Naugatuck, CT 06770
203-729-3299
FAX: 203-729-2839
e-mail: indnw@aol.com

Eileen Horndt, Director

Offers peer counseling, disability education and awareness.

4478 **Independence Unlimited**

151 New Park Avenue
Suite D
Hartford, CT 06106
860-523-5021
FAX: 860-523-5603
e-mail: clowindunl@aol.com

Candace Low, Executive Director

4479 **New Horizons**

37 Bliss Road
Unionville, CT 06085
860-675-4711
FAX: 860-675-4369

Michael Shaw, Contact

Services offered Housing and other support systems for the physically disabled

Delaware

4480 **Easter Seal Independent Living Center**

24 Reads Way
New Castle, DE 19720
302-324-4482
FAX: 302-324-4481
e-mail: rbrouill@inet.net

Ray Brouillette, Contact

4481 **Independent Living**

1800 N Broom Street
Wilmington, DE 19802
302-888-5900
FAX: 302-429-8034

Susan Cycyk, Director

Providing skilled support and caring guidance to adults with disabilities. Our case management services include: daily living skills training, medical coordination, transportation assistance, financial management, housing assistance, and vocational/educational planning.

Sliding Scale

4482 **Independent Resource Georgetown**

410 Bedford Street
Suite 37
Georgetown, DE 19947
302-854-9330
FAX: 302-854-9408
TTY:302-854-9340

4483 **Independent Resources**

52 Reads Way
New Castle, DE 19720
302-328-6704
FAX: 302-328-6705

4484 **Independent Resources Wilmington**

6 Denny Road
Suite 205
Wilmington, DE 19809
302-765-0191
FAX: 302-765-0195
TTY:302-765-0194
e-mail: fox205007@aol.com

4485 **Independent Resources: Dover**

32 W Loockerman Street
Suite 104
Dover, DE 19904
302-735-4599
FAX: 302-735-5623
TTY:302-735-5629
e-mail: djustice@independenceresources.org

Deborah Justice, Program Manager
Ray Hunt, Independent Living Specialist
John McNeal, Independent Living Specialist

4486 **Martin Luther Homes of Delaware**

822 Basin Road
Suite D
Newcastle, DE 19720
302-453-1933
FAX: 302-328-4795

Terry Olson, Administrator
Fred Naumann III, Communications

Providing a wide array of services to assist individuals and families in achieving positive life goals. Services to persons with disabilities and other special needs include community living options, training and employment options, spiritual growth and development options, training and counseling support.

District of Columbia

4487 Centers for Independent Living Program
Rehabilitation Services Department
Mary E Switzer Building
330 C Street SW
Washington, DC 20201 **202-619-3482**

Approximately 400 Independent Living Centers, most funded by this program, provide local services and programs to enable individuals with severe disabilities to live and function independently.

4488 DC Center for Independent Living
1345 Good Hope Road SE
Washington, DC 20020 **202-889-5802**
FAX: 202-889-1159
e-mail: dcil@aol.com
www.dccil.org

Richard A Simms, Executive Director

4489 Disability Rights Center
2500 G Street NW
Washington, DC 20007 **202-342-9439**
FAX: 202-337-4939
e-mail: crippower@aol.com

Susan Ferris, Contact

4490 District of Columbia Center for Independent Living
1400 Florida Avenue NE
Suite 3
Washington, DC 20002 **202-388-0033**
FAX: 202-398-3018
e-mail: dccil@aol.com

Richard A Simms, Executive Director

Florida

4491 Adult Day Training
Goodwill Industries-Suncoast
10596 Gandy Boulevard N
St Petersburg, FL 33702 **727-523-1512**
888-279-1988
FAX: 727-563-9300
www.goodwill-suncoast.org

An innovative program which uses job skills to teach self-help, daily living, communication, mobility, travel, decision-making, behavioral and social skills. This focus provides concrete, transferable experiences to help prepare individuals for greater community inclusion by achieving the highest possible degree of independence in their daily life, increasing their confidence and supporting their successful transitions to less structured, self-sufficient environments.

4492 CIL of Central Florida
1845 N Crystal Lake Drive
Lakeland, FL 33801 **863-701-1308**
FAX: 863-701-1309
e-mail: cilpolk@mpinet.net

4493 CIL of Florida Keys
88005 Overseas Highway
Suite 17
Islamorada, FL 33036 **305-852-0177**
FAX: 305-852-0121
e-mail: paulashea@aol.com

4494 Caring and Sharing Center for Independent Living
1130 94th Avenue N
Saint Petersburg, FL 33702 **727-577-0065**
FAX: 727-577-2932
TTY:727-576-5034
e-mail: cascil@mindspring.com

Michael Cook, Contact

4495 Cathedral Center for Independent Living
3599 University Boulevard S
Jacksonville, FL 32216 **904-399-4185**

Susan Hughes, Administrator
Offers comprehensive rehabilitation.

4496 Center for Independent Living in Central Florida - Advocacy Living Skills Peer Support
720 N Denning Drive
Winter Park, FL 32789 **407-623-1070**
877-891-6448
FAX: 407-623-1390
TTY:407-623-1000

Elizabeth Howe, Executive Director
Information and referral services, advocacy, living skills, peer support, employment.

4497 Center for Independent Living of Broward
8857 W McNab Road
Tamarac, FL 33321 **954-722-6400**
FAX: 954-722-9801
TTY:954-722-6400
e-mail: cilb@cilbroward.org

Karen Dickerhoof, Executive Director
Brenda Pizzio, Information/Referral Specialist

4498 Center for Independent Living of N Central Florida
3445 NE 24th Street
Ocala, FL 34470 **352-368-3788**
FAX: 352-629-0098
TTY:352-368-2969
e-mail: carol@cilncf.org
www.cilnwf.org

4499 Center for Independent Living of N Florida
1823 Buford Courtrive
Tallahassee, FL 32308 **850-575-9621**
800-226-9621
FAX: 850-575-5740
TTY:850-576-5245
e-mail: cilnf@nettally.com
www.cilnf.org

Janet Kahn, Executive Director
CILNF is a non-profit organization whose mission is to empower persons with disabilities to live independently and participate actively in their community.

4500 Center for Independent Living of NW Florida
3600 N Pace Boulevard
Pensacola, FL 32505 **850-595-5566**
877-245-2457
FAX: 850-595-5560
e-mail: cilnwf@cilnwf.org
www.cilnwf.org

Frank Cherry, Executive Director
Debbie Stanwood, Office Manager
We provide resources and services for people with disabilities in Escambia, Santa Rosa, Okaloosa and Walton Counties. Equipment loan, home modifications, ramps, art class and many other services.

4501 Center for Independent Living of S Florida

501 NE 1st Avenue
Suite 102
Miami, FL 33132
305-379-6650
FAX: 305-379-6653
e-mail: info@soflacil.org
www.soflacil.org

Kelly Greene, Executive Director
Ubaldo Alvarez, Program Manager
Jackie Anderson, Information/Referral Specialist

A community based non for profit, independent living center serving people of all ages with any type of disability. Services: Basic education, GED preperation, American sign language advocacy, peer support, information and referral, independent living skills training, housing assistance, transportation assistance, home modiifications, transition from nursing facility to the community assisatnace filing ADA complaints, accessibility surveys, diability awareness traing.

4502 Center for Independent Living of SW Florida

3626 Evans Avenue
Fort Myers, FL 33901
239-277-1447
888-343-6991
FAX: 941-227-1647
TTY:941-277-3964
e-mail: cilfl@mindspring.net
cilfl.org

Jim Zakas, Contact

4503 Center for Independent Technology and Education (CITE)

215 E New Hampshire Street
Orlando, FL 32804
407-896-3177
888-898-2483
FAX: 407-895-5255
e-mail: comcite@aol.com

Carol Adams, Executive Director

4504 Coalition for Independent Living Option

6800 Forest Hill Boulevard
W Palm Beach, FL 33413
561-966-4288
FAX: 561-641-6619
TTY:561-641-6538
e-mail: cilo2000@bellsouth.net
www.cilo.org

Shelly Gottsagen, Executive Director

Independent living centers offer peer counseling, advocacy, information and referral and independent living skills development. CILO offers teen programs, an adaptive equipment loan closet, disability sensitivity training and accessibility studies and services for people who are crime victims

4505 Independent Living Resource Center of Northeast Florida

2709 Art Museum Drive
Jacksonville, FL 32207
904-399-8484
888-427-4313
FAX: 904-396-0859
TTY:904-398-6322
e-mail: cilj@southeast.net
www.cilf.com

Marcia Randall, Executive Director
Pamela Williams, Office Manager
Andrea Williamson, Program Manager

Offers information/referral, advocacy, peer mentoring, independent living skills training, up to date ADA information, FIRI program, deaf consumer programs, interpreting services, and high school career choice. Serves Duval, Clay, Nassau, Flagler, St. Johns, Volusia, and Baker counties in Florida.

4506 Independent Living for Adult Blind

101 W State Street
Jacksonville, FL 32202
904-633-8220
FAX: 904-632-5107
e-mail: bsimpson@fccj.org

Becky Simpson, Project Coordinator

Offers services for the totally blind, legally blind and visually impaired. Services include independent living skills, training and guidance toward rehabilitation. Also provides vocational training in computers. Supported by government grants and private donations.

4507 Miami-Dade County Disability Services and Independent Living (DSAIL)

1335 NW 14th Street
Miami, FL 33125
305-547-5444
FAX: 305-547-7355

Paul Prevost, Director

Offers information and referral services serving all types of disabilities with the goal of assisting the disabled acquiring independence and control over their lives. Teaches independent living skills, job readiness and placement, home health care, sensitivity training, training in ASL and Braille, counsel people with disabilities or wide range of problems.

4508 North Central Florida Citrus County

3277 S Suncoast Boulevard
Homosassa, FL 34448
352-628-3600
FAX: 352-628-3600

Alma Warren, Excutive Director

4509 Northern Florida Center for Independent Living

572 Appleyard Drive
Suite C
Tallahassee, FL 32304
850-759-21
FAX: 850-575-5740
e-mail: janetkahn@nettally.com
www.cilnf.org

Janet Kahn, Contact

4510 SCCIL at Titusville

725 Deleon Avenue
Titusville, FL 32780
321-268-2244
FAX: 706-724-6729
TTY:706-724-6324
e-mail: kswoil@csranet.com

4511 Self-Reliance Center for Independent Living

11215 N Nebraska Avenue
Suite B3
Tampa, FL 33612
813-975-6560
FAX: 813-975-6559
e-mail: self-reliance@slef-reliance.org

Susan Stacey, Executive Director
Yvonne Epps, Administrative Assistant

Offers peer counseling, disability education and awareness, advocacy and other services to the community.

4512 Space Coast Center for Independent Living

331 Ramp Road
Cocoa Beach, FL 32931
321-784-9008
FAX: 321-784-3702
e-mail: sccil@bellsouth.net

Barbara Allard, Executive Director
Donna Taylor, Assistant Director

4513 **Suncoast Center for Independent Living**
1945 Northgate Boulevard
Sarasota, FL 34234 **941-351-9545**
FAX: 941-351-9875
TTY:941-351-9943
e-mail: scillori@aol.com

Daniela Szado, Executive Director

Offers information and referrals, advocacy, peer counseling, independent living skills training, equipment, loan and consultation on ADA laws.

4514 **Suncoast Center for Independent Living: Arcadia**
503 W Oak Street
Arcadia, FL 34266 **863-993-4142**
FAX: 863-993-4142

4515 **Tampa Lighthouse for the Blind**
1106 W Platt Street
Tampa, FL 33606 **813-251-2407**
FAX: 813-254-4305
e-mail: tpalight@gate.net
www.tampalighthouse.org

CE Olstrom, Executive Director

Our purpose is to maximize independence and provide employment opportunities for persons who are blind or visually impaired.

Georgia

4516 **Access Center for Independent Living**
430 Prior Street SE
Room 120
Gainesville, GA 30501 **770-534-6656**
FAX: 770-534-6626
TTY:770-534-6626
e-mail: remcgarry@earthlink.net
ilru.org/news/JobsACILGainesville.html

Robert E McGony, Executive Director
April McKrag, Independent Living Coordinator
Anna Robinson, Hispanic Outreach

To assist the disabled to learn the skills need to remain independent.

4517 **Bain**
1235 E Shotwell Street
PO Box 1674
Bainbridge, GA 31717 **229-246-0150**
FAX: 229-246-1715
TTY:800-255-0135
e-mail: bain@surfsouth.com

Virginia Harris, Contact

4518 **Disability Action Center for Georgia**
246 Sycamore Street
Suite 100
Decatur, GA 30030 **404-687-8890**
FAX: 404-687-8298
www.disabilitylink.org

Rebecca Ramage-Tuttle, Executive Director

4519 **Disability Connections**
170 College Street
Macon, GA 31201 **478-741-1425**
800-745-2117
FAX: 478-743-8359
e-mail: dcinfocoordinator@aol.com

Krista King, Information & Referral Coord.
Jerilyn Leverett, Executive Director

Anon profit residential center for independent living serving severving counties in center CA.

4520 **Disability LINK**
755 Commerece Drive
Suite 415
Decatur, GA 30030 **404-687-8890**
FAX: 404-687-8298
TTY:404-687-9175
e-mail: rrtuttle@disabilitylink.org

4521 **Division of Rehabilitation Services**
410 Mall Boulevard
Suite B
Savannah, GA 31406
FAX: 912-691-6816

Allen Beall, Regional Director

Vocational rehabilitation services.

4522 **Georgia Field Services Independent Living Program**
3125 Presidential Parkway
Atlanta, GA 30340 **770-452-9601**

Pat Puckett, Director

Offers disability education, attendant care registry and information on housing.

4523 **Georgia's SILC**
1431 McLendeon Drive
Suite C
Decatur, GA 30033 **770-270-6860**
FAX: 770-270-5957
TTY:770-452-7087
e-mail: silc@mindspring.com

4524 **Living Independently for Everyone (LIFE)**
17-21 E Travis Street
Savannah, GA 31406 **912-920-2419**
FAX: 912-920-0007
e-mail: hodgep@mindspring.com

Pamela Hodge, Contact

4525 **North District Independent Living Program**
311 Green Street NW
Suite 209
Gainesville, GA 30501

Sharon McCurry, Coordinator

Information and referral, advocacy, peer counseling, service coordination and ADA consultation.

4526 **Roosevelt Warm Springs Institute for Rehabilitation**
PO Box 1000
Warm Springs, GA 31830 **706-655-5000**
FAX: 706-655-5011
www.rooseveltrehab.org

Frank Ruzycki, Executive Director
Martin Harmon, Public Relations Director
Carolyn McKinley, Director Organization Dev.

Comprehensive medical rehabilitation is offered for brain injury, spinal cord injury, stroke, diabetic foot care, post-polio syndrom and rehab technology, as well as vocational rehabilitations.

4527 Southeastern PVA

US Highway 1
4010 Deans Bridge Road
Hephzibah, GA 30815 **404-921-5822**
FAX: 404-921-5822

4528 Southwest District Independent Living Program

PO Box 1606
Albany, GA 31702 **229-430-4170**
FAX: 229-430-4466

Bill Layton, Director

Offers peer counseling, disability education and awareness, attendant care registry, and information on accessible home for the disabled.

4529 Walton Option for Independent Living

948 Walton Way
Augusta, GA 30901 **706-724-6262**
FAX: 706-724-6729
TTY:706-724-6262
e-mail: tjohnson@walteroptions.org
www.waltonoptions.org

Tiffany Johnston, Contact

Services include advocacy, assistive technology services, braille instruction, community education, home modifications, orientation and mobility services, peer support, and return to work services

Hawaii

4530 Center for Independent Living: E Hawaii

400 Hualani Street
Suite 16D
Hilo, HI 96720 **808-935-3777**
FAX: 808-961-6737
e-mail: cileh@interpac.net
www.hcil.org

Laura Tobosa, Branch Coordinator

Provides an array of support services for people with all types of disabilities of any age.

4531 Hawaii Centers for Independent Living

414 Kuwili Street
Suite 102
Honolulu, HI 96817 **808-522-5400**
FAX: 808-522-5427
TTY:808-536-3739
e-mail: mobatake@diverseabilities.org
www.hcil.org

Mark Obatake, Executive Director

Living arrangments, personal care, assistive technology, mobility, acessibility, income, transportation, vacation, recreation, and interpersonal relationships are all parts of independent living In essence, the vast majority of HCIL consumers are able to make the transition to increase personal choices and a higher quality of life

4532 Kailua Kona Center for Independent Living: West Hawaii

PO Box 2197
Kealakekua, HI 96750 **808-323-2221**
FAX: 808-323-4250

Morel Martin, Branch Office Director

A nonprofit organization run by and for persons with disabilities. Information on housing referrals, financial benefits, advocacy, personal care attendants, services for elderly blind, and independent living skills counseling. Services are free to all disabled persons.

4533 Kauai Center for Independent Living

PO Box 3529
Lihue, HI 96766 **808-245-4034**
FAX: 808-245-7218
e-mail: kcil@mail.aloha.net

Humberto Blanco, Administrator
Teri Yamashiro, IL Specialist
Gordon Dodd, ILF Counselor

Offers peer counseling, disability education and attendant care registry.

4534 Maui Center for Independent Living

1446-D Lower Main Street
Wailuku, HI 96793 **808-242-4966**
FAX: 808-244-6978
e-mail: mcilogg@qte.net

Ruth Hamilton, Administrator

Offers disability education and awareness, advocacy and counseling.

Idaho

4535 American Falls Office: Living Independently for Everyone (LIFE)

223 Harrison Street
American Falls, ID 83211 **208-226-2673**
FAX: 208-226-2673
www.idaholifecenter.org

Dean Nielson, Executive Director

4536 Dawn Enterprises

PO Box 388
Blackfoot, ID 83221 **208-785-5890**
FAX: 208-785-3095
e-mail: dawnent2@if.rmci.net
www.orgsites.com/id/dawnent

Donna Butler, Executive Director

4537 Disability Action Center

1323 E Sherman Avenue
Suite 7
Coeur d'Alene, ID 83814 **208-664-9896**
800-854-9500
FAX: 208-666-1362
e-mail: dac@icehouse.net
www.dacsc.org

Michelle Portere, Independent Living Specialist
Mark Leeper, Executive Director
Amy Dreps, Independent Living Coordinator

4538 Disability Action Center NW

124 E 3rd Street
Moscow, ID 83843 **208-883-0523**
FAX: 208-883-0524
e-mail: dac@moscow.com
www2.state.id.us/silc/dacn.htm

Mark Leeper, Executive Director
Donn Lestage, Satellite Office Coordinator
Krista Kramer, Independent Living Specialist

Information and referrals, accessibility consultant, advocacy, personal care attendant registry, peer support groups, counseling and recreation opportunities and skills training. Also provides assistive technology services and information. *$45.00*

4539 Idaho Commission for the Blind and Visually Impaired

341 W Washington Street
PO Box 83720
Boise, ID 83720 **208-334-3220**
800-542-8688
FAX: 208-334-2963
e-mail: mgraham@icbvi.state.id.us
www.icbvi.state.id.us

Michael Graham, Administrator
Mike Blackaller, Rehab Services Chief

Provides medical, counseling, education, training and other services needed to prepare for the working world and independent living.

4540 Idaho Falls Office: Living Independently for Everyone (LIFE)

2120 Rollandet Avenue
Idaho Falls, ID 83402 **208-529-8610**
FAX: 208-529-6804
e-mail: eici@ida.net
www.idaholifecenter

Dean Nielson, Executive Director

4541 LINC Canyon County

317 Happy Day Boulevard
Suite 130
Caldwell, ID 83605 **208-455-5511**
FAX: 208-455-5515
e-mail: lincc3info@aol.com
www.2.state.id.us/silc/linc.htm

4542 LINC-Satellite Office

1002 Shoshone Street E
Twin Falls, ID 83301 **208-733-1712**

Dennis McDermott, Director

Offers peer counseling, disability education and information on accessible housing.

4543 Life

2110 Rollandet Avenue
Idaho Falls, ID 83402 **208-529-8610**
FAX: 208-529-6804
TTY:208-529-8610
e-mail: eici@ida.net
www.idaholifecenter.org

Dean Nielson, Executive Director

Provides peer counseling, disability education, attendant care registry and information and referral services to the disabled.

4544 Living Independence Network Corporation: Twin Falls Satellite

132 Main Avenue S
Twin Falls, ID 83301 **208-733-1712**
FAX: 208-733-7711
e-mail: mheinrich@lincidaho.org
www.lincidaho.org

Roger Howard, Executive Director
Melva Heinrich, Resource Director

A non-profit organizaition, empowers people with disabilities to achieve their desired level of independence.

4545 Living Independence Network Corporation

2500 Kootenai Street
Boise, ID 83705 **208-336-3335**
FAX: 208-384-5037
e-mail: info@lincidaho.org
www.lincidaho.org

Roger Howard, Executive Director

A non-profit organizaition, empowers people with disabilities to achieve their desired level of independence.

4546 Living Independence Network Corporation: Canyon County Satelite

2922 E Cleveland Boulevard
Suite 800
Caldwell, ID 83605 **208-454-5511**
FAX: 208-454-5515
e-mail: amausling@lincidaho.org
www.lincidaho.org

Roger Howard, Executive Director
Amber Mausling, Advocacy Director

A non-profit organizaition, empowers people with disabilities to achieve their desired level of independence.

4547 Living Independent for Everyone (LIFE): Pocatello Office

PO Box 4185
845 W Center
Pocatello, ID 83201 **208-232-2747**
FAX: 208-232-2753
e-mail: dean@if.rmci.net
www.idaholifecenter.org

4548 Living Independently for Everyone (LIFE): Blackfoot Office

67 N Maple
PO Box 86
Blackfoot, ID 83221 **208-785-9648**
FAX: 208-785-9648
e-mail: bfoot@ida.net
www.idaholifecenter.org

Dean Nielson, Executive Director
Sheila Jones, Independent Living Advisor

4549 Living Independently for Everyone: Burley

2311 Park Avenue
Suite 7
Burley, ID 83318 **208-678-7705**
FAX: 208-678-7771
TTY:208-678-7705
e-mail: lifespan@cyberhyway.net
www.idaholifecenter.org

Dean Nielson, Executive Director

4550 Southwestern Idaho Housing Authority

1108 W Finch Drive
Nampa, ID 83651 **208-467-7461**
FAX: 208-463-1772

Jeanne Troutner, Contact

Illinois

4551 Access Living of Metro Chicago

614 W Roosevelt Road
Chicago, IL 60607 **312-253-7000**
FAX: 312-253-7001
TTY:312-253-7002
e-mail: generalinfo@accessliving.org

Marca Bristo, Contact

4552 **Center for Comprehensive Services**
306 W Mill Street
Carbondale, IL 62901
618-529-3060
800-582-4227
FAX: 618-457-5372
e-mail: sandy.boston@thementornetwork.com
www.thementornetwork.com

Sandra Boston, National Director of Admissions

Post-acute rehabilitation services for adults and adolescents with acquired brain injuries. Residential, day-treatment and out-patient services tailored to individual needs.

4553 **Central Illinois Center for Independent Living**
614 W Glen Avenue
Peoria, IL 61614
309-682-3500
877-501-9808
FAX: 309-682-3989
e-mail: jmiller@cicil.org
www.cicil.org

John Miller, Executive Director
Todd Browning, Community Realtions Director

Offers peer counseling, disability education, advocacy services, independent living skills training, interpreter referral program, TTY distribution program, deaf community services, personal assistant program, community reintegration program, transition resources program, and accessibility audits.

4554 **Community Residential Alternative**
Coleman Tri-County Services
100 W Walnut Street
Harrisburg, IL 62946
618-252-3204
FAX: 618-252-0884
e-mail: cracts6@shawneelink.net

Samantha Austin, Coordinator

Six bed group home that provides a residential alternative for the developmentally disabled adult. This program is designed to promote independence in daily living skills, economic self-sufficiency, and integration into the community.

4555 **Cornerstone Services**
777 Joyce Road
Joliet, IL 60436
815-741-7603
FAX: 815-723-1177
e-mail: jhogan@cornerstoneservices.org
www.cornerstoneservices.org

James A Hogan, President/CEO
Matthew Lanove, Director of PR
Susan Murphy, Director of Human Resources

Cornerstone Services provides progressive, comprehensive services for people with disabilities, promoting choice, dignity and the opportunity to live and work in the community. Established in 1969, the agency provides developmental, vocational, residential and behavior health services.

4556 **DuPage Center for Independent Living**
739 Roosevelt Road, Suite 109
Building 8
Glen Ellyn, IL 60137
630-469-2300
FAX: 630-469-2606
e-mail: DuPagecil@aol.com
www.glen-ellyn.com/dcil

Gregg Newberry MA, Executive Director

4557 **Fox River Valley Center for Independent Living**
730 W Chicago Street
Elgin, IL 60123
847-695-5818
FAX: 847-695-5892
e-mail: frvcil@mindspring.com
www.frvcil.com

Cindy Ciancio-Wallace, CEO
Kristen Sensor, Community Outreach Coordinator

Provides services to people with disabilities in Kane, Kendall and McHenry counties. Our non-residential agency provides independent living skills training, advocacy, information and referral and housing services. Also provides technical assistance to businesses and agencies to work with people with disabilities.

4558 **Gaining Access to IL**
205 N 4th Street
PO Box 486
Effingham, IL 62401
217-342-7110
FAX: 217-347-2562

4559 **Illinois Department of Rehab Services**
623 E Adams Street
Springfield, IL 62705
217-782-9689
FAX: 217-254-7549

4560 **Illinois Valley Center for Independent Living**
12 Gunia Drive
LaSalle, IL 61301
815-224-3126
FAX: 815-224-3567
TTY:815-224-8271
e-mail: ivcil@ivnet.com
www.ivnet.com

4561 **Illinois/Iowa Center for Independent Living**
PO Box 6156
Rock Island, IL 61204
563-324-1460
FAX: 563-324-1036
e-mail: iicil@revealed.net
www.iicil.com

Elizabeth Sherwin, Contact

A non-residential service and advocacy program for people with disabilities.

4562 **Impact Center for Independent Living**
2735 E Broadway
Alton, IL 62002
618-462-1411
FAX: 618-474-5309

Dick Goodwin, Executive Director

Offers peer counseling, disability education and awareness.

4563 **Jacksonville Area Center for Independent Living**
60 E Central Park Plaza
Jacksonville, IL 62650
217-245-8371
888-317-3287
FAX: 217-245-1872
e-mail: info@jacil.org
www.jacil.org

Becky McGinnis, Executive Director
Lori Shipley, Program Director

4564 **LIFE Center for Independent Living**

2201 Eastland Drive
Suite 1
Bloomington, IL 61704 **309-663-5433**
888-543-3245
FAX: 309-663-7024
TTY:309-663-0054
e-mail: lifecil@lifcil.org
www.lifecil.org

Gail Kear, Executive Director
Karen Turner, Director Community Education

Disability advocacy, information & referral, independent living skills training, peer counseling, sign language interpreter referrals, braille & alternate formats, equipment loan. Services people with disabilities and their families and friends in DeWitt, Ford, Livingston, and McLean Counties in Illinois.

4565 **Lake County Center for Independent Living**

706 E Hawley Street
Mundelein, IL 60060 **847-949-0060**
FAX: 847-949-4445

Lorie Clark, Executive Director

Offers peer counseling, disability education and advocacy services.

4566 **Living Independently Now Center (LINC)**

120 E A Street
Belleville, IL 62220 **618-235-9988**
FAX: 618-235-9244
TTY:618-235-0451
e-mail: linccil@apic.net
www.lincinc.org

John Laker, Executive Director

4567 **Mosaic-Pontiac**

725 W Madison Street
Pontiac, IL 61764 **815-842-4166**
FAX: 815-842-4053

Rod Patterson, Executive Director

Providing a wide array of services to assist individuals and families in achieving positive life goals. Services to persons with disabilities and other special needs include community living options, training and employment options, spiritual growth and development options, training and counseling support.

4568 **Northwestern Illinois Center for Independent Living**

229 1st Avenue
Suite 2
Rock Falls, IL 61074 **815-625-7860**
888-886-4245
FAX: 815-625-7876
TTY:815-625-7863
e-mail: kfischer@essex1.com
www.incil.org

Cilvia Rivera, Program Director
Kathy Fischer, Executive Director

Provides services to people with disabilities. Services provided include information and referral, skills training, peer counseling, site accessibility surveys, personal assistant referral interpreters, and support groups.

4569 **Office of Rehabilitation Services**

Department of Human Services
100 S Grand Avenue E
Springfield, IL 62762 **217-524-7551**
800-843-6154
FAX: 217-558-4270
e-mail: ilvr@rehabnetwork.org
www.state.il.us/agency/dhs

Rob Kilbury, Associate Director

Provides medical, therapeutic and counseling services for the disabled, as well as employment services. TTY #: 800-447-6404

4570 **Opportunities for Access: A Center for Independent Living**

4206 Williamson Place
Suite 3
Mt Vernon, IL 62864 **618-244-9212**
800-938-7400
FAX: 618-244-9310
e-mail: info@ofacil.org
www.ofacil.org

Michael Spud Egbert, Executive Director

Serves, trains and provides information to persons with disabilities, family members and significant others and service providers. Services include: advocacy, information and referral, peer support, skills training, volunteer programs and other related services. Services are free. A cross disability community based, nonresidential, nonprofit organization serving Clinton, Edwards, Hamilton, Jefferson, Marion, Wabash, Washington, Wayne and White Counties in Southern Illinois.

4571 **Options Center for Independent Living: Bourbonnais**

22 Heritage Drive
Suite 107
Bourbonnais, IL 60914 **815-936-0100**
FAX: 815-936-0117
TTY:815-936-0132
e-mail: options@daily-journal.com
www.idhhc.state.il.us/signLanguage/cil.htm

Kathy Jackson, Executive Director

Promotes independent living for people with disabilities in Kankakee and Iroquis counties in Illinois. Offered free of charge are: advocacy information and referral, peer support, independent living skills training, personal assistant training and referral, community reintergration, elderly blind program, youth advocacy, free equipment/assistive technology loan, TTY training and distribution, and sign language interpreter referral.

4572 **Options Center for Independent Living: Wat seka**

130 Laird Littelfuse Road
Suite 103
Watseka, IL 60970 **815-432-1332**
FAX: 815-432-1360
TTY:815-432-4361
e-mail: options@daily-journal.com
www.idhc.state.il.us/signLanguage/cil.htm

Promotes independent living for people with disabilities in Kankakee and Iroquis counties in Illinois. Offered free of charge are: advocacy information and referral, peer support, independent living skills training, personal assistant training and referral, community reintergration, elderly blind program, youth advocacy, free equipment/assistive technology loan, TTY training and distribution, and sign language interpreter referral.

4573 **PACE Center for Independent Living**
1317 E Florida Avenue
Urbana, IL 61801 **217-344-5433**
FAX: 217-344-2414
TTY:217-344-5024
e-mail: nmch@pacecil.org
www.incil.org

Nancy McClellen-Hickey, Executive Director
Barb Pritchard, Director Programs

Services for people with disabilities, PACE supports efforts to achieve or maintain independence. *$10.00*

8-10 pages

4574 **Progress Center for Independent Living**
400 Forest Boulevard
Park Forest, IL 60466 **708-748-1630**
FAX: 708-748-1630
e-mail: progress@theramp.net

Diane Coleman, Executive Director
Nic Steehout, Program Director

Offers peer counseling, attendant registry, information and referral services, advocacy, independent living skills, paid internships, housing assistance, national headquarters of Not Dead Yet.

4575 **RAMP Regional Access & Mobility Project**
202 Market Street
Rockford, IL 61107 **815-968-7467**
FAX: 815-968-7612
e-mail: rampcil@rampcil.org
www.rampcil.org

Julie Bosma, Executive Director
Lydia Grzywa, Marketing Coordinator

Provides services and advocacy for people with disabilities. Services include information and referral, personal assistant services, sign language interpreters, 24 hour emergency sign language service, bus training, peer counseling, independent living skills training, accessibility assessments and information on the Americans with Disabilities Act (ADA) serving Boone, DeKalb, Stephenson and Winnebago counties in north central Illinois.

4576 **Southern Illinois Center for Independent Living**
100 N Glenview
PO Box 627
Carbondale, IL 62903 **618-457-3318**
FAX: 618-549-0132
e-mail: sicilccc@aol.com

Bonnie Vaughn, Director

Services include: advocacy, skills training, peer counseling, information and referral, elderly blind, deaf services, personal attendant screening, community reintegration programs, limited transportation services and supported employment services.

4577 **Soyland Access to Independent Living (SAIL)**
2545 Millikin Parkway
Suite 1305
Decatur, IL 62526 **217-876-8888**
800-358-8080
FAX: 217-876-7245
TTY:217-876-9850
e-mail: sail@midwest.net
www.incil.org

Bill Rienzle, Executive Director

4578 **Springfield Center for Independent Living**
426 W Jefferson Street
Springfield, IL 62702 **217-523-2587**
FAX: 217-523-0427
www.incil.org

Peter Robinson, Director
Pete Roberts, Contact

4579 **Stone-Hayes Center for Independent Living**
39 N Prairie Street
Galesburg, IL 61401 **309-344-1306**
888-347-4245
FAX: 309-344-1305
TTY:309-344-1269
e-mail: stonehayes@gellatinriver.net
www.incil.org

Catherine Holland, Executive Director

4580 **West Central Illinois Center for Independent Living**
406 N 24th Street
Durst Building, Suite 3
Quincy, IL 62301 **217-223-0400**
FAX: 217-223-0475
e-mail: wcicil@adams.net
www.incil.org

Madeline Bikus, Contact

4581 **Will Grundy Center for Independent Living**
2415A W Jefferson Street
Joliet, IL 60435 **815-723-2928**
FAX: 815-729-3697
e-mail: wil.grundy.c.i.l.juno.com

Pam Heavens, Director

Information and referral services.

Indiana

4582 **Assistive Technology Training & Information Center (ATTIC)**
1721 Washington Avenue
Vincennes, IN 47591 **812-886-0575**
800-962-8842
FAX: 812-886-1128
TTY:812-886-1128
e-mail: inatticl@aol.com
www.theattic.org

Pat Stewart, Executive Director

4583 **Damar Homes**
PO Box 41
Camby, IN 46113 **317-856-5201**
FAX: 317-856-2333

Greg Johnson, Executive Director

Providers of residential services: developmental center, group homes and alternative family homes.

4584 **Everybody Counts Center for Independent Living**
9111 Broadway, Suite A
Broadfield Center
Merrillville, IN 46410 **219-769-5055**
888-769-3636
FAX: 219-769-5325
TTY:219-756-3323
e-mail: ecount@netnitco.net

Teresa Torres, Executive Director
Emas Bennett, Assistant Director

4585 **Four Rivers Resource Services**

PO Box 249
Highway 59 S
Linton, IN 47441 **812-847-2231**
FAX: 812-847-8836
e-mail: fourrivers@frrs.org
www.frrs.org

Lyna Landis, Marketing Coordinator

4586 **Independent Living Center of Eastern Indiana (ILCEIN)**

WorkOne Center
3771 S A Street
Richmond, IN 47374 **765-939-9226**
877-939-9226
FAX: 765-966-3431
TTY:765-966-3431
e-mail: ilcein@ruraltek.com

Ed Bell, Executive Director
Christi Gigliotti, Administrative Director

Information and referrals for people with disabilities.

4587 **Indiana SILC, Indiana Council on Independent Living (ICOIL)**

402 W Washington Street, Suite W453
PO Box 7083
Indianapolis, IN 46207 **317-232-1303**
800-545-7763
FAX: 317-232-6478
TTY:317-232-1427
e-mail: nyoung@fssa.state.in.us

Nancy Young, Program Director
Al Tolbert, SILC Chairperson

4588 **Indianapolis Resource Center for Independent Living**

2110 N Capitol Avenue
Indianapolis, IN 46202 **317-596-6440**
FAX: 317-596-6446
e-mail: ircil@direct.net

Melissa Madill, Co-Executive Director
David Scott, Information/Referral
Emma Lewis Sullivan, Co-Executive Director

Offers advocacy, information and referral services, independent living skills training, peer counseling, supported employment services and information on the Americans with Disabilities Act.

4589 **League for the Blind and Disabled**

5800 Fairfield Avenue
Suite 210
Fort Wayne, IN 46807 **260-745-5491**
800-889-3443
FAX: 260-744-2202
TTY:800-889-3443
e-mail: 1bdfw@ctlnet.com
www.the-league.org

David Nelson, Executive Director
John Guingrich, Program Director

Peer counseling, education, advocacy services training and support, independent living skills training, assistive equipment loaner program, youth services, orientation and mobility training, information and referral, disability awareness, Braille transcription, Center for Independent living, and public education.

4590 **Martin Luther Homes of Indiana**

PO Box 7057
Terre Haute, IN 47802 **812-235-3399**
FAX: 812-235-1590
e-mail: thaute@mlhs.com
www.mlhs.com

Anita Bean, Administrator

Providing a wide array of services to assist individuals and families in achieving positive life goals. Services to persons with disabilities and other special needs include community living options, training and employment options, spiritual growth and development options, training and counseling support.

4591 **Southern Indiana Center for Independent Living**

3300 W 16th Street
Stone City Mall
Bedford, IN 47421 **812-277-9626**
FAX: 812-277-9628
e-mail: sicil@tima.com

Albert Tolbert, Executive Director
Denise Mullis, Assistant Director

4592 **Wabash Independent Living Center & Learning Center (WILL)**

Meadow Center
Suite 7J
Terre Haute, IN 47803 **812-232-9455**
877-915-9455
FAX: 812-234-1536
TTY:877-915-9455
e-mail: info@thewillcenter.org
www.thewillcenter.org

Teresa Mager, Executive Director

The WILL Center is a nonprofit community based, nonresidential organization that is run by and for people with disabilities The WILL Center provides Systems Advocacy Information and Referral Independent Living Skills Training, Assistance in fionding anf obtaining affordable housing, Infromation on the Americans with Disabilities Act, and Assistive Technology Infromation

Iowa

4593 **Black Hawk Center for Independent Living**

312 Jefferson Street
Waterloo, IA 50701 **319-291-7755**
FAX: 319-291-7781
TTY:319-232-3955
e-mail: bhcil@cedarnet.org
www.blackhawkcenter.org

Jane Nelson-Kuhn, Executive Director

4594 **Central Iowa Center for Independent Living**

655 Walnut Street
Suite 131
Des Moines, IA 50309 **515-243-1742**
888-503-2287
FAX: 515-243-5385
e-mail: cicil@raccoon.com
www.raccoon.com/~cicil

Robert Jeppesen, Director
Frank Strong, Assistant Director Programs

A non-residential, consumer controlled, community based organization assisting people with disabilities who seek to live independently within the community. Provides independent living skills training, peer support, advocacy and self advocacy training and information and referral services. Publishes a quarterly newsletter.

4595 **Hope Haven**
1800 19th Street
Rock Valley, IA 51247
712-476-2737
FAX: 712-476-2802
www.hopehaven.org

David VanNingen, Executive Director

Purpose is to assist persons with mental/physical/emotional disabilities to reach their potential based on Biblical convictions. Services group homes, supervised apartments, and vocational employment services.

4596 **Independent Living: Iowa**
20 E Market Street
Iowa City, IA 52245
319-337-3400
FAX: 319-338-8385
e-mail: connerctr@aol.com

Ethel Madison, Executive Director

An independent living center, non-profit, nonresidential, consumer run, community based. The center assists individuals with disabilities to maintain control over day to day activities and to advocate for themselves in order to achieve greater independence and full participation in an integrated society.

4597 **League of Human Dignity**
1417 1/2 W Broadway
Council Bluffs, IA 51501
712-323-6863
FAX: 712-323-6811
e-mail: cinfo@leagueofhumandignity.com
www.leagueofhumandignity.com

Christy Solomon, Director
Nancy Hansen, Secretary

4598 **Martin Luther Homes of Iowa**
445 7th Avenue SE
Waukon, IA 52172
563-568-3992
FAX: 563-568-3992

Mary Lynn ReVoir, Administrator
Fred Naumann III, Communications

Providing a wide array of services to assist individuals and families in achieving positive life goals. Services to persons with disabilities and other special needs include community living options, training and employment options, spiritual growth and development options, training and counseling support.

4599 **South Central Iowa Center for Independent Living**
500 High Avenue W e E
Suite 301
Oskaloosa, IA 52577
641-672-1867
FAX: 641-672-1867
e-mail: scicil@kdsi.net
www.welcome.to/scicil

Nika Naylor, Contact

4600 **Three Rivers Center for Independent Living**
505 6th Street
Suite 504
Sioux City, IA 51101
712-258-2657
FAX: 712-255-1065
e-mail: bjdenny@aol.com

Brenda Denney, Contact

Kansas

4601 **Coalition for Independence**
3738 State Avenue
Kansas City, KS 66102
913-321-5140
FAX: 913-321-5182
TTY:913-321-5216
e-mail: mail@cfi-kc.org
www.cfi-kc.org

Tom Lally, Executive Director
Jason Nicol, Marketing Director

Publishes monthly newsletter - Keys to Independence. State os KS designated, nonresidential, private center for independent living addressing the unmet needs of PWD.

4602 **Coalition for Independence Leavenworth County**
1281 Eisenhower
Leavenworth, KS 66048
913-250-0287
FAX: 913-250-0167
TTY:913-631-8877
e-mail: kolson@cfikc.org
www.cfi-kc.org

Kathy Olson, Independent Living Counselor

Center for Independent Living provides services for people with disabilities, family memebers and caregivers, as well as accessibility services for businesses.

4603 **Cowley County Developmental Services**
Arkansas City, KS 67005
620-442-7777

Martha Crane, Director

Offers peer counseling, attendant care registry and other services to the community.

4604 **Independence**
2001 Haskell Avenue
Lawrence, KS 66046
785-841-0333
888-824-7277
FAX: 785-841-1094
e-mail: webmaster@indpendenceinc.org
www.independenceinc.org

Susan Mikesic, Community Coordinator

Services include individual and systems advocacy, assistance obtaining benefits, technical assistance, housing, assistance with modifications for accessibility, counseling, peer support, microcomputer training, transportation, community outreach and education, business management services for persons using attendants, a resource library, independent living skills training, assistive technology, information and referral, human diversity workshops and volunteer involvement.

4605 **Independent Connection**
1710 W Schilling Road
Salina, KS 67401
755-827-9383
800-526-9731
FAX: 785-823-2015

Offers peer counseling, disability education, independent living skills training advocacy, information and referrals, attendant care registry and information on accessible housing.

4606 **Independent Living Center of Northeast Kan sas**
PO Box 292
Atchinson, KS 66002
913-367-1830
FAX: 913-367-1430
TTY:913-367-1830
e-mail: ilcnek@journey.com

4607 **Independent Living Resource Center**
3330 W Douglas Avenue
Wichita, KS 67203
316-942-6300
FAX: 316-942-2078
e-mail: jweigel@hit.net

Judy Weigel, Executive Director

4608 **Kansas Services for the Blind & Visually Impaired**
2601 SW E Circle Drive N
Topeka, KS 66606
785-296-3311
FAX: 785-291-3138

Dianne Hemphill, Administrator

Offers peer counseling, advocacy and other services to the community.

4609 **LINK**
2401 E 13th Street
Hays, KS 67601
785-625-6942
FAX: 785-625-2334
e-mail: batívell@eaglecom.net
www.linkinc.org

Brian Atwell, Director

Offers personal care attendants, independent living skills instruction, adaptive equipment, community involvement and peer support, legal advocacy, interpreting services, recreation, transportation, HCBS services, and support groups.

4610 **Osage City Resource Center for Independent Living**
PO Box 257
Osage City, KS 66523
785-528-3105
FAX: 785-528-3665
e-mail: mary@rcilinc.org

Mary Holloway, Contact

4611 **Prairie Independent Living Resource Center**
915 S Main Street
Hutchinson, KS 67501
620-663-3989
888-715-6818
FAX: 620-663-4711
e-mail: pilr@southwind.net
hubris.net/ilarc.org

Christine Owens, Director

4612 **Resource Center for Independent Living- Fort Scott**
1417 South Judson
Fort Scott, KS 66701
620-223-3594
800-580-7245
FAX: 620-224-2085

Mary Holloway, CEO

4613 **Resource Center for Independent Living - Eldorado**
615 N Main Street
Eldorado, KS 67042
316-322-7853
FAX: 316-322-7888
www.rcilinc.org

4614 **Resource Center for Independent Living - Overland Park**
9948 W 87th Street
Suite G1
Overland Park, KS 66212
913-385-9088
FAX: 913-385-1665

4615 **Resource Center for Independent Living - Atchinson**
117 N Fifith Street
Atchinson, KS 66002
913-367-5353
888-509-7245
FAX: 913-367-6373
www.rcilinc.org

Cladette Buchanan, ILC, ILS
Robin Hennigh, ILC ILS

4616 **Resource Center for Independent Living Arkansas City**
115 E 5th Avenue
Arkansas City, KS 67005
620-442-0775
FAX: 620-442-3173
e-mail: rcil@hit.net
www.rcilinc.org

4617 **Resource Center for Independent Living: Iola**
PO Box 602
Iola, KS 66749
620-365-8144
FAX: 620-365-7726

4618 **Resource Center for Independent Living: Ot tawa**
1320 Sash Street
Suite 205
Ottawa, KS 66067
785-242-1805
FAX: 785-242-1448
www.rcilinc.org

4619 **Resource Ctr. for Independent Living - Burlington**
410 Cumberland
Burlington, KS 66839
620-364-2263
FAX: 620-364-2700

4620 **Resource Ctr. for Independent Living: Emporia**
625 Merchant
Room 238
Emporia, KS 66801
620-342-1648
FAX: 620-342-1821
www.rcilinc.org

4621 **Southeast Kansas Independent Living: Yates Center**
119 W Butler
Yates Center, KS 66783
620-625-2818
FAX: 620-625-2585

4622 **Southeast Kansas Independent Living**
PO Box 1035
Parsons, KS 67357
620-421-5502
FAX: 620-421-3705
e-mail: skil@terraworld.net
www.hubris.net

4623 **Southeast Kansas Independent Living: Pittsburgh**
104 W Sixth Street
Pittsburgh, KS 66762
620-231-6780
FAX: 620-231-5920
www.hubris.com

4624 **Southeast Kansas: Chanute**
222 W Main
Suite D
Chanute, KS 66720
620-431-0757
FAX: 620-431-7274

4625 **Southeast Kansas: Fredonia**
305 N Sixth
Fredonia, KS 66736
620-378-4881
FAX: 620-378-4851

4626 **Southwest Kansas Center for Independent Living**
111 N Grant Street
Garden City, KS 67846
620-276-1900
FAX: 620-271-0200
e-mail: cilswks@gcnet.com
www.ilarc.org

Troy Horton, Contact

4627 **Three Rivers Independent Living**
PO Box 664
Wamego, KS 67804
785-456-9915
800-555-3994
FAX: 785-456-9923
e-mail: egerte@mail.midusa.net
www.threeriversinc.org

Audrey Schremmer-Philip, Executive Director

Non-profit organization that assists people with all types of disabilities, of all income levels, to reach their personal goals and live as independently as possible.

4628 **Three Rivers Independent Living Center**
PO Box 33
Clay Center, KS 67432
785-632-6117
FAX: 785-632-3105
e-mail: 3rivers@bluevalley.net
www.angelfire.com/il/threeriversilrc

Audrey Schremmer-Philip, Contact

4629 **Three Rivers Independent Living Center: Centralia**
PO Box 236
Centralia, KS 66415
785-857-3521
FAX: 785-857-3521
e-mail: 3 rivers@bluevalley.net

4630 **Three Rivers Independent Resource Center**
323 Poyntz Avenue
2nd Floor
Manhattan City, KS 66502
785-537-8985
FAX: 785-537-3435
e-mail: lori@threeriversinc.org
www.threeriversinc.org

Theresa Frazier, Administrative Assistant

4631 **Topeka Independent Living Resource Center**
501 SW Jackson Street
Suite 100
Topeka, KS 66603
785-233-4572
800-443-2207
FAX: 785-233-5072

Michael Oxford, Executive Director

Offers peer counseling, attendant care registry and disability education, independent living skills training, housing assistance, advocacy (individual and system), interpreting services and legal services.

4632 **Whole Person: Nortonville**
PO Box 117
Nortonville, KS 66066
913-886-2738
FAX: 913-886-2739

4633 **Whole Person: Olathe**
312 E Park
Suite B
Olathe, KS 66061
913-393-9805
FAX: 913-393-9814

Kentucky

4634 **Best Center for Independent Living**
624A Eastwood Avenue
Bowling Green, KY 42103
270-796-5992
FAX: 270-796-5992
e-mail: klesieur@aol.com

Karen Lesieur, Contact

4635 **Center for Accessible Living**
981 S 3rd Street
Suite 102
Louisville, KY 40203
502-589-6620
FAX: 502-589-3980
e-mail: jday@calky.org
www.calky.org

Jan Day, Executive Director

Independent living center.

4636 **Center for Accessible Living: Murray**
1304U Chestnut Street
Murray, KY 42071
279-753-7676
FAX: 270-753-7729
e-mail: jeannegal@kih.net
www.calky.org

Jeanne Gallimore, Contact

4637 **Center for Independent Living Options**
3031 Dixie Highway
Suite 103
Edgewood, KY 41017
859-341-4346
FAX: 859-341-1252
e-mail: cilo@single-point.org

4638 **Center for Independent Living: Kentucky Department for the Blind**
Independent Living Office
1210 Johnson Boulevard
Murray, KY 42071
270-759-9227
800-334-6920
FAX: 270-759-9227
e-mail: buel.stalls@mail.state.ky.us

Buel E Stalls Jr, Office Manager & IL Specialist

Offers peer counseling, attendant care registry and other services to the community as they relate to the blind community. The Murray office is an independent living regional office which covers 20 far western counties of Kentucky.

4639 **Community Alternatives**
103 Bridge Street
Frankfort, KY 40601
502-223-1736
FAX: 502-223-4404

Carol Filson, Executive Director

Offers peer counseling, education, advocacy, information and referral services.

4640 **Disability Coalition of Northern Kentucky**
36 W Pike Street
Covington, KY 41011
859-431-7668
FAX: 859-431-7688
e-mail: ger@iglou.com

Gerry Rader, Contact

4641 Independence Place
153 Patchen Drive
Suite 33
Lexington, KY 40517
859-266-2807
FAX: 859-335-0627
e-mail: cwesalb@aol.com

Wes Albright, Contact

4642 Pathfinders for Independent Living
105 E Mound Street
Harlan, KY 40831
606-573-5777
FAX: 606-573-5739
e-mail: pathfinderil@harlanonline.net

Sandra Goodwyn, Executive Director

We publish a newsletter called LifeLine 6-10 times a year. Most articles are written by Sandra Goodwyn. Editor is F.E. Goodwyn.

4643 SILC Department of Vocational Rehabilitati on
209 Saint Clair Street
Frankfort, KY 40601
502-564-4440
FAX: 502-564-6745
TTY:502-564-6742

Louisiana

4644 Baton Rouge Resources for Independent Living
5700 Florida Boulevard
Baton Rouge, LA 70806
225-272-4102
FAX: 225-216-3845

Emily Blackwell, Site Director
Shannon Breaux, Social Worker

Non-profit organization serving people with disabilites. Services include personal care attendants, independent living training, peer counseling, disability awareness training, information and referrel.

4645 Independent Living Center
401 Veterans Memorial Boulevard
Suite 100
Metairie, LA 70005
504-841-0591
FAX: 504-841-0595

Joan Meunier, Contact
Brenda Coxen, Contact

4646 New Horizons
6670 Saint Vincent Avenue
Shreveport, LA 71106
318-865-1000
FAX: 318-865-1094
e-mail: nhilc@nhilc.org
myweb.cableone.net/nhilc

Helen Moses, Contact

4647 New Horizons Independent Living Center: NE Louisiana
1900 Lamy Lane
Suite H
Monroe, LA 71201
318-323-4374
800-428-5505
FAX: 318-323-5445
e-mail: horizons@bayou.com

Vickie Ivey, Independent Living Specialist
Katherine Carnell, Office Mgr/Administrative Asst
Latoiya Smith, PCA Coordinator/Case Manager

Advocacy, information and referrals, support groups, attendant services and loan closet.

4648 New Horizons: Alexandria
3400 Jackson Street
Suite A
Alexandria, LA 71301
318-484-3596
FAX: 318-484-3640
TTY:318-487-4322
e-mail: cen53578@centuryinter.net

4649 Resources for Independent Living
1555 Poydras Street
Suite 1500
New Orleans, LA 70112
504-522-1955
FAX: 504-522-1954
e-mail: noril@aol.com

Esther Boutte, Info./Referral Program Manager

Non-profit agency that advocates for a fully accessible and integrated community and provides services for individuals with disabilities that enhance personal choice and promote social, vocational and economic opportunities. Programs include Personal Assistant Services, Independent Living Skills training, Advocacy, Peer Support, Supported Living, Deafblind services, Lending Library and Accessibility Surveys.

4650 Resources for Independent Living: Baton Rouge
5700 Flordia Boulevard
Suite 600
Baton Rouge, LA 70806
225-216-3844
FAX: 225-216-3845
TTY:225-2163844

4651 Southwest Louisiana Independence Center
3505 Fifth Avenue
Suite A-2
Lake Charles, LA 70607
337-477-7194
FAX: 337-477-7198
TTY:337-477-7196
e-mail: slic@usunwired.net

Mitch Granger, Contact

4652 Southwest Lousiana Independence Center
109 Jomela Drive
Layfayette, LA 70503
337-269-0027
888-516-5009
FAX: 337-233-7660
TTY:337-233-7660
e-mail: lafslic@eatel.net

Katherine Prejean, Program Director

4653 Volunteers of America Supported Living Program
3939 Causeway Boulevard
Suite 3200
Metairie, LA 70002
504-834-7015
FAX: 504-835-0409

Suzanne Howell, Program Director

Provides supported living services including pca, respite, skills traning, day, night, and behavior companion.

4654 W Troy Cole Independent Living Specialist New Horizons, I L Center
1900 Lamy Lane
Suite H
Monroe, LA 71201
318-323-4374
800-428-5505
FAX: 318-323-5445
e-mail: horizons@bayou.com

W Troy Cole, Independent Living Specialist

New Horizons provides the following four core services: Advocacy; Information & Referral; Peer Support; Independent Living Skills Training. Other services include: ADA Accessibility Site Surveys (for a fee); Cross disABILITY Independent Living support Groups; Housing Information; Assistive Driving Information; Personal Care Attendant Services; disABILITY Based Community Education; Medical Equipment Loan Closet; Quarterly News Letter; For other services available, please call.

Maine

4655 **Alpha One**

242 Western Avenue
Augusta, ME 04330
207-623-1115
800-499-2357
FAX: 207-623-1369
www.alphaonenow.com

Steven Tremblay, Director

Works throughout the state of Maine. The Board of Directors, staff and a network of personal and professional connections assist people with disabilities to gain access to and achieve their own independent living goals. Wherever persons are in Maine, this network creates improved and increased opportunities for people with disabilities.

4656 **Alpha One: Aroostook Branch**

PO Box 560
Mapleton, ME 04757
207-764-6466
800-974-6466
FAX: 207-764-5396
e-mail: kcrosson@alphaonenow.com
www.alphaonenow.com

Darlene Stewart, Independent Living Specialist
Ketra A Crosson OTR, Branch Manager

Committed to being a leading enterprise providing the community with information, services and products that create opportunities for people with disabilities to live independently. Offers adaptive equipment loan program, independent skills instruction, adapted driver evaluation and training, information and referral services, peer support, advocacy, access design consultation, and more.

4657 **Alpha One: Brewer Office**

41 Acme Road
Brewer, ME 04412
207-989-4968
800-300-6016
FAX: 207-989-7976

Kelley McTague, Branch Manager

Committed to being a leading enterprise providing the community with information, services and products that create opportunities for people with disabilities to live independently. Provides many services including adaptive and mobility equipment selection, peer support, advocacy, information and referral services, adapted drive evaluation and training, and consumer directed personal assistance.

4658 **Alpha One: Main Office**

127 Main Street
South Portland, ME 04106
207-767-2189
800-640-7200
FAX: 207-799-8346
www.alpha-one.org

Steven Tremblay, Director
Ketra Crosson, Branch Manager

Alpha One, directed by people with disabilities, is committed to being a leading enterprise providing the community with information, services and products that create opportunities for people with disabilities to live independently. Offer a variety of services including access design consultation, information and referrals, attendant services, independent living skills instruction and more.

4659 **Maine Mental Health Connections**

150 Union Street
Bangor, ME 04401
207-941-2897
FAX: 207-941-2996
e-mail: together@mint.net
www.mmhcommunityconnection.org

Robert J Mathien, Executive Director
Shelley Smith, Community Connections Manager
Sharon Shepard, Employment Connections Manager

Offers a variety of social, recreational, residential, vocational and personal growth opportunities as well as peer support, education and advocacy services.

4660 **Motivational Services**

PO Box 229
Augusta, ME 04332
207-626-3465
FAX: 207-626-3469
e-mail: rweiss@mocomaine.com
www.mocomaine.com

Richard Weiss PhD, Executive Director

Residential treatment, supervised apartment living, case management, supported employment, drop-in centers, and affirmative businesses.

4661 **Shalom House**

400 Congress Street, 3rd Floor
PO Box 560
Portland, ME 04112
207-874-1080
FAX: 207-874-1077
e-mail: shalomhs@gwi.net
www.gwi.net/shalomhouse

Joseph Brannigan, Executive Director

A non-profit agency providing a range of housing and community support services for adults recovering from serious mental illness. Service in the greater Portland, Maine area.

Maryland

4662 **Broadmead**

13801 York Road
Cockeysville, MD 21030
410-527-1900
FAX: 410-527-0259
e-mail: broadmead@erols.com
www.broadmead.org

Peggy Porter

A continuing care retirement community, near Baltimore, maryland, wich offers independent living, enriched living, assisted living and comprehensive care. Accredited by the American Association of Homes & Services for the Aging's Continuing Care Accrediation.

4663 Eastern Shore Center for Independent Living
9 Sunburst Center
Cambridge, MD 21613
410-221-7701
800-705-7944
FAX: 410-221-7714
TTY:410-221-7701
e-mail: escil@comcast.net
www.escil.org

Price Baum, Executive Director
Shirl Tarbox, Assistant Executive Director
Lisa Morgan, Director IL Services

Nonprofit resource center for people with disabilities to remain independent.

4664 Freedom Center
20 Rose Hill Plaza
Unit A
Frederick, MD 20702
301-846-7811
FAX: 301-846-7812
e-mail: jameygeorge@prodigy.net

4665 Housing Unlimited
4928 Wyaconda Road
Suite 15
Rockville, MD 20852
301-230-2825
FAX: 301-230-2826
e-mail: hui97@erols.com
www.handhousing.org/housingunlimited

Abe Schuchman

To address the housing crisis for adults with psychiatric disabilities who reside in Montgomery County, Maryland.

4666 Human Resources Management
American Assn. of Children's Residential Centers
51 Monroe Place
Suite 1603
Rockville, MD 20850
301-738-6460
FAX: 301-738-6461
e-mail: info@aacrc-dc.org
www.aacrc-dc.org

Bob Leiberman MA LPC, President
Elissa Malter Schwartz, Association Director
Amy Parsley, Association Assistant

One-day seminar addresses the Management of Human Resources standards in the Comprehensive Accreditation Manual for Hospitals, Behavioral Health, Long Term Care, Ambulatory and Home Care, plus standards on orientation and education, staffing and managing staff requests.

4667 Independence Now
6811 Kenilworth Avenue
Suite 504
Riverdale, MD 20737
301-277-2839
FAX: 301-277-4587
TTY:301-277-2839
e-mail: independence@innow.org

Catherine Raggio, Executive Director
Laurel James, Independent Living Services
Georgia Coffey, Benefits InfoSource Project

Center for Independent Living serving Montgomery and Prine George's Counties in Maryland.

4668 Making Choices for Independent Living
3011 Montebello Terrace
Baltimore, MD 21214
410-444-1400
FAX: 410-444-0825
e-mail: mcil@mcil-md.org
www.mcil-md.org

Frank Pinter, Executive Director

4669 Resources for Independent Living
100 N Mechanic Street
Cumberland, MD 21502
301-784-1774
FAX: 301-784-1776

Lori Magruder, Executive Director

4670 Southern Maryland Center for LIFE
30265 Oaks Road
Charlotte Hall, MD 20622
301-884-4498
FAX: 301-884-6099
TTY:800-735-2258
e-mail: cflife@us.hsanet.net

Barbara Hayden, Contact

Massachusetts

4671 AD-LIB
221 N Street
Pittsfield, MA 01201
413-442-7047
FAX: 413-443-4338

William Cavanaugh, Executive Director

Offers information and referral services, independent living skills training, peer counseling, individual and group advocacy services available to all people with disabilities. Access consultation provided to businesses, agencies and institutions in accordance to the Americans with Disabilities Act.

4672 ARC: Gateway
PO Box 428
Hyannis, MA 02601
508-771-6595
FAX: 508-775-5233

4673 American Red Cross of Cape Cod
286 S Street
Hyannis, MA 02601
508-775-1540
FAX: 508-771-2209
e-mail: capecod@cape.com
www.capecodredcross.org

Marlene Weir, Executive Director

Handicapped accessible motor service to Boston Area Hospitals from Cape Cod with pick-up for Nantucket residents.

4674 Boston Center for Independent Living
95 Berkeley Street
Suite 206
Boston, MA 02116
617-338-6665
888-338-8085
FAX: 617-338-6661
e-mail: info@bostoncil.org
wwww.bostoncil.org/home.htm

Bill Henning, Executive Director
Jimi Tierney, Deputy Director
Holly Vernon, Director of Program Services

Offers skills training, peer mentoring, advocacy training and information services to help persons with disabilities of all ages assume full control over their own life choices. Works with youth in schools to promote effective transition into adult independence. Empowers people by providing information in all aspects of daily living, including the statewide housing registry, personal care assistant program and ongoing assistance. Works with others to address social concerns effecting disabled.

4675 **Cape Organization for Rights of the Disabled (CORD)**

1019 Iyannough Road
Suite 4
Hyannis, MA 02601
508-775-8300
FAX: 508-775-7022
e-mail: bhcord@cape.com
www.cordonline.org

Bill Henning, Contact

4676 **Center for Living & Working: Milford**

76 Summer Street
Fitchburg, MA 01420
978-345-1568
FAX: 978-345-1568
e-mail: rbailey@centerlw.com
www.centerlw.org

4677 **DEAF**

215 Brighton Avenue
Allston, MA 02134
617-523-8928

Heidi Reed, Director

Multi-service agency operated by the community to provide advocacy, training and access assistance.

4678 **IL Center: Center for Living & Working**

67 Millbrook Street
WBC, 1st Floor
Worcester, MA 01606
508-363-1226
FAX: 508-363-1254
e-mail: centerlw@centerlw.org
www.centerlw.org

James H Ross, Executive Director

4679 **IL Center: Independent Living Center of the North Shore & Cape Ann (ILNSCA)**

27 Congress Street
Suite 107
Salem, MA 01970
978-741-0077
FAX: 978-741-1133
e-mail: ilcnsca@aol.com
www.ilcnsca.org

Mary M Moore, Executive Director

ILNSCA is a service and advocacy center run by and for people with disabilities. Offered services include independent living skills training, peer counseling, information and referral, and advocacy; home modification, vehicle modifications and assistive equipment limited funding; ADA technical assistance.

4680 **IL Center: Southeast Center for Independent Living**

66 Troy Street
1st Floor
Fall River, MA 02720
508-679-9210
FAX: 508-677-2377
e-mail: scil@choiceonemail.com
www.scil.org

Cheryl Finnerty, Executive Director
Lisa Pitta, Assistant Executive Director
Elaine Faria, Housing Advocate

4681 **Independence Associates**

10 Oak Street
2nd Floor
Taunton, MA 02780
508-880-5325
800-649-5568
FAX: 508-880-6311
e-mail: cgallant@iacil.org
www.iacil.org

Constance Gallant, Executive Director
Gayle B Dubois, Information & Referral Spec

We offer Advocacy Services, Information and referral, Independent living skills training, Peer counseling. Also personal care management training program.

4682 **Independent Living Center of the North Shore and Cape Ann**

583 Chestnut Street
Lynn, MA 01904
781-596-8255
FAX: 781-741-1133
e-mail: ilcnsca@aol.com
www.ilcnsca.org

Lori Stewart, Executive Director
Shawn McDuff, Community Affairs

ILCNSCA works to address individual, community-wide and broad systemic issues that affect the ability of people with disabilities to live independently in the community. The staff provides peer counseling, independent living skills training, individual advocacy, information and referral to people with disabilities, and more. These services are offered to empower individuals with disabilities and assist them in gaining the control and skills needed to live independent lives.

4683 **Independent Living Center: Massachusetts Community for the Blind**

88 Kingston Street
Boston, MA 02111
617-727-5550
FAX: 617-727-5960
e-mail: chris.crawford@mcb:bbs.pm.com

Donald Johnson, Director

Offers peer counseling and disability education.

4684 **MetroWest Center for Independent Living**

63 Fountain Street
Suite 401
Framingham, MA 01702
508-875-7883
FAX: 508-875-8359
www.mcil.org

Paul Spooner, Executive Director

Advocacy organization serving individuals with disabilities.

4685 **Northeast Independent Living Program**

20 Ballard Road
Lawrence, MA 01843
978-687-4288
FAX: 978-689-4488
e-mail: nilprogram@quest.net
www.nilp.org

Charlie Carr, Executive Director

Provides advocacy and independent living services (information and referral, peer counseling, skills training) to people with disabilities, to empowering them to live and work as independently as possible.

4686 **Renaissance Clubhouse**

176 Walker Street
Lowell, MA 01854
978-454-7944
FAX: 978-937-7867
e-mail: renclub@channel1.com
www.channel1.com/~renclub

Elaine Walker, Director
Tammy Savoie, Assistant Director

Offers daily structure, assistance wtih jobs, retirement, and housing.

4687 Stavros Center for Independent Living
691 SE Street
Amherst, MA 01002
413-256-0473
800-804-1899
FAX: 413-256-0190
www.stavros.org

James Kruidenier, Executive Director

Offers peer counseling, advocacy, skills training, information and referral, disability education/awareness, personal assistance services, services to all disabilities and deaf and hard of hearing individuals, equipment loan, assistive technology education, and related issues.

4688 Student Independent Living Experience
3 Randolph Street
Canton, MA 02021
781-828-1519
FAX: 781-821-4086

Tom Bosco, Director

Transitional living program serving adolescents with disabilities teach independent living skills.

4689 Vivienne S Thomson ILC
MDAC-555 Amory Street
Jamaica Plains, MA 02130
617-522-9840
FAX: 617-522-9839

Michigan

4690 Ann Arbor Center for Independent Living
2568 Packard Street
Ann Arbor, MI 48104
734-971-0277
FAX: 734-971-0826
TTY:734-971-0310
e-mail: cilstaff@aacil.org

Sue Probert, Information/Referral Coord.

The mission to assure equality of opportunity, independent living and the economic self-sufficiency of people with disabilities.

4691 Arc Detroit
51 W Hancock Street
Detroit, MI 48201
FAX: 313-831-7974

Shirley Moordian, Director

Advocacy for people with developmental disabilities, clerical aide training, parent outreach, mental affairs, self advocacy, newsletter. Membership dues $20 per year. Includes state and national Arc membership.

4692 Association for Retarded Citizens of Muskegon County
1145 Wesley Avenue
Muskegon, MI 49442
231-773-5355
FAX: 231-777-3507

Margaret O'Toole, Director

Offers information and referral, advocacy services and peer counseling.

4693 Bay Area Coalition for Independent Living
701 S Elmwood Street
Suite 17
Traverse City, MI 49684
269-929-4865
FAX: 269-929-5330

Mary Jean Brick, Contact

4694 Blue Water CIL
610 Woodworth
Bad Axe, MI 48413
810-269-5421
FAX: 810-269-5422

4695 Blue Water CIL: Caro
1184 Cleaver Road
Suite 1000
Caro, MI 48732
989-673-3678
FAX: 989-673-3678
e-mail: bwcil@centurytel.net

4696 Blue Water Center for Independent Living
310 Water Street
Port Huron, MI 48060
810-987-9337
FAX: 810-987-9548
e-mail: bob925@hotmail.com

Rob Devary, Director

Offers disability education, peer counseling, advocacy, transpotation, employment, substance abuse counseling, support groups and information on accessible housing.

4697 Capital Area Center for Independent Living
1048 Pierpont Drive
Suite 9-10
Lansing, MI 48911
517-334-7830
FAX: 517-334-7849
e-mail: cacil@cacil.org
www.cacil.org

Janet Del Valle, Contact

4698 Center for Handicapped Affairs
3815 W Saint Joesph
Suite D
Lansing, MI 48917
517-334-7830
FAX: 517-334-7849

4699 Center for Independent Living of Mid-Michigan
1206 James Sauage
Midland, MI 48640
989-835-4041
800-782-4160
FAX: 989-835-8121
e-mail: cilinfo@cilmn.org

Melissa Gleason, Associate Director
Melissa Davert, Executive Director
Rose Spear, Information/Referral

Comprised of over 51 percent of people with disabilities, and advocates for the rights of people with disabilities in the Mid-Michigan area. Call for information on disability issues or for assistance in obtaining services, within your community..

4700 Cristo Rey Handicappers Program
1717 N High Street
Lansing, MI 48906
517-372-4700
FAX: 517-372-8499

Tony Bevavides, Director
Cindi Benavides, Program Coordinator

Social/recreational program, outreach, support and self sufficiency services, drop in area.

4701 Disability Advocates of Kent County Living
3600 Camelot Drive SE
Grand Rapids, MI 49546
616-949-1100
FAX: 616-949-7865
e-mail: tracy@disabilityadvocates.us
www.disabilityadvocates.us

David Bulkowski, Director
Tracy Philips, Information/Referral Coord.

Offers 4 core services: Information and Referral, Advocacy, Peer Support and Independent Living Skills training for people with disabilities. Specific programs and services include accessibility and occupational therapy assessments, transitions services, assistance with personal care attendant issues, interpreter referral and other services for hearing impaired persons.

4702 **Disability Network**
3600 S Dort Highway
Suite 54
Flint, MI 48507
810-742-1800
FAX: 810-742-2400
TTY:810-742-7647
e-mail: tdn@disnetworki.org
www.disnetwork.org

Mike Zelley, President/CEO

4703 **Disability Resource Center of Southwestern Michigan**
517 E Crosstown Parkway
Kalamazoo, MI 49001
269-345-1516
800-394-7450
FAX: 269-345-0229
TTY:616-345-1516
e-mail: dshortt@drccil.org
www.drccil.org

Joel Cooper, President/CEO
Debra Shortt, Information/Referral Specialist

A Center for Independent Living offering core services in the areas of advocacy, peer support, independent living skills training, and information and referral to persons with disabilities living in the following southwestern Michigan counties: Allegan, Barry, Berrien, Calhoun, Cass, Kalamazoo, St. Joseph and Van Buren. Specialized services available through the DRC include: occupational therapy assessments; accessibility assessments, driver evaluation and training.

4704 **Grand Traverse Area Community Living Center**
935 Barlow Street
Traverse City, MI 49686
269-941-7150
FAX: 269-941-3421

Juanita Lyon, Program Director
Laura Tougas, Administrative Director

We are a training home for individuals with developmental disabilities over the age of 18

4705 **Great Lakes Center for Independent Living**
2995 E Grand Boulevard
Detroit, MI 48202
313-870-4580
FAX: 313-832-3850
e-mail: jmeece@glcil.org
www.misilc.org/partnerships.htm

Jeannie Meece, Executive Director

Independent living skills training, de-institutionalization and empowerment training for persons with disabilities.

4706 **Great Lakes/Macomb Rehabilitation Group**
4 E Alexandrine
Suite 104
Detroit, MI 48201
313-832-3371
FAX: 313-832-3850
e-mail: jlcil@home.msen.com

Jeannie Meece-Brooks, Contact

4707 **Hope Network Independent Living Program**
1550 E Beltline Avenue SE
Office 125
Grand Rapids, MI 49506
616-831-2000
FAX: 616-940-8151

Kathryn Mullarkey FSE, Manager

Postacute rehabilitation program serving adults with physical disabilities, especially spinal cord injuries, blindness, MS, brain injuries and stroke. Home adaptation, independent living skills and vocational services are highlighted. Program focus is independent living and return to work.

4708 **Jackson Center for Independent Living**
2319 W Main Street S
Suite A
Jackson, MI 49203
517-784-1723
FAX: 517-784-9921

4709 **Jewish Association for Residential Care (JARC)**
28366 Franklin Road
Southfield, MI 48034
248-352-5272
FAX: 248-352-5279
e-mail: jarc@jarc.org
www.jarc.org

Joyce Keller, Executive Director
Randee Klein, Intake Social Worker

Non-profit organizations providing residential care and support services to adults with developmental disabilities. Operates 13 licensed homes and 5 unlicensed transition homes, and supports over 60 people who live on their own. JARC aldo offers an array of services to families of children with any disability, including respite care, life planning, educatinoal and social programming, outreach, and peer support.

4710 **Kalamazoo Center for Independent Living**
4026 S Westnedge
Kalamazoo, MI 49008
269-345-1516
FAX: 269-345-0229

4711 **Lakeshore Center for Independent Living**
426 Century Lane
Holland, MI 49423
616-850-9781
800-656-5245
FAX: 616-396-3220
e-mail: aimee@egl.net

Ruth Stegeman, Executive Director
Clare Clark, Office Manager
Lorette Evans, Support Staff

Promotes personal initiative and pride among those with disabilities, fostering an integrated community of people who remove barriers to full participation.

4712 **Life Skills Services**
1608 Lake Street
Kalamazoo, MI 49001
FAX: 269-344-0285

Don Vanderkooy, Director

Offers skill development and monitoring for children and supported living and respite services for adults with developmental disabilities and/or mental illnesses.

4713 **Michigan Commission for the Blind: Detroit**
State of Michigan Plaza Building
1200 6th Avenue, 3rd Floor
Detroit, MI 48226
313-256-1524
FAX: 313-256-1519
www.mfia.state.mi.us

Charlene Edge, Contact

4714 **Michigan Commission for the Blind: Independent Living Rehabilitation Program**

411 E Genesee Avenue
Saginaw, MI 48607 **989-758-1765**
800-292-4200
FAX: 989-758-1405
www.mfia.state.mi.us

Leaman Jones, Supervisor

Rehabilitation teaching, independent living skills for persons over 55 with severe vision loss.

4715 **Midland Center for Independent Care**

1206 James Savage
Midland, MI 48640 **989-835-4041**
FAX: 989-835-8121

4716 **Oakland/Macomb Center for Independent Living**

3765 E 15 Mile Road
Sterling Heights, MI 48310 **586-268-4160**
FAX: 586-268-4720
e-mail: ricks@omcil.org
www.omcil.org

Richard Sides, Contact

4717 **Southeastern Michigan Commission for the Blind**

1200 6th Street
3rd floor, N Tower
Detroit, MI 48226 **313-256-1524**
FAX: 313-256-1519
www.michigan.gov/fia

Leamon Jones, Southeast Regional Supervisor

Vocational rehabilitation agency. Personal adjustment vocational assessment and training, job placement and follow-up services.

4718 **Superior Alliance for Independent Living (SAIL)**

129 W Baraga Avenue
Suite H
Marquette, MI 49855 **906-228-5744**
800-729-SAIL
FAX: 906-228-5573
e-mail: sail@up.net
www.sail.match.org

Amy Rosemergy, Contact

Minnesota

4719 **Accessibility Home Fund**

400 Sibley Street
Suite 300
Saint Paul, MN 55101 **651-296-7608**
800-657-3769
FAX: 651-296-8139

Barb Collins, Program Manager

Offers peer counseling, education and referral services.

4720 **Accessible Space**

2550 University Avenue W
Suite 330N
Saint Paul, MN 55114 **651-645-7271**
800-466-7722
FAX: 651-645-0541
www.accessiblespace.org

Stephen Vander Schaaf, President/CEO

Provides accessible, affordable community-based housing with support services at residential apartment sites in other states. Support services offered in Minnesota, Montana, Nevada, North Dakota and Tennessee.

4721 **Center for Independent Living**

424 W Superior Street
Suite 400
Duluth, MN 55802 **218-726-4896**
FAX: 218-726-4897
e-mail: val@accessnorth.net
www.accessnorth.net

Valerie LePorte, Branch Office Director

4722 **Center for Independent Living of NE Minnesota**

Mesabi Mall
Suite 11
Hibbing, MN 55746 **218-262-6675**
FAX: 218-262-6677
e-mail: kim@accessnorth.net
www.accessnorth.net

Kimberly Breznik, Contact

4723 **Courage Center**

3915 Golden Valley Road
Minneapolis, MN 55422 **612-588-0811**
888-846-8253
FAX: 612-520-0577
www.courage.org

Tony Lebahn, Client Services Representative

A comprehensive rehabilitation center serving both people with physical and sensory disabilities. Over 70 different services are available to children and adults with physical disabilities. Some services are physical, occupational and speech therapies, a young adult residential program, camping opportunities, driving evaluations, sports and recreation services, vocational services and much more.

4724 **Freedom Resource Center for Independent Living**

3505 Eighth Street
Suite 7
Moorhead, MN 56560 **218-236-0459**
FAX: 218-236-0510
TTY:218-236-0459
e-mail: frcilfg9@mail.corpcomm.net

4725 **Freedom Resource Center for Independent Living**

308 W Lincoln
Fergus Falls, MN 56537 **218-737-1800**
FAX: 718-737-1801
TTY:218-737-1800
e-mail: reyem@prtel.com

4726 **Independence Crossroads**

8932 Old Cedar Avenue S
Bloomington, MN 55425 **952-854-8004**
FAX: 952-854-7842
e-mail: info@independencecrossroads.org
www.independencecrossroads.org

Donna Robb, Director
Rob Olson, Counselor

Offers free information and referral, advocacy, mental health, counseling services, support groups and public education.

4727 **Independent Lifestyles: A Center for Independent Living**

519 2nd Street N
Saint Cloud, MN 56303 **320-529-9000**
FAX: 320-529-0747
e-mail: CaraR@IndependentLifestyles.org
www.macil.org/cmcil

Cara Ruff, Executive Director

4728 **Metropolitan Center for Independent Living**

1600 University Avenue W
Suite 16
St Paul, MN 55104 **651-646-8342**
FAX: 651-603-2006
e-mail: mcil@mcil-mn.org
www.mcil-mn.org

David Hancox, Director
Carol Streasick, Manager Personal Asst Services
Taylor Kearns, Manager Independent Living

MCIL provides services for people with disabilities, their families, friends, service providers and community members. Services include: information and referral (info on accessible/subsidized housing), independent living skills, peer support, system/individual advocacy (nursing home out to community living project, personal care services, ramp project (manual/video available on building ramps), transition, ADA program and support groups.

4729 **New Horizons Home Care**

600 25th Avenue S
Suite 111
Saint Cloud, MN 56301 **320-255-1882**
FAX: 320-255-5137

Courtney Salzl, Director Nursing
Brenda Fuchs, Human Resources Intake

Offers skilled nursing services RN, LPN, TV Therapy, Pediatrics, Rehabilitation Services, PT, OT, ST, Paraprofessional staff, Home Health Aides, Homemakers, Personal Care Attendents, Companions, Live-ins, Sleep overs, Respite care, Extended hours.

4730 **Options Interstate Resource Center for Independent Living**

318 Third Street NW
E Grand Forks, MN 56721 **218-773-6100**
800-726-3692
FAX: 218-773-7119
e-mail: randy@rry.net
www.macil.org/options

Randy Sorensen, Contact

4731 **Southeastern Minnesota Center for Independent Living: Red Wing**

201 E Seventh Street
Red Wing, MN 55066 **651-388-0466**
888-460-1815
FAX: 651-385-0643
www.semcil.org

4732 **Southeastern Minnesota Center for Independent Living**

2720 N Broadwayreet NW
Rochester, MN 55906 **507-285-1815**
888-460-1815
FAX: 507-288-8070
e-mail: semcil.uhhc@semcil.org
www.semcil.org

Dave Schwartzkoff, Executive Director
Laurie Brownell, Operations Manager

Offers peer counseling, disability education and referrals, support groups, independent living skills training, information and referral, home medication and housing.

4733 **Southern Minnesota Independent Living Enterprises & Services**

709 S Front Street
Mankato, MN 56001 **507-345-8590**
888-676-6498
FAX: 507-345-8429
e-mail: smiles@smilescil.org
www.smilescil.org

Alan Augustin, Director
Doug Miller, Operations Manager
Mary Mensing, Independent Living Manager

A nonprofit organization committed to providing an array of services to assist individuals with disabilities to live independently, pursue meaningful goals, and have the same opportunities and choices as all persons. Offers direct services such as: individual and systems advocacy, peer counseling, independent living skills training, transition from school to community living, information and referral, semi-independent living services, assistive technology, ramp projects, and community education.

4734 **Southwestern Center for Independent Living (SWCIL)**

109 S 5th Street
Suite 700
Marshall, MN 56258 **507-532-2221**
FAX: 507-532-2222
e-mail: swcil@swcil.com
www.swcil.com

Steven Thovson, Executive Director
Annette Swanson, Operations Manager

4735 **Vinland National Center**

PO Box 308
Loretto, MN 55357 **763-479-3555**
FAX: 763-479-2605
e-mail: vinland@mtn.org

Sue Rivard, Director

Offers peer counseling, disability education and other services to the community.

Mississippi

4736 **Alpha Home Royal Maid Association for the Blind**

PO Box 30
Hazlehurst, MS 39083
FAX: 601-894-2993
e-mail: sigworks@teclink.net

Howard Becker, Director

Offers attendant care registry, information on accessible housing and referrals.

4737 **Gulf Coast Independent Living Center**

18 JM Tatum Industrial Drive
Hattiesburg, MS 39401 **601-544-4860**
FAX: 601-582-2544

Albert Holifield, Contact

4738 **Jackson Independent Living Center**

300 Capers Avenue
Jackson, MS 39203 **601-969-3649**
800-378-9156
FAX: 601-351-1484

Bridget James, Counselor III

Provides services to consumers with severe disabilities.

4739 LIFE of Central Mississippi
754 N President Street
Suite 1
Jackson, MS 39203
601-969-4009
FAX: 800-748-9398
e-mail: lifecen@meta3.net
www.cdd-life.org/life

Christy Gilliland, Contact

4740 LIFE of Southern Mississippi
710 Katie Avenue
Hattiesburg, MS 39401
601-583-2108
800-898-8477
FAX: 601-583-1814
e-mail: hatt@netdoor.com
www.cdd-life.org

Elna Garner, Center Director

4741 Life of North Mississippi: Greenville
638 Main Street
Suite 111
Greenville, MS 38701
601-332-2220
FAX: 601-332-2261

4742 Life of North Mississippi: Tupelo
201 Jefferson Street
Suite D
Tupelo, MS 38801
601-874-4663
FAX: 662-844-6633

4743 Life of South Mississippi: Biloxi
1011 Arbor View Circle
Biloxi, MS 39532
228-435-5433
FAX: 228-435-1338

4744 Mississippi State Independent Living Center
PO Drawer 6321
Mississippi State, MS 39762
601-351-1525
FAX: 601-351-1484
www.mdrs.state.ms.us

Butch McMillian, Director

Offers peer counseling and disability education.

Missouri

4745 Access II Independent Living Center
611 W Johnson Street
Gallatin, MO 64640
660-663-2423
FAX: 660-663-2517
e-mail: access@ccp.com
www.accesii.org

Gary Maddox, Executive Director
Leslie Anderson, Program Manager

4746 Bootheel Area Independent Living Services
PO Box 326
Kennett, MO 63857
573-888-0002
FAX: 573-888-0708
e-mail: bails@jrwent.com

Kelly Barfoot, Contact

4747 Council for Extended Care of Mentally Retarded Citizens
1600 S Hanley Road
Suite 100A
Saint Louis, MO 63144
FAX: 314-781-3850

Cynthia Compton, Executive Director

Services are provided to individuals with mental retardation. Supported living arrangements are located in St. Louis. Group homes and camping services are located in Dittmer, MO.

4748 Delta Center for Independent Living
5933 Highway 94 S
Suite 107
Saint Charles, MO 63304
636-926-8761
FAX: 314-447-0341
e-mail: delta@mail.win.org

Selena Korte, Contact

4749 Disability Resource Association
420-B S Truman Boulevard
Crystal City, MO 63019
636-931-7696
FAX: 636-937-9019
e-mail: dra@disabilityresourceassociation.org

Craig Henning, Contact

4750 Disabled Citizens Alliance for Independence
PO Box 675
Viburnum, MO 65566
314-244-3315
FAX: 314-244-5609
e-mail: blake@misn.com

Juanita Hagemeier, Contact

4751 Independence Center
4380 W Pine Boulevard
Saint Louis, MO 63108
314-533-4380
FAX: 314-531-7372
www.independencecenter.org

Robert Harvey, Executive Director

Provides psychiatric rehabilitation, housing, vocational rehabilitation and evening, weekend and holiday services to adults with serious and persistent mental illnesses.

4752 Independent Living Center
1001 E 32nd Street
Suite 102
Joplin, MO 64804
417-659-8086
FAX: 417-659-8087
e-mail: ilcjoplin@joplin.com

Leatta Workman, Executive Director

4753 Independent Living Center of Southeast Missouri
809 W Pine Street
Poplar Bluff, MO 63901
573-686-2333
888-890-2333
FAX: 573-686-0733
e-mail: ilcsm@semo.org
www.ilcsm.org

Bruce Lynch, Executive Director
Jennifer Barnes, IL Manager
Suzann McKnight, PAS Manager

4754 **Independent Living Resource Center**
3620 W Truman Boulevard
Suite D
Jefferson City, MO 65109
573-556-0400
FAX: 573-556-0402
e-mail: ilrc@midamerica.net

Frank Nease, Contact

4755 **LIFE Center for Independent Living**
1109 Saint Genevieve Avenue
Farmington, MO 63640
573-756-4314
800-596-7273
FAX: 573-756-3507
e-mail: lifec@il.net

Tim Azinger, Executive Director

4756 **Life Skills Foundation**
1158 Huntsman Drive
Saint Louis, MO 63137
314-567-7705
FAX: 314-567-6539
e-mail: lifeskills@aol.com

4757 **Midland Empire Resources (MERIL)**
3715 Beck Road
Building D
St Joseph, MO 64506
816-279-8558
800-242-4326
FAX: 816-279-1550
e-mail: meril@meril.org
www.meril.org

Debbie Merritt, Executive Director
Marilyn Finney, Assistant Director
Ian Gewin, Director of PAS Services

4758 **Northeast Independent Living Services**
109 Virginia
5th Floor, Suite 560
Hannibal, MO 63401
573-221-8282
FAX: 573-221-9445
e-mail: neils@nemonet.com

Michelle Green, Executive Director

4759 **On My Own**
3102 Industrial Parkway
Nevada, MO 64772
417-667-7007
FAX: 417-667-6262
e-mail: onmyown@ipa.net

Jack Brock, Executive Director
Susie Kimmell, PAS Director
Tina Overton, Program Director

4760 **Ozark Independent Living**
109 Aid Avenue
W Plains, MO 65775
417-257-0038
FAX: 417-257-2380
TTY:888-440-7500
e-mail: ozark@townsqr.com
users.townsqr.com/ozark

Cynthia Moore, Contact

4761 **Paraquad**
311 N Lindbergh Boulevard
Saint Louis, MO 63141
314-567-1558
FAX: 314-567-1559
TTY:314-567-5552
e-mail: paraquad@paraquad.org
www.paraquad.org

Max Starkloff, President

4762 **Places for People**
4120 Lindell Boulevard
Saint Louis, MO 63108
314-535-5600
FAX: 314-535-6037

Scott Bayliff, Associate Director
Francie Broderick, Executive Director
Kelly Wilson, Operations Director

Provides individualized, high quality, and cost effective servies to adults with serious and persistent mental disorders to assist them in living, working and socializing in environments of their choice. We accept a special responsibility to serve those individuals who rely on public funding.

4763 **RAIL**
715 S Baltimore
Kirksville, MO 63501
660-627-7245
FAX: 660-627-0525
TTY:6606270614
e-mail: ritt@kymo.net
www.nemr.net

4764 **Rehabilitation Institute, Kansas City**
3011 Baltimore Avenue
Kansas City, MO 64108
816-751-7700
FAX: 816-751-7988

Ron Hendrick, President

The Rehabilitation Institute, is a licensed, non-profit medical and vocational facility, established for the sole purpose of serving children, youth and adults with disabilities. The Institute offers comprehensive inpatient and outpatient medical services for general rehabilitation, spinal cord injuries, head injuries and other disabling conditions. It is also one of the largest vocational rehabilitation centers in Missouri with extensive work evaluation, counseling and placement programs.

1947

4765 **Services for Independent Living**
1401 Hathman Place
Columbia, MO 65201
573-874-1646
800-766-1968
FAX: 573-874-3564
e-mail: sil@silcolumbia.org

Mark Stone, Executive Director
Tarzie Hart, Administrative Director

A non-residential, community-based center for independent living. Provides individualized and group services to persons with severe disabilities in the Mid-Missouri area; works to help people with disabilities achieve their highest potential in independent living and community life.

4766 **Southeastern Missouri Alliance for Independence (SEMO Alliance)**
121 S Broadview Plaza
Suite 12
Cape Girardeau, MO 63703
573-651-6464
FAX: 573-651-6565
e-mail: miki@mail.sadi.org

Maryann Gudermuth, Executive Director
Scarlett Seabaugh, Program Director

4767 **Southwest Center for Independent Living (SWCIL)**
2864 S Nettleton
Springfield, MO 65807
417-886-1188
800-676-7245
FAX: 417-886-3619
e-mail: scil@swcil.org
www.swcil.org

Ann Morris, Executive Director

Services, resources and advocacy for people with any type of disability and any age.

4768 Tri-County Center for Independent Living
1704 E Tenth Street
Suite D
Rolla, MO 65401
573-368-5933
FAX: 573-368-5991
www.rollanet.org/~tricil1

Victoria Heitxler, Contact

4769 Warrenburg Independent Living Services
123 E Gay
Suite S-2
Warrensburg, MO 64093
660-422-7883
FAX: 660-422-7895
e-mail: wils@iland.net
www.w-ils.org

Robert Honan, Contact

4770 Whole Person
301 E Armour Boulevard
Suite 430
Kansas City, MO 64111
816-561-0304
FAX: 816-753-8163
e-mail: dcrinkc@aol.com

David Robinson, Contact

Montana

4771 Living Independently for Today and Tomorrow: Glendrive
PO Box 621
Glendrive, MT 59330
406-365-4062
FAX: 406-364-4064

4772 Living Independently for Today and Tomorrow
914 Wyoming Avenue
Billings, MT 59102
406-259-5181
800-669-6319
FAX: 406-259-5259
e-mail: daves@lifft.org

David Swanson, Program Director
Larry Ketchum, Information/Referral

Offers peer mentoring, disability education and referrals, information advocacy, domestic violence information and referral, ADA services community advocacy, accessibility, equipment loan, housing referral, independent living skills and accessment pass plans, ramp, service coordination transition and personal assistance services.

4773 Miles City Chapter: Living Independently for Today and Tomorrow (LIFTT)
2200 Box Elder
Suite 2
Miles City, MT 59301
406-232-2599
FAX: 406-365-4064
e-mail: liftt@midrivers.com

Pat Lockwood, Contact

4774 Montana Independent Living Project
38 S Last Chance Gulch
PO Box 5415
Helena, MT 59604
406-442-5755
FAX: 406-442-1612
TTY:406-442-5756
e-mail: milpjim@initcio.net

James Meldrum, Executive Director

4775 North Central Independent Living Services
1120 25th Avenue NE
Black Eagle, MT 59414
406-452-9834
FAX: 406-453-3940

Tom Osborn, Director

Independent living center.

4776 North Central Independent Living Services
PO Box 229
Glasgow, MT 59230
406-228-2075
FAX: 406-228-2076
e-mail: ncils2@nemontel.net

4777 Summit Independent Living Center
700 SW Higgins Avenue
Suite 101
Missoula, MT 59803
406-728-1630
800-398-9002
FAX: 406-829-3309
www.summitilc.org

Michael Mayer, Executive Director
Becky Burke, Peer Advocate Coodinator
Jude Monson, Education Coordinator

Summit ILC helps its consumers continue to live independently in the community through a variety of individual and community services.

4778 Summit Independent Living Center: Kalipsell
275 Corporate Avenue
Suite 901
Kalispell, MT 59901
406-257-0048
FAX: 406-257-0634
e-mail: summitkl@digisys.net
www.summitilc.org

Advocacy for people with disabilities.

4779 Summit Ravalli County Independent Living Center
316 N 3rd Street
Suite 113 & 112
Hamilton, MT 59840
406-363-5242
800-398-9013
FAX: 406-375-9035
e-mail: jperkins@summitilc.org
www.summitILC.org

Joanne Perkins, Ravalli County Coordinator
Dawn Gauthier, Independent Living Specialist

Nebraska

4780 Center for Independent Living of Central Nebraska
1804 S Eddy Street
Grand Island, NE 68801
308-382-9255
877-400-1004
FAX: 308-384-9231
e-mail: scook@cilnc.org

Sid Cook, Executive Director

Offers independent living skills training, peer sharing, information and referral, housing counseling and referral, accessibility and barrier removal consultation including ADA training and technical assistance, driver education and training, assistive technology services including demonstration and equipment loan, and a free lending library of adapted toys and ability switches for children with severe disabilities. Serves all diabilities and all ages.

4781 **League of Human Dignity**
1701 P Street
Lincoln, NE 68508
402-441-7871
FAX: 402-441-7650
TTY:402-441-7871

Mike Schafer, Contact

4782 **League of Human Dignity Center for Independent Living**
5513 Center Street
Omaha, NE 68106
402-595-1256
FAX: 402-595-1410
e-mail: lhdomaha@navix.net
www.leagueofhumandignity.com

Mike Schafer, CEO
Peg Westfall, Director

Provides information and referral, independent living skills training, advocacy, case coordination, peer counseling, personal assistant services, barrier removal services, public education and awareness.

4783 **Leauge of Human Dignity Independent Living Center**
400 Elm Street
Norfolk, NE 68701
402-371-4475
FAX: 402-371-4625
TTY:402-371-4475

4784 **Martin Luther Homes of Beatrice**
722 S 12th Street
607
Beatrice, NE 68310
402-223-4066
FAX: 402-223-4951
e-mail: beatrice@mlhs.com
www.mlhs.com

Jerry Campbell, Administrator
Amky Bell, Clinical Director

Providing a wide array of services to assist individuals and families in achieving positive life goals. Services to persons with disabilities and other special needs include community living options, training and employment options, spiritual growth and development options, training and counseling support.

4785 **Martin Luther Homes of Nebraska**
220 W S 21st Street
York, NE 68467
402-362-2180
FAX: 402-362-2961
e-mail: yorkagencyMLHCentral@mlsh.com
www.mlhs.com

Jessica Schoepf, Program Director
Tim Summers, Area Progam Director
Alan Blakestad, Cheif Operating Officer

Providing a wide array of services to assist individuals and families in achieving positive life goals. Services to persons with disabilities and other special needs include community living options, training and employment options, spiritual growth and development options, training and counseling support.

4786 **Panhandle Independent Living Services**
510 S Broadway
Suite 2, PO Box 2454
Scottsbluff, NE 69363
308-635-7901
800-644-5352
FAX: 308-635-7676
e-mail: pils@bbc.net

Carolyn Foged, Executive Director

PILS Pathfinder - Quarterly newsletter that contains 8 pages. No charge to be added to our mailing list.

Nevada

4787 **Carson City Center for Independent Living**
675 Fairview Drive
Suite 224
Carson City, NV 89701
775-841-2580
FAX: 775-267-3969

Sandy Coyle, Contact

4788 **Endeavor**
6200 W Oakey Boulevard
Las Vegas, NV 89146
702-870-7050
FAX: 702-870-7649
e-mail: Handi77@aol.com
www.endeavor-nv.org

Vince Triggs, Executive Director

A community based agency providing training, advocacy, support to persons with disabilities, regardless of age or type or degree of disability, developmental child care, employment services, family respite, and supported living.

4789 **Northern Nevada Center for Independent Living: Fallon**
1919 Grimes Street
Suite B
Fallon, NV 89406
775-423-4900
FAX: 775-423-1399
TTY:775-423-4900
e-mail: nncil4@aiinc.com

4790 **Northern Nevada Center for Independent Living**
999 Pyramid Way
Sparks, NV 89431
775-353-3599
800-552-5588
FAX: 775-353-3588
e-mail: nncil3@sbcglobal.net
www.medtech-services.com

Joe Bohl, Contact

Community based, not for profit organizaiton providing quality support services that include: independent living skills training, information and referral, peer counseling, and aggressive advocacy for all people with disabilites and disability issues.

4791 **Southern Nevada Center for Independent Living: North Las Vegas**
3100 E Lake Mead Boulevard
North Las Vegas, NV 89030
702-649-3822
FAX: 702-649-5022
e-mail: sncilsocnv@aol.com

4792 **Southern Nevada Center for Independent Living (SNCIL)**
6039 Eldora
Suite F-6
Las Vegas, NV 89146
702-889-4216
FAX: 702-889-4574
e-mail: sncilnv@aol.com

Mary Evilsizer, Contact

New Hampshire

4793 **Granite State Independent Living Foundation**

PO Box 895 Drive
Franconia, NH 03580 **603-823-5772**
FAX: 603-823-5402
www.gsil.org

Larry Robinson, Director

Offers attendant care registry, disability education and referrals.

4794 **New Hampshire Technology Partnership Project: Institute on Disability**

Concord Center
Concord, NH 03301 **603-862-4320**
800-427-3338
FAX: 603-226-0389
TTY:603-224-0630
e-mail: mcschuh@cisunix.unh.edu
www.nichcy.edu/projects/technology_policy.htm

Jan Nisbet PhD, Principal Investigator
Terese Wilkomm PhD, Principal Investigator

Provides extensive training and network development focused on: (1)early intervention, (2) inclusive education, (3) supported living and employment, and (4) using alternative and augmentative communication to develop free expression and citizenship.

New Jersey

4795 **A Center for Independent Living: Alliance for Disabled in Action**

629 Amboy Avenue
Suite LL
Edison, NJ 08837 **732-738-4388**
FAX: 732-738-4416
TTY:732-388-4416
e-mail: adacil@adacil.org
www.adacil.org

Richard Ringhof, Executive Director

Serves Middlesex, Somerset and Union counties in NJ.

4796 **Camden City Independent Living Center**

2600 Mount Ephraim Avenue
Suite 415
Camden, NJ 08104 **856-966-0800**
FAX: 856-966-0832
TTY:609-966-0830
e-mail: ccilc@bellatlantic.net

Lorraine Culbertson, Contact

4797 **Center for Independent Living of S Jersey**

1200 Delsea Drive
Plaza 47, Suite 6
Westville, NJ 08093 **856-853-6490**
800-413-3791
FAX: 856-853-1466
TTY:856-853-7602
e-mail: cilsj@aol.com

Hazel Lee, Executive Director
Danuta Debicki, Administrator
Edith Gray, Independent Living Specialist

Dedicated to providing people with disabilities in Gloucester and Camden counties the opportunity to actively participate in society, to provide freedom of choice, to work, to own a home, raise a family and in general, to participate to the fullest extent in day-to-day activities. The center provides information and referrals, advocacy, peer support, and independent living skills training.

4798 **Community Action for Independent Living**

One Cornell Parkway
Springfield, NJ 07081 **973-564-7557**
FAX: 973-467-4255
e-mail: CAILnj@aol.com
www.shanj.org/Resources/directory/dirb.htm

Stanley John, Executive Director

Private, non-profit, New Jersey based agency dedicated to providing quality services to individuals with developmental disabilities and mental health issues. Designed to maintain and improve the emotional well-being and quality of life of all individuals receiving services.

4799 **Dial: Disabled Information Awareness & Liv ing**

66 Mount Prospect Avenue
Building C
Clifton, NJ 07013 **973-470-8090**
FAX: 973-470-8171
TTY:973-470-2521
e-mail: dial.inc@yahoo.com
community.nj.com/cc/dial

John Fedix Jr, Executive Director

DIAL, Inc. is a non-profit center for Independent Living offering information and referral, peer support, independent living skills training, recreation and advocacy guidance to persons with disabilities in north New Jersey Passaic and Essex counties. *$25.00*

8 pages Annually

4800 **Disabled Advocates Working for Northwest (DAWN)**

400 S Main Street
Suite 3
Wharton, NJ 07885 **973-361-5666**
888-383-DAWN
FAX: 973-361-7086
TTY:973-361-6032
e-mail: info@dawninc.org
www.dawninc.org

Carmela Slivinski, Executive Director
Roberta Schwartz, Independent Living Specialist

DAWN is nonprofit, consumer controlled, nonresidential Center for Independent Living. DAWN provides a variety of services to people with disabilities and their families to help them secure a more independent lifestyle. Services include information and referral, peer support groups, sibling support groups, Independent Living Skills training, advocacy, recreation activities for adults and youth.

4801 **Family Resource Associates**

35 Haddon Avenue
Shrewsbury, NJ 07702 **732-530-9646**
FAX: 732-747-1896

Susan Levine, Social Worker

A private, non-profit agency serving disabled and developmentally delayed children birth to 8 years old and their families. Education, therapy, parent training, counseling and support in a home-based setting is emphasized. Recreation programs and other resources are available for the community. Physical, Occupational, Speech and Developmental services Also the TECH CONNECTION provides technology access, resource information and training for all ages.Free to per hour cost depending on service.

4802 Heightened Independence and Progress

131 Main Street
Suite 120
Hackensack, NJ 07601
201-996-9100
FAX: 201-996-9422
e-mail: ber@hipcil.org

Eileen Goff, Executive Director

4803 Jersey City Chapter: Heightened Independence and Progress

2815 Kennedy Boulevard
Suite 2G
Jersey City, NJ 07306
201-413-1200
FAX: 201-413-0520
TTY:201-413-0521
e-mail: hud@hipcil.org

Kathleen Wood, Contact

4804 MOCEANS Center for Independent Living

279 Broadway
1st Floor
Long Branch, NJ 07740
732-571-4884
FAX: 732-571-4003
e-mail: moceans@moceans.org
www.moceans.org

Patricia K McShane, Executive Director
Stanley Soden, Coordinator of IL Services

Offers peer support, disability education and personal assistant services. Serving Monmouth and Ocean Counties with information and referrals, advocacy, peer support and independent living instructions.

4805 New Jersey Technology Assistive Resource Program (TARP)

New Jersey Protection & Advocacy
210 S Broad Street, Third Floor
Trenton, NJ 08608
609-777-0945
800-342-5832
FAX: 609-341-3327
TTY:609-633-7106
e-mail: gblue@njpanda.org
www.njpanda.org/tarp

Ellen Lence, Project Director

Consumer-driven program whose mission is to increase awareness of and improve access to assistive technology for all people with disabilities in the state. Provides information and referral through its 800 telephone number and Web site regarding all aspects of assistive technology.Also provides advocacy saervices.

4806 Progressive Center for Independent Living

831 Parkway Avenue
Suite B-2
Ewing, NJ 08618
609-530-0006
FAX: 609-530-1166
e-mail: susan.jacobsen@pcil.org
www.pcil.org

Susan Jacobsen, Information/Referral Specialist

To foster the independence of peple with disabilities through information and referall services, advocacy, peer support and independent living skills training.

4807 Project Freedom

223 Hutchinson Road
Robbinsville, NJ 08691
609-448-2998
FAX: 609-448-5821
e-mail: projectfreedom@aol.com
www.projectfreedom.org

Norman Smith, Associate Executive Director
Tim Doherty, Executive Director

Provides services with the goal of empowering people with disabilities to live independently; Housing Development/Administration geared to develop and administer various barrier-free apartment complexes with support services.

4808 Resources for Independent Living

1 Hospital Plaza
Riverside, NJ 08075
856-764-2745
FAX: 856-764-5573
TTY:856-461-3482
e-mail: pam@rilnj.com

Pam Reid, Executive Director

4809 Total Living Center

402 A White Horse Pike
PO Box 342
Egg Harbor City, NJ 08215
609-965-3734
FAX: 609-965-1270
e-mail: totalctr@bellatlantic.net
www.total-living-center.org

Carolyn G Silvestro, Executive Director

One of nine Independent Living Centers in New Jersey. TLC is a community-based, consumer-driven non-profit, working with cross disability population and offers information and referral, advocacy, peer counseling and life skills training. TLC works with the severely disabled population.

4810 Tri-County Independent Living Center

120 N High Street
Suite 12
Millville, NJ 08332
856-327-5177
FAX: 856-327-5153

New Mexico

4811 Ability Center

715 E Idaho
Suite 3-E
Las Cruces, NM 88001
505-526-5016
800-376-4372
FAX: 505-526-1202
e-mail: ability_center@hotmail.com

Arnulfo Hernandez, Executive Director
Sandy Lopez, Intake Specialist

4812 CASA

2301 Christine N
PO Box 36916
Albuquerque, NM 87176
505-298-7609

Francis Nye, Director

Offers peer counseling and information and referral services.

4813 CHOICES Center for Independent Living

400 N Pennsylvania
Suite 425
Roswell, NM 88201
505-627-6727
FAX: 505-627-6754
e-mail: choicesed@zianet.com

Barbara Thomson, Executive Director

4814 Independent Living Resource Center

4401-B Lomas Boulevard NE
Albuquerque, NM 87110
505-266-5022
800-260-5022
FAX: 505-266-5150
e-mail: ilrcabq@aol.com

Gil Yildiz, Executive Director
Kathy Petrella, Program Manager

Using a self-help peer approach model, ILRC staff provides services, such as, independent living skills training, peer counseling, individual and systems advocacy, information and referral and service coordination to more than 400 people with disabilities annually in the counties of Bernalillo, Valencia, Cibola, Sandoval, Torrance, Guadalupe and DeBaca. Also provides funding for home modifications, vehicle modifications, assistive technology, adaptive devices, and professional counseling.

4815 New Mexico Technology Assistance Program

New Mexico State Department of Education
Division /Vocational Rehabilitation
435 Saint Michaels Drive, Bldg D
Santa Fe, NM 87505
505-954-8533
800-866-2253
FAX: 505-954-8562
TTY:800-659-4915
e-mail: aklaus@state.nm.us
www.nmtap.com

Alan Klaus, Project Director
Caroll Cadena, Public Contact

Examines and works to eliminate barriers to obtaining assistive technology in New Mexico. Has established a statewide program for coordinating assistive technology services; is designed to assist people with disabilities to locate, secure, and maintain assistive technology.

4816 New Vistas

1205 Parkway Drive
Santa Fe, NM 87505
505-471-1001
FAX: 505-471-4427
e-mail: rgarcia@newvistas.org

Ronald Garcia, Contact

4817 San Juan Center for Independence

3535 E 30th Street
Suite 101
Farmington, NM 87402
505-566-5827
FAX: 505-566-5842
e-mail: swatson@sjci.org
www.sjci.org

Sherry Watson, Executive Director
Andy Curry, Program Director
Nancy Johnson, Contracts Manager

SJCI is a New Mexico private residential, nonprofit corporation that serves people with disabilities. The purpose of SJCI is to provide a variety of community based, consumer driven service to people with disablities to promote independence, self-residence and intergration into the community.

New York

4818 AIM

2028 Lake Road
Elmira, NY 14903
607-733-3718
FAX: 607-733-0180
TTY:607-733-7764

4819 AIM Independent Living Center

271 E 1st Street
Corning, NY 14830
607-962-8225
FAX: 607-937-5125
e-mail: aimilc@surftech.com

Maria Sweet, Director
Peter Maier, Executive Director

A non-residential resource center run by and for people with disabilities, works with individuals providing I & R, peer support, IL skills, development & advocacy. Works with the community to promote a barrier free inclusive environment.

4820 ARISE: Center for Independent Living

1065 James Street
Suite 110
Syracuse, NY 13203
315-472-3171
FAX: 315-472-9252

Melissa Weiss, Executive Director

Offers peer counseling, attendant care registry, referrals and advocacy services, computer recycling, supported employment, career ladders transition program, universal design center.

4821 ARISE: Center for Independent Living

104 W Utica Street
Oswego, NY 13126
315-342-4088
FAX: 315-342-4107
TTY:315-342-4088

4822 Access to Independence of Cortland County

37 Church Street
Cortland, NY 13045
607-753-7363
FAX: 607-756-4884
e-mail: access@odyssey.net
www.cilcortland.org

An independent living center providing resources and advocacy for all people with disabilities. Services include: peer counseling, individual and systems advocacy, independent living skills training, information and referral.

4823 Action Toward Independence Middletown

130 Dolson Avenue
Suite 35
Middletown, NY 10940
845-343-4284
FAX: 845-342-5269
e-mail: ati@warwick.net
www.actiontowardindependence.org

4824 Action Toward Independence: Monticello

33 Lakewood Avenue
Monticello, NY 12701
845-794-4228
FAX: 845-794-4475
www.actiontowardindependence.org

4825 Barrier Free Living

270 E 2nd Street
New York, NY 10009
212-677-6668
FAX: 212-539-1526
e-mail: paulf@bflnyc.org
www.bflnyc.org

Paul B Feuerstein, President/CEO
Lewis B Lokitz, COO
Tina Barth, Residence Director

Services to disabled adults include: shelter for homeless disabled men and women; non-residential domestic violence intervention counseling; homeless outreach; mental health counseling.

4826 Bergeron Health Care
15 Second Street
Dolgeville, NY 13329
315-429-8407
800-371-2778
FAX: 315-429-8862
e-mail: info@adaptivemall.com
www.adaptivemall.com

Katie Bergeron, Managing Partner

Adaptive equipment on display, strollers, wheelchairs, walkers, gait trainers, car seats, seating, tricycles, and more.

4827 Bronx Independent Living Services
3525 Decatur Avenue
Bronx, NY 10467
718-515-2800
FAX: 718-515-2844
e-mail: bobbi@bils.org

Barbara Linn, Contact

4828 Brooklyn Center for Independence of the Disabled
2044 Ocean Avenue
Suite B-3
Brooklyn, NY 11230
718-998-3000
FAX: 718-998-3743
e-mail: advocate@bcid.org
www.bcid.org

Sharon Shapiro-Lacks, Contact

4829 Buffalo Independent Living Center
3108 Main Street
Buffalo, NY 14214
716-836-0822
FAX: 716-835-3967

Douglas Usiak

A nonprofit, cross-disability, consumer/citizen directed services and advocacy organization for persons with disabilities in Western New York. Its main purpose is to assist and educate persons with disabilities to take control of the events and processes that influence their daily lives. Services include: transportation, peer counseling, interpreters of the deaf, blind/deaf instruction, housing and architectural consultation.

4830 Capital District Center for Independence
855 Central Avenue
Suite 110
Albany, NY 12206
518-459-6422
FAX: 518-459-7847
e-mail: cdci@nobleharbor.com
cdci@cdciweb.com

Laurel Lei Kelley, Executive Director

An independent living center.

4831 Catskill Center for Independence
Route 23 Southside
PO Box 1247
Oneonta, NY 13820
607-432-8000
FAX: 607-432-6907
e-mail: ccfi@wpe.com
www.wpe.com/~ccfi

Chris Zachmeyer, Executive Director

One of 35 community-based independent living centers located throughout the state of New York. As an advocacy agency, we provide a vareity of services to people with disabilities, their friends and family members. In addition, we provide advocacy, training, and technical assistance to our community members, organizations, businesses and state and local governments in a variety of disability related areas. Serves Otsego, Delaware and Schoharie counties.

4832 Center for Independence of the Disabled of New York (CIDNY)
841 Broadway
Suite 205
New York, NY 07152
212-674-2300
FAX: 212-254-5953
TTY:212-674-5619
e-mail: info@cindy.org
www.cidny.org

Susan Sheer, Executive Director
Sharon Shapiro-Lacks, Deputy Director
Charles Nolan, Training Education Coordinator

4833 Center for Independent Living: Action Towards Independence
2927 Route 6
Slate Hill, NY 10973
845-355-2030
FAX: 845-355-2060
e-mail: ati@warwick.net

Nancy Horton, Co-Director
Margaret Jeffries, Co-Director

Information, referral, case management, transportation and system and individual advocacy, architectural barrier removal consultations, peer support, independent living skills development and parenting classes.

4834 DD Center/St.Lukes: Roosevelt Hospital Center
1000 10th Avenue
New York, NY 10019
212-523-6230
FAX: 212-523-6241

Dr. Steven Wolf, Director

4835 Directions in Independent Living
512 W State Street
Olean, NY 14760
585-373-4602
FAX: 585-373-4604
e-mail: oleanilc@yahoo.com

Leonard X Liquori, Executive Director

4836 Finger Lakes Independence Center
609 W Clinton Street
Suite 112
Ithaca, NY 14850
607-272-2433
FAX: 607-272-0902
e-mail: flic@clarityconnect.com
www.fliconline.org

Lenore Schwager, Executive Director

Offers peer counseling, attendant care registry, information on accessible housing and referrals.

4837 Genesee Region Independent Living Center
61 Swan Street
Batavia, NY 14020
585-343-4524
FAX: 585-343-6656

Ann Bell, Executive Director

Offers: Advocacy, peer counseling, benefits advisement (information and assistance), support groups, loan closet, transportation (ten passenger lift equipped van), library - books, tapes and brochures on various aspects of disabilities, also closed circuit TV print enlarger, and a print scanner with synthesized speech, architectural barrier consultations, independent living skills instruction, community education and information and referral.

4838 Glens Falls Independent Living Center

71 Glenwood Avenue
Queensbury, NY 12804
518-792-3537
FAX: 518-792-0979
e-mail: gfile@adelphia.net
www.gfilc.com

Patrick Doyle, Executive Director

Offers standard ILC core services. Programs include Center for Assistive Computer Technology; Capital District Regional TRAID Center; and monthly consumer luncheons; Polly's House - Center for Therapeutic Arts.

4839 Harlem Independent Living Center

5-15 W 125th Street
New York, NY 10027
212-369-2371
800-673-2371
FAX: 212-369-9283
e-mail: harlemilc@aol.com
www.proyectovision.net/english/about/harlemci

Christina Curryas, Executive Director

A non-profit agency that advocates for people with disabilities by assisting with the application process of housing, benefits, etc. Our services are free of charge.

4840 Herkimer Resource Center for Independent Living

401 E German Street
Steuben Center, 2nd Floor
Herkimer, NY 13350
315-866-7246
FAX: 315-866-7280
e-mail: dannym_13350@yahoo.com
www.rcil.com

Danny McLain, Advocacy Coordinator
Kathy Brown, Information Resource Coordinator
Ann Abramczyk, Coordinator ADAC

RCIL's varied services are consumer-driected. With expertise in law and services assistance is available not only to persons with disabilities, but the community at large. Advocacy, independent living skills training, peer counseling information and referral, benefits advisement and a coalition of support services to persons with Alzheimer's disease and related dementias and to the families, caregivers and professionals involved with them.

4841 Independent Living

5 Washington Terrace
Newburgh, NY 12550
845-565-1162
FAX: 845-565-0567
e-mail: ilid@frontiernet.net

Doug Hovey, Contact

4842 Independent Living Center of the Hudson Valley

160 Fairview Avenue
Hudson, NY 12534
518-828-4886
518-828-6293
FAX: 518-828-2592
TTY:518-828-6293
www.ilusa.com

Denise Figueroa, Excutive Director
Karen Garofallou, Director
Vincent Reiter, Personal Assistance Services

4843 Independent Living Center of the Hudson Valley

Troy Atrium
Broadway & Fourth Street
Troy, NY 12180
518-274-0701
FAX: 518-274-7944
e-mail: dfigny@aol.com
www.ilusa.com/ilchv

Denise Figueroa, Contact

4844 Long Island Center for Independent Living

3601 Hempstead Turnpike
Suite 208
Levittown, NY 11756
516-731-7385
FAX: 516-796-0529
TTY:516-796-0135
e-mail: licil@aol.com
www.members.aol.com/licil/prof/index.htm

Joan Lynch, Program Manager (CDPAP)
Therese Aprile, Director Advocacy
Marc Miller, Resource Specialist

Offers peer counseling, information and referral services and other services to te community. Benefits, advisement, advocacy, counseling, attendant care referral, housing referral, equipment loan bank, transportation service, consumer directed personal assistant program (CDPAP).

4845 Massena Independent Living Center

156 Center Street
Massena, NY 13662
315-764-9442
FAX: 315-764-9464
e-mail: mindepli@twny.rr.com

Jeff Reifensnyder, Executive Director

Provides a variety of non-residential direct services as well as educating the public through community awareness campaigns. Also seeks to address the current appropriate unmet needs of persons experiencing a disability - primarily in St Lawrence and Franklin Counties.

4846 Minority Outreach Project

200 Hamliton Avenue
White Plains, NY 10607
914-682-3926
FAX: 914-682-0926

4847 Nassau County Office for the Physically Challenged

1550 Franklin Avenue
Mineola, NY 11501
516-571-3119
FAX: 516-571-6150

Don Dreyer, Director

This agency serves as the ADA compliance coordinating office for all Nassau County governmental facilities, programs and services. It also serves in an advisory capacity to local, regional and national policy-making organizations, planning committees and legislative bodies and conducts advocacy as well as direct programs and services to enhance inclusion by people with disabilities to employment, consumerism and transportation.

4848 Niagara Frontier Center for Independent Living

1522 Main Street
Niagara Falls, NY 14305
716-282-4730
FAX: 716-284-0829

Kathleen , Executive Director

Offers peer counseling, referrals and disability education.

4849 North Country Center for Independence: Tupper Lake

38 Barry Avenue
Tupper Lake, NY 12986
518-359-3291
FAX: 518-359-3291

4850 North Country Center for Independence: Plattsburgh

102 Sharron Avenue
Plattsburgh, NY
518-563-9058
FAX: 518-563-0292
TTY:518-563-9058
e-mail: andrew@ncci-online.com
www.ncci-online.com

4851 **Northern Regional Center for Independent Living**

7594 State Street
Lowville, NY 13367
315-376-8696
FAX: 315-376-8986
TTY:315-376-8696

4852 **Northern Regional Center for Independent Living**

165 Mechanic Street
Watertown, NY 13601
315-785-8703
800-585-8703
FAX: 315-785-8704
e-mail: nrcil@nrcil.org
www.ncil.org

Aileen Geiling, Contact

4853 **Options for Independence: Auburn**

75 Genesee Street
Auburn, NY 13021
315-253-9786
800-496-9148
FAX: 315-255-0836
e-mail: opforind.@aol.com
www.optionsforindependence.org

Guy Thomas Cosentino, Executive Director
Crystal Purcell, Seneca County Coordinator
Rosemarie Homick, Peer Advocate

Offers peer counseling, disability education and information on accessible housing and information regarding the Americans with Disabilities Act.

4854 **Options for Independence: Seneca Falls**

55 Fall Street
Seneca Falls, NY 13148
315-568-2724
FAX: 315-568-1844
e-mail: opforind.@aol.com
www.optionsforindependence.org

Guy Thomas Cosentino, Executive Director
Crystal Purcell, Seneca County Coordinator
Rosemarie Homick, Peer Advocate

Offers peer counseling, disability education and information on accessible housing and information regarding the Americans with Disabilities Act.

4855 **Queens Independent Living Center**

14040 Queens Boulevard
Jamaica, NY 11435
718-658-2526
FAX: 718-658-5295

Robin S Shaikun, Executive Director

Provides resources, individual advocacy and systems advocacy to ensure independence and the civil rights of people with disabilities through peer counseling, education and referrals.

4856 **Regional Center for Independent Living**

1641 E Avenue
Rochester, NY 14610
585-442-6470
FAX: 585-271-8558
TTY:7164426470
e-mail: rcil@rcil.org
www.rcil.org

4857 **Resource Center for Accessible Living**

592 Ulster Avenue
Kingston, NY 12401
845-331-0541
FAX: 845-331-2076
TTY:845-331-8680
e-mail: rcal@ulster.net

Joan Gundersen, Executive Director

4858 **Resource Center for Independent Living**

401-409 Columbia Street
PO Box 210
Utica, NY 13503
315-797-4642
FAX: 315-797-4747
TTY:315-797-5837
e-mail: rcil@rcil.com

Burt Danovitz PhD, Executive Director
Rose Marie Roberts CRC, Associate Dir. Consumer Svcs.
Wendy Gagliardo, Associate Director Admin. Svcs.

A nonresidential, nonprofit agency which administers a wide range of independent living and advocacy services for and with people with disabilities. As part of the Independent Living Movement, we believe that the basic right of contributing to and participating in society as a self-determining individual must extend to all citizens. All Center services are consumer directed and aimed to increase individual rights, options and achievements.

4859 **Resource Center for Independent Living: Amsterdam**

2540 Riverfront Center
Amsterdam, NY 12010
518-842-3561
FAX: 518-842-0905

Ramon Rodriguez, Program Director
Marybeth Wojcik, Program Assistant

Peer counseling, advocacy, independent living skills training, information and referral services, self-advocacy training, ADA consultation, home and community based services, community education, disability benefits, advisement and more. All programs and services are available in English and Spanish.

4860 **Rockland Independent Living Center**

238 N Main Street
Spring Valley, NY 10977
845-426-0707
FAX: 845-426-0989
e-mail: LJO@MHV.NET
www.roldirect.com

Lorraine Jackson-Ordia, Contact

4861 **SILO**

3180 Express Drive S
Central Islip, NY 11722
516-348-0207
FAX: 516-348-0262

4862 **SILO: Islandia**

20 Oval Drive
Islandia, NY 11722
631-348-7655
FAX: 631-348-0262

4863 **Saratoga County Options for Independent Living**

8 Butler Place
Saratoga Springs, NY 12866
518-584-8202
FAX: 518-584-1195
TTY:518-584-4752

Teena Willard, Assistant Director
Dawn Lincoln, Advocate
Pat Doyle, ER Director

4864 **Southern Tier Independence Center**

24 Prospect Avenue
Binghamton, NY 13901
607-724-2111
FAX: 607-722-5646
e-mail: stic@stic-cil.org
www.stic-cil.org

Maria Dibble, Executive Director

Offers supported employment, consumer directed personel assistance, assistive technology services, sign language interpreters, ADA training/consultation, servive coordinator, peer counseling, advocacy.

4865 Southwestern Independent Living Center
843 N Main Street
Jamestown, NY 14701
716-661-3010
FAX: 716-661-3011

Marie Carrubba, Executive Director

Offers disability education, advocacy and information on accessible housing, wheelchair or acessible transportation, interpreting services, brulling, IL skills training, peer support.

4866 Staten Island Center for Independent Living
470 Castleton Avenue
Staten Island, NY 10301
718-720-9016
FAX: 718-720-9664
e-mail: dorothy.doran@verizon.net
community.silive.com/cc/sicil

Dorothy Doran, Executive Director

4867 Suffolk Independent Living Organization (SILO)
745 Waverly Avenue
Holtsville, NY 11742
631-654-8007
FAX: 631-654-8077
TTY:631-654-8076
e-mail: suffolkilc1@aol.com

June Roberts, Executive Director

4868 Taconic Resources for Independence
82 Washington Street
Suite 214
Poughkeepsie, NY 12601
845-452-3913
FAX: 845-485-3196
TTY:845-485-8110
e-mail: trionline@taconicresources.net
www.taconicresources.net

Bryan Cranna, Executive Director

A center for independent living, benefits advisement information, and referral, advocacy, independent living skills, peer counseling, parent advocacy, sign language interpreters.

4869 Visions/Services for the Blind & Visually Impaired
500 Greewich Street
Third Floor
New York, NY 10013
212-425-2255
FAX: 212-425-7114
e-mail: info@visionsvcb.org
www.visionsvcb.org

Nancy Miller, Executive Director

4870 Westchester County Independent Living Center
200 Hamilton Avenue
White Plains, NY 10601
914-328-0441
FAX: 914-682-8518

Joseph Bravo, Executive Director

Offers peer counseling, attendant care registry and referrals.

4871 Westchester Disabled on the Move
984 N Broadway
Suite L-01
Yonkers, NY 10701
914-968-4717
FAX: 914-968-6137
e-mail: info@wdom.org
wdom.org

Melvyn R Tanzman, Executive Director
Scott Smith, Program Director

Full range of independent living services including housing search and acquisition assistance, ADA compliance, services to high school students with disabilities.

4872 Wiswall Center for Independent Living
71 Glenwood Avenue
Queensbury, NY 12804
518-792-3537
FAX: 518-792-0979
e-mail: cil@interpcs.net

Patrick Doyle Jr, Contact

North Carolina

4873 Center for Accessible Housing
North Carolina State University
PO Box 8613
Raleigh, NC 27695
919-515-3015
FAX: 919-515-3023
e-mail: cahd@ncsu.edu

Established in 1989, the Center improves the quality and availability of housing for people with disabilities. The center provides assistance and information to individuals and industry through research, collaborative efforts with manufacturers, training and information services.

4874 Disability Awareness Network
609 Country Club Drive
Suite C
Greenville, NC 27834
252-355-5272
FAX: 252-353-5160
e-mail: DAWNpittco@aol.com

Marty Silverthorne, Contact

Information and referral for diabled persons; peer counseling for diabled persons; advocacy on ADA issues; independent living skills and training.

4875 Joy A Shabazz Center for Independent Living
620 S Elm Street
Suite 309
Grennsboro, NC 27406
336-272-0501
FAX: 336-272-0572
e-mail: tap99@bellsouth.net
www.advocacyproject.org

4876 Live Independently Networking Center
PO Box 1135
Newton, NC 28658
828-464-0331
FAX: 828-464-7375
e-mail: linc@twave.net
www.dimenet.com/dimeweb/il.htm

Donavon Kirby, Deputy Director

Private, nonprofit, federally funded center for independent living located in Western North Carolina.

4877 Live Independently Networking Center: Hickory
2830 16th Street NE
Hickory, NC 28601
828-464-0331
FAX: 828-464-7375

4878 Pathways for the Future
525 Mineral Springs Drive
Sylva, NC 28779
828-631-1167
FAX: 828-631-1169
e-mail: pathways@dnet.net
www.pathwayscil.org

Aimee Speers, Program Development Coordinator

Dedicated to increasing independence, changing attitudes, promoting equal access and building a peer support network in Western North Carolina through the use of community education, independent living services and advocacy. Quarterly newsletter is published. Call or write to Pathways to add your name to the mailing list for Pathfinder.

4879 Programs for Accessible Living
5701 Executive Center Drive
Suite 320
Charlotte, NC 28212
704-537-0550
FAX: 704-566-0507

Julia Sain, Executive Director

Offers information and referrals, peer counseling for people with disabilities, advocacy and independent living skills classes. PAL helps people with disabilities achieve and maintain their independence in the community.

4880 Western Alliance Center for Independent Living
30 London Road
Asheville, NC 28803
828-274-0444
FAX: 828-274-4461
e-mail: ashcilnc@bellsouth.net
www.westernalliance.org

Bart Floyd, Site Coordinator

Core: Information and Referral, Peer Counseling, Independent Living Skills Training and Advocacy. Counties served: Buncombe, Henderson, Madison, McDowell, Polk, Rutherford and Transylvania.

North Dakota

4881 Dakota Center for Independent Living
3111 E Broadway Avenue
Bismarck, ND 58501
701-222-3636
FAX: 701-222-0511
TTY:701-222-3636
e-mail: raptor@dcil.com
www.dakotacil.org

Robert Gomez, Contact

4882 Dakota Center for Independent Living: Dickinson
40 1st Avenue W
Suite 203
Dickinson, ND 58601
701-483-4363
FAX: 701-483-4361
e-mail: dcil@ndsupernet.com

Kim Johnson, Coordinator

4883 Fraser
2902 S University Drive
Fargo, ND 58103
701-232-3301
FAX: 701-237-5775
e-mail: fraser@fraserltd.org
www.fraserltd.org

Sandra Leyland, Executive Director

4884 Freedom Resource Center for Independent Living
2701 Ninth Avenue SW
Fargo, ND 58103
701-478-0459
800-450-0459
FAX: 701-478-0510
e-mail: freedom@fargocity.com
www.macil.org/freedom

Nate Aalgaard, Executive Director
Bobbi Franks, Information Specialist

Work toward equility and inclusion for people with disabilities throuigh programs of empowerment, community education and systems change. We serve eighteen counties, ten in North Dakota and eight in Minnesota. A quarterly newsletter, Freedom Focus, is published

4885 Independence CIL
300 3rd Avenue SW
Suite F
Minot, ND 58701
701-839-4724
800-377-5114
FAX: 701-838-1677
TTY:701-839-6561
e-mail: life@minot.ndak.net

Stephen Repnow, Executive Director
Trisha Jessen, Outreach Coordinator
Cheryl Johnson, Peer Support

A resource center for independent living.

Ohio

4886 Ability Center of Defiance
516 Perry Street
Defiance, OH 43512
419-782-9231
FAX: 419-782-9231
e-mail: dsteffel@abilitycenter.org

4887 Ability Center of Greater Toledo
5605 Monroe Street
Sylvania, OH 43560
419-885-5733
FAX: 419-882-4813
e-mail: shellypc@yahoo.com
www.abilitycenter.org

Timothy Harrington, Contact

4888 Access Center for Independent Living
35 S Jefferson
Dayton, OH 45402
937-341-5202
FAX: 937-341-5217
TTY:937-341-5215
e-mail: roy@acils.com
www.acils.com

Roy Puston, Interim Executive Director

Offers peer counseling, disability education and other services to the community.

4889 Fairfield Center for Disabilities and Cerebral Palsy
681 E 6th Avenue
Lancaster, OH 43130
740-653-5501
FAX: 740-653-6046

Edwin Payne, Board Secretary

Adult Day Program and Transportation.

4890 Help Foundation
3622 Prospect Avenue
Cleveland, OH 44115
216-432-4810
FAX: 216-361-2608
e-mail: helpfoundation@worldnet.att.net

Daniel Rice, COO
Patricia Schwartz, Quality Resurance Director
Pam Cypher, Director HELP Six Chimneys

Offers disability education and referrals as well as subsidized housing and independent living services at several locations. Program support services to adults with mental retardation and other developmental disabilities. Serving, Northeast Ohio.

4891 **Independent Living Center of Central Ohio**

1 Marion Avenue
Suite 115C
Mansfield, OH 44903

419-526-6770
FAX: 419-526-6870
e-mail: ilcnco@aol.com

Jonnie Fisher, Contact

4892 **Linking Employment Ability Potential: Independent Living Center**

2100 N Ridge Road
Elyria, OH 44035

440-324-3444
FAX: 440-324-2112
TTY:440-324-2113
e-mail: leap@kellnet.com
www.ohiosilc.org/about/cils.html#leap_cil

Elsie Danevich, Contact

4893 **Mid-Ohio Board for an Independent Living Environment (MOBILE)**

690 S High Street
Columbus, OH 43206

614-443-5936
FAX: 614-443-5954
TTY:614-443-5957
e-mail: bev@infinet.com
www.ohiosilc.org/about/cils.html

Beverly Rackett, Executive Director

Offers information and research, advocacy, independent living skills training, peer support, disability awareness training and accessibility design standards technical assistance.

4894 **Rehabilitation Service of North Central Ohio**

270 Sterkel Boulevard
Mansfield, OH 44907

419-756-1133
800-589-1133
FAX: 419-756-6544
e-mail: rehabvp@richnet.net
www.therehabcenter.org

Eric R Weber, President/CEO
Linda Williams, VP Medical Rehab Services
Linda Kafer, VP Behavioral Health Services

Private nonprofit organization providing coordinated, team-oriented comprehensive outpatient rehabilitation services to children and adults of all ages. Serves 8 counties in N/C Ohio. Four umbrella areas of service include medical rehabilitation services, vocational rehabilitation services, behavioral health service and drug and alcohol addiction services. Medical rehabilitation services include physical therapy, occupational therapy, speech therapy and audiology.

4895 **Samuel W Bell Home for the Sightless**

1507 Elm Street
Cincinnati, OH 45210

513-241-0720
FAX: 513-241-2560

Louis Hoff, Director

Offers a residential home for the totally blind and legally blind adults, male and female.

4896 **Services for Independent Living**

25100 Euclid Avenue
Suite 105
Cleveland, OH 44117

216-731-1529
FAX: 216-731-3083
e-mail: sil@stratos.net

Jamy Zadel, Services Coordinator

Offers support ADA, consultation and education, advocacy, transitional education services, independent living skills training, information and referrals.

4897 **Society for Equal Access: Independent Living Center**

821 Anola Avenue
Suite B
Dover, OH 44622

330-343-3668
888-213-4452
FAX: 330-343-3721
TTY:330-602-2557
e-mail: ilc@tusco.net
gmntrico4u.org/counties/tscarawas/sfeailc.htm

Julie A Ronald, Executive Director
Ruthanne Fulmer, Advocate
Jerome Geisinger, Independent Skills Specialist

The Society works with individuals to become more independent. Our agency assists with peer support, advocacy, information and referral, independent living skills and transportation. Our goal is to move those with challenges in the direction ofn independence.

4898 **Tri-County Independent Living Center**

680 E Market Street
Suite 205
Akron, OH 44304

330-762-0007
FAX: 330-762-7416
TTY:800-750-0750
e-mail: rose@tcilc.tnet.com

Rose Juriga, Contact

4899 **United Cerebral Palsy of Central Ohio**

440 Industrial Mile Road
Columbus, OH 43228

614-279-0109
800-670-9146
FAX: 614-279-2527
e-mail: ucpco@mindspring.com
www.ucpofcentralohio.org

Aviana Adams, Manager
Kathy Streblo, Executive Director

UCP central ohio provides exceptional program and support services designed to promote self reliance, present choices, and improve the quality of life for central ohiosans with disabilities and aging conditions.

4900 **United Cerebral Palsy of Columbus and Franklin County**

440 Industrial Mile Road
Columbus, OH 43228

614-279-0109
FAX: 614-279-2527
e-mail: uspoco@prodiax.net

Mark Guthry, Executive Director
Karen D Osborne, Development Director

The mission of the organization is to encourage and facilitate growth of self-sufficient, productive and participating citizens who are differently-abled. Services are individually tailored to the consumer.

Oklahoma

4901 **Ability Resources**

823 S Detroit
Suite 110
Tulsa, OK 74120

918-592-1235
FAX: 918-592-5651

Carla Lawson, Director

Offers disability education, peer counseling and referrals, assistive technology lending library, job readiness training, employment placement, nursing home outreach, literacy tutoring, ADA training and technical assistance.

4902 **Green County Independent Living Resource Center**
4100 SE Adams Road
Suite C106
Bartlesville, OK 07152
918-335-1314
800-559-0567
FAX: 918-333-1814
e-mail: gcilrc@aol.com

Brandi Johnson, Administrative Assistant
Judy Viles, Executive Director
Tammy Williams, Independent Skills Specialist

Independent living skills training, information and referrals, advocacy, a loan library of adaptive equipment and books. Services available to all individuals with disabilities and their family members who reside in Northeastern Oklahoma.

4903 **Oklahomans for Independent Living**
321 S 3rd
Suite 2
McAlester, OK 74501
918-426-6220
FAX: 918-426-3245
e-mail: mikew@icok.net
www.icok.net

Mike Ward, Executive Director
Pam Pulchny, Associate Director

OIL is a resource center for people with disabilities. Its mission is to encourage individuals of all ages, with all type of disabilities, to increase their personal independence, empowerment, and self determination, and to achieve full integration and participation in their work, community and school.

4904 **Progressive Independence**
121 N Porter Avenue
Norman, OK 73071
405-321-3203
800-801-3203
FAX: 405-321-7601
e-mail: progind@telepath.com
www.progind.org

Jeff Hughes, Executive Director
Joseph S Mecham, AT Program Manager
Debbie Fidler, IL Programs Manager

Preovides four cores services of Information & Referral, Individaul& Systems Advocacy, Peer Counseling, and Skills Training; in addition, offers accessible computer lab, short term DME loans, ande benefits counseling for SSI/SSDI.

4905 **Sandra Beasley Independent Living Center**
705 S Oakwood Road
Suite B1
Enid, OK 73703
580-237-8508
800-375-4358
FAX: 580-233-6403
e-mail: sbilcdirector@coxinet.net

Frieda Kliewer, Executive Director
Kathy Miller, Service Coordinator

An independent living center which offers independent living skills training, peer counseling, attendant care registry, ADA consultation, advocacy services and an equipment Loan Closet.

Oregon

4906 **Central Oregon Resources for Independent Living**
20436 Clay Pigeon Court
PO Box 9425
Bend, OR 97702
541-388-8103
FAX: 541-388-1226
TTY:541-388-8103
e-mail: donstew@bendnet.com

Don Stewart, Contact

4907 **Columbia Gorge Center**
2940 Thomsen Road
Hood River, OR 97031
541-386-2376
FAX: 541-386-7788
www.CGC-direct.com

Patty Elkins, Director
CJ Webb, Client Services Coordinator
Sarah Smutz, Client Services Coordinator

Provides residential and vocational services for people with disabilities in the community.

4908 **Eastern Oregon Center for Independent Living**
144 S Oregon
PO Box 173
Ontario, OR 97914
541-889-3119
FAX: 541-889-4573
e-mail: eocil@eocil.org
www.eocil.org

4909 **HASL Independent Abilities Center**
1252 Redwood Avenue
Grants Pass, OR 97527
541-479-4275
800-758-4275
FAX: 541-479-7261
e-mail: hasl1@qwest.net

Don Drake, Chairman Board of Directors
Tina Sayre, Executive Director

To promote public awareness of the special needs and legal rights of individuals with cross-disabilities; to facilitate their integration into society and provide support through advocacy, peer counseling, skills training and information and referral to encourage independence.

4910 **Independent Living Resources**
2410 SE 11th Avenue
Portland, OR 97214
503-232-7411
FAX: 503-232-7480
TTY:503-232-8404
e-mail: ilred1@yahoo.com
www.irl.org

Suzanne Westwood, Contact

4911 **Laurel Hill Center Independent Living Program**
2145 Centennial Plaza
Eugene, OR 97401
FAX: 541-345-9218

Mary Alice Brown PhD, Executive Director

Offers vocational evaluation, training and job placement services; socialization and independent living skills training and support; serving adults with psychiatric and/or physical disabilities.

4912 Oregon Commission for the Blind
535 SE 12th Avenue
Portland, OR 97214
503-731-3221
FAX: 503-731-3230
e-mail: linda.mock@state.or.us
www.cfb.state.or.us

Linda Mock, Administrator

4913 Progressive Options
715 SW Hubert Street
Suite D
Newport, OR 97365
541-574-0384
FAX: 541-574-1927
e-mail: progop541@earthlink.net
www.progressive-options.org

4914 SPOKES Unlimited
415 Main Street
Klamath Falls, OR 97601
541-883-7547
FAX: 541-885-2469
www.spokesunlimited.org

Wendy Howard, Program Coordinator

4915 Umpqua Valley Disabilities Network
PO Box 507
Roseburg, OR 97470
541-672-6336
FAX: 541-672-8606
TTY:541-440-2882
e-mail: uvdn@jeffnet.org

Tricia Hoelscher, Contact

Pennsylvania

4916 Abilities in Motion
416 Blair Avenue
Reading, PA 19601
610-376-0010
888-376-0120
888-376-0120
FAX: 610-376-0021
TTY:610-228-2301
e-mail: aimcil@netcarrier.com
www.abilitiesinmotion.org

John Tassone, Director CIL Services
Beth Hennigan, Attendant Care Program Director

Free services to individuals with disabilities and their families.

4917 Anthracite Region Center for Independent Living
44 W Broad Street
Hazleton, PA 18201
570-455-9800
FAX: 570-455-1731
TTY:570-455-9800
e-mail: arcil@intergrafix.net

Shirley Ray, Contact

4918 Brian's House
1300 S Concord Road
W Chester, PA 19382
610-399-1175
FAX: 610-399-1828
e-mail: nnelson@woods.org
www.brianshouse.org

Lori Plunkett, Executive Director
Nancy Nelson, Director Development

Residential care in a variety of homes and apartments for people with a range of development disabilities. Cost varies with needs. Also year-round recreation programs, vocational training and employment programs.

4919 Center for Independent Living Opportunities
3450 Industrial Drive
York, PA 17402
717-840-9653
800-956-0099
FAX: 717-840-9748
TTY:717-840-9653
e-mail: cilo@yorkinternet.net

Vicki Cuscino, Executive Director
Mindy Demorest, IL Program Manager

4920 Center for Independent Living of South Central Pennsylvania
17th Street & 9th Avenue
Station Mall, Lot 30
Altoona, PA 16602
800-237-9009
FAX: 814-949-1909
e-mail: cilscpa@penn.com
www.cilscpa.org

David Brown, Srvc Coordinator/Skills Trainer
Howard Ermin Jr, Independent Living Specialist

The Center is a non-profit tax exempt community based organization, non-residential in nature. Programs are consumer controlled, accessible to the public and focusing on the individual. CILSCPA stresses the importance of utilizing community resources in meeting independent living needs in South Central PA. The Center provides services to people with disabilities and their families in Bedford, Blair, Cambria, Fulton, Huntingdon, Indiana and Somerset counties.

4921 Center for Independent Living of Central Pennsylvania
207 House AvenueRoad
Suite 107
Camp Hill, PA 17011
717-731-1900
800-323-6060
FAX: 717-731-8150
TTY:717-731-1077
e-mail: theobraddy@cilcp.org
www.cilcp.org

Theotis Braddy, Director
Janetta Green, Assistant Director
Ann Neimer, IL Program Manager

Offers information and referral services, sign language classes, independent living skills, and advocacy.

4922 Center for Independent Living of N Central Pennsylvania
210 Market Street
Suite A
Williamsport, PA 17701
717-327-9070
800-984-7492
FAX: 717-327-8610
e-mail: cilcp@aol.com

George Morton, Contact

4923 Center for Independent Living of SW Pennysylvania
7110 Penn Avenue
Pittsburgh, PA 15208
412-371-7700
FAX: 412-371-6230
TTY:412-371-7700

4924 Community Resources for Independence
2222 Filmore Avenue
Erie, PA 16506
814-838-7222
FAX: 814-838-5104
TTY:814-838-8115
e-mail: cri@cri.org
www.crinet.org

Timothy Finegan, Contact

4925 **Freedom Valley Disability Enablement**
3607 Chapel Road
Newtown Square, PA 19073 610-353-6640
800-423-4754
FAX: 610-353-6753
TTY:610-353-6753

Ann Cope, Contact

4926 **Lehigh Valley Center for Independent Living**
435 Allentown Drive
Allentown, PA 18109 610-770-9781
FAX: 610-770-9801

Amy C Beck, Executive Director

Advocacy services, information and referral, peer support, independent living skills services, housing search assistance, and refurbished computer program.

4927 **Liberty Resources**
1341 N Delaware Avenue
Suite 105
Philadelphia, PA 19125 215-634-2000
FAX: 215-634-6628

David J Schultheis, Comptroller

Provides lists of accessible housing and attendants, courses in independent living, recreational programs, equipment referrals and loans. Recently a merger with Liberty Center for Independent Living, has enabled this center to offer a wider spectrum of services for the disabled throughout the northeastern and southeastern Pennsylvania.

4928 **Life and Independence for Today**
503 Arch Street Extension
Saint Marys, PA 15857 814-781-3050
FAX: 814-781-1917
TTY:814-781-1917
e-mail: lift@penn.com

Robert Mecca, Contact

4929 **Northeastern Pennsylvania Center for Independent Living**
431 Wyoming Avenue
Scranton, PA 18503 570-344-7211
FAX: 570-344-7218

Daniel P Loftus, Executive Director

Offers information and referral services.

4930 **Pennsylvania's Initiative on Assistive Technology (PIAT) - Temple University**
1301 Cecil B Moore Avenue
423 Ritter Annex
Philadelphia, PA 19122 215-204-5966
800-204-7428
FAX: 215-204-9371
TTY:215-204-1356
e-mail: piat@astro.ocis.temple.edu
www.temple.edu/instituteondisabilities/piat

Amy S Goldman, Public Contact

Focuses on the creation of a consumer responsive system, supported by combined public and private resources, through which Pennsylvanians with disabilities have access to the assistive technology services and supports.

4931 **Three Rivers Center for Independent Living**
7110 Penn Avenue
Pittsburgh, PA 15208 412-371-7700
800-633-4583
FAX: 412-371-9430
trfn.clpgh.org/trcil

WD Chrisner III, President

Offers peer counseling, information and referral services, housing data and referral service, assistive technology program, deinstitutionalization program, consumer-controlled personal assistance program, independent living skills training, advocacy and accessibility consultants.

Sliding Fee

4932 **Tri-County Partnership for Independent Living**
69 E Beau Street
Washington, PA 15301 724-627-8826
FAX: 401-738-1083
e-mail: doug@tripil.com

Kathleen Kleinmann, Director

Offers peer counseling, disability education and information on accessible housing.

4933 **Voices for Independence**
3711 W 12th Street
Suite 3
Erie, PA 16505 814-838-9890
FAX: 814-838-9779
TTY:814-838-3702
e-mail: Shona@erie.net

Shona Eakin, Contact

Rhode Island

4934 **Blackstone Valley Center**
115 Manton Street
Pawtucket, RI 02861 401-727-0150
FAX: 401-727-0153
e-mail: contact@bucriarc.org
www.bvcriarc.org/contact99.html

Peter Holden, Executive Coordinator
Barbara Lindsay, Development Director

4935 **Franklin Court Assisted Living**
180 Franklin Street
Bristol, RI 02809 401-253-3679
www.seniorlivingresidences.com

Offers local seniors an affordable assisted living option with first-rate services and gracious accommodations.

4936 **IN-SIGHT Independent Living**
43 Jefferson Boulevard
Warwick, RI 02888 401-941-3322
FAX: 401-941-3356

Judith Smith, Contact

4937 **Ocean State Center for Independent Living**
1944 Warwick Avenue
Warwick, RI 02889 401-738-1013
FAX: 401-738-1083
TTY:401-738-1015
www.oscil.org

Lorna Ricci, Director

Information and referral services.

4938 Ocean State Center for Independent Living
59 W Shore Road
Warwick, RI 02889
401-738-1015
FAX: 401-738-1083
e-mail: oscil@rida.net
www.oscil.org

Lorna Ricci, Contact

4939 PARI Independent Living Center
500 Prospect Street
Suite 18
Pawtucket, RI 02860
401-725-1966
FAX: 401-725-2104
www.pari-ilc.org

Leo Canuel MA, Executive Director

Offers information and referral services, personal care attendant services, home modifications, advocacy services and peer counseling, independent living skills training, and recycled equipment.

4940 Rhode Island Assistive Technology Access Partnership (ATAP),RI Department of Human Services
Office of Rehabilitation Services
40 Fountain Street
Providence, RI 02903
401-421-7005
800-752-8088
FAX: 401-421-9259
TTY:401-421-7016
e-mail: reginac@ors.state.ri.us
www.atap.state.ri.us

Regina Connor, Project Director

Statewide partnership of organizations, each with a targeted focus, working together with a consumer council to remove barriers and increase access to assistive technology for individuals with disabilities of all ages.

South Carolina

4941 Coastal Disability Access
1021 Third Avenue
Conway, SC 29526
843-488-1309
FAX: 843-488-0994
e-mail: cdaspecial1@aol.com

Jessica Keith-Avinger, Volunteer Coordinator
Barbara Cole, Independent Living Specialist

Provides information and referral, advocacy, independent living skills training, and peer support for Harry, Georgetown, and Marion counties.

4942 Disability Action Center
3126 Beltline Boulevard
Columbia, SC 29204
803-779-5121
FAX: 803-779-5114
e-mail: dacdirect1@aol.com

Kathy Pelletier, Executive Director

4943 Disability Action Center Greenville
618 E Washington Street
Greenville, SC 29601
864-235-1421
FAX: 803-235-2056

4944 Graham Street Community Resources
306 Graham Street
Florence, SC 29501
843-665-6674
FAX: 843-665-6675

4945 South Carolina Assistive Technology Program (SCATP)
USC School Of Medicine
Center for Disability Resources
Columbia, SC 29208
803-935-5263
FAX: 803-935-5342
e-mail: jjendron@usit.net
www.sc.edu/scatp.net/jjendron

Evelyn Evans, Project Director

Catalyst for uniting assistive technology services statewide into an easily accessible system that is responsive to the needs of all South Carolinians with disabilities.

4946 South Carolina Independent Living Council
810 Dutch Square Boulevard
Suite 214
Columbia, SC 29210
803-731-1607
877-217-2331
FAX: 803-731-1439
e-mail: scilcdee@aol.com

Maris Burton, Executive Director
DeeAnn Jones, Executive Assistant

The SC Independent Living Council's mission is to jointly (with the DSUs) develop uses for Part B funding throughout the state. These monies can be used to: develop Centers for Independent Living; outreach to unserved and underserved populations; conduct needs assessments and research; make recommendation to policy makers regarding the delivery of IL services and provide resources for direct services.

South Dakota

4947 Aberdeen Communication Service for the Deaf
1719 Fourth Avenue SE
Aberdeen, SD 57401
605-626-2668
FAX: 605-626-3089
e-mail: csdabr@iw.net
www.c-s-d.org

Nancy Schlichenmayer, Contact

4948 Adjustment Training Center
612 10th Avenue SE
Aberdeen, SD 57401
605-229-0263
FAX: 605-225-3455

Rob Wanous, Director

Offers peer counseling, attendant care registry and referrals.

4949 Black Hills Workshop & Training Center
PO Box 2104
Rapid City, SD 57702
605-343-4550
FAX: 605-343-0879
e-mail: dennisp@bhws.com
www.bhws.com

Dennis Popp, CEO
Colleen Ronning, VP

Offers job placement, housing options, case coordination, supported employment and supported living for all disability groups, as well as specialized services for head trauma victims.

4950 **Communication Service for the Deaf (CSD)**

102 N Krohn Place
Sioux Falls, SD 57103
605-367-5760
800-642-6410
FAX: 605-367-5958
e-mail: info@c-s-d.org
www.c-s-d.org

Benjamin J Soukup, CEO

Since 1975, CSD has provided a variety of services to deaf and hard of hearing individuals. From relay services to community interpreting, advocacy to education, CSD promotes self-actualization, professional growth, independence and greater access for our consumers across the country.

4951 **Communication Service for the Deaf: Yankton**

231 Broadway Street
Suite C6
Yankton, SD 57078
605-668-9759
FAX: 605-668-6712
TTY:605-668-9759
e-mail: kmerril@iw.net

4952 **Communication Service for the Deaf: Rapid City**

150 Knollwood Drive
Rapid City, SD 57701
605-394-2544
888-304-2311
FAX: 605-394-6609
e-mail: bcudmore@c-s-d.org

Brenda Cudmore, Unit Director
Jennifer Taylor, Community Service Specialist
Summer Patchen, Community Service Specialist

4953 **Native American Advocacy Project**

PO Box 527
Winner, SD 57580
605-842-3977
FAX: 605-842-3983
e-mail: admin@sdnaap.org
www.sdnaap.org

Marla Bull Bear, Contact

4954 **Opportunities for Independent Living**

100 S Maple Street
Suite 205
Watertown, SD 57201
605-626-2976
FAX: 605-229-3954

Jeff Kisecker, Director

Offers peer counseling, attendant care registry and other services to the community.

4955 **Prairie Freedom Center for Independent Living of Yankton**

413 W 15th
Suite 107
Yankton, SD 57078
605-668-2940
FAX: 605-668-3060
TTY:605-668-2940
e-mail: pfcily@willinet.net

4956 **Prairie Freedom Center for Independent Living**

PO Box 282
Madison, SD 57042
605-256-5070
FAX: 605-256-5071
e-mail: freedom1@hcpd.com

4957 **Prairie Freedom Center for Independent Living**

301 S Garfield Avenue
Suite 8
Sioux Falls, SD 57104
605-367-5630
800-947-3770
FAX: 605-367-5639
e-mail: prairie@ideasign.com

Char Crisp, Director

Mission: To empower individuals with disabilities who choose to live independently.

4958 **South Dakota Assistive Technology Project**

DakotaLink
21 S Central
Pierre, SD 57501
605-224-5336
800-244-5336
FAX: 605-224-8320
e-mail: dvogel@tie.net
dakotalink.tie.net/BrochureNAg.htm

Dave Vogel, Public Contact

Works with consumers, state and private agencies, and organizations providing services to, or advocating for, people with disabilities to identify and eliminate barriers to individuals receiving assistive technology devices or services in a timely manner. Uses a mobile unit, outreach coordinators, rehabilitation technicians, and training programs.

4959 **Western Resources for dis-ABLED Independence**

36 E Chicago Street
Rapid City, SD 57701
605-394-1930
800-226-3938
FAX: 605-394-1933
e-mail: wrdi@dtgnet.com

Glade Jones, Executive Director

Offers peer counseling, disability education and advocacy services, independent living skills training, information and referral services, home modifications and adaptive devices.

Tennessee

4960 **Center for Independent Living of Middle Tennessee**

480 Craighead Street
Suite 200
Nashville, TN 37204
615-292-5803
FAX: 615-383-1176
e-mail: cilmt@tndisability.org
www.cil-mt.org

Tom Hopton, Contact
Floyd Stewart, Contact

A community-based nonresidential program of services designed to assist persons with disabilities gain independence and to assist the community in eliminating barriers to independence.

4961 **Disability Resource Center**

900 E Hill Avenue
Suite 120
Knoxville, TN 37915
865-637-3666
FAX: 865-637-5616
e-mail: drc@korrnet.org
www.korrnet.org/drc

Cathy Randall, Contact

4962 Jackson Center for Independent Living
231-D N Parkway
Jackson, TN 38305
731-668-2211
FAX: 731-668-0406
TTY:901-668-1772
e-mail: jcil@usit.net
www.j-cil.com

Glen Barr, Contact

4963 Memphis Center for Independent Living
163 N Angelus Street
Memphis, TN 38104
901-726-6404
FAX: 901-726-6521
e-mail: mcil@mcil.org
www.mcil.org

Deborah Cunningham, Executive Director

Offers peer counseling, disability education and information and referral services.

4964 Nashville Center for Independent Living
480 Craighead Street
Suite 200
Nashville, TN 37204
615-292-5803
FAX: 615-383-1176
e-mail: cilmt@tndisability.org
www.cil-mt.org

Tom Hopton, Contact
Floyd Stewart, Contact

4965 Tennessee Technology Access Project (TTAP)
Cordell Hull Building,5th Floor
425 5th Avenue N
Nashville, TN 37243
615-532-3122
800-732-5059
FAX: 615-532-4685
TTY:615-741-4566
e-mail: kwright@mail.state.tn.us
www.state.tn.us/mental/ttap.html

Kevin R Wright, Project Director

Emphasizes the implementation and pursuit of systems change and advocacy activities by developing an information/communication network, working with state agency policy values and developing alternate funding mechanisms. Involves consumers, and facilitates interagency cooperation and interaction with the private sector.

4966 Tri-State Resource and Advocacy
5708 Uptain Road
Suite 350
Chattanooga, TN 37411
423-892-4774
FAX: 423-892-9866
TTY:423-892-4774
e-mail: 4trac@bellsouth.net

Mark Woolfall, Executive Director

Texas

4967 ABLE Center for Independent Living
3641 N Dixie
Odessa, TX 79762
432-580-3439
FAX: 432-580-0280
e-mail: jerik4able@aol.com

Jeri Kounce, Executive Director
Jacki Campbell, Indep. Living Spec./Peer Couns.
Samuel Aguilar, Indep. Living Spec./Peer Couns.

Non-residential, nonprofit organization, guided by the philosophy of consumer choice, to assist people with disabilities achieve and maintain independent lifestyle.

4968 Austin Resource Center for Independent Living
825 E Rundberg Lane
Suite A-1
Austin, TX 78753
512-832-6349
FAX: 512-832-1869
e-mail: arcil@arcil.com
www.arcil.com

Ronald Rocha, Executive Director

4969 Austin Resource Center: Round Rock
301 Hesters Crossing
Suite 210
Round Rock, TX 78781
512-828-4624
FAX: 512-828-4625
TTY:512-828-4624
e-mail: roundrock@arcil.com
www.arcil.com

4970 Austin Resource Center: San Marcos
618 S Guadalupe Street
Suite 103
San Marcos, TX 78666
512-396-5790
FAX: 512-396-5794
TTY:512-396-5790
e-mail: sanmarcos@arcil.com
www.arcil.com

Laurie Wills, Independent Living Skills Coord.
Nancy Clarke, Community Advocacy Coordinator
Cheryl Harwood, Parent Training Coordinator

Provides advocacy services, info and refferal, independent living skills and life skills classes. Other services include peer support and social and leisure activities and some community services.

4971 Brazoria County Center for Independent Living
1101 D E Mulberry
Angleton, TX 77515
979-849-7060
FAX: 979-849-8465
TTY:979-849-7060
e-mail: bccil@neosoft.com
www.barrier-freeliving.org

4972 Center Serving Persons with Mental Retardation
3550 W Dallas
PO Box 130564
Houston, TX 77019
713-525-8401
FAX: 713-523-0340
e-mail: agarms@cri-usa.org
www.cri-usa.org

4973 Coalition for Barrier Free Living
7000 Regency Square Boulevard
Suite 160
Houston, TX 77036
713-974-4621
FAX: 713-974-6927

4974 Council on Independent Living
4905 Center Park Boulevard
San Antonio, TX 78218
210-599-7711
FAX: 210-599-7815

4975 Crockett Resource Center for Independent Living
1020 E Loop 304
Crockett, TX 75835
936-544-2811
800-784-8710
FAX: 936-544-7315
e-mail: crcil@sat.net

Cynthia Cook, Executive Director

Provides independent living services to cross-disability groups to increase their personal self-determination and minimize dependence on others. Maintain comprehensive information on availability of resources and provides referrals to such resources. Provides instruction to assist people with disabilities to gain skills that would empower them to live independently. Peer counseling, advocacy - both individual and community by assisting to obtain support services to make changes in society.

4976 Houston Center for Independent Living

7000 Regency Square Boulevard
Suite 160
Houston, TX 77036 **713-654-1864**
FAX: 713-974-6927

Sandra Bookman, Director

Information on accessible housing, advocacy services and peer counseling.

4977 Independent Life Styles

1917 Augusta Drive
PO Box 571874
Houston, TX 77257 **713-861-4266**

Peter Simmons, Director

Offers peer counseling, advocacy and other services to the community.

4978 Independent Living Research Utilization Project

Institute for Rehabilitation & Research
2323 S Shepherd Drive
Suite 1000
Houston, TX 77019 **713-520-0232**
FAX: 713-520-5785
e-mail: ilru@ilru.org
www.ilru.org

Lex Frieden, Director

ILRU is a national center for information, training, research and technical assistance in independent living. Its goal is to expand the body of knowledge in independent living and to improve utilization of results of research programs and demonstration projects in this field. ILRU is a program of The Institute for Rehabilitation and Research, a nationally recognized medical rehabilitation facility for persons with disabilities. TTY phone number: (713) 520-5136.

4979 LIFE Independent Living Center

3212 34th
Lubbock, TX 79410 **806-795-5433**
FAX: 806-781-5607
TTY:806-795-5509

Rich Van Hersch, Contact

4980 LIFE/ Run Centers for Independent Living

1001 W Tenth Avenue
Amarillo, TX 79101 **806-372-7556**
FAX: 806-372-2045
e-mail: chinan3@aol.com

Nancy Penland, Coordinator

4981 Martin Luther Homes of Texas

324 S Loop 123 - Business
Seguin, TX 78155 **830-372-2525**
FAX: 830-372-3076

Barbara Hokum, Administrator
Fred Naumann III, Communications

Providing a wide array of services to assist individuals and families in achieving positive life goals. Services to persons with disabilities and other special needs include community living options, training and employment options, spiritual growth and development options, training and counseling support.

4982 Office for Students with Disabilities University of Texas at Arlington

300 W 1st Street
PO Box 19355
Arlington, TX 76019 **817-272-3364**
FAX: 817-272-1447
e-mail: dianne@uta.edu
www.uta.edu/disability

Dianne Hengst, Director
Ron Venable, Assistant Director

Offers disability counseling and academic accomodation for UTA community.

4983 Palestine Resource Center for Independent Living

421 Avenue A
Palestine, TX 75801 **903-729-7505**
888-326-5166
FAX: 903-729-7540
e-mail: prscil@risecom.net

Cheryl Bass, Executive Director

Provides independent living services to cross-disability groups to increase their personal self-determination and minimize dependence on others. Maintain comprehensive information on availability of resources and provides referrals to such resources. Provides instruction to assist people with disabilities to gain skills that would empower them to live independently. Peer counseling, advocacy - both individual and community by assisting to obtain support services to make changes in society.

4984 Panhandle Action Center for Independent Living Skills

3608 S Washington Street
Amarillo, TX 79110 **806-374-1400**
FAX: 806-374-4550

Leanne Wesley, Director

Offers peer counseling, attendant care registry and information on accessible housing.

4985 REACH of Dallas Resource Center on Independent Living

8625 King George Drive
Suite 210
Dallas, TX 75235 **214-630-4796**
FAX: 214-630-6390
e-mail: reachdallas@reachcils.org
www.reachcils.org

Charlotte Stewart, Executive Director
Susie Reukema, Assistant Director

Information and referral services, peer counseling, independent living skills training, loaner adaptive equipment, advocacy assistance, social, recreational activities and ADA technical assistance.

4986 REACH of Denton Resource Center on Independent Living

405 S Elm
Suite 202
Denton, TX 76201 **940-383-1062**
FAX: 940-383-2742
e-mail: reachden@reachcils.org
www.reachcils.org

Becky Teal, Office Manager

4987 **REACH/Resource Center on Independent Living**
1205 Lake Street
Fort Worth, TX 76102 **817-870-9082**
FAX: 817-870-9086
e-mail: reachftw@reachcils.org
www.reachcils.org

Charlotte Stewart, Executive Director
Anne Ancy, Case Manager

Information and referral services, peer counseling, independent living skills training, loaner equipment, advocacy assistance, ADA technical assistance and social/recreational activities.

4988 **SAILS**
1028 S Alamo
San Antonio, TX 78210 **210-281-1878**
FAX: 210-281-1759
TTY:210-281-1878

Julie Faneaza, Executive Director
Gloria Bank, Assisatnt Executive Director
Mary Blake, ILPC

Center for independent living non residential providing advocacy, including skill training, peer support, information and refferal services.

4989 **San Antonio Independent Living Services**
5101 San Pedro
San Antonio, TX 78212 **210-734-9971**
FAX: 210-785-3400

4990 **Southeast Texas Living Independent for Everyone (SETLIFE)**
780 S Fourth Street
Beaumont, TX 77701 **409-832-2599**
FAX: 409-838-4499
e-mail: setlife@sat.net

Nancy Comeaux, Contact

4991 **Texas Rehabilitation Commission Independent Living Services**
4900 N Lamar Boulevard
Austin, TX 78751 **512-424-4136**
FAX: 512-424-4982
e-mail: terryshelden@rehab.state.tx.us

Terry Sheldon, Program Specialist

Provides technical assistance and other support services to the state's Independent Living Council, Independent Living Centers and Independent Living Counseling programs.

4992 **VAIL: Brownsville**
2685 N Corea
Brownsville, TX 78520 **956-541-0468**
FAX: 956-541-6036

4993 **VOLAR Center for Independent Living**
8929 Viscount
Suite 101
El Paso, TX 79925 **915-591-0800**
FAX: 915-591-3506
TTY:915-591-0800
e-mail: volar1whc.net
www.volarcil.org

Luis Enrique Chew, Contact

4994 **Valley Associates for Independent Living (VAIL)**
PO Box 5035
McAllen, TX 78502 **956-781-7733**
FAX: 956-781-7735
e-mail: valleyassociation@earthlink.net

Laura Sexton, Interim Executive Director
Doresdo Jay-Pang, Deputy Director

Utah

4995 **Active Re-Entry**
451 S Carbon Avenue
Suite 931
Price, UT 84501 **435-637-4950**
FAX: 435-637-4952

Nancy Bentley, Director

Offers information and referral services.

4996 **Active Re-Entry: Vernal**
PO Box 122
Vernal, UT 84532 **435-789-4021**
FAX: 435-789-1031
TTY:435-259-3909

4997 **Central Utah Independent Living Center**
491 N Freedom Boulevard
Provo, UT 84501 **801-373-5044**
FAX: 801-373-5094

4998 **OPTIONS for Independence**
Northern Utah Center for Independent Living
1095 N Main Street
Logan, UT 84341 **435-753-5353**
800-753-2344
FAX: 435-753-5390
e-mail: jbiggs@optionind.org
www.optionsind.org

Helen Roth, Executive Director
Paula Bartholomew, IL Coordinator
Theresa Christensen, IL Coordinator

Information and referral, systems change advocacy, individual advocacy, peer counseling, independent living skills training, PAS registry, assistive technology assessment and acquisition and recreation for people with disabilities.

4999 **Options for Independence: Brigham**
862 S Main Street
Suite 9
Brigham City, UT 84302 **435-723-2171**
FAX: 435-723-9618
TTY:435-723-2171
e-mail: paulab@brigham.net
www.rrci.com

Paula Bartholomew, Independent Living Coordinator

5000 **Red Rock Center for Independence**
515 W 300 N
Suite A
Saint George, UT 84770 **435-673-7501**
FAX: 435-673-8808
e-mail: gowens@rrci.org
www.rrci.org

Garry Owens, Executive Director

5001 **Red Rock Center for Independence: Fillmore**
PO Box 531
Fillmore, UT 84631 **435-619-7724**
FAX: 435-691-7724

5002 Red Rock Independent Living Center: Minersville
PO Box 168
Minersville, UT 84752 435-843-7353
FAX: 435-843-7359

5003 Tri-County Independent Living Center
705 40th Street
S Ogden, UT 84403 801-612-3215
866-734-5678
FAX: 801-612-3732
e-mail: vickie@tri-county-ilc.com
www.tri-county-ilc.com

Sandra Meehan, Executive Director
Vickie Brenchley, Deputy Director/Office Manager

The mission of the Tri-County ILC is to enhance independence for all people with disabilities. Publishes a free quarterly newsletter.

5004 Utah Assistive Technology Program (UTAP) Utah State University
Center Persons with Disabilities
6855 Old Main Hill
Logan, UT 84322 435-797-3824
FAX: 435-797-2355
TTY:435-797-7089
e-mail: meblair@cc.usu.edu
www.uatpat.org

Martin E Blair, Program Director

Provides expertise, resources, and a structure to enhance and expand AT services provided by private and public agencies in Utah. Occcurs through monitoring, coordination, information dissemination, empowering individuals, the identification and removal of barriers, and expanding state resources.

5005 Utah Independent Living Center
764 S 200 W
Salt Lake City, UT 84101 801-359-2444
FAX: 801-466-2363

Debra Mair, Director

Offers information and referral services.

5006 Utah Independent Living Center: Tooele
33 S Main Street
Tooele, UT 84074 435-843-7353
FAX: 435-843-7359

Vermont

5007 Vermont Assistive Technology Project: Department of Aging & Disabilities
103 S Main Street
Weeks Building
Waterbury, VT 05671 502-241-2620
800-750-6355
FAX: 802-241-2174
e-mail: lynnec@dad.state.vt.us
www.dad.state.vt.us/

Lynne Cleveland, Project Director

Encompasses a state coordinating council for assistive technology issues, regional centers for demonstration, trial and technical support with computer and augmentative communication equipment and regional seating and positioning centers.

5008 Vermont Center for Independent Living: Burlington
59-63- Pearl Street
Burlington, VT 05401 802-862-0234
FAX: 802-258-2651

5009 Vermont Center for Independent Living: Brattleboro
167 Main Street
Suite 207
Brattleboro, VT 05301 802-254-6851
FAX: 802-258-2651
TTY:802-254-8867
e-mail: bratvcil@together.net
www.vcil.com

5010 Vermont Center for Independent Living
11 E State Street
Montpelier, VT 05602 802-229-0501
800-639-1522
FAX: 802-229-0503
e-mail: vcil@vcil.org
www.vcil.org

Deborah Lisi-Baker, Executive Director
Dhiresha Blose, Director of Development

Information and referral services, peer advocacy counseling, home modification funding, community advocacy and independent living services and cibil rights advocacy.

5011 Vermont Center for Independent Living: Bennington
532 Main Street
Bennington, VT 05201 802-447-0574
FAX: 802-442-4052
TTY:802-442-1878
e-mail: vcilbenn@together.com
www.vcil.com

Virginia

5012 Access Independence
403 B S Loudoun Street
Winchester, VA 22601 540-662-4452
FAX: 540-662-4474
e-mail: askai@accessindependence.org
www.accessindependence.org

Kim Schick, Executive Director
Joan Davis, Manager Operations

Offers support services to persons with disabilities to assist in maintaining or increasing their independence and self-determination. Includes housing assistance, independent living skills training, information, referral services, assistance and representative payee and advocacy.

5013 Appalachian Independence Center
230 Charwood Drive
Abingdon, VA 24210 276-628-2979
FAX: 276-628-4931

Greg Morrell, Executive Director
Charley Barry, Program Director
Donna Buckland, Operations Director

A nonprofit center for independent living serving people with disabilities in Southwestern Virginia. Services include peer counseling, independent living skills training, information and referrals, accessible transportation, community education, technical assistance and individual and systems advocacy.

5014 Blu Ridge Independent Living Center: Low Moor

PO Box 7
Room 631
Low Moor, VA 24457
540-862-0252
FAX: 540-862-0252
TTY:540-862-0252

5015 Blue Ridge Independent Living Center - Troutville

US Route 11 N
Troutville, VA 24175
540-966-4951
FAX: 540-342-9505

5016 Blue Ridge Independent Living Center

1502-B Williamson Road NE
Roanoke, VA 24012
540-342-1231
FAX: 540-342-9505
e-mail: kmichalski@brilc.org
www.brilc.org

Karen Michalski-Karney, Executive Director
Sara Ingram, Program Services Director
Gordon Davidson, Community Services Director

Offers independent living skills training, peer counseling, support groups, advocacy, information and referral, technical assistance, community education and housing assistance.

5017 Blue Ridge Independent Living Center: Christianburg

215 Roanoke Street
Christianburg, VA 24073
540-381-8829
FAX: 540-381-8829

5018 Central Virgina Independent Living Center

1845 Fort Mahone
Suite A
Petersburgh, VA 23805
804-862-9338
FAX: 804-862-6177

5019 Central Virginia Independent Living Center

2900 W Broad Street
Richmond, VA 23230
804-353-6503
FAX: 804-358-5606
TTY:804-353-6503

Sandra Wagner, Director

Information and referral services.

5020 Clinch Independent Living Services

PO Box 2741
Grundy, VA 24614
276-935-6088
800-597-2322
FAX: 276-935-6342
e-mail: cils@netscope.net

Betty Bevins, Executive Director
Barbara Crouse, Administrative Assistant

Nonprofit organization providing information and referral, peer counseling, advocacy and independent living skills training to persons with disabilities.

5021 Colonial Area: PENCIL

151 Kristiansand Drive
Suite 109
Williamsburg, VA 23188
757-564-1880
FAX: 757-564-1285

5022 DisAbility Resource Center

409 Progress Street
Fredericksburg, VA 22401
540-373-2559
800-648-6324
FAX: 540-373-8126
e-mail: drc@drc-fredericksburg.org
www.drc-fredericksburg.org

Robert J Boyd III, Executive Director
Anne Sullivan, Office Manager

5023 Eastern Shore Center for Independent Living

4376 Lankford Highway
Suite 3
Exmore, VA 23350
757-414-0100
FAX: 757-414-0205
TTY:757-414-0080

Althea Pittman, Exeuctive Director

5024 Endependence Center of Northern Virginia

3100 Clarendon Boulevard
Arlington, VA 22201
703-525-3268
FAX: 703-525-3585
e-mail: info@ecnv.org
www.ecnv.org

Michael Cooper, Contact

5025 Equal Access Center for Independence

4031 University Drive
Suite 301
Fairfax, VA 22030
703-934-2020
FAX: 703-277-7730
e-mail: drc@patriot.net

5026 Independence Empowerment Center

9001 Digges Road
Suite 103
Manasses, VA 20108
703-257-5400
FAX: 703-257-5043
e-mail: iecinc@starpower.net
www.empower.org

Bill Ward, Executive Director
Lisa Fletcher, Community Services Program Coor.

5027 Independence Resource Center

201 W Main Street
Apartment 8
Charlottesville, VA 22902
434-981-7723
FAX: 434-971-8242
e-mail: ircl@comcilin.net

Tom Vandover, Director

Information and referral services.

5028 Independent Living Center Network: Department of the Visually Handicapped

1809 Staples Mill Road
Suite 300
Richmond, VA 23230
804-355-7900
FAX: 804-355-9297

Bob Burton, Director

Information and referral services.

5029 Junction Center for Independent Living

548 Park Avenue NW
Norton, VA 24273
276-679-5989
FAX: 276-679-5969

5030 Junction Center for Independent Living

247 W Morgan Avenue
Pennington Gap, VA 24277
s40-546-5093
FAX: 276-546-3360
e-mail: jcil1@bellatlantic.net

Gwen Gillenwater, Executive Director
Sam Smith, Assistant Director

A private non-profit community-based, non-residential organization that is consumer directed and controlled. Services provided to people with disabilities include advocacy, peer counseling, independent living, skills training and information and referral. Our goal is total community inclusion for everyone - including people with diabilities.

5031 Lynchburg Area Center for Independent Living

500 Alleghany Avenue
Suite 520
Lynchburg, VA 24501
434-528-4971
FAX: 434-528-4976
e-mail: lacil@lacil.org
www.lacil.org

Walter Sabin, Executive Director
Dana Jackson, Administrative Asst/Finance

5032 National Council on Independent Living

1916 Wilson Boulevard
Suite 209
Arlington, VA 22201
703-525-3406
FAX: 703-525-3409
TTY:703-525-4153
e-mail: ncil@ncil.org
www.ncil.org

Anne Marie Hughey, Executive Director
Kelly Buckland, NCIL VP

Advances the independent living philosophy and advocates for the human rights of and services for people with disabilities to further their full integration and participation in society. The National Council on Independent Living (NCIL) is the oldest cross disability, grassroots organization run by and for people with disabilities.

5033 Peidmont Independent Living Center

816 B W Main Street
Danville, VA 24616
434-797-2567
FAX: 434-797-2568
e-mail: pilc@gamewood.com

5034 Peninsula Center for Independent Living

2021 A Cunningham Drive
Suite 2
Hampton, VA 23666
757-827-0275
FAX: 757-827-0655
e-mail: iepcil@aol.com
www.ilusa.com/links/ilcenters.htm#VA

Ralph Shelman, Contact

5035 Valley Associates for Independent Living (VAIL)

1791-A South High Street
Harrisonburg, VA 22801
540-433-6513
888-242-8245
FAX: 540-433-6313
e-mail: vail@govail.org
www.govail.org

VAIL is a not-for-profit, private Center for Independent Living providing advocacy, information and referral, independent living skills training, supported employment, and peer counseling to individuals with disabilities in our planning district.

5036 Valley Associates for Independent Living (VAIL)

1791 A S High Street
Harrisburg, VA 22801
540-433-6513
FAX: 540-433-6513
e-mail: vail@govail.org
www.govail.org

5037 Valley Associates for Independent Living: Lexington

7 McDowell Street
Suite A
Lexington, VA 24450
540-464-5454
FAX: 540-433-6313

5038 Woodrow Wilson Independent Living Skills Training Program

PO Box 1500
Fishersville, VA 22939
540-332-7103
800-345-9972
FAX: 540-332-7330
e-mail: clemencb@wwrc.state.va.us
www.wwrc.net

Dane DeMoss, Director

Information & referral services. Six week Virginia residential programs and evaluation services.

Washington

5039 Center for Independence

407 14th Avenue SE
PO Box 1247
Puyallup, WA 98372
253-845-5187
FAX: 253-848-0798
TTY:253-848-0798
e-mail: cfi@goodsamhealth.org

Jim Lindley, Director
Kimberly Rinehardt-Dodd, Independent Living Specialist

The Center For Independence is a resource organization dedicated to serving individuals with disabilities to more fully access and participate in the community through outreach, advocacy and skills development. We participate in community activities that address civil and equal rights issues, peer counseling and monitoring, individual advocacy, independent living skills development and information referral.

5040 Coalition of Responsible Disabled

612 N Maple Street
Spokane, WA 99201
509-326-6355
FAX: 509-327-2420
e-mail: elecord@cet.com
www.rip-cord.org

Linda Schappals- McClain, Executive Director

5041 Community Service Center for the Deaf and Hard of Hearing

1609 19th Avenue
Seattle, WA 98122
206-322-4996
800-301-0006
FAX: 206-720-3251
TTY:206-568-1234
e-mail: cscdhh@aol.com
www.cscdhh.org

Kenneth Puckett, Executive Director

Community information and referral services; interpreter referral services such as sign language interpreting, real time captioning, relay interpreting, oral interpreting; 9-1-1/TTY eduction program; communication access advocacy; and community education.

5042 **Community Services for the Blind and Partially Sighted**

9709 3rd Avenue NE
Suite 100
Seattle, WA 98115
206-525-5556
800-458-4888
FAX: 206-525-0422
e-mail: csbps@csbps.com
www.csbps.com

June Mansfield, President/CEO
Michael Walker, VP Marketing/Communications

Founded in 1965 as an independent nonprofit, CSBPS works to restore, maintain, and enhance the independence and well-being of people with impaired vision. Programs include professional counseling and support; safe travel and orientation training; instruction in independent living skills; low vision clinic and low vision rehavilitation; one-on-one volunteer services, education, information and referral, assistive technology center; and an adaptive aids retail, and online store.

5043 **Designs for Independent Living**

819 S Hatch
Spokane, WA 99202
509-535-9696

Gloria Caryl, Contact

5044 **DisAbility Resource Center**

607 SE Everett Mall Way
Suite 17
Everett, WA 98208
425-347-5768
FAX: 425-710-0767
e-mail: ilsc@richpoor.com
www.wa-ilsc.org

Sarajane Siegfriedt, Executive Director

5045 **DisAbility Resources of Southwest Washington**

5501 109th Court
Suite N
Vancouver, WA 98662
360-694-6790
FAX: 360-694-6910
e-mail: ilrswwa@lqwest.net

Jim Baker, Executive Director
Angela Hartford, Administrative Technician
Scott Anfinson, Independent Living Specialist

To promote the philosophy of independent living by creating opportunities, encouraging choices, advancing equal access and furthering the level of independence for all people with disabilities.

5046 **Disability Resource Network (dNET)**

16315 N 87th Street
Suite B3
Redmond, WA 98052
425-558-0993
800-216-3335
FAX: 425-558-4773
e-mail: dnetredmond@hotmail.com
www.wccd.org/dnet.htm

Gladys Springborn-Brannigan, Manager
Robert Blumenfeld, Employment/Access Specialist

Redmond office of the Washington Coalition Citizens with Disabilities serving East King County. dNET provides independent living skills training, information and referral, peer groups, advocacy, health insurance advising, employment assistance and access reviews.

5047 **Epilepsy Foundation of Washington**

3800 Aurora Avenue N
Suite 370
Seattle, WA 98103
206-547-4551
800-752-3509
FAX: 206-547-4557
e-mail: mail@epilepsyfoundationwash.org
www.epilepsyfoundationwash.org

Joel Neier, Executive Director
Malanie Redman, Director Epilepsy Services

Epilepsy Foundation Washington works to ensure that people with sizures are able to particiapte in all life expirences. This is supported through education, advocacy and direct services.

5048 **Everett Coalition of People with Disabilities**

1301 Hewitt Avenue
Everett, WA 98201
425-742-8533

5049 **Greater Lakes Mental Healthcare**

9330 59th Avenue SW
Lakewood, WA 98499
253-581-7020
FAX: 254-620-5140
www.glmhc.org

Richard J Towell, President/CEO
Madelaine A Thompson, Director Development
Jane-Ellen Delgado, Community Relations/Marketing

Greater Lakes Mental Healthcare is a premier behavioral healthcare facility in the Pacific Northwest helping individuals develop solutions for successful living. Greater Lakes provides a wide range of confidential professional counseling services for all ages.

5050 **Independent Lifestyles Services**

422 N Pine Street
Ellensburg, WA 98926
509-962-9620
FAX: 509-933-1571
e-mail: ils@televar.com

Noelle Blazevich, Contact

5051 **Independent Living Center of SW Washington**

PO Box 2129
Vancouver, WA 98668
FAX: 253-848-0798

Morris Gielser, Director

Offers peer counseling, referral and advocacy services.

5052 **Independent Living Service Center**

607 SE Everett Mall Way
Suite E
Everett, WA 98208
206-347-5768
800-315-3583
FAX: 206-710-0767
e-mail: ilsc@richpoor.net

5053 **Kitsap Community Resources**

1201 Park Avenue
Bremerton, WA 98337
360-377-0053
FAX: 360-792-8708

Larry Eyer, Executive Director

KCR provides services to low-income residents of Kitsap County. These services include emergency housing, WIC nutrition and health, Head Start preschool, employment and training. Information and referral services.

5054 **Lilac Blind Foundation**
1212 N Howard Street
Spokane, WA 99201
509-328-9116
800-422-7893
FAX: 509-328-8965
e-mail: info@lilacblindfoundation.org
www.lilacblindfoundation.org

Cherly L Martin, Director

5055 **Resource Center for the Handicapped**
20150 45th Avenue NE
Seattle, WA 98155
206-364-8179
FAX: 425-271-1096

Jeff Sykes, Director
Information and referral services.

5056 **Tacoma Area Coalition of Individuals with Disabilities**
6315 S 19th Street
Tacoma, WA 98466
253-565-9000
877-538-2243
FAX: 253-565-5578
e-mail: tacid@tacid.org
www.tacid.org

Chris Ensor, Executive Director
Offers information and referral services.

5057 **Washington Coalition for Citizens with Disabilities (WCCD)**
4649 Sunnyside N
Suite 100
Seattle, WA 98103
206-545-7055
FAX: 206-545-7059
e-mail: wccd@premieer1.net

JoAnn Fritsche, Contact

West Virginia

5058 **Appalachian Center for Independent Living**
Elk Office Center
4710 Chimney Drive
Suite C
Charleston, WV 25302
304-965-0376
800-642-3003
FAX: 304-965-0377

Larry E Paxton, Executive Director
Vicky L Robinson, Executive Secretary
Provides services and formation to handicapped persons including professional and peer counseling, advocacy, referral, housing, transportation, support groups, build wheelchair ramps, mobility equipment loan, attendant care, older blind services and skills training.

5059 **Division of Rehabilitation Services: Staff Library**
PO Box 1004
Institute, WV 25112
304-766-4644
800-642-8207
FAX: 304-766-4913
e-mail: carolc@mail.drs.state.wv.us

Carol R Johnson-Cyrus, Librarian
Specialized library with information on disabilities and the rehabilitation there of special collections: Deaf and hard of hearing, Visually impaired/blinf, Wellness Center, Literacy and career. The library has assistive devices such as CCTV, scanner and enhancement software. Also braille magazines, large print, talking books, magazines on cassette, descriptive videos, captioned media program, newspapers, magazines/journals, video, computers with internet access, fax, and a copier.

5060 **Mountain State Center for Independent Living**
329 Prince Street
Beckley, WV 25801
304-255-0122
FAX: 304-255-0157

5061 **Mountain State Center for Independent Living**
821 4th Avenue
Huntington, WV 25701
304-525-3324
FAX: 304-525-3360
e-mail: mtstcil@mtstcil.org
www.mtstcil.org

Anne Weeks, President/CEO

5062 **Northern West Virginia Center for Independent Living**
601-3 E Brockway Avenue
Suite A&B
Morgantown, WV 26505
304-296-6013
FAX: 301-292-5217
e-mail: nwvcil@labyrinth.net

Jan Desey, Executive Director
Madeline Miralles, Administrative Assistant
Independent living services to persons with disabilities including skills training, peer counseling, orientation and mobility training, advocacy and self-help training, community based systems advocacy, disability awareness training, ADA consultation, technical assistance and information and referrals are provided.

Wisconsin

5063 **Access to Independence**
2345 Atwood Avenue
Madison, WI 53704
608-242-8484
800-362-9877
FAX: 608-242-0383
TTY:608-242-8485
e-mail: ati@chorus.net

Wendy Hecht, Executive Director
An Independent Living Center serving people with disabilities. Services include: information and referral, housing counseling, advocacy, deaf services, assistive technology, peer support, independent living skills training, and volunteer opportunities, among others.

5064 **Center for Independent Living of Western Wisconsin**
2920 Schneider Avenue E
Menomonie, WI 54751
715-233-1070
800-228-3287
FAX: 715-233-1083
e-mail: cilww@cilww.com
www.cilww.com

Tim Sheehan, Director

5065 Great Rivers Independent Living Services
4328 Mormon Coulee Road
La Crosse, WI 54601
608-787-1148
FAX: 608-787-1148
e-mail: advocacy@greatrivers.org
www.greatrivers.com

Kathie Knoble-Iverson, Contact

5066 Independence First
121 Wisconsin Street
Waukesha, WI 53186
262-521-1664
FAX: 414-291-7525

5067 Independence First
600 W Virginia Street
Suite 301
Milwaukee, WI 53204
414-291-7520
FAX: 414-291-7525
e-mail: info@independencefirst.org
www.independencefirst.org

Lee Schulz, Executive Director
Karen Avery, Associate Director

Serves individuals with disabilities in the metro-Milwaukee four county area. Services include advocacy, independent living skills training, information/referral, peer counseling, youth camp and personal assistance services.

5068 Independence First: West Bend
735 S Main Street
W Bend, WI 53095
262-306-6717
FAX: 262-521-1664

5069 Independent Living Resources
149 E Mill Street
Suite A
Richland Center, WI 53581
608-647-8053
877-471-2095
FAX: 608-647-7783
www.ilresources.org

5070 Inspiration Ministries
Corner Route 67/Cty F
PO Box 948
Walworth, WI 53184
262-275-6131
FAX: 262-275-3355
e-mail: inspirationministries@elknet.net
www.inspirationministries.org

David Rowland, President
Tim Schnake, VP Resident Services

Formerly known as Christian League for the Handicapped.The ministry is a caring Christian community who enable and encourage people with disabilities. We address physical, mental and spiritual needs through accessible residential accommodations, work opportunities and integration into the local community and its churches. 160 acre campus including residential apartments, a work center, a Christian bookstore and gift shop, and a retreat center/summer camp (Inspiration Center).

5071 Mid-state Independent Living Consultants
10101 Market Street
Suite B
Monisee, WI 54455
715-241-6927
FAX: 715-241-8168
www.tznet.com/comn/firstcall/database/xr0iuvf

5072 Mid-state Independent Living Consultants: Stevens Point
201 C W Clark Street
Stevens Point, WI 54481
715-344-4210
800-382-8484
FAX: 715-344-4414

Julie Krueger, Executive Director

5073 North Country Independent Living
2231 Catlin Avenue
PO Box 1245
Superior, WI 54880
715-392-9118
800-924-1220
FAX: 715-392-4636

John Novsainc, Director

5074 North Country Independent Living: Ashland
201 Main Street
Ashland, WI 54806
715-682-5676
FAX: 715-682-3144

5075 Options for Independent Living
555 Country Club Road
PO Box 11967
Green Bay, WI 54807
920-490-0500
888-485-1515
888-465-1515
FAX: 920-490-0700

Thomas J Diedrick, Director
Kathryn C Barry, Assistant Director

Provides independent living core services including: peer counseling, information and referral, IL skills training, advocacy - individual and systems, and housing referrals. Rehabilitation technology services provided include: home evaluations, vehicle evaluations, computer evaluations, deaf/hard of hearing equipment evaluations and ADA Title III Technical Assistance and benefits counseling.

5076 Options for Independent Living: Fond du Lac
151 E First Street
Fond du Lac, WI 54935
920-907-8440
FAX: 920-907-8441

5077 Society's Assets
5200 Washington Avenue
Suite 225
Racine, WI 53406
262-637-9128
FAX: 262-637-8646
e-mail: info@sai-inc.org
www.saintinc.org

Bruce Nelsen, Executive Director
Karen Olufs, Director Indepedent Living
Jean Rumachik, Director Home Care Services

Society's Assets assists people with disabilities to live as indpendently as possible. A non-profit human services agency, Society's Assets provides information and referal, independent living skills training, peer support, advocacy, and supportive home care. Home health care is provided by SAI Home Health Care. The agency serves 5 counties in southeastern Wisconsin and also provides information about interpreters, employment, benefits, home modifications, assistive equipment and accessibility.

Fees vary

5078 Society's Assets: Elkhorn
35 S Wisconsin Street
Elkhorn, WI 53121
262-723-8181
FAX: 262-723-8184

5079 Society's Assets: Kenosha
5727 Sixth Avenue
Kenosha, WI 53140
262-657-3999
FAX: 262-657-1672

Wyoming

5080 LifeQuest: Interdisciplinary Rehabilitation
339 W Loucks Street
Sheridan, WY 82801
307-674-4462
800-684-2289
FAX: 307-674-5117

Shannon Trierweiler, Manager

Multi-disciplines organization dedicated to the highest possible economic and social independence for persons with disabilities. Extensive referral service, specialized employment placement, occupational therapy, psychological services, evaluation services, and coordination of external services as needed to meet client plans and objectives.

5081 Rehabilitation Enterprises of N Eastern Wyoming
35 Fairgrounds Road
New Castle, WY 82701
307-746-4733
FAX: 307-746-9071

Larry W Samson, President/CEO
Jeff Holsinger, Director Operations

Committed to enhancing personal and community relationships, providing opportunities for growth, and helping people with varying abilities achieve their personal goals.

5082 Rehabilitation Enterprises of North Eastern Wyoming
1969 S Sheridan Avenue
Sheridain, WY 82801
307-672-7481
FAX: 307-674-5117

Larry W Samson, President/CEO
Jeff Holsinger, Director Operations

Committed to enhancing personal and community relationships, providing opportunities for growth, and helping people with varying abilities achieve their personal goals.

5083 Wyoming Independent Living Rehabilitation
305 W First Street
Casper, WY 82601
307-266-6956
800-736-8322
FAX: 307-266-6959
e-mail: dpotter@trib.com
w3.trib.com/~dpotter

Ken Hoff, Director

Creates opportunities for severly disabled individuals to live more independently, direct services, advocacy, home modifications and independent living skills.

5084 Wyoming Services for Independent Living
190 Custer Street
Lander, WY 82520
307-332-4889
FAX: 307-332-2491
e-mail: wwcil@rmisp.com

Carol Fontaine, Contact

Associations & Referral Agencies

5085 AIDS Legal Council of Chicago

188 W Randolph
Suite 2400
Chicago, IL 60601
312-427-8990
FAX: 312-427-8419
e-mail: info@aidslegal.com
www.aidslegal.com

Justin Hayford, Case Manager

Legal advice and services for persons who are HIV positive or have AIDS, and their companions, families, etc., regarding HIV-related legal matters.

5086 AIDSLAW of Louisiana

Greater New Orleans Foundation
2515 Canal Street
New Orleans, LA 70119
504-581-6363
FAX: 504-821-8326

Gregory Ben Johnson

Second year of funding for new legal agency serving persons affected by HIV/AIDS.

5087 Advocacy

7800 Shoal Creek Boulevard
Suite 171-E
Austin, TX 78757
512-454-4816
800-252-9108
FAX: 512-323-0902
e-mail: infoai@advocacyinc.org
www.advocacyinc.org

Jonas Schwartz, Policy Services Manager

Advocacy, Inc advocates for, protects and advances the legal, human and service rights of people with disabilities throughout the state of Texas.

5088 Center for Disability and Elder Law

710 N Lake Shore Drive
 # 3
Chicago, IL 60611
FAX: 312-908-0866

Jann Dragswich, Executive Director
Miriam Seitz, Executive Manager

Provides legal services at no cost to low income persons with disabilities in Cook County. LCD staff screen applicants to determine if they meet the financial, disability and geographical eligibility requirements for service.

5089 Chicago Lawyers' Committee for Civil Rights Under Law

100 N LaSalle Street
Suite 600
Chicago, IL 60604
312-630-9744
FAX: 312-630-1127
e-mail: clccrul@aol.com
www.clccrul.org

Provides legal services to individuals and groups with civil rights problems through class action and law reform cases. Also provides technical assistance to community groups. Spanish-speaking staff available. Individual cases and walk-ins are not accepted. Wheelchair accessible.

5090 DNA People's Legal Services

PO Box 987
Shiprock, NM 87420
505-368-3200
FAX: 505-368-3212
www.dnalegalservices.org/dnalegalservices

Brigitte Thomas, Managing Attorney
Elsie Shorthair, Office Manager

Offers legal assistance to Native Americans.

5091 Disability Rights Education and Defense Fund

2212 6th Street
Berkeley, CA 94710
510-644-2555
FAX: 510-841-8645
e-mail: dredf@dredf.org
www.dredf.org

Susan Henderson, Managing Director

Nonprofit organization dedicated to advancing the civil rights of individuals with disabilities through legislation, litigation, informal and formal advocacy and education and training of lawyers, advocates and clients with respect to disability issues. DREDF also provides training, advocacy, technical assistance and referrals for parents of disabled children.

5092 Equal Employment Advisory Council

1015 15th Street NW
Suite 1200
Washington, DC 20005
202-789-8600
FAX: 202-789-2291

A nonprofit association for the purpose of monitoring federal equal employment litigation and filing amicus curiae briefs in precedent-setting cases. Also file comments on equal opportunity employment and affirmative action regulatory proposals and monitors judicial developments.

5093 Guardianship Services Associates

41-A S Boulevard
Oak Park, IL 60302
708-386-5398
FAX: 708-386-5970
e-mail: GSAoakpark@aol.com

Robert R Wohlgemuth, Director

Information and counseling on guardianship issues. Can provide direct assistance in obtaining guardianship for disabled adults. Also provides information and direct assistance on durable powers of attorney. Can assume appointment as guardian in selected cases.

5094 Judge David L Bazelon Center for Mental Health Law

1101 15th Street NW
Suite 1212
Washington, DC 20005
202-467-5730
FAX: 202-223-0409
e-mail: info@bazelon.org
www.bazelon.org

Robert Bernstein, Executive Director

National litigation and technical assistance center for advocates for people with mental disabilities. Offers a website with advocacy resources and a variety of publications, handbooks, issue papers and manuals to help advocate for, implement, enforce and comply with federal laws and court orders on involuntary outpatient commitment, discrimination based on a label of mental disability, fair housing, criminalization, custody relinquishment for access to children's mental health care.

5095 Legal Action Center

236 Massachusetts Avenue NE
Suite 505
Washington, DC 20002 **202-544-5478**
FAX: 202-544-5712
e-mail: lacdc@lac-dc.org

Ellen Weber, Senior VP

Provides technical assistance and education programs on ADA issues related to individuals with drug and alcohol abuse and HIV disease and legal assistance to individuals who have faced discrimination on the basis of these disabilities.

5096 Legal Center

455 Sherman Street
Suite 130
Denver, CO 80203 **303-722-0300**
800-288-1376
FAX: 303-722-0720
e-mail: tlcmail@thelegalcenter.org
www.thelegalcenter.org

Mary Anne Harvey, Executive Director

The Legal center uses the legal system to protect and promote the rights of people with disabilities and older people in Colorado through direct legal representation, advocacy, education and legislative analysis. We are also the State Ombudsman for nursing homes and assisted living facilities. Call for a free publications and products list.

5097 Legal Center for the Elderly and Disabled

2862 Arden Way
Suite 200
Sacramento, CA 95825 **916-488-5298**
FAX: 916-973-3199
e-mail: jonellison@sbrglobal.net
www.iced.org

Jon Ellison, Executive Director
Carol Pasch, Office Manager

Free civil legal services for low-income people over sixty and permanently disabled persons under sixty, specializing in social security, medical benefits elder law, disability rights and housing in North Central California.

5098 National Center for State Courts

300 Newport Avenue
Williamsburg, VA 23185 **757-259-7575**
800-877-1233
FAX: 757-564-2028
www.ncsconline.org

Deborah White, HR Director

Develops a national clearinghouse and resource center for local and state courts to focus on requirements and methods of compliances with ADA.

5099 National Center for Youth Law

405 15th Street
15th Floor
Oakland, CA 94612 **510-835-8098**
FAX: 510-835-8099
e-mail: info@youthlaw.org
www.youthlaw.org

Support services to legal services attorneys and child advocates on SSI (Supplemental Security Income) disability benefits for children.

5100 National Right to Work Legal Defense and Education Foundation

8001 Braddock Road
Suite 600
Springfield, VA 22160 **703-321-9820**
800-336-3600
FAX: 703-321-9613
e-mail: infoAnrtw.org
www.nrtw.org

Reed Larson, President
Stefan Gleason, VP

Provides free legal aid to employees whose human and civil rights are being violated by compulsory unionism abuses.

5101 REACH/Resource Center on Independent Living

617 7th Avenue
Suite 304
Fort Worth, TX 76104
FAX: 817-877-1622
e-mail: reachdal@fiberramp.net
www.reachcil.org/rchftw.php4

Charlotte Stewart, Director
Anne Ancy, Case Manager

Information and referral services, peer counseling, independent living skills training, loaner equipment, advocacy assistance, ADA technical assistance and social/recreational activities.

5102 Winifred Law Opportunity Center

106 E 2nd Avenue
Indianola, IA 50125 **515-961-5341**
FAX: 515-961-5002

Diane M Griffith MS, Executive Director

Resources for the Disabled

5103 AACD Legal Series

American Counseling Association
5999 Stevenson Avenue
Alexandria, VA 22304 **800-347-6647**
800-473-2329
FAX: 703-823-6862
www.counseling.org

Offering three volumes: Preparing for Court Appearances; Documentation in Counseling Records; and The Counselor and The Law.

3 Volumes

5104 ADA Mandate for Social Change

Paul H Brookes Publishing Company
PO Box 10624
Baltimore, MD 21285
800-638-3775
FAX: 410-337-8539

This timely book moves a large step beyond detailing the legislative requirements of the ADA by focusing on the changes the ADA is generating for persons with disabilities.
$32.00

320 pages Paperback 1993
ISBN 1-557661-17-0

5105 **Americans with Disabilities Act Manual**

American Bar Association
740 15th Street NW
9th Floor
Washington, DC 20005 **202-662-1581**
800-285-2221
FAX: 202-662-1032
e-mail: hammillj@staff.abanet.org
www.abanet.org/disability

John Hammill, Publications Coordinator
Amy Allbright, Managing Editor

An in-depth analysis of the legal and practical implications of the ADA using non-technical language. *$20.00*

5106 **Americans with Disabilities Act: Selected Resources for Deaf**

Gallaudet University Bookstore
11030 S Langley Avenue
Chicago, IL 60628 **202-651-5488**
800-621-2736
FAX: 202-651-5489

This resource identifies programs and publications specific to the ADA and deafness and also lists ADA materials and programs for people with any disability. *$1.00*

5107 **Approaching Equality**

TJ Publishers
817 Silver Spring Avenue
Suite 206
Silver Spring, MD 20910 **301-585-4440**
800-999-1168
FAX: 301-585-5930
e-mail: TJPubinc@aol.com

Angela K Thames, President
Jerald A Murphy, VP

Public education laws guarantee special education for all deaf children, but may find the special education system confusing, or are unsure of their rights under current laws. For anyone with an interest in education, advocacy and the deaf community, this book reviews dramatic developments in education of deaf children, youth and adults since COED's 1988 report, Toward Equality. *$12.95*

112 pages
ISBN 0-93266 -39-6

5108 **Assessment of the Feasibility of Contracting with a Nominee Agency**

Mississippi State University
PO Box 6189
Mississippi State, MS 39762 **662-325-2001**
800-675-7782
FAX: 662-325-8989
www.blind.msstate.edu

Kelly Schaefer, Publications Manager

Only five State Licensing Agencies currently utilize nominee agreements. This study compared the Pennsylvania program with four states that utilize nominee agencies and four states that do not. Results and recommendations compared state and national data from Federal FY 1991-1993. *$20.00*

152 pages Paperback

5109 **Bluebook: Explanation of the Contents of the ADA**

Disability Rights Education and Defense Fund
2212 6th Street
Berkeley, CA 94710 **510-644-2555**
FAX: 510-841-8645
e-mail: dredf@dredf.org
www.dredf.org

Susan Henderson, Managing Director

Written in narrative form for both professionals and lay people, DREDF's bluebook offers detailed, thorough analysis of all of the law's provisions, encompassing ADA legislative history, the statute and regulations. Available in alternative formats. *$100.00*

214 pages

5110 **Can America Afford to Grow Old?**

Brookings Institution
1775 Massachusetts Avenue NW
Washington, DC 20036 **202-797-6252**
FAX: 202-797-6004
e-mail: bibooks@brookings.edu
www.brookings.edu

Social security laws and regulations. *$8.95*

144 pages Paperback
ISBN 0-815700-43-1

5111 **Childcare and the ADA**

Eastern Washington University
705 W 1st Avenue
Room 223
Spokane, WA 99201 **509-623-4213**
FAX: 509-623-4230
e-mail: susan.vanmeter@mail.ewu.edu

Nancy Ashworth, Director Child Development

Provides information on how childcare providers must comply with the ADA. Eight videotapes plus an instructional manual with examples of situations and problems. *$85.00*

Set

5112 **Complying with the Americans with Disabilities Act**

Greenwood Publishing Group
88 Post Road W
Suite 5007
Westport, CT 06880 **203-226-3571**
FAX: 203-222-1502
www.greenwood.com

A guidebook for management and people with disabilities. Hardcover.

280 pages $52.95 - $57.95
ISBN 0-899307-14-0

5113 **Convicting the Innocent**

Brookline Books
PO Box 1047
Cambridge, MA 02238 **617-868-0360**
800-666-2665
FAX: 617-868-1772
e-mail: brooklinebks@delphi.com
www.brooklinebooks.com

Exposes the dirtiest secret of American Law Enforcement: the process of subjecting innocent citizens- often poor or mentally impaired- to inquisitions to elicit confessions which often result in wrongful convictions. These thoughtful and compassionate essays analyze scandals nationwide, spotlighting the Richard Lapointe case featured on 60 minutes. Contributes include Pulitzer Prize winners William Styron, Arthur Miller, and Richard Ofshe. *$16.95*

220 pages Paperback
ISBN 1-57129 -21-4

5114 **Council for Disability Rights**

205 W Randolph Street
Suite 1645
Chicago, IL 60606 **312-444-9484**
FAX: 312-444-1977
TTY:312-444-1967
e-mail: cdrights@interaccess.com
www.disabilityrights.org

Jo Holzer, Executive Director

Promotes human rights of persons with disabilities and their families. Offers a job preparation and placement service, legal referrals, information services, education advocacy services, disability awareness training, and mediation services.

5115 Court-Related Needs of the Elderly and Persons with Disabilities

Mental Health Commission
2700 Martin Luther King Avenue SE
Washington, DC 20032 **202-373-7595**
FAX: 202-373-7982

This book features the ground-breaking recommendations from the national Conference on the Court-Related Needs of the Elderly and Persons with Disabilities, funded by the States Justice Institute and co-sponsored by the American Bar Association and National Judicial College. Accompanying the recommendations are detailed commentaries and extensive background research papers organized around issues. *$20.00*

276 pages

5116 Criminal Law Handbook on Psychiatric & Psychological Evidence & Testimony

ABA Commission on Mental & Physical Disability Law
740 15th Street NW
9th Floor
Washington, DC 20005 **202-662-1581**
800-285-2221
FAX: 202-662-1032
e-mail: hammillj@staff.abanet.org
www.abanet.org/disability

John Hammill, Publications Coordinator
Amy Allbright, Managing Editor

Provides lawyers, judges, and forensic experts with comprehensive in-depth treatment of psychiatric and psychological evidence and testimony keyed to specific mental health law standards. *$60.00*

278 pages
ISBN 1-570738-49-1

5117 Critical Issues in the Lives of People with Severe Disabilities

Paul H Brookes Publishing Company
PO Box 10624
Baltimore, MD 21285
800-638-3775
FAX: 410-337-8539

This comprehensive book explores the values, practices and empirical research that have guided legal and practical decisions concerning the lives of people with severe disabilities in the past. *$90.00*

704 pages Hardcover 1991
ISBN 1-557660-48-4

5118 Dealing with Mental Incapacity

Center for Public Representation
PO Box 260049
Madison, WI 53726 **608-251-4008**
800-369-0388
FAX: 606-251-1263
e-mail: cpr@lawmail.law.wisc.edu
www.law.wisc.edu/pal

This manual contains a comprehensive introduction to the problem of guardianship as well as chapters of financial and health care planning tools, guardianship under Wisconsin law, protective placement and Watts reviews. *$19.95*

5119 Dimensions of State Mental Health Policy

Greenwood Publishing Group
88 Post Road W
Suite 5007
Westport, CT 06880 **203-226-3571**
FAX: 203-222-1502
www.greenwood.com

Introduces students to the emerging field of state mental health policy. Hardcover.

320 pages $59.95 - $65
ISBN 0-275932-52-4

5120 Disability Law in the United States

William Hein & Company
1285 Main Street
Buffalo, NY 14209 **716-675-3555**
800-828-7571
FAX: 716-883-8100
e-mail: mail@wshein.com
www.wshein.com

Customer Service Department

Offers thousands of pages of information on the laws and legislation affecting the disabled in the United States. Its purpose is to provide a clear and comprehensive mandate to end discrimination against individuals with disabilities and to bring disabled persons into the economic and social mid-stream of American Life. *$650.00*

5750 pages
ISBN 0-899417-97-3

5121 Disability Rights Now

Disability Rights Education and Defense Fund
2212 6th Street
Berkeley, CA 94710 **510-644-2555**
FAX: 510-841-8645
e-mail: dredf@dredf.org
www.dredf.org

Susan Henderson, Managing Director

Free quarterly publication describing the activities of the Disability Rights Education and Defense Fund, available in alternative formats.

Quarterly

5122 Education of the Handicapped: Laws, Legislative Histories and Administrative Documents

William Hein & Company
1285 Main Street
Buffalo, NY 14209
800-828-7571
FAX: 716-883-8100
e-mail: mail@wshein.com
www.wshein.com

Focuses upon elementary and secondary Education Act of 1965 and its amendment, Education For All Handicapped Children Act of 1975 and its amendments and acts providing services for the blind, deaf, mentally retarded, etc. Hardcover. *$2850.00*

55 Volume set
ISBN 0-899411-57-6

5123 Ethical and Legal Issues in School Counseling

American Counseling Association
5999 Stevenson Avenue
Alexandria, VA 22304
800-347-6647
800-473-2329
FAX: 703-823-6862
www.counseling.org

This comprehensive text is filled with answers to many of the most controversial and challenging questions faced by the professional every day. This text helps avoid ethical violations and provides thorough information on: confidentiality, privacy, privileged communication, access to school records, using group techniques ethically, computerized record keeping and reporting unethical practices. *$24.95*

341 pages paperback 1988
ISBN 1-556200-55-2

5124 Families Forward: Health Care Resource Guide for Children with Special Care Needs

Center for Public Representation
PO Box 260049
Madison, WI 53726
608-251-4008
800-369-0388
FAX: 606-251-1263
e-mail: cpr@lawmail.law.wisc.edu
www.law.wisc.edu/pal/famfrwd.htm

Extensive resource material: health insurance, HMOs, dealing with medical debt, services to keep your child at home and more. *$10.00*

ISBN 0-932622-54-2

5125 Federal Laws of the Mentally Handicapped: Laws, Legislative Histories and Admin. Documents

William Hein & Company
1285 Main Street
Buffalo, NY 14209
800-828-7571
FAX: 716-883-8100
e-mail: mail@wshein.com
www.wshein.com

Chronological compilation of all relevant federal laws dealing with the mentally handicapped along with supporting documentation necessary to create a complete legislative history. *$2200.00*

42 Volume/Set
ISBN 0-899411-06-1

5126 Formed Families: Adoption of Children with Handicaps

Haworth Press
10 Alice Street
Binghamton, NY 13904
607-722-5857
800-429-6784
FAX: 607-722-6362
e-mail: orders@haworthpress.com
www.haworthpress.com

Laraine Masters Glidden PhD, Editor

Provides broad coverage of the issues relating to the adoption of children with handicaps. Concerned professionals can find here all the answers about clinical programs, legal issues, estimates of frequency, and important factors related to positive and negative outcomes of these adoptions. *$74.95*

242 pages Hardcover 1990
ISBN 0-866569-14-6

5127 Free Appropriate Public Education

Love Publishing Company
9101 E Kenyon Avenue
Denver, CO 80222
303-221-7333
FAX: 303-221-7444
e-mail: lovepublishing@compuserve.com

Information on significant legislation regarding the handicapped. Laws are discussed with attention to their impact on the child, the parents, the public schools and higher education. *$44.95*

ISBN 0-89108 -11-5

5128 Handbook on Mental Disability Law

ABA Commission on Mental & Physical Disability Law
740 15th Street NW
9th Floor
Washington, DC 20005
202-662-1581
800-285-2221
FAX: 202-662-1032
e-mail: hammillj@staff.abanet.org
www.abanet.org/disability

John Hammill, Publications Coordinator
Amy Allbright, Managing Editor

Intended for attorneys and judges new to mental disability law, mental health professionals and advocates, and law students, this handbook covers (1) mental disability terms and definitions; (2) ADA-related mental health issues involving employment, housing/zoning, education, insurance, federal entitlements; (3) civil and criminal commitment and incompetency; (4) institutional rights; (5) professional liability concerns; (6) sexually violent predators; (7) rights in jails and prison. *$45.00*

5129 Health Care Quality Improvement Act of 1986

William Hein & Company
1285 Main Street
Buffalo, NY 14209
716-882-2600
800-828-7571
FAX: 716-883-8100
e-mail: mail@wshein.com
www.wshein.com

In order to encourage more stringent peer review by doctors and hospitals, and to protect reporting physicians and institutions from retaliatory lawsuits, Congress enacted The Health Care Quality Improvement Act. The Act was also intended to address the increasing incidence of medical malpractice and to prevent the ease with which incompetent practitioners moved from state to state. Hardcover. *$75.00*

730 pages
ISBN 0-899416-93-4

5130 Housing and Transportation of the Handicapped

William Hein & Company
1285 Main Street
Buffalo, NY 14209
716-882-2600
800-828-7571
FAX: 716-883-8100
e-mail: mail@wshein.com
www.wshein.com

National laws, recognizing the problems encountered by the handicapped in the areas of Housing and Transportation and providing assistance in an effort to surmount those problems. Hardcover or microfilm. *$1850.00*

250 documents
ISBN 0-899412-47-5

5131 Human Resource Management and the Americans with Disabilities Act

Greenwood Publishing Group
88 Post Road W
Suite 5007
Westport, CT 06880 **203-226-3571**
FAX: 203-222-1502
www.greenwood.com

John G Veres III, Editor
Ronald R Sims, Editor

Concrete advice for human resource professionals on how to cope with the vague, often obscure provisions of the Americans with Disabilities Act.

232 pages $59.95 - $62.95
ISBN 0-899308-57-0

5132 International Handbook on Mental Health Policy

Greenwood Publishing Group
88 Post Road W
Suite 5007
Westport, CT 06880 **203-226-3571**
FAX: 203-222-1502
www.greenwood.com

The first major reference book for academics and practitioners that provides a systematic survey and analysis of mental health policies in twenty representative countries.

512 pages $110 - $125
ISBN 0-313275-67-X

5133 Knowing Your Rights

AARP Fulfillment
601 E Street NW
Washington, DC 20049 **202-434-2277**
800-424-3410
FAX: 202-434-3443
e-mail: member@aarp.org
www.aarp.org

Describes how changes in Medicare's reimbursement policies are designed to reduce health care costs and suggests steps that Medicare beneficiaries, their families and friends can take to assure that they continue to receive quality care under the Prospective Payment System.

19 pages

5134 Law Center Newsletter

Public Interest Law Center of Philadelphia
125 S 9th Street
Philadelphia, PA 19107 **215-922-6854**

Information on mental health, foster care and public education. Provides all updates concerning the law in these areas.

5135 Legal Center

455 Sherman Street
Suite 130
Denver, CO 80203 **303-722-0300**
800-288-1376
FAX: 303-722-0720
e-mail: tlcmail@thelegalcenter.org
www.thelegalcenter.org

Mary Anne Harvey, Executive Director

The Legal center uses the legal system to protect and promote the rights of people with disabilities and older people in Colorado through direct legal representation, advocacy, education and legislative analysis. We are also the State Ombudsman for nursing homes and assisted living facilities. Call for a free publications and products list.

5136 Legal Rights of Persons with Disabilities: An Analysis of Federal Law

LRP Publications
PO Box 24668
West Palm Beach, FL 33416 **215-784-0941**
800-341-7874
FAX: 215-784-9639
e-mail: custserve@lrp.com
www.lrp.com

Gary Bagin, Director Communications

A comprehensive analysis of the rights accorded individuals with disabilities under federal law covering such issues as: Definitions of individuals with disabilities, reasonable accomidations, architectural barriers, access to transportation and communication services, education and newborns. *$185.00*

1536 pages
ISBN 0-934753-46-6

5137 Legislative Network for Nurses

Business Publishers
8737 Colesville Road
Suite 1100
Silver Spring, MD 20910
800-274-6737
FAX: 301-587-4530
e-mail: bpinews@bpinews.com
www.bpinews.com

Leonard A Eiserer, Publisher
Sarah Spencer, Editor

Provides up-to-date information on the nursing shortage, nurse training programs, AIDS and Hepatitis B, unionization, registered care technologies, compensation, child care, home health care staffing and much more. *$286.00*

8 pages Newsl./BiMonth

5138 Madness in the Streets

Free Press
135 S Mount Zion Road
Lebanon, IN 46052
800-323-7445
FAX: 800-882-8583

How psychiatry and the law abandoned the mentally ill. *$24.95*

436 pages
ISBN 0-02915 -80-8

5139 Making News: How to Get News Coverage of Disability Rights Issues

Advocado Press
PO Box 145
Louisville, KY 40201 **502-894-9492**
FAX: 502-899-9562
e-mail: office@advocadopress.org
www.advocadopress.org

Mary Johnson, Editor

This book gives examples and tips on how to fight back and get on the front pages, lead the newscasts and influence public debate. *$10.95*

165 pages
ISBN 0-96270 -43-4

5140 **Medicare and Medicaid Patient and Program Protection Act of 1987**

William Hein & Company
1285 Main Street
Buffalo, NY 14209
716-882-2600
800-828-7571
FAX: 716-883-8100
e-mail: mail@wshein.com
www.wshein.com

This act enables the Department of Health and Human Services to protect Medicare and Medicaid patients and federal health care programs from censured practitioners. Hardcover. *$185.00*

3 Volumes
ISBN 0-899416-95-0

5141 **Mental & Physical Disability Law Reporter**

American Bar Association
740 15th Street NW
9th Floor
Washington, DC 20005
202-662-1581
800-285-2221
FAX: 202-662-1032
e-mail: hammillj@staff.abanet.org
www.abanet.org/disability

John Hammill, Publications Coordinator
Amy Allbright, Managing Editor

Contains over 2,000 summanes per year of federal and state court decisions and legislation that affect persons with mental and physical disabilities. Includes bylined articles by experts in the field regarding disability law developments and trends. *$374.00*

150+ pages BiMonthly

5142 **Mental Disabilities and the Americans with Disabilities Act**

Greenwood Publishing Group
88 Post Road W
Suite 5007
Westport, CT 06880
203-226-3571
FAX: 203-222-1502
www.greenwood.com

A clear, practical compliance guide, written by a psychologist, to help organizations conform to provisions on mental disabilities in the Americans with Disabilities Act. Hardcover.

216 pages $45 - $49.95 1997
ISBN 0-899308-26-0

5143 **Mental Disabilities and the Americans with Disabilities Act**

ABA Commission on Mental & Physical Disability Law
740 15th Street NW
9th Floor
Washington, DC 20005
202-662-1581
800-285-2221
FAX: 202-662-1032
e-mail: hammillj@staff.abanet.org
www.abanet.org/disability

John Hammill, Publications Coordinator
Amy Allbright, Managing Editor

Written for lawyers, advocates, teachers, consumers, employers, and employees, this ADA handbook examines the ADA from the legal and non-legal practitioner's point of view. In six parts, the handbook covers ADA Titles I, II, and III provides case law summaries of ADA court decisions affecting individuals with mental disabilities including mental illness, developmental disabilities, learning disabilities, substance abuse, and organic brain injuries. *$40.00*

5144 **Mental Health Law News**

Interwood Publications
3 Interwood Place
 # 20241
Cincinnati, OH 45220
513-221-375

Frank Bardack, Marketing Director/Editor

Mental health case law summaries — malpractice, patient rights, discrimination, alcoholism, guardianship, negligence, professional liability, commitment, drug dependency and conservatorship. *$99.00*

6 pages Monthly Nwslttr
ISSN 0889-01 0

5145 **Mental Health Law Reporter**

Business Publishers
8737 Colesville Road
Suite 1100
Silver Spring, MD 20910
301-587-6300
800-274-6737
FAX: 301-589-8493
e-mail: custserv@bpinews.com
www.bpinews.com

Leonard A Eiserer, Publisher
Bonnie Becker, Editor

Brings you the most timely, focused and thorough information on the legal issues that concern mental health practitioners in mental health litigation. Topics include: malpractice litigation, patient-therapist confidentiality, sexual victimization of patients, the insanity defense, social security administrative case law and much more. *$286.00*

8 pages Monthly

5146 **Mentally Disabled and the Law**

William Hein & Company
1285 Main Street
Buffalo, NY 14209
716-882-2600
800-828-7571
FAX: 716-883-8100
e-mail: mail@wshein.com
www.wshein.com

Offers information on treatment rights, the provider-patient relationship, and the rights of the mentally disabled persons in the community. *$85.00*

867 pages
ISBN 0-910059-05-5

5147 **NAD Broadcaster**

National Association of the Deaf
814 Thayer Avenue
Silver Spring, MD 20910
301-587-1788
FAX: 301-587-1791
TTY:301-587-1789
e-mail: nadinfo@nad.org
www.nad.org

Dawn Bradley, Editor

National newspaper published 11 times a year by the nation's largest organization safeguarding the accessbility and civil rights of 28 million deaf and hard of hearing Americans in education, employment, health care, and telecommunications. Membership: individual $30 per year. *$7.00*

5148 **National Focus**

PO Box 37485
Phoenix, AZ 85069
602-943-6044
FAX: 602-866-9206

Offers information on disabilities issues and legal information for the disabled.

5149 **No Longer Disabled: The Federal Courts**

Greenwood Publishing Group
88 Post Road W
Suite 5007
Westport, CT 06880
203-226-3571
FAX: 203-222-1502
www.greenwood.com

This book is a case study of judicial policy making. It focuses on the role of adjudication in the making and refining of federal policy.

208 pages $45 - $55
ISBN 0-313254-24-9

5150 **Opening the Courthouse Door: An ADA Access Guide for State Courts**

American Bar Association
740 15th Street NW
9th Floor
Washington, DC 20005
202-662-1581
800-285-2221
FAX: 202-662-1032
e-mail: hammillj@staff.abanet.org
www.abanet.org/disability

John Hammill, Publications Coordinator
Amy Allbright, Managing Editor

Practical, step-by-step guide explains how to comply with the public access provisions of the ADA in the courthouse. The centerpiece of the guide is a series of action steps. *$12.00*

5151 **Operation Help: A Mental Health Advocate's Guide to Medicaid**

Nat'l Council for Community Behavioral Healthcare
12300 Twinbrook Parkway
Suite 320
Rockville, MD 20852
301-984-6200
FAX: 301-881-7159
www.nccbh.org

This book explains the Medicaid entitlement program in easy-to-read language and focuses on the needs of your clients. *$17.00*

5152 **PAL News**

Parent Professional Advocacy League
56 Temple Place
Suite 664
Boston, MA 02111
617-542-7860
800-537-0446
FAX: 617-542-7832
e-mail: pal@fcsn.org
www.ppal.net

Donna Welles, Director
Lisa Lambert, Assistant Director

Offers information on medical and technological updates in the area of research on birth defects, support groups and family resources for persons with disabled children.

Quarterly

5153 **Power of Attorney for Health Care**

Center for Public Representation
PO Box 260049
Madison, WI 53726
608-251-4008
800-369-0388
FAX: 606-251-1263

Discusses Wisconsin law regarding medical decisions, the Cruzan case and ethical considerations in addition to legal implications and advantages of this document. Book tells how to create a personalized Power Of Attorney document, including language for the Special Provisions portion. *$49.95*

132 pages
ISBN 0-93262 -38-0

5154 **Toward Independence**

National Council on Disability
1331 F Street NW
Suite 850
Washington, DC 20004
202-272-2004
FAX: 202-272-2022
TTY:202-272-2074

Mark Quigley, Communications Director

A 1986 report to the U.S. Congress on the federal laws and programs serving people with disabilities, and recommendations for legislation.

5155 **US Department of Health and Human Services Office for Civil Rights**

200 Independence Avenue SW
Room 509F HHH Building
Washington, DC 20201
800-368-1019
FAX: 202-619-3818

Enforces the Rehabilitation Act of 1973, which prohibits discrimination against handicapped persons by recipients of federal funding.

5156 **US Department of Labor**

200 Constitution Avenue NW
Washington, DC 20210
202-693-5000
FAX: 202-219-7312

Offers publications to assist employers in determining and achieving workplace accessibility.

5157 **US Department of Labor Office of Federal Contract Compliance Programs**

Regional Office
230 S Dearborn Street
Room 570
Chicago, IL 60604
312-596-7010
FAX: 312-596-7037

Investigates complaints brought under section 504 of the Rehabilitation Act of 1973 against federal contractors.

5158 **Washington Watch**

United Cerebral Palsy Association
3135 8th Street NE
Washington, DC 20017
202-269-1500
800-USE-5UCP
FAX: 202-526-0519
TTY:202-973-7197
e-mail: webmaster@ucpdc.org
www.ucpa.org

Susanna L Gorton, Editor

Dependable, timely information on national legislative and regulatory issues affecting people with disabilities and their families. *$25.00*

4 pages BiWeekly

5159 **William S Hein & Company**

1285 Main Street
Buffalo, NY 14209
716-675-3555
800-828-7571
FAX: 716-883-8100
e-mail: mail@wshein.com
www.wshein.com

Offers a catalog of periodicals, publications and reprints, microforms and government publications on medical, handicapped and health law.

5160 **Word from Washington**

United Cerebral Palsy Association
3135 8th Street NE
Washington, DC 20017

202-269-1500
800-USA-5UCP
FAX: 202-526-0519
TTY:202-973-7197
e-mail: webmaster@ucpdc.org
www.ucpa.org

Akua Kouyate

Provides information on national legislation and regulatory affairs, updates on disability and social service fields.
$25.00

24-36 pages Quarterly

Alabama

5161 **Alabama Institute for Deaf and Blind Library and Resource Center**

705 S Street
PO Box 698
Talladega, AL 35160
256-761-3337
800-848-4722
FAX: 256-761-3561
e-mail: tlacy@aidb.state.al.us
www.aidb.org

Teresa Lacy, Librarian

Book collection includes discs, cassettes, Braille and large print. Also closed-circuit TV and magnifiers. Offers Braille production and binding.

5162 **Alabama Radio Reading Service Network (ARR)**

650 11th Street S
Birmingham, AL 35233
205-934-6576
800-444-9246
FAX: 205-934-5075
e-mail: philip@wbhm.org
www.wbhm.org

Philip Habesh, Director

Services and readings are broadcast over a subcarrier service of public radio WBHM. This is a statewide station devoted to Alabama's blind and handicapped community.

5163 **Alabama Regional Library for the Blind and Physically Handicapped**

Alabama Public Library Service
6030 Monticello Drive
Montgomery, AL 36130
334-213-3906
800-392-5671
FAX: 334-213-3993
e-mail: fzaleski@apls.state.al.us
www.apls.state.al.us

Fara Zaleski, Regional Librarian

Recreational reading in special format for persons unable to use standard print. Reference materials offered include materials on blindness and other handicaps, films, local subjects and authors.

5164 **Houston-Love Memorial Library**

212 W Burdeshaw Street
PO Box 1369
Dothan, AL 36302
334-793-9767
FAX: 334-793-6645

Myrtis Merrow, Librarian

Offers magnifiers, summer reading programs and more for the blind and physically handicapped. Scanner, software, jaws for Windows.

5165 **Huntsville Subregional Library for the Blind & Physically Handicapped**

PO Box 443
915 Monroe Street
Huntsville, AL 35804
256-532-5980
FAX: 256-532-5994
e-mail: bphdept@hpl.lib.al.us
www.hpl.lib.al.us/main.html

Joyce Smith, Librarian

Talking books for people who are blind or disabled offering reference materials on the blind and other disabilities, large-print photocopier, thermaform duplicator and more.

5166 **Library for the Blind & Handicapped Public Library: Anniston/Calhoun Counties**

PO Box 308
Anniston, AL 36202
256-237-8503
FAX: 256-238-0474
e-mail: library@quicklink.net

Deenie Culver, Librarian

Reference materials on blindness, cassettes, large print books and discs.

5167 **Multipurpose Arthritis & Musculoskeletal Diseases Center: UAB**

Tinsley Harrison Tower
Birmingham, AL 35294
205-934-5306
FAX: 205-934-1564

Dr. Robert Kimberly MD, Director

Arthritis and related rheumatic disorders are studied.

5168 **Research for Rett Foundation**

PO Box 50347
Mobile, AL 36605
251-479-8293
800-422-7388
FAX: 251-479-8293

Patty Cofer, President
Anna Luce, Executive Director

National not-for-profit voluntary organization dedicated to raising funds for critical ongoing medical research into Rett Syndrome, hosting medical research symposia, and funding grant applications. Committed to expanding public awareness of and encouraging Rett Syndrome research within the National Institute of Child Health and Human Development. Provides a variety of educational mateials including brochures and fact sheets.

5169 **Technology Assistance for Special Consumers**

PO Box 443
Huntsville, AL 35804
205-532-5950
FAX: 256-532-5994
TTY:205-532-5996
e-mail: tasc@traveller.com
tasc.ataccess.org

Pam Harnden, Contact

Offers reference materials on the blind and other disabilities, large-print photocopier, thermaform duplicator and more. Provides the Library of Congress talking book services for persons with disabilities. Braille transcribing of short materials (not books).

5170 **Tuscaloosa Subregional Library for the Blind & Physically Handicapped**

1801 River Road
Tuscaloosa, AL 35401
205-345-5820
FAX: 205-752-8300

Barbara Jordan, Librarian

Provide talking books to patrons who are unable to use standard print because of a visual or physical limitation. Deliver playback equipment to qualified patrons. Provides reference and referral service to this special population also.

Alaska

5171 **Alaska State Library Talking Book Center**
344 W 3rd Avenue
Suite 125
Anchorage, AK 99501 **907-269-6569**
800-776-6566
FAX: 907-269-6580
e-mail: patience_frederiksen@eed.state.ak.us
www.eed.state.ak.us

Patricia Meek

Offers reference materials on blindness and other handicaps, native language materials, local subjects and authors. Small and large print collection available.

Arizona

5172 **Arizona Braille and Talking Book Library**
1030 N 32nd Street
Phoenix, AZ 85008 **602-255-5578**
FAX: 602-255-4312
e-mail: btbl@lib.az.us
www.lib.az.us/braille

Linda Montgomery, Director

Closed-circuit TV, summer reading programs, volunteer-produced cassette books, braille writer, films, large-print photocopier and more.

5173 **Books for the Blind of Arizona**
6120 E 5th Street
Unit A107
Tucson, AZ 85711 **602-792-9153**
FAX: 520-886-9839

Betty Evans, Chairperson

Offers large print photocopier, textbooks, recreational, career, vocational, braille books, talking books, cassettes, large print books and more for the visually impaired K-12, college students and adults.

5174 **Center for Neurodevelopmental Studies**
5430 W Glenn Drive
Glendale, AZ 85301 **623-915-0345**
e-mail: cns@netwrx.com
www.cirs.org

Lorna Jean King, Director, Emeritus

Effective treatment methods for autism and developmental disabilities are subjects researched and studied at the Center.

5175 **Flagstaff City-Coconino County Public Library**
300 W Aspen Avenue
Flagstaff, AZ 86001 **928-779-7670**
FAX: 928-774-9573
e-mail: colguin@fpl.lib.az.us

Christina Olguin, Librarian

Reference materials on blindness and other handicaps, Braille writer, magnifiers and large-print photocopier. Large-type books, closed captioned videos, adapters and books on tape.

5176 **Fountain Hills Lioness Braille Service**
PO Box 18332
Fountain Hills, AZ 85269 **480-837-3961**

Jean Hauck, Chairperson

Braille and large print books on the subjects of recreation, career and vocations, religion, novels and cookbooks for the visually impaired.

5177 **Harrington Arthritis Research Center**
1800 E Van Buren Street
Phoenix, AZ 85006 **602-254-0377**
FAX: 602-253-4817
e-mail: info@harcaz.org
www.harcaz.org

John Theobald, President/ CEO

Research into the various areas of arthritis, including assistive devices, joint repair and replacement, medical treatment and early detection and prevention.

5178 **Prescott Public Library**
215 E Goodwin Street
Prescott, AZ 86303 **928-777-1500**
FAX: 928-445-1851
www.prescottlib.lib.az.us

Katherine Kujawa, Adult Services Librarian

Large print, Braille and audio books; magnifiers; text to voice scanner; talking book machine application; toy library for children with special needs; special needs product catalogs; home book delivery; descriptive videos; 43 point PC monitor.

5179 **Special Needs Center/Phoenix Public Library**
12 E McDowell Road
Phoenix, AZ 85004 **602-261-8690**
TTY:602-254-8205
www.phoenixlibrary.org

Mary Roatch, Supervisor

Offers talking books and records, braille books and magazines, large print books, video print enlarger, video magnifier and VersaBraille software with synthetic speech for the blind, visually handicapped, physically/mentally handicapped and speech and hearing impaired children and adults.

5180 **WAHEC Medical Library Consortium**
Bullhead Community Hospital
2735 Silver Creek Road
Bullhead City, AZ 86442 **928-763-1505**
FAX: 928-704-6759

Kathleen Stanley, Medical Library Co.

Medical library management.

5181 **World Research Foundation**
41 Bell Rock Plaza
Sedona, AZ 86351 **928-284-3300**
FAX: 928-284-3530
e-mail: info@wrf.org
www.wrf.org

Large research library of alternative medicine; offers a computer search and printout of specific health issues for a nominal fee.

Arkansas

5182 **Arkansas Regional Library for the Blind and Physically Handicapped**
One Capitol Mall
Little Rock, AR 72201 **501-682-1155**
FAX: 501-682-1529
TTY:501-682-1002
e-mail: jhall@asl.lib.ar.us

John D Hall, Director

Public library books in recorded or braille format. Popular fiction and nonfiction books for all ages, books and players are on free loan, sent to patrons by mail and may be returned postage free. Anyone who cannot see well enough to read regular print with glasses on or who has a disability that makes it difficult to hold a book or turn the pages is eligible.

5183 Educational Services for the Visually Impaired

2600 W Markham Street
PO Box 668
Little Rock, AR 72203 **501-296-1815**
FAX: 501-663-3536

David Beavers, Director

Offers textbooks, braille books and more to the visually impaired grades K-12 in the Arizona area.

5184 Library for the Blind and Physically Handicapped SW Region of Arkansas

220 E Main Street
PO Box 668
Magnolia, AR 71753 **870-234-0399**
866-234-8273
FAX: 870-234-5077
e-mail: lbph@hotmail.com

Susan Walker, Supervisor

A free library service that serves adults and children who meet the eligiblity requirements, offers free loan of cassette machine and recorded books, which meet the reading preferences of a highly diverse clientele.

5185 Northwest Ozarks Regional Library for the Blind and Handicapped

217 E Dickson S
Fayetteville, AR 72701 **479-442-6243**
FAX: 479-442-6254
www.uark.edu

Rachel Anne Ames, Librarian

Offers a summer reading program, closed-circuit TV, magnifiers, braille writers and large print books.

California

5186 Association of Visual Science Librarians

University of California
School of Optometry
Berkeley, CA 94720 **501-642-1020**

Bette Anton, President

Promotes information services in ophthalmology and optometry. Conducts institutes, workshops, and training courses for professional personnel and provides legislative consultation.

5187 Autism Research Institute

4182 Adams Avenue
San Diego, CA 92116 **619-281-7165**
FAX: 619-563-6840
e-mail: autismresearchinstitute.com
www.autismresearchinstitute.com

B Rimland PhD, Director

Conducts research on the causes, diagnosis, and treatment of autism and publishes a quarterly newsletter that reviews worldwide research. Literature on causes and treatment available. Refers patients and families to health care professionals and clinics. Request publication list and sample newsletter, Autism Research Review.

5188 Books Aloud

PO Box 5731
San Jose, CA 95150 **408-277-4839**
FAX: 408-277-4818
e-mail: booksaloud@juno.com
www.booksaloud.org

David Rich, Director

Loands books on tape at no fees to visually, physically, and learning impaired people of all ages. Over 4,500 titles available.

5189 Braille Institute Library

741 N Vermont Avenue
Los Angeles, CA 90029 **323-660-3880**
800-808-2555
FAX: 323-663-0867
e-mail: dls@brailib.org
www.braillelibrary.org

Dr. Henry C Chang, Librarian

Cassettes, braille, reference materials on blindness and other disabilities. Reading lab area with closed-circuit TV, Kurzweil Personal Reader (scanner), and typewriters. Field visits and interlibrary loans of books on cassettes, braille or other medium.

5190 Braille Institute Orange County Center

527 N Dale Avenue
Anaheim, CA 92801 **714-821-5000**
800-272-4553
FAX: 714-527-7621
www.brailleinstitute.org

Offers services, publications, information and programs free of charge to blind and visually impaired persons of all ages.

5191 Braille Institute Santa Barbara Center

2031 De La Vina Street
Santa Barbara, CA 93105 **805-682-6222**
FAX: 805-569-2048

Offers programs, services and information for persons with visual impairments.

5192 Braille Institute Sight Center

741 N Vermont Avenue
Los Angeles, CA 90029 **323-663-1111**
e-mail: bils@brailib.org
www.brailleinstitue.org

Dr. Henry Chang, Librarian

Offers help, programs, services and information to the blind and visually impaired children and adults.

5193 Braille Institute Youth Center

3450 Cahuenga Boulevard W
Los Angeles, CA 90068 **323-851-5695**

Offers various youth programs and services for the blind and visually impaired youngster.

5194 Broadcast Services for the Blind

214 Van Ness Avenue
San Francisco, CA 94102 **415-431-1481**
FAX: 415-863-7568
TTY:415-431-4572

Randy Scott, Director

Offers radio broadcasting, braille books, cassettes, records, and more for the visually handicapped in the nine San Francisco Bay Area major cities.

5195 California State Library: Braille and Talking Book Library

900 N Street
Sacramento, CA 95814 **916-654-0640**
800-952-5666
FAX: 916-654-1119
e-mail: btbl@library.ca.gov
www.library.ca.gov/html/pubser05.cfm

Donine Hedrick, Program Manager
Pam Ryan, Librarian

Provides library services to people in Northern California who are unable to read standard print books because of visual or physical disabilities. Braille and talking books, magazines, machines, catalogs and postage are provided free to qualified appicants. The service is conducted by mail.

5196 Clearinghouse for Specialized Media and Technology

California Department of Education
1430 N Street
Room 3410
Sacramento, CA 95814 **916-445-5103**
FAX: 916-323-9732
e-mail: rbrawley@cde.ca.gov
www.cde.ca.gov/csmt

Rod Brawley, Consultant

Assists schools and students in the identification and acquisition of textbooks, reference books and study materials in aural media, Braille, large print and electronic media access technology.

5197 Fresno County Free Library Blind and Handicapped Services

770 N San Pablo Avenue
Fresno, CA 93728 **559-488-3217**
800-742-1011
FAX: 559-488-1971
TTY:559-488-1971
e-mail: weisenbe@sjvls.lib.ca.us

Wendy Eisenberg, Librarian

Magnifiers, home visits, volunteer-produced cassette books, discs and cassettes.

5198 Glaucoma Research Foundation

490 Post Street
Suite 2538
San Francisco, CA 94102 **415-986-3162**
800-826-6693
FAX: 415-986-3763
e-mail: info@glacoma.org
www.glaucoma.org

Robert N Shaffer MD, Chairman
Yuko Madono, Outreach/Public Relations

Clinical and laboratory studies of glaucoma.

5199 Herrick Health Sciences Library

Alta Bates Medical Center
2001 Dwight Way
Berkeley, CA 94704 **510-204-4444**
FAX: 510-204-3521

Laurie Bagley, Librarian

Information on rehabilitation, psychiatry and psychoanalysis.

5200 Kuzell Institute for Arthritis and Infectious Diseases

Medical Research Institute of San Francisco
2200 Webster Street
R305
San Francisco, CA 94115 **415-561-1734**
FAX: 415-441-8548

Lowell S Young, Director

One of seven units comprising the Medical Research Institute of San Francisco that offers basic and applied research in arthritis and related diseases.

5201 Multipurpose Arthritis & Musculoskeletal Diseases Center

University of California, San Diego
9500 Gilman Drive
La Jolla, CA 92093 **858-552-7439**
FAX: 858-534-5475

Dr. Dennis Carson, Co-Director

Causes and treatment of arthritis.

5202 New Beginnings: The Blind Children's Center

4120 Marathon Street
Los Angeles, CA 90029 **323-664-2153**
800-222-3566
FAX: 323-665-3228
blindchildrenscenter.org

The purpose of the Center is to turn initial fears into hope. Helps children and their families become independent by creating a climate of safety and trust. Children learn to develop self confidence and to master a wide range of skills. Services include an infant stimulation program, educational preschool, interdisciplinary assessment services, family services, correspondence program, toll free national hotline and a publication and research service.

5203 Research & Training Center on Mental Health for Hard of Hearing Persons

California School of Professional Psychology
6215 Ferris Square
Suite 140
San Diego, CA 92121 **619-282-4443**
800-HEA-R619
FAX: 800-642-0266

Raymond J Trybus PhD, Director
Thomas J Goulder PhD, Associate Director

Funded by the National Institute on Disability and Rehabilitation Research, this training center aims to address issues of psychological relevance to persons who are hard of hearing or late deafened (as distinct from prelingually, culturally deaf persons). Also serves as information clearinghouse on this topic.

5204 Rosalind Russell Medical Research Center for Arthritis

350 Parnassus Avenue
Room 600
San Francisco, CA 94143 **415-476-1141**
FAX: 415-476-3526
www.ucsf.edu

Ephraim P Engelman MD, Director

Arthritis research and its probable causes.

5205 San Francisco Public Library for the Blind and Print Handicapped

100 Larkin Street
San Francisco, CA 94102 **415-557-4253**
FAX: 415-557-4375
e-mail: lbphmgr@sfpl.lib.org
www.sfol.org

Martin Maqid, Librarian

Foreign-language books on cassette, children's books on cassettes and more.

5206 **San Jose State University Library**
One Washington Square
San Jose, CA 95192 **408-924-2805**
FAX: 408-924-2701
e-mail: sliu@email.sisu.edu

Susana Liu, Reference Librarian

Information on physical disabilities, accessibility and learning disabilities.

Colorado

5207 **AMC Cancer Research Center**
1600 Pierce Street
Denver, CO 80214 **303-233-7419**
800-525-3777
FAX: 303-239-3340

Provides trained counselors who provide understanding and support for cancer patients; information and referral services; and screening programs.

5208 **Boulder Public Library**
1000 Canyon Boulevard
Boulder, CO 80302 **303-441-3100**
www.boulder.lib.co.us

Marcelee Gralapp, Director
Randy Smith, Assistant Director

Offers braille books, cassettes, talking books, large print photocopier, large print books and more for the visually impaired.

5209 **Colorado Library for the Blind and Physically Handicapped**
Colorado Talking Book Library
180 Sheridan Boulevard
Denver, CO 80226 **303-727-9277**
800-685-2136
FAX: 303-727-9281
e-mail: ctbl.info@cde.state.co.us
www.cde.state.co.us/ctbl

Barbara Goral, Librarian

Offers reference materials on blindness and other handicaps, children's print/braille books, cassettes, large print books, and volunteer-produced cassette books and magazines.

5210 **National Jewish Medical & Research Center**
1400 Jackson Street
Denver, CO 80206 **303-388-4461**
800-222-5864
e-mail: allstetterw@njc.org
www.njc.org

William Allstetter, Media Relations Manager

The only medical center in the country whose research and patient care resources are dedicated to respiratory and immunologic diseases.

Connecticut

5211 **Connecticut Assistive Technology Project**
Connecticut Department of Social Services
Bureau of Rehabilitation Services
25 Sigourney Street, 11th Floor
Hartford, CT 06106 **860-424-4881**
800-537-2549
FAX: 860-424-4850
TTY:860-424-4839
e-mail: cttap@aol.com
www.techact.uconn.edu

Judith Fein, NIDRR Officer

Single point of entry, advocacy, information and referral, peer counseling, and access to objective expert advice and consultation for people with disabilities.

5212 **Connecticut Braille Association**
664 Oakwood Avenue
W Hartford, CT 06110 **860-953-9692**

Anne Murphy, Executive Secretary

Offers textbooks, cassettes, large print books, braille books and more.

5213 **Connecticut State Library**
198 W Street
Rocky Hill, CT 06067 **860-566-2151**
800-842-4516
FAX: 860-566-6669
e-mail: lbph@cslib.org

Carol Taylor, Librarian

Discs, cassettes, braille, reference materials on blindness and other handicaps, closed-circuit TV and large-print photocopier.

5214 **Prevent Blindness Connecticut**
1275 Washington Street
Middletown, CT 06457 **860-628-0347**
800-850-2020
FAX: 860-347-0613

The mission of Prevent Blindness Connecticut is to save sight and prevent blindness through eye screenings, education, safety activities and research.

5215 **Yale University: Vision Research Center**
330 Cedar Street
New Haven, CT 06510 **203-785-4640**
FAX: 203-785-6123

Marvin Sears, Prin/ Investigator

Vision including studies on growth and development.

Delaware

5216 **Delaware Assistive Technology Initiative Center for Applied Science and Engineering**
University of Delaware
Alfred I duPont Hospital
Wilmington, DE 19899 **302-651-6790**
800-870-3284
FAX: 302-651-6793
TTY:302-651-6794
e-mail: dati@asel.udel.edu
www.asel.udel.edu/dati

Sonja Rathel, Project Coordinator

Project has established county resource centers in each of Delaware's three counties. These centers serve as information and equipment resource sites, offering short-term equipment loans, training and demonstration workshops and regular informational mailings.

5217 **Delaware Library for the Blind and Physically Handicapped**

43 S Dupont Highway
Dover, DE 19901 **302-739-4748**
800-282-8676
FAX: 302-739-6787
e-mail: debph@lib.de.us

John Phillos, Regional Librarian

Books on cassette and playback equipment are provided to patrons who are unable to read regular printed books.

5218 **Rehabilitation Engineering Library**

321 E 11th Street
Wilmington, DE 19801 **302-657-5601**
FAX: 302-654-5815

Robert Rodgers

Rehabilitation engineering and physical disabilities.

District of Columbia

5219 **District of Columbia Public Library: Services to the Deaf Community**

901 G Street NW
Room 215
Washington, DC 20001 **202-727-2145**
FAX: 202-727-1129
e-mail: library_deaf_dc@yahoo.com
www.dclibrary.org

Janice Rosen, Librarian

Offers reference services through TTY, signers for library programs, sign language classes, information about deafness, print and non-print materials for persons who have hearing disabilities. Book talks on deaf culture are held once a month

5220 **District of Columbia Regional Library for the Blind and Physically Handicapped**

901 G Street NW
Room 215
Washington, DC 20001 **202-727-2142**
FAX: 202-727-1129
TTY:202-727-2145
e-mail: lbphb_2000@yahoo.com
www.dclibrary.org

Grace J Lyons, Librarian

Regional library/RPH is network library in the Library of Congress, National Library Services for the Blind and Physically Handicapped.

5221 **Georgetown University Child Development Center**

3307 M Street Avenue NW
Suite 401
Washington, DC 20007 **202-944-2130**
FAX: 202-687-8899
TTY:202-687-5503

5222 **National Institute on Disability and Rehabilitation Research**

400 Maryland Avenue SW
Washington, DC 20202 **202-205-8134**
800-872-5327
TTY:2022054475

William J Ryan, Acting Director

A national leader in sponsoring research. Mission is to generate, disseminate and promote new knowledge to improve the options available to disabled persons.

1978

5223 **Senior Center for the Hearing Impaired**

1510 9th Street NW
Washington, DC 20001 **202-232-4288**
FAX: 202-667-9781

Angela Jones, Director
Alma Beasley, Administrative Assistant

Offers daily programs, activities, counseling, noon meals, and transportation for deaf and hard of hearing seniors, 60 and older, living in the District of Columbia.

5224 **University Legal Services AT Program**

300 I Street NE
Suite 200
Washington, DC 20002 **202-547-0198**
FAX: 202-547-2662
TTY:202-547-2657
e-mail: atpdc@uls-dc.com

Alicia C Johns, Principal Investigator
Carol Cohen, NIDRR Officer

Designed to empower individuals with disabilities; to promote consumer involvement and advocacy, and provide information, referral and training as they relate to accessing assistive technology services and devices; and to identify and improve access to funding resources.

Florida

5225 **Brevard County Talking Books Library**

308 Forrest Avenue
Cocoa, FL 32922 **321-633-1810**
FAX: 321-633-1838
e-mail: kbriley@brev.org

Kay Briley, Librarian

Offers reference materials on blindness and other handicaps. Subregional library for the blind and physically handicapped, assistive reading devices collection, reference materials on blindness and other handicaps; CCTV, phonic ear, reading edge and LOUD-R assistive listening devices available.

5226 **Broward County Talking Book Library**

100 S Andrews Avenue
Ft. Lauderdale, FL 33301 **954-357-7397**
FAX: 954-357-5548
www.klas.com/AnnouncementsBroward.html

Barbara Kelly, Librarian

Reference materials on blindness and other handicaps, films, closed-circuit TV, discs, cassettes and a book discussion group is offered.

5227 **Dade County Talking Book Library**
Miami-Dade Public Library System
150 NE 79th Street
Miami, FL 33138 **305-751-8687**
800-451-9544
FAX: 305-757-8401
e-mail: talkingbooks@mdpls.org

Barbara Moyer, Librarian

Library services for people with disabilities.

5228 **Florida Division of Blind Services**
Regional Library
420 Platt Street
Daytona Beach, FL 32114 **386-258-8692**
FAX: 850-239-6069
TTY:800-226-6079
e-mail: weberd@mail.firn.edu

Donald John Weber, Librarian

Discs, cassettes, closed-circuit TV, large-print photocopier, films, children's books on cassettes and more.

5229 **Florida Instructional Materials Center for the Visually Handicapped**
5002 N Lois Avenue
Tampa, FL 33614 **813-872-5281**
800-282-9193
FAX: 813-872-5284

Suzanne Dalton, Supervisor

Operates a clearinghouse depository and production center for braille, large print and recorded texts. Provides assistance in assessment of materials and specialized apparatus, organizes volunteers for material production and more for the visually handicapped.

5230 **Hillsborough County Talking Book Library Tampa-Hillsborough County Public Library**
900 N Ashely Street
Tampa, FL 33602 **813-264-3831**
FAX: 813-273-3641
TTY:813-273-3610
e-mail: myersl@scfn.thpl.lib.fl.us
www.hcplc.org/hcplc/liblocales/tbl

Kurt Jasielonis

5231 **Lee County Library System: Talking Books Library**
13240 N Cleveland Avenue
 # 5-6
North Fort Myers, FL 33903 **239-995-2665**
800-854-8195
FAX: 239-995-1681
TTY:941-995-2665
www.lee-county.com/library/progserv/sscvs/tb.

Provides free books and magazines to Lee County residents of all ages who have any disability that prevents them from reading printed material. Books are played on special players provided free by the National Library Service. Circulates low tech assistive aids and devices for temporary loan to Lee County Library card holders. Directs people to assistive technology and disability related resources.

5232 **Louis de la Parte Florida Mental Health Institute Research Library**
13301 Bruce B Downs Boulevard
Tampa, FL 33612 **813-974-4471**
FAX: 813-974-7242
e-mail: library@fmhi.usf.edu
www.fmhi.usf.edu

Information offered on mental illness, autism and pervasive development disabilities mental health research and archives management.

5233 **Orange County Library System: Audio-Visual Department**
101 E Central Boulevard
Orlando, FL 32801 **407-425-4694**
FAX: 407-425-6779
TTY:407-425-5668

Sally Fry

5234 **Pearlman Biomedical Research Institute**
Mt. Sinani Medical Center
4300 Alton Road
Miami Beach, FL 33140 **305-674-2121**
FAX: 305-674-2198

Dr. William Abraham, Director

Pulmonary medicine, arthritis, sleep disorders and gynecology departments of research.

5235 **Pinellas Talking Book Library for the Blind and Physically Handicapped**
1330 Cleveland Street
Clearwater, FL 33755 **727-441-9958**
FAX: 727-441-9068
TTY:813-538-8949
e-mail: mstevenson@pplc.us
www.pplc.us/tbl/

Marilyn Stevenson, Talking Book Librarian
Harriet Thompson, Outreach Librarian
Marianne Morawetz, Reader Advisor

5236 **Subregional Talking Book Library**
Jacksonville Public Library
1755 Edgewood Avenue W
Suite 1
Jacksonville, FL 32208 **904-765-5588**
FAX: 904-768-7404
TTY:904-768-7822
e-mail: arthurs@mail.firn.edu

Laurie Baumgardner, Department Head
Nkoyo Ross, Librarian

Offers cassettes, reference materials on blindness and other handicaps, children's braille books, descriptive videos, and some assistive devices.

5237 **Talking Book Service: Mantatee County Central Library**
6081 26th Street W
Bradenton, FL 34207 **941-742-5914**
FAX: 941-751-7098

Patricia Schubert, Librarian

Offers children's books on disc and cassette and more reference materials for the blind and physically handicapped.

5238 **Talking Books Library for the Blind and Physically Handicapped**
Palm Beach County Library Annex
7950 Central Ind Drive
Suite 104
Riviera Beach, FL 33404 **561-775-8274**
FAX: 561-845-4640

Pat Mistretta, Librarian

Library services for people with disabilities.

5239 **Talking Books/Homebound Services**

Brevard County Library System
308 Forrest Avenue
Cocoa, FL 32922 **321-633-1810**
FAX: 321-633-1838
e-mail: kbriley@brev.org

Kay Briley, Librarian

Offers reference materials on blindness and other handicaps. Subregional library for the blind and physically handicapped, assistive reading devices collection, reference materials on blindness and other handicaps; CCTV, phonic ear, reading edge and LOUD-R assistive listening devices available.

5240 **University of Miami: Bascom Palmer Eye Institute**

Department of Ophthalmalogy
1638 NW 10th Avenue
Miami, FL 33136 **305-326-6031**
FAX: 305-326-6306

John G Clarkson MD, Chairman

Clinical and basic research into blindness and visual impairments.

5241 **University of Miami: Mailman Center for Child Development**

PO Box 016820
Miami, FL 33101 **305-585-2703**
FAX: 305-547-6309

Dr. Robert Stempfel Jr, Director

Focuses on birth defects and children's illnesses.

5242 **West Florida Regional Library**

200 W Gregory Street
Pensacola, FL 32501 **850-435-1760**
FAX: 850-432-9582

Martha Lazor, Librarian

Offers children's print/braille books.

Georgia

5243 **Albany Talking Book Center**

Dougherty County Public Library
300 Pine Avenue
Albany, GA 31701 **229-420-3220**
FAX: 229-420-3240

Kathryn Sinquefield, Librarian

Offers discs, cassettes, reference materials on blindness and other handicaps, large-print photocopiers, summer reading programs, cassette books and more.

5244 **Athens Regional Library Talking Book Center**

2025 Baxter Street
Athens, GA 30606 **706-613-3655**
FAX: 706-613-3660

Paige Burns, Manager

Discs, cassettes, large print books, reference materials on blindness, descriptive videos, films, closed-circuit TV, magnifiers, braille writer, summer reading programs, cassette books and magazines and more.

5245 **Augusta Talking Book Center**

425 9th Street
Augusta, GA 30901 **706-821-2625**
FAX: 706-724-5403
e-mail: gswint@csra,net

Gary Swint, Librarian

Discs, cassettes, braille writer, films, large print books, summer reading program, magnifiers and reference materials on blindness and other handicaps.

5246 **Bainbridge Subregional Library for the Blind & Physically Handicapped**

SW Georgia Regional Library
301 S Monroe Street
Bainbridge, GA 39819 **229-248-2680**
800-795-2680
FAX: 229-248-2670
e-mail: lbph@mail.decatur.public.lib.ga.us
www.swgrl.org

Susan Whittle, Librarian
Kathy Hutchins, Supervisor
Priscilla Southall, Library Assistant

Cassettes, large print books, summer reading programs, closed-circuit TV, magnifiers and more.

5247 **Division of Birth Defects and Genetic Diseases**

4770 Buford Highway
Chamblee, GA 30341 **404-498-3800**
FAX: 404-498-3041

Muin J Khoury MD

5248 **Emory Autism Resource Center**

Emory University
718 Gatewood Road
Atlanta, GA 30322 **404-727-3360**
FAX: 404-727-8350

Offers on-line bulletin boards which are relevant to autism.

5249 **Emory University Laboratory for Ophthalmic Research**

1365B Clifton Road
Atlanta, GA 30322 **404-778-4456**
e-mail: pbennet@emory.edu

Henry F Edelhauser, Director

Various studies into the aspects of blindness.

5250 **Georgia Library for the Blind and Physically Handicapped**

1150 Murphy Avenue SW
Atlanta, GA 30310 **404-756-4619**
800-248-6701
FAX: 404-756-4618

Linda Stetson, Director

Discs, cassettes, braille, films, closed-circuit TV, braille writer, large-print photocopier, cassette books and magazines.

5251 **Hall County Library: East Hall Branch and Special Needs Library**

2434 Old Cornelia Highway
Gainesville, GA 30507 **770-531-2500**
FAX: 770-532-2502
e-mail: kevans@mail.hall.public.lib.ga.us
www.hall.public.lib.ga.us

Kathy Evans, Branch Manager

Summer reading programs, braille writer, magnifiers, scanners and readers, audio described videos, closed captioned videos, closed-circuit TV, large-print photocopier, cassette books and magazines, large print books, children's books on cassette, home visits and other reference materials on blindness and other handicaps.

5252 Lafayette Subregional Library for the Blind and Physically Handicapped

305 S Duke Street
PO Box 707
La Fayette, GA 30728 **706-638-1958**
888-506-0509
FAX: 706-638-4028
e-mail: stubblec@yahoo.com
www.walker.public.lib.ga.us

Charles H Stubblefield, Library Manager

Summer reading programs, magnifiers, closed-circuit TV, large-print photocopier, cassette books and magazines, children's books on cassette, home visits and other reference materials on blindness and other handicaps.

5253 Library for the Blind and Physically Handicapped

Live Oak Public Libraries
2708 Mechanics Avenue
Savannah, GA 31404 **912-354-5864**
FAX: 912-354-5534
e-mail: lbphsav@liveoakpl.org
www.liveoakpl.org

Linda Stokes, Librarian

Braille writer, magnifiers, closed-circuit TV, cassette books and magazines, children's books on cassette, home visits and other reference materials on blindness and other handicaps.

5254 Macon Library for the Blind and Physically Handicapped

Washington Memorial Library
1180 Washington Avenue
Macon, GA 31201 **478-743-3345**
800-805-7613
FAX: 478-742-3161
e-mail: sherrilr@mail-bibb.public.lib.ga.us

Rebecca Sherrill, Librarian

Summer reading programs, braille writer, magnifiers, closed-circuit TV, large-print photocopier, cassette books and magazines, children's books on cassette, home visits and other reference materials on blindness and other handicaps.

5255 Oconee Regional Library

Bellevue Avenue
PO Box 100
Dublin, GA 31040 **478-275-5382**
FAX: 478-272-0524

Betty Schild, Director
Linda Kight, Special Service Manager

Summer reading programs, braille writer, magnifiers, closed-circuit TV, large-print photocopier, cassette books and magazines, children's books on cassette, home visits and other reference materials on blindness and other handicaps.

5256 Rome Subregional Library for the Blind and Physically Handicapped

205 Riverside Parkway NE
Rome, GA 30161 **706-236-4618**
888-263-0769
FAX: 706-236-4631
e-mail: dianam@mail.floyd.public.lib
www.floyd.public.lib.ga.us/tbc.html

Diana Mills, Librarian

5257 South Georgia Regional Library-Valdosta Talking Book Center

300 Woodrow Wilson Drive
Valdosta, GA 31602 **229-333-7658**
FAX: 229-333-0774
e-mail: djernigan@sgrl.org

Diane Jernigan, Manager

Summer reading programs, Braille writer, magnifiers, closed-circuit TV, large print photocopier, cassette books and magazines, children's books on cassette, home visits and other reference materials on blindness and other handicaps.

5258 Subregional Library for the Blind and Physically Handicapped

1120 Bradley Drive
Columbus, GA 31906 **706-649-0780**
FAX: 706-649-1259
e-mail: slbph@mail.museogee.public.lib.ga.us

Dorothy Bowen, Librarian

Braille writer, magnifiers, closed-circuit TV, large-print photocopier, cassette books and magazines, children's books on cassette, home visits and other reference materials on blindness and other handicaps.

5259 Talking Book Center Brunswick-Glynn County Regional Library

606 O Street
Brunswick, GA 31520 **912-267-1212**
FAX: 912-267-9597
e-mail: ransomb@mail.glynn.public.lib.ga.us

Betty Ransom, Librarian

Hawaii

5260 Assistive Technology Resource Centers of Hawaii (ATRC)

414 Kuwili Street
Suite 104
Honolulu, HI 96817 **808-532-7110**
800-645-3007
FAX: 808-532-7120
TTY:808-532-7110
e-mail: atrc@atrc.org
www.atrc.org

Provides information and training on assistive technology devices, services, and funding resources. Conducts presentations and demonstrations in the community to increase AT awareness and promote self-advocacy among people with disabilities.

5261 Hawaii State Library for the Blind and Physically Handicapped

402 Kapahulu Avenue
Honolulu, HI 96815 **808-733-8444**
800-559-4096
FAX: 808-733-8449
e-mail: olbcirc@state.lib.hi.us
www.librarieshawaii.org

Fusako Miyashiro, Managing Librarian
Betty J Kingery, Librarian

Supported by the Hawaii State Public Library System and the National Library Service for the Blind and Physically Handicapped, Library of Congress. Staff with knowledge of sign language; Special interest periodicals; Books on deafness and sign language; captioned media; High interest/low vocabulary books. Special Services: Radio Reading Service, Talking Books Reader's Club, educational and cultural programs, machine lending agency. Braille, cassette and large type. Regional and National service.

Idaho

5262 **Idaho Assistive Technology Project**
University of Idaho
129 W 3rd Street
Moscow, ID 83843
208-885-3559
800-432-8324
FAX: 208-885-3628
e-mail: rseiler@uidaho.edu
www.educ.uidaho.edu/idatech

Sue House, Information Specialist

Project engages in systems change activities, training, materials development, information dissemination and advocacy activities directed at increasing the availability of assistive devices and services to Idahoans who have disabilities.

5263 **Idaho State Library: Talking Book Library**
325 W State Street
Boise, ID 83702
208-334-2117
800-233-4931
FAX: 208-334-4016
e-mail: ksalmon@isl.state.id.us
www.lili.org/isl

Andrea R Testi, Regional Librarian

Offers talking books and magazines, large print materials, braille, equipment and accessories. Available to all residents of Idaho who are visually impaired and/or have disabilities which disallows the use of print material.

Illinois

5264 **Catholic Guild for the Blind**
180 N Michigan Avenue
Suite 1700
Chicago, IL 60601
312-236-8569
FAX: 312-236-8128
e-mail: guild@guildfortheblind.org
www.guildfortheblind.org

Jodi Jasek, Consumer Product Center Coord.

Offers assistive devices for sale, provides computer assistive traing. Offers audio and braille transcription, sponsers seminars on a wide arrange of topics and provides weekly sales information via telephone.

5265 **Chicago Public Library Talking Book Center**
400 S State Street 5 N
Chicago, IL 60605
312-747-4001
800-757-4654
FAX: 312-747-1609
e-mail: mgrady@ch.publib.org

Mamie Grady, Librarian

Summer reading programs, Braille writer, closed-circuit TV, large print photocopier, cassette books and magazines, children's books on cassette, home visits and other reference materials on blindness and other handicaps. Three assistive technology centers designed and equipped for the blind and visually impaired, funded by the National Library Service for the Blind and Handicapped, a division of the Library of Congress. All services FREE!

5266 **Department of Ophthalmology/Eye and Ear Infirmary**
1855 W Taylor Street
Chicago, IL 60612
312-996-6590
FAX: 312-996-7770

Adrienne Adelman, Administrative Secretary

Offers help, support, information and research for persons with vision problems, including Retinitis Pigmentosa.

5267 **Horizons for the Blind**
2 N Williams Street
Crystal Lake, IL 60014
815-444-8800
FAX: 815-444-8830
e-mail: mail@horizons-blind.org
www.horizons-blind.org

Mission is to improve the quality of life for people who are blind or visually impaired by increasing accessibility to culture, education, recreation and consumer information on a national basis.

1977

5268 **Illinois Early Childhood Intervention Clearinghouse**
830 S Spring Street
Springfield, IL 62704
217-522-4655
800-852-4302
FAX: 217-522-4670
e-mail: clearinghouse@eosinc.com
www.eiclearinghouse.org

Chet Brandt, Project Director
Patricia Taylor, Project Associate

Free lending library of materials related to early childhood and disability. Books, audiovisuals and articles available. Computerized database with more than 31,000 items available to Illinois residents.

5269 **Illinois Regional Library for the Blind and Physically Handicapped**
1055 W Roosevelt Road
Chicago, IL 60608
312-746-9210
800-331-2351
FAX: 773-746-9192

Shawn Thomas, Reference Librarian
Barbara Perkins, Acting Director

Summer reading programs, braille writer, magnifiers, closed-circuit TV, large-print photocopier, cassette books and magazines, descriptive videos, children's books on cassette, home visits and other reference materials on blindness and other handicaps.

5270 **Mid-Illinois Talking Book Center**
515 York
Quincy, IL 62301
217-224-6619
800-537-1274
FAX: 217-224-9818
e-mail: lbell@alliancelibrarysystem.com
www.mitbc.org

Lori Bell, Director

Subregional library provides Talking book and Braille Book program to eligible persons unable to use standard print materials due to visual or physical disabilities. Includes cassette books and magazines; summer reading program.

5271 **National Eye Research Foundation (NERF)**

910 Skokie Boulevard
Suite 207A
Northbrook, IL 60062 **847-564-4652**
800-621-2258
FAX: 847-564-0807
e-mail: nerf1955@aol.com
www.eyemac.com/nerf

Dedicated to improving eye care for the public and meeting the professional nees of eye care practitioners; sponsors eye research projects on contact lens applications and eye care problems. Special study sections in such fields as orthokertology, primary eyecare, pediatrics, and through continuing education programs. Provides eye care information for the public and professionals. Educational materials including pamphlets. Program activities include education and referrals.

5272 **National Lekotek Center**

2100 Ridge Avenue
Evanston, IL 60201 **847-328-0001**
800-366-7529
FAX: 847-328-5514
e-mail: lekotek@lekotek.org
www.lekotek.org

Helen McCarthy, Executive Director

Toy library and play-centered programs for children with special needs and their families with branches in 17 states. Sliding fee scale. Lekotek also has a Toy Resource Helpline that provides individualized assistances in the selection of toys and play materials and general resources for families with children with disabilities.

5273 **Northwestern University Multipurpose Arthritis & Musculoskeletal Center**

303 E Chicago Avenue
Chicago, IL 60611 **312-908-8171**
FAX: 312-503-0994

Dr. Richard Pope, Head

Conducts biomedical, educational and health services research into musculoskeletal diseases.

5274 **Rehabilitation Institute of Chicago Learning Resource Center**

345 E Superior Street
Chicago, IL 60611 **312-908-6000**
FAX: 312-908-1369

Elizabeth DeLaHunt, Coordinator

Offers information on rehabilitation and physical disabilities.

5275 **Skokie Accessible Library Services**

Skokie Public Library
5215 Oakton Street
Skokie, IL 60077 **847-673-7774**
FAX: 847-673-7797
e-mail: tellus@skokie.lib.il.us
www.skokie.lib.il.us

Gary Gustin, Program Manager
Patricia Grobs, Coordinator of Community Service

Library services for people with disabilities, including electronic aids, materials in special formats, programs and special services, and access to the North Suburban Library System.

5276 **Southern Illinois Talking Book Center**

607 S Greenbriar Road
Carterville, IL 62918 **618-985-8375**
800-455-2665
FAX: 618-985-4211
e-mail: dbrawley@shawls.lib.il.us
www.shawls.lib.il.us/docs/bhp/bhpindex.html

Diana Sussman, Director

Library service, recorded books & magazines for people with difficulty reading print due to visual or physical limitations or reading disability (all ages), reference/referral, descriptive videos, newsline newspaper service, presentations/in-service. Free.

5277 **University of Illinois at Chicago: Lions of Illinois Eye Research Institute**

UIC Eye Center
1905 W Taylor Street
Chicago, IL 60612 **312-996-8937**
FAX: 312-996-7770

Prf. Jose Pulrdo, Head

Visual impairments and blindness research, including glaucoma studies.

5278 **Voices of Vision Talking Book Center at DuPage Library System**

127 S 1st Street
Geneva, IL 60134 **630-208-0398**
800-227-0625
FAX: 630-208-0399
e-mail: kodean@dupagels.lib.il.us
www.dupagels.lib.il.us/pages/voices.html

Karen Odean, Director

Provides library service to persons who are unable to use standard printed material because of visual or physical disabilities. Part of the Illinois network of Talking Book Libraries. The service is free to those who are eligable. Provides books and magazines on audio-cassettes. Special playback equipment needed to use the books is also loaned. Braille books and magazines are also available. The collection includes popular books, classics and magazines.

Indiana

5279 **Allen County Public Library**

900 Webster Street
PO Box 2270
Fort Wayne, IN 46801 **260-421-1200**
FAX: 260-241-1386
e-mail: sfortriede@acpl.lib.in.us

Joyce Misner, Librarian

Summer reading programs, braille writer, magnifiers, closed-circuit TV, large-print photocopier, cassette books and magazines, children's books on cassette, home visits and other reference materials on blindness and other handicaps.

5280 **Bartholomew County Public Library**

5th at Lafayette
Columbus, IN 47201 **812-376-9253**
FAX: 812-379-1275

Wilma Perry, Librarian

Summer reading programs, braille writer, magnifiers, closed-circuit TV, large-print photocopier, cassette books and magazines, children's books on cassette, home visits and other reference materials on blindness and other handicaps.

5281 **Elkhart Public Library**
300 S Second Street
Elkhart, IN 46516 **574-522-2665**
FAX: 574-293-9213

Pat Ciancio, Librarian

Summer reading programs, braille writer, magnifiers, closed-circuit TV, large-print photocopier, cassette books and magazines, children's books on cassette, home visits and other reference materials on blindness and other handicaps.

5282 **Indiana Resource Center for Autism**
Indiana Institute on Disability and Community
2853 E 10th Street
Bloomington, IN 47408 **812-855-6508**
FAX: 812-855-9630
e-mail: prattc@indiana.edu
www.iidc.indiana.edu/irca

The Indiana Resource Center for Autism staff conduct outreach training and consultations, engage in research and develop and disseminate information focused on building the capicity of local communities, organizations, agencies and families to support children and adults across the autism spectrum in typical work, school, home and community settings. Please check our website for our complete list of publications.

5283 **Indiana University: Multipurpose Arthritis Center**
School of Medicine, Rheumatology Division
105 Jordan Hall
Bloomington, IN 47405 **812-855-8118**
FAX: 812-855-4436

Dr. Kenneth Brandt, Contact
Talmage Bosin, Director

Integral unit of the Division of Rheumatology, this department researches the causes and treatment of arthritis. Offers programs for health care providers and promotes cost-efficient care methods through community demonstration projects.

5284 **Lake County Public Library Talking Books Service**
1919 W 81st Avenue
Merrillville, IN 46410 **219-769-7800**
FAX: 219-769-0690
e-mail: tbooks@lakeco.lib.in.us

Renee Lewis

Large-print books, descriptive videos, braille writer, magnifiers, closed-circuit TV, large-print photocopier, cassette books and magazines, children's books on cassette, and other reference materials on blindness and other handicaps.

5285 **Northwest Indiana Subregional Library for Blind and Physically Handicapped**
1919 W 81st Avenue
Merrillville, IN 46410 **219-769-3541**
FAX: 219-769-0690

Renee Lewis

Summer reading programs, braille writer, magnifiers, closed-circuit TV, large-print photocopier, cassette books and magazines, children's books on cassette, home visits and other reference materials on blindness and other handicaps.

5286 **Special Services Division: Indiana State Library**
140 N Senate Avenue
Indianapolis, IN 46204 **317-232-3682**
800-622-4970
FAX: 317-232-3728
e-mail: lbph@statelib.lib.in.us
www.statelib.lib.in.us

Lissa Shanahan, Librarian

Circulates a collection of braille, recorded, and large print books and magazines and the special equipment needed to play the recorded materials to anyone in Indiana who cannot read regular print due to a visual or physical disability.

5287 **St. Joseph Hospital Rehabilitation Center**
700 Broadway
Fort Wayne, IN 46802 **260-425-3740**
FAX: 260-425-3741

Robert Archer RN LSW, Case Manager

Information offered on rehabilitation.

5288 **Talking Books Service Evansville Vanderburgh County Public Library**
22 SE Fifth Street
Evansville, IN 47708 **812-428-8235**
FAX: 812-428-8215
e-mail: tbs@evans.evcpl.lib.in.us

Barbara Shanks

Iowa

5289 **Iowa Department for the Blind Library**
524 4th Street
Des Moines, IA 50309 **515-281-1333**
FAX: 515-281-1378
e-mail: library@blind.state.ia.us
www.blind.state.ia.us

Karen Kenninger, Program Administrator

Summer reading programs, large print, disc, Braille and cassette books and magazines, descriptive videos and reference materials on blindness and other handicaps.

5290 **Library Commission for the Blind**
524 4th Street
Des Moines, IA 50309 **515-281-1333**
FAX: 515-281-1378
e-mail: library@blind.state.ia.us
www.blind.state.ia.us

Karen Kenninger, Program Administrator

Summer reading programs, Braille writer, magnifiers, closed-circuit TV, large print photocopier, cassette books and magazines, children's books on cassette and other reference materials on blindness and other handicaps.

5291 **University of Iowa Birth Defects and Genetic Disorders Unit**
2614 JCP
Iowa City, IA 52242 **319-335-9901**
FAX: 319-356-3347

Val Sheffield MD

Kansas

5292 **CKLS Headquarters**
1409 Williams
Great Bend, KS 67530 **620-792-2409**
FAX: 620-793-7270
e-mail: cenks@ink.org

Jerri Robinson, Librarian

Summer reading programs, braille writer, magnifiers, closed-circuit TV, large-print photocopier, cassette books and magazines, children's books on cassette, home visits and other reference materials on blindness and other handicaps.

5293 Center for the Improvement of Human Functioning

3100 N Hillside Avenue
Wichita, KS 67219 **316-682-3100**
FAX: 316-682-5054
e-mail: staff@brightspot.org

Hugh Riordan, President

Medical, research, and educational facility specializing in the treatment of chronic illness.

5294 Kansas State Library

ESU Memorial Union
1200 Commercial Street
Emporia, KS 66801
FAX: 620-343-7124
e-mail: ksst16lb@ink.org

2aroline Lang, Librarian

Summer reading programs, braille writer, magnifiers, closed-circuit TV, large-print photocopier, cassette books and magazines, children's books on cassette, home visits and other reference materials on blindness and other handicaps.

5295 Manhattan Public Library

629 Poyntz Avenue
Manhattan, KS 66502 **785-776-4741**
FAX: 785-776-1545
e-mail: annp@manhattan.lib.ks.us
www.manhattan.lib.ks.us

Ann Pearce, Librarian

Summer reading programs, Braille writer, magnifiers, closed-circuit TV, large-print photocopier, cassette books and magazines, children's books on cassette, home visits and other reference materials on blindness and other disabilities.

5296 Northwest Kansas Library System Talking Books

2 Washington Street
PO Box 446
Norton, KS 67654 **785-877-5148**
FAX: 785-877-5697
e-mail: tbook@ruraltel.net
www.skyways.lib.ks.us/kansas/KLS/talking/ksl_

Clarice Howard, Librarian

Offers books on disc and cassette. Library of Congress talking book and program for qualified individuals. Also offers descriptive videos to eligible persons.

5297 South Central Kansas Library System

Talking Bookz/SCKLS
901 N Main
Hutchinson, KS 67501 **620-663-5441**
800-234-0529
FAX: 620-663-1215
e-mail: ksocha@holsck.org
skyways.lib.ks.us/sckls

Karen Socha, Librarian

Summer reading programs, Braille writer, closed-circuit TV, large-print photocopier, cassette books and magazines, children's books on cassette, home visits and other reference materials on blindness and other handicaps.

5298 Topeka & Shawnee County Public Library Talking Book Service

1515 SW 10th Avenue
Topeka, KS 66604 **785-231-0574**
800-432-2925
FAX: 785-231-0579
e-mail: tbooks@tscpl.lib.ks.us
www.tscpl.org

Suzanne Bundy, Librarian

Summer reading programs, braille writer, magnifiers, closed-circuit TV, large-print photocopier, cassette books and magazines, children's books on cassette, home visits and other reference materials on blindness and other handicaps.

5299 Wichita Public Library

223 S Main
Wichita, KS 67202 **316-262-0611**
FAX: 316-262-4540

Brad Reha, Librarian

Summer reading programs, braille writer, magnifiers, closed-circuit TV, large-print photocopier, cassette books and magazines, children's books on cassette, home visits and other reference materials on blindness and other handicaps.

5300 Wichita Public Library/Talking Book Service

223 S Main Street
Wichita, KS 67202 **316-264-8308**
FAX: 316-262-4540

Brad Reha, Librarian

Furnish recorded reading material (books and magazines) for visually and physically challenged citizens.

Kentucky

5301 EnTech: Enabling Technologies of Kentuckiana

301 York Street
Louisville, KY 40203 **502-574-1637**
800-890-1840
FAX: 502-582-2448
e-mail: entech@iglou.com
kyblind.state.ky.us/personne.asp

Sherrill Williams, Program Director
Donna Jentes, Technology Specialist
April Kerr, Contact

Assistive technology resource and demonstration center, serving persons of all ages and disabilities in Western Kentucky and Southern Indiana. Services include: assistive technology information, demonstration, evaluation, training, technical support and short-term loan of equipment.

5302 Kentucky Library for the Blind and Physically Handicapped

300 Coffee Tree Road
PO Box 818
Frankfort, KY 40602 **502-564-8300**
800-372-2968
FAX: 502-564-5773
e-mail: ktbl.mail@kdlc.net
www.nfb.org/states/library.htm

Richard Feindel, Librarian

Braille book and magazines, large-print photocopier, cassette books and magazines, children's books on cassette, and other reference materials on blindness and other handicaps.

5303 **Louisville Free Public Library**
301 York Street
Louisville, KY 40203 **502-574-1625**
FAX: 502-574-1657
e-mail: denning@lfpf.org

Tom Denning, Coord, Special Adult Services

Summer reading programs, braille writer, magnifiers, closed-circuit TV, large-print photocopier, cassette books and magazines, children's books on cassette, home visits and other reference materials on blindness and other handicaps.

Louisiana

5304 **Central Louisiana State Hospital Medical and Professional Library**
PO Box 5031
Pineville, LA 71361 **318-484-6200**
FAX: 318-484-6284

Carol Benton McGee, Librarian

Information offered on psychiatry, psychology and mental health.

5305 **Louisiana State Library**
760 N Fouth Street
Baton Rouge, LA 70802 **225-342-4944**
800-543-4702
FAX: 225-342-6817
e-mail: sbph@pelican.state.lib.la.us

Elizabhet H Perkins, Regional Librarian
Leola H Walker, Library Manager

Summer reading programs, braille writer, magnifiers, closed-circuit TV, large-print photocopier, cassette books and magazines, children's books on cassette. Descriptive videoss and other reference materials on blindness and other handicaps.

5306 **Louisiana State Library: Section for the Blind and Physically Handicapped**
701 N 4th Street
Baton Rouge, LA 70802 **225-924-2484**
800-543-4702
FAX: 504-342-3547

Jennifer Anjier, Librarian

Summer reading programs, braille writer, magnifiers, closed-circuit TV, large-print photocopier, cassette books and magazines, children's books on cassette and other reference materials on blindness and other handicaps. Louisiana Hotlines - quarterly newsletter.

5307 **Louisiana State University Genetics Section of Pediatrics**
533 Bolivar Street
New Orleans, LA 70112 **504-568-6151**
FAX: 504-568-8500
www.medschool.lsuhsc.edu/genetics

TF Thurman MD, Director

Maine

5308 **Bangor Public Library**
145 Harlow Street
Bangor, ME 04401 **207-947-8336**
FAX: 207-945-6694
e-mail: bpill@bpl.lib.me.us
www.bpl.lib.me.us

Judith Leighton, Librarian

Summer reading programs, braille writer, magnifiers, closed-circuit TV, large-print photocopier, cassette books and magazines, children's books on cassette, home visits and other reference materials on blindness and other handicaps.

5309 **Cary Library**
107 Main Street
Houlton, ME 04730 **207-532-1302**
FAX: 207-532-4350

Norma Watson, Librarian

Summer reading programs, braille writer, magnifiers, closed-circuit TV, large-print photocopier, cassette books and magazines, children's books on cassette, home visits and other reference materials on blindness and other handicaps.

5310 **Lewiston Public Library**
200 Lisbon Street
Lewiston, ME 04240 **207-784-0135**
FAX: 207-784-3011
e-mail: lplweb@lplonline.org

Muriel Landry, Librarian

Summer reading programs, braille writer, magnifiers, closed-circuit T.V., large-print photocopier, cassette books and magazines, children's books on cassette, home visits and other reference materials on blindness and other handicaps.

5311 **Maine State Library**
64 State House Station
Augusta, ME 04333 **207-287-5650**
FAX: 207-287-5624
e-mail: benitad@ursus3.ursus.maine.edu

Benita Davis, Cooridinator Special Services

Summer reading programs, cassette books and magazines, children's books on cassette, home visits and other reference materials on blindness and other handicaps.

Newsl./BiAnnual

5312 **New England Regional Genetics Group**
PO Box 682
Gorham, ME 04038 **207-839-5324**
FAX: 207-839-8637

Ms. A Merrill Henderson, Coordinator

Human genetic services and educational planning pertaining to birth defects.

5313 **Portland Public Library**
5 Monument Square
Portland, ME 04101 **207-871-1700**
FAX: 207-871-1703
www.portlandlibrary.com

Sheldon Kaye, Librarian

Summer reading programs, braille writer, magnifiers, closed-circuit T.V., large-print photocopier, cassette books and magazines, children's books on cassette, home visits and other reference materials on blindness and other handicaps.

5314 Waterville Public Library

73 Elm Street
Waterville, ME 04901 **207-873-4779**
FAX: 207-873-4779

Meta Vigue, Librarian

Summer reading programs, braille writer, magnifiers, closed-circuit T.V., large-print photocopier, cassette books and magazines, children's books on cassette, home visits and other reference materials on blindness and other handicaps.

Maryland

5315 Friends of Libraries for Deaf Action

2930 Craiglawn Road
Silver Spring, MD 20904
FAX: 301-572-4134
TTY:301-572-5168
e-mail: folda86@aol.com
www.folda.net

Alice L Hagemeyer, Founder

FOLDA is a public service of Library for Deaf Action. FOLDA has no membership dues. FOLDA encourages the deaf community to become involved in activities of their local public library and its friends. Some public libraries have FOLDA's copy of THE RED NOTEBOOK, an information service in the form of a regularly updated loose-leaf binder containing deaf fact sheets, library reprints and announcements. Check website to keep up with library access for the public on hearing loss and deaf culture.

5316 Johns Hopkins University Dana Center for Preventive Ophthalmology

Wilmer Ophthalmology Institute
600 N Wolfe Street, Wilmer 120
Baltimore, MD 21287 **410-955-2436**
FAX: 410-955-2542
e-mail: hquigley@jhmi.edu

Harry A Quigley, Director

5317 Johns Hopkins University: Asthma and Allergy Center

5501 Hopkins Bayview Circle
Baltimore, MD 21224 **410-550-2101**
FAX: 410-550-2090

Dr. Lawrence Lichtenstein, Director

Studies of allergic diseases and individuals with allergic disease, pulmonary diseases and diseases involving inflammation and immunological processes.

5318 Maryland State Library for the Blind and Physically Handicapped

415 Park Avenue
Baltimore, MD 21201
800-964-9209
FAX: 410-333-2095
TTY:800-934-2541

Gillian Lewis, Librarian

Summer reading programs, cassette books and magazines, children's books on cassette, and other reference materials on blindness and other handicaps.

5319 Montgomery County Department of Public Libraries/Special Needs Library

6400 Democracy Boulevard
Bethesda, MD 20817 **240-777-0960**
TTY:301-897-2217

Charlette Stinnett, Head Librarian
Susan F Cohen, Assistant Head Librarian
Charlette Stinnett, Agency Manager

Serves the library information and reading needs of people with disabilities, family members, students and service providers. Some of its services include books, periodicals, and videos on disability issues, adaptive technology, community information; the National Library for the Blind and Physically Handicapped Talking Book program; large print books; and computer room with adaptive technology.

5320 National Epilepsy Library (NEL)

Epilepsy Foundation
4351 Garden City Drive
Landover, MD 20785 **301-457-3700**
800-332-4050
FAX: 301-577-4941
e-mail: postmaster@efa.org
www.epilpsyfoundation.org

Cecille Jech, Manager, NEL Library

Contains information about epilepsy and seizure disorders and serves physicians and other health professionals. Provides in-house bibliographic database (ESDI), searches and documents delivery and interlibrary loans. Maintains the Albert and Ellen Grass Archives.

5321 National Rehabilitation Information Center (NARIC)

1010 Wayne Avenue
Suite 800
Silver Spring, MD 20910 **301-562-2400**
800-346-2742
FAX: 301-562-2401
TTY:301-495-5626
e-mail: naricinfo@kra.com
www.naric.com

A national disability and rehabilitation library and information center that collects and disseminates the results of NIDRR-funded research projects. The collection, which also includes commercially published books, journals, articles and audiovisuals, grows at a rate of 300 documents a month. NARIC currently has more than 50,000 documents on all aspects of disability and rehabilitation. Searchable web page includes 5 databases and a calendar of events.

5322 Social Security Library

US Social Security Administration
PO Box 17330
Baltimore, MD 21235
800-772-1213
www.ssa.gov

Leo Hollenbeack, Reference Librarian

Information on social security and disability insurance.

5323 Warren Grant Magnuson Clinical Center

Building 10-Room 1C255
9000 Rockville Pike
Bethesda, MD 20892 **301-496-2563**
FAX: 301-402-0664
www.cc.nih.gov

Established in 1953 as the research hospital of the National Institutes of Health. Designed so that patient care facilities are close to research laboratories so new findings of basic and clinical scientists can be quickly applied to the treatment of patients. Upon referral by physicians, patients are admitted to NIH clinical studies.

Massachusetts

5324 **Boston University Arthritis Center**

715 Albany Street
4th Floor
Boston, MA 02118 **617-638-7083**
FAX: 617-638-7032

Aubrey Milunsky, Director

5325 **Boston University Center for Human Genetics**

715 Albany Street
4th Floor
Boston, MA 02118 **617-638-7083**
FAX: 617-638-7092

Aubrey Milunsky MD, Director

Offers research into genetic disorders and growth disorders.

5326 **Boston University Robert Dawson Evans Memorial Dept. of Clinical Research**

75 E Newton Street
Boston, MA 02118 **617-638-7250**
FAX: 617-638-8728

Dr. Joseph Loscalzo, Director

Integral unit of the University Hospital specializing in arthritis and connective tissue studies.

5327 **Braille and Talking Book Library, Perkins School for the Blind**

175 N Beacon Street
Watertown, MA 02472 **617-972-7240**
800-852-3133
FAX: 617-972-7363
e-mail: library@perkins.org
www.perkins.org

Kim Charlson, Director

Provides free books on tape and Braille to persons who cannot read printed material because of a physical disability such as blindness, visual impairment, physical impairment or learning disability. Serves Massachusetts. For Braille, also serves New Hampshire, Rhode Island, Maine and Vermont.

5328 **Brigham and Women's Hospital: Asthma and Allergic Disease Research Center**

75 Francis Street
Boston, MA 02115 **617-732-8201**
FAX: 617-730-2858
e-mail: arc@partners.org

K Frank Austen MD, Director

Integral unit of the hospital focusing research attention on asthma and allergy related disorders.

5329 **Brigham and Women's Hospital: Robert B Brigham Multipurpose Arthritis Center**

75 Francis Street
Boston, MA 02115 **617-732-5500**
FAX: 617-432-0979

Dr. Matthew Liang, Director

Research studies into arthritis and rheumatic diseases.

5330 **Caption Center**

Media Access Group at WGBH
125 Western Avenue
Boston, MA 02134 **617-300-3600**
FAX: 617-300-1020
e-mail: caption@wgbh.org
www.wgbh.org/caption

Lori Kay, Director

Has been pioneering and delivering accessible media to disabled adults, students and their families, teachers and friends for over 30 years. Each year, the Center captions more than 10,000 hours worth of broadcast and cable programs, feature films, large-format and IMAX films, home videos, music videos, DVDs, teleconferences and CD-Roms.

1972

5331 **Center for Interdisciplinary Research on Immunologic Diseases**

Children's Hospital Medical Center
300 Longwood Avenue
Boston, MA 02115 **617-355-6524**
FAX: 617-730-0449
e-mail: sundel@al.tch.harvard.edu
www,tch.harvard.edu

Fred S Rosen MD, Prin. Investigator

Organizational research unit of the Children's Hospital that focuses on the causes, prevention and treatments of asthma, infections and allergies.

5332 **Harvard University Howe Laboratory of Ophthalmology**

Massachusetts Eye & Ear Infirmary
243 Charles Street
Boston, MA 02114 **617-573-5520**
FAX: 617-573-3444

Development ophthalmology and eye research.

5333 **Laboure College Library**

2120 Dorchester Avenue
Boston, MA 02124 **617-296-8300**
FAX: 617-296-7947
e-mail: admit@labourecollege.org
www.laboure.edu

Linda Brierley, Director

Offers information on physical disabilities, independent living, peer counseling and advocacy.

5334 **Massachusetts Rehabilitation Commission Library**

27-43 Wormwood Street
Boston, MA 02210 **617-727-2172**
FAX: 617-727-1354
TTY:617-727-9063

Elmer C Bartels, Commissioner

Library and information science, rehabilitation and the handicapped.

5335 **Schepens Eye Research Institute**

20 Staniford Street
Boston, MA 02114 **617-912-0100**
FAX: 617-912-0110
e-mail: geninfo@@vision.eri.harvard.edu
www.eri.harvard.edu/default/htm

J Wayne Streilein MD, President

Prominent center for research on eye, vision, and blinding diseases; dedicated to research that improves the understanding, management, and prevention of eye diseases and visual deficiencies; fosters collaboration among its faculty members; trains young scientists and clinicians from around the world; promotes communication with scientists in allied fields; leader in the worldwide dispersion of basic scientific knowledge of vision.

5336 **Talking Book Library at Worcester Public Library**

3 Salem Square
Worcester, MA 01608 **508-799-1730**
800-762-0085
FAX: 508-799-1676
e-mail: talkbook@cwmars.org

James L Izatt, Librarian
Barbara Figurski, Librarian

Summer reading programs, adapted computers, Braille writer, magnifiers, closed-circuit TV, large print books, cassette books and magazines, children's books on cassette, reference materials on blindness and other disabilities.

Michigan

5337 **Artificial Language Laboratory**

405 Computer Center
Michigan State University
E Lansing, MI 48824 **517-353-5399**
FAX: 517-353-4766
e-mail: artlang@msu.edu
www.msu.edu/~artlang

Dr. John Eulenberg, Director
Katie Smith, Manager

Multidisciplinary research center in the Audiology & Speech Science department, Michigan State University. Its basic research program includes speech analysis and synthesis. Applied research is carried out on computer-based systems for persons who are blind and for persons with cerebral palsy and head injury. The laboratory develops physical, cognitive and linguistic assessment technology.

5338 **Burger School for the Autistic**

30922 Beechwood Street
Garden City, MI 48135 **734-762-8420**
FAX: 734-762-8533
www.resa.net

Mary O'Niell, Director Secondary Unit
Barbara Masten, Director Intermediate Unit
Judy Gapp, Director Childrens Unit

Burger school for students with autism is the largest public school in the United States that specializes in the education of students with autism.

5339 **Glaucoma Laser Trabeculoplasty Study**

Sinai Hospital of Detroit
29275 Northwestern Highway
Southfield, MI 48034 **248-493-5157**

Hugh Beckman, Chairman

Examines the effectiveness and safety of the treatments of glaucoma.

5340 **Grand Traverse Area Library for the Blind and Physically Handicapped**

1610 Woodmere
Traverse City, MI 49684 **231-932-8558**
FAX: 800-932-8578
TTY:616-922-0901

Evelyn Welty

5341 **Kent District Library for the Blind and Physically Handicapped**

775 Ball Avenue NE
Grand Rapids, MI 49503
FAX: 616-774-3250
e-mail: kdlsc@lakeland.lib.mi.us
www.kentlibrary.lib.mi.us

Claudya Muller, Director

Summer reading programs, braille writer, magnifiers, large-print photocopier, cassette books and magazines, children's books on cassette, and other reference materials on blindness and other handicaps.

5342 **Library of Michigan Service for the Blind**

PO Box 30007
Lansing, MI 48909 **517-373-5614**
FAX: 517-373-5865
e-mail: info@sbph.libomich.lib.mi.us

Maggie Bacon, Manager

Braille writer, magnifiers, closed-circuit T.V., large-print photocopier, cassette books and magazines, children's books on cassette, and other reference materials on blindness and other handicaps.

5343 **Macomb Library for the Blind and Physically Handicapped**

16480 Hall Road
Clinton Township, MI 48038 **586-286-1580**
FAX: 586-286-0634
e-mail: macbld@libcoop.net
www.macomb.lib.mi.us/macspe

Beverlee Babcock, Librarian

Summer reading programs, braille writer, closed-circuit T.V., large-print books, cassette books and magazines, children's books on cassette, home visits and other reference materials on blindness and other handicaps, descriptive videos and bifokal kits.

5344 **Michigan Capital Medical Center John W Chi Memorial Medical Library**

2727 S Pennsylvania Avenue
Lansing, MI 48910 **517-377-8332**
FAX: 517-334-2939

Judith Barnes, Information Resources Coord.

Extensive consumer health and patient education collection in books, videotapes, pamphlets. Open to the public.

5345 **Michigan's Assistive Technology Resource**

1023 S US 27
St Johns, MI 48879 **989-224-0333**
800-274-7426
FAX: 989-224-0330
e-mail: matr@match.org
www.matr.org

Maryann Jones, Coordinator
Jeff Diedrich, Director

Michigan's Assistive Technology Resource (MATR) is a comprehensive support center located in St Johns, Michigan. The overall purpose of MATR is to provide information services, support materials, technical assistance and training to local and intermediate school districts in Michigan to increase their capacity to address the needs of students with disabilities for assistive technology.

5346 **Mideastern Michigan Library Co-op**
G-4195 W Pasadena Avenue
Flint, MI 48504 **810-232-7119**
FAX: 810-732-1715
e-mail: cnash@genesse.freeret.org
www.falcon.edu/libraries

Carolyn Nash, Librarian

Summer reading programs, braille writer, magnifiers, closed-circuit T.V., large-print photocopier, cassette books and magazines, children's books on cassette, home visits and other reference materials on blindness and other handicaps.

5347 **Muskegon County Library for the Blind**
97 E Apple Avenue
Muskegon, MI 49442 **231-724-6257**
FAX: 231-724-6675
e-mail: mclsm@llcoop.org
www.lakeland.lib.mi.us

Sheila Miller, Librarian

Braille typewriter, magnifiers, closed-circuit TV, large-print photocopier, cassette books and magazines, children's books on cassette, home visits and other reference materials on blindness and other handicaps, The Reading Edge, and large print books.

5348 **Northland Library Cooperative**
316 E Chisholm
Alpena, MI 49707 **989-356-1622**
FAX: 989-354-3939
e-mail: nlclbph@northland.lib.mi.us

Bryon Sitler, Director

Summer reading programs, Braille writer, magnifiers, closed-circuit TV, large-print photocopier, cassette books and magazines, children's books on cassette and other reference materials on blindness and other handicaps.

5349 **Oakland County Library for the Blind and Physically Handicapped**
1200 N Telegraph Dept 482
Pontiac, MI 48341 **248-858-5050**
800-774-4542
FAX: 248-858-9313
e-mail: oakllbph@oakland.lib.mi.us
www.co.oakland.mi.us/lvpi

David Conklin, Librarian

5350 **St. Clair County Library Special Technologies Alternative Resources (S.T.A.R.)**
210 McMorran Boulevard
Port Huron, MI 48060 **810-987-3600**
800-272-8570
FAX: 810-987-6768
e-mail: star@sccl.lib.mi.us
www.sccl.lib.mi.us/star.html

Mary Jo Koch, Subregional Librarian

Offers library services to the blind, deaf and blind, visually disabled, phsyically disabled, and reading disabled.

5351 **University of Michigan: Orthopaedic Research Laboratories**
400 N Ingalls Building
Ann Arbor, MI 48109 **734-763-6784**
FAX: 734-747-0003

Dr. SA Goldstein, Director

Develops and studies the causes and treatments for arthritis including new devices and assistive aids.

5352 **Upper Peninsula Library for the Blind**
1615 Presque Isle Avenue
Marquette, MI 49855 **906-228-7697**
800-562-8985
FAX: 906-228-5627
e-mail: rruff@uproc.lib.mi.us

Ruth Ruff, Librarian

Summer reading programs, braille writer, magnifiers, closed-circuit T.V., large-print photocopier, cassette books and magazines, children's books on cassette, home visits and other reference materials on blindness and other handicaps.

5353 **Washtenaw County Library for the Blind & Physically Handicapped**
4133 Washtenaw Avenue
Ann Arbor, MI 48108 **734-971-6059**
FAX: 734-971-3892
www.ewashtenaw.org/government/departments/lib

Mary Udoji, Director

Michigan Subregional Library, Library of Congress National Library Service network. General library service for persons unable to use standard print materials for various physical reasons. Lends audio books and listening equipment, large type books, descriptive videos. Provides reference information and programs. Kurzweil scanner with components which convert standard print to Braille, large type or audio and closed circuit TV magnifier on site.

5354 **Wayne County Regional Library for the Blind**
30555 Michigian Avenue
Westland, MI 48186 **734-727-7300**
888-968-2737
FAX: 734-727-7333
TTY:313-326-3008
e-mail: wcrlbph@wayneregional.lib.mi.us
wayneregional.lib.mi.us

Frederick R Howkins, Director

Summer reading programs, braille writer, magnifiers, closed-circuit T.V., large-print photocopier, cassette books and magazines, children's books on cassette, and other reference materials on blindness and other handicaps.

5355 **Wayne State University: CS Mott Center for Human Genetics and Development**
275 E Hancock Street
Detroit, MI 48201 **313-577-4603**
FAX: 313-577-8554

Dr. Ernest Abel, Director

Human growth and development disorders.

Minnesota

5356 **Century College**
3300 Century Avenue N
White Bear Lake, MN 55110 **651-779-3300**
800-228-1978
FAX: 651-779-5779
www.centurycollege.net

Ed Haddon, Faculty
Jill Gebhardt, Public Relations

Programs of study - Orthotic Practitioner, Orthotic Technician, Prosethetic Practitioner, Prosthetic Technician. In addition, Century College offers more than 50 other programs in liberal arts, career and occupational programs.

5357 **Communication Center/Minnesota State Services for the Blind**

2200 University Avenue W
Suite 240
St Paul, MN 55114
651-642-0500
800-652-9000
FAX: 651-649-5927
e-mail: chamilto@ssb.state.mn.us

Chuk Hamilton, Director

Special library service for the blind and physically handicapped providing tape and Braille transcription of textbooks and vocational materials; Minnesota Radio Talking Book providing current newspaper, magazines and best selling books; Dial-in-News, a touch tone phone accessed newspaper service; Library of Congress cassette and phonograph talking book equipment; repair services for special audio reading equipment, with most services free to Minnesota Residents.

5358 **Duluth Public Library**

520 W Superior Street
Duluth, MN 55802
218-723-3800
FAX: 218-723-3822
www.duluth.lib.mn.us/

Randall Vogt, Coordinator

Adapted access to Apple computer, adapted toys and adapted library equipment.

5359 **Minnesota Library for the Blind and Physically Handicapped**

Highway 298
PO Box 68
Faribault, MN 55021
800-722-0550
FAX: 507-333-4832
e-mail: libblnd@sate.mn.us

Nancy Walton, Program Director
Rene Perrance, Librarian

Provides books and magazines in Braille, large print, records, and cassettes to qualified residents of Minnesota who have a visual or physical impairment, including reading disabilities due to an organic cause certified by a Medical Doctor, that prevents residents from reading standard print or physically handling a book. Equipment for in-house use include magnifiers, braillers, listening equipment, and CCTV. Reference collection for in-house use only on visual impairment topics.

5360 **Special U**

University of Minnesota
Box 721-UMHC
Minneapolis, MN 55455
612-626-3087
800-276-8642
FAX: 612-624-0997
e-mail: kdwb-var@umn.edu
www.peds.umn.edu/peds-adol/

Brings together comprehensive sources of information related to youth with chronic or disabling conditions and their families. Topics include psychosocial issues, disability awareness, developmental processes, family, sexuality, education, employment, independent living, cultural issues, gender issues, service delivery, professional issues, advocacy and legal issues, and health issues. Special focus on transition from childhood to adolesecence to adulthood.

Mississippi

5361 **Mississippi Library Commission**

5455 Executive Plaza
Jackson, MS 39206
601-354-7208
FAX: 601-354-6077
TTY:601-354-6411
e-mail: tbbs@mls.lib.ms.us
www.mlc.lib.ms.us

Rahya Puckett, Librarian

Summer reading programs, braille writer, magnifiers, closed-circuit T.V., large-print photocopier, cassette books and magazines, children's books on cassette, home visits and other reference materials on blindness and other handicaps.

5362 **Mississippi Library Commission\Talking Book and Braille Services**

5455 Executive Plaza
Jackson, MS 39206
601-366-5112
800-446-0892
FAX: 601-731-3405
e-mail: tbbs@mlc.lib.ms.us
www.mlc.lib.ms.us

Rahye Puckett, Coordinator

Library service for the print handicapped braille, cassette and disc materials (books & periodicals) for children and adults. Large print RG production (copier & printer), braille embosser and other handicaps.

Missouri

5363 **Assemblies of God National Center for the Blind - Adriene Resource Center for Blind Children**

Whitney Library for the Blind
1445 Boonville Avenue
Springfield, MO 65802
417-862-2781
FAX: 417-862-5120
e-mail: blind@ag.org
www.blind.ag.org

Paul Weingartner, National Director

Offers Braille and cassette lending library, Braille and cassette Sunday School materials for all ages, Braille and cassette periodicals, resource assistance, and resources for blind children and children of blind parents.

5364 **Church of the Nazarene**

Nazarene Publishing House
2923 Troost Avenue
Kansas City, MO 64141
816-931-1900
FAX: 816-531-0923
www.nazarene.org

Offers braille and large print books. Also offers a lending library and cassettes for the blind.

5365 **Judevine Center for Autism**

1101 Olivette Executive P
St. Louis, MO 63132
314-432-6200
FAX: 314-432-8894
e-mail: judevine@judevine.org
www.judevine.org

Lois Blackwell, Director

Evaluations and Assessments, Parent and Professional Training Programs, Consultations, Workshops, Seminars, Family Support, Clinical Therapies, Adult Programs and Support, Residential Services.

5366 **Lutheran Library for the Blind**

Lutheran Church: Missouri Synod
1333 S Kirkwood Road
Saint Louis, MO 63122
314-965-9000
800-433-3954
FAX: 314-965-0959
e-mail: ic_borchele@icms.org
www.blindmission.org

Lynne Borchelt, Administrative Assistant

Offers Christian books in braille and large print books and cassettes for the blind and visually impaired, on loan, as well as Christian periodicals in braille, large print and cassette tape.

5367 **University of Missouri: Columbia Arthritis Center**

MA427 Health Sciences Center
1 Hospital Drive
Columbia, MO 65212
573-882-8738
FAX: 573-884-3996

Gordon C Sharp MD, Director

Research into arthritis and rheumatic diseases.

5368 **Wolfner Library for the Blind**

PO Box 387
Jefferson City, MO 65102
573-751-8720
800-392-2614
FAX: 573-526-2985
TTY:800-347-1379
e-mail: wolfner@mailsos.state.mo.us

Sara Parker, State Librarian

Free library service in alternate formats, braille, recorded, large print. For any Missouri resident who cannot read standard print, due to a physical disability. Summer reading programs, braille writer, magnifiers, closed-circuit T.V., large-print photocopier, cassette books and magazines, children's books on cassette, home visits and other reference materials on blindness and other handicaps.

Montana

5369 **MonTECH University of Montanta**

Rural Institute on Disabilities
634 Eddy Avenue
Missoula, MT 59812
406-243-5676
800-732-0323
FAX: 406-243-4730
TTY:406-243-5676
e-mail: montech@selway.umt.edu
http://ruralinstitute.umt.edu/HDC/montech.htm

Gail McGregor, Project Director

Develops a comprehensive statewide system of technology-related assistance to ensure that all Montanans with disabilites have equitable access to the assistive technology devices and services they need.

5370 **Montana State Library**

1515 E Sixth Avenue
PO Box 201800
Helena, MT 59620
406-444-2064
800-332-3400
FAX: 406-444-0266
TTY:406-444-5431
e-mail: cbriggs@msl.state.mt.us
www.msl.state.mt.us/tbl

Christie Briggs, Supervisor

Over 50,000 titles on 4-track cassette, WebBraille, Web0pac, WebBlud, summer reading programs, braille writer, magnifiers, closed-circuit T.V., large-print photocopier, cassette books and magazines, children's books on cassette, home visits and other reference materials on blindness and other handicaps. Large print and Braille services to blind, low vision, physically handicapped and reading disabled citizens of Montana.

5371 **Montana State Library\Talking Book Library**

1515 E 6th Avenue
Helena, MT 59601
406-444-3115
800-332-3400
www.msl.state.mt.us

Sandra Jarbie, Librarian

Summer reading programs, braille writer, magnifiers, large-print photocopier, cassette books and magazines, children's books on cassette, and other reference materials on blindness and other handicaps.

Nebraska

5372 **Martin Luther Home Society Resource Center**

804 J Street
Suite 305
Lincoln, NE 68508
800-443-4899
FAX: 402-434-3253
e-mail: mlhs_MEINTS@compuserve.com
www.mlhs.com

Alice Meints, Resource Center Director
Fred Naumann III, Communications Dir.

Provides materials and opportunities for consultation with individuals and communities assisting persons with special needs.

5373 **Nebraska Assistive Technology Partnership - Nebraska Department of Education**

5143 S 48th Street
Suite C
Lincoln, NE 68516
402-471-0734
888-806-6287
FAX: 402-471-6052
TTY:402-471-0735
e-mail: atp@atp.state.ne.us
www.nde.state.ne.us/ATP/

Mark Schultz, Project Director
Nancy Noha, Public Contact

Provides statewide assistive technology and home modification services for Nebraskans of all ages and disabilities.

5374 **Nebraska Library Commission: Talking Book and Braille Service**

Talking Book and Braille Service
1200 N Street
Suite 120
Lincoln, NE 68508
800-742-7691
FAX: 402-471-6244
e-mail: readadv@nlc.state.ne.us
www.nlc.state.ne.us/tbbs/tbbs1.html

Dave Oertli, Program Director

Summer reading programs, braille writer, magnifiers, closed-circuit T.V., large-print photocopier, cassette books and magazines, children's books on cassette, home visits and other reference materials on blindness and other handicaps.

Nevada

5375 **Las Vegas-Clark County Library District**

1401 E Flamingo Road
Las Vegas, NV 89119 **702-382-3493**
FAX: 702-733-1567

Mary Anne Morton, Librarian

Summer reading programs, braille writer, magnifiers, closed-circuit T.V., large-print photocopier, cassette books and magazines, children's books on cassette, home visits and other reference materials on blindness and other handicaps.

5376 **Nevada State Library and Archives**

Capitol Complex
Carson City, NV 89710 **775-687-5469**
FAX: 775-687-8311
TTY:702-687-8338
e-mail: putnam@equinox.unr.edu

Kevin E Putnam, Librarian

Summer reading programs, braille writer, magnifiers, closed-circuit T.V., large-print photocopier, cassette books and magazines, children's books on cassette, home visits and other reference materials on blindness and other handicaps.

New Hampshire

5377 **New Hampshire State Library: Library Services to Persons with Disabilities**

117 Pleasant Street
Concord, NH 03301 **603-271-3429**
FAX: 603-271-8370
e-mail: gilbreth@library.state.nh.us
www.state.nh.us/nhsl/talkbks/index.html

Donna Gilbreth, Librarian

Regional Library for National Library Service for the Blind & Physically Handicapped offers cassette books and magazines, children's books on cassette, home visits, descriptive videos, large print books, and other reference materials on blindness and other handicaps.

New Jersey

5378 **Children's Specialized Hospital Medical Library - Parent Resource Center**

150 New Providence Road
Mountainside, NJ 07092 **908-233-3720**
FAX: 908-301-5576

Contains some 3,000 books, and journals specializing in nursing, pediatrics, child neurology, and rehabilitation. Also provides a Parent Resource Center, a special collection of books, videos and pamphlets designed to meet the information needs of parents and families, as well as the local community.

5379 **Christopher & Dana Reeve Paralysis Resource Center**

636 Morris Tunrpike
Suite 3A
Short Hills, NJ 07078 **973-467-8270**
800-539-7309
FAX: 973-467-9845
e-mail: prc@crpf.org
www.paralysis.org

Sheila Fitzgibbon, Librarian
Linda LoCasale, Director Operations
Joseph Canose, Director

A national clearinghouse for information, referral and educational materials on paralysis.

5380 **Eye Institute of New Jersey**

New Jersey Medical School
90 Bergen Street
Newark, NJ 07103 **973-972-2036**
FAX: 973-972-2068
community.nj.com/cc/eyeinstituteofnewjersey

Marshall S Klein, Director

Ophthamology, including research into cornea, retina and neuro-ophthamalogy.

5381 **Mycoclonus Research Foundation**

200 Old Palisade Road
Suite 17D
Fort Lee, NJ 07024 **201-585-0770**
FAX: 201-585-0770

Supports clinical and basic research into the cause and treatment of myoclonus; four international workshops facilitated the sharing of information by physicians, scientists, and investigators active in the field, resulted in three publications; supports promising research projects, clinical neurological fellows, with special emphasis on posthypoxic myoclonus and encourages all who are interested in futhering the understanding, treatment, and cure of myoclonus.

5382 **New Jersey Center for Outreach and Services for the Autism Community (COSAC)**

1450 Parkside Avenue
Suite 22
Ewing, NJ 08638 **609-883-8100**
800-428-8476
FAX: 609-883-5509
e-mail: information@njcosac.org
www.njcosac.org

Paul A Potito, Executive Director

Purpose is to assist families, individuals and agencies concerned with the welfare and education of children and adults with autism and other pervasive development disorders.

5383 **New Jersey Library for the Blind and Handicapped**

2300 Stuyvesant Avenue
PO Box 501
Trenton, NJ 08625 **609-530-4000**
800-792-8322
FAX: 609-530-6384
TTY:877-882-5593
e-mail: njlbh@njstatelib.org
www2.njstatelib.org/lbh/index.htm

Deborah Toomey, Director
Luz Sanchez, Hispanic Services
Karen Messick, Children's Services

Summer reading programs, braille writer, magnifiers, closed-circuit T.V., large-print, cassette, braille books and magazines, children's books on cassette, and other reference materials on blindness and other handicaps. Provides reading material on audio, cassette, large print and Braille to eligible NJ residents.

New Mexico

5384 New Mexico State Library for the Blind and Physically Handicapped

325 Don Gaspar Avenue
Santa Fe, NM 87501 **505-954-8539**
800-866-2253
FAX: 505-827-3888
TTY:800-659-4915
e-mail: jbrewstr@stlib.state.nm.us
www.stlib.state.nm.us

Glee Wenzel, Librarian

Summer reading programs, braille writer, magnifiers, closed-circuit T.V., large-print photocopier, cassette books and magazines, children's books on cassette, home visits and other reference materials on blindness and other handicaps.

New York

5385 Braille Book Bank

National Braille Association
3 Townline Circle
Rochester, NY 14623 **585-427-8260**
FAX: 585-427-0263
e-mail: nbaoffice@compuserve.com
www.nationalbraille.org

Contains over 1800 Braille titles and Braille music scores. Copies produced on demand and sold below cost. Catalog available on request.

5386 Center on Human Policy

Syracuse University
805 S Crouse Avenue
Syracuse, NY 13244 **315-443-3851**
800-894-0826
FAX: 315-443-4338
e-mail: thechp@sued.syr.edu
thechp.syr.edu

Steve Taylor, Director
Rachael Zubal-Ruggieri, Information Coordinator

The Center on Human Policy is a Syracuse University-based policy, research and advocacy organization involved in the national movement to ensure the rights of people with disabilities.

5387 DREAMMS for Kids

273 Ringwood Road
Freeville, NY 13068 **607-539-3027**
FAX: 607-539-9930

An educational technology and parent service agency, founded in 1988 by parents of a Down Syndrome child. DREAMMS is committed to increasing the use of computers, assistive technologies, and quality instructional technology for special needs students in school and homes throughout the country.

5388 Eastern Paralyzed Veterans Association

75-20 Astoria Boulevard
Flushing, NY 11370 **718-397-4181**
800-444-0120
FAX: 718-803-0414
e-mail: info@epva.org
www.epva.org

Angela Wu, Library Director

Library offering information on physical disabilities, spinal cord injury and rehabilitation. Also provides literature searches on specific topics. Association news and free publications on architecture and barrier-free designs, legislation and other current events affecting Americans with Disabilities.

5389 Ehrman Medical Library

New York University Medical Center
550 1st Avenue
New York, NY 10016 **212-263-5372**
FAX: 212-263-6534

Barbara Schiffer, Librarian

Statistics, reports and evaluation.

5390 Foundation Center

79 Fifth Avenue
Department ZE
New York, NY 10003 **212-620-4230**
800-424-9836
FAX: 212-691-1828
www.fdncenter.org

Thomas Buckman, President

The Center disseminates current information on foundation and corporate giving through our national collections in New York City and Washington D.C., our field offices in San Francisco and our network of over 180 cooperating libraries in all 50 states and abroad.

5391 Helen Keller National Center

111 Middle Neck Road
Sands Point, NY 11050 **516-944-8900**
800-225-0411
FAX: 516-944-7302
e-mail: hkncdir@aol.com
www.helenkeller.org/national

Joseph McNulty, Executive Director

Provides evaluation and training in vocational skills, adaptive technology and computer skills, orientation and mobility, independent living, communication, speech-language skills, creative arts, fitness and leisure activities.

5392 Helen Keller Worldwide

90 Washington Street
New York, NY 10006 **212-766-5266**
FAX: 212-532-5860

John M Palmer, Executive Director

Nonprofit organization for the blind.

5393 Institute for Basic Research in Developmental Disabilities

1050 Forest Hill Road
Staten Island, NY 10314 **718-494-0600**
FAX: 718-494-0837

Conducts research into neurodegenerative diseases, Alzheimer's disease, developmental disabilities, fragile X syndrome, Down's Syndrome, autism, epilepsy and basic science issues underlying all developmental disabilities.

5394 Institute for Visual Sciences

1 E 71st Street
New York, NY 10021 **212-249-1140**

Francis L'Esperance, Chairman

Ophthalmology with emphasis on the development of care for the eye.

5395 **JGB Cassette Library International**

15 W 65th Street
New York, NY 10023 **212-769-6331**
FAX: 212-769-6266
e-mail: bemass@aol.com

Bruce Massis

Summer reading programs, braille writer, magnifiers, closed-circuit T.V., large-print photocopier, cassette books and magazines, children's books on cassette, home visits and other reference materials on blindness and other handicaps.

5396 **Monroe Developmental Center**

620 Westfall Road
Rochester, NY 14620 **585-461-8970**
FAX: 585-473-1963
e-mail: folwelbe@nysomr.emi.com

Steve Jarose, Staff Development

Information on mental retardation and developmental disabilities.

5397 **Nassau Library System**

900 Jerusalem Avenue
Uniondale, NY 11553 **516-292-8920**
FAX: 516-481-4777
e-mail: nls@lilrc.org

Dorothy Pruyear, Librarian

Summer reading programs, braille writer, magnifiers, closed-circuit T.V., large-print photocopier, cassette books and magazines, children's books on cassette, home visits and other reference materials on blindness and other handicaps.

5398 **New York Public Library: Andrew Heiskell Library for the Blind and Physically Handicapped**

40 W 20th Street
New York, NY 10011 **212-206-5400**
FAX: 212-206-5418
TTY:212-206-5458
e-mail: ablgph@nypl.org
www.nypl.org/branch/lb/

Kathleen Rowan, Reglional Librarian

By mail and on-site offers talking books and braille books to eligible patrons in New York City and Long Island. Additional on-site services include large-print books, books on tape, descriptive videos, class visits, programs, and assistive devices such as closed circuit televisions and Karzweil Personal Readers

5399 **New York State Talking Book & Braille Library**

Empire State Plaza CEC
Albany, NY 12230 **518-474-5935**
FAX: 518-474-5786
TTY:518-474-7121
e-mail: tbbl@mail.nysed.gov
www.suffolk.lib.ny.us

Jane Somers, Director

Books on audio cassette, cassette players, braille books, summer reading programs, braille writer, magnifiers, closed-circuit T.V., large-print photocopier, cassette books and magazines, children's books on cassette, reference materials on blindness and other handicaps.

5400 **Postgraduate Center for Mental Health**

124 E 28th Street
New York, NY 10016 **212-689-7700**
FAX: 212-696-1679

Leona Mackler, Director

Information on mental health.

5401 **Rehabilitation Research Library**

Human Resources Center
Albertson, NY 11507 **516-741-2010**
FAX: 516-746-3298

Amnon Tishler, Research Librarian

Information on rehabilitation and occupational rehabilitation.

5402 **State University of New York Health Sciences Center**

450 Clarkson Avenue
PO Box 32
Brooklyn, NY 11203 **718-778-5332**
FAX: 718-778-5397

Adolf Christ, Director

Child psychiatry research programs.

5403 **Suffolk Cooperative Library System: Long Island Talking Book Library**

627 N Sunrise Highway
Bellport, NY 11713 **631-286-1600**
FAX: 631-286-1647
e-mail: lbph@suffolk.lib.ny.us
www.litbl.org

Valerie Lewis, Librarian

Talking book services, assistive device center, disability reference, information and referral services for local libraries, organizations and residents.

5404 **Wallace Memorial Library**

Rochester Institute of Technology
1 Lomb Memorial Drive
Rochester, NY 14623 **585-475-2562**
FAX: 585-475-7007
TTY:716-475-2760
wally.rit.edu

Joan Naturale, Special Needs Ref. Librarian

Information on physical disabilities and deafness.

5405 **Xavier Society for the Blind**

154 E 23rd Street
New York, NY 10010 **212-473-7800**
800-637-9193

Fr Alfred E Ceruana, Executive Director

Provides spiritual and inspirational reading material to visually impaired persons in suitable format: braille, large print and cassette, throughout U.S. and Canada. Services are provided both by way of regular periodical publications sent through the mail and non-returnable; and by means of a lending library where books are returned. All services are provided free.

North Carolina

5406 **Autism Society of North Carolina**

Autism Society of North Carolina Bookstore
505 Oberlin Road
Suite 230
Raleigh, NC 27605 **919-743-0204**
800-442-2762
FAX: 919-743-0208
e-mail: dcoffey@autismsociety-nc.org
www.autismsociety-nc.org

Darla Coffey, Bookstore Manager

One of the largest autism-specific bookstores in the US. All proceeds are used to provide services to people with autism and their families.

5407 Great Smokies Diagnostic Laboratory
63 Zillicoa Street
Asheville, NC 28801
800-522-4762
FAX: 828-252-9303
e-mail: cs@gsdl.com
www.gsdl.com

Functional testing assesses the dynamic inter-relationshp of physiological systems.

1986

5408 North Carolina Library for the Blind and Physically Handicapped
1811 Capital Boulevard
Raleigh, NC 27604
919-676-2288
800-662-7726
FAX: 919-733-6910
e-mail: ncleph@ncsl.dcr.state.nc.us

Francine Martin, Librarian

Free loan of large print, braille, and cassette tape books and magazines and specialized playback equipment to registered eligible North Carolinians. Call for an application form. Collection contains general fiction and nonfiction titles. Registered borrowers may subscribe to receive descriptive videos for a one time fee.

5409 Pediatric Rheumatoid Clinic
Duke Medical Center
Box 3212
Durham, NC 27710
919-684-6575
FAX: 919-681-8943

Dr. Deborah Kredich, Chairman

Clinical and laboratory pediatric rheumatoid studies.

5410 University of North Carolina at Chapel Hill: Brain Research Center
CB 7250
Chapel Hill, NC 27599
919-966-2405
FAX: 919-966-1844

Kunihiko Suzuki MD, Director

North Dakota

5411 North Dakota State Library Talking Book Services
604 E Boulevard Avenue
Department 250
Bismarck, ND 58505
701-328-1408
800-843-9948
FAX: 701-328-2040
TTY:800-892-8622
e-mail: tbooks@state.nd.us.
ndsl.lib.state.nd.us

Terri Wilhelm, Talking Book Manager

Ohio

5412 Case Western Reserve University
10900 Euclid Avenue
Cleveland, OH 44106
216-368-2000
e-mail: webmaster@po.cwru.edu
www.cwru.edu

Jeanne O'Malley Teeter, Manager

Programs which encompass the arts and sciences, engineering, health sciences, law, management, and social work.

5413 Case Western Reserve University Northeast Ohio Multipurpose Arthritis Center
University Hospitals of Cleveland
2074 Abington Road
Cleveland, OH 44106
216-844-7242
FAX: 216-844-5172

Dr. Roland Moskowitz, Director

Basic and clinical research into the causes, diagnosis and treatment of arthritis.

5414 Cleveland FES Center
11000 Cedar Avenue
Cleveland, OH 44106
216-231-3257
800-666-2353
FAX: 216-231-3258
e-mail: info@fesc.org
www.fesc.org

Jeanne O'Malley Teeter, Communications Director

Research and development center on functional electrical stimulation. Houses the FES Information Center, a resource center with a library. Publications, newsletters and videotapes for persons with disabilities and others interested in electrical stimulation are offered.

5415 Cleveland Public Library
17121 Lake Shore Boulevard
Cleveland, OH 44110
216-623-2911
FAX: 330-623-7036
e-mail: lbphmgr1@library.cpl.org
www.cpi.org

Barbara Mates, Librarian

Summer reading programs, braille writer, magnifiers, closed-circuit T.V., large-print photocopier, cassette books and magazines, children's books on cassette, and other reference materials on blindness and other handicaps.

5416 Clovernook Center for the Blind and Visually Impaired
7000 Hamilton Avenue
Cincinnati, OH 45231
513-522-3860
888-234-7156
FAX: 513-728-3946
e-mail: clovernook@clovernook.org
www.clovernook.org

Carol Friedman, Intake Specialist
Joshua Howard, Community Relations Associate

Clovernook promotes independence and fosters the highest quality of life for people with visual impairments, including those with multiple disabilities. The Center provides comprehensive rehabilitation services including training and support for independent living, orientation and mobility instruction, vocational training, job placement, counseling, low vision assessment, computer training, recreation, and youth services. Headquarters located in Cincinatti, Ohio.

5417 Ohio Regional Library for the Blind and Physically Handicapped
800 Vine Street
Library Square
Cincinnati, OH 45202
800-582-0335
FAX: 513-369-3111
TTY:513-369-6072
e-mail: ifbaplch.lib.oh.us
plch.lib.oh.us

Donna Foust, Librarian

Summer reading programs, braille writer, magnifiers, closed-circuit T.V., large-print photocopier, cassette books and magazines, children's books on cassette, and other reference materials on blindness and other handicaps.

5418 State Library of Ohio: Talking Book Program

274 E 1st Avenue
Columbus, OH 43201 **614-644-6895**
FAX: 614-995-2186

Judith Bow

A machine-lending agency for the visually impaired.

5419 University Affiliated Cincinnati Center for Developmental Disabilities

University of Cincinnati UAP
3333 Burnet Avenue
Pavilion Building
Cincinnati, OH 45229 **513-636-7361**
e-mail: oopes0@chmcc.org
www.chmcc.org

Sonya Oppenheimer MD, Executive Director

Oklahoma

5420 Oklahoma Library for the Blind & Physically Handicapped

300 NE 18th Street
Oklahoma City, OK 73105 **405-521-3514**
FAX: 405-521-4582
e-mail: library@drs.state.ok.us
www.library.state.ok.us

Geraldine Adams, Librarian Director

Braille writer, magnifiers, closed-circuit T.V., large-print photocopier, cassette books and magazines, children's books on cassette, home visits and other reference materials on blindness and other handicaps.

5421 Oklahoma Medical Research Foundation

825 NE 13th Street
Oklahoma City, OK 73104 **405-271-6673**
FAX: 405-271-3980

J Donald Capra MD, President

Focuses on arthritis and muscoloskeletal disease research.

5422 Tulsa City-County Library System: Outreach Services

400 Civic Center
Tulsa, OK 74103 **918-596-7922**
FAX: 918-596-7941
e-mail: astephe@tulsalibrary.org
www.tulsalibrary.org

Amy Stephens, Librarian

Homebound delivery of library services for the physically disabled.

Oregon

5423 Oregon Health Sciences University, Elks' Children's Eye Clinic

Casey Eye Institute
3375 SW Terwilliger
Boulevard
Portland, OR 97201 **503-494-7672**
FAX: 503-494-5347
e-mail: Roystere@ohsu.edu
www.oregonelks.org/ECEC.htm

Earl A Palmer MD, Director
Eleen Reyster, Clinic Manager

The elks children's eye clinic is the major charitable project of the Oregon State Elks association. The clinic would not be possible without the organization's dedication and commitment to providing eye care for babies and children.

5424 Oregon Talking Book & Braille Services

250 Winter Street NE
Salem, OR 97301 **541-737-6145**
800-452-0292
FAX: 503-588-7119
TTY:503-378-4276
e-mail: carolynn.m.avery@state.or.us
www.osl.state.or.us/home/tbabs/tbabsac.htm

Carolynn Avery, Regional Librarian

We serve the blind and physically handicapped. Cassette books and magazines, Braille books-magazines, for children and adults. Descriptive videos. Audiocassette machines are provided free of charge. Call us for an application.

5425 Talking Book & Braille Services Oregon State Library

State Library Building
Salem, OR 97310 **503-378-3849**
FAX: 503-588-7119
e-mail: tbabs@sparkie.osl.state.or.us
www.osl.state.or.us/home/tbabs

Donna Bensen, Librarian

Braille writer, magnifiers, large-print photocopier, cassette books and magazines, children's books on cassette and braille books.

Pennsylvania

5426 Carnegie Library of Pittsburgh Library for the Blind & Physically Handicapped

Leonard C Staisey Building
4724 Baum Boulevard
Pittsburgh, PA 15213 **412-687-2440**
800-242-0586
FAX: 412-687-2442
e-mail: clbph@clpgh.org
www.clpgh.org/clp/LBPH

Sue Murdock, Director
Kathleen Kappel, Assistant Director

Loans recorded books/magazines and playback equipment, large print books and described videos to western PA residents unable to use standard printed materials due to a visual, physical, or physically-based reading disability.

5427 Free Library of Philadelphia: Library for the Blind and Physically Handicapped

919 Walnut Street
Philadelphia, PA 19107 **215-683-3213**
800-222-1754
FAX: 215-683-3211
e-mail: flpblind@library.phila.gov

Vickie Lange Collins, Administrator
Richard Riddell, Technical Services Manager
Reneee Snowten, Public Services Manager

Summer reading programs for children and teens. Closed-circuit T.V.for enlarging print for low vision; computers with screen readers and large print; cassette books and magazines; braille books and magazines; and descriptive videos for the blind and visually impaired.

5428 Pennsylvania College of Optometry Eye Institute
1200 W Godfrey Avenue
Philadelphia, PA 19141 215-276-6000
FAX: 215-276-1329

Eugene Wayne, Director

5429 Reading Rehabilitation Hospital
RR 1 Box 250
Reading, PA 19607 610-926-4017
FAX: 610-796-6303

Margaret Hsieh, Librarian

Information on physical disabilities, stroke, head injuries, aging and spinal cord injuries.

5430 Recorded Periodicals
Associated Services for the Blind
919 Walnut Street
Philadelphia, PA 19107 215-627-0600
FAX: 215-922-0692
e-mail: pjohnson@asb.org
www.asb.org

Patricia C Johnson, CEO

A service of Associated Services for the Blind. 26 magazines are available on cassette through this subscription service. A magazine list can be sent, in both large print and on audio cassette. *$18.00*

Rhode Island

5431 Regional Library for the Blind and Physically Handicapped
Talking Books Plus
1 Capitol Hill
Providence, RI 02908 401-222-2080
FAX: 401-277-4195
www.lori.state.ri.us/tbp/summary.php

Richard Leduc, Librarian

Offers talking book services for the blind and physically handicapped. Collection includes reference materials, braille printer, braille writer, large-print books, adaptive computer workstations and referrals to appropriate agencies/programs for other services.

5432 Rhode Island Department of State Library for the Blind and Physically Handicapped
One Capital Hill
Providence, RI 02908 401-277-2726
FAX: 401-277-4195
e-mail: richard@dsl.rhilinet.gov

Richard Ledue, Librarian

Offers information and services for the visually impaired including reference materials, braille printers, braille writers, large-print books and more.

South Carolina

5433 Medical University of South Carolina Arthritis Clinical/Research Center
96 Jonathan Lucas Street
Box 250623
Charleston, SC 29425 843-792-1991
FAX: 843-792-7121

Richard M Silver, Director

Offers patient care services and basic and clinical research on various types of arthritis and connective tissue diseases.

5434 South Carolina State Library
301 Gervais Street
PO Box 821
Columbia, SC 29202 803-734-0470
FAX: 803-737-9983
TTY:803-734-7298
e-mail: guynell@leo.scsl.state.sc.us
www.state.sc.us./scsl

Guynell Williams, Librarian

Summer reading programs, braille writer, magnifiers, closed-circuit T.V., large-print photocopier, cassette books and magazines, children's books on cassette, home visits and other reference materials on blindness and other handicaps.

South Dakota

5435 South Dakota State Library
800 Governors Drive
Pierre, SD 57501 605-224-8641
FAX: 605-773-4950
TTY:605-773-4950
e-mail: darn@stlib.state.sd.us

Daniel Boyd, Librarian

Summer reading programs, braille writer, magnifiers, closed-circuit T.V., large-print photocopier, cassette books and magazines, children's books on cassette, home visits and other reference materials on blindness and other handicaps.

Tennessee

5436 Tennessee Library for the Blind and Physically Handicapped
403 7th Avenue N
Nashville, TN 37243 615-741-3915
800-342-3308
FAX: 615-532-8856
e-mail: tlbph@state.tn.us

Ruth Hemphill, Director
Janie Murphree, Assistant Director

Offers free public library services to those unable to hold, read or turn the pages of ordinary books and magazines due to physical or visual impairment or reading disabilities. Special library materials are provided by the Library of Congress, and free mailing privileges for these materials is provided through the US Post Office. Playback equipment is provided along with books on cassette, in Braille and in large print.

Texas

5437 Baylor College of Medicine Birth Defects Center
6621 Fannin Street
Houston, TX 77030 713-770-3013
FAX: 713-770-4294

Frank Greenberg MD, Director

5438 Baylor College of Medicine: Cullen Eye Institute

6501 Fannin
Houston, TX 77030 **713-798-3200**
FAX: 713-798-4364

Dan B Jones MD, Chairman

Research activities focus on restoring vision and preventing blindness through a better understanding of the disease.

5439 Brown-Heatly Library

4900 N Lamar Boulevard
Austin, TX 78751 **512-424-4240**
FAX: 512-424-4245
e-mail: library@rehab.state.tx.us
www.rehab.statetx.us/library.html

Geneva Davis, Librarian
Judy Reinhart, Assistant Librarian

Houses a collection of books, audio and video tapes and periodicals focusing on rehabilitation, disabilities, employment skills and practices and management for the Texas Rehabilitation Commission. Houses materials on developmental and other disabilities, assessment and evaluation for the Texas Interagency on Early Childhood Intervention.

5440 Center for Research on Women with Disabilities

3400 Richmond Avenue
Suite B
Houston, TX 77046 **713-960-0505**
800-442-7693
FAX: 713-961-3555
e-mail: mnosek@bcm.tmc.edu
www.bcm.tmc.edu/crowd/

Margaret Nosek,PhD, Executive Director

Research organization dedicated to conducting research and promoting, developeing, and disseminating information to expand the life choices of women with disabilities. Conducts research and training activities on issues related to the health, independence and community integration of women and men with physical disabilities. The center has a database of psychosocial behaviors of women with disabilities.

5441 Christian Education for the Blind

7205 Church Park Drive
PO Box 331388
Fort Worth, TX 76163 **817-292-7562**

Roger Dyer, Director

Offers braille and large print books and cassettes for the visually impaired.

5442 Houston Public Library: Access Center

500 McKinney
1st Floor
Houston, TX 77002 **713-224-2976**
TTY:713-247-3546
e-mail: kcurry@htp.lib.tx.us
www.hpl.lib.tx.us/hpl/disabled.html

Kemo Curry, Supervisor

Offers full library services to the visually and hearing impaired in Houston, TX at no charge. Houses unique and critical services for its users including online access to the Internet in a private and secure area.

5443 Talking Book Program/Texas State Library

Talking Book Program
PO Box 12927
Austin, TX 78711 **512-463-5460**
800-252-9605
FAX: 512-463-5436
e-mail: tbp.services@tsl.state.tx.us

Dale Propp, Director
Renulfo Ramirez, Administrative Services Lib.

Provides reading materials in special formats to Texas residents who cannot read conventional printed matter because of visual or physical limitations, whether permanent or temporary. The service is free and materials are sent through the mail free. Books and magazines are available in cassette, braille, recorded disk and large print formats. A Disabilities Reference Center can answer questions on topics related to disabilities.

5444 University of Texas Southwestern Medical Center/Allergy & Immunology

5323 Harry Hines Boulevard
Dallas, TX 75235 **214-648-3004**
FAX: 214-648-6377

Paul Bergstresser MD, Principal Investor

5445 University of Texas at Austin Library

Austin, TX 78712 **512-475-7348**

e-mail: www@lib.utexas.edu
www.lib.utexas.edu

Ann Neville, Coordinator

Provides access to information for all users, including those with disabilities, in accordance with the overall mission of the General Libraries of the University of Texas at Austin.

Utah

5446 Family Resource Library/Center for Persons with Disabilities

1780 N Research Parkway
Suite 112
North Logan, UT 84341 **801-752-0238**
FAX: 435-753-9750
TTY:801-753-9750
e-mail: cope@cc.usu.edu

Marilyn Thomas, President
Julia Burnham, Executive Director

Not-for-profit service organization dedicated to collecting materials containing practical information for families of persons with disabilities. Serves persons with disabilities and their famlies in Utah, Idaho, Wyoming and Nevada. Educational materials include books, booklets, videotapes and audiotapes.

5447 Utah State Library Division: Program for the Blind and Disabled

250 N 1950 W
Suite A
Salt Lake City, UT 84116 **801-715-6789**
FAX: 801-715-6767
e-mail: blind@utah.gov
www.library.utah.gov

Gerald Buttars, Librarian

Summer reading programs, Braille embosser, cassette books and magazines, children's books on cassette and other reference materials on blindness and other handicaps, descriptive videos, Braille books, large print books and radio reading service.

Vermont

5448 **Vermont Department of Libraries/Special Services Unit**
578 Paine Turnpike N
Berlin, VT 05602
802-828-3273
800-479-1711
FAX: 802-828-2199
e-mail: ssu@dol.state.vt.us

S Francis Woods, Librarian
Jennifer Hart, Assistant Librarian

Service consists of reading material in large print and in talking book formats. The book collection consists of cassettes and large print. Special collections include: childrens print/braille books, reference materials on blindness, and descriptive videos.

Virginia

5449 **Alexandria Library Talking Book Service**
826 Slaters Lane
Alexandria, VA 22314
703-519-5900
FAX: 703-823-4524
TTY:703-519-5809
e-mail: emccaffr@lea.eda
www.alexandria.lib.va.us

Patricia Bates, Librarian

Summer reading programs, braille writer, magnifiers, closed-circuit T.V., large-print photocopier, cassette books and magazines, children's books on cassette, home visits and other reference materials on blindness and other handicaps.

5450 **Arlington County Department of Libraries**
1015 N Quincy Street
Arlington, VA 22201
703-358-6548
FAX: 703-534-1240
TTY:703-358-6320

Roxanne Barnes, Librarian

Summer reading programs, braille writer, magnifiers, closed-circuit T.V., large-print photocopier, cassette books and magazines, children's books on cassette, home visits and other reference materials on blindness and other handicaps.

5451 **Braille Circulating Library for the Blind**
2700 Stuart Avenue
Richmond, VA 23220
804-359-3743
FAX: 804-359-4777
e-mail: brailleCL@aol.com

Robert Gordon, Executive Director

Offers library materials for the blind and visually impaired on a free-loan basis. Serves the entire USA and 41 foreign countries with cassette tapes, reel to reel tapes, braille books, large print books along with talking book records.

5452 **Central Rappahannock Regional Library**
1201 Caroline Street
Fredericksburg, VA 22401
540-372-1160
FAX: 540-373-9411
TTY:540-371-9165
e-mail: nschiff@hq.crrl.org

Nancy Schiff, Librarian

Offers reference materials on blindness and other disabilities.

5453 **Council for Exceptional Children**
1110 N Glebe Road
Suite 300
Arlington, VA 22201
703-620-3660
FAX: 703-264-9494
www.cec.sped.org

Janice Burdick, President

Members are teachers, college faculty members, administrators, supervisors and others concerned with the education and welfare of visually handicapped and blind children and youth. This is a division of the Council For Exceptional Children.

5454 **Hampton Subregional Library for the Blind**
4207 Victoria Boulevard
Hampton, VA 23669
757-727-1149
FAX: 757-727-1047
e-mail: swoolard@leo.vsla.edu

Mary Sue Woolard, Librarian

Summer reading programs, braille writer, magnifiers, closed-circuit T.V., large-print photocopier, cassette books and magazines, children's books on cassette, home visits and other reference materials on blindness and other handicaps.

5455 **James Branch Cabell Library**
Virginia Commonwealth University
901 Park Avenue
PO Box 842033
Richmond, VA 23284
804-828-1110
866-828-2665
FAX: 804-828-0151

Sally Jacobs, Reference Librarian

Provides individualized orientations and assistance with library research and equipment.

5456 **Newport News Public Library System**
112 Main Street
Newport News, VA 23601
757-591-7418
FAX: 757-591-7425
e-mail: shalswin@leo.vsla.edu

Sue Balswin, Librarian

Summer reading programs, braille writer, magnifiers, closed-circuit T.V., large-print photocopier, cassette books and magazines, children's books on cassette, home visits and other reference materials on blindness and other handicaps.

5457 **Northern Virginia Resource Center for Deaf and Hard of Hearing Persons**
3951 Pender Drive
Suite 130
Fairfax, VA 22030
703-352-9055
FAX: 703-352-9058
e-mail: info@nvrc.org
www.nvrc.org

Cheryl A Heppner, Executive Director
Gay Nagy, Outreach Manager

Empowering deaf and hard of hearing individuals and their families through education, advocacy and community involvement.

5458 **Roanoke City Public Library System**
2607 Salem Turnpike NW
Roanoke, VA 24017
540-853-2621
FAX: 540-853-1030

Rebecca Cooper, Librarian

Summer reading programs, braille writer, magnifiers, closed-circuit T.V., large-print photocopier, cassette books and magazines, children's books on cassette, home visits and other reference materials on blindness and other handicaps.

5459 Special Services/Talking Books
2501 Sherwood Hall Lane
Alexandria, VA 22306 **703-765-3645**
FAX: 703-765-5893
e-mail: sjapikse@leo.vsld.edu
www.co.fairfax.va.us/library/homepage.ht

Jeanette Studley, Manager

Offers talking books, TDD access, assistive devices such as decoders for three-week loans, support groups for people who are visually impaired, library program interpreters available with four weeks advance notice, adapted computer work station with braille printer and assistive listening devices.

5460 Staunton Public Library Talking Book Center
One Churchville Avenue
Staunton, VA 24401 **540-332-3902**
800-995-6215
FAX: 540-332-3906
e-mail: talkingbooks@ci.staunton.va.us

Oakley Pearson, Librarian

Offers free library service by circulating recorded books, magazines, and playback equipment to individuals unable to use standard print materials because of visual or physical impairment.

5461 University of Virginia Health System General Clinical Research Group
PO Box 800787
Charlottesville, VA 22908 **434-924-2394**
FAX: 434-924-9960
e-mail: GCRC@Virginia.EDU
gcrc.med.virginia.edu

Eugene J Barrett, Program Director

Provides investigators with the specialized resources necessary to conduct advanced clinical research. The facility includes ten inpatient beds, skilled research nurses, a core assay laboratory, a metabolic kitchen, outpatient facilities, computing and statistical consultants and facilities, and sleep and exercise physiology laboratories.

1968

5462 Virginia Autism Resource Center
PO Box 1250
Winchester, VA 22604 **540-542-1723**
877-667-7771
877- -
FAX: 540-667-5481
e-mail: info@varc.org
www.grafton.org/vaautismresourc.htm

Carol Schall, Director
Brenda Whitlock, Administrative Specialist

Provides training, individual case consultation, materials and information to families and professionals working with individuals with autism in Virginia.

1983

5463 Virginia Beach Public Library Special Services Library
930 Independence Boulevard
Virginia Beach, VA 23455 **757-464-9175**
FAX: 757-460-7606

Susan Head, Librarian

A public library for people with visual and physical disabilities, braille writer, magnifiers, closed-circuit T.V., large-print photocopier, cassette books and magazines, children's books on cassette, and other reference materials on blindness and other disabilities.

5464 Virginia Chapter of the Arthtitis Foundation
3805 Cutshaw Avenue
Suite 200
Richmond, VA 23230 **804-359-1700**
800-456-4687
FAX: 804-359-4900
e-mail: info.va@arthritis.org
www.arthritis.org/Communities/Chapters/

Provides free information, services and counseling to the public. Services include assistance in locating and accessing government and other health care programs for persons with arthritis, referral to doctors specializing in the treatment of arthritis, free literature about the different types of arthritis and counseling for people with arthritis and their families.

5465 Virginia State Library for the Visually and Physically Handicapped
395 Azalea Avenue
Richmond, VA 23227 **804-371-3661**
FAX: 804-371-3508

Barbara McCarthy, Director

Summer reading programs, braille writer, magnifiers, closed-circuit T.V., large-print photocopier, cassette books and magazines, children's books on cassette, home visits and other reference materials on blindness and other handicaps.

Washington

5466 Meridian Valley Clinical Laboratory
801 SW 16th Streeteet
Suite 126
Renton, WA 98055 **253-271-8689**
800-234-6825
FAX: 253-271-8674
e-mail: meridian@meridianvalleylab.com
www.meridianvalleylab.com

5467 Ophthalmic Research Laboratory Eye Institute
Swedish Hospital Medical Center
747 Summit Avenue
Seattle, WA 98104 **206-386-6000**
FAX: 206-386-2625

Dr. Brian Godell, Director

Color vision physiology, vision disorders and blindness research.

5468 Washington Talking Book and Braille Library
2021 9th Avenue
Seattle, WA 98121 **206-464-1011**
FAX: 206-464-0247
TTY:206-464-6930
e-mail: wtbbl@spl.lib.wa.us
www.spl.org/wtbbl/wtbbl.html

Jan Ames, Librarian

Summer reading programs, braille writer, magnifiers, closed-circuit T.V., large-print photocopier, cassette books and magazines, children's books, and other reference materials on blindness and other handicaps, online catalog, reference station with assistive devices and a radio reading service.

West Virginia

5469 **Autism Services Center**
605 9th Street
PO Box 507
Huntington, WV 25710 **304-525-8014**
FAX: 304-525-8026
www.autismservices.com

Ruth C Sullivan PhD, Executive Director

Provides developmental disabilities services with a specialty in autism. Services include case management, residential, personal care, assessments and evaluations, supported employment, independent living and family support.

1979

5470 **Cabell County Public Library/Talking Book Department/Subregional Library for the Blind**
455 9th Street Plaza
Huntington, WV 25701 **304-528-5700**
FAX: 304-528-5866
e-mail: tbooks@cabell.lib.wv.us
cabell.lib.wv.us

Donna Cushman, Coordinator

Summer reading programs, Braille writer, magnifiers, closed-circuit TV, cassette books and magazines, children's books on cassette reference materials on blindness and other handicaps, enlargers and Arkenstone Reader.

5471 **Kanawha County Public Library**
123 Capitol Street
Charleston, WV 25301 **304-348-7770**
FAX: 304-348-6530

Reference, Librarian

Summer reading programs, large print PC option, magnifiers, large type books, cassette books, and magazines, children's books on cassette, home visits and other reference materials on blindness and other handicaps

5472 **Ohio County Public Library Services for the Blind and Physically Handicapped**
52 16th Street
Whelling, WV 26033 **304-232-0244**
FAX: 304-232-6848

Lori Nicholson

5473 **Talking Book Department, Parkersburg and Wood County Public Library**
3100 Emerson Avenue
Parkersburg, WV 26104 **304-420-4587**
800-642-8674
FAX: 304-420-4589
e-mail: hickmanm@hp9k.park.lib.wv.us

Michael Hickman, Coordinator Services

Services for the bind and physically handicapped. Library of Congress Talking Book Program.

5474 **West Virginia Autism Training Center**
Marshall Univ. College of Educational & Human Serv
400 Hal Greer Boulevard
Suite 316
Huntington, WV 25755 **304-696-2332**
800-344-5115
www.marshall.edu/coe/atc/

Provides education, training, and treatment programs for W Virginians who have Autism, Pervasive Devolopmental Disorders or Asperger's disease and have formally been registered with the Center.

5475 **West Virginia Library Commission**
1900 Kanawha Boulevard E
Charleston, WV 25305 **304-588-2041**
FAX: 304-558-2044
e-mail: fesenmf@mars.wr1c.wvnet.edu
www.librarycommision.lib.wv.us

Francis Fesenmainer, Librarian

Summer reading programs, braille writer, magnifiers, closed-circuit T.V., large-print photocopier, cassette books and magazines, children's books on cassette, home visits and other reference materials on blindness and other handicaps.

5476 **West Virginia School for the Blind Library**
301 E Main Street
Romney, WV 26757 **304-822-3521**
FAX: 304-822-4896
e-mail: cjohn@access.mountain.net

Cynthia Johnson, Librarian

Summer reading programs, braille writer, magnifiers, closed-circuit T.V., large-print photocopier, cassette books and magazines, children's books on cassette, home visits and other reference materials on blindness and other handicaps.

Wisconsin

5477 **Brown County Library**
515 Pine Street
Green Bay, WI 54301 **920-448-4400**
FAX: 920-448-4376
TTY:9204484350
e-mail: BC_Library@co.brown.wi.us
www.co.brown.wi.us/library/

Angela Basten, Librarian

Summer reading programs, braille writer, magnifiers, closed-circuit TV, large-print photocopier, cassette books and magazines, children's books on cassette, home visits and other reference materials on blindness and other handicaps.

5478 **Eye Institute of the Medical College of Wisconsin and Froedtert Hospital**
8700 W Wisconsin Avenue
Milwaukee, WI 53226 **414-456-2020**
e-mail: eyecare@mcw.edu

Richard Schultz MD, Director

A full service academic ophthalmology program.

1976

5479 **Trace Center**
University of Wisconsin-Madison
5901 Research Park Boulevard
Madison, WI 53719 **608-263-5776**
FAX: 608-262-8848
TTY:608-263-5408
e-mail: info@trace.wisc.edu
www.trace.wisc.edu

Nancy Gores, Public Information Coordinator

Research and development center at the University of Wisconsin-Madison that focuses on making off-the-shelf technologies and systems more usable for everyone. Trace is designated as the Rehabilitation Engineering Research Center (RERC) on information technology access and it also a partner with Gallaudet University in the RERC on universal telecommunications access and Trace's work is in great part funded throught the National Institute on Disability and Rehabilitaiton Research (NIDRR).

5480 Wisconsin Regional Library for the Blind & Physically Handicapped

813 W Wells Street
Milwaukee, WI 53233 **414-286-3045**
800-242-8822
FAX: 414-286-3102
TTY:414-286-3548
e-mail: mvalne@mpl.org
www.dpi.state.wi.us/dltcl/rll/lbphinfo.html

Marsha Valance, Regional Librarian
Constance Pirtle, Assistant Librarian

Circulates recorded materials, playback equipment and braille materials to print-handicapped Wisconsin residents.

Wyoming

5481 Wyoming Services for the Visually Impaired

Wyoming Department of Education
2300 Capitol Avennue
Hathaway Building, 2nd Floor
Cheyenne, WY 82002 **307-777-7675**
FAX: 307-777-6234

Kent Jensen

Eligible readers of Wyoming receive library service from the regional library in Salt Lake City, Utah.

5482 Wyoming's New Options in Technology (WYNOT) - University of Wyoming

Wyoming Institute for Disabilities
1465 N Fourth Street, Suite 111
Laramie, WY 82072 **307-766-2051**
800-861-4312
FAX: 307-721-2084
e-mail: wynot.uw@uwyo.edu
wind.uwyo.edu/wind/community/wynotinfo.htm

Kathy Laurin, Public Contact

Designed to develop and implement a consumer oriented statewide system of technology-related assistance for people with disabilities of all ages.

AIDS

5483 AIDS 2nd Edition

JB Lippincott
227 E Washington Square
Philadelphia, PA 19106
301-521-8300
800-777-2295
FAX: 301-824-7390

Gives the latest information on AIDS covering basic science considerations, clinical aspects and public health issues. *$55.00*

474 pages

5484 AIDS Alert

American Health Consultants
3525 Piedmont Road
Building 6, Suite 400
Atlanta, GA 30305
404-262-7436
800-688-2421
FAX: 800-850-1232
e-mail: customerservice@ahcpub.com
www.ahcpub.com

Glen Harris, Managing Editor

Source of AIDS news and advice for health care professionals. Covers up-to-the-minute developments and guidance on the entire spectrum of AIDS challenges, including treatment, education, precautions, screening, diagnosis and policy. *$467.00*

12 pages Monthly
ISSN 0887-02 2

5485 AIDS Disease State Management Resource

PO Box 740056
Atlanta, GA 30374
404-262-7436
FAX: 800-284-3291
e-mail: customerservices@ahcpub.com
www.ahcpub.com

Milo Falcon, Managing Editor

Provides staff and patient education materials on HIV/AIDS. *$299.00*

Paperback

5486 AIDS, What Does it Mean to You?

Walker Publishing Company
435 Hudson Street
New York, NY 10014
212-727-8300
800-289-2553
FAX: 212-727-0984
e-mail: orders@walkerbooks.com

Researchers have been working frantically to solve the puzzle of AIDS - a disease that has taken the lives of thousands of men and women during the past ten years. *$13.95*

128 pages Cloth/Hardcover
ISBN 0-802782-02-7

5487 AIDS: The HIV Myth

St. Martin's Press
175 5th Avenue
New York, NY 10010
212-674-5151
www.stmartins.com

Challenges the theory that AIDS is caused by a virus called HIV. Puts forward the view that in the rush to identify the cause of an apparently new disease, a harmless passenger virus was leapt upon as the sole culprit.

1989
ISBN 0-333489-30-6

5488 APLA Update

AIDS Project Los Angeles
550 N Larchmount
Suite 202
Los Angeles, CA 90004
323-993-1600
FAX: 323-993-1392

Presents news about AIDS and programs of AIDS Project Los Angeles to people affected by the disease.

20 pages

5489 Questions and Answers: The ADA and Persons with HIV/AIDS

US Department of Justice
950 Pennsylvania Avenue NW DRS-NYAV
Washington, DC 20530
202-307-0663
800-574-0301
FAX: 202-307-1197
www.ada.gov

A 16-page publication explaining the requirements for employers, businesses and nonprofit agencies that serve the public, and state and local governments to avoid discriminating against persons with HIV/AIDS.

5490 Surviving AIDS

HarperCollins
1350 Avenue of the Americas
New York, NY 10019
212-261-6500
virusmyth.net/aids/books/mcbsurv.htm

Author tells the story of how he and hundreds of others also diagnosed with AIDS have beaten the odds. Profiles thirteen long-term survivors and brings into focus the courage, drama, and humor that has helped them to answer the question Why am I alive? Includes photographs.

254 pages 1990
ISBN 0-060161-48-5

5491 World Without AIDS: The Controvertial Holistic Health

HarperCollins
1350 Avenue of the Americas
New York, NY 10019
212-261-6500

A convincing argument that conventional medicine approaches do not 'cure' disease, which outlines how AIDS can be treated using methods of naturopathic medicine. Also includes an appendix outlining 21 ways to strengthen the immune system.

288 pages Paperback 1988
ISBN 0-722516-32-0

Children & Young Adults

5492 ABCD Newsletter Volume Reprints

Birth Defect Research for Children
930 Woodcock Road
Suite 225
Orlando, FL 32803
407-895-0802
FAX: 407-895-0824
e-mail: staff@birthdefects.org
www.birthdefects.org

Betty Mekdeci, Executive Director

Offers a variety of reprints from the ABCD newsletter on birth defects

Monthly

5493 ACPOC News

6300 N River Road
Suite 727
Rosemont, IL 60018
847-698-1637
FAX: 847-823-0536
e-mail: raymond@aaos.org
www.acpoc.org

Sheril King, Executive Director

Quarterly publication from the Association of Children's Prosthetic/Orthotic Clinics. Included with membership.

35-40 pages Quarterly

5494 ADHD with Comorbid Disorders: Clinical Assessment and Management

Guilford Press
72 Spring Street
New York, NY 10012
212-431-9800
800-365-7006
FAX: 212-966-6708
www.guilford.com

James M Swanson, Author

$44.00

Cloth
ISBN 1-572304-78-2

5495 AT for Infants and Toddlers with Disabilities

Idaho Assistive Technology Project
129 W 3rd Street
Moscow, ID 83843
208-885-3559
800-432-8324
FAX: 208-885-3628
e-mail: rseiler@uidaho.edu
www.educ.uidaho.edu/idatech

$5.00

68 pages

5496 Adolescent in Family Therapy: Breaking the Cycle of Conflict and Control

Guilford Press
72 Spring Street
New York, NY 10012
212-431-9800
800-365-7006
FAX: 212-966-6708
www.guilford.com

Presenting a developmentally grounded approach, Joseph Micucci shows how troubled teenagers and their parents can be helped to use family relationships as catalysts for growth and change. Filled with case examples and clinical advice, the book describes specific family intervention strategies for eating disorders, depression, underachievement, stress caused by psychotic symptoms and other conditions. Also in cloth at $40.00 (ISBN# 1-57230-389-1) *$23.00*

336 pages Paper 1900
ISBN 1-572305-88-6

5497 Assistive Technology for School Age

Idaho Assistive Technology Project
129 W 3rd Street
Moscow, ID 83843
208-885-3559
800-432-8324
FAX: 208-885-3628
e-mail: rseiler@uidaho.edu
www.educ.uidaho.edu/idatech

$5.00

84 pages

5498 Autism Research Review

Autism Research Institute
4182 Adams Avenue
San Diego, CA 92116
619-281-7165
FAX: 619-563-6840
www.autism.com/ari/index.html

B Rimland PhD, Director

$18.00

8 pages Quarterly

5499 Belonging

Dial Books
375 Hudson Street
New York, NY 10014
212-366-2000
FAX: 212-414-3394

Meg attended special schools for the blind until she was ready for high school. She decided that she wanted to go to a regular high school. She and her mother practiced her walks to school and studied the layout of the building prior to school starting, but Meg was unprepared for the trip when there were 1,500 students. She adjusted quickly to the crowds and the pace of the new school.

200 pages Hardcover
ISBN 0-80370 -30-1

5500 Best Toys, Books, Videos & Software for Kids: Kid-Tested Classic and New Products

Exceptional Parent Library
120 Sylvan Avenue, Suite 10
PO Box 1807
Englewood Cliffs, NJ 07632
800-535-1910
FAX: 201-947-9376
e-mail: eplibrary@aol.com
www.eplibrary.com

Ron Richards, Executive Director

Aims to take the guesswork out of finding the best products for kids from infancy to age ten. Reviews over one-thousand products that have been tested by kids and evaluated by experts. *$12.00*

5501 **Birth Defect News**

Birth Defect Research for Children
930 Woodcock Road
Suite 225
Orlando, FL 32803 **407-895-0802**
FAX: 407-895-0824
e-mail: staff@birthdefects.org
www.birthdefects.org

Betty Mekdeci, Executive Director

Offers updated information on the association activities, events and updates regarding birth defects and environmental exposures.

Monthly

5502 **Burnish Me Bright**

Pantheon Books
1540 Broadway
New York, NY 10036 **212-782-9000**
800-638-6460
FAX: 212-302-7985
www.randomhouse.com/pantheon/

Hilaire, a famous mime, had retired to a small village to live out his life. He met frail Auguste, who was unable to speak, and immediately he saw the potential for this agile and physically expressive youth to become a mime.

80 pages Hardcover 1970

5503 **Bus Girl: Selected Poems**

Brookline Books
PO Box 97
Newton Upper Falls, MA 02464 **617-558-8010**
800-666-2665
FAX: 617-558-8011
e-mail: brbooks@yahoo.com
www.brooklinebooks.com

Poems written over several decades by a young woman with Down Syndrome. *$14.95*

144 pages Paperback
ISBN 1-57129 -41-9

5504 **But I'm Ready to Go**

Bradbury Press
8306 Aurora Avenue N
Seattle, WA 98103 **206-524-4910**
800-257-5755

Judy always had a problem learning math and performing skills that required good motor control.

230 pages Hardcover
ISBN 0-87888 -07-7

5505 **Camping Magazine**

5000 State Road 67 N
Martinsville, IN 46151 **765-342-8456**
800-428-2267
FAX: 765-342-2065
www.acacamps.org

Kim Bruno, Communications/Development Spec
Peg Smith, Executive Director

Bi-monthly periodical published by the American Camping Association. *$24.95*

45-76 pages Bi-monthly

5506 **Camps 2003: A Directory of Camps & Summer Programs for Children and Youth with Disablities**

Resources for Children with Special Needs
116 E 16th Street
5th Floor
New York, NY 10003 **212-667-4650**
FAX: 212-254-4070
e-mail: info@resourcesnyc.org
www.resourcesnyc.org

Karen Schlesinger, Executive Director
Dianne Littwin, Director Publications

Yearly publication from Resources for Children with Special Needs, Inc. *$22.00*

308 pages Yearly
ISBN 0-967836-57-3

5507 **Caring for Children with Chronic Illness**

Springer Publishing Company
536 Broadway
New York, NY 10012 **212-431-4370**
877-687-7476
FAX: 212-941-7842
e-mail: marketing@springerpub.com
www.springerpub.com

Annette Imperati, Marketing/Sales Director

A critical look at the current medical, social, and psychological framework for providing care to children with chronic illnesses. Emphasizing the need to create integrated, interdisciplinary approaches, it discusses issues such as the roles of families, professionals, and institutions in providing health care, the impact of a child's illness on various family structures, financing care, the special problems of chronically ill children as they become adolescents and more. *$36.95*

320 pages Hardcover
ISBN 0-82615 -00-1

5508 **Child Who Never Grew Up**

Exceptional Parent Library
120 Sylvan Avenue, Suite 10
PO Box 1807
Englewood Cliffs, NJ 07632
800-535-1910
FAX: 201-947-9376
e-mail: eplibrary@aol.com
www.eplibrary.com

Offers Pearl Buck's inspiring account of her struggle to understand and help her daughter with mental retardation. *$14.95*

112 pages 1992
ISBN 0-933149-49-2

5509 **Child and Adolescent Therapy: Cognitive-Be havioral Procedures, Second Edition**

Guilford Press
72 Spring Street
New York, NY 10012 **212-431-9800**
800-365-7006
FAX: 212-966-6708
www.guilford.com

Incorporating significant developments in treatment procedures, theory and clinical research, new chapters in this second edition examine the current status of empirically supported interventions and developmental issues specific to work with adolescents. *$45.00*

432 pages Cloth 1900
ISBN 1-572305-56-8

5510 **Child's Courage, A Doctor's Devotion: Triumph Over Head Trauma**

Special Needs Project
324 State Street
Suite H
Santa Barbara, CA 93101
800-333-6867
FAX: 805-962-5087
www.specialneeds.com

Information for nonprofessionals about head trauma. Tells the story of young Mike Mahanes' injury in a car accident and his recovery aided by a positive parent-professional relationship. *$6.95*

164 pages 1985

ISBN 0-932620-48-5

5511 **Childhood Ear Infections: What Every Parent Should Know**

North Atlantic Books
1456 4th Street
Berkley, CA 94710
510-559-8277
FAX: 510-559-8279
www.northatlanticbooks.com

A guide to helping control and eliminate ear infections in children. Other topics include the use of antibiotics, the unnecessary removal of adenoids, and the implantation of tubes into the ear drums. Gives causes of middle ear infections, discusses concerns about common treatments, and encourages alternative treatments.

1992

ISBN 1-556430-89-2

5512 **Children Who Vary from the Normal Type: Special Education in Boston, 1838-1930**

Gallaudet University Press
11030 S Langley Avenue
Chicago, IL 60628
800-621-2736
FAX: 800-621-8476
TTY:800-621-9347
gupress.gallaudet.edu

Identifies Boston as both typical of and a national leader in Special Education programs, tracing its history with an eye towards the future. *$49.95*

220 pages Hardcover

5513 **Commonly Asked Questions About Child Care Centers and the Americans with Disabilities Act**

US Department of Justice
950 Pennsylvania Avenue NW DRS-NYAV
Washington, DC 20530
202-307-0663
800-574-0301
FAX: 202-307-1197
www.ada.gov

A 13-page publication explaining how the requirements of the ADA apply to Child Care Centers. The document also describes some of the Department of Justice's ongoing enforcement efforts in the child care area and it provides a resource list on sources of information on the ADA.

5514 **Communication Coloring Book**

Speech Bin
1965 25th Avenue
Vero Beach, FL 32960
772-770-0007
800-477-3324
FAX: 772-770-0006
www.speechbin.com

Jan J Binney, VP

Publisher and distributor of books and materials for professionals in rehabilitation, speech-language pathology, special education and related fields and persons interested in communication disorders and related disabilities. Major product lines include professional and children's books, computer software, diagnostic tests, instructional games and materials for children and adults and specialty items. *$14.95*

48 pages

ISBN 0-93785 -53-0

5515 **Complete IEP Guide: How to Advocate for Yo ur Special Ed Child**

Spina Bifida Association of America
4590 MacArthur Boulevard NW
Suite 250
Washington, DC 20007
202-944-3285
800-621-3141
FAX: 202-944-3295
e-mail: sbaa@sbaa.org
www.sbaa.org

This all-in-one guide will help you understand special education law, identify your child's needs, prepare for meetings, develop the IEP and resolve disputes. *$28.95*

5516 **Coping When a Parent Has Multiple Sclerosis**

Rosen Publishing Group
29 E 21st Street
New York, NY 10010
212-777-3017
800-237-9932
FAX: 888-436-4643
e-mail: triciab@rosenpub.com
www.rosenpub.com

Tricia Bauer, Director Special Markets

Explains to young people how living with a parent who has Multiple Sclerosis will affect their lives. Hardcover. *$19.95*

128 pages

ISBN 0-823914-06-2

5517 **Coping for Kids Who Stutter**

Speech Bin
1965 25th Avenue
Vero Beach, FL 32960
772-770-0007
800-477-3324
FAX: 772-770-0006
www.speechbin.com

Jan J Binney, Senior Editor

Informative book for children and adults about stuttering and how to manage it. *$15.95*

32 pages

ISBN 0-93785 -43-2

5518 **Coping with Being Physically Challenged**

Rosen Publishing Group
29 E 21st Street
New York, NY 10010
718-851-4859
FAX: 888-436-4643
e-mail: rosenpub@tribeca.ios.com

Ratto deals with strong emotions, such as general anger and depression, which affect these young adults and their families. The author shows them how to deal and cope on a day-to-day basis. *$15.95*

ISBN 0-82391 -44-9

5519 Coping with Special Needs Classmates

Rosen Publishing Group
29 E 21st Street
New York, NY 10010
212-777-3017
800-237-9932
FAX: 888-436-4643
e-mail: rosenpub@tribeca.ios.com

Tricia Bauer, Director Special Markets

Special needs classmates include people who are physically different, disfigured or challenged, emotionally disturbed, or those who have learning disabilities. The author offers guidance on how to get past discomfort or fear of confrontation with someone who seems very different, but is, in reality, not so different after all. Hardcover. *$17.95*

128 pages
ISBN 0-823915-98-0

5520 Coping with a Learning Disability

Rosen Publishing Group
29 E 21st Street
New York, NY 10010
212-777-3017
800-237-9932
FAX: 888-436-4643
e-mail: rosenpub@tribeca.ios.com

Tricia Bauer, Director Special Markets

Being a teen with a learning disorder does not have to be a devastating experience. The authors discuss family, personal, and peer emotional reactions. Biographies of famous people with learning disorders provide positive role models and special education is discussed. Hardcover. *$17.95*

128 pages
ISBN 0-823928-87-X

5521 Coping with a Physically Challenged Brother or Sister

Rosen Publishing Group
29 E 21st Street
New York, NY 10010
212-777-3017
800-237-9932
FAX: 888-436-4643
e-mail: rosenpub@tribeca.ios.com

Tricia Bauer, Director Special Needs

Dealing with a relative who is born physically challenged or who suffers a personal tragedy is one of the biggest adjustments in life. This book shows step-by-step methods of coping with these emotions so the reader may learn how to have a happy life once again. Hardcover. *$17.95*

ISBN 0-823914-92-5

5522 Deenie

Bradbury Press
135 S Mount Zion Road
Lebanon, IN 46052
800-257-5755
FAX: 800-882-8583

Deenie, a beautiful thirteen-year-old girl, had a mother who was pushing her to become a model. The agency representatives told Deenie she had the looks but walked differently. Deenie's main wish was to become a cheerleader. Her close friend, Janet, made the cheerleading squad but Deenie didn't make the final list. After this her gym teacher noticed her posture and called her family. After seeing therapists, the diagnosis of adolescent idiopathic scoliosis was made.

159 pages Hardcover
ISBN 0-02711 -20-6

5523 Determined to Win: Children Living with Allergies and Asthma

Gareth Stevens
1555 N Rivercenter Drive
Milwaukee, WI 53212
414-225-0333
800-542-2595
FAX: 414-332-3567
www.gsinc.com

Claire Messier, Marketing Associate

Isabell, a six year old girl, has been living with allergies and asthma almost her entire life. With proper medical care and a determined attitude, she leads an active life. *$15.95*

48 pages
ISBN 0-83681 -75-9

5524 Don't Feel Sorry for Paul

JB Lippincott
E Washington Square
Philadelphia, PA 19105
FAX: 215-824-7390

Paul is seven but was born with deformities of both hands and feet. Paul must wear a prosthesis on both feet so that he can walk. He has a third prosthesis for his right hand. The third prosthesis has a pair of hooks Paul uses as fingers.

94 pages Hardcover
ISBN 0-39731 -88-0

5525 Enabling Romance: A Guide to Love, Sex & Relationships for the Disabled

Spina Bifida Association of America
4590 Macarthur Boulevard NW
Suite 250
Washington, DC 20007
202-944-3285
800-621-3141
FAX: 202-944-3295
e-mail: sbaa@sbaa.org
www.sbaa.org

An uncensored, illustrated guide to intimacy and sexual expression for persons with physical disabilities. *$15.95*

5526 Every Second Child

Keats Publishing
1221 Avenue of the Americas
New York, NY 10020
212-512-2000
800-323-4900
www.mcgraw-hill.com/

Linus Pauling, Designer

A thorough investigation of the crucial role of nutrition in preventing infant crib death.

1981
ISBN 0-879832-50-9

5527 Family Therapy for ADHD: Treating Children , Adolescents and Adults

Guilford Press
72 Spring Street
New York, NY 10012
212-431-9800
800-365-7006
FAX: 212-966-6708
www.guilford.com

$40.00

Cloth
ISBN 1-572304-38-3

5528 Feed Your Kids Right

McGraw-Hill Company
1221 Aveune of the Americas
New York, NY 10020 **212-512-2000**
www.mcgraw-hill.com

Covers most of the health problems associated with childhood and the more natural methods of treating them.

1979
ISBN 0-070584-96-6

5529 Follow My Leader

Puffin
375 Hudson Street
New York, NY 10014 **212-366-2000**
800-328-7327
FAX: 212-366-2666
www.puffin.co.uk

Robert Greiner, Illustrator

Jimmy was an active eleven year old. One of his friends found a firecracker with a short fuse. Although the boys advised him not to light it, Mike set it off. When the fuse started to burn, Mike threw the firecracker even though Jimmy was near by. The explosion occurred in Jimmy's face, blinding him. At first he was very bitter toward Mike and his blindness, but he soon found that with the help of his tutor and his friends he could learn braille and use a cane.

191 pages Hardcover 1994
ISBN 0-140364-85-4

5530 For Siblings Only

Family Resource Associates
35 Haddon Avenue
Shrewsbury, NJ 07702 **732-747-5310**
FAX: 732-747-1896

Sue Levine, Social Worker

A newsletter for brothers and sisters, aged 4 through 10, whose sibling has a disablilty. Includes stories, library resources, activities and discussion of feelings. $12/year for families, $20/year for professionals. *$12.00*

12 pages Quarterly

5531 Funology Fables: Stories for Phonology Learning

Speech Bin
1965 25th Avenue
Vero Beach, FL 32960 **772-770-0007**
800-477-3324
FAX: 772-770-0006
www.speechbin.com

Talking Tales develop children's language skills and enhance their phonological competence. *$45.00*

264 pages
ISBN 0-93785 -59-9

5532 Getting a Grip on ADD: A Kid's Guide to Understanding & Coping with ADD

Educational Media Corporation
4256 Central Avenue NE
Box 21311
Minneapolis, MN 55421 **763-781-0088**
800-966-3382
FAX: 763-781-7753
educationalmedia.com

Don, Sorenson
President

Free catalog of resources.

64 pages Yearly

5533 Goldilocks and the Three Bears in Signed English

Gallaudet University Press
11030 S Langley Avenue
Chicago, IL 60628
800-621-2736
FAX: 800-621-8476
TTY:800-621-9347
gupress.gallaudet.edu

Harry Bornstein, Co-Author
Karen L Saulnier, Co-Author

The classic story is told again but with a twist. Full color illustrations show the Bears, Goldilocks and the text. Includes line drawings that show the story in Signed English. *$15.95*

48 pages Hardcover

5534 Guide to ACA Accredited Camps

American Camping Association
5000 State Road 67 N
Martinsville, IN 46151 **765-342-8456**
800-428-2267
FAX: 765-349-6357
e-mail: bookstore@ACAcamps.org
www.acacamps.org

Melody Snider, Director Bookstore/Distribution

A national listing of accredited camping programs. Listed by: special clientele, specific disabilities, camp name, activities. *$10.95*

Quarterly

5535 Guide to Summer Camps & Summer Schools

Porter Sargent Publishers
11 Beacon Street
Suite 1400
Boston, MA 02108 **617-523-1670**
800-342-7470
FAX: 617-523-1021
e-mail: orders@portersargent.com
www.portersargent.com

Daniel McKeever, Senior Editor
Leslie Weston, Production Manager

Covers the broad spectrum of recreational and educational summer opportunities in the USA and abroad. Current facts from 1300 camps and schools, as well as specialized programs for those with special needs or learning disabilities make the Guide a comprehensive resource. *$ 45.00*

640 pages Biennially 1954
ISBN 0-875581-45-5

5536 Handbook of Infant Mental Health

Guilford Press
72 Spring Street
New York, NY 10012 **212-431-9800**
800-365-7006
FAX: 212-966-6708
www.guilford.com

$65.00

Cloth
ISBN 1-572305-15-0

5537 Help for the Hyperactive Child: A Good Sense Guide for Parents

Professional Books
680 W Forrest Avenue
PO Box 3246
Jackson, TN 38303 **731-423-5400**

A large-print, easy-to-read book for parents and children that simply describes options and approaches to dealing with what have come to be known as hyperactivity, attention defecit disorder, and other behavior and learning problems.

245 pages Paperback 1991
ISBN 0-933478-18-6

5538 Helping Children Understand Disabilities

Brookline Books
PO Box 1046
Cambridge, MA 02238 **617-868-0360**
800-666-2665
FAX: 617-868-1772
e-mail: brooklinebks@delphi.com
www.brooklinebooks.com

Examines children's literature as a vehicle to help children, parents and teachers understand important issues relating to the effects of disability on children. Using the child as narrator, Quicke demonstrates how to use popular children's fiction to explore taboo areas and stimulate discussion by children and adults. *$10.95*

Hardcover
ISBN 0-91479 -09-3

5539 How to Raise a Healthy Child...In Spite of Your Doctor

Ballantine Books
4958 Main Street
Appartment 1
Downers Grove, IL 60515 **630-663-1472**
www.randomhouse.com/BB/

A practical and informative guide that demystifies medical treatment for children, helps parents determine what ailments require an office visit and which can be dealt with at home, and calms parents' fears with sound advice on childhood illnesses. Advises parents on home diagnosis and treatment of colds, flus, childhood illnesses, vision and hearing problems, and allergies.

1990
ISBN 0-345342-76-3

5540 Howie Helps Himself

Exceptional Parent Library
120 Sylvan Avenue, Suite 10
PO Box 1807
Englewood Cliffs, NJ 07632
800-535-1910
FAX: 201-947-9376
e-mail: eplibrary@aol.com
www.eplibrary.com

Joe Lasker, Illustrator

Designed to help the child with a disability and the sibling identify with some of the joys, stresses and strains of a disability. *$13.95*

32 pages 1987
ISBN 0-807534-22-6

5541 I'm Tougher Than Asthma!

Albert Whitman & Company
6340 Oakton Street
Morton Grove, IL 60053 **847-581-0033**
800-255-7675
FAX: 847-581-0039
e-mail: mail@awhitmanco.com
www.albertwhitman.com

Joe Boyd, President
Joe Campbell, Customer Service

Eight-year-old Siri loves to sing. play baseball, and catch toads. She won't let her asthma stop her! In her own words (with a little help from Dad), she tells how she was first diagnosed with asthma at age three and how she is learning to understand and manage her disease. *$ 6.95*

32 pages Paperback 1996
ISBN 0-807534-75-7

5542 I'm the Big Sister Now

Exceptional Parent Library
120 Sylvan Avenue, Suite 10
PO Box 1807
Englewood Cliffs, NJ 07632
800-535-1910
FAX: 201-947-9376
e-mail: eplibrary@aol.com
www.eplibrary.com

Nine-year old Michelle describes the joys and challenges of living with her older sister, Amy, who has severe cerebral palsy. A true story, recommended for ages six to ten. *$13.95*

32 pages Hardcover 1989
ISBN 0-807534-58-7

5543 Ideas for Kids on the Go

Accent Books & Products
PO Box 700
Bloomington, IL 61702 **309-378-2961**
800-787-8444
FAX: 309-378-4420
e-mail: acmtlvng@aol.com

Raymond C Cheever, Publisher
Betty Garee, Editor

This guide shows kids with physical disabilities how to go for it! Lists products and where to get them, and includes tips from others for having fun and getting ahead. Ages 1-18. *$6.95*

69 pages Paperback
ISBN 0-91570 -17-5

5544 Infant & Toddler Health Sourcebook

Omnigraphics
615 Griswold Street
Detroit, MI 48226
800-234-1340
FAX: 800-875-1340
www.omnigraphics.com

Paul Rogers, Publicity Associate
Georgiann Lauginger, Customer Service Manager

Includes information on the mental and physical development of infants, including nutrition and common pediatric disorders. *$78.00*

600 pages 1900

5545 It isn't Fair!: Siblings of Children with Disabilities

Greenwood Publishing Group
88 Post Road W
Suite 5007
Westport, CT 06880
203-226-3571
FAX: 203-222-1502
www.greenwood.com

This book presents a wide range of perspectives on the relationship of siblings to children with disabilities. These perspectives are written in the first person by parents, young adult siblings, younger siblings, and professionals.

200 pages $39.95 - $45
ISBN 0-897893-32-8

5546 JRA and Me

American Juvenile Arthritis Organization
1330 W Peachtree Street
PO Box 7669
Atlanta, GA 30326
404-872-7100
800-283-7800
FAX: 404-872-9559
e-mail: help@arthritis.org
www.arthritis.org

A workbook for school-aged children who have juvenile arthritis. This book offers a variety of educational games, puzzles and worksheets to teach children about their illness and how to take care of themselves. *$7.85*

57 pages

5547 Jason & Nordic Publishers

PO Box 441
Hollidaysburg, PA 16648
814-696-2920
FAX: 814-696-4250
e-mail: turtlbks@nb.net
www.jasonandnordic.com

Richard S McPhee, Director

Turtle Books for children with disabilities present heroes who look like them, have problems like theirs, have similar doubts and feelings in non-threatening, fun stories. They are motivational, bridge the gap and promote understanding among peers and siblings. 12 children's books (grades preK-3) plus Sensitivity and Awareness Guide containing lesson plans, activities, background information keyed to the series. Disabilities include: Down syndrome, cerebral palsy, blindness, deafness and more.

5548 Jazz Man

Atheneum
135 S Mount Zion Road
Lebanon, IN 46052
FAX: 800-882-8583

Zeke and his family moved to Harlem from the South and lived in a walk-up tenement. He didn't go to school; instead, he watched out the window all day, especially at the yellow room. The yellow room came to be inhabited by the Jazz Man, who played all day and night to the whole family's delight.

42 pages Paperback

5549 Joey and Sam

Exceptional Parent Library
120 Sylvan Avenue, Suite 10
PO Box 1807
Englewood Cliffs, NJ 07632
800-535-1910
FAX: 201-947-9376
e-mail: eplibrary@aol.com
www.eplibrary.com

Franz Borowitz, Illustrator
Edward Ritvo, Contributor

A heartwarming story about autism, a family and a brother's love. *$9.95*

Hardcover 1993
ISBN 1-882388-06-2

5550 Josh: A Boy with Dyslexia

Waterfront Books
85 Crescent Road
Burlington, VT 05401
802-658-7477
800-639-6063
FAX: 612-337-5050

The reader is taken into the heart and mind of a boy with LD as he struggles to live down the stigma of his learning differences and earns both respect and friendship from his peers. Also includes information on the characteristics of dyslexia and a list of organizations that deal with learning differences. *$7.95*

100 pages 1988
ISBN 0-91452 -18-2

5551 Jumpin' Johnny Get Back to Work, A Child's Guide to ADHD/Hyperactivity

25 Van Zant Street
Suite 15-5
E Norwalk, CT 06855
203-838-5010
FAX: 203-866-6108
e-mail: CACLD@optonline.net
www.CACLD.org

Beryl Kaufman, Executive Director

Written primarily for elementary age youngsters with ADHD to help them understand their disability. Also valuable as an educational tool for parents, siblings, friends and classmates. Includes two pages on medication. *$12.50*

24 pages

5552 Keeping Childhood

Alliance for Parental Involvement in Education
PO Box 59
E Chatham, NY 12060
518-392-6900
FAX: 518-392-6900

Understanding the anthropological views of child development. *$12.00*

5553 Kid Kare News

3101 SW Sam Jackson Park Road
Portland, OR 97201
FAX: 503-241-5090
www.shrinershq.org

Barbara Flaherty, New Patient Coordinator
Sonia Bouchard, Rehabilitation Services Manager
Kerry Grindeland, Care Coordination Manager

Bi-annual publication from the Shriners Hospital for Children in Portland, Oregon. Free. Produced by the medical staff.

5554 Kid-Friendly Parenting with Deaf and Hard of Hearing Children: A Treasury of Fun Activities

Gallaudet University Press
11030 S Langley Avenue
Chicago, IL 60628
800-621-2736
FAX: 800-621-8476
TTY:800-621-9347
gupress.gallaudet.edu

Denise Chapman, Co-Author
Daria Medwid, Co-Author

Scores of activities, parenting techniques and insights by experts, both hearing and deaf, to help parents of deaf and hard of hearing children. Activities are designed to promote better behavior and educate. *$24.95*

382 pages Softcover

5555 **Kidz Korner**

Children's Hopes & Dreams Wish Foundation
280 Route 46
Dover, NJ 07801 **973-361-7366**
800-437-3262
FAX: 973-361-6627
e-mail: chdfdover@juno.com
www.childrenswishes.org

6 pages Monthly

5556 **Kitten Who Couldn't Purr**

William Morrow & Company
1350 Avenue of the Americas
New York, NY 10019 **212-261-6500**
FAX: 212-261-6925

Jonathan the kitten doesn't know how to purr to say thank you, so he sets off to find someone to teach him. *$12.95*

32 pages

5557 **Language and the Developing Child**

International Dyslexia Association
Chester Building
Suite 382
Baltimore, MD 21286
800-ABC-D123
FAX: 410-296-0232
www.interdys.org

This collection of papers introduces a new generation of teachers, clinicians and parents to the work of one of the key figures in the search for the causes and treatment of dyslexia. *$15.00*

5558 **Let's Talk About Having Asthma**

Rosen Publishing Group's PowerKids Press
29 E 21st Street
New York, NY 10010 **212-777-3017**
800-237-9932
FAX: 888-436-4643
e-mail: rosenpub@tribeca.ios.com

This book talks about the cause and treatments for asthma as well as the precautions sufferers should take. Recommended for grades K-4. *$13.95*

ISBN 0-823950-32-8

5559 **Living with Asthma**

Walker Publishing Company
435 Hudson Street
New York, NY 10014 **212-727-8300**
800-289-2553
FAX: 212-727-0984
e-mail: orders@walkerbooks.com
www.walkerbooks.com

Up-to-date guide for children with asthma as well as the parents of sufferers. *$14.95*

112 pages Library Binding 1900
ISBN 0-613260-43-0

5560 **Lollipop Lunch**

Speech Bin
1965 25th Avenue
Vero Beach, FL 32960 **772-770-0007**
800-477-3324
FAX: 772-770-0006
www.speechbin.com

Cleverly illustrated stories and activities for phonological and language development. *$19.95*

128 pages
ISBN 0-93785 -54-8

5561 **Loop the Loop**

William Morrow & Company
1350 Avenue of the Americas
New York, NY 10019 **212-974-3100**
FAX: 212-974-3188
www.williammorrow.com

Anne has never met anyone like Mrs. Simpson. She travels in a wheelchair and performs fabulous yo-yo tricks. *$14.00*

32 pages

5562 **Luke Has Asthma, Too**

Waterfront Books
85 Crescent Road
Burlington, VT 05401 **802-658-7477**
800-639-6063
FAX: 612-337-5050

This gentle book will make for good reading with children whether they have asthma or not. The story shows that asthma can be managed in a calm fashion. The child who has moderate asthma can now have a normal life, taking part in all sports and special activities. For the more than two million families who have children with asthma, this is an important message.

32 pages Paperback 1988
ISBN 0-91452 -06-9

5563 **Lynda Madaras Talks to Teens About Aids**

Waterfront Books
85 Crescent Road
Burlington, VT 05401 **802-658-7477**

Guide for parents, teachers and young people about the subject of AIDS. Especially for fourteen to nineteen-year-olds. Preface shows parents and teachers how to use the book with youngsters.

106 pages Hardcover 1988
ISBN 1-557040-10-9

5564 **Mandy**

William Morrow & Company
1350 Avenue of the Americas
New York, NY 10019 **212-974-3100**
FAX: 212-261-6595
www.williammorrow.com

Told from the point of view of a deaf child, this warm picture book is neither saccharine nor preachy. Mandy has never heard anyone speak or sing. It is from her close relationship with her grandmother that the small girl learns about the world through lip-reading, facial expression, gesture, touch and sign. *$14.95*

32 pages

5565 **Me, Too**

JB Lippincott
227 E Washington Square
Philadelphia, PA 19106 **215-238-4200**
800-777-2295
FAX: 215-824-7390

Lydia and Lornie were twins. Lydia was a bright twelve year old who vowed to spend her summer vacation teaching her retarded sister, Lornie, how to be normal.

158 pages Hardcover

ISBN 0-39731 -85-X

5566 **Mine for Keeps**

Little, Brown & Company
1271 Avenue of the Americas
New York, NY 10020 **212-522-7200**
800-343-9204
FAX: 212-522-7989

Lewis Parker, Illustrator

Sarah Jean Copeland was born with cerebral palsy. At four years of age she was placed in a school for handicapped children but made such good progress that she could return home. Coming home for Sarah meant a new school, and new adjustments to her parents, two sisters, and her brother. At first Sarah was scared and didn't think she could do all the things she needed to do, but she soon learned her fears were not well-founded.

186 pages Paperback 1988

ISBN 0-316528-00-5

5567 **My Book for Kids with Cancer: A Child's Autobiography of Hope**

Waterfront Books
85 Crescent Road
Burlington, VT 05401 **802-658-7477**
800-639-6063
FAX: 612-337-5050

Tim Gaes, Illustrator

Frustrated because he couldn't find any books about kids who survived cancer, Jason decided to write his own. This book is a poignant, true story of courage and hope which describes his successful battle against the disease. *$12.95*

32 pages 1987

ISBN 0-937603-04-X

5568 **My Buddy**

Exceptional Parent Library
120 Sylvan Avenue, Suite 10
PO Box 1807
Englewood Cliffs, NJ 07632
800-535-1910
FAX: 201-947-9376
e-mail: eplibrary@aol.com
www.eplibrary.com

Story focuses on the friendship between a boy with a disability and his loyal golden retriever. *$5.95*

Library Binding 1999

ISBN 0-785799-24-9

5569 **My Signing Book of Numbers**

Gallaudet University Press
800 Florida Avenue NE
Washington, DC 20002 **202-651-5000**
800-621-2736
FAX: 202-651-5489
TTY:888-630-9347

Dan Wallace, Marketing Manager

This full-color book helps children learn their numbers in sign language. Each two-page spread of this delightfully illustrated book has the appropriate number of things or creatures for the numbers 0 through 20. *$14.95*

56 pages Hardcover

ISBN 0-93032 -37-8

5570 **Natural Child Care: A Complete Guide to Safe Holistic Remedies for Infants and Children**

Crown Publishing Group
1540 Broadway
New York, NY 10036 **212-782-9000**
FAX: 212-302-7985

Devoted to raising children by natural, holistic, drug-free methods, this comprehensive guide includes charts showing the uses of sixty readily available medicinal herbs.

Paperback 1989

ISBN 0-517568-31-4

5571 **Negotiating the Special Education Maze: A Guide for Parents and Teachers**

Spina Bifida Association of America
4590 MacArthur Boulevard
Suite 250
Washington, DC 20007 **202-944-3285**
800-621-3141
FAX: 202-944-3295
e-mail: sbaa@sbaa.org
www.sbaa.org

An excellent aid for the development of an effective special education program. *$19.00*

5572 **New Language of Toys: Teaching Communicati on Skills to Children with Special Needs**

Spina Bifida Association of America
4590 MacArthur Boulevard NW
Suite 250
Washington, DC 20007 **202-944-3285**
800-621-3141
FAX: 202-944-3295
e-mail: sbaa@sbaa.org
www.sbaa.org

A guide for parents and teachers and a reader-friendly resource guide that provides a wealth of information on how play activities affect a child's language development and where to get the toys and materials to use in these activities. *$19.00*

5573 **New York Families for Autistic Children**

95-16 Pitkin Avenue
Ozone Park, NY 11417 **718-641-3441**
FAX: 718-641-4452

5574 **Nick Joins In**

Spina Bifida Association of America
4590 Macarthur Boulevard NW
Suite 250
Washington, DC 20007 **202-994-3285**
800-621-3141
FAX: 202-944-3295
e-mail: sbaa@sbaa.org
www.sbaa.org

When Nick, who is in a wheelchair, enters a regular classroom for the first time, he realizes that he has much to contribute. *$17.00*

5575 **Nursery Rhymes from Mother Goose**

Gallaudet University Press
800 Florida Avenue NE
Washington, DC 20002 **202-651-5000**
FAX: 202-651-5704
TTY:888-630-8347

Dan Wallace, Marketing Manager

Each complete nursery rhyme is presented in Signed English and delightfully illustrated in full color. *$14.95*

64 pages

ISBN 0-93032 -99-8

5576 **On Our Own Terms: Children Living with Physical Disabilities**

Gareth Stevens
1555 N River Center Drive
Milwaukee, WI 53212 **414-225-0333**
800-542-2595
FAX: 414-225-0377

Meet Kicki, a three-year-old with Spina Bifida, battling to walk for the first time. Meet Annelie, nine years old, learning to walk again after a bad car accident. Face the physical challenges with her. *$13.95*

48 pages

ISBN 1-555329-42-X

5577 **One Day at a Time: Children Living with Leukemia**

Gareth Stevens
1555 N Rivercenter Drive
Milwaukee, WI 53212 **414-225-0333**
800-542-2595
FAX: 414-225-0377
beta.healthlinkusa.com/bookpage/184_27.html

Claire Messier, Marketing Associate

Focus on Hanna, two years old, and 3 year old Frederick. Both diagnosed with Leukemia and follows them as they are treated for their illness. Includes such daily routines as eating breakfast, washing and playing. *$16.95*

56 pages Hardcover

ISBN 1-55532 -13-6

5578 **Out of the Corner of My Eye**

American Foundation for the Blind/AFB Press
PO Box 1020
Sewickley, PA 15143 **412-741-1142**
800-232-3044
FAX: 412-741-0609
e-mail: afborders@abdintl.com
www.afb.org

A personal account of students' vision loss and subsequent adjustment that is full of practical advice and cheerful encouragement, told by an 87 year old retired college teacher who has maintained her independence and zest for life. *$14.95*

ISBN 0-891281-93-2

5579 **Parent Teacher Packet**

Spina Bifida Association of America
4590 MacArthur Boulevard NW
Suite 250
Washington, DC 20007 **202-944-3285**
800-621-3141
FAX: 202-944-3295
e-mail: sbaa@sbaa.org
www.sbaa.org

Includes educational material, learning disabilities literature, children's book, social development and the person with spina bifida and one copy of each fact sheet. *$14.00*

5580 **Pinballs**

Harpercollins
10 E 53rd Street
Cellar 1
New York, NY 10022 **212-207-7042**
800-242-7737
FAX: 212-207-7203

The story of three children who are placed in foster care: Harvey, whose two broken legs were crushed when his drunken father ran over him in a car; Thomas J., who was left at the door of an eighty-year-old couple as a toddler; and Carlie, a street-wise kid who caused trouble at home with her many step fathers. The children were defiant at first, than the fine Mason home began to take effect. The children first began to like each other and then faced their problems.

136 pages Hardcover 1993

ISBN 0-064401-98-7

5581 **Please Don't Say Hello**

Human Sciences Press
233 Spring Street
New York, NY 10013 **212-229-2859**
800-221-9369
FAX: 212-463-0742

Paul and his family moved into a new neighborhood. Paul's brother was autistic. The children thought that Eddie was retarded until they learned that there were skills that he could do better than they could. *$10.95*

47 pages Paperback

ISBN 0-89885 -99-8

5582 **Princess Pooh**

Spina Bifida Association of America
4590 Macarthur Boulevard NW
Suite 250
Washington, DC 20007 **202-944-3285**
800-621-3141
FAX: 202-944-3295
e-mail: sbaa@sbaa.org
www.sbaa.org

Jealous of her weelchair bound sister's supposed privileges, Patty Jean borrows her sister's throne for an afternoon. She discovers that wheelchairs are not as much fun as she thought. For elementary age children. *$17.00*

32 pages 1989

5583 **Quad City Deaf & Hard of Hearing Youth Group: Tomorrow's Leaders for our Community**

Independent Living Research Utilization ILRU
2323 S Shepherd Drive
Suite 1000
Houston, TX 77019 **713-520-0232**
FAX: 713-520-5785
www.ilru.org

IICIL staff see this program as a way to develop young leaders for themovement. Emphasis is given to providing oppportunities for memebers of the youth group to develop skills in planning and organizing activities.

10 pages

5584 **Raising a Child Who Has a Physical Disability**

Exceptional Parent Library
120 Sylvan Avenue, Suite 10
PO Box 1807
Englewood Cliffs, NJ 07632
800-535-1910
FAX: 201-947-9376
e-mail: eplibrary@aol.com
www.eplibrary.com

The author draws on her personal experience with her own daughters to cover everything from dealing with medications, diet, and hygiene to developing positive self-esteem and choosing clothing, in this encouraging book that offers practical advice on every as[ect of loving and living with a special needs child. *$12.95*

228 pages 1995
ISBN 0-471042-40-4

5585 **Rajesh**

Atheneum
135 S Mount Zion Road
Lebanon, IN 46052
FAX: 800-882-8583

Rajesh, a student in a headstart program, was born without complete legs and must wear two prostheses to walk. When Rajesh first attended school he found that older children teased him. After he explained about his legs to the class, his classmates began to accept him.

32 pages Hardcover
ISBN 0-68931 -74-9

5586 **Reading, Writing and Speech Problems in Children**

International Dyslexia Association
Chester Building
Suite 382
Baltimore, MD 21286
800-ABC-D123
FAX: 410-296-0232
www.interdys.org

A tribute to the man who more than any other aroused the attention of the scientific community and who provided the sound educational principles on which much teaching of dyslexics today is based. *$27.00*

ISBN 0-89079 -79-1

5587 **Reflections on Growing Up Disabled**

Council for Exceptional Children
1110 N Glebe Road
Suite 300
Arlington, VA 22201
703-620-3660
FAX: 703-264-9494
www.cec.sped.org

Janice Burdick, President

Understand how it feels to be a disabled person in school by tuning in to the first-hand accounts of people who have disabilities. *$10.00*

112 pages

5588 **Rehab Update**

New England Medical Center
750 Washington Street
Suite 75 K-R
Boston, MA 02111
617-636-5000
FAX: 617-636-4269

Vincent Licenziato, Training Coordinator

Reports on causes and consequences of injuries among children and adolescents. Focus on rehabilitation research, family adjustment, special education, and violence prevention. Special attention on brain injury among youth.

8 pages BiAnnual

5589 **Ride the Red Cycle**

Houghton Mifflin
222 Berkely Street
Boston, MA 02116
617-351-5000
800-225-3362
www.hmco.com

Jerome Johnson is nine, but due to brain damage he can't walk and his speech is hard to understand. Jerome gets around in a wheelchair, but he knows that if he could get a tricycle he could go where and when he wanted. His parents not only agreed to buy him the cycle, but his dad built up the pedals and added a seat with a back and a seatbelt to hold Jerome.

34 pages Hardcover
ISBN 0-39529 -83-6

5590 **Rolling Along with Goldilocks and the Thre e Bears**

Spina Bifida Association of America
4590 Macarthur Boulevard NW
Suite 250
Washington, DC 20007
202-944-3285
800-621-3141
FAX: 202-944-3295
e-mail: sbaa@sbaa.org
www.sbaa.org

The familiar fairytale with a special needs twist. Ages 3-7. *$17.00*

5591 **Rose-Colored Glasses**

Human Sciences Press
233 Spring Street
New York, NY 10013
212-229-2859
800-221-9369
FAX: 212-463-0742

After a vacation, Deborah was excited about going back to school. Renewing old friendships, she met a classmate who seemed stuck up. Deborah learned that Melanie was in a recent accident resulting in impaired vision. She did not wish to wear her glasses, which were rose-colored and very funny looking. With Deborah's help, Miss Davis, the teacher showed a blurry film and then had Melanie speak about her impaired vision. When Melanie began to participate in the class they accepted her. *$16.95*

30 pages Hardcover
ISBN 0-87705 -08-8

5592 **Seeing-Children Living with Blindness**

Gareth Stevens
1555 N RiverCenter Drive
Milwaukee, WI 53212
414-225-0333
800-341-3569
FAX: 414-225-0377

Go with Thomas to a special school for children who can't see, where you will meet Andrew, Kate, Jordan, Katherine, Peter and Kent. Read what they told Thomas about being blind, about daily life, their feelings, the funny things, and the sad. *$10.95*

ISBN 1-555329-15-2

5593 **Self-Control Games & Workbook**

Western Psychological Services
12031 Wilshire Boulevard
Los Angeles, CA 90025
310-478-2061
800-648-8857
FAX: 310-478-7838

This game is designed to teach self-control in academic and social situations. Addresses a total of 24 impulsive, inattentive and hyperactive behaviors. The companion workbook reinforces the use of positive self-statements, and problem-solving techniques, instead of expressing anger. *$62.50*

Game TCGS

5594 **Sleeping Beauty**

Gallaudet University Press
800 Florida Avenue NE
Washington, DC 20002
202-651-5000
800-621-2736
FAX: 800-660-8476
TTY:888-630-9347

Dan Wallace, Marketing Manager

The popular fairytale of the princess put to sleep for a hundred years is presented with beautiful full color illustrations and selected sentences in American Sign Language. *$14.95*

64 pages
ISBN 0-93032 -97-1

5595 **Solve Your Child's Sleep Problems**

Simon & Schuster
100 Front Street
Riverside, NJ 07085
800-323-7445
www.simonsays.com

Offers advice and concrete help when lullabies are not enough to luu your child into dreamland. Based on the authors research as director of Boston's Center for Pediatric Sleep Disorders at Children's Hospital. Guide to common sleeping problems from ages one to six. Detailed case histories on night walking, difficulty sleeping, and more serious disorders such as sleep apnea and sleepwalking help illustrate a wide variety of problems and thier solutions.

251 pages Paperback 1986
ISBN 0-671620-99-1

5596 **Solving the Puzzle of the Hyperactive Child**

Professional Books
211 N Sycamore
Newtown, PA 18940
215-504-1700
FAX: 215-860-5374

An excellent book which summarizes the many things that can make children hard to raise and provides workable solutions.

1987

5597 **Somebody Called Me a Retard Today...and My Heart Felt Sad**

Walker Publishing Company
435 Hudson Street
New York, NY 10014
212-727-8300
800-289-2553
FAX: 212-727-0984
e-mail: orders@walkerbooks.com
www.walkerbooks.com

David Garner, Illustrator

A simple, moving story that empowers mentally challenged children and sensitizes everyone to the need to celebrate the differences in all of us. *$14.85*

24 pages Cloth/Hardcover
ISBN 0-802781-97-7

5598 **Son-Rise: The Miracle Continues**

2080 S Undermountain Road
Sheffield, MA 01257
413-229-2100
800-562-7171
FAX: 413-229-3202
e-mail: sonrise@option.org
www.son-rise.org

Part One is the astonishing record of Raun Kaufman's development from an autistic and retarded child into a loving, brilliant youngster who shows no traces of his former condition. Part Two follows Raun's development after the age of four, teaching the limitless possibilities of the Son-Rise Program. Part Three shares moving accounts of five other ordinary families who became extraordinary when they used the Son-Rise Program to reach their own unreachable children. *$12.95*

343 pages
ISBN 0-915811-53-7

5599 **Sorrow's Song**

Atlantic-Little Brown
34 Beacon Street
Boston, MA 02108
800-343-9204
FAX: 800-286-9471
www.twbookmark.com

Sorrow never learned to talk. Her parents had taken her to all the specialists to find out why she couldn't talk, but no reason was ever found.

150 pages Hardcover
ISBN 0-31612 -97-4

5600 **Sound Connections for the Adolescent**

Speech Bin
1965 25th Avenue
Vero Beach, FL 32960
772-770-0007
800-477-3324
FAX: 772-770-0006
www.speechbin.com

A resource to help older elementary and secondary students understand their sound systems an how it functions. It targets skills critical for academic achievement: phonological awareness, phonemic relationships, phonemic processing, listening and memory and teaches linguistic rules they need to succeed. *$19.95*

Paperback

5601 **Special Education Report**

Aspen Publishers
7201 McKinney Circle
Frederick, MD 21704
301-417-7591
800-638-8437
FAX: 301-695-7931
e-mail: customer.service@aspenpubl.com
www.aspenpublishers.com

Published biweekly, Special Education Report is the independent news service on law, policy and funding of programs for disabled children. *$16.00*

8-12 pages Newsletter

5602 **Special Format Books for Children and Youth Ages 3-19**

New York State Library
Cultural Education Center
Albany, NY 12230
518-474-5935
800-342-3688
www.nysl.nysed.gov/tbbl/index.html

Jane Somers, Director

5603 Special Format Books for Children and Youth: Ages 3-19.Serving New York City/Long Island

Ney York Public Library
476 5th Avenue
New York, NY 10018 **212-206-5400**
e-mail: pleclerc@nypl.org
www.nypl.org

Paul LeClerc, President

5604 Steps to Independence: Teaching Everyday S kills to Children with Special Needs

Spina Bifida Association of America
4590 MacArthur Boulevard NW
Suite 250
Washington, DC 20007 **202-944-3285**
800-621-3141
FAX: 202-944-3295
e-mail: sbaa@sbaa.org
www.sbaa.org

A guide to help parents teach life skills to their disabled child. *$28.00*

5605 Straight Talk About Psychiatric Medications for Kids

Guilford Press
72 Spring Street
New York, NY 10012 **212-431-9800**
FAX: 212-966-6708
www.guilford.com

Also in cloth at $29.95 (ISBN# 1-57230-404-9 *$35.00*

280 pages Paperback 1998
ISBN 1-572302-04-6

5606 Students with Learning Disabilities

McGraw-Hill, School Publishing
220 E Danieldale Road
DeSoto, TX 75115 **972-224-1111**
800-442-9685
FAX: 972-228-1982
mhschool.com

A comprehensive text which introduces students to the entire field of learning disabilities.

512 pages

5607 Superkids

Superkids
60 Clyde Street
Newton, MA 02460
www.super-kids.org

Non-profit organization and newsletter for families and friends of children with limb differences. It is published twice a year and is free to interested families and professionals. Offers timely information and support to those affected by limb differences.

5608 Talkable Tales

Speech Bin
1965 25th Avenue
Vero Beach, FL 32960 **772-770-0007**
800-477-3324
FAX: 772-770-0006
www.speechbin.com

Jan J Binney, Senior Editor

Read-a-rebus stories and pictures targeting most consonant phonemes for K-5 children. *$25.95*

128 pages
ISBN 0-93783 -44-0

5609 Teen Mental Health Book

Omnigraphics
615 Griswold Street
Detroit, MI 48226
800-234-1340
FAX: 800-875-1340
www.omnigraphics.com

Georgiann Lauginiger, Customer Service Manager

Health tips for teens about mental health and mental illness, including facts about depression, suicide, addictive disorders, eating disorders, obsessive-compulsive disorders, panic attacks, phobias, schizophrenia, aggression, violence and more. *$48.00*

250 pages Hardcover 1900
ISBN 0-780804-42-2

5610 Tempered Wind

Atheneum
135 S Mount Zion Road
Lebanon, IN 46052
FAX: 800-882-8583

Gabrielle was a dwarf and was never out of her house until her parents died and she was sent from one aunt to the next. At age thirteen she was enrolled in school for the first time. The children teased her about being a dwarf, and although she excelled academically, she failed socially. After three years in school an illness forced her aunt to take Gabrielle to the doctor. The doctor's prognosis was grim and led Gabrielle's aunt to tell her that she would have to find a job.

210 pages Hardcover
ISBN 0-68931 -39-X

5611 Texas Families

7701 N Lamar Boulevard
Suite 505
Austin, TX 78752 **512-407-8844**
866-893-3264
FAX: 512-407-8266
e-mail: info@txffcmh.org
www.txffcmh.org

Patti Derr, Executive Director
Pat Calley, Board Chair
SG Barron, Director of Operations

A quarterly publication from Texas Federation of Families for Children's Mental Health. Free.

8 pages Quarterly

5612 Thinking Big

William Morrow & Company
1350 Avenue of the Americas
New York, NY 10019 **212-974-3100**
FAX: 212-261-6595
www.williammorrow.com

Eight-year-old Jaime's lively personality shines through in this perceptive photo essay which explains what being a dwarf means physically and then presents Jaime's world at home and at school from her viewpoint. *$15.95*

48 pages

5613 Tourette Syndrome Association Children's Newsletter

42-40 Bell Boulevard
Bayside, NY 11361 **718-224-2999**
800-237-0717
FAX: 718-279-9596
e-mail: ts@tsa-usa.org
www.tsa-usa.org

Fred Cook, Chair
Judit Ungar, President

National, nonprofit membership organization. Mission is to identify the cause of, find the cure for, and control the effects of this disorder. A growing number of local chapters nationwide provide educational materials, seminars, conferences and support groups for over 35,000 members.

5614 Trouble with Explosives

Bradbury Press
135 S Mount Zion Road
Lebanon, IN 46052
800-257-5755
FAX: 800-882-8583

Polly moved regularly with her family, changing schools almost every year. This was especially difficult as she couldn't pronounce her explosive name, Polly Banks, without stuttering.

117 pages Hardcover
ISBN 0-87888 -94-1

5615 Understanding Cub Scouts with Disabilities

Boy Scouts of America
1325 W Walnut Hill Lane
Irving, TX 75038
214-351-1010
800-323-0732

Manual on how to teach and understand boy scouts with handicaps.

10 pages

5616 Vegetarian Baby: A Sensible Guide for Parents

McBooks Press
ID Booth Building
520 N Meadow Street
Ithaca, NY 14850
607-272-2114
888-266-5711
FAX: 607-273-6068
e-mail: mcbooks@mcbooks.com
www.mcbooks.com

Tom Parker, Illustrator

Gives information on the basics of a healthy diet, how to prepare vegetarian foods, and when to introduce different types of foods; includes recipes.

224 pages Paperback 1980
ISBN 0-935526-02-1

5617 Views from Our Shoes

Spina Bifida Association of America
4590 MacArthur Boulevard
Washington, DC 20007
202-944-3285
800-621-3141
FAX: 202-944-3295
e-mail: sbaa@sbaa.org
www.sbaa.org

Siblings share what it is like to have a brother or sister with a disability. Age 9 and up. *$17.00*

106 pages Paperback

5618 We Laugh, We Love, We Cry: Children Living with Mental Retardation

Gareth Stevens
1555 N River Center Drive
Milwaukee, WI 53212
414-225-0333
800-524-2595
FAX: 414-225-0377

Two sisters, Asa and Anna Karin, are mentally retarded. They find it hard to understand things quickly, so learning to walk and talk has been slow work for them. With help from their parents, friends and teachers and their doctors, they are both learning to do the things that most of us are not lucky enough to learn easily. *$13.95*

48 pages
ISBN 1-555329-14-4

5619 What About Me? Growing Up with a Developmentally Disabled Sibling

Plenum Publishing Corporation
233 Spring Street
Floor 7
New York, NY 10013
212-620-8000
800-221-9369
FAX: 212-463-0742
e-mail: info@plenum.com
www.enotalone.com/books/ASIN/073820630X.html

Includes a personal account of a physician's experiences as the older brother of an autistic sibling, discussion of family approachs to handicaps, and a review of research on family factors and adjustments of the nonimpaired siblings, along with an analysis of family coping and defenses patterened on the Adult Children of Alcoholics model. *$24.95*

296 pages Hardcover 1994
ISBN 0-30644 -50-2

5620 What Happens Next?

Exceptional Parent Library- Star Bright Books
120 Sylvan Avenue, Suite 10
PO Box 1807
Englewood Cliffs, NJ 07632
800-535-1910
FAX: 201-947-9376
e-mail: eplibrary@aol.com
www.eplibrary.com

Photo-flap book where babies lift the sturdy flap, page by page, to find out what happens next. *$4.95*

14 pages Hardcover 1996
ISBN 1-887734-10-4

5621 What It's Like to be Me

Friendship Press
PO Box 37844
Cincinnati, OH 45222
513-948-8733
FAX: 513-761-3722
www.ncccusa.org

Nancy Kennedy, Customer Service

This was written and illustrated entirely by children with handicapped conditions. These contributions invite the reader to set aside any pity or prejudices and listen. Black and white, and color drawings and photographs make this book visually appealing, enjoyable for all ages. *$10.95*

5622 What's a Virus, Anyway? The Kid's Book About AIDS

Waterfront Books
85 Crescent Road
Burlington, VT 05401
802-658-7477

A simple introduction to help adults talk with children about the subject of AIDS. Includes children's drawings and questions and provides basic information in a manner appropriate for 4-10 years old. *$8.95*

67 pages

5623 Wheels for Walking

Little, Brown & Company
1271 Avenue of the Americas
New York, NY 10020
212-522-7200
800-343-9204
FAX: 212-522-7989

Sally tried to accept the rules and regulations set up by her family. As a teenager she didn't understand why her parents doubted her judgement. Sally rebelled and insisted on going on a trip with her boyfriend. Although the weekend was innocent, it ended in a car accident that left her a quadriplegic.

195 pages Hardcover 1988
ISBN 0-451152-35-2

5624 You Can Control Asthma: A Book for Families

Asthma and Allergy Foundation of America
1125 15th Street NW
Suite 502
Washington, DC 20005 **202-466-7643**
FAX: 202-466-8940
e-mail: info@aafa.org
www.aafa.org

Workbook to help families learn everything one needs to know about asthma. Learn how to keep episodes from starting, what to do when an asthma episode starts, how to use peak flow meters, spacers, and inhalers through the use of pictures, captions, and activities. *$5.50*

61 pages 1987

5625 You Can Control Asthma: A Book for Kids

Asthma and Allergy Foundation of America
1125 15th Street NW
Suite 502
Washington, DC 20005 **202-466-7643**
FAX: 202-466-8940
e-mail: info@aafa.org
www.aafa.org

Workbook to help kids, six to twelve, to make choices and to feel more in control of their asthma. Learn how to keep episodes from starting, what to do when an asthma episode starts, how to use peak flow meters, spacers, and inhalers through the use of pictures, captions, and activities. *$5.50*

45 pages 1987

5626 You Seem Like a Regular Kid to Me

American Foundation for the Blind/AFB Press
PO Box 1020
Sewickley, PA 15143 **412-741-1142**
800-232-3044
FAX: 412-741-0609
e-mail: afborders@abdintl.com
www.afb.org

An interview with Jane, a blind child, tells other children what it's like to be blind. Jane explains how she gets around, takes care of herself, does her school work, spends her leisure time and even pays for things when she can't see money.

16 pages
ISBN 0-891289-21-6

Community

5627 A Commitment to Inclusion: Outreach to Unserved/Underserved Populations

Independent Living Research Utilization ILRU
2323 S Shepherd Drive
Suite 1000
Houston, TX 77019 **713-520-0232**
FAX: 713-520-5785
www.ilru.org

Carol Bradley describes Independent Living Resource Center San francisco's community organizing/outreach approach to serving under-represented consumers. This organization successfully reaches persons with pychiatric disabilities, environmental illness/multiple chemical sensitivities, chronic fatigue immune deficiency syndrome, learning disabilities, institutionalized persons, Chinese, Latinos, deaf/hard of hearing, and lesbian/bisexual populations.

10 pages

5628 A World Awaits You

Mobility International USA
PO Box 10767
Eugene, OR 97440 **541-343-1284**
FAX: 541-343-6812
e-mail: info@miusa.org
www.miusa.org

Susan Sygall, Executive Director
Pamela Houston, Public Relations Coordinator
Tracy Scharn, Editor

A yearly publication from Mobility International USA. Free.

44 pages Yearly

5629 Advocacy-Oriented Peer Support: Moving from Talk to Action

Independent Living Research Utilization ILRU
2323 S Shepherd Drive
Suite 1000
Houston, TX 77019 **713-520-0232**
FAX: 713-520-5785
www.ilru.org

This month's Readings examines how staff at centers for independent living can identify and support potential leaders who will move beyond talking about their problems to making changes in their communities.

10 pages

5630 Annual Community Awards Booklet

National Organization on Disability
910 16th Street NW
Suite 600
Washington, DC 20006 **202-293-5960**
FAX: 202-293-7999
e-mail: ability@nod.org
www.nod.org

Alan Reich, President
Brewster Thackeray, VP, Communications
John Hershey, Advice and Resource Manager

Information on disability programs in communities across the nation.

5631 Arc Connection Newsletter

Arc of Tennessee
44 Vantage Way
Suite 550
Nashville, TN 37228 **615-248-5878**
800-835-7077
FAX: 615-248-5879
e-mail: pcooper@thearctn.org
www.thearctn.org

Quarterly publication from the ARC of Tennessee. *$10.00*

12 pages Quarterly

5632 Asthma and Allergy Answers: A Patient Education Library

Asthma and Allergy Foundation of America
1125 15th Street NW
Suite 502
Washington, DC 20005 **202-466-7643**
FAX: 202-466-8940
e-mail: info@aafa.org
www.aafa.org

A resource tool has information on more than 40 topics of interest to patients. These reproducible camera ready Answers are written in a patient friendly questions and answer format. There is space to personalize these handy patient education materials with your practice or facility information. *$50.00*

5633 California Community Care News

Charles W Skoien Jr
1924 Alhambra Boulevard
PO Box 163270
Sacramento, CA 95816 **916-455-0723**
FAX: 916-455-7201
e-mail: sncnews@aol.com

Charles W Skoien Jr, Editor/Publisher

Forum for the exchange of ideas, information and opinions among clients, families and service providers. Information regarding services and assisted living programs for the elderly, mentally ill and disabled. *$45.00*

24 pages Monthly

5634 Community Recreation and People with Disabilities: Strategies for Inclusion

Brookes Publishing
PO Box 10624
Baltimore, MD 21285 **410-337-9580**
800-638-3775
FAX: 410-337-8539
e-mail: custserv@brookespublishing.com
www.brookespublishing.com

Offers creative ideas and new techniques for including people with disabilities in community recreation programs. *$39.00*

368 pages Paperback 1997
ISBN 1-55766 -59-2

5635 Crossing the River: Creating a Conceptual Revolution in Community & Disability

Brookline Books
PO Box 1047
Cambridge, MA 02238 **617-868-0360**
800-666-2665
FAX: 617-868-1772
e-mail: brooklinebks@delphi.com
www.brooklinebooks.com

For persons with disabilities, a new conception of care is beginning to emerge—a conception seeking to embed these persons in a web of personal relationships, and to involve them in the dynamics of their community. Schwartz explores the promise, potential, and limits of this new direction. *$24.95*

238 pages Paperback
ISBN 0-91479 -82-4

5636 Culture and the Restructuring of Community Mental Health

Greenwood Publishing Group
88 Post Road W
Suite 5007
Westport, CT 06880 **203-226-3571**
FAX: 203-222-1502
www.greenwood.com

Examines treatment, organizational planning and research issues and offers a critique of the theoretical and programmatic aspects of providing mental health services to traditionally underserved populations. $45.00-$52.95.

168 pages Hardcover
ISBN 0-313268-87-8

5637 Disablement in the Community

Oxford University Press
2001 Evans Road
Cary, NC 27513 **212-726-6000**
800-451-7556
FAX: 919-677-1303
www.oup-usa.org

This book shows how the knowledge of the epidemiology of disablement can help planners, service providers, patients and voluntary organizations choose strategies for community care. *$39.95*

248 pages Illustrated

5638 Empowering Youth

Independent Living Research Utilization ILRU
2323 S Shepherd Drive
Suite 1000
Houston, TX 77019 **713-520-0232**
FAX: 713-520-5785
www.ilru.org

The Disabilities Network of Eastern Connecticut recognized that in order for young people to take on leadership roles and bring about change in their communities, they needed support in establishing their own identities. DNEC's innovative program demonstrates how they combined peer support and hands-on advocacy projects to empower teens to become leaders.

10 pages

5639 Free and User Supported Software for the IBM PC: A Resource Guide

McFarland & Company
PO Box 611
Jefferson, NC 28640 **336-246-4460**
800-253-2187
FAX: 336-246-5018
www.mcfarlandpub.com

A selection of word processing, database management, spreadsheets, and graphics programs are described and evaluated. Describes how the program works and its strengths and weaknesses. Rating charts cover such aspects as ease of use, ease of learning, documentation, and general utility. *$27.50*

224 pages Paperback
ISBN 0-89950 -99-0

5640 HealthViews

New Orleans VA Medical Center
1601 Perdido Street
New Orleans, LA 70112 **504-568-0811**
800-935-8387
FAX: 504-589-5210
e-mail: Stacie.Rivera@med.va.gov
www.va.gov

John D Church, Jr, Medical Center Director
Fernando Rivera, Assoc Medical Center Director
Sam Lucero, Special Assistant to Director

A teaching hospital, providing a full range of patient care services, with state-of-the-art technology as well as education and research. Comprehensive health care is provided through primary care, tetiary care, and long-term care in areas of medicine, surgery, psychiatry, physical medicine and rehabilitation, neurology, oncology, dentistry, geriatrics, and extended care.

quarterly

5641 Home and Community Care for Chronically Ill Children

Oxford University Press
2001 Evans Road
Cary, NC 27513
212-726-6000
800-451-7556
FAX: 919-677-1303
www.oup-usa.org

This book lays common ground for all who have reason and responsibility to enhance the capability of families to care for their ill children over the long term at home. *$32.95*

192 pages

5642 Housing, Support, and Community

Brookes Publishing
PO Box 10624
Baltimore, MD 21285
410-337-9580
800-638-3775
FAX: 410-337-8539
e-mail: custserv@brookespublishing.com
www.brookespublishing.com

Choices and strategies for adults with disabilities. *$ 32.00*

416 pages Paperback
ISBN 1-55766 -90-5

5643 Inclusive Child Care for Infants and Toddlers: Meeting Individual and Special Needs

Brookes Publishing
PO Box 10624
Baltimore, MD 21285
410-337-9580
800-638-3775
FAX: 410-337-8539
e-mail: custserv@brookespublishing.com
www.brookespublishing.com

This book gives child care providers the practical guidance they need to serve infants and toddlers with and without disabilities in inclusive settings. It offers information and helpful advice on handling daily care tasks, teaching responsively, meeting individual needs, developing rapport with parents, understanding toddlers' behavior, working with IFSPs, and maintaining high standards of care. *$34.95*

400 pages Paperback 1997
ISBN 1-55766 -96-7

5644 Independence & Transition to Community Living: The Role of Independent Living Centers

Independent Living Research Utilization ILRU
2323 S Shepherd Drive
Suite 1000
Houston, TX 77019
713-520-0232
FAX: 713-520-5785
www.ilru.org

This publication covers important information on why we all should make assistance to people living in nursing homes a priority. Just as important, this is an excellent summary of all the facts - quality of life, health, and costs - which support deinstitutionalization.

10 pages

5645 Independent Living Matters

DisAbility Resources of Southwest Washington
5501 109th Court
Suite N
Vancouver, WA 98662
360-694-6790
FAX: 360-694-6910
e-mail: ilrswwa@lqwest.net

Jim Baker, Executive Director
Angela Hartford, Editor/Administrative Technician
Scott Anfinson, Independent Living Specialist

To promote the philosophy of independent living by creating opportunities, encouraging choices, advancing equal access and furthering the level of independence for all people with disabilities.

8-10 pages Quarterly

5646 Lifelong Leisure Skills and Lifestyles for Persons with Developmental Disabilities

Brookes Publishing
PO Box 10624
Baltimore, MD 21285
410-337-9580
800-638-3775
FAX: 410-337-8539
e-mail: custserv@brookespublishing.com
www.brookespublishing.com

This instructional manual offers ideas and detailed examples that describe how to guide individuals of all ages through popular activities using adaptations that foster skill acquisition and inclusion. Some of the concepts explored are home-school-community collaboration, choice making and the dignity of risk, and leisure skill acquisition for the life span. *$35.00*

352 pages Paperback
ISBN 1-55766 -47-2

5647 Living in the Community

Independent Living Research Utilization ILRU
2323 S Shepherd Drive
Suite 1000
Houston, TX 77019
713-520-0232
FAX: 713-520-5785
www.ilru.org

James, Lori, and Jamey describe the elements of their successful program to move people out of nursing homes and into the community: providing funding for deposits, first month's rent and other neccessities, including assistive technology; providing training and the other core services before and after consumers leave the nursing home; developing relationships with housing and other service providers.

10 pages

5648 Loud, Proud and Passionate

Mobility International USA
PO Box 10767
Eugene, OR 97440
541-343-1284
FAX: 541-343-6812
e-mail: info@miusa.org
www.miusa.org

Susan Sygall, Executive Director
Pamela Houston, Public Relations Coordinator
Tracy Scharn, Project Assistant

A resource book for international development and women's organization about including women with disabilities in projects in the community. Informs women sith disabilities about the efforts and successes of their peers worldwide. *$30.00*

5649 NSEE Quarterly

9001 Braddock Road
Suite 380
Springfield, VA 22151
703-426-4268
800-803-4170
FAX: 703-426-8400
e-mail: info@nsee.org
www.nsee.org

Charles Walker, Executive Director

Quarterly publication from the National Society for Experiential Education.

16 pages Quarterly

5650 National Registry of Community Mental Health Services

Nat'l Council for Community Behavioral Healthcare
12300 Twinbrook Parkway
Suite 320
Rockville, MD 20852
301-984-6200
FAX: 301-881-7159
www.nccbh.org

Lists more than 1,900 agencies in all 50 states giving names, addresses and phones. *$59.00*

5651 Northwest Media

326 W 12th Avenue
Eugene, OR 97401
541-343-6636
800-777-6636
FAX: 541-343-0177
e-mail: nwm@northwestmedia.com
www.sociallearning.com

Lee White, President

Northwest Media is an independent publishing company that focuses on independent living and foster care products.

5652 Our Own Road

Aquarius Health Care Videos
5 Powderhouse Lane
PO Box 1159
Sherborn, MA 01770
508-651-2963
FAX: 508-650-4216
e-mail: aqvideos@tiac.net
www.aquariusproductions.com

Leslie Kussmonn, President

This video shows the disabled helping other people who are disabled and portrays the sense of pride they get from helping others. This multicultural program features many different healing techniques, and teaches the importance of helping those who are disabled become independent and productive. *$99.00*

5653 Parc Views

PO Box 3418
Peoria, IL 61612
309-691-3800
FAX: 309-689-3613
www.peoriaarc.org

Anne Follis, Editor

Quarterly publication from Peoria ARC, free with donation.

5654 Part Two: A Preview of Independence and Transition to Community Living

Independent Living Research Utilization ILRU
2323 S Shepherd Drive
Suite 1000
Houston, TX 77019
713-520-0232
FAX: 713-520-5785
www.ilru.org

This publication covers important strategies for helping people leave nursing homes. It includes several important recommendations which CIL leaders and staffs will find useful in organizing transition activities.

10 pages

5655 Perspective

900 Varnum Street NE
Washington, DC 20017
202-636-2950
FAX: 202-636-2996
e-mail: arcdc@juno.com
www.arcdc.net

Mary Durso, Social Worker
Tasha Kluseman, Manager Employment Services
Monita Short-Ellis, Manger Commerical Services

Bi-annual publication from the Arc of the District of Columbia.

4 pages Bi-annual

5656 Positive Behavioral Support: Including People with Difficult Behavior in the Community

Brookes Publishing
PO Box 10624
Baltimore, MD 21285
410-337-9580
800-638-3775
FAX: 410-337-8539
e-mail: custserv@brookespublishing.com
www.brookespublishing.com

This text demonstrates how people with challenging behavior can be fully included at home, at school, and in the community. Offers intervention techniques and explores the planning and assistance needed to implement nonaversive inclusion strategies. *$37.95*

528 pages Paperback
ISBN 1-55766 -28-2

5657 Prevention in Community Mental Health

Brookline Books
PO Box 1046
Cambridge, MA 02238
617-868-0360
800-666-2665
FAX: 617-868-1772
e-mail: brooklinebks@delphi.com
www.brooklinebooks.com

Describes prevention programs written through a collaborative effort between university researchers and community practitioners. The result is theoretical and practical perspectives in each chapter which provide explicit examples of how prevention focused community mental health networks operate and evaluate efforts. *$27.95*

ISBN 0-91479 -70-0

5658 Resourceful Woman

Rehabilitation Institute of Chicago
345 E Superior Street
Chicago, IL 60611
312-238-1051
FAX: 312-238-1205
TTY:312-908-8523
e-mail: hrcwd@rehabchicago.org
rehabchicago.org

Judy Panko Reis, Director
Kristi Kirchner, MD, Medical Director
Linda E Miller, Domestic Violence Coordinator

National, not-for-profit, general health and service center providing accessible medical services for women with disabilities. Conducts research into health issues concerning disabled women and offers educational resources for healthcare professionals and women with disabilities. Provides materials and educational opportunities through its library and resource center, newsletter, information sheets, brochures, videos and free seminars for women and their healthcare providers.

yearly

5659 Strengthening the Roles of Independent Living Centers Through Implementing Legal Services

Independent Living Research Utilization ILRU
2323 S Shepherd Drive
Suite 1000
Houston, TX 77019
713-520-0232
FAX: 713-520-5785
www.ilru.org

Featuring the Disability Law Clinic at Community Resources for Independence (CRI) in Northern California.

10 pages

5660 **Supporting Young Adults Who are Deaf-Blind in Their Communities**

Brookes Publishing
PO Box 10624
Baltimore, MD 21285 **410-337-9580**
800-638-3775
FAX: 410-337-8539
e-mail: custserv@brookespublishing.com
www.brookespublishing.com

A Transition Planning Guide for Service Providers, Families, and Friends. This handbook stresses the importance of person-centered planning in helping individuals who are deaf-blind make the transition from school to adult life. *$39.95*

384 pages Paperback
ISBN 1-55766 -61-8

5661 **Transitioning Exceptional Children and Youth Into the Community**

Haworth Press
10 Alice Street
Binghamton, NY 13904 **607-722-5857**
800-429-6784
FAX: 607-722-6362
e-mail: orders@haworthpress.com
www.haworthpress.com

Focusing on the dynamic process of mainstreaming exceptional children and youth into the community, experts examine some of the exciting technological advances made to accompany the social changes enacted over the years. *$44.95*

202 pages Hardcover
ISBN 0-866567-33-X

5662 **Transitions to Adult Life**

Books on Special Children
PO Box 305
Congers, NY 10920 **845-638-1236**
FAX: 845-638-0847
e-mail: irene@boscbooks.com

Transition programs that can help severely handicapped people become participating, contributing members of the community. *$ 37.00*

385 pages Softcover

Elderly

5663 **Abstracts in Social Gerontology: Current Literature on Aging**

National Council on the Aging
600 Maryland Avenue SW
Washington, DC 20024 **202-554-5981**
FAX: 202-479-0735

Detailed abstracts are provided for recent major journal articles, books, reports and other materials on many facets of aging, including: adult education, demography, family relations, institutional care and work attitudes.

5664 **Activities in Action**

Haworth Press
10 Alice Street
Binghamton, NY 13904 **607-722-5857**
800-429-6784
FAX: 607-722-6362
e-mail: orders@haworthpress.com
www.haworthpress.com

An invaluable resource which serves as a catalyst for professional and personal growth and provides a national forum on geriatric and activity issues. *$74.95*

98 pages Hardcover
ISBN 1-560241-32-2

5665 **Activities with Developmentally Disabled Elderly and Older Adults**

Haworth Press
10 Alice Street
Binghamton, NY 13904 **607-722-5857**
800-429-6784
FAX: 607-722-6362
e-mail: orders@haworthpress.com
www.haworthpress.com

Learn how to effectively plan and deliver activities for a growing number of older people with developmental disabilities. It aims to stimulate interest and continued support for recreation program development and implementation among developmental disability and aging service systems. *$59.95*

156 pages Hardcover
ISBN 1-560240-92-X

5666 **Aging & Vision News**

Lighthouse International
111 E 59 Street
New York, NY 10022 **212-821-9737**
800-829-0500
FAX: 212-821-9706
e-mail: info@lighthouse.org
www.lighthouse.org

Joanna Mellor, VP Information Services

Intended for professionals engaged in research, education or service delivery in the field of vision and aging.

6-12 pages BiAnnually

5667 **Aging Eye and Low Vision**

Lighthouse International
111 E 59 Street
New York, NY 10022 **212-821-9737**
800-829-0500
FAX: 212-821-9706
e-mail: info@lighthouse.org

Joanna Mellor, VP Information Services

A study guide for physicians on common age-related vision disorders.

5668 **Aging News Alert**

CD Publications
8204 Fenton Street
Silver Spring, MD 20910 **301-588-2280**
800-666-6380
FAX: 301-588-6385
e-mail: cdpubs@clark.net
www.cdpublications.com/seniors/ana.htm

Publishes short articles on legislation and other federal action affecting elderly people. *$237.00*

16-18 pages Weekly
ISSN 1050-31 8

5669 **Aging Process: Therapeutic Implications**

Lippincott, Williams & Wilkins
227 E Washington Square
Philadelphia, PA 19106
215-238-4200
800-777-2295
FAX: 301-824-7390
www.lpub.com

Experts examine the physiological and biological aspects of aging that impinge upon drug disposition and medical therapeutics.

352 pages

5670 **Aging Research & Training News**

Business Publishers
8737 Colesville Road
Suite 1100
Silver Spring, MD 20910
800-274-6737
FAX: 301-587-4530
e-mail: bpinews@bpinews.com
www.bpinews.com

Leonard A Eiserer, Publisher
Nancy Aldrich, Editor
Katie Johnson, Marketing Manager

Essential information on aging education and staff training, funding and grant oppurtunities, the National Institute on Aging, medical and scientific research, ans statistical measures in geveontology and genetics. *$282.00*

10 pages Monthly

5671 **Aging and Family Therapy: Practitioner Perspectives on Golden Pond**

Haworth Press
10 Alice Street
Binghamton, NY 13904
607-722-5857
800-429-6784
FAX: 607-722-6362
e-mail: orders@haworthpress.com
www.haworthpress.com

Here are creative strategies for use in therapy with older adults and their families. This significant new book provides practitioners with information, insight, reference tools, and other sources that will contribute to more effective intervention with the elderly and their families. *$74.95*

244 pages Hardcover
ISBN 0-866567-78-X

5672 **Aging and Our Families**

Human Sciences Press
233 Spring Street
New York, NY 10013
212-229-2859
800-221-9369
FAX: 212-463-0742

Handbook for family caregivers. *$18.95*

132 pages Paperback
ISBN 0-89885 -41-5

5673 **Aging and Vision News**

National Center for Vision and Aging
111 E 59th Street
New York, NY 10022
212-821-9200
800-829-0500
FAX: 212-821-9707
TTY:212-821-9713

3x Year

5674 **Aging in the Designed Environment**

Haworth Press
10 Alice Street
Binghamton, NY 13904
607-722-5857
800-429-6784
FAX: 607-722-6362
e-mail: orders@haworthpress.com
www.haworthpress.com

The key sourcebook for physical and occupational therapists developing and implementing environmental designs for the aging. *$ 74.95*

133 pages
ISBN 1-560240-31-8

5675 **Aging with a Disability**

Special Needs Project
324 State Street
Suite H
Santa Barbara, CA 93101
800-333-6867
FAX: 805-962-5087
www.specialneeds.com

This unique and recent book discusses the role of family, financial resources and the American health care system in the life of aging adults with developmental disabilities. $32.95

5676 **Assistive Technology for Older Persons**

Idaho Assistive Technology Project
129 W 3rd Street
Moscow, ID 83843
208-885-3559
800-432-8324
FAX: 208-885-3628
e-mail: rseiler@uidaho.edu
www.educ.uidaho.edu/idatech

$5.00

60 pages

5677 **Beat the Nursing Home Trap: A Consumer's Guide to Assisted Living and Long Term Care**

NOLO
950 Parker Street
Berkeley, CA 94710
510-549-1976
800-955-4775
FAX: 510-548-5902
www.nolo.com

Maira Dizgalvis, Trade Customer Service Manager
Susan McConnell, Director Sales
Natasha Kaluza, Sales Assistant

Don't guess. Use this book to figure out how to choose a nursing home, or find a viable alternative. Covers how to get the most out of Medicare and other benefit programs. *$21.95*

336 pages paperback
ISBN 0-873375-15-7

5678 **CAPSule**

Children of Aging Parents
1609 Woodbourne Road
Suite 302A
Levittown, PA 19057
215-945-6900
800-227-7294
FAX: 215-945-8720
e-mail: caps4caregivers@aol.com
www.caps4caregivers.org

Nancy Harven, Administrative Assistant

Provides practical information for family caregivers. CAPS is a nonprofit organization serving the family caregivers of the elderly with information and referrals, a network of support groups and public information as well as a newsletter quarterly. *$25.00*

12 pages Quarterly 1984

5679 **California Financial Power of Attorney**

NOLO
950 Parker Street
Berkeley, CA 94710 **510-549-1976**
800-955-4775
FAX: 510-548-5902
www.nolo.com

Maira Dizgalvis, Trade Customer Service Manager
Susan McConnell, Director Sales
Natasha Kaluza, Sales Assistant

A plain-English book packed with forms and instructions to give a trusted person the legal authority to handle your financial affairs.

paperback

5680 **Caring for Alzheimer's Patients**

Plenum Publishing Corporation
233 Spring Street
New York, NY 10013 **212-229-2859**
800-221-9369
FAX: 212-463-0742
e-mail: info@plenum.com

This handbook is designed for families, friends, and health-care professionals coping with the myriad of problems encountered by those afflicted with Alzheimer's disease. *$22.95*

308 pages Cloth
ISBN 3-06431 -98-

5681 **Caring for Those You Love: A Guide to Compassionate Care for the Aged**

Horizon Publishers
50 S 500 W
Bountiful, UT 84010 **801-295-9451**
800-453-0812
FAX: 801-295-0196

This book is a practical guide to coping with special problems of the aged and infirm, and examines the many challenges of caring for the elderly on a personal and family level. *$12.98*

ISBN 0-88290 -70-9

5682 **Caring for the Disabled Elderly**

Brookings Institution
1775 Massachusetts Avenue NW
Washington, DC 20036 **202-797-6252**
FAX: 202-797-6004
e-mail: bibooks@brookings.edu
www.brookings.edu

Financial information for the elderly. *$31.95*

318 pages Cloth
ISBN 0-815774-97-4

5683 **Chronically Disabled Elderly in Society**

Greenwood Publishing Group
88 Post Road W
Suite 5007
Westport, CT 06880 **203-226-3571**
FAX: 203-222-1502
www.greenwood.com

This timely work increases awareness of and knowledge about problems of societal living among the chronically disabled elderly, with implications for policy makers, educational institutions, advocacy groups, families and individuals. Hardcover.

160 pages $52.95 - $55
ISBN 0-313291-09-8

5684 **Communication Disorders in Aging**

Gallaudet University Press
800 Florida Avenue NE
Washington, DC 20002 **202-651-5000**
800-451-1073
FAX: 202-651-5489

This text presents contemporary practices in the medical and clinical assessment of the aged, reviews clinical evaluation techniques, and provides a comprehensive discussion of neurological imaging techniques. *$39.95*

528 pages Hardcover

5685 **Coping and Caring: Living with Alzheimer's Disease**

AARP Fulfillment
601 E Street NW
Washington, DC 20049 **202-434-2277**
800-424-3410
FAX: 202-434-3443
e-mail: member@aarp.org
www.aarp.org

Addresses the questions: What is Alzheimer's? How does the disease progress? How long does it last? How can families cope?

24 pages

5686 **Directory of Self-Help/Mutual Aid Support Groups for Older People**

Lighthouse International
111 E 59 Street
New York, NY 10022 **212-821-9737**
800-829-0500
FAX: 212-821-9706
e-mail: info@lighthouse.org

Joanna Mellor, VP Information Services

State-by-state listings of over 650 support groups for older people with impaired vision, plus listings of state commissions for the blind, self-help clearinghouses, vision rehabilitation agencies, and national resource organizations. *$10.00*

5687 **Domestic Mistreatment of the Elderly: Towards Prevention**

AARP Fulfillment
601 E Street NW
Washington, DC 20049 **202-434-2277**
800-424-3410
FAX: 202-434-3443
e-mail: member@aarp.org
www.aarp.org

This comprehensive publication addresses the problem of mistreatment or neglect in the home.

39 pages

5688 **Early Story of Alzheimer's Disease**

Lippincott, Williams & Wilkins
227 E Washington Square
Philadelphia, PA 19106 **215-238-4200**
800-777-2295
FAX: 301-824-7390
www.lpub.com

Translation of the historical papers by Alos Alzheimer. *$58.50*

160 pages Illustrated
ISBN 0-88167 -68-4

5689 Elder Abuse

Human Sciences Press
233 Spring Street
New York, NY 10013
212-229-2859
800-221-9369
FAX: 212-463-0742

Practice, policy and laws for abuse on the aging.

232 pages Cloth
ISBN 0-89885 -15-6

5690 Elder Care

Center for Public Representation
PO Box 260049
Madison, WI 53726
608-251-4008
800-369-0388
FAX: 608-251-1263
www.law.wisc.edu/pal

A compendium of alternatives for providing and financing long-term care. This practical guide provides the most comprehensive and comforting information to help navigate a number of consumer mine fields. *$16.95*

224 pages
ISBN 0-87337 -13-5

5691 Exercise and the Older Adult

Kendall/Hunt Publishing Company
1900 Association Drive
Reston, VA 20191
703-476-3400
800-213-7193
FAX: 703-476-9527
e-mail: aaalf@aahperd.org
www.aahperd.org

Jan A Seaman MBA PED, Executive Director

The latest information on physical activity for the older adults is in this textbook. Biomechanics, exercise physiology, health issues, sensory-motor function and measurement are covered by leading experts in the field. Other topics addressed include low-impact aerobics, strength development, exercise and activities for the frail elderly. *$35.00*

202 pages
ISBN 0-787210-04-8

5692 Falling in Old Age

Springer Publishing Company
536 Broadway
New York, NY 10012
212-431-4370
877-687-7476
FAX: 212-941-7842
e-mail: marketing@springerpub.com
www.springerpub.com

Annette Imperati, Marketing/Sales Director

Presented are practical techniques for the prevention of falls and for determining and correcting the causes.

5693 Family Carebook

CAREsource Program Development
505 Seattle Tower
Seattle, WA 98101
206-625-9128
800-448-5213
FAX: 206-682-2901
e-mail: service@caresource.com
www.caresource.com

Guide to aging, the special needs of older adults, and the demands of providing care and support. Experts explain potential conflicts, planning opportunities and strategies for success. Six guides. *$49.95*

475 pages Paperback
ISBN 1-87886 -12-5

5694 Functional Fitness Assessment for Adults

American Alliance for Health, Phys. Ed. & Dance
1900 Association Drive
Reston, VA 20191
703-476-3400
FAX: 703-476-9527
e-mail: aaalf@aahperd.org

This field test assesses the functional fitness of adults over 60 years of age. It is designed to serve the larger population through field based measurement techniques that can be used in a facility where older persons live and can be conducted by personnel not necessarily trained for clinical responsibilities. *$7.50*

24 pages
ISBN 0-88314 -47-6

5695 Handbook of Assistive Devices for the Handicapped Elderly

Haworth Press
10 Alice Street
Binghamton, NY 13904
607-722-5857
800-429-6784
FAX: 607-722-6362
e-mail: orders@haworthpress.com
www.haworthpress.com

Concise yet comprehensive reference of assistive devices for handicapped elders. *$34.95*

77 pages Hardcover
ISBN 0-866561-52-8

5696 Handbook on Ethnicity, Aging and Mental Health

Greenwood Publishing Group
88 Post Road W
Suite 5007
Westport, CT 06880
203-226-3571
FAX: 203-222-1502
www.greenwood.com

State-of-the-art reference by leading experts and first book-length appraisal of research, practices and policies concerning mental health needs of the ethnic elderly in America. $95-$99.50.

376 pages Hardcover
ISBN 0-313282-04-8

5697 Health Care of the Aged

Haworth Press
10 Alice Street
Binghamton, NY 13904
607-722-5857
800-429-6784
FAX: 607-722-6362
e-mail: orders@haworthpress.com
www.haworthpress.com

Focusing on the need for developing new service delivery models for the aged, this book examines fiscal, political, and social criteria influencing this challenge of the 1990's. The aged are caught in the sweeping changes currently occurring in the financing, organizing and delivery of human health care services. *$74.95*

183 pages Hardcover
ISBN 1-560240-65-2

5698 Health Promotion and Disease Prevention

Lippincott, Williams & Wilkins
227 E Washington Square
Philadelphia, PA 19106
215-238-4200
800-777-2295
FAX: 301-824-7390
www.lpub.com

Professional directory offering information on health care and rehabilitation for the elderly. *$87.00*

218 pages
ISBN 0-88167 -90-0

5699 **International Health Guide for Senior Citizen Travelers**

Pilot Books
PO Box 2102
Greenport, NY 11944
631-477-1094
FAX: 631-477-0978

Covers essential pre-departure health planning; advice on specific health concerns; disease prevention and more. *$4.95*

5700 **Managing Aging and Human Services Agencies**

Springer Publishing Company
536 Broadway
New York, NY 10012
212-431-4370
877-687-7476
FAX: 212-941-7842
e-mail: marketing@springerpub.com
www.springerpub.com

Annette Imperati, Marketing/Sales Director

Offers specialized information for the human resources professional who works with the elderly. *$27.95*

160 pages

5701 **Mastering the Medicare Maze**

Center for Public Representation
PO Box 260049
Madison, WI 53726
608-251-4008
800-369-0388
FAX: 606-251-1263

This book provides simple explanations of how to appeal denied Medicare claims. Less than 3% of Medicare claims are ever appealed. But of those that are, over 60% are successful in returning dollars to beneficiaries. With simple instructions, this book tells you how to do it and includes all the necessary forms. *$9.95*

128 pages
ISBN 0-93262 -40-2

5702 **Medicare Maximization**

Center for Public Representation
PO Box 260049
Madison, WI 53726
608-251-4008
800-369-0388
FAX: 606-251-1263
e-mail: cpr@lawmail.law.wisc.edu
www.law.wisc.edu/pal

This manual for nursing homes provides information on Medicare billing procedures, Medicare coverage guidelines - Part A and Part B as well as Medicare Bed Certification for nursing homes. Chapters with examples and exercises give you the knowledge to maximize Medicare reimbursements. *$39.95*

150 pages
ISBN 0-93262 -34-8

5703 **Mentally Impaired Elderly: Strategies and Interventions to Maintain Function**

Haworth Press
10 Alice Street
Binghamton, NY 13904
607-722-5857
800-429-6784
FAX: 607-722-6362
e-mail: orders@haworthpress.com
www.haworthpress.com

S Harrington-Miller, Advertising

Provides effective support and sensitive care for the most vulnerable segment of the elderly population, those with mental impairment. *$74.95*

171 pages Hardcover
ISBN 1-560241-68-3

5704 **Mirrored Lives: Aging Children and Elderly Parents**

Greenwood Publishing Group
88 Post Road W
Suite 5007
Westport, CT 06880
203-226-3571
FAX: 203-222-1502
www.greenwood.com

Discusses geriatric decline connected to nonterminal illness in old age. Koch takes a sensitive but thorough look at the declining years of his father. $19.95-$21.95.

240 pages Hardcover
ISBN 0-275936-71-6

5705 **Now Where Did I Put My Keys?**

AARP Fulfillment
601 E Street NW
Washington, DC 20049
202-434-2277
800-424-3410
FAX: 202-434-3443
e-mail: member@aarp.org
www.aarp.org

Your copies of this brochure won't last long on your information counter.

5706 **Older & Wiser: A Workbook for Coping with Aging**

New Harbinger Publications
5674 Shattuck Avenue
Oakland, CA 94609
510-652-0215
800-748-6273
FAX: 510-652-5472
e-mail: customerservice@newharbinger.com

This compassion guide teaches the practical skills and elicits personal insight necessary to meet the demands of aging in our society. *$12.95*

300 pages
ISBN 1-87923 -10-5

5707 **Older Adults with Developmental Disabilities: Optimizing Choice and Change**

Brookes Publishing
PO Box 10624
Baltimore, MD 21285
410-337-9580
800-638-3775
FAX: 410-337-8539
e-mail: custserv@brookespublishing.com
www.brookespublishing.com

$37.00

416 pages Paperback
ISBN 1-55766 -20-0

5708 **On Your Behalf**

CAREsource Program Development
505 Seattle Tower
Seattle, WA 98101
206-625-9128
800-448-5213
FAX: 206-682-2901
e-mail: service@caresource.com
www.caresource.com

This book takes the mystery out of very important sets of legal options. It gives lay people as well as advisors, service providers, and caregivers the information they need to understand their options and the importance of individual choice.

16 pages Books & Video
ISBN 1-87886 -14-1

5709 Operation Help: A Mental Health Advocate Guide to Medicaid

Nat'l Council for Community Behavioral Healthcare
12300 Twinbrook Parkway
Suite 320
Rockville, MD 20852 **301-984-6200**
FAX: 301-881-7159
www.nccbh.org

Explains the Medicaid entitlement program in easy-to-understand language and focuses on the needs of adults with serious mental illness, children with serious emotional disturbance and elderly persons who need mental health care. *$17.00*

5710 Perspective on Aging

National Council on the Aging
600 Maryland Avenue SW
Washington, DC 20024 **202-554-5981**
FAX: 202-479-0735

Explores significant developments in the field of aging, including disabilities, through opinion articles, profiles and book reviews. *$4.00*

5711 Perspectives on Prevention and Treatment of Cancer in the Elderly

Lippincott, Williams & Wilkins
227 E Washington Square
Philadelphia, PA 19106 **215-238-4200**
800-777-2295
FAX: 301-824-7390
www.lpub.com

This book presents an exchange of ideas and information on the complexities of cancer and aging. Clinicians and investigators from a wide range of pertinent disciplines highlight the issues unique to the elderly patient in cancer prevention, diagnosis and treatment. *$113.00*

360 pages

5712 Prescriptions for Independence

American Foundation for the Blind/AFB Press
PO Box 1020
Sewickley, PA 15143 **412-741-1142**
800-232-3044
FAX: 412-741-0609
e-mail: afborders@abdintl.com
www.afb.org

Easy-to-read manual on how older visually impaired persons can pursue their interests and activities in community residences, senior centers, long-term care facilities and other community settings. Paperback. *$29.95*

ISBN 0-891282-44-0

5713 Rehabilitation in the Aging

Lippincott, Williams & Wilkins
227 E Washington Square
Philadelphia, PA 19106 **215-238-4200**
800-777-2295
FAX: 301-824-7390
www.lpub.com

This volume provides the physician with a comprehensive approach to the medical and rehabilitative management of geriatric patients. *$82.50*

390 pages

5714 Respiratory Health Association

301 Sicomac Avenue
Wykoff, NJ 07481 **201-447-8508**

Edward Duffie, President

Offers eight-day cruises for people with respiratory conditions to Bermuda and Alaska at least twice a year.

5715 Senior Citizens and the Law

Center for Public Representation
PO Box 260049
Madison, WI 53726 **608-251-4008**
800-369-0388
FAX: 606-251-1263
e-mail: cpr@lawmail.law.wisc.edu
www.law.wisc.edu

An introduction to legal problems facing the elderly in Wisconsin. This edition discusses legal problems associated with Social Security, Medicare, SSI, guardianship and its alternatives, community-based services, probate, taxes, private health insurance and consumer protection. *$5.00*

ISBN 0-936226-15-1

5716 Sharing Solutions: A Newsletter for Support Groups

Lighthouse International
111 E 59 Street
New York, NY 10022 **212-821-9737**
800-829-0500
FAX: 212-821-9706
e-mail: info@lighthouse.org
www.lighthouse.org

Joanna Mellor, VP Information Services

A newsletter for members and leaders of support groups for older adults with impaired vision. The letter provides a forum for support groups members to network and share information, printed in a very large type format.

5717 So Many of My Friends Have Moved Away or Died

AARP Fulfillment
601 E Street NW
Washington, DC 20049 **202-434-2277**
800-424-3410
FAX: 202-434-3443
e-mail: member@aarp.org
www.aarp.org

A typical problem faced by older persons, discussion focuses on coping with the loss of old friends and finding new ones.

5718 Social Security Bulletin

US Social Security Administration
4301 Connecticut Avenue NW
Room 209
Washington, DC 20008
800-772-1213
FAX: 202-282-7219
www.ssa.gov/policy

Reports on results of research and analysis pertinent to the Social Security and SSI programs. *$16.00*

Monthly

5719 Social Security, Medicare, and Pensions

NOLO
950 Parker Street
Berkeley, CA 94710 **510-549-1976**
800-955-4775
FAX: 510-548-5902
www.nolo.com

Maira Dizgalvis, Trade Customer Service Manager
Susan McConnell, Director Sales
Natasha Kaluza, Sales Assistant

A plain-speaking guide explaining the ins and outs of the Social Security system; retirement, disability and benefits for dependents and survivors. *$24.95*

320 pages paperback
ISBN 0-873374-87-8

5720 **Successful Models of Community Long Term Care Services for the Elderly**

Haworth Press
10 Alice Street
Binghamton, NY 13904
607-722-5857
800-429-6784
FAX: 607-722-6362
e-mail: orders@haworthpress.com
www.haworthpress.com

S Harroington-Miller, Advertising

Experienced practitioners provide examples of successful community-based long term care service programs for the elderly. *$ 74.95*

174 pages
ISBN 0-866569-87-1

5721 **Therapeutic Interventions in Alzheimer**

Aspen Publishers
200 Orchard Ridge Drive
Gaithersburg, MD 20878
301-698-7100
800-234-1660
FAX: 301-695-7931
www.aspenpublishers.com

A program of functional skills for activities of daily living. Hardcover. *$65.00*

256 pages
ISBN 0-834209-30-6

5722 **Topics in Geriatric Rehabilitation**

Aspen Publishers
200 Orchard Ridge Road
Gaithersburg, MD 20878
301-698-7100
800-638-8437
FAX: 301-695-7931
www.aspenpublishers.com

Peer-review journal presenting clinical, basic and applied research as well as theoretical information. Published quarterly. *$ 86.00*

90 pages

5723 **Unloving Care**

Harper Collins Publishers/Basic Books
10 E 53rd Street
New York, NY 10022
212-207-7042
800-242-7737
FAX: 212-207-7203

A leading public health expert gives a definitive account of what nursing homes are really like. *$9.95*

305 pages
ISBN 0-46508 -81-3

5724 **Vision and Aging: Issues in Social Work Practice**

Haworth Press
10 Alice Street
Binghamton, NY 13904
607-722-5857
800-429-6784
FAX: 607-722-6362
e-mail: orders@haworthpress.com
www.haworthpress.com

S Harrington-Miller, Advertising

Responds to the needs of the growing population of blind or severely disabled elderly. *$74.95*

196 pages Hardcover
ISBN 1-560241-99-3

5725 **Visually Impaired Seniors as Senior Companions: A Reference Guide**

American Foundation for the Blind/AFB Press
PO Box 1020
Sewickley, PA 15143
412-741-1142
800-232-3044
FAX: 412-741-0609
e-mail: afborders@abdintl.com
www.afb.org

This useful guide describes the Senior Companion Program that is intended to broaden opportunities for older persons with disabilities. Appendix includes training materials, evaluation forms, recruitment and public relations information. *$15.00*

108 pages Paperback
ISBN 0-891282-38-6

5726 **Work, Health and Income Among the Elderly**

Brookings Institution
1775 Massachusetts Avenue NW
Washington, DC 20036
202-797-6252
FAX: 202-797-6004
e-mail: bibooks@brookings.edu
www.brookings.edu

Employment, health and financial information for the elderly. *$26.95*

318 pages Cloth
ISBN 0-815774-97-4

Employment

5727 **A Guide for People with Disabilities Seeking Employment**

US Department of Justice
950 Pennsylvania Avenue NW DRS-NYAV
Washington, DC 20530
202-307-0663
800-574-0301
FAX: 202-307-1197
www.ada.gov

A 2-page pamplet for people with disabilities providing a general explanation of the employment provisions of the ADA and how to file a complaint with the Equal Employment Opportunity Commission.

5728 **ADA Questions and Answers**

US Department of Justice
950 Pennsylvania Avenue NW DRS-NYAV
Washington, DC 20530
202-307-0663
800-574-0301
FAX: 202-307-1197
www.ada.gov

A 31-page booklet giving an overview of the ADA's requirements affecting employers, businesses, nonprofit service agencies, and state and local governments programs, including public transportation.

5729 **ANCOR Wage and Hour Handbook**

American Network of Community Options & Resources
1101 King Street
Suite 380
Alexandria, VA 22314
703-535-7850
FAX: 703-535-7860
e-mail: ancor@ancor.org
www.ancor.org

Renee L Pietrangelo, CEO
Suellen Galbraith, Director Public Policy

This useful publication contains the latest rules and interpretations from the U.S. Department of Labor relative to employment in residential support services for people with disabilities, including copies of enforcement policies and letters of interpretation. It outlines in detail when exemptions from miniimum wage and overtime rules can be applied,a nd when and how employees may be paid on a salary basis. Sample staffing patterns are provided.

121 pages

5730 Americans with Disabilities Department of Justice

Consumer Information Center
Department 577A
Pueblo, CO 81009
719-948-3334
888-878-3256
FAX: 719-948-9724
e-mail: catalog.pueblo@gsa.gov

Michael Clark, Public Affairs

Explains how civil rights of persons with disabilities are protected at work and in public places.

5731 Americans with Disabilities Act: Questions and Answers

Federal Consumer Information Center
Department 513 J
Pueblo, CO 81009
888-878-3256
FAX: 719-948-9724
e-mail: catalog.pueblo@gsa.gov
www.pueblo.gsa.gov

Judi Mahaney, Public Affairs

Explains how the Civil Rights of Persons with disabilities are protected at work and in public places. Free.

5732 Career Education for Handicapped Individuals

McGraw-Hill, School Publishing
220 E Danieldale Road
DeSoto, TX 75115
972-224-1111
800-442-9685
FAX: 972-228-1982
mhschool.com

Based on a life-centered career education program that goes beyond elementary school level to include handicapped people of all ages.

454 pages

5733 Disability Under the Fair Employment & Housing Act: What You Should Know About the Law

California Department of Fair Employment & Housing
2014 T Street
Suite 210
Sacramento, CA 95814
916-227-2873
800-884-1684
FAX: 916-227-2870
www.dfeh.ca.gov

Dia S Poole, Deputy Director Public Affairs

$12.90

ISSN 9311-5126

5734 Discrimination is Against the Law

California Department of Fair Employment & Housing
2014 T Street
Suite 210
Sacramento, CA 95814
916-227-2873
800-884-1684
FAX: 916-227-2870
www.dfeh.ca.gov

Dia S Poole, Deputy Director Public Affairs

$12.90

ISSN 9311-5114

5735 Earning a Living

Accent Books & Products
PO Box 700
Bloomington, IL 61702
309-378-2961
800-787-8444
FAX: 309-378-4420
e-mail: acmtlvng@aol.com

Raymond C Cheever, Publisher
Betty Garee, Editor

Discusses how to prepare a person for a career, what to say in an interview, and gives examples of both home businesses and jobs away from home. Tells how to modify a worksite and how to be successful on the job. *$9.50*

88 pages Paperback

ISBN 0-91570 -23-0

5736 Employee Complaint Handling: Tested Techniques for Human Resource Managers

Greenwood Publishing Group
88 Post Road W
Suite 5007
Westport, CT 06880
203-226-3571
FAX: 203-222-1502
www.greenwood.com

Examines issues of human relations and communications as well as those of legal and ethical concerns. *$59.95*

208 pages Hardcover

ISBN 0-899304-33-8

5737 Employment Discrimination Based on Disability

California Department of Fair Employment & Housing
2014 T Street
Suite 210
Sacramento, CA 95814
916-227-2873
800-884-1684
FAX: 916-227-2870
www.dfeh.ca.gov

Dia S Poole, Deputy Director Public Affairs

$12.90

ISSN 9311-8413

5738 Employment in the Mainstream

Mainstream
3 Bethesda Metro Center
Suite 830
Bethesda, MD 20814
301-891-8777
800-247-1380
FAX: 301-891-8778
e-mail: info@mainstreaminc.org
www.mainstreaminc.org

David Pichette, Executive Director
Fritz Rumpel, Editor

Reports on issues, ideas, problems and solutions in employing persons with any kind of physical or mental disability. Quarterly magazine. *$25.00*

32 pages

5739 **Good Employee Is Capable, Conscientious, Productive**

American Foundation for the Blind/AFB Press
PO Box 1020
Sewickley, PA 15143
412-741-1142
800-232-3044
FAX: 412-741-0609
e-mail: afborders@abdintl.com
www.afb.org

Answers employers' questions about the blind and visually handicapped and provides assurance to employees with visual impairments can get to work, perform their jobs safely and require little in the way of special training.

ISBN 0-891289-19-4

5740 **Guide to Successful Employment for Individuals with Autism**

Brookes Publishing
PO Box 10624
Baltimore, MD 21285
410-337-9585
800-638-3775
FAX: 410-337-8539
e-mail: custserv@brookespublishing.com
www.brookespublishing.com

Describing all aspects of job placement, this book details strategies for assessing workers, networking for job opportunities, and tailoring job supports to each individual. Also illustrates how to help individuals with autism become productive workers, and with detailed descriptions of specific jobs help provide ideas for employment. *$ 32.95*

336 pages Paperback
ISBN 1-55766 -71-5

5741 **Handbook of Career Planning for Special Needs Students**

Pro-Ed Publications
8700 Shoal Creek Boulevard
Austin, TX 78757
512-451-3246
800-897-3202
FAX: 512-451-8542
e-mail: info@proedinc.com
www.proedinc.com

The practitioner's guide will show you how to help special needs adolescents and young adults overcome barriers to employment by identifying goals and problems, assessing interests and aptitudes, involving client families and developing communication skills. *$46.00*

358 pages Hardcover
ISBN 0-890797-06-4

5742 **Job Hunting Tips for the So-Called Handicapped**

Special Needs Project
324 State Street
Suite H
Santa Barbara, CA 93101
800-333-6867
FAX: 805-962-5087
www.specialneeds.com

Richard Bolles

This nifty booklet from the guru of job hunting himself is sincere, useful and careful brief. *$4.95*

5743 **Job Search People**

JIST Publishing
8902 Otis Avenue
Indianapolis, IN 46216
317-613-4200
800-648-5478
FAX: 800-547-8329
e-mail: info@jist.com
www.jist.com

Tom Abeel, VP Marketing
Barry Newborn, Director Sales

FREE catalog! Foster self-directed attitudes and behaviors with products focused on career planning, job search, career development, job retention, and life skills. Includes career assessments, occupational references, interactive workbooks, instructional videos, multimedia software, intructor's guides, and training. $4.95-$995.

176 pages Yearly 1983

5744 **Keys to the Workplace: Skills and Supports for People with with Disabilities**

Brookes Publishing
PO Box 10624
Baltimore, MD 21285
410-337-9585
800-638-3775
FAX: 410-337-8539
e-mail: custserv@brookespublishing.com
www.brookespublishing.com

This manual gives employment professionals step-by-step instructions for helping people with developmental disabilities find appropriate and fulfilling employment. Introduced here is the Seven-Phase Sequence, which fosters the natural supports that are vital to long-term job satisfaction and success. *$26.95*

304 pages Paperback 1997
ISBN 1-55766 -76-2

5745 **Let Community Employment be the Goal for Individuals with Autism**

Autism Society of North Carolina Bookstore
505 Oberlin Road
Suite 230
Raleigh, NC 27605
919-743-0204
800-442-2762
FAX: 919-743-0208
e-mail: dcoffey@autismsociety-nc.org
www.autismsociety-nc.org

Darla Coffey, Bookstore Manager

A guide designed for people who are responsible for preparing individuals with autism to enter the work force. *$7.00*

5746 **Making the Workplace Accessible: Guidelines, Costs and Resources**

Spina Bifida Association of America
4590 MacArthur Boulevard NW
Suite 250
Washington, DC 20007
202-944-3285
800-621-3141
FAX: 202-944-3295
e-mail: sbaa@sbaa.org
www.sbaa.org

Fritz Rumpel, Editor

A 20 page reference guide on how to provide physical access to persons with disabilities in a cost effective manner. *$9.00*

5747 **Marketing Your Abilities: A Guide for the Disabled Job-Seeker**

Mainstream
3 Bethesda Metro Center
Suite 830
Bethesda, MD 20814 **301-951-6122**
FAX: 301-654-6714
e-mail: info@mainstreaminc.org

A publication designed to assist the individual with a disability in conducting a successful job search. Major topics include how to write an effective resume and how to give a good interview. *$ 4.95*

24 pages

5748 **Meeting the Needs of Employees with Disabilities**

Resources for Rehabilitation
33 Bedford Street
Suite 19A
Lexington, MA 02420 **781-368-9094**
FAX: 781-368-9096

Susan Greenblatt

Provides information to help people with disabilities retain or obtain employment. Information on government programs and laws, supported employment, training programs, environmental adaptations and the transition from school to work are included. Chapters on mobility impairment, vision impairment and hearing and speech impairments. *$ 47.95*

167 pages Biennial
ISBN 0-92971 -13-5

5749 **Mental Health in the Workplace: An Employer's & Manager's Guide**

Greenwood Publishing Group
88 Post Road W
Suite 5007
Westport, CT 06880 **203-226-3571**
FAX: 203-222-1502
www.greenwood.com

A guide to the impact of mental health issues on the workplace, with special attention to complying with provisions of the Americas with Disabilities Act. *$59.95*

296 pages $59.95 - $67.95
ISBN 0-899307-03-5

5750 **Model Program Operation Manual: Business Enterprise Program Supervisors**

Mississippi State University
PO Box 6189
Mississippi State, MS 39762 **662-325-2001**
800-675-7782
FAX: 662-325-8989
www.blind.msstate.edu

Kelly Schaefer, Publications Manager

This monograph serves as a Model Program Operation Manual for Business Enterprise Program Supervisors who administer Randolph-Sheppard vending facilities under the Randolph-Sheppard Act. A wide variety of topics are covered including the role of the State Committee of Blind Venders, the role and responsibilities of the Vending Facility Operator, model qualification, for potential Facility Managers, guidelines for location of vending facilities and policies for closing vending facilities. *$20.00*

199 pages Paperback

5751 **More Than a Job: Securing Satisfying Careers for People with Disabilities**

Brookes Publishing
PO Box 10624
Baltimore, MD 21285 **410-337-9585**
800-638-3775
FAX: 410-337-8539
e-mail: custserv@brookespublishing.com
www.brookespublishing.com

This text shows employment professionals how to transform job placement into career counseling for people with physical and developmental disabilities. Issues such as transition from school to adult life, transportation, social relationships, and community access are also discussed. *$34.95*

368 pages Paperback 1998
ISBN 1-55766 -28-9

5752 **Paraplegics and Quadriplegics**

Mainstream
3 Bethesda Metro Center
Suite 830
Bethesda, MD 20814 **301-951-6122**
800-247-1380
FAX: 301-654-6714
e-mail: info@mainstreaminc.org

Mainstreaming paraplegics and quadriplegics into the workplace. *$2.50*

12 pages

5753 **People with Hearing Loss and the Workplace Guide for Employers/ADA Compliances**

Self Help for Hard of Hearing People
7910 Woodmont Avenue
Suite 1200
Bethesda, MD 20814
FAX: 301-913-9413
e-mail: national@shhh.org

Nancy Macklin, Business Manager

A guide for both people with hearing loss and their employers to learn about accommodations under the law. Includes employment guidelines, resource list of manufacturers and case studies. *$15.00*

40 pages Paperback

5754 **Planning Reasonable Accomodations: A Cost Effective Guide in a Legal Framework**

Spina Bifida Association of America
4590 MacArthur Boulevard NW
Suite 250
Washington, DC 20007 **202-944-3285**
800-621-3141
FAX: 202-944-3295
e-mail: sbaa@sbaa.org
www.sbaa.org

Fritz Rumpel, Editor

A 24 page reference guide on the reasonable accomodations process under the ADA. *$9.00*

5755 **Project LINK Guidebook**

Mainstream
3 Bethesda Metro Center
Suite 830
Bethesda, MD 20814 **301-951-6122**
800-247-1380
FAX: 301-654-6714
e-mail: info@mainstreaminc.org

A manual for operating an employment services program for persons with disabilities. *$49.95*

78 pages

5756 Providing Employment Support for People with Long-Term Mental Illness

Brookes Publishing
PO Box 10624
Baltimore, MD 21285
410-337-9585
800-638-3775
FAX: 410-337-8539
e-mail: custserv@brookespublishing.com
www.brookespublishing.com

Choices, resources, and practical strategies. Topics covered include natural supports, behavior management, Social Security issues, vocational barriers to productive employment, and workers' rights under the Americans with Disabilities Act. Also includes detailed discussions of specific psychiatric diagnoses vocational assessment and career development, crisis intervention, interdisciplinary support models, and more. *$30.95*

352 pages Paperback
ISBN 1-55766 -90-1

5757 Questions and Answers: The ADA and Hiring Police Officers

US Department of Justice
950 Pennsylvania Avenue NW DRS-NYAV
Washington, DC 20530
202-307-0663
800-574-0301
FAX: 202-307-1197
www.ada.gov

A 5-page publication providing information on ADA requirements for interviewing and hiring police officers.

5758 Supported Employment for Disabled People

Human Sciences Press
233 Spring Street
New York, NY 10013
212-229-2859
800-221-9369
FAX: 212-463-0742

Highlights the major features of supported employment. Contributions offer service providers in social work, education and mental health much-needed information. *$38.95*

288 pages Cloth
ISBN 0-89885 -46-6

5759 Survey of Direct Labor Workers Who Are Blind & Employed by NIB

Mississippi State University
PO Box 6189
Mississippi State, MS 39762
662-325-2001
800-675-7782
FAX: 662-325-8989
www.blind.msstate.edu

Kelly Schaefer, Publications Manager

This report is a follow-up to surveys by National Industries for the Blind in 1983 and 1987 and summarizes the results of a national survey of approximately 500 legally blind direct labor workers. *$10.00*

101 pages Paperback

5760 Understanding and Accommodating Physical Disabilities: Desk Reference

Greenwood Publishing Group
88 Post Road W
Suite 5007
Westport, CT 06880
203-226-3571
FAX: 203-222-1502
www.greenwood.com

Medical conditions that qualify as disabilities under the American's with Disabilities Act are explained in non-medical terminology. Hardcover.

200 pages $52.95 - $55
ISBN 0-899308-14-7

5761 Vocational Counseling for Special Populations

Chrisann Schire-Geist
2600 S First Street
Springfield, IL 62704
217-789-8980
800-258-8980
FAX: 217-789-9130
e-mail: books@ccthomas.com
www.ccthomas.com

$36.95

172 pages Paperback
ISBN 0-398056-50-1

5762 Vocational Training and Employment of the Autistic Adolescent

Charles C Thomas
2600 S First Street
Springfield, IL 62704
217-789-8980
800-258-8980
FAX: 217-789-9130
e-mail: books@ccthomas.com
www.ccthomas.com

Professionals and parents are now advocating, demanding and arranging that persons receive vocational training and equal rights for the disabled. Also available in paper edition. *$41.95*

182 pages Cloth
ISBN 0-398058-01-6

5763 WORK

64511 Via Real
Suite 9
Carpintera, CA 93013
805-566-9000
FAX: 805-566-9070

Kathy Webb, Executive Director

Vocational and residential training and support services for adults with developmental disabilities.

5764 Working Together: Workplace Culture, Employment and Disabilities

Brookline Books
PO Box 1046
Cambridge, MA 02238
617-868-0360
800-666-2665
FAX: 617-868-1772
e-mail: brooklinebks@delphi.com
www.brooklinebooks.com

Presents a new approach to assisting individuals with significant disabilities achieve meaningful careers, the book stresses partnerships between work, service providers and natural support systems to achieve positive employment outcomes. *$27.95*

Paperback
ISBN 0-91479 -88-3

General Disabilities

5765 A Christian Approach to Overcoming Disability: A Doctor's Story

Haworth Press
10 Alice Street
Binghamton, NY 13904
607-722-5857
800-429-6784
FAX: 607-722-6362
e-mail: orders@haworthpress.com
www.haworthpress.com

S Harrington-Miller, Advertising

This is the personal account of a Christian physician who changed her career specialty from obstetrics and gynecology when she was diagnosed with a genetic disease that would cause her to become blind. Dr. Elaine Eng offers faith-based and psychological techniques for coping with disability.
$29.95

174 pages Hardcover
ISBN 0-789022-57-5

5766 A Guide to Disability Rights Law

US Department of Justice
950 Pennsylvania Avenue NW DRS-NYAV
Washington, DC 20530
202-307-0663
800-574-0301
FAX: 202-307-1197
www.ada.gov

A 21-page booklet providing a brief description of the ADA, the Telecommunications Act, Fair Housing Act, Air Carrier Access Act, Voting Accessibility for the Elderly and Handicapped Act, National Voter Registration Act, Civil Rights of Institutionalized Persons Act, Individuals with Disabilities in Education Act, Rehabilitation Act, Architectural Barriers Act, and the federal agencies to contact for more information.

5767 A Guidebook on Consumer-Controlled Housing for Minnesotans with Disabilities

Arc Minnesota
770 Transfer Road
Suite 26
Saint Paul, MN 55114
651-523-0823
800-582-5256
FAX: 651-523-0829
e-mail: mail@arcminnesota.com
www.arcminnesota.com

Mike Gude, Administrative Assistant
$10.00

8 pages
ISBN 0-965040-41-0

5768 A World Awaits You

PO Box 10767
Eugene, OR 97440
541-343-1284
FAX: 541-343-6812
e-mail: info@miusa.org
www.miusa.org

Susan Sygall, Executive Director
Michele Scheib, Manager NCDE
Tracy Scharn, Project Assistant

Free publication from Mobility International USA.

44 pages Yearly

5769 AAPD News

American Association of People with Disabilities
1819 H Street NW
Suite 330
Washington, DC 20006
202-457-0046
800-840-8844
FAX: 202-457-0473
e-mail: aapd@aol.com
www.aapd-dc.org

Anelie Bush, Editor

Quarterly

5770 ABC of Asthma, Allergies & Lupus

Global Health Solutions
8472 A Tyco Road
Vienna, VA 22182
703-848-2333
800-759-3999
FAX: 703-848-0028
e-mail: shipping@watercure.com
www.watercure.com

Kristin Swan, Secretary
Joy Barber, Secretary
$17.00

240 pages 1900
ISBN 0-962994-26-x

5771 ADA Guide for Small Businesses

US Department of Justice
950 Pennsylvania Avenue NW DRS-NYAV
Washington, DC 20530
202-307-0663
800-574-0301
FAX: 202-307-1197
www.ada.gov

A 15-page booklet for businesses that provide goods and services to the public. This publication explains basic ADA requirements, illustrates ways to make facilities accessible, and provides information about tax credits and deductions.

5772 ADA Guide for Small Towns

US Department of Justice
950 Pennsylvania Avenue NW DRS-NYAV
Washington, DC 20530
202-307-0663
800-574-0301
FAX: 202-307-1197
www.ada.gov

A 21-page guide that presents an informal overview of some basic ADA requirements and provides cost-effective tips on how small towns can comply with the ADA.

5773 ADA Information Services

US Department of Justice
950 Pennsylvania Avenue NW DRS-NYAV
Washington, DC 20530
202-307-0663
800-574-0301
FAX: 202-307-1197
www.ada.gov

A 2-page list with the telephone numbers and internet addresses of federal agencies and other organizations that provide information and technical assistance to the public about the ADA.

5774 ADA Pipeline

ADA Technical Assistance Program
490 Tenth Street
Atlanta, GA 30318
404-385-0636
800-949-4232
FAX: 404-385-0641
e-mail: sedbtac@catea.org
www.sedbtac.org

Amy Oliveras, Administrative Assistant
Mary Morder, Alternative Format Coordinator
Shelley Kaplan, Director

16 pages Quarterly

5775 ADA Questions and Answers

US Department of Justice
950 Pennsylvania Avenue NW DRS-NYAV
Washington, DC 20530
202-307-0663
800-574-0301
FAX: 202-307-1197
www.ada.gov

A 31-page booklet giving an overview of the ADA's requirements affecting employers, businesses, nonprofit service agencies, and state and local governments programs, including public transportation.

5776 ADA Tax Incentive Packet for Business

US Department of Justice
950 Pennsylvania Avenue NW DRS-NYAV
Washington, DC 20530
202-307-0663
800-574-0301
FAX: 202-307-1197
www.ada.gov

A 13-page packet of information to help businesses understand and take advantage of the tax credit and deduction available for complying with the ADA.

5777 ADA and City Governments: Common Problems

US Department of Justice
950 Pennsylvania Avenue NW DRS-NYAV
Washington, DC 20530
202-307-0663
800-574-0301
FAX: 202-307-1197
www.ada.gov

A 9-page document that contains a sampling of common problems shared by city governments of all sizes, provides examples of common deficiencies and explains how these problems affect persons with disabilities.

5778 ADA-TA: A Technical Assistance Update from the Department of Justice

US Department of Justice
950 Pennsylvania Avenue NW DRS-NYAV
Washington, DC 20530
202-307-0663
800-574-0301
FAX: 202-307-1197
www.ada.gov

A serial publication that answers Common Questions about ADA requirements and provides Design Details illustrating particular design requirements. The first edition addresses Readily Achievable Barrier Removal and Van Accessible Packing Spaces.

5779 AID Bulletin

Project AID Resource Center
PO Box 5190
Kent, OH 44242
330-672-2672
FAX: 330-672-4724

Alex Boros PhD, Director AID
J Sue Adams, Senior Counselor

Has the latest news on upcoming conferences, literature, developments in programs and/or services for disabled persons who are substance abusers. Offers articles on their experiences, ideas and questions of others in this field which includes providers and consumers. *$7.50*

5780 ARC's Government Report

Arc of the District of Columbia
900 Varnum Street NE
Washington, DC 20017
202-636-2950
FAX; 202-636-2996
e-mail: arcdc@juno.com
www.arcdc.net

Reports on government activities related to individuals with disabilities with a focus on persons with mental retardation. *$ 50.00*

5781 ARCA Newsletter

ARCA - Dakota County Technical College
1300 145th Street E
Rosemount, MN 55068
651-423-8000
800-548-5502
FAX: 651-423-8775

Offers information on support groups, conventions, books, manuscripts and programs for the rehabilitation professional and the disabled.

Monthly

5782 Accent on Living Magazine

Cheever Publishing
PO Box 700
Bloomington, IL 61702
309-378-2961
800-787-8444
FAX: 309-378-4420

Julie Cheever, Marketing Manager

A magazine published for forty four years, serves physically disabled people, general interest, includes, travel, home modification etc. *$12.00*

112 pages Quarterly

5783 Access Design Services: CILs as Experts

Independent Living Research Utilization ILRU
2323 S Shepherd Drive
Suite 1000
Houston, TX 77019
713-520-0232
FAX: 713-520-5785
www.ilru.org

Featuring the Access Design Services of Alpha One in Maine, this month's Readings is another of the winners of the recent competition for innovative CIL programs.

10 pages

5784 Access Info

Access to Independence
2345 Atwood Avenue
Madison, WI 53704
608-242-8484
800-362-9877
FAX: 608-242-0383
TTY:608-242-8485

Frank Martin, Editor

Covers news, features and resources for people with disabilities living in the Madison, Wisconsin area.

16-20 pages Quarterly

5785 Access for 911 and Telephone Emergency Services

US Department of Justice
950 Pennsylvania Avenue NW DRS-NYAV
Washington, DC 20530
202-307-0663
800-574-0301
FAX: 202-307-1197
www.ada.gov

A 10-page publication explaining the requirements for direct, equal access to 911 for persons who use teletypewriters (TTYs).

5786 **Accessible Gardening for People with Physical Disabilities**

Spina Bifida Association of America
4590 MacArthur Boulevard NW
Suite 250
Washington, DC 20007 **202-944-3285**
800-621-3141
FAX: 202-944-3295
e-mail: sbaa@sbaa.org
www.sbaa.org

Presents all the information and practical know-how necessary for designing, planting, and maintaining a garden that suits the special needs of young and older gardeners. Dozens of mail-order sources are provided for the many tools, seeds, plants, and other materials discussed. From measuring for planter boxes to selecting suitable tools and plants, the author thoroughly describes how to garden in a variety of situations. *$19.95*

300 pages Paperback 1994
ISBN 0-933149-56-5

5787 **Achieving Diversity at Independence**

Independent Living Research Utilization ILRU
2323 S Shepherd Drive
Suite 1000
Houston, TX 77019 **713-520-0232**
FAX: 713-520-5785
www.ilru.org

10 pages

5788 **Acu-Yoga: The Acupressure Stress Management Book**

Japan Publications
419 Occidental Avenue S
PO Box 3092
Seattle, WA 98114 **206-622-7443**

Handbook describing the origin, practice and benefits of acupression and yoga. *$22.00*

1981
ISBN 0-870404-89-x

5789 **Acupuncture: Is it for You?**

Harper & Row
10 E 53rd Street
New York, NY 10022 **212-207-7042**
800-242-7737
FAX: 212-207-7203

1973

5790 **Ad Lib Drop-In Center: Consumer Management, Ownership and Empowerment**

Independent Living Research Utilization ILRU
2323 S Shepherd Drive
Suite 1000
Houston, TX 77019 **713-520-0232**
FAX: 713-520-5785
www.ilru.org

Joe describes how Ad Lib ensured consumer control in their Drop-In Center: the DIC came about because of consumer input, and consumers are involved in planning the program; members can choose to become volunteers or paid staff members. All of the staff at the DIC are consumers; and active consumer advisory board helps develop policies and programs and provides input to the Ad Lib board.

10 pages

5791 **Adaptive Baby Care Equipment Video and Book**

Through the Looking Glass
2198 Sixth Street
Suite 100
Berkeley, CA 94710 **510-848-1112**
800-644-2666
FAX: 510-848-4445
e-mail: TLG@lookingglass.org
www.lookingglass.org

Includes Adaptive Baby care Equipment: Guide Lines; Prototypes and Resources, plus a twelve minute video. Available in braille, large print or cassette. *$79.00*

5792 **Adaptive Baby Care Equipment: Guidelines, Prototypes & Resources**

Through the Looking Glass
2198 Sixth Street
Suite 100
Berkeley, CA 94710 **510-848-1112**
800-644-2666
FAX: 510-848-4445
e-mail: TLG@lookingglass.org
www.lookingglass.org

K Vensand
J Rogers
C Tuleja

Available in braille, large print or cassette. *$30.00*

86 pages

5793 **Adaptive Tracks**

Adaptive Sports Center
PO Box 1639
Crested Butte, CO 81224 **970-349-2296**
866-349-2296
FAX: 970-349-4950
e-mail: info@adaptivesports.org
www.adaptivesports.org

Christopher Hensley, Director

6 pages Quarterly

5794 **Adobe News**

Santa Barbara Foundation
15 E Carrilla Street
Santa Barbara, CA 93101 **805-263-1873**
805-966-2345

8 pages Bi-Annually

5795 **Adults Incorporated Annual Report**

3420 University Avenue
Waterloo, IA 50701 **319-236-0901**
888-879-1365
FAX: 319-236-3701
e-mail: ainc@cedarnet.org
www.cedarnet.org/ainc

Donna Davis, Editor
Mark Witmer, Editor

Free upon request.

12 pages Yearly

5796 **Advocate**

Arc Massachusetts
217 S Street
Waltham, MA 02453 **781-891-6270**
FAX: 781-891-6271
e-mail: arcmass@arcmass.org
www.arcmass.org

$20.00

8-12 pages Quarterly

5797 Ageless Body, Timeless Mind

Harmony Books
231 Broad Street
Nevada City, CA 95959
530-265-9564
www.harmonybookstore.com

1993
ISBN 0-517592-57-6

5798 Alcoholism Sourcebook

Omnigraphics
615 Griswold Street
Detroit, MI 48226
800-234-1340
FAX: 800-875-1340
www.omnigraphics.com

Karen Bellenir, Editor
Georgiann Lauginiger, Customer Service Manager

Provides information on the disorders which may result from alcohol abuse. *$78.00*

650 pages 1900
ISBN 0-780803-25-6

5799 Alerter

San Diego Area Chapter of the Arthritis Foundation
9089 Clairemont Mesa Boulevard
Suite 104
San Diego, CA 92123
858-492-1090
800-422-8885
FAX: 858-492-9248
e-mail: cchase@arthritis.org
www.arthritis.org

Chris Chase, Programs & Services Coordinator

Offers chapter updates, information on activities and events, resources and medical research for members.

5800 Alexander Technique

St. Martin's Press
175 Fifth Avenue
New York, NY 10010
212-674-5151
800-221-7945
FAX: 212-420-9314

Guide that shows the correct and incorrect positions to use for exercises.

1991

5801 Allergies Sourcebook, 2nd Edition

Omnigraphics
615 Griswold Street
Detroit, MI 48226
800-234-1340
FAX: 800-875-1340
www.omnigraphics.com

Includes information on the causes of allergies, identification, treatments and statistics. *$78.00*

650 pages 1900
ISBN 0-780803-76-0

5802 American Herb Association Newsletter

14648 Pear Tree Lane
PO Box 353
Nevada City, CA 95959
530-265-9552
FAX: 530-274-3140
www.ahaherb.com

Information on many different herbs and herb usues. *$20.00*

5803 American Journal of Audiology

American Speech-Language-Hearing Association
10801 Rockville Pike
Rockville, MD 20852
301-897-5700
800-638-8255
FAX: 301-897-7348
e-mail: info@asha.org
www.asha.org

John E Bernthal, President
Frederick T Spahr PhD, Executive Director
Joanne Jessen, Publications Director

Articles concern screening, assesment, and treatment techniques; prevention; professional issues; supervision; and administration; and may appear in the form of clinical forums, clinical recveiws, letters to the editor, or research reports that emphasize clinical practice.

5804 Americans with Disabilities Act Checklist for New Lodging Facilities

US Department of Justice
950 Pennsylvania Avenue NW DRS-NYAV
Washington, DC 20530
202-307-0663
800-574-0301
FAX: 202-307-1197
www.ada.gov

This 34-page checklist is a self-help survey that owners, franchisors, and managers of lodging facilities can use to identy ADA mistkes at their facilities.

5805 Americans with Disabilities Act Guide for Places of Lodging: Serving Guests Who Are Blind

US Department of Justice
950 Pennsylvania Avenue NW DRS-NYAV
Washington, DC 20530
202-307-0663
800-574-0301
FAX: 202-307-1197
www.ada.gov

A 12-page publication explaining what hotels, motels, and other places of transient lodging can do to accommodate guests who are blind or have low vision.

5806 Anesthesia

Advocado Press
PO Box 145
Louisville, KY 40201
502-894-9492
FAX: 502-899-9562
e-mail: office@advocadopress.org
www.advocadopress.org

$14.95

96 pages
ISBN 0-962706-46-9

5807 Answering Your Questions About Spina Bifid a

Spina Bifida Association of America
4590 Macarthur Boulevard NW
Suite 250
Washington, DC 20007
202-944-3285
800-621-3141
FAX: 202-944-3295
e-mail: sbaa@sbaa.org
www.sbaa.org

Provides information to help you understand the basic medical, educational and socail issues which commonly affect people with spina bifida. *$8.00*

5808 Aphasia

Federal Government
31 Center Drive MSC2320
Bethesda, MD 20892
800-241-1044
FAX: 301-402-0018
e-mail: nidcdinfo@nidcd.nih.gov
www.aphasia.org/NAAfactsheet.html

This fact sheet explains who has aphasia, the causes of aphasia, how aphasia is diagnosed and treated, and what research is being conducted on aphasia.

5809 Arc Connection Newsletter

Arc of Tennessee
44 Vantage Way
Suite 550
Nashville, TN 37228
615-248-5878
800-835-7077
FAX: 615-248-5879
e-mail: pcooper@thearctn.org
www.thearctn.org

Walter Rogers, Executive Director
Peggy Cooper, Associate Director

The Arc of Tennessee is a nonprofit organization that offers advocacy, information, referral and support to people with mental retardation or a related developmental disability and their families. This is their publication. It is free to members. *$10.00*

12 pages Quarterly

5810 Arc Light

Arc of Arizona
5610 S Central Avenue
Phoenix, AZ 85040
602-243-1787
800-252-9054
FAX: 602-268-7483
e-mail: Arcofarizona@aol.com
www.arcofarizona.org

Quarterly

5811 Aromatherapy Book: Applications and Inhalations

North Atlantic Books
1456 Fourth Street
Berkeley, CA 94710
510-559-8277
FAX: 510-559-8279
e-mail: info@northatlanticbooks.com
www.northatlanticbooks.com

Considered a bible for those interested in aromatherapy. *$18.95*

1992
ISBN 1-556430-73-6

5812 Aromatherapy for Common Ailments

Simon & Schuster
100 Front Street
Riverside, NJ 08075
800-323-7445
FAX: 800-943-9831
www.simonsays.com

Explains aromatherapy with emphasis on medicinal uses.

96 pages 1991
ISBN 0-671731-34-3

5813 Aromatherapy to Heal and Tend the Body

Lotus Press
PO Box 325
Twin Lakes, WI 53181
262-889-8561
800-824-6369
FAX: 262-889-2461
e-mail: lotuspress@lotuspress.com
www.lotuspress.com

Santosh Krinsky, President

Explains the history of aromatherapy. *$10.95*

1988
ISBN 0-941524-42-6

5814 Art of Aromatherapy

Destiny Books
1 Park Street
PO Box 388
Rochester, VT 05767
802-767-3174
FAX: 802-767-3174

Jessica Dudley, Sales Associate

Reference book on essential oils. *$14.95*

328 pages Paperback 1987
ISBN 0-892810-01-7

5815 Arthritis Bible

Healing Arts Press
One Park Street
Rochester, VT 05767
802-767-3174
800-246-8648
FAX: 802-767-3726
e-mail: orders@innertraditions.com
www.InnerTraditions.com

Jessica Dudley, Sales Associate

A comprehensive guide to the alternative therapies and conventional treatments for Arthritic diseases including Osteoarthritis, Rheumatoid Arthritis, Gout, Fibromyalgia and more. *$14.95*

272 pages
ISBN 0-892818-25-5

5816 Assistive Technology News

South Carolina Assistive Technology Project
School Of Medicine, CDR
University Of South Carolina
Columbia, SC 29208
803-935-5263
FAX: 803-935-5342
e-mail: jjendron@usit.net
www.sc.edu/scatp/

Evelyn Evans, Editor
Janet Jendron, Editor
Mary Alice Bechtler, Editor

7-8 pages Bi-annually

5817 Asthma & Allergy Advocate Newsletter

Academy of Allergy, Asthma, Immunology
611 E Wells Street
Milwaukee, WI 53202
414-272-6071
800-822-2762
FAX: 414-272-6070
e-mail: info@aaaai.org
www.aaaai.org

Offers tips and medical information on allergies and asthmatic conditions including the newest treatments and public awareness news. *$6.00*

4 pages Quarterly

5818 **Attending to America: Personal Assistance for Independent Living**

World Institute on Disability
510 16th Street
Suite 100
Oakland, CA 94612 **510-763-4100**
FAX: 510-763-4109
e-mail: wid@wid.org
www.wid.org

This unique 1987 report explores the then-current publicly provided personal assistance system in the US. It contains policy recommendations and action steps, a definition of terms, a directory of attendant service programs in the US and a bibliography. *$20.00*

190 pages Paperback

5819 **Attitudes Toward Persons with Disabilities**

Springer Publishing Company
536 Broadway
New York, NY 10012 **212-431-4370**
877-687-7476
FAX: 212-941-7842
e-mail: marketing@springerpub.com
www.springerpub.com

Annette Imperati, Marketing/Sales Director

This volume examines what is known of people's complex and multifaceted attitudes toward persons with disabilities. Divided into five areas of concern: theory, origin of attitudes, attitude measurement, attitudes of specific groups and attitude change. *$38.95*

352 pages Hardcover
ISBN 0-82616 -90-1

5820 **Augmentative and Alternative Communication**

Brookes Publishing
49 the Downey W
Suite 308
Tronto, ON M3C-3 **416-385-0351**
800-638-3775
FAX: 416-385-0352
e-mail: secretariat@issac-online.org
www.jadea.dk/baggrund.htm

Nancy Christie, Executive Director

Management of Severe Communication Disorders in Children and Adults, 2nd edition. This textbook contains the most recent information available on implementing augmentative and alternative communication (AAC), explaining principles and procedures of AAC assessment and offering intervention techniques. *$59.95*

592 pages Hardcover 1998
ISBN 1-55766 -33-5

5821 **Authoritative Guide to Self- Help Resource in Mental Health**

Guilford Press
72 Spring Street
New York, NY 10012 **212-431-9800**
800-365-7006
FAX: 212-966-6708
www.guilford.com

Linda F Campbell PhD, Author
Thomas P Smith PsyD, Author
Robert Sommer PhD, Author

Reviews and rates 600+ self-help books, autobiographies, and popular films, and evaluates hundreds of Internet sites. Addresses 28 of the most prevalent clinical disorders and life challenges- from ADHD, Alzheimer's, and anxiety disorders, to marital problems, mood disorders and weight management. Also in cloth at $45.00 (ISBN# 1-57230-506-1) *$25.00*

377 pages Paperback 1900
ISBN 1-572305-80-0

5822 **AwareNews**

Services for Independent Living
25100 Euclid Avenue
Suite 105
Cleveland, OH 44117 **216-731-1529**
FAX: 216-731-3083
e-mail: sil@stratos.net

Molly Thomas, Services Coordinator

12 pages Quarterly

5823 **Awareness Through Movement: Health Exercises for Personal Growth**

Harper & Row
10 E 53rd Street
New York, NY 10022 **212-207-7002**
800-242-7737
FAX: 212-207-7145

Explores renewed health and increased sensory awareness through the Feldenkrais method. Provides paths for people of every age to integrate physical and mental develpment into a new, invigorating wholeness. Indtroduces a modern-day, practical program for the perennial ideal of a healthy mind and a healthy body, avoiding mystical components or pupil to master abtruse theories.

173 pages Paperback 1972
ISBN 0-060623-45-4

5824 **Babycare Assistive Technology**

Through the Looking Glass
2198 Sixth Street
Suite 100
Berkeley, CA 94710 **510-848-1112**
800-644-2666
FAX: 510-848-4445
e-mail: TLG@lookingglass.org
www.lookingglass.org

C Tuleja
A DeMoss

Available in braille, large print or cassette. *$2.00*

8 pages

5825 **Babycare Assistive Technology for Parents with Physical Disabilties**

Through the Looking Glass
2198 Sixth Street
Suite 100
Berkeley, CA 94710 **510-848-1112**
800-644-2666
FAX: 510-848-4445
e-mail: TLG@lookingglass.org
www.lookingglass.org

M Kirshbaum

Relational, systems and Cultural perspectives. Available in braille, large print or cassette. *$2.00*

7 pages

5826 **Babyface: A Story of Heart and Bones**

Spina Bifida Association of America
4590 Macarthur Boulevard NW
Suite 250
Washington, DC 20007 **202-944-3285**
800-621-3141
FAX: 202-944-3295
e-mail: sbaa@sbaa.org
www.sbaa.org

A must read for families that seek insight into coping with a chronic condition. Many useful resources provided. *$32.90*

5827 **Bach Flower Therapy: Theory and Practice**

Inner Traditions
1 Park Street
POBox 388
Rochester, VT 05767 **802-767-3174**

Contemporary study of Bach's techniques, intended for practitioners and lay readers alike. Includes lists of symptoms to facilitate diagnosis, ans aims to provide an understanding of psychosomatic elements in relation to physical complaints.

1988
ISBN 0-892812-39-7

5828 **Balancing Act**

Vestibular Disorders Association
PO Box 4467
Portalnd, OR 97208 **503-229-7705**
800-837-8428
FAX: 503-229-8064
e-mail: veda@vestibular.org
www.vestibular.org

Lisa Haven, Editor
Connie Pilcher, Editor

$15.00

1901
ISBN 0-963261-15-0

5829 **Be Sick Well: A Healthy Approach to Chronic Illness**

New Harbinger Publications
5674 Shattuck Avenue
Oakland, CA 94609 **510-652-0215**
800-748-6273
FAX: 510-652-5472
e-mail: customerservice@newharbinger.com
www.newharbinger.com

Makes the distinction between disease - what is objective and measurable - and illness, the subjective, unmeasurable experience of being sick. *$11.95*

188 pages Hardcover 1991
ISBN 1-879237-08-3

5830 **Beliefs, Values, and Principles of Self Advocacy**

Brookline Books
PO Box 1047
Cambridge, MA 02238 **617-868-0360**
800-666-2665
FAX: 617-868-1772
e-mail: brooklinebks@delphi.com
www.brooklinebooks.com

Written by self-advocates around the world, they tell about the beliefs, values, and principles important to them, and the empowerment and personal growth they experience through self-advocacy. *$7.00*

48 pages Paperback
ISBN 0-57129 -22-2

5831 **Beliefs: Pathways to Health and Well Being**

Metamorphous Press
PO Box 10616
Portland, OR 97296 **503-228-4972**
FAX: 503-223-9117
www.metamodels.com/meta/bks/hea1.htm

Explores behavioral technologies and belief change strategies that can alter beliefs that support unhealthy habbits such as smoking, overeating, and drug use. Also covers the changing of thinking processes that create phobias and unreasonable fears, retraining the immune system to eliminate allergies and to deal optinally with cancer, AIDS, and other diseases. Includes strategies to transform unhealthy beliefs into lifelong constructs of wellness.

5832 **Bench Marks**

Govennor's Council on Developmental Disabilities
1717 W Jefferson Street
Site Code 0742
Phoenix, AZ 85007 **602-542-4049**
800-889-5893
FAX: 602-542-5320
e-mail: mward@mail.dc.state.us

Micheal Ward, Executive Director

Quarterly

5833 **Between Heaven and Earth: A Guide to Chinese Medicine**

Ballantine Books
1540 Braodway
New York, NY 10022 **212-782-9000**
FAX: 212-302-7985
www.randomhouse.com

Researches areas of Chinese medicine.

1991

5834 **Beyond Antibiotics: Healthier Options for Families**

North Atlantic Books
1456 4th Street
Berkley, CA 94710 **510-559-8277**
FAX: 510-559-8279
e-mail: info@northatlanticbooks.com
www.northatlanticbooks.com

An overview of ways to boost immunity and avoid antibiotics. Provides a range of alternative health measures, including vitamins and herbal medicines. *$16.95*

Paperback 1992
ISBN 1-556431-34-1

5835 **Beyond Gentle Teaching**

Autism Society of North Carolina Bookstore
505 Oberlin Road
Suite 230
Raleigh, NC 27605 **919-743-0204**
800-442-2762
FAX: 919-743-0208
e-mail: dcoffey@autismsociety-nc.org
www.autismsociety-nc.org

Darla Coffey, Bookstore Manager

A nonaversive approach to helping those in need, caregivers. *$35.00*

5836 **Body Awareness in Action: A Study of the Alexander Technique**

Schocken Books
201 E 50th Street
New York, NY 10019 **212-261-6500**
FAX: 212-261-6785
www.towardsfreedom.com/books/body.html

J McVicker Hunt, Illustrator

206 pages 1979
ISBN 0-805206-28-0

5837 **Body Electric: Electromagnetism and the Foundation of Life**

William Morrow & Company
1350 Avenue of the Americas
New York, NY 10019 **212-261-6500**
FAX: 212-261-6795

Maria D Guarnaschelli, Editor
David Bell, Illustrator

Explores the role of electricity in healing, challenging the traditional mechanistic model of the body. Includes research, scientific and medical politics, and new discoveries and possibilities for fighting disease and harnessing the body's healing powers.

368 pages Hardcover 1987
ISBN 0-688069-71-1

5838 Body Reflexology: Healing at Your Fingertips

Parker Publishing Company
1501 Broadway
 # 2605
New York, NY 10036 **212-719-9777**

Features step-by-step instructions of how to send healing flows of energy through the body to relieve back pain, headaches, arthritis, and other afflictions. Illustrated.

343 pages Hardcover 1995
ISBN 0-132997-36-3

5839 Body Silent: The Different World of the Disabled

WW Norton & Company
324 State Street
Suite H - Special Needs Project
Santa Barbara, CA 93101
800-333-6867
FAX: 805-962-5087
www.specialneeds.com/store/

The author's personal account of his progressive and terminal loss of muscle function caused by a spinal tumor, resulting in quadripilegia. Includes society's fears, myths, and misunderstandings about disability and the damage they inflict. *$9.95*

256 pages 1901
ISBN 0-393320-42-1

5840 Body of Knowledge/Hellerwork

406 Berry Street
Mt. Shasta, CA 96067 **530-926-2500**

Information, referral directory, training and certification.

5841 Body/Mind Purification Program

Simon & Schuster
100 Front Street
Riverside, NJ 08075
800-323-7445
FAX: 800-943-9831
www.simonsays.com

Guide to detoxification and a clean, healthy diet.

Paperback 1991
ISBN 0-671685-26-0

5842 Book of Massage: The Complete Step-By-Step Guide to Eastern and Western Techniques

Simon & Schuster
100 Front Street
Riverside, NJ 08075
800-323-7445
FAX: 212-605-4872
www.simonsays.com

Anthony Porter, Contributor

Step-by-step instructional guide to the relaxing and healing skills of the hands, from massage to shiatsu and reflexology.

191 pages 1984
ISBN 0-671541-39-0

5843 Brain Allergies: The Psychonutrient Connection

Keats Publishing
27 Pine Street
PO Box 876
New Canaan, CT 06840 **203-966-8721**
800-323-4900

$15.00

245 pages Hardcover 1987
ISBN 0-879833-28-9

5844 Breaking Ground

Tennessee Council on Developmental Disabilities
500 Deaderick Street
Andrew Jackson Building 13th Floor
Nashville, TN 37243 **615-532-6615**
FAX: 615-532-6964
e-mail: tnddc@state.tn.us
www.state.tn.us/cdd

20 pages Quarterly

5845 Breaking New Ground News Note

Purdue University
1146 ABE Building
Purdue University
W Lafayette, IN 47907 **765-494-5088**
800-825-4264
FAX: 765-496-1356
e-mail: bng@ecn.purdue.edu
engineering.purdue.edu/CEM/News/2002/cem_news

Paul Jones, Coordinator

News, practical ideas and success stories of and for farmers with physical disabilities.

12-16 pages Quarterly

5846 Breaking New Ground Resource Center

Purdue University
1146 ABE Building
W Lafayette, IN 47907 **765-494-5088**
800-825-4264
FAX: 765-496-1356
e-mail: bng@ecn.purdue.edu
www.agrability.org

William Field, Director
Paul Jones, Information Specialist

A resource center devoted to helping farmers and ranchers with physical disabilities. Several resource materials and a free newsletter are available to anyone.

5847 Breathe Free

Lotus Press
PO Box 325
Twin Lakes, WI 53181 **262-889-8561**
800-824-6369
FAX: 262-889-2461
e-mail: lotuspress@lotuspress.com
www.lotuspress.com

Santosn Krinsky, President

A nutritional and herbal medicine self-help guide to treating a full range of respiratory conditions, including colds and flu.

179 pages 1998
ISBN 0-914955-07-1

5848 Bridge Newsletter

Arizona Bridge to Independent Living
1229 E Washington Street
Pheonix, AZ 85034
602-256-2245
800-280-2245
FAX: 602-254-6407
e-mail: azbridge@abil.org
www.abil.org

12 pages Monthly

5849 Brown University Long Term Care Advisor

Manisses Communications Group
208 Governor Street
Providence, RI 02906
401-831-6020
800-333-7771
FAX: 401-861-6370
e-mail: manisses@manisses.com
www.manisses.com

Fraser Lang, Publisher

Contains practical reports for health care professionals working in long-term care facilities. Published monthly. *$329.00*

8 pages Newsletter

ISSN 1088-92 8

5850 Building Bridges: Including People with Disabilities in International Programs

Mobility International USA
PO Box 10767
Eugene, OR 97440
541-343-1284
FAX: 541-343-6812
e-mail: info@miusa.org
www.miusa.org

Susan Sygall, Executive Director
Pamela Houston, Public Relations Coordinator
Tracy Scharn, Project Assistant

Features more than 200 pages of suggestions and creative ideas for including, recruiting and accommodating people with disabilities in international programs. This third edition contains expanded and updated information, as well as new chapters on cross-cultural issues in disability, volunteer service programs and legal issues for international advisors. Available in alternative formats. *$20.00*

1998

ISBN 1-880034-36-0

5851 Bulletin of the Association on the Handicapped

Assoc. on Handicapped Student Service Program
PO Box 21192
Columbus, OH 43221
614-365-5216
FAX: 614-365-6718

Membership journal including Association news, articles and sections such as Literature in Review and Speak Out. *$16.00*

5852 Bush Fellows News

Bush Foundation
E-900 First National Bank Building
332 Minnesota Street
Saint Paul, MN 55101
651-227-0891
FAX: 651-297-6485
e-mail: kkleppe@bushfoundation.org
www.bushfoundation.org

Kelly Kleppe, Editor

24-32 pages Quarterly

5853 CDR Reports

Council for Disability Rights
205 W Randolph Street
Suite 1645
Chicago, IL 60606
312-444-9484
FAX: 312-444-1977
e-mail: cdrights@interaccess.com
www.disabilityrights.org

Jo Holzer, Executive Director/Editor
Bruce Moore, Employment Specialist

$15.00

8 pages Monthly

5854 California Financial Power of Attorney

NOLO
950 Parker Street
Berkeley, CA 94710
510-549-1976
800-955-4775
FAX: 510-548-5902
www.nolo.com

Maira Dizgalvis, Trade Customer Service Manager
Susan McConnell, Director Sales
Natasha Kaluza, Sales Assistant

A plain-English book packed with forms and instructions to give a trusted person the legal authority to handle your financial affairs.

paperback

5855 Center for Libraries and Educational Improvement

400 Maryland Avenue SW
Washington, DC 20202
202-260-2226
FAX: 202-401-0689

Malcolm Davis, Acting Director

Administers the Library Services Construction Act, which authorizes grants to the states for library services to the physically handicapped.

5856 Centers for Disease Control Public Health Service

US Department of Health and Human Services
MS C09 1600 Clifton Road NE
Atlanta, GA 30333
404-639-3311

Publishes an annually updated list of infectious and communicable diseases transmitted through the handling of food in accordance with Section 103 of Title I.

5857 Centurion

Delaware Commision of Veterans Affairs
Robbins Building
802 Silver Lake Boulevard,Suite 100
Dover, DE 19904
302-739-2792
800-344-9900
FAX: 302-739-2794
e-mail: adavila@state.de.us
www.state.de.us

Quarterly

5858 Charting a Hero's Journey

International Partnership for Service-Learning
815 2nd Avenue
Suite 315
New York, NY 10017
212-986-0989
FAX: 212-986-5039
e-mail: info@ipsl.org
www.ipsl.org

Linda A Chisholm, President
Sarah Callahan, Coordinator of Special Projects

A guide to the writing of a journal for college students engaged in study abroad, off-campus study. and/or service-learning. *$ 23.95*

328 pages

ISBN 0-970198-42-6

5859 Chesity

Spina Bifida Association of America
4590 Macarthur Boulevard NW
Suite 250
Washington, DC 20007
202-944-3285
800-621-3141
FAX: 202-944-3295
e-mail: sbaa@sbaa.org
www.sbaa.org

5860 Chinese Herbal Medicine

Shambhala Publications
PO Box 308
Boston, MA 02117
617-424-0030
FAX: 617-236-1563
e-mail: editors@shambhala.com
www.shambhala.com

Gives an in-depth look into herbal medicine.

176 pages

ISBN 0-877733-98-8

5861 Choosing a Wheelchair: A Guide for Optimal Independence

Patient-Centered Guides
101 Morris Street
Sebastopol, CA 95472
707-829-0515
800-294-4747
FAX: 800-997-9901
e-mail: order@oreilly.com
www.patientcenters.com

Linda Lamb, Editor
Shawnde Paull, Marketing

With the right wheelchair, quality of life increases dramatically and even people with severe disabilities can have a considerable degree of independence and activity. Choosing the wrong chair can indeed the tantamount to confinement. This book describes technology, options, and the selection process to help you identify the chair than can provide you with optimal independence. *$9.95*

186 pages Paperback

ISBN 1-565924-11-8

5862 Closing the Gap

PO Box 68
Henderson, MN 56044
507-248-3294
FAX: 507-248-3810
e-mail: info@closingthegap.com
www.closingthegap.com

Megan Turek, Editor

Explores use of microcomputers as personal and educational tools for persons with disabilities.

36+ pages BiMonthly

5863 College Student's Guide to Merit and Other No-Need Funding 2002-2004

Reference Service Press
5000 Windplay Drive
Suite 4
El Dorado Hills, CA 95762
916-939-9620
FAX: 916-939-9626
e-mail: findaid@aol.com
www.rspfunding.com

Gail Ann Schlachter, Author

More than 1,200 funding opportunities for currently-enrolled or returning college students are described in this directory. *$32.00*

450 pages

ISBN 1-588410-41-2

5864 Color Therapy

Aurora Press
300 Catron Street
Suite B
Santa Fe, NM 87501
505-989-9804

Guide to daily uses.

5865 Common Cold and Common Sense

Simon & Schuster Mail Order
100 Front Street
Riverside, NJ 08075
800-323-7445
FAX: 800-943-9831

A practical approach to treating colds and flu based on diet and nutrition.

1981

5866 Commonly Asked Questions About the ADA and Law Enforcement

US Department of Justice
950 Pennsylvania Avenue NW DRS-NYAV
Washington, DC 20530
202-307-0663
800-574-0301
FAX: 202-307-1197
www.ada.gov

A 13-page publication explaining ADA requirements for ensuring that people with disabilities receive the same law enforcement services and protections as provided to others.

5867 Commuique/Newspaper

National Association of School Psychologist
4340 EW Highway
Suite 402
Bethesda, MD 20814
301-657-0270
FAX: 301-657-0275
e-mail: inealis@naspweb.org
www.nasponline.org

$45.00

50 pages Monthly

5868 Communicating at the End oF the Twentieth Century: Innovative Computer Programs

Independent Living Research Utilization ILRU
2323 S Shepherd Drive
Suite 1000
Houston, TX 77019
713-520-0232
FAX: 713-520-5785
www.ilru.org

This month's readings features two more of the winners in last year's Innovative CIL competitions. Steve brown of the Institute on Disability culture has combined the submissions of MetroWest Center for Independent Living and Pathways for the future, Inc. into an article that looks at how centers can use their independence.

10 pages

5869 **Communication Outlook**

Artificial Language Laboratory
405 Computer Center
Michigan State University
E Lansing, MI 48824 **517-353-0870**
FAX: 517-353-4766
e-mail: artling@msu.edu
www.msu.edu/~artlang

Caroline Watt, Editor
Katie Smith, Editor

Communication Outlook (CO) is an international quarterly magazine, which focuses on the techniques and technology of augmentative and alternative communication. CO provides information on technological developments for persons experiencing communication handicaps due to neurological, sensory or neuromuscular conditions. *$18.00*

32 pages Quarterly

5870 **Communication in Autism**

Federal Government
31 Center Drive MSC2320
Bethesda, MD 20892
800-241-1044
FAX: 301-402-0018
e-mail: nidcdinfo@nidcd.nih.gov
www.nidcd.nih.org

Describes what is autism, who is affected be autism, the communication problems with autism, how are the speech and language problems of autism treated, and what research is being conducted to improve the communication of individuals with autism.

5871 **Communique**

Michigan Association for Deaf, Hearing and Speech
2929 Covington Court
Suite 200
Lansing, MI 48912 **517-487-0066**
800-968-7327
FAX: 517-487-2586
e-mail: yourear@msu.edu
www.madhs.org

4-8 pages Bi-Annually

5872 **Community Connections Newsletter**

Mental Health Association of NY State
194 Washington Avenue
Suite 415
Albany, NY 12210 **518-434-0439**
800-766-6177
FAX: 518-427-8676
e-mail: infocenter@mhanys.org
www.mhany.org

Quarterly

5873 **Community Services Reporter**

National Assoc. of State Directors of DD Services
113 Oronoco Street
Alexandria, VA 22314 **703-683-4202**
FAX: 703-683-8773
e-mail: lsarigoi@nasddds.org
www.nasddds.org/index.shtml

Leyla Sarigor, State Policy Analyst

Reports exclusively on state and local policy and programmatic initiatives affecting people with developmental disabilities, including; person-centered planning models, quality assurance activities, managed care initiatives, state reorganizations, waiting list reduction initiatives, community-living options, and key state legislation, including an annual nationwide summary of newly enacted state laws. *$ 95.00*

8 pages Yearly

5874 **Complete Aromatherapy Handbook: Essential Oils for Radiant Health**

Sterling Press
420 W 1700 S
Salt Lake City, UT 84115 **801-486-4641**
FAX: 801-467-2221

Describes the history of aromatherapy.

1991

5875 **Complete Guide To Mercury Toxicity from De ntal Fillings**

Environmental Dental Association
16905 Avenidia De Acacias
PO Box 2184
Rancho Santa Fe, CA 92067 **858-586-1208**
800-388-2184
FAX: 858-756-7843
e-mail: info@enviormentaldental.com
www.enviormentaldental.com

191 pages
ISBN 0-944796-36-2

5876 **Complete Guide to Health and Nutrition**

Delacorte Press
1540 Broadway
New York, NY 10036 **212-782-9000**
FAX: 212-302-7985

Explores the nurtitional field.

5877 **Computer and Web Resources for People with Disabilities**

Hunter House Publishers
1515 1/2 Park Street
PO Box 2914
Alameda, CA **510-865-5282**
800-266-5592
FAX: 510-865-4295
e-mail: sales@hunterhouse.com
www.hunterhouse.com

Earlita K Chenault, Publicity Coordinator

Part One describes conventional and assistive technologies and gives strategies for accessing the Internet. Part Two features easy-to-use charts organized by key access concerns, and provides detailed descriptions of software, hardware, and communication aids. Part Three is a gold mine of Web resources, publications, support organizations, government programs, and technology vendors. *$27.95*

ISBN 0-897933-01-X

5878 **Constellations**

Minnesota STAR Program
50 Sherburne Avenue
Suite 309
St Paul, MN 55155 **651-296-2771**
800-657-3862
FAX: 651-282-6671
e-mail: star.program@state.mn.us
www.admin.state.mn.us/assistivetechnology

Chuck Rassbach, Executive Director

Free quarterly publication from the Minnesota STAR Program.

8 pages Quarterly

5879 **Consumer Buyer's Guide for Independent Living**

American Occupational Therapy Association (AOTA)
4720 Montgomery Lane
Bethesda, MD 20814
301-654-7655
800-OHE-LP4U
FAX: 301-652-7711

Cheryl Hager, Marketing Director

A buyer's directory of products and publications for the general public listing suppliers' names, addresses and telephone numbers. This directory lists AOTA publications on numerous topics (back pain, Alzheimers, Carpal Tunnel Syndrome, etc.) and suppliers of equipment to assist in activities of daily living for individuals with disabilities.

60 pages Annual

5880 **Consumer Information Catalog**

Consumer Information Center
Pueblo, CO 81009
888-878-8256
FAX: 719-948-9724
e-mail: catalog.pueblo@gsa.gov
www.pueblo.gsa.gov

Judi Mahaney, Media Specialist

The Consumer Information Center publishes the free, quarterly Consumer Information Catalog. The catalog lists over 200 selected booklets of consumer interest published by more than 40 agencies of the federal government. Topics covered includes employment and education, children, cars, small business, housing, health, nutrition, money management, federal programs and more. Nearly half of the publications listed are available for free; the remainder are moderately priced.

5881 **Coping with Your Allergies**

Simon & Schuster
100 Front Street
Riverside, NJ 08075
800-323-7445
FAX: 800-943-9831
www.simonsays.com

1986

ISBN 0-671601-99-7

5882 **Coping+Plus: Dimensions of Disability**

Greenwood Publishing Group
88 Post Road W
Suite 5007
Westport, CT 06880
203-226-3571
FAX: 203-222-1502
www.greenwood.com

Everyone can learn new or more effective coping skills and strategies to deal with times of loss, crisis and disability. $55-$59.95

280 pages Hardcover

ISBN 0-275945-44-8

5883 **Council News**

Northern Nevada Center for Independent Living
999 Pyramid Way
Sparks, NV 86431
775-353-3599
FAX: 775-353-3588
e-mail: nncil@sbcglobal.net

12 pages Quarterly

5884 **Cox-2 Connection**

Healing Arts Press
One Park Street
Rochester, VT 05767
802-767-3174
800-246-8648
FAX: 802-767-3726
e-mail: orders@innertraditions.com
www.InnerTraditions.com

Jessica Dudley, Sales Associate

$12.95

176 pages

ISBN 0-892819-84-7

5885 **Creating Wholeness: Self-Healing Workbook Using Dynamic Relaxation, Images and Thoughts**

Plenum Publishing Corporation
233 Spring Street
Floor 7
New York, NY 10013
212-620-8000
FAX: 212-463-0742

232 pages

ISBN 0-306441-72-1

5886 **Creative Care Package Catalog**

Centering Corporation
1531 N Saddle Creek Road
Omaha, NE 68104
402-553-1200
FAX: 402-533-0507
e-mail: j1200@aol.com
www.centering.org

Janet Sieff, Editor

A full catalog of all our available bereavement resources. We are a small, non-profit organization providing help to families in crisis situations.

32 pages BiAnnually

5887 **Cross Currents**

Jeremy P Tarcher
375 Hudson Street
New York, NY 10014
212-366-2000

Describes electromagmetism and how it is used in medicine.

Paperback 1991

ISBN 0-874776-09-0

5888 **DAV Magazine**

DAV Magazine
807 Maine Avenue SW
Washington, DC 20024
202-554-3501
FAX: 202-554-3581
e-mail: feedback@davmail.org
www.dav.com

Davides Autry, Editor
David Gorman, Executive Director

Reports the news, activities and programs of the organization and its members.

5889 **DRS Connection**

Disabled Resource Services
424 Pine Street
Suite 101
Fort Collins, CO 80524
970-482-2700
FAX: 970-407-7072
e-mail: drs@lymis.com
www.drs@fortnet.org

4 pages Quaterly

5890 Deaf Parents and Their Hearing Children

Through the Looking Glass
2198 Sixth Street
Suite 100
Berkeley, CA 94710 **510-848-1112**
800-644-2666
FAX: 510-848-4445
e-mail: TLG@lookingglass.org
www.lookingglass.org

J L Singleton
M D Tittle

$2.00

8 pages

5891 Demand Response Transportation Through a Rural ILC

Independent Living Research Utilization ILRU
2323 S Shepherd Drive
Suite 1000
Houston, TX 77019 **713-520-0232**
FAX: 713-520-5785
www.ilru.org

Oklahomans for Independent Living's transportation program was selected as exemplary becuase they marketed it by emphasizing people with disabilities as economic constituency.

10 pages

5892 Dental Amalgam Syndrome (DAMS) Newsletter

725-9 Tramway Lane NE
Albuquerque, NM 87122 **505-291-8239**
FAX: 505-294-3339

Dedicated to informing the public about the potential risks of mercury in dental amalgam fillings.

5893 Detecting Your Hidden Allergies

Professional Books/Future Health
211 N Sycamore
Newtown, PA 18940 **215-504-1700**
FAX: 215-860-5374
e-mail: FH@futurehealth.org
www.futurehealth.org

$10.95

232 pages Papperback 1988
ISBN 0-933478-15-1

5894 Determined to Win The Inspirational Story of Paradymic Athlete Jean Driscoll

Spina Bifida Association of America
4590 Macarthur Boulevard NW
Suite 250
Washington, DC 20007 **202-944-3285**
800-621-3141
FAX: 202-944-3295
e-mail: sbaa@sbaa.org
www.sbaa.org

$21.00

5895 Developing Organized Coalitions and Strategic Plans

Independent Living Research Utilization ILRU
2323 S Shepherd Drive
Suite 1000
Houston, TX 77019 **713-520-0232**
FAX: 713-520-5785
www.ilru.org

10 pages

5896 Dictionary of Developmental Disabilities Terminology

Brookes Publishing
PO Box 10624
Baltimore, MD 21285 **410-337-9580**
800-638-3775
FAX: 410-337-8539
e-mail: custserv@brookesopublishing.com
www.brookespublishing.com

Barbara Y Whitman MSW PhD, Editor
Carla Laszewski MSW

With more than 3,000 easy-to-understand entries, this dictionary provides thorough explanations of terms associated with developmental disabilities and disorders. *$55.95*

368 pages Hardcover 1996
ISBN 1-557662-45-2

5897 Directory of Financial Aids for Women

Reference Service Press
5000 Windplay Drive
Suite 4
El Dorado Hills, CA 95762 **916-939-9620**
FAX: 916-939-9626
e-mail: findaid@aol.com
www.rspfunding.com

Gail Ann Schlachter, Author

Funding programs listed support study, research, travel, training, career development, or innovative effort at any level; descriptions of more than 1,700 funding programs - representing billions of dollars in financial aid set aside for women; also an annotated bibliography of 60 key directories that identify even more financial aid opportunities and a set of indexes that let you search the directory by title, sponser, researching, tenability, subject, and deadline. *$45.00*

578 pages Biennial 1999
ISBN 1-588410-00-5

5898 Directory of Members

American Network of Community Options & Resources
1101 King Street
Suite 380
Alexandria, VA 22314 **703-535-7850**
FAX: 703-535-7860
e-mail: ancor@ancor.org
www.ancor.org

Renee L Pietrangelo, CEO
Suellen Galbraith, Director Public Policy

The Directory lists over 600 agencies that provide residential services and supports in 48 states and the District of Columbia. The listings include the name of the Executive Directors, the name, address, and phone number of the agency, describe the types of services that are provided and how many individuals receive services from that agency. *$25.00*

189 pages

5899 Disabilities Sourcebook

Omnigraphics
615 Griswold Street
Detroit, MI 48226
800-234-1340
FAX: 800-875-1340
www.omnigraphics.com

Paul Rogers, Publicity Associate
Georgiann Lauginger, Customer Service Manager

$78.00

616 pages 1900
ISBN 0-780803-89-2

5900 Disability Awareness Guide

Central Iowa Center for Independent Living
655 Walnut Street
Suite 131
Des Moines, IA 50309
515-243-1742
FAX: 515-243-5385
e-mail: cicil@raccoon.com
www.raccoon.com/-cicil

Robert Jeppesen, Director
Frank Strong, Assistant Director Programs

The Disability Awareness Guide contains information about our center; who we are and what we do. It also contains the telephone numbers of local and national agencies and resources available for people with disabilities.

5901 Disability Bookshop Catalog

PO Box 129
Vancouver, WA 98666
360-694-2462
800-637-2256
FAX: 360-696-3210
e-mail: twinpeak@pacifier.com
disabilitybookshop.virtualave.net/

Offers more than 400 hard-to-find titles covering a wide range of health topics for the general public, and matters of interest to people with disabilities. Catalog. *$4.00*

40 pages

5902 Disability Culture Perspective on Early Intervention

Through the Looking Glass
2198 Sixth Street
Suite 100
Berkeley, CA 94710
510-848-1112
800-644-2666
FAX: 510-848-4445
e-mail: TLG@lookingglass.org
www.lookingglass.org

M Kirshbaum

For parents with physical or cognitive disabilities and their families. Available in braille, large print or cassette. *$2.00*

12 pages

5903 Disability Rights Movement

Children's Press
Sherman Turnpike
Danbury, CT 06813
800-621-1115
FAX: 800-374-4329

Elena Rockman, Marketing Manager

Author Deborah Kent illuminates both the history of the National Disability Rights Movement and the inspiring personal stories of individuals with various disabilities. *$18.00*

32 pages Hardcover
ISBN 0-53106 -32-3

5904 Disabled People's International's Fifth World Assembly As Reported by Two US Participant

Independent Living Research Utilization ILRU
2323 S Shepherd Drive
Suite 1000
Houston, TX 77019
713-520-0232
FAX: 713-520-5785
www.ilru.org

This report describes the international conference on independent living held in Mexico City in December 1998 as experienced by staff members from two U.S. centers. Kaye Beneke interviewed Luis Chew and Marco Antonio Coronado for htis edition of Readings in Independent Living.

10 pages

5905 Disabled We Stand

Brookline Books
PO Box 1046
Cambridge, MA 02238
617-868-0360
800-666-2665
FAX: 617-868-1772
e-mail: brooklinebks@delphi.com
www.brooklinebooks.com

This book is impassioned, often angry, but also hopeful and practical, suggesting a series of actions that will lead to constructive change. It is imbued with spirit and energy of disabled people who are determined to take their lives into their own hands. *$10.95*

Paperback
ISBN 0-25331 -80-0

5906 Disabled, the Media, and the Information Age

Greenwood Publishing Group
88 Post Road W
Suite 5007
Westport, CT 06880
203-226-3571
FAX: 203-222-1502
www.greenwood.com

A short and easy-to-read overview of how disabled Americans have been portrayed by the media and how images and the role of the handicapped are changing. *$55.00*

264 pages Hardcover
ISBN 0-313284-72-5

5907 Discovery Newsletter

North Dakota State Library Talking Book Services
604 E Boulevard Avenue
Department 250
Bismarck, ND 58505
701-328-1408
800-843-9948
FAX: 701-328-2040
e-mail: tbooks@state.nd.us
ndsl.lib.state.nd.us/DisabilityServices.html

Terri Wilhelm, Manager Talking Books

6 pages Bi-Annually

5908 Diverse Abilities: An Outcome of Organizational Collab. & Oper. Integration

Independent Living Research Utilization ILRU
2323 S Shepherd Drive
Suite 1000
Houston, TX 77019
713-520-0232
FAX: 713-520-5785
www.ilru.org

Hawaii Centers for independent Living collaborated with other non-profit agencies to reduce costs and expand services. Although the resulting platform organization, DiverseAbilities, is still in its infancy, Mark Obatake, executive director of HCIL and one of this months authors, believes that the processthey went through in developing the collaboration has value for centers and SILCs.

10 pages

5909 EP Resource Guide

Exceptional Parent Library
120 Sylvan Avenue, Suite 10
PO Box 1807
Englewood Cliffs, NJ 07632
800-535-1910
FAX: 201-947-9376
e-mail: eplibrary@aol.com
www.eplibrary.com

Lists directories of national organizations, associations, products and services. *$9.95*

5910 **ESCIL Update Newsletter**

Eastern Shore Center for Independent Living
9 Sunburst Center
Cambridge, MD 21613 **410-221-7701**
800-705-7944
FAX: 410-221-7714
e-mail: escil@comcast.net
www.escil.org

Price Baum, Executive Director
Shirl Tarbox, Assistant Executive Director
Lisa Morgan, Director IL Services

6 pages Quarterly

5911 **Easy Things to Make Things Simple: Do It Yourself Modifications for Disabled Persons**

Brookline Books
PO Box 1047
Cambridge, MA 02238 **617-495-3682**
800-666-2665
FAX: 617-868-1772
e-mail: brooklinebks@delphi.com
www.brooklinebooks.com

This book aims at older adults and others with physical limitations who require adaptations for safer and easier living in the kitchen, bathroom, bedroom, yard, and garden. The adaptations can be done inexpensively, from common materials. Large print format and detailed diagrams, plus special sections with advice caregivers . *$15.95*

160 pages Paperback
ISBN 1-571290-24-9

5912 **Eating Out: Your Guide to More Enjoyable Dining**

Plume
375 Hudson Street
New York, NY 10014 **212-366-2000**

In this book, a nationally recognized expert on diabetes nutrition, shows you how eating out can be fun, without fear of weight gain or an uncontrolled rise in blood sugar. *$4.95*

272 pages Paperback 1900
ISBN 0-452279-76-3

5913 **Educational Care**

Educators Publishing Service
31 Smith Place
Cambridge, MA 02138 **617-367-2700**
800-225-5750
FAX: 617-547-0412
www.epsbooks.com

This book, written for both parents and teachers, is based on the view that education should be a system of care that is able to look after the specific needs of individual students. Using case studies, it analyzes various types of learning disorders and then suggests ways to help students with these problems. *$31.50*

325 pages
ISBN 0-838819-87-7

5914 **Effective Strategies for Interacting with Policy-Makers**

Independent Living Research Utilization ILRU
2323 S Shepherd Drive
Suite 1000
Houston, TX 77019 **713-520-0232**
FAX: 713-520-5785
www.ilru.org

10 pages

5915 **Encyclopedia of Natural Medicine**

Prima Publishing
3000 Lava Ridge Court
PO Box 1260
Rocklin, CA 95677 **916-787-7000**
800-632-8676
FAX: 916-787-7001
e-mail: websupportlife@primapub.com
www.primapublishing.com

An authoritative guide to naturapathic medicine outlining the basic principles of health and how they can be used to treat over sixty health conditions, including candidiasis. Includes self-help approaches using diet, nutrition, and herbal medicine. *$24.95*

1991
ISBN 0-761511-57-1

5916 **Enforcing the ADA: A Status Report from th e Department of Justice**

US Department of Justice
950 Pennsylvania Avenue NW DRS-NYAV
Washington, DC 20530 **202-307-0663**
800-574-0301
FAX: 202-307-1197
www.ada.gov

A quarterly report providing timely information about ADA cases and settlements, building codes that meet ADA accessibility standards, and ADA technical assistance activities. The most current issue of the Status Report is available by Fax.

5917 **EveryBody's Different: Understanding and Changing Our Reactions to Disabilities**

Brookes Publishing
PO Box 10624
Baltimore, MD 21285 **410-337-9580**
800-638-3775
FAX: 410-337-8539
e-mail: custserv@brookespublishing.com
www.brookespublishing.com

This book discusses the emotions, questions, fears, and stereotypes that people without disabilities sometimes experience when they interact with people who do have disabilities. The author teaches readers to become more at ease with the concept of disability and to communicate more effectively with each other. Features activities and exercises that encourage self-examination, helping people to create more enriching personal relationships and work toward a fully inclusive society.

Paperback 1998
ISBN 1-55766 -59-9

5918 **Everybody's Guide to Homeopathic Medicines**

Jeremy P Tarcher
375 Hudson Street
New York, NY 10014 **212-366-2000**

Covers alternative treatments in homeopathic medicines.

375 pages 1997
ISBN 0-874778-43-3

5919 Everyday Social Interaction: A Program for People with Disabilities, 2nd Edition

Brookes Publishing
PO Box 10624
Baltimore, MD 21285 **410-337-9580**
800-638-3775
FAX: 410-337-8539
e-mail: custserv@brookespublishing.com
www.brookespublishing.com

This source guides teachers and human services professionals in helping people with disabilities acquire social interaction skills and develop satisfying relationships. Included is a checklist and task analyses that shows how complex skills can be broken down into major components for easy performance monitoring accompanied by tips on social courtesies, rewards, praise, and criticism. *$41.95*

342 pages Paperback
ISBN 1-55766-58-4

5920 Explore Your Options

Kansas Department on Aging
New England Building
503 S Kansas
Topeka, KS 66603 **785-296-4986**
800-432-3535
FAX: 785-296-0256
www.agingKansas.org

Yearly

5921 Families Magazine

New Jersey Developmental Disabilities Council
20 W State Street, 7th Floor
PO Box 700
Trenton, NJ 08625 **609-292-3745**
800-216-1199
FAX: 609-292-7114
TTY:609-777-3238
e-mail: njddc@njddc.org
www.njddc.org

Ethan Ellis, Executive Director/Editor
Norman Reim, Managing Editor

Quarterly magazine for people with disabilities, their families and the public, features family profiles, news, columns and the New Jersey Family support councils newsletter.

Quarterly

5922 Families, Illness & Disability

Through the Looking Glass
2198 Sixth Street
Suite 100
Berkeley, CA 94710 **510-848-1112**
800-644-2666
FAX: 510-848-4445
e-mail: TLG@lookingglass.org
www.lookingglass.org

J Rolland

$35.00

320 pages

5923 Family Context and Disability Culture Reframing: Through the Looking Glass

Through the Looking Glass
2198 Sixth Street
Suite 100
Berkeley, CA 94710 **510-848-1112**
800-644-2666
FAX: 510-848-4445
e-mail: TLG@lookingglass.org
www.lookingglass.org

M Kirshbaum

Available in braille, large print or cassette. *$2.00*

5 pages

5924 Farmington Valley ARC

10 Tower Lane
Avon, CT 06001 **860-693-6662**
FAX: 860-693-8662

Lynn Flerri, President
Tom Thompson, Executive Director

The official newsletter containing information, new ideas, progress and more on the Farmington Valley Association for Retarded and Handicapped Citizens.

5925 Fedcap News

Fedcap Rehabilitation Services
211 W 14th Street
New York, NY 10011 **212-727-4200**
FAX: 212-727-4374
e-mail: info@fedcap.org
www.fedcap.org

Susan Jourad, Director Community Relations

A publication from Fedcap Rehabilitation Services.

12 pages

5926 Final Report: Adapting Through the Looking Glass

Through the Looking Glass
2198 Sixth Street
Suite 100
Berkeley, CA 94710 **510-848-1112**
800-644-2666
FAX: 510-848-4445
e-mail: TLG@lookingglass.org
www.lookingglass.org

P Preston
M Lou

Adapting Through the Looking Glass intervention model for deaf parents and their children. Available in braille, large print or cassette. *$2.00*

24 pages

5927 Final Report: Challenges and Strategies of Disabled Parents: Findings from a Survey

Through the Looking Glass
2198 Sixth Street
Suite 100
Berkeley, CA 94710 **510-848-1112**
800-644-2666
FAX: 510-848-4445
e-mail: TLG@lookingglass.org
www.lookingglass.org

L Toms Barker
V Maralani

Available in braille, large print or cassette. *$25.00*

24 pages

5928 Financial Aid for Research and Creative Ac tivities Abroad

Reference Service Press
5000 Windplay Drive
Suite 4
El Dorado Hills, CA 95762 **916-939-9620**
FAX: 916-939-9626
e-mail: findaid@aol.com
www.rspfunding.com

Gail Ann Schlachter, Author

Described here are 1,200 funding programs (scholarships, fellowships, grants, etc.) available to support research, professional, or creative activities abroad. *$45.00*

378 pages

ISBN 1-588410-82-5

5929 **Financial Aid for Study and Training Abroa d**

Reference Service Press
5000 Windplay Drive
Suite 4
El Dorado Hills, CA 95762 **916-939-9620**
FAX: 916-939-9626
e-mail: findaid@aol.com
www.rspfunding.com

Gail Ann Schlachter, Author

This directory, which Children's Bookwatch calls invaluable describes more than 1,100 financial aid opportunities available to support study abroad. *$39.50*

398 pages

ISBN 1-588410-31-5

5930 **Focus Newsletter**

Arc Minnesota
770 Transfer Road
Suite 26
Saint Paul, MN 55114 **651-523-0823**
800-582-5256
FAX: 651-523-0829
e-mail: mail@arcminnesota.com
www.arcminnesota.com

Mike Gude, Editor

8 pages

5931 **Fosters Botanical and Herb Reviews**

B&H Reviews
PO Box 106
Eureka Springs, AK 72632
FAX: 479-253-7442

5932 **Four-Ingredient Cookbook**

Laurel Designs
5 Laurel Avenue
Belvedere, CA 94920
FAX: 415-435-1451
e-mail: laureld@ncal.verio.com

Janet Sawyer, Owner
Lynn Montoya, Owner

Simple, easy to follow recipes, each containing four ingredients. Particularly suited to persons with limited physical ability. Includes 400 recipes, appetizers to desserts. *$9.00*

5933 **Free Yourself From Pain**

Pocket Books
100 Front Street
Suite 158
Riverside, NJ 08075
800-323-7445
FAX: 800-943-9831

This self-help book for managing chronic pain and depression includes several chapters illustrating the use of imagery for pain control.

1992

5934 **Freedom Press**

Freedom Resource Center for Independent Living
2701 Ninth Avenue SW
Fargo, ND 58103 **701-478-0459**
800-450-0459
FAX: 701-478-0510
e-mail: freedom@fargocity.com
www.macil.org/freedom

Nate Aalgaard, Executive Director
Bobbi Franks, Information Specialist

Quarterly

5935 **Freedom from Headaches**

Simon & Schuster Mail Order
100 Front Street
Riverside, NJ 08075
800-323-7445
FAX: 800-943-9831

Covers the causes, treatments, and different varieties of headaches.

236 pages 1986

ISBN 0-671254-04-9

5936 **Freedom of Movement: IL History and Philosophy**

Independent Living Research Utilization ILRU
2323 S Shepherd Drive
Suite 1000
Houston, TX 77019 **713-520-0232**
FAX: 713-520-5785
www.ilru.org

10 pages

5937 **Frequently Asked Questions About Multiple Chemical Sensitivity**

Independent Living Research Utilization ILRU
2323 S Shepherd Drive
Suite 1000
Houston, TX 77019 **713-520-0232**
FAX: 713-520-5785
www.ilru.org

This FAQ covers important information about multiple chemical sensitivity and environmental illness. The FAQ describes the conditions, recommends strategies for improving access, and lists resources for CILs and other organizations. As the fact sheet states, centers must set an example in assuring that all people can enter their offices.

10 pages

5938 **Gastrointestinal Health**

Harper Perennial
10 E 53rd Street
New York, NY 10022 **212-207-7000**
FAX: 212-209-7145
www.harpercollins.com

Comprehensive self-help guide for treating a full range of gastrointestinal disorders using diet and nutrition.

1992

5939 **General Guidelines for Disability Policy Change Agents**

Independent Living Research Utilization ILRU
2323 S Shepherd Drive
Suite 1000
Houston, TX 77019 **713-520-0232**
FAX: 713-520-5785
www.ilru.org

10 pages

5940 **Genetic Disorders Sourcebook**

Omnigraphics
615 Griswold Street
Detroit, MI 48226
800-234-1340
FAX: 800-875-1340
www.omnigraphics.com

Kathy Massimini, Editor

Provides information on hereditary diseases and disorders. *$7800.00*

650 pages 1900

ISBN 0-789892-41-1

5941 **Getting Better**

Vestibular Disorders Association
PO Box 4467
Portland, OR 97208
503-229-7705
800-837-8428
FAX: 503-229-8064
e-mail: veda@vestibular.org
www.vestibular.org

Dr. Lisa Haven, Executive Director
Connie Pilcher, Outreach Coordinator

A non-profit organization dedicated to providing education and support to people with inner ear balance/dizziness disorder and their families and people who help them. *$25.00*

Quarterly

ISBN 0-963261-17-7

5942 **Getting Life**

Avacado Press
PO Box 145
Louisville, KY 40201
502-894-9492
FAX: 502-899-9562
e-mail: office@avocadopress.org
www.advocadopress.org

$16.00

304 pages

ISBN 0-962706-48-5

5943 **Getting the Most Out of Consultation Services**

Independent Living Research Utilization ILRU
2323 S Shepherd Drive
Suite 1000
Houston, TX 77019
713-520-0232
FAX: 713-520-5785
www.ilru.org

A practical, nuts-and-bolts approach to help make working with a consultant a positive, helpful experience for independent living centers.

10 pages

5944 **Grief: What it is and What You Can Do**

Centering Corporation
1531 N Saddle Creek Road
Omaha, NE 68104
402-553-1200
FAX: 402-533-0507
e-mail: j1200@aol.com
www.centering.org

General grief information for all grief issues. *$3.50*

32 pages Paperback

5945 **Guide to Hydrocephalus**

Spina Bifida Association of America
4590 Macarthur Boulevard NW
Suite 250
Washington, DC 20007
202-994-3285
800-621-3141
FAX: 202-944-3295
e-mail: sbaa@sbaa.org
www.sbaa.org

information to help you understand the circustances that surround you and make the job advocacy and easier one. *$8.00*

5946 **Guide to Polarity Therapy: The Gentle Art of Hands-on Healing**

North Atlantic Books
1456 Fourth Street
Berekley, CA 94710
510-559-8277
FAX: 510-559-8279

Explains the theory of polarity therapy and basic techniques.

180 pages 1991

ISBN 1-556433-29-8

5947 **Guidelines on Disability**

US Department of Housing & Urban Development
451 Seventh Street SW
Washington, DC 20410
202-708-1112
TTY:202-708-1455

Contains information on housing and accessibility for persons with disabilities.

5948 **Guidlines for Spina Bifida & Health Care S ervices Throughout Life**

Spina Bifida Association of America
4590 Macarthur Boulevard NW
Suite 250
Washington, DC 20007
202-944-3285
800-621-3141
FAX: 202-944-3295
e-mail: sbaa@sbaa.org
www.sbaa.org

These guidelines are designed to help people who have spina bifida expirence a greater sense of purpose and place in society. *$ 19.00*

5949 **Guild Audio Library**

JGB Audio Library for the Blind
15 W 65th Street
New York, NY 10023
212-769-6331
800-284-4422
FAX: 212-769-6266
e-mail: info@JGB.org
www.JGB.org

Peter Williamson, Director
Ken Satnley, Manager

5950 **Guild Briefs**

Catholic Guild for The Blind
180 N Michigan Avenue
Suite 1700
Chicago, IL 60601
312-236-8569
FAX: 312-236-8128
e-mail: guild@guildfortheblind.org
www.guildfortheblind.org

Bi-Annually

5951 Hand and Foot Reflexology: A Self-Help Guide

Simon & Schuster
100 Front Street
Riverside, NJ 08075
800-323-7445
FAX: 800-943-9831
www.simonsays.com

Comprehensive encyclopedia of personal reflexology.

1987
ISBN 0-671763-19-9

5952 Handbook of Mental Disorders Among Black Americans

Greenwood Publishing Group
88 Post Road W
Suite 5007
Westport, CT 06880 203-226-3571
FAX: 203-222-1502
www.greenwood.com

In addition to providing a wealth of new data on the mental health status of black communities, this handbook presents analyses of specific social, structural, and cultural conditions that affect the lives of individual Black Americans. $55-$65.

352 pages Hardcover
ISBN 0-313263-30-2

5953 Handbook of Services for the Handicapped

Greenwood Publishing Group
88 Post Road W
Suite 5007
Westport, CT 06880 203-226-3571
FAX: 203-222-1502
www.greenwood.com

A handy reference book offering information and services for disabled individuals. $59.95-$65.00.

291 pages Hardcover
ISBN 0-313213-85-2

5954 Handbook on Mental Health Policy in the United States

Greenwood Publishing Group
88 Post Road W
Suite 5007
Westport, CT 06880 203-226-3571
FAX: 203-222-1502
www.greenwood.com

Covers the historical, policy and administrative aspects of public mental health care. *$95.00*

563 pages $95 - $99.50
ISBN 0-313250-09-0

5955 Head First: The Biology of Hope

Thorndike Press
375 Hudson Street
New York, NY 10014 212-366-2000

Helps patients to see the positive sides of all situations.

368 pages 1990
ISBN 0-140139-65-6

5956 Headache Newsletter

19 Mantua Road
Mount Royal, NJ 08061 856-423-0258
800-255-2243
FAX: 856-423-0082
e-mail: achehq@talley.com
www.achenet.org

$20.00

Quarterly

5957 Healing Herbs

Rodale Press
33 E Minor Street
Emmaus, PA 18098 610-967-5171
FAX: 610-967-8963
www.rodale.com

Covers everything from growing the herbs to home remedies.

5958 Healing Without Fear

Healing Arts Press
One Park Street
Rochester, VT 05767 802-767-3174
800-246-8648
FAX: 802-767-3726
e-mail: orders@innertraditions.com
www.InnerTraditions.com

Jessica Dudley, Sales Associate

How to overcome your fear of doctors, hospitals and the health care system and find your way to true healing. *$14.95*

192 pages
ISBN 0-892819-92-8

5959 Healing Yourself: a Step-by-Step Program for Better Health Through Imagery

Pocket Books
100 Front Street
Riverside, NJ 08087
800-323-7445
FAX: 800-943-9831
www.simonsays.com

5960 Health Affairs

Project HOPE
7500 Old Georgetown Road
Suite 600
Bethesda, MD 20814 301-656-7401
FAX: 301-654-2845
www.healthaffairs.org

Don Metz, Executive Editor
Judie Tucker, Manager Customer Service

Multidisciplinary journal of health-care policy with articles on health-care cost, practices, innovations and new data. *$ 95.00*

30 pages Bi-Monthly 1981

5961 Hearing, Speech and Deafness Center (HSDC)

Hearing, Speech & Deafness Center (HSDC)
1625 19th Avenue
Seattle, WA 98122 206-323-5770
FAX: 206-328-6871
e-mail: hsdc@hsdc.org
www.hsdc.org

We foster and integrated approach to communication issues by providing services that address the impact of hearing loss, speech challenges and deafness on the individual, family, workplace and community, and by promoting community awareness and accessibility. A United Way funded, non-profit agency, building community through communication since 1937.

5962 **Heart of the Mind**

Real People Press
Box F
Moab, UT 84532 **435-259-7578**
FAX: 435-259-4042
e-mail: realpoep@lasal.net
www.realpeoplepress.com

Susan Ossana, Office Manager

Provides common NLP problems and several new techniques.

5963 **Herbs for the Mind: What Science Tells Us about Nature's Remedies for Depression, Stress...**

Guilford Press
72 Spring Street
New York, NY 10012 **212-431-9800**
800-365-7006
FAX: 212-966-6708
e-mail: info@guilford.com
www.guilford.com

Translates hard data into the accessible answers consumers need to make informed decisions on taking St. John's wort for depression, kava for stress or anxiety, valerian for insomnia or ginko for memory loss. *$14.95*

278 pages Paperback 1900
ISBN 1-572304-76-6

5964 **High School Senior's Guide to Merit and Ot her No-Need Funding**

Reference Service Press
5000 Windplay Drive
Suite 4
El Dorado Hills, CA 95762 **916-939-9620**
FAX: 916-939-9626
e-mail: findaid@aol.com
www.rspfunding.com

Gail Ann Schlachter, Author

Here's your guide to 1,100 funding programs that never look at income level when making awards to college bound high school seniors. *$29.95*

400 pages
ISBN 1-588410-44-X

5965 **Homeopathic Medicines at Home: Natural Remedies for Everyday Ailments and Minor Injuries**

Jeremy P Tarcher
375 Hudson Street
New York, NY 10014 **212-366-2000**

book.realbuy.ws/0874771951.html

Guide for common ailments and their cures.

5966 **Hormone Replacement Therapy, Yes or No: How to Make an Informed Decision**

Nutrition Encounter
61 Bahama Reef
Novato, CA 94948 **415-883-5154**

e-mail: sikam@earthlink.net
www.bettykamen.com

Safe, non-toxic and medically valid alternatives to conventional hormone replacement treatment for menopausal symptoms and osteoporosis.

1993

5967 **Hospice Alternative**

Harper Collins Publishers/Basic Books
10 E 53rd Street
New York, NY 10022 **212-207-7042**
800-242-7737
FAX: 212-207-7203

An account of the hospice experience. An innovative and humane way of caring for the terminally ill. *$8.95*

256 pages
ISBN 0-46503 -61-0

5968 **Housing and Independence: How Innovative CILs are Assisting Housing for Disabled People**

Independent Living Research Utilization ILRU
2323 S Shepherd Drive
Suite 1000
Houston, TX 77019 **713-520-0232**
FAX: 713-520-5785
www.ilru.org

This month's Readings is the first of many publications which will feature the winners of the Innovative CILs competition. This article is a compilation of the four winning essays as well as telephone interviews with the key staff members at each of the centers.

10 pages

5969 **How to Conduct an Assessment**

FSSI
3905 Huntington Drive
Amarillo, TX 79104 **806-853-1114**
FAX: 806-353-1114
e-mail: webamster@winfssi.com
www.winfssi.com

5970 **How to File a Title III Complaint**

US Department of Justice
950 Pennsylvania Avenue NW DRS-NYAV
Washington, DC 20530 **202-307-0663**
800-574-0301
FAX: 202-307-1197
www.ada.gov

This publication details the procedure for filing a complaint under Title III of the ADA.

5971 **How to Live Longer with a Disability**

Accent Books & Products
PO Box 700
Bloomington, IL 61702 **309-378-2961**
800-787-8444
FAX: 309-378-4420
e-mail: acmtlvng@aol.com

Raymond C Cheever, Publisher
Betty Garee, Editor

Eleven chapters to help you enjoy every aspect of your life, and live easier and happier. Includes sexuality and disability, getting more from the medical community and benefit programs. Co-authored by Robert Mauro, sociologist and Elle Becker, counselor and psychologist, both disabled. *$11.50*

266 pages Paperback
ISBN 0-19570 -38-8

5972 **How to Outsmart Your Allergies**

Asthma and Allergy Foundation of America
1125 15th Street NW
Suite 502
Washington, DC 20005
202-466-7643
FAX: 202-466-8940
e-mail: info@aafa.org
www.aafa.org

Colorful poster that will enhance any office or waiting room while educating patients. Contains innovative and factual tips for avoiding allergens and reducing or eliminating allergic symptoms. The poster depicts common allergens in an appealing format. *$1.00*

5973 **How to Pay for Your Degree in Business & Related Fields 2002-2004**

Reference Service Press
5000 Windplay Drive
Suite 4
El Dorado Hills, CA 95762
916-939-9620
FAX: 916-939-9626
e-mail: findaid@aol.com
www.rspfunding.com

Gail Ann Schlachter, Author

If you need funding for an undergraduate or graduate degree in business or related fields, this is the directory to use (500+ funding programs described). *$30.00*

290 pages
ISBN 1-588410-49-8

5974 **How to Pay for Your Degree in Education & Related Fields 2002-2004**

Reference Service Press
5000 Windplay Drive
Suite 4
El Dorado Hills, CA 95762
916-939-9620
FAX: 916-939-9626
e-mail: findaid@aol.com
www.rspfunding.com

Gail Ann Schlachter, Author

Here's hundreds of funding opportunities available to support undergraduate and graduate students preparing for a career in education, guidance etc. *$30.00*

250 pages
ISBN 1-588410-63-3

5975 **IAL News**

International Association of Laryngectomees
8900 Thornton Road E
Box 99311
Stockton, CA 95209
866-425-3678
FAX: 209-472-0516
e-mail: ial@larynxlink.com

Focuses on rehabilitation and well-being of persons who have had laryngectomy surgery.

5976 **If I Only Knew What to Say or Do**

AARP Fulfillment
601 E Street NW
Washington, DC 20049
202-434-2277
800-424-3410
FAX: 202-434-3443
e-mail: member@aarp.org
www.aarp.org

Provides a concise discussion of how to help a friend in crisis. Learn what to say and what not to say.

5977 **If it Weren't for the Honor: I'd Rather Have Walked**

Accent Books & Products
PO Box 700
Bloomington, IL 61702
309-378-2961
800-787-8444
FAX: 309-378-4420
e-mail: acmtlvng@aol.com

Raymond C Cheever, Publisher
Betty Garee, Editor

Revealing, often humorous, highly interesting and important reading. This book offers an account told by the author who was on the scene and actually saw and participated in many events that paved the way for progress for all those with disabilities. *$14.50*

262 pages Paperback
ISBN 0-91570 -41-8

5978 **Imagery in Healing Shamanism and Modern Medicine**

Shambhala Publications
PO Box 308
Boston, MA 02117
617-424-0030
FAX: 617-236-1563
e-mail: editors@shambhala.com
www.shambhala.com

Patients use self imagery to fight sickness and pain throughout their lives. *$15.95*

272 pages 1902
ISBN 1-570629-34-x

5979 **Imagine That**

Innovative Res. for Cognitive & Physical Challenes
1400 Dixon Avenue
Lafayette, CO 80026
303-665-7789
FAX: 303-665-2648
e-mail: caroline@imaginecolorado.org
www.imaginecolorado.org

Gary Stebick, Editor
Caroline Siegfried, Executive Assistant

For people of all ages with cognitive, developmental, physical & health related needs, so they may live lives of independence & quality in their homes and communities.

12-16 pages quarterly

5980 **InTouch Networks: National Radio Reading Service**

JGB Audio Library for the Blind
15 W 65th Street
New York, NY 10023
212-769-6331
800-284-4422
FAX: 212-769-6266
e-mail: info@JGB.org
www.JGB.org

Peter Williamson, Director
Ken Stanley, Manager

5981 **Independence**

Easter Seales Volusia and Flagler Ceounties, FL
1219 Dunn Avenue
Daytona Beach, FL 32114
386-255-4568
877-255-4568
FAX: 386-258-7677
e-mail: info@eseals-vf.org
http://www.easterseals-volusiaflagler.org

Penny Young, Communications Director

4-6 pages Quarterly

5982 **Independent Living Centers and Managed Care: Results of an ILRU Study on Involvement**

Independent Living Research Utilization ILRU
2323 S Shepherd Drive
Suite 1000
Houston, TX 77019 **713-520-0232**
FAX: 713-520-5785
www.ilru.org

This month's Readings presents findings from an ILRU study of roles centers are taking vis-a-vis managed care. Initiated in spring 1998, we asked Drew Batavia to take the lead in conducting this study for us. We were interested in collecting data on frequency with which centers are contacted by consumers with managed care problems. This is a study that will need to be repeated periodically as our experiences with managed care evolves. Meanwhile, here are the initial findings.

10 pages

5983 **Independent Living Challenges the Blues**

Independent Living Research Utilization ILRU
2323 S Shepherd Drive
Suite 1000
Houston, TX 77019 **713-520-0232**
FAX: 713-520-5785
www.ilru.org

Patricia's article highlights the Georgia SILC's health care advocacy efforts: the Georgia legislature passed a bill enabling Georgia Bleu to convert to for-profit status without a distribution of assets to similar nonprofit corporations; the Georgia SILC joined other health care advocates in filing a class action law suit to challenge the legality of the conversion; the Georgia SILC continues advocacy efforts to involve people with disabilities in developing and monitoring health care policy.

10 pages

5984 **Independent Living Office**

Department of Housing & Urban Development (HUD)
451 7th Street SW
Washington, DC 20410 **202-708-1422**

This office within HUD is charged with encouraging the construction of housing that is accessible to handicapped persons. The Office of Independent Living encourages modifications of apartments and other dwellings so that handicapped persons can enter without assistance.

5985 **Information Services for People with Developmental Disabilities**

Greenwood Publishing Group
88 Post Road W
Suite 5007
Westport, CT 06880 **203-226-3571**
FAX: 203-222-1502
www.greenwood.com

Linda Lucas Walling, Editor
Marilyn M Irwin, Editor

Overviews the information needs of people with developmental disabilities and tells librarians how to meet them. $65.oo-$75.00.

368 pages Hardcover
ISBN 0-313287-80-5

5986 **Informed Touch**

Healing Arts Press
One Park Street
Rochester, VT 05767 **802-767-3174**
800-246-8648
FAX: 802-767-3726
e-mail: orders@innertraditions.com
www.InnerTraditions.com

Jessica Dudley, Sales Associate

A Clinician's guide to the evaluation and treatment of myofascial disorders. *$30.00*

224 pages
ISBN 0-892817-40-2

5987 **Innovative Programs: An Example of How CILs Can Put Their Work in the Context of**

Culture
2323 S Shepherd Drive
Suite 1000
Houston, TX 77019 **713-520-0232**
FAX: 713-520-5785
www.ilru.org

Another winner in the innovative CIL competition- Steve Brown describes the Talking Books Program of Southeast Alaska Independent Living, discussing their efforts to record the oral history and life experiances of people with disabilities in the larger context of disability culture.

10 pages

5988 **International Ventilator Users Network**

Gazette International Networking Institute
4207 Lindell Boulevard
Suite 110
Saint Louis, MO 63108 **314-534-0475**
FAX: 314-534-5070
e-mail: gini_intl@msn.com
www.post-polio.org/ivun

Joan L Headley, Executive Director
Judith R Fischer, Editor

IVUN is a worldwide network of ventilator users and health professionals experienced in and committed to home care and long term mechanical ventilation. IVUN News, a quarterly newsletter, offers articles on family adjustments, equipment, techniques, travel, ethical issues, medical topics, and resources. Also publishes the annual iVUN resource directory, listing ventilator users, health professionals, equipment manufacturers and vendors, as well as other related organizations. *$ 17.00*

8 pages Quarterly

5989 **Introduction to Spina Bifida**

Spina Bifida Association of America
4590 Macarthur Boulevard NW
Suite 250
Washington, DC 20007 **202-944-3285**
800-621-3141
FAX: 202-944-3295
e-mail: sbaa@sbaa.org
www.sbaa.org

An aid for parents, family and nonmediacl people who care for a child with spina bifida. *$7.00*

5990 **It Feels Good to be in Control**

Accent Books & Products
PO Box 700
Bloomington, IL 61702 **309-378-2961**
800-787-8444
FAX: 309-378-4420
e-mail: acmtlvng@aol.com

Raymond C Cheever, Publisher
Betty Garee, Editor

Understanding yourself can make almost anything work better, your health, your personal relationships, your happiness, you name it. This small book could be the best medicine and the most inexpensive a person could ever have. *$4.50*

18 pages Paperback
ISBN 0-91570 -39-6

5991 Journal of the Association for Persons with Severe Handicaps

29 W Susquehanna Avenue
Suite 210
Baltimore, MD 21204
410-828-8274
FAX: 410-828-6706
e-mail: info@tash.org
www.tash.org

Provides contemporary articles on specialized topics of interest to TASH members and others in the field of development disabilities. *$25.00*

Quarterly

5992 Just Like Everyone Else

World Institute on Disability
510 16th Street
Suite 100
Oakland, CA 94612
510-763-4100
FAX: 510-763-4109
e-mail: wid@wid.org
www.wid.org

The oversize-format publication, intended for general audiences, provides perspective, inspiration and information about the Independent Living Movement and the Americans with Disabilities Act. *$5.00*

16 pages

5993 Kaleidoscope: Exploring the Experience of Disability Through Literature & the Fine Arts

United Disability Services
701 S Main Street
Akron, OH 44311
330-762-9755
FAX: 330-762-0912
TTY:330-379-3349
e-mail: mshiplett@udsakron.org
www.udsakron.org

Mildred Shiplett, Editorial Coordinator
Gail Willmott, Senior Editor
Phyllis Boerner, Publication Director

This magazine explores the experiences of disability through the lens of creative arts. Unlike rehabilitation, advocacy or independent living journals, this journal challenges and transcends stereotypical, patronizing and sentimental attitudes about disability. Offers a variety of articles, fiction, art and poetry relating to issues of disability, literature and the fine arts. *$10.00*

64 pages BiAnnually

5994 Keep the Promise: Managed Care and People with Disabilities

American Network of Community Options & Resource
1101 King Street
Suite 380
Alexandria, VA 22314
703-535-7850
FAX: 703-535-7860
e-mail: ancor@ancor.org
www.ancor.org

Renee L Pietrangelo, CEO
Suellen Galbraith, Director Public Policy

This publication presents a detailed review of the process and the lessons learned. Details a way for all stake holders to work together for a state or local system.

119 pages $18 - $22

5995 Keeping Our Families Together

Through the Looking Glass
2198 Sixth Street
Suite 100
Berkeley, CA 94710
510-848-1112
800-644-2666
FAX: 510-848-4445
e-mail: TLG@lookingglass.org
www.lookingglass.org

P Preston
M Jakobson

Report of the National Task Force on parents with disabilities and their families. Available in braille, large print or cassette. *$2.00*

12 pages

5996 Keys to Independence

Coalition for Independence
1281 Eisenhower
Leavenwoth, KS 66048
913-250-0287
FAX: 913-250-0167
e-mail: kolson@cfikc.org
www.cfikc.org

Bi-Monthly

5997 Kids Get Arthiritis Too!

American Juvenile Athritis Organization (AJAO)
1330 W Peachtree Street
PO Box 7669
Atlanta, GA 30309
404-872-7100
800-283-7800
FAX: 404-872-9559
e-mail: help@arthritis.org
www.arthritis.org

8 pages Quarterly

5998 Killing Pain Without Prescription

Harper Perennial
10 E 53rd Street
New York, NY 10022
212-207-7000
FAX: 212-207-7145
www.harpercollins.com

An outline of treatments to deal with chronic pain, including diet, nutrition, applied kinesiology, osteopathy, and bodywork. Also includes a resource guide of organizations offering help nationwide.

Paperback 1982
ISBN 0-064635-62-7

5999 LDA Newsbriefs

Learning Disabilities Association of America
4156 Library Road
Pittsburgh, PA 15234
412-341-1515
FAX: 412-344-0224
e-mail: info@ldaamerica.org
www.ldaamerica.org

Jane Browning, National Executive Director

Articles of interest to all persons concerned with learning disabilities. *$15.00*

24 pages BiMonthly 1965

6000 Laugh with Accent, #3

Accent Books & Products
PO Box 700
Bloomington, IL 61702
309-378-2961
800-787-8444
FAX: 309-378-4420
e-mail: acmtlvng@aol.com

Raymond C Cheever, Publisher
Betty Garee, Editor

These special cartoons prove laughter is the best medicine of all. It's when the laughter stops that we become truly disabled, say readers. *$3.50*

89 pages Paperback
ISBN 0-91570 -16-7

6001 Learn About the ADA in Your Local Library

US Department of Justice
950 Pennsylvania Avenue NW DRS-NYAV
Washington, DC 20530 **202-307-0663**
800-574-0301
FAX: 202-307-1197
www.ada.gov

A 10-page annotated list of 95 ADA publications and one videotape that are available in 15,000 public libraries throughout the country.

6002 Learning to Listen: Positive Approaches & People with Difficult Behavior

Brookes Publishing
PO Box 10624
Baltimore, MD 21285 **410-337-9580**
800-638-3775
FAX: 410-337-8539
e-mail: custserv@brookespublishing.com
www.brookespublishing.com

This book describes how the interactive process of learning to listen provides practical alternatives to overly controlling behavior modification techniques. Includes compelling and detailed case studies that illustrate possible positive approaches and reveal how people with disabilities can take control of their lives. *$27.00*

288 pages Paperback
ISBN 1-55766 -64-2

6003 Life After Trauma: A Workbook for Healing

Guilford Press
72 Spring Street
New York, NY 10012 **212-431-9800**
800-365-7006
FAX: 212-966-6708
www.guilford.com

$18.95

352 pages Paperback 1999
ISBN 1-572302-39-9

6004 Life Planning Workbook

Exceptional Parent Library
120 Sylvan Avenue, Suite 10
PO Box 1807
Englewood Cliffs, NJ 07632
800-535-1910
FAX: 201-947-9376
e-mail: eplibrary@aol.com
www.eplibrary.com

A hands-on guide to help parents provide for the future security and happiness of their child with a disability after their death. *$24.95*

6005 Life Skills for Vocational Success

Workshops
4244 Third Avenue S
Birmingham, AL 35222 **208-592-9683**
FAX: 205-592-9687

$35.00

250 pages

6006 LifeLines

Disabled & Alone/Life Services for the Handicapped
352 Park Avenue S
11th Floor
New York, NY 10010 **212-532-6740**
800-995-0066
FAX: 212-532-3588
e-mail: info@disabledandalone.org
www.disabledandalone.org

Roslyn Brilliant, Executive Director

Newsletter providing current and valuable information about lifetime care and planning for persons with disabilities and their families and the organizations serving them. Free upon request.

4-10 pages BiAnnual

6007 Livin'

Lehigh Valley Center for Independent Living
435 Allentown Drive
Allentown, PA 18109 **610-770-9781**
FAX: 610-770-9801

Amy C Beck, Executive Director

4 pages Quarterly

6008 Living in a State of Stuck

Brookline Books
PO Box 1046
Cambridge, MA 02238 **617-868-0360**
800-666-2665
FAX: 617-868-1772
e-mail: brooklinebks@delphi.com
www.brooklinebooks.com

Offers explanations on how adaptive technologies affect the lives of people with disabilities. *$24.95*

3rd ed., paper
ISBN 1-571290-27-3

6009 Living the Therapeutic Touch: Healing as Lifestyle

Quest Books
1926 N Main Street
PO Box 270
Wheaton, IL 60189 **630-668-1571**
FAX: 630-668-4976

How to do Therapeutic Touch.

201 pages Hardcover 1987
ISBN 0-396090-25-7

6010 Love: Where to Find It, How to Keep It

Accent Books & Products
PO Box 700
Bloomington, IL 61702 **309-378-2961**
800-787-8444
FAX: 309-378-4420
e-mail: acmtlvng@aol.com

Raymond C Cheever, Publisher
Betty Garee, Editor

Offers ideas such as how to meet other single people, avoid the wrong type; communications skills and much more for the disabled person wanting to date. *$6.95*

104 pages Paperback
ISBN 0-91570 -31-0

6011 Lupus: Alternative Therapies That Work

Healing Arts Press
One Park Street
Rochester, VT 05767
802-767-3174
800-246-8648
FAX: 802-767-3726
e-mail: orders@innertraditions.com
www.InnerTraditions.com

Jessica Dudley, Sales Associate

$14.95

256 pages
ISBN 0-892818-89-1

6012 MAGIC Touch

MAGIC Foundation for Children's Growth
6645 W N Avenue
Oak Park, IL 60302
708-383-0808
800-362-4423
FAX: 708-383-0899
e-mail: mary@magicfoundation.org
www.magicfoundation.org

Dianne Andrews, Executive Director

Provides support and education regarding growth disorders in children and related adult disorders, including adult GHD. Dedicated to helping children whose physical growth is affected be a medical problem by assiating families of afflicted children through local support groups, public education/awareness, newsletters, specialty divisions and programs for the children.

36-40 pages Quarterly

6013 MOOSE: A Very Special Person

Brookline Books
PO Box 1046
Cambridge, MA 02238
617-868-0360
800-666-2665
FAX: 617-868-1772
e-mail: brooklinebks@delphi.com
www.brooklinebooks.com

Moose, which in very human terms, teaches us that each of us is different and that we have our own unique capacity for loving, sharing, enjoying and learning. *$10.95*

Paperback
ISBN 0-91479 -73-5

6014 Mainstream Magazine

2973 Beech Street
San Diego, CA 92102
619-234-3138
FAX: 619-234-3155
e-mail: editor@mainstream.mag.com
www.mainstream-mag.com

Cyndi Jones, Publisher

The authoritative, national voice of people with disabilities, publishes in-depth reports on employment, education, new products and technology, legislation and disability rights advocacy, recreation and travel, disability arts and culture, plus personality profiles and challenging commentary. *$24.00*

Monthly

6015 Making Informed Medical Decisions: Where to Look and How to Use What You Find

Patient-Centered Guides
101 Morris Street
Sebastopol, CA 95472
707-829-0515
800-998-9938
FAX: 707-829-0104
www.patientcenters.com

You are involved in healthcare decisions-whether you want to be or not. Making Informed Medical Decisions acts like a friendly reference librarian, explaining: tips for researching for someone else; medical journal articles; statistics and risk; standard treatment options; clinical trial; making an ally of your doctor; and determining your own best course. Authors Oster, Thomas, and Joseff-a pateint advocate, medical librarian, and medical doctor-also share examples and stories. *$17.95*

280 pages Paperback
ISBN 1-565924-59-2

6016 Making News

Avacado Press
PO Box 145
Louisville, KY 40201
502-894-9492
FAX: 502-899-9562
e-mail: office@advocadopress.org
www.advocadopress.org

$8.00

165 pages
ISBN 0-962706-43-4

6017 Making Wise Decisions for Long-Term Care

AARP Fulfillment
601 E Street NW
Washington, DC 20049
202-434-2277
800-424-3410
FAX: 202-434-3443
e-mail: member@aarp.org
www.aarp.org

Here's a comprehensive consumer education effort in the area of long-term care.

28 pages

6018 Managing Pain before it Manages You

Guilford Press
72 Spring Street
New York, NY 10012
212-431-9800
800-365-7006
FAX: 212-966-6708
www.guilford.com

$19.95

224 pages Paperback 1994
ISBN 0-898622-24-7

6019 Managing Your Symptoms

Vestibular Disorders Association
PO Box 4467
Portland, OR 97208
503-229-7705
800-837-8428
FAX: 503-229-8064
e-mail: veda@vestibular.org
www.vestibular.org

$25.00

ISBN 0-963261-16-9

6020 Marriage & Disability

Accent Books & Products
PO Box 700
Bloomington, IL 61702 **309-378-2961**
800-787-8444
FAX: 309-378-4420
e-mail: acmtlvng@aol.com

Raymond C Cheever, Publisher
Betty Garee, Editor

This guide can help you make the right decision and it can help smooth the way to a happier life. *$7.95*

Paperback
ISBN 0-91570 -34-5

6021 Massage Book

Random House
1540 Braodway
New York, NY 10022 **212-782-9000**
800-726-0600
FAX: 212-302-7985

Hailed as the 'classic book' on massage.

1972

6022 Massage Magazine

NOAH Publishing Company
638 2nd Street
Kenyon, MN 55946 **507-789-6161**

Covers the art and science of massage, bodywork and related healing arts.

BiMonthly

6023 Matheny Matters

Matheny School and Hospital
PO Box 339
Peapack, NJ 07977 **908-234-0011**
FAX: 908-719-2137
e-mail: info@matheny.org
www.matheny.org

Steven Proctor, President
Gabor Barabas MD, Medical Director
Gary E Eddey MD, Director of Medicine & Dentistry

A publication from the Matheny School and Hospital.

3 times a year

6024 Matrix and Matrix Regulation Basis for an Holistic Theory in Medicine

Karl Haug International
2937 Ne Flanders Street
Portalnd, OR 97323 **503-287-6775**

221 pages 1991
ISBN 2-804340-00-7

6025 Medical Aspects Of Disability Second Editi on A Handbook For The Rehabilitation Professional

Springer Publishing Company
536 Braodway
New York, NY 10012 **212-431-4370**
877-687-7476
877-687-7976
FAX: 212-941-7842
e-mail: marketing@springerpub.com
www.springerpub.com

Annette Imperati, Marketing/Sales Director

$62.92

744 pages
ISBN 0-826179-71-1

6026 Medical Herbalism

Bergner Communications
PO Box 20512
Boulder, CO 80308 **303-541-9552**

e-mail: bergner@concentric.com
http://www.medherb.com

Paul Bergner, Editor

Newsletter written by physicians and is published six times a year.

6027 Meditative Mind

Jeremy P Tarcher
375 Hudson Street
New York, NY 10014 **212-366-2000**

Describes how various differant religous organizations use meditation. *$12.95*

1995
ISBN 0-874778-33-6

6028 Mending the Body, Mending the Mind

Bantam
1540 Broadway
New York, NY 10036 **212-782-9000**
FAX: 212-302-7985

6029 Meniere's Disease: What You Need To Know

Vestibular Disorders Association
PO Box 4467
Portland, OR 97208 **503-229-7705**
800-837-8428
FAX: 503-229-8064

$34.95

Quarterly
ISBN 0-963261-11-8

6030 Menopause Self-Help Book

Celestial Arts
PO Box 7123
Berkley, CA 94707 **510-559-1600**
800-841-2665
FAX: 510-559-1629
e-mail: order@tenspeed.com
www.tenspeedpress.com

An easy-to-understand workbook on how to approach menopause; explains what menopause is and explores the many natural treatments available and gives the pros and cons of estrogen replacement therapy. Resources are listed. *$18.95*

224 pages 1990
ISBN 0-890875-92-8

6031 Menopause without Medicine

Hunter House
1515 1/2 Park Street
PO Box 2914
Alameda, CA **510-865-5282**
800-266-5592
FAX: 510-865-4295
e-mail: sales@hunterhouse.com
www.hunterhouse.com

JoAnne Retzlaff, Sales/Marketing Associate
Christina Sverdrup, Customer Service Manager

Research on nutrition, exercise, and osteoporosis, including good news about the body's ability to rebuild bone later in life; describes how women can best prepare their minds and bodies for the transition of menopause, and explains how women can prevent osteoporosis and control the disturbing symptoms of hot flashes, insomnia, fatigue, and weight gain. *$15.95*

368 pages

ISBN 0-897932-81-1

6032 Menopause: A Second Spring 3rd Edition

Blue Poppy Press
5441 Western Avenue
Suite 2
Boulder, CO 80301 **303-447-8372**
800-487-9296
FAX: 303-245-8362
acupuncture.com/Acup/menop-hlm.htm

The first book-length decription of the traditional Chinese medical view of menopause, menopausal syndrome, and postmenopausal disorders. Extensive sections on self-help, preventative therapies, and remedial treatment of specific problems, as well as a complete TCM explanation of menopausal symptoms.

175 pages 1993

ISBN 0-936185-47-3

6033 Mental Retardation

Allyn & Bacon
75 Arlington Street
Suite 300
Boston, MA 02116 **617-848-6000**
800-852-8024
FAX: 617-848-7490
www.ablongman.com

Examines mental retardation within a larger social context. Provides an understanding of how social and legal events have shaped the lives of mentally retarded people.

224 pages Paper 1986

ISBN 0-135765-21-8

6034 Mental Retardation, Third Edition

McGraw-Hill, School Publishing
220 E Danieldale Road
DeSoto, TX 75115 **972-224-1111**
800-442-9685
FAX: 972-228-1982
mhschool.com

Combines significant findings from the most current research, focusing on a unique relationship between the special educator and the learner with mental retardation.

656 pages Casebound

6035 Mental Retardation: A Life-Cycle Approach

McGraw-Hill, School Publishing
220 E Danieldale Road
DeSoto, TX 75115 **972-224-1111**
800-442-9685
FAX: 972-228-1982
mhschool.com

This text considers the needs of the retarded individual at every stage of life.

512 pages

6036 Mental and Physical Disability Law Reporter

ABA Commission on Mental & Physical Disability Law
740 15th Street NW
9th Floor
Washington, DC 20005 **202-662-1581**
FAX: 202-662-1032
e-mail: hammillj@staff.abanet.org
www.abanet.org/disability

John Hammill, Publications Coordinator
Amy Allbright, Managing Editor

Contains over 2,000 a summanes per year of federal and state court decisions and legislation that affect persons with mental and physical disabilities. Includes bylined articles by experts in the field regarding disability law developments and trends. *$374.00*

150+ pages Bimonthly 1976

6037 Mercury Poisoning from Dental Amalgam: A Hazard to Human Brain

Bio-Probe
5508 Edgewater Drive
PO Box 608010
Orlando, FL 32860 **407-290-9670**
www.bioprobe.com

Provides scientific evidence that mercury vapor released from amalgam fillings can be transported directly to the brain through the valveless venous system and from the mucous membranes of the nasal cavity along the olfactory nnerves to the brain. Fully referenced. *$20.00*

213 pages 1986

ISBN 0-941011-01-1

6038 Midtown Sweep: Grassroots Advocacy at its Best

Independent Living Research Utilization ILRU
2323 S Shepherd Drive
Suite 1000
Houston, TX 77019 **713-520-0232**
FAX: 713-520-5785
www.ilru.org

Josie, Janetta, and Linda describe the steps their center's advocacy group have taken to ensure enforcement of the ADA: target one neighborhood; survey and collect information on businesses that are inaccessible; send letters offering to work with the businesses to help them become accessible and providing information on tax incentives; file lawsuits against businesses that do not respond; involve the media.

10 pages

6039 Miles Away and Still Caring: A Guide for Long Distance Caregivers

AARP Fulfillment
601 E Street NW
Washington, DC 20049 **202-434-2277**
800-424-3410
FAX: 202-434-3443
e-mail: member@aarp.org
www.aarp.org

This is one of the most helpful and frequently requested publications. Helps people who must coordinate the care of a loved one from a long distance.

18 pages

6040 Mind Over Mood: Change How You Feel By Changing the Way You Think

Guilford Press
72 Spring Street
New York, NY 10012 **212-431-9800**
800-365-7006
FAX: 212-966-6708
www.guilford.com

$21.00

243 pages Paperback 1995
ISBN 0-898621-28-3

6041 Missing Diagnosis

Missing Diagnosis
2614 Highland Avenue S
PO Box 26508
Birmingham, AL 35205 **205-326-0642**

A comprehensive overview of candidiasis and how to treat it by a pioneer in the field.

175 pages 1985
ISBN 0-961575-80-8

6042 Mississippi Message

Arc of Mississippi
7 Lakeland Circle
Suite 600
Jackson, MS 39216 **601-982-1180**
800-717-1180
FAX: 601-982-5792
e-mail: arcms@arcms.org
www.arcms.org

Cindy Dittis, Community Outreach

Quarterly

6043 Mother Father Deaf: Living between Sound and Silence

Through the Looking Glass
2198 Sixth Street
Suite 100
Berkeley, CA 94710 **510-848-1112**
800-644-2666
FAX: 510-848-4445
e-mail: TLG@lookingglass.org
www.lookingglass.org

P Preston

$18.00

278 pages

6044 Mother to Be

Through the Looking Glass
2198 Sixth Street
Suite 100
Berkeley, CA 94710 **510-848-1112**
800-644-2666
FAX: 510-848-4445
e-mail: TLG@lookingglass.org
www.lookingglass.org

J Rogers
M Matsumura

Guide to pregnancy and birth for women with disabilities. *$34.00*

410 pages

6045 Mothers with Visual Impairments Who Are Raising Young Children

Through the Looking Glass
2198 Sixth Street
Suite 100
Berkeley, CA 94710 **510-848-1112**
800-644-2666
FAX: 510-848-4445
e-mail: TLG@lookingglass.org
www.lookingglass.org

C Conley-Jung
R Olkin

Available in braille, large print or cassette. *$2.00*

16 pages

6046 Multiple Sclerosis

Healing Arts Press
One Park Street
Rochester, VT 05767 **802-767-3174**
800-246-8648
FAX: 802-767-3726
e-mail: orders@innertraditions.com
www.InnerTraditions.com

Jessica Dudley, Sales Associate

A self-help guide to its management. Includes information on promising new natural treatments, diet, exercise and more. *$12.95*

272 pages
ISBN 0-892812-42-7

6047 Multiple Sclerosis and Having A Baby

Healing Arts Press
One Park Street
Rochester, VT 05767 **802-767-3174**
800-246-8648
FAX: 802-767-3726
e-mail: orders@innertraditions.com
www.InnerTraditions.com

Jessica Dudley, Sales Associate

Everything you need to know about conception, pregnancy and parenthood. *$12.95*

160 pages
ISBN 0-892817-88-7

6048 Myotherapy

Ballantine Books
1540 Broadway
New York, NY 10022 **212-751-2600**
FAX: 212-572-4949

Myotherapy explained as a technique.

1985

6049 NBA Bulletin

National Braille Association
3 Townline Circle
Rochester, NY 14623 **585-427-8260**
FAX: 585-427-0263
e-mail: nbaoffice@compuserve.com
www.nationalbraille.org

Quarterly publication from the National Braille Association. *$50.00*

28-32 pages Quarterly

6050 NCD Bulletin

National Council on Disability
1331 F Street NW
Suite 850
Washington, DC 20004
202-272-2004
FAX: 202-272-2022
www.ncd.gov

Mark Quigley, Communication Director

Reports on the latest issues and news affecting people with disabilities.

2 pages Monthly

6051 NOD E-Newsletter

National Organization on Disability
910 16th Street NW
Suite 600
Washington, DC 20006
202-293-5960
FAX: 202-293-7999
e-mail: ability@nod.org
www.nod.org

Alan Reich, President
Brewster Thackeray, VP, Communications
John Hershey, Advice and Resource Manager

Monthly E-Newsletter from the National Organization on Disability. Free.

3 pages Monthly

6052 NORD Resource Guide

National Organization for Rare Disorders
PO Box 1968
Danbury, CT 06813
203-744-0100
800-999-6673
FAX: 203-798-2291
TTY:203-746-6927
e-mail: orphan@rarediseases.org
www.rarediseases.org

Mary Dunkle, Senior Director/Communications

Book providing information on more than 1,200 organizations, support groups and government agencies offering help to people with rare diseases.

6053 National Hookup

ISC
16 Liberty Street
Larkspur, CA 94939
415-924-3549
FAX: 415-927-9556
e-mail: russab@earthlink.net

Russ Bohlke, Executive Secretary

Newsletter published by ISC, a national organization of people with physical disabilities. *$6.00*

12 pages BiMonthly 1950

6054 National Network of Learning Disabled Adults

808 N 82nd Street
Suite F2
Scottsdale, AZ 85257
480-941-5112

Bill Butler, VP

Offers general information, software, articles and products for the learning disabled.

6055 Natural Health Bulletin

Princeton Educational Publishers
117 Cuttermill Road
Great Neck, NY 11021
516-482-3800

Carlson Wade, Editor

Diet and nutrition, physical fitness lifestyle, attitude, developments in natural and preventive medicine.

4 pages Monthly

6056 Natural Menopause: Guide to a Woman's Most Misunderstood Passage

Addison-Wesley Publishing Company
75 Arlington Street
Suite 300
Boston, MA 02116
617-848-6000
FAX: 617-848-6034
www.awprofessional.com

Assists women in making a decision about Hormone Replacement Therapy and explores diet, exercise, and other alternatives in relieving the symptoms of menopause. *$15.00*

1992
ISBN 0-201479-87-7

6057 Negotiating the Disability Maze

Charles C Thomas
2600 S First Street
Springfield, IL 62704
217-789-8980
800-258-8980
FAX: 217-789-9130
e-mail: books@ccthomas.com
www.ccthomas.com

This book has been designed and written to furnish people from diverse backgrounds with important information regarding education of children with disabilities. The authors are as thorough as they are explicit. They analyze the concepts, translate the jargon, and outline the characteristics of various disabilities. Also avalable in cloth edition. *$36.95*

206 pages Paperback
ISBN 0-398066-64-7

6058 Neurophysiology of Enlightenment

Neuroscene Press

Provides scientific research on Maharishi Transcendental Meditation. The Unified Field of Natural Law, phsyiological changes associated with transccendence, perfect health, and ideal behavior through the Maharishi Vedic approach to Health program, reversing the aging process, and the physiological basis for world peace, are discussed. *$12.00*

386 pages paperback 1986

6059 New Horizons in Sexuality

Accent Books & Products
PO Box 700
Bloomington, IL 61702
309-378-2961
800-787-8444
FAX: 309-378-4420
e-mail: acmtlvng@aol.com

Raymond C Cheever, Publisher
Betty Garee, Editor

This manual helps both males and females progress toward a satisfying post-injury relationship. *$7.95*

50 pages Paperback
ISBN 0-91570 -42-6

6060 New Menopausal Years the Wise Woman Way

Ash Tree Publishing
PO Box 64
Woodstock, NY 12498
845-246-8081
800-431-1579
FAX: 845-246-8081
www.ashtreepublishing.com

Susun Weed, Editor in Chief

This book focuses on various aspects of women's health including osteoporosis, and reviews a wide range of remedies from massage and energy work to supplements and medication.

228 pages 1992

ISBN 0-961462-04-3

6061 New Mobility

23815 Stuart Ranch Road
Malibu, CA 90265
310-317-4522
800-543-4116
FAX: 310-317-9644
www.newmobility.com

Sam Maddox, Publisher
Barry Corbet, Editor

The full-service, full-color lifestyle magazine for the disability community. The award-winning magazine is contemporary, witty and candid. Produced by professional journalists and visual artists, the magazine's voice is uncompromising and unsentimental, yet practical, knowing and friendly. The magazine covers issues that matter to readers: medical news, and cure research; jobs, benefits and civil rights; sports, recreation and travel; product news, technology and innovation.

ISSN 1065-21 4

6062 New No Pill: No Risk Birth Control

Wiley Publishing
605 3rd Avenue
New York, NY 10158
212-850-6000
FAX: 212-850-6088

Cathy Kenneally, Illustrator

The latest in natural family planning and contraception without drugs, chemicals, IUDs or barrier devices.

Hardcover 1986

ISBN 0-892563-00-1

6063 New Voices: Self Advocacy By People with Disabilities

Brookline Books
PO Box 1047
Cambridge, MA 02238
617-868-0360
800-666-2665
FAX: 617-868-1772
e-mail: brooklinebks@delphi.com
www.brooklinebooks.com

A collection of original papers many by self advocates themselves that vividly illustrate the dynamic, ever-growing self-advocacy movement (persons with disabilities speaking out and seeking better non-institutional living situations, social and political equality and decent jobs at reasonable pay. *$29.95*

274 pages Paperback

ISBN 1-57129 -04-4

6064 News from Advocates for Deaf-Blind

National Family Association for Deaf-Blind
111 Middle Neck Road
Sands Point, NY 11050
516-944-8900
800-225-0411
FAX: 516-944-7302
e-mail: NFADB@aol.com
www.NFADB.org

Mary Fox, Administrative Assistant

A membership organization which provide resources, education, advocacy, referrals and support for families with children who are deaf-blind; professionals in the field; and individuals who are deaf-blind.

20 pages TriAnnual

6065 NewsLine

Federation for Children with Special Needs
56 Temple Place
Suite 664
Boston, MA 02111
617-542-7860
800-537-0446
FAX: 617-542-7832
e-mail: pal@fcsn.org
www.ppal.net

Donna Welles, Director
Lisa Lambert, Asistant Director

Offers information for parents and families on resources, medical updates, activities, fund-raising events and association news for their disabled children.

Quarterly

6066 Newsletter of PA's AT Lending Library

Temple University Institute on Disabilities
1301 Cecil B Moore Avenue
Philadelphia, PA 19122
215-204-1356
800-204-7428
FAX: 215-204-9371
TTY:800-750-7428
e-mail: piat@temple.edu
http://disabilities.temple.edu

Amy Goldman, Project Director
Sandra McNally, Editor

Newsletter from the Assistive Technology Lending Library in Pennsylvania. It is published quarterly and is free of charge.

4-8 pages Quarterly

6067 Nine Nineteen News

Free Library of Philadelphia Library
919 Walnut Street
Philadelphia, PA 19107
215-683-3213
800-222-1754
FAX: 215-683-3211
e-mail: flpblind@library.phila.gov

4 pages Quarterly

6068 Nolo's Guide to Social Security Disability

NOLO
950 Parker Street
Berkeley, CA 94710
510-549-1976
800-955-4775
FAX: 510-548-5902
www.nolo.com

Maira Dizgalvis, Trade Customer Service Manager
Susan McConnell, Director Sales
Natasha Kaluza, Sales Assistant

Not many bureaucratic programs are as large- and as confusing- as Social Security disability. This book shows you the ins and outs of the system. *$29.95*

350 pages paperback

ISBN 0-873375-74-2

6069 Nutritional Action Health Letter: Center for Science in the Public Interest

1875 Connecticut Avenue NW
Suite 300
Washington, DC 20009
202-332-9110
FAX: 202-265-4954
e-mail: cspi@cspinet.org
www.cspinet.org

6070 Nutritional Desk Reference

Keats Publishing
27 Pine Street
PO Box 876
New Canaan, CT 06840 **203-966-8721**
800-323-4900

6071 Nutritional Influences on Illness 2nd Edition

Third Line Press
4751 Viviana Drive
Tarzana, CA 91356 **818-996-0076**
tlp@third-line.com

Nutritional Influences on Illness is a comprehensive summary of the world's knowledge concerning the relationship between dietary and nutrtional factors and illness. This book does not try to promote any particular school of thought. Instead of the author telling readers his opinion as to what research says, he makes it easy for them to see data for themselves and then form their own opinions.

504 pages
ISBN 0-879835-31-1

6072 OT Practice

American Occupational Therapy Association
164 Rollins Avenue
Suite 301
Rockville, MD 20852 **301-951-9070**
800-877-1383
FAX: 301-652-7711

Jeanette Bair, Executive Director

Offers information on conferences, books, resources, materials and information and referral services for persons with disabilities.

6073 Obesity Sourcebook

Omnigraphics
615 Griswold Street
Detroit, MI 48226
800-234-1340
FAX: 800-875-1340
www.omnigraphics.com

Wilma Caldwell, Editor

Discusses diseases and other problems associated with obesity. *$48.00*

400 pages 1900
ISBN 0-780803-33-7

6074 Occupational Therapy Strategies and Adaptations for Independent Daily Living

Haworth Press
10 Alice Street
Binghamton, NY 13904 **607-722-5857**
800-429-6784
FAX: 607-722-6362
e-mail: orders@haworthpress.com
www.haworthpress.com

S Harrington-Miller, Advertising

This contains clinical expertise of some fourteen authors or author teams addressing the issue of occupational therapy to assist in independent daily living. Also available as hardcover. *$74.95*

186 pages Softcover
ISBN 0-866563-50-4

6075 On the Edge of Deaf Culture: An Annotated Bibliography of Hearing Children/Deaf Parents

Through the Looking Glass
2198 Sixth Street
Suite 100
Berkeley, CA 94710 **510-848-1112**
800-644-2666
FAX: 510-848-4445
e-mail: TLG@lookingglass.org
www.lookingglass.org

T Bull

$35.00

360 pages

6076 One Hundred Fifty Most-Asked Questions About Menopause

Hearst Books
959 Eighth Avenue
New York, NY 10019 **212-649-2000**
e-mail: hearstbooks@hearst.com
www.hearstbooks.com

This book provides the plain facts on a host of topics including: the pros and cons of hormone replacement therapy; choosing the right doctor; how to de-stress your life; and twelve tips to make the most of a physician visit.

1993

6077 Options

People Against Cancer
PO Box 10
Otho, IA 50569 **515-972-4444**
FAX: 515-972-4415
e-mail: info@PeopleAgainstCAncer.com
www.peopleagainstcancer.com

8 pages Quarterly

6078 Oregon Clarion

Oregon Developmental Disability Council
540 24th Place NE
Salem, OR 97301 **503-945-9941**
800-292-4154
FAX: 503-945-9947
e-mail: ocdd@ocdd.org
www.ocdd.org

Michael T Bailey, Editor
Bill Lynch, Acting Executive Director

A quarterly publication from the Oregon Developmental Disability Council.

6079 Organ Transplants: Making the Most of Your Gift of Life

Patient-Centered Guides
101 Morris Street
Sebastopol, CA 95472 **707-829-0515**
800-998-9938
FAX: 707-829-0104
www.patientcenters.com

Linda Lamb, Editor
Shawnde Paull, Marketing

Over 64,000 people in the US are awaiting an organ transplant. Although transplant surgeries are now fairly routine and can give their recipients the gift of new life, the road to getting a transplant can be long and harrowing. Living with immunosuppressive drugs and strong emotional responses can also be more challenging than families imagine. Medical journalist Robert Finn answers the concerns of these families, with the latest facts about transplantation - as well as the stories behind them. *$19.95*

326 pages Paperback
ISBN 1-565926-34-X

6080 Orphan Disease Update

NORD
55 Kenosia Avenue
PO Box 1968
Danbury, CT 06813 **203-744-0100**
800-999-6673
FAX: 203-798-2291
TTY:203-797-9590
e-mail: orphan@rarediseases.org
www.rarediseases.org

James Broatch, Chair
Carolyn Asbury PhD, Vice Chair

Publication of NORD, a unique federation of voluntary health organizations dedicated to helping people with rare orphan diseases and assisting the organizations that serve them. NORD is committed to the identification, treatment and cure of rare disorders through programs of education, advocacy, research and service.

6081 Orthotics and Prosthetics Almanac

Orthotics and Prosthetics National Office
1650 King Street
Suite 500
Alexandria, VA 22314 **703-836-7114**
FAX: 703-836-0838
e-mail: opalmanac@aol.com
www.aopanet.org

Stacey L Bell, Editor-in-Chief

Features articles covering current professional, patient care, government, business and National Office activities affecting the orthotics and prosthetics profession and industry. *$40.00*

80 pages Monthly
ISSN 1061-46 1

6082 Osteoporosis Sourcebook

Omnigraphics
615 Griswold Street
Detroit, MI 48226
800-234-1340
FAX: 800-875-1340
www.omnigraphics.com

Allan R Cook, Editor

Discusses causes, risk factors, treatments and traditional and non-traditional pain management issues concerning osteoporosis. *$ 78.00*

600 pages 1900
ISBN 0-780802-39-X

6083 Our Bodies, Ourselves for the New Century: A Book by and for Women

Simon & Schuster
100 Front Street
Riverside, NJ 08075
800-323-7445
FAX: 800-943-9831

Health refernce for women of all ages and ethnic groups, covering such issues as managed care and the insurance industry, breast cancer treatment options, and recent developments in contraception. Includes 150 photographs and charts and graphs throughout.

780 pages Hardcover 1998
ISBN 0-684842-31-9

6084 Overcoming Binge Eating

Guilford Press
72 Spring Street
New York, NY 10012 **212-431-9800**
800-365-7006
FAX: 212-966-6708
www.guilford.com

$16.95

247 pages Paperback 1995
ISBN 0-898621-79-8

6085 PALAESTRA

Challenge Publications, Limited
PO Box 508
Macomb, IL 61455 **309-833-1902**
FAX: 309-833-1902
e-mail: challpub@macomb.com
www.palaestra.com

Julian Stein, Associate Editor
David Beaver, Editor In Chief

A quarterly publication from PALAESTRA. *$19.95*

64 pages Quarterly

6086 PDF News

Parkinson's Disease Foundation
833 Washington Boulevard
Chicago, IL 60607 **312-733-1893**
FAX: 312-733-1896
e-mail: pdfchgo@enteract.com
PDF@info.org

Lewis P Rowland MD, President
Robin Elliot, Executive Director

8-12 pages Quarterly

6087 PIRS Hotsheet

Placer Independent Resource Services
11768 Atwood Road
Suite 29
Auburn, CA 95603 **530-885-6100**
FAX: 530-885-3032
e-mail: tmiller@pirs.org
www.pirs.org

Monthly publication from Placer Independent Resource Services that is provided free of charge to constituents.

6 pages Monthly

6088 Pacing Yourself

Accent Books & Products
PO Box 700
Bloomington, IL 61702 **309-378-2961**
800-787-8444
FAX: 309-378-4420
e-mail: acmtlvng@aol.com

Raymond C Cheever, Publisher
Betty Garee, Editor

A guide loaded with ideas and tips on starting the day, housekeeping, meal preparation, parenting and socializing. Also includes information on how to group errands and manage household chores, improve posture to make movement easier, and much more. *$10.95*

141 pages Paperback
ISBN 0-91570 -31-0

6089 Parenting with a Disability

Through the Looking Glass
2198 Sixth Street
Suite 100
Berkeley, CA 94710 **510-848-1112**
800-644-2666
FAX: 510-848-4445
e-mail: TLG@lookingglass.org
www.lookingglass.org

International newsletter. Available in braille, large print or cassette.

3 per year

6090 Partnering with Public Health: Funding & Advocacy Opportunities for CILs and SILCs

Independent Living Research Utilization ILRU
2323 S Shepherd Drive
Suite 1000
Houston, TX 77019 **713-520-0232**
FAX: 713-520-5785
www.ilru.org

Laura Rauscher discusses how CILs and SCILs can use funding from the Centers for Disease Control and partnerships with public health agencies to provide innovative programs promoting the health of people with disabilities.

10 pages

6091 Partners in Everyday Communicative Exchanges

Brookes Publishing
PO Box 10624
Baltimore, MD 21285 **410-337-9580**
800-638-3775
FAX: 410-337-8539
e-mail: custserv@brookespublishing.com
www.brookespublishing.com

A Guide to Promoting Intervention Involving people with Severe Intellectual Disability. This book helps improve communication with people with severe disabilities using practical forms, numerous examples, and illustrative case studies. *$43.00*

192 pages Paperback
ISBN 1-55766 -41-X

6092 Pause: Positive Approaches to Menopause

Plume
375 Hudson Street
New York, NY 10014 **212-366-2000**

Gives a symptom-by-symptom breakdown of the physical changes that women experience as well as advice on how to choose the right treatment and make the right lifestyle adjustments. Barbach also offers the most up-to-date and pratical ways to make the 'third third' of a woman's life healthier and more productive.

320 pages 1993
ISBN 0-452281-10-5

6093 Peer Counseling: Advocacy-Oriented Peer Support —Part One

Independent Living Research Utilization ILRU
2323 S Shepherd Drive
Suite 1000
Houston, TX 77019 **713-520-0232**
FAX: 713-520-5785
www.ilru.org

This month's Readings examines how peer support from the point of view of how in talking to each other and sharing life experiences, we help to form groups that are making changes around the world.

10 pages

6094 Peer Counseling: Roles, Functions, Bounderies

Independent Living Research Utilization ILRU
2323 S Shepherd Drive
Suite 1000
Houston, TX 77019 **713-520-0232**
FAX: 713-520-5785
www.ilru.org

In this article, the following points were discussed: Describing peer support as counseling suggests safeguards and expectations which cannot be provided by nonprofessionals; the purpose of peer counseling is to promote the independent living philosophy and encourage consumers to embrace it; peer counseling cannot and is not intended to help individuals deal with intense emotional stress, whether it is related to their disability or to something else.

10 pages

6095 Peer Mentor Volunteers: Empowering People for Change

Independent Living Research Utilization ILRU
2323 S Shepherd Drive
Suite 1000
Houston, TX 77019 **713-520-0232**
FAX: 713-520-5785
www.ilru.org

Arizona Bridge to Independent Living (ABIL) in phoenix, featured inthis issue, is another winner in the innovative CIL program competition.

10 pages

6096 People with Disabilities & Abuse: Implications for Center for Independent Living

Independent Living Research Utilization ILRU
2323 S Shepherd Drive
Suite 1000
Houston, TX 77019 **713-520-0232**
FAX: 713-520-5785
www.ilru.org

10 pages

6097 People with Disabilities Magazine

New Jersey Devlopmental Disabilities Council
20 W State Street, 7th Floor
PO Box 700
Trenton, NJ 08625 **609-292-3745**
800-216-1199
FAX: 609-292-7114
TTY:609-777-3238
e-mail: njddc@njddc.org
www.njddc.org

Ethan Ellis, Director/Editor
Susan Richmond, Assistant Director
Norman Reim, Communications

A free magazine for people with disabilities, their families and the public about disability topics such as personal assistance, deinstitutionalization, health care and community living. Published by the New Jersey Developmental Disabilities council, a federally funded advocacy and policy advisory body. The council has 30 members - 15 consumer/product volunteers and 15 professionals.

48 pages Quarterly

6098 **People with Disabilities Who Challenge the System**

Brookes Publishing
PO Box 10624
Baltimore, MD 21285
800-638-3775
FAX: 410-337-8539
e-mail: custserv@brookespublishing.com
www.brookespublishing.com

Helpful forms, tables, and case studies plus an emphasis on self-determination point the way to the development of supports so that people who are deaf-blind, have severe to profound physical and cognitive disabilities, or have serious behavior problems can be fully included in the classroom, workplace, and community. *$34.00*

464 pages Paperback
ISBN 1-55766 -29-0

6099 **People's Voice**

Independence CIL
300 Third Avenue SW
Suite F
Minot, ND 58701
701-839-4724
800-377-5114
FAX: 701-838-1677

8 pages Quarterly

6100 **Personal Perspectives on Personal Assistance Services**

World Institute on Disability
510 16th Street
Suite 100
Oakland, CA 94612
510-763-4100
FAX: 510-763-4109
e-mail: wid@wid.org
www.wid.org

This collection of personal essays explores a wide range of perspectives on Personal Assistance Services. Family issues and PAS concerns for people with various different disabilities, of different ages and as members of minority groups are addressed. *$5.00*

80 pages Paperback

6101 **Perspectives**

National Assoc. of State Directors of DD Services
113 Oronoco Street
Alexandria, VA 22314
703-683-4202
FAX: 703-683-8773

Provides a concise summary of national policy developments and initiatives affecting persons with devlopmental disabilities and the programs that serve them. From bills pending before Congress, to the growth in Medicaid-funded services, to changes in federal-state Medicaid policies and the shift of responsibility from Washington to the states, keeps readers in tune with the latest national issues shaping publically funded disability services. *$95.00*

Monthly

6102 **Place to Live**

Accent Books & Products
PO Box 700
Bloomington, IL 61702
309-378-2961
800-787-8444
FAX: 309-378-4420
e-mail: acmtlvng@aol.com

Raymond C Cheever, Publisher
Betty Garee, Editor

Many disabled people have found that group housing or accessible apartments are the best alternative to living in a nursing home. These articles tell about some of the alternatives people have found so they can live independently. Just one idea might be the answer for better living for you. *$4.95*

64 pages Paperback
ISBN 0-91570 -30-2

6103 **Plan Ahead: Do What You Can**

Spina Bifida Association of America
4590 Macarthur Boulevard NW
Suite 250
Washington, DC 20007
202-994-3285
800-621-3141
FAX: 202-944-3295
e-mail: sbaa@sbaa.org
www.sbaa.org

Folic aciid information for women at risk for recurrence. *$15.00*

6104 **Pollen Calendar**

Asthma and Allergy Foundation of America
1125 15th Street NW
Suite 502
Washington, DC 20005
202-466-7643
FAX: 202-466-8940
e-mail: info@aafa.org
www.aafa.org

Color poster of the US shows types of pollens and when they appear in each region. *$3.00*

6105 **Potent Self: A Guide to Spontaneity**

Harper & Row
10 E 53rd Street
New York, NY 10022
212-207-7024
800-242-7737
FAX: 212-207-7203

Explanation of the revolutionary theory behind the Feldenkrais method.

1992

6106 **Practice of Aromatherapy**

Inner Traditions
One Park Street
Rochester, VT 05767
802-767-3174
800-246-8648
FAX: 802-767-3726
e-mail: orders@innertraditions.com
www.InnerTraditions.com

The classic manual provides detailed evidence for the efficacy of plant medicine. *$16.95*

280 pages
ISBN 0-892813-98-9

6107 **Premenstrual Syndrome Self-Help Book**

Celestial Arts
PO Box 7123
Berkley, CA
510-559-1600
FAX: 510-559-1629
www.tenspeedpress.com

Every month, 10 to 15 million women experience symptoms such as irritability, anxiety, mood swings, depression, weight gain, breast tenderness, bloating, and more. Dr. Lark gives a complete step-by-step plan to help women cope with, and overcome PMS. *$16.95*

240 pages 1993
ISBN 0-890875-87-1

6108 Proceedings

AHEAD
PO Box 21192
Columbus, OH 43221
617-287-3880
FAX: 617-287-3881
TTY:617-287-3882
e-mail: aagad@postbox.acs.ohio-state.edu
www.ahead.org

National conferences, innovative programs, research, evaluation services, auxiliary aids, career information and other vital information.

6109 Protecting Against Latex Allergy

Spina Bifida Association of America
4590 Macarthur Boulevard NW
Suite 250
Washington, DC 20007
202-944-3285
800-621-3141
FAX: 202-944-3295
e-mail: sbaa@sbaa.org
www.sbaa.org

Because awareness and proper action may help prevent an allergic reation, learning about latex allergy is especially important for parents, health care workers and anyone who is exposed to latex regulary. *$20.00*

6110 Psychological & Social Impact of Disabilit y

Springer Publishing Company
536 Broadway
New York, NY 10012
212-431-4370
877-687-7476
FAX: 212-941-7842
e-mail: marketing@springerpub.com
www.springerpub.com

Annette Imperati, Marketing/Sales Director

$49.95

488 pages

ISBN 0-826122-13-2

6111 Psychology and Health

Springer Publishing Company
536 Broadway
New York, NY 10012
212-431-4370
877-687-7476
FAX: 212-941-7842
e-mail: marketing@springerpub.com
www.springerpub.com

Annette Imperati, Marketing/Sales Director

Content of this book spans a wide range of clinical conditions, including somatization disorders, chronic pain, migraine, anxiety and cancer. *$29.95*

256 pages

6112 Psychology of Disability

Springer Publishing Company
536 Broadway
New York, NY 10012
212-431-4370
877-687-7476
FAX: 212-941-7842
e-mail: marketing@springerpub.com
www.springerpub.com

Annette Imperati, Marketing/Sales Director

Reactions to the disabled. *$27.95*

288 pages

ISBN 0-82613 -40-1

6113 Public Law 101-336

US Department of Justice
950 Pennsylvania Avenue NW DRS-NYAV
Washington, DC 20530
202-307-0663
800-574-0301
FAX: 202-307-1197
www.ada.gov

Text of the Americans with Disabilities Act, as enacted on July 26, 1990.

6114 Public Policy Report

Nat'l Council for Community Behavioral Healthcare
12300 Twinbrook Parkway
Suite 320
Rockville, MD 20852
301-984-6200
FAX: 301-881-7159
www.nccbh.org

Information on promoting advocacy, action and association for people with mental disabilities.

Monthly

6115 Public Technology

US Department of Transportation
Urban Mass Transportation Admin
Washington, DC 20016
202-366-4000

One of a series of reports concerned with improving transportation for elderly and disabled persons.

28 pages

6116 Quality Care Newsletter

National Association for Continence
PO Box 176
Charleston, SC 29402
843-377-0900
800-252-3337
FAX: 843-377-0905
e-mail: memberservices@nafc.org
www.nafc.org

Rachel Coker, Editor

Newsletter from NAFC. *$25.00*

14-16 pages Quarterly

6117 Quality of Life for Persons with Disabilities

Brookline Books
PO Box 1046
Cambridge, MA 02238
617-868-0360
800-666-2665
FAX: 617-868-1772
e-mail: brooklinebks@delphi.com
www.brooklinebooks.com

Quality of life generally refers to a person's subjective experience of his or her life and focuses attention on how the individual with a disabling condition experiences the world. This book presents a comprehensive and international view of this concept as applied to a broad range of settings in which persons with disabilities live, work and play. *$35.00*

Paperback

ISBN 0-91479 -92-1

6118 Quantum Healing

Bantam Books
1540 Broadway
New York, NY 10022
212-782-9000
FAX: 212-302-7985
www.randomhouse.com

$14.95

1990

ISBN 0-553348-69-8

6119 REACHing Out Newsletter

8625 King George Drive
Suite 210
Dallas, TX 75235
214-630-4796
FAX: 214-630-6390
e-mail: reachdallas@reachcils.org
www.reachcils.org

Charlotte Stewart, Executive Director
Susie Reukema, Assistant Director

Quarterly newsletter from REACH of Dallas Resource Center on Independent Living.

24 pages

6120 RSP Funding for Engineering Students 2002- 2004

Reference Service Press
5000 Windplay Drive
Suite 4
El Dorado Hills, CA 95762
916-939-9620
FAX: 916-939-9626
e-mail: findaid@aol.com
www.rspfunding.com

Gail Ann Schlachter, Author

Use this directory to identify the 700 biggest and best funding opportunities available to support undergraduate or graduate studies in engineering. *$30.00*

230 pages
ISBN 1-588410-45-5

6121 RSP Funding for Nursing Students & Nurses 2002-2004

Reference Service Press
5000 Windplay Drive
Suite 4
El Dorado Hills, CA 95762
916-939-9620
FAX: 916-939-9626
e-mail: findaid@aol.com
www.rspfunding.com

Gail Ann Schlachter, Author

Described in detail are 500+ funding opportunities available for nursing students (at any level) and nurses for study, research, professional, or other activities. *$30.00*

189 pages
ISBN 1-588410-46-3

6122 RTC Connection

Research and Training Center
University of Wisconsin - Stout
Menomonie, WI 54751
715-232-2236
FAX: 715-232-2251
e-mail: menz@uwstout.edu
www.rtc.uwstout.edu

Julie Larson, Program Assistant

Bi-annual reports on disability and rehabilitation research and policy topics.

Newsletter

6123 Ragged Edge

Advocado Press
POx 145
Louisville, KY 40201
502-894-9492
FAX: 502-899-9562
e-mail: office@advocadopress.org
www.advocadopress.org

$18.95

38 pages
ISBN 0-962706-45-0

6124 Ragged Edge: The Disability Experience

Advocado Press
PO Box 145
Louisville, KY 40201
502-894-9492
FAX: 502-899-9562
e-mail: office@advocadopress.orgom
www.advocadopress.org

Barrett Shaw, Editor

Anthology of writing from the pages of the first 15 years of The Disability Rag. *$18.95*

245 pages
ISBN 0-96270 -45-0

6125 Reaching Out

REACH of Denton Resource Center
405 S Elm
Suite 202
Denton, TX 76201
940-383-1062
FAX: 940-383-2742
e-mail: reachdes@reachcils.org
www.reachcils.org

Quarterly

6126 Referral Directory of Social Services in Metropolitan Washington

Prevent Child Abuse of Metropolitan Washington
PO Box 57194
Washington, DC 20037
202-223-0020
FAX: 202-296-4046
e-mail: pcamw@juno.com
www.pcamw.org

Kendra Dunn, Executive Director

$50.00

500 pages Bi-Annually

6127 Rehabilitation Counseling: Profession & Pr actice

Springer Publishing Company
536 Broadway
New York, NY 10012
212-431-4370
877-687-7476
877-687-7976
FAX: 212-941-7842
e-mail: marketing@springerpub.com
www.springerpub.com

Annette Imperati, Marketing/Sales Director

$49.95

392 pages
ISBN 0-826195-10-5

6128 Rehabilitation Gazette

Gazette International Networking Institute
4207 Lindell Boulevard
Suite 110
Saint Louis, MO 63108
314-534-0475
FAX: 314-534-5070
e-mail: gini_intl@msn.com
www.post-polio.org

International journal of independent living for people with disabilities. *$12.00*

8 pages Bi-Annually

6129 Relaxation: A Comprehensive Manual for Adults and Children with Special Needs

Research Press
2612 N Mattis Avenue
Champaign, IL 61822
217-325-3273
800-519-2707
FAX: 217-352-1221
e-mail: rp@researchpress.com
www.researchpress.com

Gail Salyards, Marketing Services Manager

This unique contribution to the field of relaxation training presents: self relaxation techniques designed for adults, methods for teaching relaxation to adults and older children, and procedures for teaching relaxation to young children and children with developmental disabilities. The clear, concise text is supplemented by over 100 helpful illustrations. *$16.95*

108 pages Paperback
ISBN 0-878221-86-7

6130 Resources for People with Disabilities and Chronic Conditions

Resources for Rehabilitation
33 Bedford Street
Suite 19A
Lexington, MA 02420
781-890-6371
FAX: 781-861-7517

Susan Greenblatt

A comprehensive resource directory that helps people with disabilities and chronic conditions achieve their maximum level of independence. Chapters on spinal cord injuries, low back pain, diabetes, hearing and speech impairments, epilepsy, multiple sclerosis. Describes organizations, products and publications. *$49.95*

215 pages Biennial
ISBN 0-92971 -12-7

6131 Role Portrayal and Stereotyping on Television

Greenwood Publishing Group
88 Post Road W
Suite 5007
Westport, CT 06880
203-226-3571
FAX: 203-222-1502
www.greenwood.com

Nancy Signorielli, Author

An annotated bibliography of studies relating to women, minorities, aging, health and handicaps.

214 pages $55 - $59.95
ISBN 0-313248-55-9

6132 Rolfing: The Intergration of Human Structures

Harper & Row
10 E 53rd Street
New York, NY 10022
212-207-7042
800-242-7737
FAX: 212-207-7203
www.harpercollins.com

$27.50

Harcover 1977
ISBN 0-930422-10-4

6133 SCI/LIFE

National Spinal Cord Injury Association
6701 Democracy Boulevard
Suite 300-9
Bethesda, MD 20817
301-214-4006
800-962-9629
FAX: 301-588-9414
e-mail: Info@spinalcord.org
www.spinalcord.org

Charles W Haynes, Publisher
J Charles Haynes JD, Publisher
Thomas H Countee Jr, Esq, Editor in Chief

SCI/LIFE is dedicated to the presentation of news concerning people with spinal cord injuries caused by trauma or disease. *$38.00*

39 pages Quarterly

6134 School Psychology Review

National Association of School Psychologists
4340 EW Highway
Suite 402
Bethesda, MD 20814
301-657-0270
FAX: 301-657-0275
e-mail: inealis@naspweb.org
www.nasponline.org

$75.00

2150 pages Qyarterly

6135 Screening in Chronic Disease

Oxford University Press
2001 Evans Road
Cary, NC 27513
212-726-6000
800-451-7556
FAX: 919-677-1303
www.oup-usa.org

Early detection, or screening, is a common strategy for controlling chronic disease, but little information has been available to help determine which screening procedures are worthwhile, until this textbook. *$42.50*

256 pages

6136 See A Bone

Facts on File
132 W 31 Street
17th Floor
New York, NY 10001
212-907-8800
800-322-8755
FAX: 212-967-9196
e-mail: jchambers@factsonfile.com
www.factsonfile.com

$65.00

352 pages
ISBN 0-816042-80-2

6137 Serving Adults with Cognitive Disabilities

Independent Living Research Utilization ILRU
2323 S Shepherd Drive
Suite 1000
Houston, TX 77019
713-520-0232
FAX: 713-520-5785
www.ilru.org

Darrel, Tyrone and Susan of Arizona Bridge to Independent Living (ABIL) describe the success of their Community Living Options Program for adults with developmental disabilities in this months readings.

10 pages

6138 Setebaid Sentinel

Setebaid Services
PO Box 196
Winfield, PA 17889
570-524-9090
FAX: 570-523-0769
e-mail: info@setebaidservices.org
www.setebaidservices.org

Mark Moyer, Executive Director
Diane Facer, Office Assistant

4-8 pages Bi-Annually

6139 Seven Weeks to a Healthy Stomach

Simon & Schuster
100 Front Street
Riverside, NJ 08075
800-323-7445
FAX: 800-943-9831
www.simonsays.com

A seven-week program to restore the gastrointestinal tract to optimal health, using diet, nutrition, and herbal medicine.

Hardcover 1990
ISBN 0-671682-34-2

6140 Sexual Adjustment

Accent Books & Products
PO Box 700
Bloomington, IL 61702
309-378-2961
800-787-8444
FAX: 309-378-4420
e-mail: acmtlvng@aol.com

Raymond C Cheever, Publisher
Betty Garee, Editor

Essential information concerning sexual adjustment for the paraplegic male. *$4.95*

73 pages Paperback
ISBN 0-19570 -00-0

6141 Sexuality and Disabilities: A Guide for Human Service Practitioners

Haworth Press
10 Alice Street
Binghamton, NY 13904
607-722-5857
800-429-6784
FAX: 607-722-6362
e-mail: orders@haworthpress.com
www.haworthpress.com

Jackie Blakeslee, Advertising
Romel W Mackelpranf DSW, Editor
Deborah Valentine, Editor

This book addresses persons with physical, sensory, intellectual and cognitive disabilities and their concerns in the areas of intimacy, family issues, sexuality and sexual functioning. *$74.95*

159 pages Hardcover
ISBN 1-560243-75-9

6142 Sibling Forum

Family Resource Associates
35 Haddon Avenue
Shrewsbury, NJ 07702
732-747-5310
FAX: 732-747-1896

Susan Levine, Social Worker

A newsletter for brothers and sisters, aged 10 through teen, whose sibling has a disablilty. Includes input from readers, library resources and discussion of feelings. $12/year for families, $20/year for professionals. *$12.00*

8-12 pages Quarterly

6143 Silver Dental Fillings: The Toxic Time Bomb

Aurora Press
300 Catron Street
Suite B
Santa Fe, NM 87504
505-989-9804

$16.95

1986
ISBN 0-943358-24-8

6144 Simon Foundation for Continence

PO Box 815
Wilmette, IL 60091
847-864-3913
800-23S-IMON
FAX: 847-864-9758
www.simonfoundation.org

Cheryle B Gartley, President

Publishes items of interest to people with bladder or bowel incontinence, including medical articles, helpful devices, publications and a pen pal list.

6145 Sinus Survival

Jeremy P Tarcher
8552 E Dry Creek Place
Englewoodes, CO 80112
888-434-0033
FAX: 303-221-5320

Self-help manual for sufferers of bronchitis, sinusitis, allergies, and colds.

6146 Sixty Days of Low-Fat, Low-Cost Meals in Minutes

John Wiley and Son
605 3rd Avenue
New York, NY 10158
212-850-6000
FAX: 212-850-6088

Leigh Anne Godfreg, Sales Coordinator

A great way to get patients on the road to healthy eating. It contains 150 recipes complete with facts on lowering calories, fat, salt and cholesterol. It contains complete menu plans for 60 days and recipes that use ingredients you can find anywhere. *$12.95*

294 pages Paperback
ISBN 1-56561 -10-5

6147 Social Perceptions of People with Disabilities in History

Charles C Thomas
2600 S First Street
Springfield, IL 62704
217-789-8980
800-258-8980
FAX: 217-789-9130
e-mail: books@ccthomas.com
www.ccthomas.com

This book helps to develop a social history on disabilities by providing a multidisciplinary overview of images of people with disabilities in Western history; promotion the exchange of cross-disciplinary information on disabled people from art, literature, original data, and historical works. With the growing interest in people with disabilities and the recent passage of the American Disability Act, this book will be of interest to special educators, humanities students, and social scientists. *$49.95*

324 pages Paperback 1998
ISBN 0-398068-38-0

6148 **Socialization Games for Persons with Disabilities**

Nevalyn F Nevil, Marna L Beatty & David Moxley
2600 S First Street
Springfield, IL 62704
217-789-8980
800-258-8980
FAX: 217-789-9130
e-mail: books@ccthomas.com
www.ccthomas.com

This book is a compilation of practical suggestions and games with easy-to-follow guide lines that provide a solid foundation for the encouragement of positive social behavior. *$47.95*

176 pages Paperback 1997

ISBN 0-398067-46-5

6149 **Solving the Puzzle of Chronic Fatigue**

Life Sciences Press
1216 S 1580 W
Suite A
Orem, UT 84058
801-224-6228
800-336-6308
e-mail: info@essentialscience.net
www.insight-books.com/new/0943685117.html

Although primarily a book about CFS, this comprehensive study also provides a detailed overview of candidiasis, including its causes and best approaches for treatment. *$14.95*

190 pages 1992

ISBN 0-943685-11-7

6150 **Sometimes You Just Want to Feel Like a Human Being**

Brookes Publishing
PO Box 10624
Baltimore, MD 21285
410-337-9580
800-638-3775
FAX: 410-337-8539
e-mail: custserv@brookespublishing.com
www.brookespublishing.com

Case studies of empowering psychotherapy with people with disabilities. This text reveals how counseling can be beneficial to individuals with disabilities of all kinds, including autism, mental retardation, sensory impairment, cerebral palsy, or HIV infection. *$ 26.95*

272 pages Paperback

ISBN 1-55766 -96-0

6151 **Son-Rise: The Miracle Continues**

2080 S Undermountain Road
Sheffield, MA 01257
413-229-2100
800-562-7171
FAX: 413-229-3202
e-mail: sonrise@option.org
www.son-rise.org

Part One is the astonishing record of Raun Kaufman's development from an autistic and retarded child into a loving, brilliant youngster who shows no traces of his former condition. Part Two follows Raun's development after the age of four and teaches us much about love and limitless possibilities. Part Three shares moving accounts of five other ordinary families who became extraordinary when they used the Son-Rise program to reach their own unreachable children. *$12.95*

343 pages Paperback

ISBN 0-915811-53-7

6152 **Source of Help and Hope Newsletter**

Arthritis Foundation
Central Pennsylvania Chapter
PO Box 668
Camp Hill, PA 17001
717-763-0900
800-776-0746
FAX: 717-763-0903
www.arthritis.org

Offers information on activities and events of the Chapter.

3x Year

6153 **Space Coast CIL News**

Space Coast Center for Independent Living
331 Ramp Road
Cocoa Beach, FL 32931
321-784-9008
FAX: 321-784-3702
TTY:321-784-9008
e-mail: agrau@bellsouth.net

Anna Grau, Ind. Living Services Coordinator

Non-profit organization that provides services which enable people with disabilities to live as independently as possible.

12 pages Quarterly

6154 **Special Care in Dentistry**

Academy of Dentistry for Persons with Disabilities
211 E Chicago Avenue
5th Floor
Chicago, IL 60611
312-440-2661
FAX: 312-440-2824
e-mail: fosccdzz@worldnet.att.net
www.specialdentistry.org

$125.00

48 pages BiMonthly

6155 **Special Edge**

Resources in Special Education
J Street
Sacramento, CA 95814
916-568-7058
800-869-4337
FAX: 916-492-9995
e-mail: rise@wested.org

Provides education news, collaborative programs, amendments to the laws, tools for accommodations, resource information, a calendar of events, and more.

BiMonthly

6156 **Spectrum Aquatics Catalog**

Spectrum Aquatics
7100 Spectrum Lane
Missoula, MT 59808
406-543-5309
800-776-5309
FAX: 406-728-7143
e-mail: info@spectrumaquatics.com
www.spectrumaquatics.com

Yearly

6157 **Spud Tech Notes**

Idaho Assistive Technology Project
129 W 3rd Street
Moscow, ID 83843
208-885-3559
800-432-8324
FAX: 208-885-3628
e-mail: rseiler@uidaho.edu
www.educ.uidaho.edu/idatech

Bi-annually

6158 Staying Healthy with Nutrition

Celestial Arts
PO Box 7123
Berkeley, CA 94707 **510-559-1600**
FAX: 510-559-1629
www.tenspeedpress.com

Guide to nutrition, proper dieting, and the mind and body.

1200 pages 1992
ISBN 0-890874-81-6

6159 Sterilization of People with Mental Disabilities

Greenwood Publishing Group
88 Post Road W
Suite 5007
Westport, CT 06880 **203-226-3571**
FAX: 203-222-1502
www.greenwood.com

An examination of the medical and legal trends in sterilization with an emphasis on people with disabilities. Hardcover.

280 pages $59.95 - $65
ISBN 0-865692-25-4

6160 Strategies and Adaptations in Working with Parents with Intellectual Disabilities

Through the Looking Glass
2198 Sixth Street
Suite 100
Berkeley, CA 94710 **510-848-1112**
800-644-2666
FAX: 510-848-4445
e-mail: TLG@lookingglass.org
www.lookingglass.org

K Corbus
S Hansen

$5.00

11 pages

6161 Strides Magazine

N America Riding for the Handicapped Association
PO Box 33150
Denver, CO 80233 **303-452-1212**
800-369-7433
FAX: 303-252-4610
e-mail: narha@narha.org
www.narha.org

Michael Kaufmann, Editor/Dir of Communications
Andrea Spridgen, Customer Service/Editor

NARHA's monthly publication. *$35.00*

42 pages Quarterly

6162 Substance Abuse and Physical Disability

Haworth Press
10 Alice Street
Binghamton, NY 13904 **607-722-5857**
800-429-6784
FAX: 607-722-6362
e-mail: orders@haworthpress.com
www.haworthpress.com

This book offers information on alcohol and drug abuse being a contributing factor in traumatic and disabling injuries. *$ 74.95*

289 pages Hardcover
ISBN 1-560242-89-2

6163 Summeries of Legal Precedents and Law Review Articles concern Parents with Disabilities

Through the Looking Glass
2198 Sixth Street
Suite 100
Berkeley, CA 94710 **510-848-1112**
800-644-2666
FAX: 510-848-4445
e-mail: TLG@lookingglass.org
www.lookingglass.org

L Baer
D Taube

Available in braille, large print or cassette. *$25.00*

24 pages

6164 TASH Connections

29 W Susquehanna Avenue
Suite 210
Baltimore, MD 21204 **410-828-8274**
800-482-8274
FAX: 410-828-6706
e-mail: info@tash.org
www.tash.org

International advocacy association of/for people with disabilities.

November

6165 TECH Watch

Tech Connection
35 Hudson Avenue
Shrewsbury, NJ 07702 **732-747-5310**
732-747-1896
e-mail: tecconn@aol.com
www.techconnection.org

8 pages Quarterly

6166 Taking Charge

Spina Bifida Association of America
4590 Macarthur Boulevard NW
Suite 250
Washington, DC 20007 **202-944-3285**
800-621-3141
FAX: 202-944-3295
e-mail: sbaa@sbaa.org
www.sbaa.org

Teenagers talk about life and physical disabilities. *$ 7.95*

6167 Teaching Dressing Skills: Buttons, Bows and More

Therapro
225 Arlington Street
Framingham, MA 01702 **508-872-9494**
800-257-5376
FAX: 508-875-2062
e-mail: info@theraproducts.com
www.theraproducts.com

Teaches us how to teach children and adults of varying abilities how to tie shoes, button buttons, use zippers and put on/remove clothing. Developed by an experienced occupational therapist, these methods have been successfully used with many children. Each task is broken down with each step clearly illustrated and specific verbal directions given to avoid confusion and to eliminate verbalization that can distract the learner. *$9.95*

5 pages Pamphlets

6168 **Telecommunication Relay Services**

Ferderal Government
31 Center Drive MSC2320
Bethesda, MD 20832
800-241-1044
FAX: 301-402-0018
e-mail: nidcdinfo@nidcd.nih.gov
www.nidcd.nih.org

This telecommunication relay services fact sheet explains what the service is how the relay service allows people who are deaf, har-of-hearing or speech impaired to communicate through a communications assiatnt with people who use a standard telephone.

6169 **Three Rivers News**

Carnegie Library of Pitts. Library for the Blind
Leonard C Staisey Building
4724 Baum Boulevard
Pittsburgh, PA 15213 **412-687-2440**
800-242-0586
FAX: 412-687-2442
e-mail: clbph@clpgh.org
www.clpgh.org/clp/LBPH

Sue Murdock, Director
Kathleen Kappel, Editor

Loans recorded books/magazines and playback equipment, large print books and described videos to western PA residents unable to use standard printed materials due to a visual, physical, or physically-based reading disability.

12 pages Quarterly

6170 **Title II & III Regulation Amendment Regarding Detectable Warnings**

US Department of Justice
950 Pennsylvania Avenue NW DRS-NYAV
Washington, DC 20530 **202-307-0663**
800-574-0301
FAX: 202-307-1197
www.ada.gov

This document suspends the requirements for detectable warnings at curb ramps, hazardous vehicular areas, and reflecting pools.

6171 **Title II Complaint Form**

US Department of Justice
950 Pennsylvania Avenue NW DRS-NYAV
Washington, DC 20530 **202-307-0663**
800-574-0301
FAX: 202-307-1197
www.ada.gov

Standard form for filing a complaint under Title II of the ADA or Section 504 of the Rehabilitation Act of 1973.

6172 **Title II Highlights**

US Department of Justice
950 Pennsylvania Avenue NW DRS-NYAV
Washington, DC 20530 **202-307-0663**
800-574-0301
FAX: 202-307-1197
www.ada.gov

An 8-page outline of the key requirements of the ADA for state and local governments.

6173 **Title II Technical Assistance Manual and Supplements**

US Department of Justice
950 Pennsylvania Avenue NW DRS-NYAV
Washington, DC 20530 **202-307-0663**
800-574-0301
FAX: 202-307-1197
www.ada.gov

A 56-page manual explaining what state and local governments must do to ensure that their services, programs, and activities are provided to the public in a non-discriminatory manner. Give practical examples.

6174 **Title III Technical Assistance Manual and Supplement**

US Department of Justice
950 Pennsylvania Avenue NW DRS-NYAV
Washington, DC 20530 **202-307-0663**
800-574-0301
FAX: 202-307-1197
www.ada.gov

A 12-page outline of the key requirements of the ADA for businesses and nonproft service agencies.

6175 **To Live with Grace and Dignity**

World Institute on Disability
510 16th Street
Suite 100
Oakland, CA 94612 **510-763-4100**
FAX: 510-763-4109
e-mail: wid@wid.org
www.wid.org

This unique book combines photographs and essays to allow the reader to enter some of the real day to day relationships that develop between individuals with disabilities and their personal assistants. Looking at and listening to what these relationships are all about is what motivated and inspired this book, says author Lydia Gans. The individuals included in this book represent a wide range of ages, disabilities and cultural backgrounds. *$26.00*

72 pages Paperback

6176 **Touch/Ability Connects People with Disabilities & Alternative Health Care Pract.**

Independent Living Research Utilization ILRU
2323 S Shepherd Drive
Suite 1000
Houston, TX 77019 **713-520-0232**
FAX: 713-520-5785
www.ilru.org

The people at DIRECT center for Independence and Touch/Ability in Tuscon, Arizona, have collaborated to develop a wellness program that makes alternative health care choices available to people with disabilities. The Touch/Ability Wellness program was selected as one of last year's winners in the Innovative CILs competition because of this outcome of increased options open to people with disabilities.

10 pages

6177 **Training Module: Adaptive Baby Care Equipment**

Through the Looking Glass
2198 Sixth Street
Suite 100
Berkeley, CA 94710 **510-848-1112**
800-644-2666
FAX: 510-848-4445
e-mail: TLG@lookingglass.org
www.lookingglass.org

Curriculum for OT programs includes Adaptive Baby Care Equipment Video and Book. *$250.00*

6178 Treatment for Chronic Depression

Guilford Press
72 Spring Street
New York, NY 10012
212-431-9800
800-365-7006
FAX: 212-966-6708
www.guilford.com

$39.00

Cloth

ISBN 1-572305-27-4

6179 US Role in International Disability Activities: A History

World Institute on Disability
510 16th Street
Suite 100
Oakland, CA 94612
510-763-4100
FAX: 510-763-4109
e-mail: wid@wid.org
www.wid.org

This study was undertaken to present an initial introduction to US involvement in the field of international rehabilitation and disability. *$12.00*

169 pages Paperback

6180 Usher Syndrome

Federal Government
31 Center Drive MSC2320
Bethesda, MD 20892
800-241-1044
FAX: 301-402-0018
e-mail: nidcdinfo@nidcd.nih.gov
www.nidcd.nih.org

Explains what is Usher Syndrome, who is affected by Usher syndrome, what causes Usher syndrome, how is Usher syndrome treated, and what research is being conducted on Usher syndrome.

6181 Vaccines: Are They Really Safe and Effective?

New Atlantean Press
PO Box 9638
Santa Fe, NM 87504
505-983-1856

Evaluates 'mandated' and many newer vaccines to determine their safety and both short- and long-term effects.

1902

ISBN 1-881217-30-2

6182 Vibrational Medicine

Bear & Company
One Park Street
Rochester, VT 05767
802-767-3174
800-246-8648
FAX: 802-767-3726
e-mail: orders@innertraditions.com
www.InnerTraditions.com

608 pages

ISBN 1-879181-58-4

6183 Vision, Values & Vitality: Bringing IL Principles to Mental Health Peer Support

Independent Living Research Utilization ILRU
2323 S Shepherd Drive
Suite 1000
Houston, TX 77019
713-520-0232
FAX: 713-520-5785
www.ilru.org

Frederick Moe
Cindy Perkins
Pat Spiller

Frederick, Cindy, and Pat describe the technical assistance GSIL provides to drop-in centers to enable them to become consumer-controlled peer support centers.

10 pages

6184 Visions & Values

Idaho Council on Developmental Disabilities
802 W Bannock Street
#308
Boise, ID 83702
800-544-2433
FAX: 208-334-3417
e-mail: msword@icdd.state.id.us
www.state.id.us/icdd

Marilyn B Sword, Executive Director/Editor

A quarterly publication from the Idaho Council on Developmental Disabilities.

6185 Vitamin C: Who Needs It?

Arlington Press
191 Harrison Avenue
Brooklynam, NY 11206
718-486-7474
FAX: 718-504-4927
e-mail: info@arlingtonpress.com
www.arlingtonpress.com

An informational book on the nutritional benefits of vitamin C.

1993

ISBN 0-944353-04-5

6186 WA & NEWS

Wheelchair Access
PO Box 12
Glenmoore, PA 19343
610-942-3266
FAX: 610-942-0282
e-mail: info@waccess.org
www.waccess.org

Frank Gomez, Publisher

Features wheelchair accessible houses and apartments for rent or for sale. Currently the newsletter includes ads from all states. Ads received from any State will be accepted free of charge. Featured also are ads of wheelchairs, vans, equipment, etc., for sale. Complete ad information and more is listed in the Web site. A free copy of WA & NEWS sent upon request. *$12.00*

20 pages Monthly

6187 Walking Tomorrow

Christopher Reeve Paralysis Foundation
500 Morris Avenue
Springfield, NJ 07081
973-379-6299
800-252-0292
FAX: 973-912-9433
e-mail: paralysis@aol.com
www.paralysis.com

A newsletter offering medical and technological updates for people with physical disabilities, including paralysis.

Quarterly

6188 Walton Independent

Walton Rehabilitation Hospital
1355 Independence Drive
Augusta, GA 30901
706-823-8511
866-492-5866
FAX: 706-724-5752
e-mail: postmaster@wrh.org
www.wrh.org

Deb Bergmann, Editor

A publication from the Walton Rehabilitation Hospital. Published three times a year, and it is free.

40 pages 3 times yearly

6189 We Can Speak for Ourselves: Self Advocacy by Mentally Handicapped People

Brookline Books
PO Box 1047
Cambridge, MA 02238 **617-868-0360**
800-666-2665
FAX: 617-868-1772
e-mail: brooklinebks@delphi.com
www.brooklinebooks.com

Practical advice and support for parents, group resident workers, and others interested in fostering self-advocacy for people with developmental disabilities. *$10.00*

246 pages Paperback
ISBN 0-25336 -65-9

6190 Weiner's Herbal

Quantum Books
Four Cambridge Center
Cambridge, MA 02142 **617-494-5042**
FAX: 617-577-7282
e-mail: orders@quantumbk.com
www.quantumbooks.com

A-Z index covering all aspects of herbs.

Paperback 1980
ISBN 0-812825-86-1

6191 What Psychotherapists Should Know about Disabilty

Through the Looking Glass
2198 Sixth Street
Suite 100
Berkeley, CA 94710 **510-848-1112**
800-644-2666
FAX: 510-848-4445
e-mail: TLG@lookingglass.org
www.lookingglass.org

R Olkin
$24.00

368 pages

6192 What You Need To Know

Vestibular Disorders Association
PO Box 4467
Portland, OR 97208 **503-229-7705**
800-837-8428
FAX: 503-229-8064

$24.95

Quarterly
ISBN 0-963261-13-4

6193 What Your Doctors Won't Tell You

Harper Perennial
10 E 53rd Street
New York, NY 10022 **212-207-7000**
FAX: 212-207-7145
www.harpercollins.com

A look at the world of alternative medicine, with a comprehensive chapter on constipation, and the illnesses it can contribute to. Also provides a treatment program based diet, nutritional supplements, herbal medicine, and colonic irrigation.

32 pages 1994
ISBN 1-883619-11-4

6194 What's Line

Alabama Public Library Service
6030 Monticello Drive
Montgomery, AL 36130 **334-213-3906**
800-392-5671
FAX: 334-213-3993
e-mail: fzaleski@apls.state.al.us
www.apls.state.al.us

4 pages Quarterly

6195 Wheelin' Around

6614 W Sweetwater Avenue
Glendale, AZ 85304 **623-776-8830**
800-456-1371
FAX: 623-412-9920
e-mail: info@wheelerscanrentals.com
www.wheelersvanrentals.com

Tammy Smith, Manager

A quarterly publication. Free.

6196 Women with Physical Disabilities: Achievin g & Maintaining Health & Well-Being

Spina Bifida Association of America
4590 MacArthur Boulevard NW
Suite 250
Washington, DC 20007 **202-944-3285**
800-621-3141
FAX: 202-944-3295
e-mail: sbaa@sbaa.org
www.sbaa.org

Introduces the critical concept of womens health in the context of physical disabilities. *$42.00*

6197 Women's Health Alert

Addison-Wesley Publishing Company
75 Arlington Street
Suite 300
Boston, MA 02116 **617-848-6000**
FAX: 617-848-6034
www.awprofessional.com

This book provides up-to-date information on the practice of female medicine with data and statistics that can help a woman make wise decisions about her health. Information on hormone-replacement therapy and osteoporosis are detailed.

1991

6198 Work in the Context of Disability Culture

Independent Living Research Utilization ILRU
2323 S Shepherd Drive
Suite 1000
Houston, TX 77019 **713-520-0232**
FAX: 713-520-5785
www.ilru.org

Another winner in the innovative CIL competition-Steve Brown describes the Talking Books Program of Southeast Alaska Independent Living, discussing their efforts to record the oral history and life experiences of people with disabilities in the larger context of the disability culture.

10 pages

6199 **Working with Your Doctor: Getting the Healthcare You Deserve**

Patient-Centered Guides
101 Morris Street
Sebastopol, CA 95472
707-829-0515
800-998-9938
FAX: 707-829-0104
e-mail: health@oreilly.com
www.patientcenters.com

Linda Lamb, Editor
Shawnde Paull, Marketing
Kerri Bonasch, Sales/Marketing Manager

Working with Your Doctor shows how to form a satisfying partnership with your doctor in a rapidly changing healthcare environment. It contains in-depth and practical information on how to find the right doctor, communicate clearly, ask about tests and treatments, seek opinions, take action when wronged, and deal effectively with managed care. This book is a great primer for patient empowerment. *$15.95*

377 pages Paperback
ISBN 1-565922-73-5

6200 **World of Options**

Mobility International USA
PO Box 10767
Eugene, OR 97440
541-343-1284
FAX: 541-343-6812
e-mail: info@miusa.org
www.miusa.org

Susan Sygall, Executive Director
Pamela Houston, Public Relations Coordinator
Tracy Scharn, Project Assistant

A guide to international, educational exchange, community service and travel for persons with disabilities. *$16.00*

338 pages
ISBN 1-880034-01-8

6201 **World of Options: A Guide to International Educational Exchange**

Mobility International USA
PO Box 10767
Eugene, OR 97440
541-343-1284
FAX: 541-343-6812
e-mail: info@miusa.org
www.miusa.org

Susan Sygall, Executive Director
Pamela Houston, Public Relations Coordinator
Tracy Scharn, Project Assistant

A Guide to International Educational Exchange, Community Service and Travel for People with Disabilities includes information travel and international programs, as well as personal experience stories from people with disabilities who have had successful international experiences. *$45.00*

600 pages 1997
ISBN 1-880034-24-7

6202 **You May Be Able to Adopt**

Through the Looking Glass
2198 Sixth Street
Suite 100
Berkeley, CA 94710
510-848-1112
800-644-2666
FAX: 510-848-4445
e-mail: TLG@lookingglass.org
www.lookingglass.org

L Toms Barker
M Kirshbaum

A guide to the adoption process for prospective mothers with disabilities and their partners. Available in braille, large print or cassette. *$10.00*

112 pages

6203 **Young Person's Guide to Spina Bifida**

Spina Bifida Association of America
4590 Macarthur Boulevard NW
Suite 250
Washington, DC 20007
202-944-3285
800-621-3141
FAX: 202-944-3295
e-mail: sbaa@sbaa.org
www.sbaa.org

Gives practical tips and suggestions for becoming independent and managing your health. *$19.00*

6204 **Your Body's Many Cries for Water**

Global Health Solutions
8472 A Tyco Road
Vienna, VA 22182
703-848-2333
800-759-3999
FAX: 703-848-0028
e-mail: shipping@watercure.com
www.watercure.com

Kristin Swan, Secretary
Joy Barber, Secretary

Global Health Solutions provides materials by Dr F Batmanghelidj. He writes about dehydration and traces many illnesses to the fact that we do not drink enough water. The ability of the body to heal itself is greatly impaired by inadequate water consumption. *$ 14.95*

182 pages
ISBN 0-962994-23-5

6205 **Your Fertility Signals**

Smooth Stone Press
PO Box 19875
St. Louis, MO 63144
314-968-2596
FAX: 314-968-2821

Naturally, cooperatively, and effectively achieve or prevent pregnancy, reduce or eliminate contraceptive use, enhance intimacy in your relationship, and possibly choose your baby's sex.

159 pages Paperback 1991
ISBN 0-961940-10-7

6206 **Your Inner Physician and You: CranioSacral Therapy SomatoEmotional Release**

North Atlantic Books
1456 Forth Street
Berkeley, CA 94710
510-559-8277
FAX: 510-559-8279
www.northatlanticbooks.com

163 pages 1997
ISBN 1-556432-46-1

Hearing Impaired

6207 **ASHA Leader**

American Speech-Language-Hearing Association
10801 Rockville Pike
Rockville, MD 20852
301-897-5700
800-638-8255
FAX: 301-897-7348
e-mail: actioncenter@asha.org
www.asha.org

Joanne K Jessen, Publications Director
John E Bernthal, President
Frederick T Spahr PhD, Executive Director

Association publication containing news, notices of events and activities and information for members on issues facing the profession of audiology and speech-language pathology. *$80.00*

35 pages 2 x month

6208 **Adult Bible Lessons for the Deaf**

LifeWay Christian Resources Southern Baptist Conv.
127 9th Avenue N
Nashville, TN 37234
615-251-2000
800-458-2772
FAX: 651-251-5764
e-mail: specialed@lifeway.com
www.lifeway.com

Omar Fernandez, Manager

Bible study lessons for every three months written by and for persons who are deaf. Based on the Family Bible Series (International Sunday School Lessons).

Quarterly

6209 **Advanced Sign Language Vocabulary: A Resource Text for Educators**

2600 S 1st Street
Springfield, IL 62704
217-789-8980
800-258-8980
FAX: 217-789-9130
e-mail: books@ccthomas.com
www.ccthomas.com

A resource text for educators, interpreters, parents and sign language instructors. *$46.95*

202 pages Paperback
ISBN 0-398057-22-2

6210 **American Annals of the Deaf**

PO Box 1778
St Augustine, FL 32086
904-810-5200
FAX: 904-810-5525
e-mail: email@ceasd.org
www.ceasd.org

Joe Finnegan, Executive Director
Barbara Raimondo, Government Relations Liaison
Mike Bello, Treasurer

Quarterly publication from the Conference of Educational Administrators Serving the Deaf.

Quarterly

6211 **American Journal of Speech-Language Pathology**

American Speech-Language-Hearing Association
10801 Rockville Pike
Rockville, MD 20852
301-897-5700
800-638-8255
FAX: 301-897-7348
e-mail: info@asha.org
www.asha.org

John E Bernthal, President
Frederick T Spahr PhD, Executive Director
Joanne Jessen, Publications Director

6212 **American Sign Language (ASL): Quick Facts**

Federal Government
31 Center Drive MSC2320
Bethesda, MD 20892
800-241-1044
FAX: 301-402-0018
e-mail: nidcdinfo@nidcd.nih.gov
www.nidcd.nih.gov

Ouick facts on what is ASL, where did it orginate, how it compares with spoken language, and why has ASL become a first language for many deaf people.

6213 **American Sign Language Handshape Dictionary**

Gallaudet University Press
11030 S Langley Avenue
Chicago, IL 60628
800-621-2736
FAX: 800-621-8476
TTY:800-621-9347
gupress.gallaudet.edu

Richard A Tennant, Co-Author
Marianne Gluszak Brown, Co-Author

More than 1,600 sign illustrations arranged by handshape for easy identification. Allows readers to look up signs they have seen without needing to know their English meaning beforehand, complemented by a complete English index cross-referenced to every sign. *$35.00*

408 pages Hardcover

6214 **American Sign Language Phrase Book**

TJ Publishers
817 Silver Spring Avenue
Suite 206
Silver Spring, MD 20910
301-585-4440
800-999-1168
FAX: 301-585-5930
e-mail: TJPubinc@aol.com

Angela K Thames, President
Jerald A Murphy, VP

The author provides interesting, realistic and meaningful situations. Sign language is learned through novel remarks cleverly organized around everyday topics. *$18.95*

362 pages Softcover
ISBN 0-80923 -00-5

6215 **American Sign Language: A Look at Its Structure & Community**

TJ Publishers
817 Silver Spring Avenue
Suite 206
Silver Spring, MD 20910
301-585-4440
800-999-1168
FAX: 301-585-5930
e-mail: TJPubinc@aol.com

Angela K Thames, President
Jerald A Murphy, VP

Answers basic questions about American Sign Language. What is it? What is its history? Who uses it? What is the deaf community? *$3.95*

22 pages Softcover
ISBN 0-93266 -01-9

6216 **Anna's Silent World**

JB Lippincott
227 E Washington Square
Philadelphia, PA 19106 **215-238-4200**
800-777-2295
FAX: 215-824-7390

Anna was a hearing impaired child who lived in New York City with her family. The text followed Anna through a hearing evaluation, speech therapy, and her participation in a class for hearing impaired children.

48 pages Hardcover
ISBN 0-39731 -39-5

6217 **At Home Among Strangers**

TJ Publishers
817 Silver Spring Avenue
Suite 206
Silver Spring, MD 20910 **301-585-4440**
800-999-1168
FAX: 301-585-5930
e-mail: TJPubinc@aol.com

Angela K Thames, President
Jerald A Murphy, Executive Assistant

Discusses deaf culture and its uniqueness in two sections: the first describes the deaf community - its development, structure and culture; the second explains Schein's theory of deaf community development. *$24.95*

254 pages Hardcover
ISBN 0-930323-51-3

6218 **Auditory Processing Disorders in Children: What Does It Mean?**

Federal Government
31 Center Drive MSC2320
Bethesda, MD 20892
800-241-1044
FAX: 301-402-0018
e-mail: nidcdinfo@nidcd.nih.gov
www.nidcd.nih.gov

This fact sheet describes what is auditory processing disorder, what causes APD diffculty, what are the symtoms, how is it diagnosed, what treatments are available, and current research into the rehabilitation of child language disorders which will help us better understand the nature of auditory processing disorders.

6219 **Auricle**

Auditory-Verbal International
2121 Eisenhower Avenue
Suite 402
Alexandria, VA 22314 **703-739-1049**
FAX: 703-739-0395
TTY:703-739-0874
e-mail: audiverb@aol.com
www.auditory-verbal.org

Sara Blair Lake, Executive Director/CEO
Tom Lucches, President

To provide the choice of listening and speaking as the way of life for children and adults who are deaf or hard of hearing.

Quarterly

6220 **BPPV**

Vestibular Disorder Association
P.O. Box 4467
Portland, OR 97208 **503-229-7705**
800-837-8428
FAX: 503-229-8064
e-mail: veda@vestibular.org
www.vestibular.org

Lisa Haven, Editor
Connie Pilcher, Outreach Coordinator

1900

6221 **Basic Course in Manual Communication**

Gallaudet University Bookstore
11030 S Langley Avenue
Chicago, IL 60628 **202-651-5488**
800-621-2736
FAX: 202-651-5489

Teach your students manual communication - that living, changing, growing language of signs. *$11.95*

158 pages Softcover

6222 **Basic Vocabulary: ASL for Parents and Children**

TJ Publishers
817 Silver Spring Avenue
Suite 206
Silver Spring, MD 20910 **301-585-4440**
800-999-1168
FAX: 301-585-5930
e-mail: TJPubinc@aol.com

Angela K Thames, President
Jerald A Murphy, VP

Carefully selected words and signs include those that children use every day. Alphabetically organized vocabulary incorporates developmental lists helpful to both deaf and hearing children and over 1000 clear sign language illustrations. *$8.95*

240 pages Softcover
ISBN 0-93266 -00-0

6223 **Ben's Story: A Deaf Child's Right to Sign**

TJ Publishers
817 Silver Spring Avenue
Suite 206
Silver Spring, MD 20910 **301-585-4440**
800-999-1168
FAX: 301-585-5930
e-mail: TJPubinc@aol.com

Angela K Thames, President
Jerald A Murphy, Executive Assistant

This is a mother's story of how she responded to the diagnosis of her son's deafness and how she struggled to have her son educated using sign language. *$7.95*

267 pages Softcover
ISBN 0-930323-47-5

6224 **Between Friends**

Beltone Electronics Corporation
4201 W Victoria Street
Chicago, IL 60646 **773-583-3600**
FAX: 773-583-1361

Renee Rockoff, Editor

For hearing aid wearers: quizzes, jokes, health, recipes and financial items.

6 pages

6225 Book of Name Signs

Gallaudet University Bookstore
11030 S Langley Avenue
Chicago, IL 60628
202-651-5488
800-621-2736
FAX: 202-651-5489

Discusses the rules for American Sign Language name sign formation and their appropriate use. *$12.95*

112 pages

6226 Bridges Beyond Sound

Brookes Publishing
PO Box 10624
Baltimore, MD 21285
410-337-9580
800-638-3775
FAX: 410-337-8539
e-mail: custserv@brookespublishing.com
www.brookespublishing.com

An instructional workbook on understanding and including students with a hearing loss. Supplement to the Bridges Beyond Sound videotape. Besides the videotape script, background information on hearing loss, discussion questions, activities, and reproducible worksheets are included. *$33.00*

176 pages Spiral-bound

ISBN 1-55766 -26-6

6227 Bulletin Newsletter

806 W Adams Boulevard
Los Angeles, CA 90007
213-748-5481
800-522-4582
FAX: 213-749-1651
e-mail: mmartindale@jtc.org
www.jtc.org

Barbara F Hecht PhD, President
Mary Ann Bell, VP Development & Communications
Jack Cooper, Editor

Bi-annual publication from the John Tracy Clinic.

8 pages Bi-annually

6228 CSD Spectrum

Communication Service for the Deaf (CSD)
102 N Krohn Place
Sioux Falls, SD 57103
605-367-5760
800-642-6410
FAX: 605-367-5958
e-mail: info@c-s-d.org
www.c-s-d.org

Marvin Miller, Author/Editor

A free quarterly publication from CSD.

Quarterly

6229 Captions for Deaf and Hard-of-Hearing View ers

Federal Government
31 Center Drive MSC2320
Bethesda, MD 20892
800-241-1044
FAX: 301-402-0018
e-mail: nidcdinfo@nidcdnih.gov
www.nidcd.nih.gov

This fact sheet explains what are the captions, current research studying caption features, speeds, and the effects od visula impairments on reading captions, ans offers additional resources.

6230 Changing the Rules

TJ Publishers
817 Silver Spring Avenue
Suite 206
Silver Spring, MD 20910
301-585-4440
800-999-1168
FAX: 301-585-5930
e-mail: TJPubinc@aol.com

Angela K Thames, President
Jerald A Murphy, VP

Like many deaf adults, Frank Bowe was mainstreamed in the small Pennsylvania town where he was raised. This is a humorous and poignant account of the obstacles that shaped this leading disability rights activist. Bowe's account of coming of age and personal growth, the discovery of signed language and an insider's view of the equal rights movement is a compelling record of one man's struggle with the challenges of profound deafness. *$8.95*

204 pages Hardcover

ISBN 0-93266 -31-0

6231 Chelsea: The Story of a Signal Dog

Gallaudet University Bookstore
800 Florida Avenue NE
Washington, DC 20002
202-651-5000
800-451-1073
FAX: 202-651-5489

This is a story of a young deaf couple and their Belgian sheepdog, who acts as their ears. It explains how these dogs are trained and paired with their new owners. *$18.95*

169 pages

6232 Children of a Lesser God

Gallaudet University Bookstore
11030 S Langley Avenue
Chicago, IL 60628
202-651-5488
800-621-2736
FAX: 202-651-5489

The play that won the hearts of thousands. This is a story of a deaf woman who refuses to succumb to the hearing people's image of what a deaf person should be. *$4.50*

91 pages Softcover

6233 Choices in Deafness

Woodbine House
6510 Bells Mill Road
Bethesda, MD 20817
301-897-3570
800-843-7323
FAX: 301-897-5838
www.woodbinehouse.com

A useful aid in choosing the appropriate communication option for a child with a hearing loss. Experts present the following communication options: Auditory-Verbal Approach, Bilingual-Bicultural Approach, Cued Speech, Oral Approach, and Total Communication. This new edition explains medical causes of hearing loss, the diagnostic process, audiological assessment, and cochlear implants. Children and parents also offer their personal experiences. *$16.95*

275 pages Paperback

ISBN 0-933149-85-9

6234 Clerc: The Story of His Early Years

TJ Publishers
817 Silver Spring Avenue
Suite 206
Silver Spring, MD 20910
301-585-4440
800-999-1168
FAX: 301-585-5930
e-mail: TJPubinc@aol.com

Angela K Thames, President
Jerald A Murphy, VP

This imaginative tale recounts the youthful history of Laurent Clerc, the deaf teacher who helped Thomas Gallaudet establish schools for the deaf in the 19th century. Early experiences influenced the teaching methods Clerc developed in later life and young adults will relish identifying with the hero of this entertaining story. *$9.95*

208 pages Softcover
ISBN 0-93032 -23-8

6235 **Client Assistance Program: Arizona**

3839 N 3rd Street
Suite 209
Phoenix, AZ 85012 **602-274-6287**
FAX: 602-274-6779

John Guiterrez, Director

6236 **Cochlear Implants**

Federal Government
31 Center Dirve MSC2320
Bethesda, MD 20892
800-241-1044
FAX: 301-402-0018
e-mail: nidcdinfo@nidcd.nih.gov
www.nidcd.nih.gov

This fact sheet explains what is a cochlear implant, how it works, who gets cochlear implants, how someone receives a cochlear impant and what the future holds for cochlear impants.

6237 **Cochlear Implants and Children**

Alexander Graham Bell Association
3417 Volta Place NW
Washington, DC 20007 **202-337-5220**
FAX: 202-337-8314
e-mail: info@agbell.org
www.agbell.org

Designed to educate readers about cochlear implants, including surgery, the importance of rehabilitation and the significance of parents' and professionals' roles. *$42.95*

189 pages Paperback

6238 **Cochlear Implants for Kids**

Alexander Graham Bell Association
3417 Volta Place NW
Washington, DC 20007 **202-337-5220**
FAX: 202-337-8314
e-mail: info@agbell.org
www.agbell.org

Designed to educate readers about cochlear implants, including surgery, the importance of rehabilitation and the significance of parents' and professionals' roles. *$42.95*

404 pages Paperback

6239 **Cognition, Education and Deafness**

Gallaudet University Press
800 Florida Avenue NE
Washington, DC 20002 **202-651-5000**
800-451-1073
FAX: 202-651-5489

The work of 54 authors is gathered in this definitive collection of current research on deafness and cognition. The articles are grouped into seven sections: cognition, problem solving, thinking processes, language development, reading methodologies, measurement of potential, and intervention programs. *$21.95*

260 pages Hardcover

6240 **College and Career Programs for the Deaf**

Gallaudet University Bookstore
11030 S Langley Avenue
Chicago, IL 60628 **202-651-5488**
800-621-2736
FAX: 202-651-5489

Which college is the right one for you? This is a guide to colleges in the United States and Canada that offer special programs for deaf students. *$12.95*

108 pages Softcover

6241 **Come Sign with Us: Sign Language Activities for Children**

TJ Publishers
817 Silver Spring Avenue
Suite 206
Silver Spring, MD 20910 **301-585-4440**
800-999-1168
FAX: 301-585-5930
e-mail: TJPubinc@aol.com

Angela K Thames, President
Jerald A Murphy, VP

Illustrated activities manual contains more than 300 line drawings of adults and children signing familiar words, phrases and sentences using ASL in English word order. *$29.95*

144 pages Softcover
ISBN 0-930321-56-3

6242 **Communicating with Deaf People: An Introduction**

Gallaudet University Bookstore
800 Florida Avenue NE
Washington, DC 20002 **202-651-5000**
800-451-1073
FAX: 202-651-5489

This illustrated publication introduces the various ways deaf people can communicate, including gesture and facial expression, speech-reading, fingerspelling and other manual communication systems. *$2.00*

20 pages

6243 **Communication Options for Children Who are Deaf or Hard-of-Hearing**

Federal Government
31 Center Drive MCS2320
Bethesda, MD 20892
800-241-1044
FAX: 301-402-0018
e-mail: midcdinfo@nidcd.nih.gov
www.nidcd.nih.gov

Explains how hearing loss or deafness is identified in newborns, how later onset of hearing loss is identified in young children, what causes hearing loss or deafness in newborns, what communication options are available to deaf and har-of-hearing children, and how your family can particiapte in research related hereditary deafness, hearing impairment, or intervention strategies.

6244 **Communique**

Michigan Association for Deaf, Hearing and Speech
2929 Covington Court
Suite 200
Lansing, MI 48912 **517-487-0066**
800-968-7327
FAX: 517-487-2586
e-mail: yourear@msu.edu
www.madhs.org

4-8 pages Bi-annually

6245 Comprehensive Reference Manual for Signers and Interpreters

Charles C Thomas
2600 S First Street
Springfield, IL 62704
217-789-8980
800-258-8980
FAX: 217-789-9130
e-mail: books@ccthomas.com
www.ccthomas.com

Manual for signers. *$47.95*

314 pages Paperback
ISBN 0-398059-19-5

6246 Comprehensive Signed English Dictionary

Gallaudet University Press
11030 S Langley Avenue
Chicago, IL 60628
800-621-2736
FAX: 800-621-8476
TTY:800-621-9347
gupress.gallaudet.edu

Harry Bornstein, Co-Author
Karen L Saulnier, Co-Author
Lillian B Hamilton, Co-Author

This complete dictionary has over 3,100 signs, including signs reflecting lively and contemporary vocabulary. *$35.00*

464 pages Hardcover

6247 Connect

Hearing, Speech & Deafness Center (HSDC)
1620 18th Avenue
Seattle, WA 98122
206-323-5770
FAX: 206-328-6871
e-mail: hsdc@hsdc.org
www.hsdc.org

David Stoner, Editor
Suisie Burdick, Deputy Director

The Center's mission to enrich the lives of all adults and childrenwho experience hearing loss, speech and language impairments, or who are Deaf, by providing professional services and technology and by promoting community awareness and accessibility. A not-for-profit United Way Agency building community through communications since 1937. Call V/TTY.

8 pages Quarterly

6248 Connect Newsletter

Hearing, Speech & Deafness Center (HSDC)
1625 19th Avenue
Seattle, WA 98122
206-323-5773
FAX: 206-328-6871
e-mail: hsdc@hsdc.org
www.hsdc.org

8 pages Bi-annually

6249 Conversational Sign Language II

Harris Communications
15155 Technology Drive
Eden Prairie, MN 55344
952-906-1180
800-825-6758
FAX: 952-906-1099
e-mail: mail@harriscomm.com
www.harriscomm.com

Bill Williams, National Sales Manager

This book presents English words and their American Sign Language equivalents. *$12.95*

218 pages Paperback
ISBN 0-913580-00-7

6250 Coping with the Multi-Handicapped Hearing Impaired: A Practical Approach

Charles C Thomas
2600 S First Street
Springfield, IL 62704
217-789-8980
800-258-8980
FAX: 217-789-9130
e-mail: books@ccthomas.com
www.ccthomas.com

Professional text offers suggestions on how to deal with the multi-handicapped deaf person. Also available in cloth.

90 pages $20.95
ISBN 0-398063-33-8

6251 Deaf Catholic

International Catholic Deaf Association
1030 LaGrange Road #9
LaGrange, IL 60525
FAX: 708-579-5847
TTY:708-579-5817
e-mail: icdaus@ameritech.com

Richard Kush, Editor

Quarterly publication from the International Catholic Deaf Association. *$15.00*

16 pages Quarterly

6252 Deaf Empowerment: Emergence, Struggle and Rhetoric

Gallaudet University Press
11030 S Langley Avenue
Chicago, IL 60628
800-621-2736
FAX: 800-621-8476
TTY:800-621-9347
gupress.gallaudet.edu

The story of the Deaf social movement, from its beginnings in the mid 1800s through its growth and strengthening in the late 20th century, much of it due to rhetoric and tactics adopted from other social movements. *$34.95*

192 pages Hardcover

6253 Deaf Heritage: A Narrative History

Gallaudet University Bookstore
11030 S Langley Avenue
Chicago, IL 60628
202-651-5488
800-621-2736
FAX: 202-651-5489

This in-depth history of deaf America contains pictures, illustrations, vignettes, and biographical profiles. *$21.95*

500 pages Paperback

6254 Deaf History Unveiled: Interpretations from the New Scholarship

Gallaudet University Press
11030 S Langley Avenue
Chicago, IL 60628
800-621-2736
FAX: 800-621-8476
TTY:800-621-9347
gupress.gallaudet.edu

John Vickrey Van Cleve, Editor

An all-star cast of historians explores the new themes driving Deaf History, including comparisons with other minority cultures and the social paternalism that affects deaf communities around the globe. *$27.50*

316 pages Softcover

6255 Deaf Like Me

Gallaudet University Press
800 Florida Avenue NE
Washington, DC 20002
202-651-5000
800-451-1073
FAX: 202-651-5489

Written by the uncle and father of a deaf girl, this is an account of parents coming to terms with deafness. This paperback edition contains a special epilogue by Lynn Spradley, grown and in her twenties, as she reflects on her growing-up years with the advantage of hindsight. *$10.95*

292 pages Softcover

6256 Deaf in America: Voices from a Culture

TJ Publishers
817 Silver Spring Avenue
Suite 206
Silver Spring, MD 20910
301-585-4440
800-999-1168
FAX: 301-585-5930
e-mail: TJPubinc@aol.com

Angela K Thames, President
Jerald A Murphy, VP

Now available in paperback, this book opens deaf culture to outsiders, inviting readers to imagine and understand a world of silence. This book shares the joy and satisfaction many people have with their lives and shows that deafness may not be the handicap most hearing people think. *$12.95*

134 pages Softcover
ISBN 0-67419 -24-1

6257 Deaf-Blind Perspective

Teaching Research
345 Monmouth Avenue
Monmouth, OR 97361
800-438-9376
FAX: 503-838-8150
e-mail: dblink@tr.wou.edu
www.tr.wou.edu/dblink

John Reiman PhD, Director

6258 Discovering Sign Language

Gallaudet University Press
800 Florida Avenue NE
Washington, DC 20002
202-651-5000
800-451-1073
FAX: 202-651-5489

Here is a book of information about deaf people and sign communication. *$6.95*

104 pages Softcover

6259 EASE

Telecommunications for the Deaf (TDI)
8630 Fenton Street
Suite 604
Silver Spring, MD 20910
301-589-3786
FAX: 301-589-3797
e-mail: info@tdi-online.org
www.tdi-online.org

Claude L Stout, Executive Director
James D House, Member Service/Public Rel. Dir.

Training package for 911 professionals.

48 pages

6260 Effectiveness of Cochlear Implants and Tactile Aids for Deaf Children

Alexander Graham Bell Association
3417 Volta Place NW
Washington, DC 20007
202-337-5220
FAX: 202-337-8314
e-mail: info@agbell.org
www.agbell.org

This monograph presents a fascinating study to evaluate differences in the rate of change in speech perception, speech production and spoken language skills among children using the Nucleus 22-channel cochlear implant, tactile aids and conventional hearing aids. This monograph also offers teaching strategies in perception, lipreading and spoken language. *$13.95*

232 pages Paperback

6261 Encyclopedia of Deafness and Hearing Disorders

Gallaudet University Bookstore
800 Florida Avenue NE
Washington, DC 20002
202-651-5000
800-451-1073
FAX: 202-651-5489

Presents the most current information on deafness and hearing disorders in an authoritative A-to-Z compendium. *$45.00*

278 pages

6262 Expressive and Receptive Fingerspelling

Gallaudet University Bookstore
800 Florida Avenue NE
Washington, DC 20002
202-651-5000
800-451-1073
FAX: 202-651-5489

Here is a new and meaningful way for adults to increase their comfort with fingerspelling. The system is based on the principles of phonetics rather than letters of the English alphabet. *$2.50*

42 pages Softcover

6263 Flute Song Magic

TJ Publishers
817 Silver Spring Avenue
Suite 206
Silver Spring, MD 20910
301-585-4440
800-999-1168
FAX: 301-585-5930
e-mail: TJPubinc@aol.com

Angela K Thames, President
Jerald A Murphy, Executive Assistant

Gallaudet student Andrea Shettle created a memorable fantasy world, Nevlin, where it is forbidden to talk with people below one's class. An improbable friendship leads the High Noble Flutir to discover that friendship and individuality defy class limitations. *$ 2.95*

218 pages Softcover
ISBN 0-380762-25-0

6264 For Hearing People Only

Harris Communications
15155 Technology Drive
Eden Prairie, MN 55344
952-906-1180
800-825-6758
FAX: 952-906-1099
e-mail: mail@harriscomm.com
www.harriscomm.com

Bill Williams, National Sales Manager

A book that answers some of the questions hearing people ask about deaf culture. Also availible in hardcover. *$19.95*

336 pages Paperback
ISBN 0-963401-61-0

6265 From Gesture to Language in Hearing and Deaf Children

Gallaudet University Press
11030 S Langley Avenue
Chicago, IL 60628
800-621-2736
FAX: 800-621-8476
TTY:800-621-9347
gupress.gallaudet.edu

Virginia Volterra, Editor
Carol J Erting, Editor

In 21 essays on communicative gesturing in the first two years of life, this vital collection demonstrates the importance of gesture in a child's transition to a linguistic system. *$34.95*

358 pages Softcover

6266 GA and SK Etiquette

Gallaudet University Bookstore
800 Florida Avenue NE
Washington, DC 20002
202-651-5000
800-451-1073
FAX: 202-651-5489

This booklet presents guidelines for proper usage of the TDD. It includes everything you wanted to know about sending and receiving TDD calls. *$8.95*

53 pages

6267 GA-SK

Telecommunications for the Deaf
8630 Fenton Street
Suite 604
Silver Spring, MD 20910
301-589-3786
FAX: 301-589-3797
e-mail: info@tdi-online.org
www.tdi-online.org

Claude L Stout, Executive Director
James D House, Member Service/Public Rel. Dir.

Promoting equal access to telecommunications and media for people who are deaf, late-deafened, hard-of-hearing or deaf-blind through consumer education and involvement; technical assistance and consulting; applications of exisiting and emerging technologies; networking and collaboration; uniformity of standards; and national policy development and advocacy.

48 pages Quarterly

6268 Gallaudet Survival Guide to Signing

Harris Communications
15155 Technology Drive
Eden Prairie, MN 55344
952-906-1180
800-825-6758
FAX: 952-906-1099
e-mail: mail@harriscomm.com
www.harriscomm.com

Bill Williams, National Sales Manager

Features 500 of the most frequently used signs with clear illustrations and descriptions for each one. *$6.95*

203 pages Paperback
ISBN 0-930323-67-x

6269 Growing Together: Information for Parents of Deaf Children

Gallaudet University Bookstore
800 Florida Avenue NE
Washington, DC 20002
202-651-5000
800-451-1073
FAX: 202-651-5489

This publication answers questions often asked by parents of children with a hearing loss. *$8.00*

92 pages

6270 Handtalk Zoo

MacMillan Publishing Company
135 S Mount Zion Road
Lebanon, IN 46052
800-257-5755
FAX: 800-882-8583

Wonderful photographs are used to show children at the zoo communicating with sign language.

28 pages Hardcover
ISBN 0-02700 -01-0

6271 Hearing Aids

Federal Government
31 Center Drive MSC2320
Bethesda, MD 20892
800-241-1044
FAX: 301-402-0018
e-mail: nidcdinfo@nidcd.nih.gov
www.nidcd.nih.gov

Explains what is a hearing aid, how can hearing aids help, what to expect from hearing aids, what questions to ask before buying hearing aids, tips for taking care of hearing aids, and what research is being done on hearing aids.

6272 Hearing Impaired Employee

Allyn & Bacon
75 Arlington Street
Suite 300
Boston, MA 02116
617-848-6000
FAX: 617-848-7490
www.ablongman.com

An invaluable aid for both large and small firms for employment agencies and counselors and for all firms, schools and associations providing equipment or services for the hearing impaired.

1991
ISBN 0-887441-08-4

6273 Hearing Loss: The Journal of Self Help for Hard of Hearing People

Self Help for Hard of Hearing People
7910 Woodmont Avenue
Suite 1200
Bethesda, MD 20814
301-657-2248
FAX: 301-913-9413
TTY:301-657-2249
e-mail: national@shhh.org
www.shhh.org

Bonnie Sporren, Business Manager

SHHH, a non-profit, educational organization is dedicated to the well-being of people of all ages and communication styles who do not hear well. SHHH is the largest international consumer organization of its kind. SHHH offers a nationwide support network of chapters and groups, a bi-monthly magazine, discounted publications and resource materials for members, an annual convention, state and regional conferences and more. *$25.00*

40 pages BiMonthly

6274 Hearing, Speech & Deafness Center (HSDC)

1620 18th Avenue
Seattle, WA 98122
206-323-5770
FAX: 206-328-6871
e-mail: hsdc@hsdc.org
www.hsdc.org

Susie Burdick, Development/Marketing Director
David Stoner, Editor

Mission is to enrich the lives of all adults and children who experience hearing loss, speech and language impairments, or who are deaf, by providing professional services and technology, and by promoting community awareness and accessibility. A not-for-profit United Way Agency.

16 pages Yearly 1937

6275 Hearing-Impaired Children and Youth with Developmental Disabilities

Gallaudet University Bookstore
800 Florida Avenue NE
Washington, DC 20002
202-651-5000
800-451-1073
FAX: 202-651-5489

The insights of 24 experts help clarify relationships between hearing impairment and developmental difficulties and propose interdisciplinary cooperation as an approach to the problems created. *$29.95*

416 pages

6276 Hollywood Speaks

Gallaudet University Bookstore
800 Florida Avenue NE
Washington, DC 20002
202-651-5000
800-451-1073
FAX: 202-651-5489

How deafness has been treated in movies and how it provides yet another window onto social history in addition to a fresh angle from which to view Hollywood. *$24.95*

167 pages Hardcover

6277 How You Gonna Get to Heaven if You Can't Talk with Jesus?

TJ Publishers
817 Silver Spring Avenue
Suite 206
Silver Spring, MD 20910
301-585-4440
800-999-1168
FAX: 301-585-5930
e-mail: TJPubinc@aol.com

Angela K Thames, President
Jerald A Murphy, VP

This collection of articles examines deaf culture and its relationship, profiling sociolinguistic and anthropological perspectives in research on American deaf society and culture. *$4.50*

78 pages Softcover
ISBN 0-93266 -15-9

6278 I Have a Sister, My Sister is Deaf

TJ Publishers
817 Silver Spring Avenue
Suite 206
Silver Spring, MD 20910
301-585-4440
800-999-1168
FAX: 301-585-5930
e-mail: TJPubinc@aol.com

Angela K Thames, President
Jerald A Murphy, VP

An emphatic, affirmative look at the relationship between siblings, as a young deaf child is affectionately described by her older sister. This Coretta Scott King Honor Award winner helps young children develop an understanding that deaf children share the same interests as hearing children. *$5.95*

32 pages Softcover
ISBN 0-06443 -59-6

6279 I Was #87: A Deaf Woman's Ordeal of Misdiagnosis, Institutionalization and Abuse

Gallaudet University Press
11030 S Langley Avenue
Chicago, IL 60628
800-621-2736
FAX: 800-621-8476
TTY:800-621-9347
gupress.gallaudet.edu

Anne M Bolander, Co-Author
Adair N Renning, Co-Author

Misdiagnosed as mentally retarded, a deaf woman emerges from six torturous years at an institution for unwanted children and a lifetime of abuse and neglect to tell her remarkable, sobering story. *$24.95*

232 pages Hardcover

6280 In This Sign

Gallaudet University Bookstore
800 Florida Avenue NE
Washington, DC 20002
202-651-5000
800-451-1073
FAX: 202-651-5489

This modern classic follows a family of deaf parents and their hearing child through several decades of growth and pain, tragedy and triumph. *$10.95*

275 pages Softcover

6281 Innovative Practices for Teaching Sign Language Interpreters

Gallaudet University Press
11030 S Langley Avenue
Chicago, IL 60628
800-621-2736
FAX: 800-621-8476
TTY:800-621-9347
gupress.gallaudet.edu

Cynthia B Roy, Editor

Six experts draw upon the new understanding of sign language interpreting as a discourse between two languages and cultures. Develops bold, original techniques for training interpreters. *$34.95*

200 pages Hardcover

6282 Intermediate Conversational Sign Language

TJ Publishers
817 Silver Spring Avenue
Suite 206
Silver Spring, MD 20910
301-585-4440
800-999-1168
FAX: 301-585-5930
e-mail: TJPubinc@aol.com

Angela K Thames, President
Jerald A Murphy, VP

Unique approach to using American Sign Language and English in a bilingual setting. Each of the 25 lessons includes an introductory paragraph, glossed vocabulary review, translation exercises, grammatical notes, substitution drills and activities. *$21.95*

400 pages Softcover
ISBN 7-91358 -79-1

6283 International Directory of Periodicals Related to Deafness

Gallaudet University Bookstore
800 Florida Avenue NE
Washington, DC 20002 **202-651-5000**
800-451-1073
FAX: 202-651-5489

This one-of-a-kind directory has useful information on more than 500 magazines and journals related to deafness. The entries come from all over the world. *$10.00*

150 pages

6284 International Telephone Directory

Gallaudet University Bookstore
800 Florida Avenue NE
Washington, DC 20002 **202-651-5000**
800-451-1073
FAX: 202-651-5489

Almost 12,000 TDD numbers for Telecommunications for the Deaf, members and organizations serving deaf people. *$20.00*

190 pages Softcover

6285 Interpretation: A Sociolinguistic Model

Gallaudet University Bookstore
800 Florida Avenue NE
Washington, DC 20002 **202-651-5000**
800-451-1073
FAX: 202-651-5489

This text presents a sociolinguistically sensitive model of the interpretation process. The model applies to interpretation in any two languages although this one focuses on ASL and English. *$16.95*

199 pages

6286 Interpreting: An Introduction, Revised Edition

TJ Publishers
817 Silver Spring Avenue
Suite 206
Silver Spring, MD 20910 **301-585-4440**
800-999-1168
FAX: 301-585-5930
e-mail: TJPubinc@aol.com

Angela K Thames, President
Jerald A Murphy, VP

This text is written by a practicing interpreter and includes information on history, terminology, research, competence, setting and a comprehensive bibliography. *$22.50*

244 pages Softcover
ISBN 0-91688 -01-9

6287 Journal

Academy of Rehabilitative Audiology
PO Box 26532
Minneapolis, MN 55426 **952-920-0484**
FAX: 952-920-6098
e-mail: ara@incnet.com
www.audrehab.org

Jodell Newman Ryan PhD, President
Sheila Pratt PhD, President-Elect
Frances Laven MS, Executive Director

Yearly publication from the Academy of Rehabilitative Audiology.

Yearly

6288 Journal of Speech, Language and Hearing Re search

American Speech-Language-Hearing Association
10801 Rockville Pike
Rockville, MD 20852 **301-897-5700**
800-638-8255
FAX: 301-897-7348
e-mail: irc@asha.org
www.asha.org

John E Berntah;, President
Frederick T Spahr PhD, Executive Director
Joanne Jessen, Publications Director

Pertains broadly to studies of the processess and disorders of hearing, language, and speech diagnosis and treatment of such disorders.

6289 Journal of the American Deafness and Rehabilitation Association

JADARA
6212 Ferris Square
San Diego, CA 92121 **619-558-7444**

Articles of interest to professionals providing services to deaf people, with special emphasis on research-practice interactions and on mental health issues. *$46.00*

6290 Joy of Signing

Gallaudet University Bookstore
800 Florida Avenue NE
Washington, DC 20002 **202-651-5000**
800-451-1073
FAX: 202-651-5489

This manual on signing includes illustrations, information on sign origins, practice sentences, and step-by-step descriptions of hand positions and movements. *$16.95*

336 pages Hardcover

6291 Joy of Signing Puzzle Book

Harris Communications
15155 Technology Drive
Eden Prairie, MN 55344 **952-906-1180**
800-825-6758
FAX: 952-906-1099
e-mail: mail@harriscomm.com
www.harriscomm.com

Bill Williams, National Sales Manager

Whether you are learning sign language to communicate with a family member, co-worker, student or friend, this puzzle book makes the learning fun and interesting. *$3.95*

57 pages Paperback
ISBN 0-882435-38-8

6292 Keys to Raising a Deaf Child

Barron's Educational Series
250 Wireless Boulevard
Hauppauge, NY 11788 **631-434-3311**
800-645-3476
FAX: 631-434-3723
e-mail: info@barronseduc.com
www.barronseduc.com

Lonny Stein , Director Marketing

Two educators offer positive advice and encouragement on helping children adapt to deafness. They show how problems related to deafness can be overcome so that the child interacts as a social and intellectual equal with children who can hear. The authors recommend bimodal communication - having the child, parents and other non-deaf family members combine sign language and speech as a first step in normal communication. *$6.95*

208 pages Paperback
ISBN 0-764107-23-2

6293 **LSDC News**

DC Public Library, Services to the Deaf
901 G Street NW
Room 215
Washington, DC 20001 **202-727-2145**
FAX: 202-727-1129
e-mail: library_deaf_dc@yahoo.com
www.dclibrary.org

Janice Rosen, Librarian

Newsletter

5-6 pages Quarterly

6294 **Language, Speech and Hearing Services in School**

American Speech-Language-Hearing Association
10801 Rockville Pike
Rockville, MD 20852 **301-897-5700**
800-638-8255
FAX: 301-897-7348
e-mail: irc@asha.org
www.asha.org/asha

John E Bernthal, President
Frederick T Spahr PhD, Executive Director
Joanne Jessen, Publications Director

Professional journal for clinicians, audiologists and speech-language pathologists. *$30.00*

6295 **Legal Right: The Guide for Deaf and Hard of Hearing People**

Gallaudet University Press
11030 S Langley Avenue
Chicago, IL 60628
800-621-2736
FAX: 800-621-8476
TTY:800-621-9347
gupress.gallaudet.edu

This revised fifth edition is in easy-to-understand language, offering the latest state and federal statues and administrative procedures that prohibit discrimination against the deaf, hard of hearing and other physically challenged people. *$24.95*

264 pages Softcover

6296 **Life Without Pain**

Addison-Wesley Publishing Company
75 Arlington Street
Suite 300
Boston, MA 02116 **617-848-6000**
FAX: 617-848-6034
www.awprofessional.com

A self-help approach for eliminationg chronic pain, including back pain, using diet, nutrition, exercise, and mind/body techniques.

1987

6297 **Linguistics of ASL: An Introduction**

Gallaudet University Press
11030 S Langley Avenue
Chicago, IL 60628
800-621-2736
FAX: 800-621-8476
TTY:800-621-9347
gupress.gallaudet.edu

Clayton Valli, Co-Author
Ceil Lucas, Co-Author

An introduction to the struture of American Sign Language, featuring all the linguistic disciplines plus practice exercises. *$ 60.00*

460 pages Hardcover

6298 **Lisa and Her Soundless World**

Human Sciences Press
233 Spring Street
New York, NY 10013 **212-229-2859**
800-221-9369
FAX: 212-463-0742

Describes the impact deafness has on communication and functioning in a hearing world. Lisa, born with a severe hearing loss, was not diagnosed as hearing impaired until her parents were worried about her lack of speech and other children had rejected her. *$18.95*

30 pages Hardcover
ISBN 0-87705 -04-6

6299 **Listen to Me**

Alexander Graham Bell Association
3417 Volta Place NW
Washington, DC 20007 **202-337-5220**
FAX: 202-337-8314
e-mail: info@agbell.org
www.agbell.org

Entertaining wookbook contains exercises that help adults who are hard of hearing learn to listen and concentrate. *$9.95*

65 pages Paperback

6300 **Listening and Talking**

Alexander Graham Bell Association
3417 Volta Place NW
Washington, DC 20007 **202-337-5220**
FAX: 202-337-8314
e-mail: info@agbell.org
www.agbell.org

This research-based text for professionals promotes communication by developing language, audition and speech in early intervention programs for young children with hearing loss. *$25.95*

191 pages Paperback

6301 **Literature Journal**

Gallaudet University Bookstore
800 Florida Avenue NE
Washington, DC 20002 **202-651-5000**
800-451-1073
FAX: 202-651-5489

This book includes extensive examples of student and teacher entries taken from actual journals of deaf high school students. *$7.95*

44 pages

6302 **Loss for Words**

Gallaudet University Bookstore
11030 S Langley Avenue
Chicago, IL 60628 **202-651-5488**
800-621-2736
FAX: 202-651-5489

She was an interpreter for her parents at four, a virtual head of household at eight, teacher and helper for her little sisters, buffer between her family and the world. Here is a daughter's account of growing up with loving parents, both of whom are deaf. *$11.00*

208 pages Paperback

6303 **Mask of Benevolence: Disabling the Deaf Community**

Gallaudet University Bookstore
800 Florida Avenue NE
Washington, DC 20002
202-651-5000
800-451-1073
FAX: 202-651-5489

Dr. Harlan Lane does not view deafness as a handicap but rather a different state from hearing. Deaf people are a societal minority and should be treasured, not eradicated. *$23.00*

310 pages

6304 **Matthew Pinkowski's Special Summer**

TJ Publishers
817 Silver Spring Avenue
Suite 206
Silver Spring, MD 20910
301-585-4440
800-999-1168
FAX: 301-585-5930
e-mail: TJPubinc@aol.com

Angela K Thames, President
Jerald A Murphy, Executive Assistant

Matthew Pinkowski meets an unlikely crew of friends - Sandy, the acrobat; Tommy, her brother who moves and learns slowly; and Laura, a deaf girl visiting an overprotective aunt and uncle. In solving a mystery together, the friends learn to expect the best of people. It is a funny, genuine story about a memorable summer. *$5.95*

150 pages Softcover
ISBN 0-930323-82-3

6305 **My First Book of Sign**

TJ Publishers
817 Silver Spring Avenue
Suite 206
Silver Spring, MD 20910
301-585-4440
800-999-1168
FAX: 301-585-5930
e-mail: TJPubinc@aol.com

Angela K Thames, President
Jerald A Murphy, VP

Full-color book gives alphabetically grouped signs for 150 words most frequently used by young children. *$14.95*

76 pages Hardcover
ISBN 0-93032 -20-3

6306 **Newsletter of American Hearing Research Foundation**

American Hearing Research Foundation
8 S Michigan Avenue
Suite 814
Chicago, IL 60603
312-726-9670
FAX: 312-726-9695
e-mail: blederer@american-hearing.org
www.american-hearing.org

William Lederer, Executive Director
Lorraine L Koch, Assistant Director

Concerned with hearing research and education. Only if one can afford to pay, a suggested appropriate donation of $15 for cover postage and printing.

6-8 pages TriAnnual

6307 **Outsiders in a Hearing World**

Gallaudet University Bookstore
800 Florida Avenue NE
Washington, DC 20002
202-651-5000
800-451-1073
FAX: 202-651-5489

An introduction to the social world of deaf people. The author gives a sociologists view of what it's like to be deaf. *$19.95*

240 pages Softcover

6308 **Paws for Silence**

International Hearing Dog
5901 E 89th Avenue
Henderson, CO 80640
303-287-3277
FAX: 303-287-3425
e-mail: ihdi@aol.com
www.ihdi.org

Valerie Foss-Brugger, President/Director

Publication from International hearing dog.

4-8 pages Quarterly

6309 **Perigee Visual Dictionary of Signing**

Harris Communications
15155 Technology Drive
Eden Prairie, MN 55344
952-906-1180
800-825-6758
FAX: 952-906-1099
e-mail: mail@harriscomm.com
www.harriscomm.com

Bill Williams, National Sales Manager

An A-to-Z guide to American Sign Language vocabulary. *$15.95*

450 pages Paperback
ISBN 0-399519-52-1

6310 **Perspective: Parent-Child Folio**

Gallaudet University Bookstore
800 Florida Avenue NE
Washington, DC 20002
202-651-5000
800-451-1073
FAX: 202-651-5489

Ranging from table conversation to bedtime reading, the seven articles collected here emphasize family communications while providing important information for parents about deafness and deaf culture. *$5.95*

29 pages

6311 **Perspectives: Whole Language Folio**

Gallaudet University Bookstore
800 Florida Avenue NE
Washington, DC 20002
202-651-5000
800-451-1073
FAX: 202-651-5489

The 19 articles in this collection offer practical help to teachers seeking to emphasize whole language strategies in their classroom. *$9.95*

64 pages

6312 **Phone of Our Own: The Deaf Insurrection Against Ma Bell**

Gallaudet University Press
11030 S Langley Avenue
Chicago, IL 60628
202-651-5488
800-621-2736
FAX: 202-651-5489
TTY:800-621-9347
gupress.gallaudet.edu

A recount of the history of the teletypewriter, from the three deaf engineers who developed the acoustic coupler that made mass communication on TTY's feasible, through the deaf community's twenty-year struggle against the government and AT&T to have TTY's produced and distributed. *$29.95*

304 pages Hardcover

6313 **Place of Their Own: Creating the Deaf Community in America**

TJ Publishers
817 Silver Spring Avenue
Suite 206
Silver Spring, MD 20910
301-585-4440
800-999-1168
FAX: 301-585-5930
e-mail: TJPubinc@aol.com

Angela K Thames, President
Jerald A Murphy, VP

Traces development of American deaf society to show how deaf people developed a common language and sense of community. Views deafness as the distinguishing characteristic of a distinct culture. *$16.95*

212 pages Paperback
ISBN 0-930324-91-

6314 **PreReading Strategies**

Gallaudet University Bookstore
800 Florida Avenue NE
Washington, DC 20002
202-651-5000
800-451-1073
FAX: 202-651-5489

Here is a wealth of good advice for preparing students to understand what they read, building comprehension and enjoyment. *$8.95*

65 pages

6315 **Psychology of Deafness**

Longman Publishing Group
10 Bank Street
9th Floor
White Plains, NY 10606
914-993-5000
FAX: 914-421-5598

Roth Wilkofsky, Systems Contact

Portrays hearing impairments as a psychological variable causing life experiences of the deaf to consistently differ from those of the non-deaf. Covers all levels of hearing loss, from prelingual and profound deafness to partial and mild hearing loss. Demonstrates how and why a hearing loss creates psychological stress no matter what its degree.

292 pages Hardcover
ISBN 0-801303-22-2

6316 **Registry of Interpreters for the Deaf**

8630 Fenton Street
Suite 324
Silver Spring, MD 20910
301-608-0050
FAX: 301-608-0508
e-mail: pr@rid.org
www.rid.org

Membership association for sign language interpreters; promoting national certification, professional development and training, and quality assurance through ethical practices system.

Monthly

6317 **Religious Signing: A Comprehensive Guide for All Faiths**

TJ Publishers
817 Silver Spring Avenue
Suite 206
Silver Spring, MD 20910
301-585-4440
800-999-1168
FAX: 301-585-5930
e-mail: TJPubinc@aol.com
www.agbell.org

Angela K Thames, President
Jerald A Murphy, VP

Contains over 500 religious signs for all denominations and their meanings illustrated by clear upper torso illustrations that show movements of hand, body and face. Includes a section on signing favorite verses, prayers and blessings. *$17.95*

219 pages Paperback
ISBN 0-553344-44-

6318 **Seeing Voices: A Journey into the World of the Deaf**

TJ Publishers
817 Silver Spring Avenue
Suite 206
Silver Spring, MD 20910
301-585-4440
800-999-1168
FAX: 301-585-5930
e-mail: TJPubinc@aol.com

Angela K Thames, President
Jerald A Murphy, VP

Well known for his exploration of how people respond to neurological impairments, Dr Sacks explores the world of the deaf and discovers how deaf people respond to their loss of hearing and how they develop language. A highly readable introduction to deaf people, deaf culture and American Sign Language. *$11.00*

186 pages Softcover
ISBN 0-06097 -47-1

6319 **Sign Language Coloring Books**

Gallaudet University Bookstore
800 Florida Avenue NE
Washington, DC 20002
202-651-5000
800-451-1073
FAX: 202-651-5489

A mischievous mouse and a spinning top, a doll on the sofa, a hobo clown with this friend the elephant: these coloring books are a FUNtastic way for children to learn to sign, fingerspell, read and write. *$4.50*

6320 **Sign Language Feelings**

Gallaudet University Bookstore
800 Florida Avenue NE
Washington, DC 20002
202-651-5000
800-451-1073
FAX: 202-651-5489

Worksheets teach signs for happy, sad and all of the feelings in between. *$4.50*

6321 **Sign Language Interpreters and Interpreting**

Gallaudet University Bookstore
800 Florida Avenue NE
Washington, DC 20002
202-651-5000
800-451-1073
FAX: 202-651-5489

This monograph presents articles about personal characteristics and abilities of interpreters, the effects of lag time on interpreter errors, and the interpretation of register. *$15.95*

161 pages

6322 **Sign with Me Books**

Gallaudet University Bookstore
11030 S Langley Avenue
Chicago, IL 60628
202-651-5488
800-621-2736
FAX: 202-651-5489

Bold, colorful pictures and accurate diagrams make it fun for beginners to learn everyday signs. Titles in this series include ABC Sign With Me; Colors Sign With Me; Weather Sign With Me; and 1,2,3 Sign With Me. *$3.95*

Per Title

6323 **Signed English Starter**

Harris Communications
15155 Technology Drive
Eden Prairie, MN 55344
952-906-1180
800-825-6758
FAX: 952-906-1099
e-mail: mail@harriscomm.com
www.harriscomm.com

Bill Williams, National Sales Manager

The first book to use when learning Signed English. *$13.95*

208 pages Paperback
ISBN 0-913580-82-1

6324 **Signing for Reading Success**

Gallaudet University Bookstore
800 Florida Avenue NE
Washington, DC 20002
202-651-5000
800-451-1073
FAX: 202-651-5489

This booklet provides summaries of four research students on the usefulness of signing for reading achievement. *$3.95*

24 pages Softcover

6325 **Signing: How to Speak with Your Hands**

TJ Publishers
817 Silver Spring Avenue
Suite 206
Silver Spring, MD 20910
301-585-4440
800-999-1168
FAX: 301-585-5930
e-mail: TJPubinc@aol.com

Angela K Thames, President
Jerald A Murphy, VP

Presents 1,200 basic signs with clear illustrations in logical topical groupings. Linguistic principles are described at the beginning of each chapter, giving insight into the rules which govern American Sign Language. *$17.95*

248 pages Paperback
ISBN 0-553375-39-3

6326 **Signs Across America**

TJ Publishers
817 Silver Spring Avenue
Suite 206
Silver Spring, MD 20910
301-585-4440
800-999-1168
FAX: 301-585-5930
e-mail: TJPubinc@aol.com

Angela K Thames, President
Jerald A Murphy, VP

A look at regional variations in ASL. Signs for selected words collected from 25 different states. More than 1,200 signs illustrated in the text. *$19.95*

285 pages Paperback
ISBN 0-913589-61-

6327 **Signs Everywhere**

Harris Communications
15155 Technology Drive
Eden Prairie, MN 55344
952-906-1180
800-825-6758
FAX: 952-906-1099
e-mail: mail@harriscomm.com
www.harriscomm.com

Bill Williams, National Sales Manager

This books includes signs for towns, cities, states and provinces. *$14.95*

254 pages Paperback
ISBN 0-916708-05-5

6328 **Signs for Computing Terminology**

Gallaudet University Bookstore
11030 S Langley Avenue
Chicago, IL 60628
202-651-5488
800-621-2736
FAX: 202-651-5489

This sign reference will facilitate communication among deaf persons involved with computers by providing a significant vocabulary base for the computing field of today and tomorrow. *$12.95*

182 pages Softcover

6329 **Signs for Me: Basic Sign Vocabulary for Children, Parents & Teachers**

TJ Publishers
817 Silver Spring Avenue
Suite 206
Silver Spring, MD 20910
301-585-4440
800-999-1168
FAX: 301-585-5930
e-mail: TJPubinc@aol.com

Angela K Thames, President
Jerald A Murphy, VP

Sign language vocabulary for preschool and elementary school children introduces household items, animals, family members, actions, emotions, safety concerns and other concepts. *$12.95*

112 pages Softcover
ISBN 0-91503 -27-8

6330 **Signs for Sexuality: A Resource Manual**

Gallaudet University Bookstore
800 Florida Avenue NE
Washington, DC 20002
202-651-5000
800-451-1073
FAX: 202-651-5489

An important book for those who want to listen to and talk with other people about feelings, loving and caring. *$24.95*

122 pages Softcover

6331 **Signs of the Times**

Gallaudet University Press
11030 S Langley Avenue
Chicago, IL 60628
800-621-2736
FAX: 800-621-8476
TTY:800-621-9347
gupress.gallaudet.edu

An excellent beginner's contact signing book that fills the gap between sign language dictionaries and American Sign Language text. Designed for use as a classroom text. *$24.95*

448 pages Softcover

6332 **Simultaneous Communication, ASL, and Other Communication Modes**

Gallaudet University Bookstore
800 Florida Avenue NE
Washington, DC 20002
202-651-5000
800-451-1073
FAX: 202-651-5489

This monograph presents four major articles that examine issues surrounding communications in an educational environment. *$ 15.95*

236 pages

6333 **Sing Praise Hymnal**

Broadman and Holman
127 9th Avenue S
Nashville, TN 37203
615-251-2000
800-458-2772
FAX: 651-251-5764
www.bssb.com/lwc

A song book for the deaf. *$6.95*

6334 **Spring Dell Center**

6040 Radio Station Road
La Plata, MD 20646
301-934-4561
FAX: 301-870-2439

Melissa Tyner, Transportation Director

Since 1967, Spring Dell center has been, bridging the gap to enhance the lives of developmentally disabled people. Spring Dell's goal is to empower people in every aspect of their lives through the implementation of two programs, employment/vocational services and residential services including transportation. Spring Dell offers transportation door-to-door for persons with developmental disabilities, including day care programs, supportive environment, residential and any other transportation

6335 **Store @ HDSC Product Catalog**

Hearing, Speech & Deafness Center (HDSC)
1625 19th Avenue
Seattle, WA 98122
206-323-5770
FAX: 206-328-6871
e-mail: hsdc@hsdc.org
www.hsdc.org

32 pages Yearly

6336 **TDI National Directory & Resource Guide: Blue Book**

Telecommunications for the Deaf
8630 Fenton Street
Suite 604
Silver Spring, MD 20910
301-589-3786
FAX: 301-589-3797
e-mail: info@tdi-online.org
www.tdi-online.org

Claude L Stout, Executive Director
James D House, Member Service/Public Rel. Dir.

$27.00

639 pages Annual

6337 **Teaching Social Skills to Hearing-Impaired Students**

Alexander Graham Bell Association
3417 Volta Place NW
Washington, DC 20007
202-337-5220
FAX: 202-337-8314
e-mail: info@agbell.org
www.agbell.org

This book provides teachers and parents with a comprehensive, clearly presented hands-on program to develop social skills in children and young adults who are deaf or hard of hearing. *$21.95*

203 pages

6338 **Telephone Communication and Hearing Impaired**

Taylor & Francis
47 Runway Drive
Suite G
Levittown, PA 19057
215-625-8900
FAX: 215-625-2940

This is a practical book containing valuable information for audiologists, teachers and others concerned with rehabilitation of the hearing impaired.

200 pages Illustrated
ISBN 0-85066 -18-3

6339 **Theoretical Issues in Sign Language Research**

Gallaudet University Bookstore
11030 S Langley Avenue
Chicago, IL 60628
202-651-5488
800-621-2736
FAX: 202-651-5489

These volumes are an outgrowth of a conference held at the University of Rochester in 1986, dealing with the four traditional core areas of phonology, morphology, syntax and semantics. *$29.95*

338 pages

6340 **They Grow in Silence**

Taylor & Francis
47 Runway Drive
 # G
Levittown, PA 19057
FAX: 215-785-5515

Gives a comprehensive picture of the deaf child in society, not only looking at the individual but also, at the related problems for the family, community and the professional. Only by the examination of such a broad perspective can questions on the position and circumstances of the deaf child be fully considered.

223 pages Paper
ISBN 0-85066 -54-6

6341 **Tinnitus Today**

American Tinnitus Association
PO Box 5
Portland, OR 97207
503-248-9985
800-634-8978
FAX: 503-248-0024
e-mail: tinnitus@ata.org
www.ata.org

Cherly McGinnis MBA, Executive Director
Barbara Sanders, Editor

Published quarterly by the American Tinnitus Association. Also available online. Online ISSN# is 1530-6569. *$25.00*

28 pages Quarterly

6342 **US Government TTY Directory**

Consumer Information Center
Department 627F
Pueblo, CO 81009

e-mail: catalog.pueblo@gsa.gov

Judi Mahoney, Public Affairs

Gives details on how to use the Federal Relay Service and which agencies and congressional offices have text telephone devices.

6343 **Understanding Deafness Socially**

Charles C Thomas
2600 S First Street
Springfield, IL 62704
217-789-8980
800-258-8980
FAX: 217-789-9130
e-mail: books@ccthomas.com
www.ccthomas.com

A look at the social difficulties of being hearing impaired in a hearing society. Also available in cloth. *$29.95*

168 pages Softcover
ISBN 0-398065-70-5

6344 **Upstate Update**

New York State Talking Book & Braille Library
Empire State Plaza CEC
Albany, NY 12230
518-474-5935
FAX: 518-474-5786
TTY:518-474-7121
e-mail: tbbl@mail.nysed.gov
www.suffolk.lib.ny.us

Jane Somers, Director
Peter Douglas, Editor

Books on audio cassette, cassette players, braille books, summer reading programs, braille writer, magnifiers, closed-circuit T.V., large-print photocopier, cassette books and magazines, children's books on cassette, reference materials on blindness and other handicaps.

4 pages Quarterly

6345 **Very Special Friend**

TJ Publishers
817 Silver Spring Avenue
Suite 206
Silver Spring, MD 20910
301-585-4440
800-999-1168
FAX: 301-585-5930
e-mail: TJPubinc@aol.com

Angela K Thames, President
Jerald A Murphy, VP

Six year old Frannie finds a very special friend who talks in sign language. She learns to sign and the two become best friends. *$9.95*

32 pages Hardcover
ISBN 0-93032 -55-6

6346 **Vision**

National Catholic Office of the Deaf
7202 Buchanan Street
Landover Hills, MD 20784
301-577-1684
FAX: 301-577-1690
e-mail: ncod@erols.com

Arvilla Rank, Executive Director/Editor

Published as a pastoral service for the deaf and hard of hearing. Provides information to members and others working in ministry. Prepares an annual gathering called Pastoral Week meeting in January. Price: $15.00 per year, $25 for 2 years; Foreign: $17 per year; $27 for 2 years.

16 pages TriAnnual

6347 **Volta Review**

Alexander Graham Bell Association
3417 Volta Place NW
Washington, DC 20007
202-337-5220
FAX: 202-337-8314
e-mail: info@agbell.org
www.agbell.org

Professionally refereed journal that publishes articles and research on education, rehabilitation and communicative development of people who have hearing impairments. Also includes subscription to Valta Voices, up-to-date magazine, bimonthly. *$62.00*

Quarterly

6348 **Volta Voices**

Alexander Graham Bell Association
3417 Volta Place NW
Washington, DC 20007
202-337-5220
FAX: 202-337-8314
e-mail: info@agbell.org
www.agbell.org

Contains Association news and educates readers on the abilities and needs of children and adults who are deaf or hard of hearing. Includes subscription to The Valta Review, published four times a year. *$62.00*

6349 **We CAN Hear and Speak**

Alexander Graham Bell Association
3417 Volta Place NW
Washington, DC 20007
202-337-5220
FAX: 202-337-8314
e-mail: info@agbell.org
www.agbell.org

Written by parents for families of children who are deaf or hard of hearing, this work describes auditory-verbal terminology and approaches and contains personal narratives written by parents and their children who are deaf or hard of hearing. *$24.95*

171 pages Paperback

6350 **Week the World Heard Gallaudet**

Gallaudet University Press
800 Florida Avenue NE
Washington, DC 20002
202-651-5488
800-451-1073
FAX: 202-651-5489
e-mail: gupress@gallaudet.edu
gupress.gallaudet.edu/homeSLSorder.html

This day-to-day description of the events surrounding the Deaf President Now movement at Gallaudet University includes full color and black and white photographs and interviews with people involved in the events of that week.

192 pages

6351 **Wheelers Accessible Van Rentals**

6614 W Sweetwater Avenue
Glendale, AZ 85304
623-776-8830
800-456-1371
FAX: 623-412-9920
e-mail: info@wheelersvanrentals.com
www.wheelersvanrentals.com

Tammy Smith, Manager

Daily, weekly and monthly rentals. Locations throughout the US.

6352 **When the Mind Hears**

Gallaudet University Bookstore
800 Florida Avenue NE
Washington, DC 20002 **202-651-5000**
800-451-1073
FAX: 202-651-5489

Comprehensive history of the deaf and their relationship with hearing academic communities. *$19.95*

414 pages Paperback

6353 **You and Your Hearing Impaired Child: A Self-Instructional Parents Guide**

TJ Publishers
817 Silver Spring Avenue
Suite 206
Silver Spring, MD 20910 **301-585-4440**
800-999-1168
FAX: 301-585-5930
e-mail: TJPubinc@aol.com

Angela K Thames, President
Jerald A Murphy, VP

Designed specifically for parents who have children newly diagnosed as hearing impaired. Provides vital information on hearing impairment, setting limits, behavior management, nonverbal behavior and much more. *$17.95*

142 pages Softcover
ISBN 0-93032 -40-8

Music

6354 **Braille Book Bank, Music Catalog**

National Braille Association
3 Townline Circle
Rochester, NY 14623 **585-427-8260**
e-mail: nbaoffice@compuserve.com
www.nationalbraille.org

Offers hundreds of musical titles in print form, braille and on cassette.

62 pages

6355 **Clinically Adapted Instruments for the Multiply Handicapped**

MMB Music
3526 Washington Avenue
Saint Louis, MO 63103 **314-531-9635**
800-543-3771
FAX: 314-531-8384
e-mail: info@mmbmusic.com
www.mmbmusic.com

A very unique book containing one hundred adapted and original instrument designs, descriptions and results of extensive practical applications. *$14.50*

192 pages Paperback 1980
ISBN 0-918812-13-5

6356 **Creative Arts Resources Catalog**

MMB Music
3526 Washington Avenue
Contemporary Arts Building
Saint Louis, MO 63103 **314-531-9635**
800-343-3771
FAX: 314-531-8384
e-mail: mlg@mmbmusic.com
www.mmbmusic.com

Marcie Lee Goldberg, VP Sales/Marketing

Publisher and distributor of creative arts therapy materials in the areas of music, dance, art, drama, and poetry. Free catalog contains hundreds of books, recordings, and videos.

6357 **Guide to the Selection of Musical Instruments**

MMB Music
3526 Washington Avenue
Saint Louis, MO 63103 **314-531-9635**
800-543-3771
FAX: 314-531-8384
e-mail: info@mmbmusic.com

A marvelous resource book to aid therapists teaching disabled to play musical instruments. *$7.75*

6358 **Mainstreaming Exceptional Learners in Music**

Pearson Education
One Lake Street
Upper Saddle River, NJ 07458 **201-236-7000**
FAX: 201-236-6549
www.pearsoneducation.com

This complete introduction provides present and future music educators and therapists with the information necessary to understand the individual differences of the variety of students designated exceptional.

224 pages 1990
ISBN 0-135453-51-8

6359 **Music Therapy for the Developmentally Disabled**

Pro-Ed Publications
8700 Shoal Creek Boulevard
Austin, TX 78757 **512-451-3246**
800-897-3202
FAX: 512-451-8542
e-mail: info@proedinc.com
www.proedinc.com

Included are practical guidelines, case samples and step-by-step instructions that enable a music therapist to bring about dramatic improvements in developmentally disabled adults and children. *$40.00*

269 pages Hardcover
ISBN 0-890791-90-2

6360 **Music for the Hearing Impaired**

MMB Music
3526 Washington Avenue
Saint Louis, MO 63103 **314-531-9635**
800-543-3771
FAX: 314-531-8384
e-mail: info@mmbmusic.com

A resource manual and curriculum guide. It is the product of a four-year developmental music program, placing emphasis on the needs of those with severe and profound losses. *$29.95*

6361 **Music: Physician for Times to Come**

Quest Books
1926 N Main Street
PO Box 270
Wheaton, IL 60189 **630-668-1571**
FAX: 630-668-4976

A resource guide for various types of music and their theraputic oputcome.

365 pages 1900
ISBN 0-835607-88-7

6362 Teaching Basic Guitar Skills to Special Learners

MMB Music
3526 Washington Avenue
Saint Louis, MO 63103
314-531-9635
800-543-3771
FAX: 314-531-8384
e-mail: info@mmbmusic.com

The first-of-its-kind guitar book for use with persons who have difficulty learning to play via traditional methods. *$16.00*

Parenting: General

6363 AEPS Family Report: For Children Ages Three to Six

Brookes Publishing
PO Box 10624
Baltimore, MD 21285
410-337-9580
800-638-3775
FAX: 410-337-8539
e-mail: custserv@brookespublishing.com
www.brookespublishing.com

This is a 64-item questionnaire that asks parents to rank their child's abilities on specific skills. In packages of 10 paperback. *$23.00*

28 pages Saddle-stiched
ISBN 1-557662-50-9

6364 AT for Parents with Disabilities

Idaho Assistive Technology Project
129 W 3rd Street
Moscow, ID 83843
208-885-3559
800-432-8324
FAX: 208-885-3628
e-mail: rseiler@uidaho.edu
www.educ.uidaho.edu/idatech

$5.00

80 pages

6365 Alternative Approach to Allergies

Harper Perennial
10 E 53rd Street
New York, NY 10022
212-207-7000
FAX: 212-207-7145
www.harpercollins.com

A comprehensive guide to staying well and allergy-free by a pioneer in the field of environmental medicine.

6366 Awareness Through Movement

Harper Perennial
10 E 53rd Street
New York, NY 10022
212-207-7000
FAX: 212-207-7145
www.harpercollins.com

A genuine self-help guide to improved posture, flexibility, breathing, health, and functioning through twelve easy-to-follow Awareness through Movement lessons.

1977

6367 Baby Book for the Developmentally Challenged Child

Exceptional Parent Library
120 Sylvan Avenue, Suite 10
PO Box 1807
Englewood Cliffs, NJ 07632
800-535-1910
FAX: 201-947-9376
e-mail: eplibrary@aol.com
www.eplibrary.com

This baby book is for parents to write milestones for their developmentally challenged child. It incorporates the usual baby book features with very special sections covering any special needs child. *$25.00*

48 pages Hardcover

6368 Back Care Basics: A Doctor's Gentle Yoga Program for Back and Neck Pain Relief

Rodmell Press
2147 Blake Street
Berkley, CA 94704
510-841-3123

Offers a gentle and effective approach to back rehabilitation without drugs or surgery. Uses the therapeutic techniques of Iyengar-style yoga.

1992

6369 Backyards and Butterflies

Brookline Books
PO Box 1047
Cambridge, MA 02238
617-868-0360
800-666-2665
FAX: 617-868-1772
e-mail: brooklinebks@delphi.com
www.brooklinebooks.com

Backyards And Butterflies: Ways to Include Children with Disabilities In Out Door Activites is a wonderful illustrated book with dozens of imaginative ways parents can include children with physical disabilities in outdoor activities. Offers clear concise, how-to directions for constructing homemaode toys, utensils, and other items that can be enjoyed outside safely and comfortably *$14.95*

72 pages Paperback
ISBN 1-57129 -11-7

6370 Behavior Problems

Research Press
PO Box 9177
Champaign, IL 61826
217-352-3273
800-519-2707
FAX: 217-352-1221
e-mail: rp@researchpress.com
www.researchpress.com

Russell Pence, VP Marketing

A practical book that provides effective techniques for solving behavior problems that are characteristic of children with developmental disabilities. Numerous charts and examples accompanied by helpful illustrations make this book an invaluable resource for parents, special education teachers and residential staff. *$12.95*

80 pages Paperback
ISBN 0-878221-70-0

6371 Books on Special Children

BOSC
PO Box 305
Congers, NY 10920
845-638-1236
FAX: 845-638-0847
e-mail: irene@boscbooks.com
www.boscbooks.com

Irene Slovak, Owner

Distributes books by mail to professionals and parents of handicapped children. The BOSC Directory contains facilities for people with learning disabilities (all disabilities, published annually)

300+ pages Hardcover

ISBN O-G61386-08-8

6372 Brain Allergies: The Psychonutrient

Keats Publishing
27 Pine Street
PO Box 876
New Canaan, CT 06840 **203-966-8721**
800-323-4900

A comprehensive look at the role nutrition and orthomolecular medicine can play in treating brain allergies, including a self-help protocol and a special appendix for physicians.

6373 Brothers, Sisters, and Special Needs

Brookes Publishing
PO Box 10624
Baltimore, MD 21285 **410-337-9580**
800-638-3775
FAX: 410-337-8539
e-mail: custserv@brookespublishing.com
www.brookespublishing.com

Information and activities for helping young siblings of children with chronic illnesses and developmental disabilities. *$30.00*

224 pages Paperback

ISBN 1-55766 -43-3

6374 Building the Healing Partnership: Parents, Professionals and Children

Brookline Books
PO Box 1046
Cambridge, MA 02238 **617-868-0360**
800-666-2665
FAX: 617-868-1772
e-mail: brooklinebks@delphi.com
www.brooklinebooks.com

Successful programs understand that the disabled child's needs must be considered in the context of a family. This book was specifically written for practitioner's who must work with families but who have insufficient training in family systems assessment and intervention. It is a valuable blend of theory and practice with pointers for applying the principles. *$24.95*

Paperback

ISBN 0-91479 -63-8

6375 Children with Disabilitie

Brookes Publishing
PO Box 10624
Baltimore, MD 21285 **410-337-9580**
800-638-3775
FAX: 410-337-8539
e-mail: custserv@brookespublishing.com
www.brookespublishing.com

Mark L Batshaw MD, Editor

Extensive coverage of genetics, heredity, pre- and postnatal development, specific disabilities, family roles, and intervention. Features chapters on substance abuse, HIV and AIDS, Down syndrome, fragile X syndrome, behavior management, transitions to adulthood, and health care in the 21st century. Also reveals the causes of many conditions that can lead to developmental disabilities. *$69.95*

912 pages Hardcover

ISBN 1-557665-81-8

6376 Children with Facial Difference

Woodbine House
6510 Bells Mill Road
Bethesda, MD 20817 **301-897-3570**
800-843-7323
FAX: 301-897-5838
www.woodbinehouse.com

The first guide for parents about their child's congenital craniofacial anomaly - a condition that affects the appearance and function of the head and face. This accessible book discusses conditions such as cleft lip, cleft palate, and Teacher Collins, Apert, and Crouzon syndromes, and more. Parents learn about the diagnostic process, interdisciplinary treatment approach, education, speech and language issues, and how to help their child and family adjust emotionally. *$ 16.95*

361 pages Paperback 1996

ISBN 0-933149-61-1

6377 Children with Mental Retardation

Woodbine House
6510 Bells Mill Road
Bethesda, MD 20817 **301-897-3570**
800-843-7323
FAX: 301-897-5838
www.woodbinehouse.com

A book for parents of children with mild to moderate mental retardation, whether or not they have a diagnosed syndrome or condition. It provides a complete and compassionate introduction to their child's medical, therapeutic, and educational needs, and discusses the emotional impact on the family. New parents can rely on Children with Mental Retardation to provide that solid foundation and confidence they need to help their child reach his or her highest potential. *$14.95*

437 pages Paperback

ISBN 0-933149-39-5

6378 Conditional Love: Parents' Attitudes Toward Handicapped Children

Greenwood Publishing Group
88 Post Road W
Suite 5007
Westport, CT 06880 **203-226-3571**
FAX: 203-222-1502
www.greenwood.com

Offers parents information on understanding disabled children and mainstreaming them into their normal family life. *$49.95*

312 pages

ISBN 0-89789 -24-7

6379 Coordinacion De Servicios Centrado En La Familia

Brookline Books
PO Box 1047
Cambridge, MA 02238 **617-868-0360**
800-666-2665
FAX: 617-868-1772
e-mail: brooklinebks@delphi.com
www.brooklinebooks.com

This book, translated into Spanish from the English original, is designed to orient and educate parents about issues of service coordination, to assist families in caring for an infant or toddler with developmental delays or disabilities. *$7.00*

34 pages Paperback

ISBN 0-91479 -90-5

6380 Creative Play Activities for Children with Disabilities

Human Kinetics
PO Box 5076
Champaign, IL 61825
800-747-4457
FAX: 217-351-2674
e-mail: orders@hkusa.com
www.humankinetics.com

Contains 250 games and activities designed to help children with all types of disabilities grow through play. Each chapter focuses on a particular world or activity theme. Themes include exploring the world of the senses, active games, building and creating, imaginative outdoor fun and water play, and group games and activities. *$16.95*

232 pages
ISBN 0-873229-33-9

6381 Delicate Threads

Woodbine House
6510 Bells Mill Road
Bethesda, MD 20817
301-897-3570
800-843-7323
FAX: 301-897-5838
www.woodbinehouse.com

How do friendships between children with and without disabilities develop? How do they compare to friendships between typically developing children? What happens to these friendships over time? In Delicate Threads, author Debbie staub helps to answer these questions through careful observations of friendships between seven pairs of children - each including a child with a moderate to severe disability - who are classmates in an inclusive Pacific Northwest elementary school. *$16.95*

250 pages Paperback
ISBN 0-933149-90-5

6382 Detecting Your Hidden Allergies

Professional Books/Future Health
211 N Sycamore
Newtown, PA 18940
215-504-1700
FAX: 215-860-5374

Gives specific instructions on how to use an elimination diet to determine food allergies.

6383 Developing Personal Safety Skills in Children with Disabilities

Brookes Publishing
PO Box 10624
Baltimore, MD 21285
410-337-9580
800-638-3775
FAX: 410-337-8539
e-mail: custserv@brookespublishing.com
www.brookespublishing.com

A guide for teachers, parents, and caregivers, this volume explores the issue of personal safety for children with disabilities and offers strategies for empowering and protecting them at home and in school. Recognizing that children with disabilities are vulnerable to abuse, this work explores why children with disabilities need personal safety skills, offers, curriculum ideas and exercises, and advocates the development of self-esteem and assertiveness so that children can protect themselves. *$34.00*

220 pages Paperback
ISBN 1-557661-84-7

6384 Developmental Disabilities in Infancy and Childhood, 2nd Edition

Brookes Publishing
PO Box 10624
Baltimore, MD 21285
410-337-9580
800-638-3775
FAX: 410-337-8539
e-mail: custserv@brookespublishing.com
www.brookespublishing.com

This two volume set explores advances in assessment and treatment, retains a clinical focus, and incorporates recent developments in research and theory. Can be purchased individually or as a set (Vol. 1: Neurodevelopmental Diagnosis and Treatment Vol. 2: The Spectrum of Developmental Disabilities). *$210.00*

Hardcover
ISBN 1-55766O-CA-P

6385 Dictionary of Developmental Disabilities Terminology

Brookes Publishing
PO Box 10624
Baltimore, MD 21285
410-337-9580
800-638-3775
FAX: 410-337-8539
e-mail: custserv@brookespublishing.com
www.brookespublishing.com

Answers thousands of questions for medical or human services professionals, parents or advocates of children with disabilities, or students preparing for their careers. Provides thorough explanations of the most common terms associated with disabilities. *$ 55.95*

368 pages Hardcover
ISBN 1-557662-45-2

6386 Dr. Braly's Food Allergy and Nutrition Revolution

Keats Publishing
27 Pine Street
PO Box 876
New Canaan, CT 06840
203-966-8721
800-323-4900

Research on food allergies, testing methods, and a detailed treatment method based upon diet and nutrition; includes treatment protocols for some forty illnesses linked to food allergies.

510 pages 1992
ISBN 0-879835-90-7

6387 Everday Social Interaction

Brookes Publishing
PO Box 10624
Baltimore, MD 21285
410-337-9580
800-638-3775
FAX: 410-337-8539
e-mail: custserv@brookespublishing.com
www.brookespublishing.com

Useful strategies for assessing needs and setting objectives, along with helpful teaching techniques, are accompanied by tips on social courtesies, rewards, praise, and criticism. Checklists and task analyses that show how complex skills can be broken down into major components for easy performance monitoring are also included. *$41.95*

342 pages Paperback
ISBN 1-55766 -58-4

6388 Exceptional Children

Council for Exceptional Children
1110 N Glebe Road
Suite 300
Arlington, VA 22201
703-620-3660
FAX: 703-264-9494
www.cec.sped.org

Janice Burdick, President

Articles include research, literature surveys and position papers concerning exceptional children, special education and mainstreaming. *$58.00*

96 pages BiMonthly

6389 Exceptional Parent Magazine

Psy-Ed Corp
555 Kinderkamack Road
Oradell, NJ 07649
201-634-6550
877-372-7368
FAX: 740-302-5866
e-mail: epedit@aol.com
www.eparent.com

Bridget Lyne, Managing Editor

Addresses concerns of raising, treating or teaching children or young adults with disabilities, for parents and professionals. *$39.95*

100 pages Monthly
ISSN 0046-91 7

6390 Face of Inclusion

Special Needs Project
324 State Street
Suite H
Santa Barbara, CA 93101
800-333-6867
FAX: 805-962-5087
e-mail: eplibrary@aol.com
www.eplibrary.com

A unique and moving parents' perspective of inclusion for administrators, teachers, and parents of children with disabilities. *$99.00*

6391 Family Interventions Throughout Disability

Springer Publishing Company
536 Broadway
New York, NY 10012
212-431-4370
877-687-7476
FAX: 212-941-7842
e-mail: marketing@springerpub.com
www.springerpub.com

Annette Imperati, Marketing/Sales Director

Family attitudes throughout chronic illness and disability. *$31.95*

320 pages
ISBN 0-82615 -80-4

6392 Family-Centered Service Coordination: A Manual for Parents

Brookline Books
PO Box 1047
Cambridge, MA 02238
617-868-0360
800-666-2665
FAX: 617-868-1772
e-mail: brooklinebks@delphi.com
www.brooklinebooks.com

A manual designed to orient and educate parents about issues of service coordination, to assist families in caring for an infant or toddler with developmental delays or disabilities. *$7.00*

34 pages Paperback
ISBN 0-91479 -90-5

6393 Fertility Awareness Handbook

Hunter House Publishers
1515 1/2 Park Street
PO Box 2914
Alameda, CA 94501
510-865-5282

Provides noninvasive and side-effect free natural family planning methods that teach you how to be more in touch with your body, more secure in your lovemaking, and more in control of your health and sexual well-being.

1992

6394 Free Yourself From Pain

Bresler Center
115 S Topanga Canyon Boulevard
Suite 158
Topanga, CA 90290
310-455-3634

This self help book for managing chronic pain and depression includes several chapters illustrating the use of guided imagery for pain control.

1992

6395 Getting Our Heads Together

Thoms Rehabilitation Hospital
68 Sweeten Creek Road
Asheville, NC 28803
828-274-2400
FAX: 828-274-9452

Kathi Petersen, Dir. of Planning & Communication
Edgardo Diez MD, Medical Director Brain Injury
Kathy Price, Director Admissions

A handbook for families of head injured patients - available in Spanish as well as English. *$4.00*

40 pages Paperback

6396 Growing Up Gifted

McGraw-Hill, School Publishing
220 E Danieldale Road
DeSoto, TX 75115
972-224-1111
800-442-9685
FAX: 972-228-1982
mhschool.com

A book that develops the potential of children at home and at school.

512 pages

6397 Handbook About Care in the Home

AARP Fulfillment
601 E Street NW
Washington, DC 20049
202-434-2277
800-424-3410
FAX: 202-434-3443
e-mail: member@aarp.org
www.aarp.org

Offers valuable information for the disabled.

24 pages

6398 How to Deal with Back Pain and Rheumatoid Joint Pain

Global Health Solutions
8472 A Tyco Road
Vienna, VA 22182
703-848-2333
800-759-3999
FAX: 703-848-0028
e-mail: shipping@watercure.com
www.watercure.com

Kristin Swan, Secretary
Joy Barber, Secretary

The physiology of pain production and its direct relationship to chronic regional dehydration of some joint spaces is explained: Special movements that would create vacuum in the disc spaces and draw water and the displaced discs into the vertebral joints are demonstrated.

6399 Human Kinetics

1607 N Market Street
PO Box 5076
Champaign, IL 61825 **217-351-5076**
FAX: 217-351-2674
www.humankinetics.com

6400 Infant Development and Risk

Brookes Publishing
PO Box 10624
Baltimore, MD 21285 **410-337-9585**
800-638-3775
FAX: 410-337-8539
e-mail: custserv@brookespublishing.com
www.brookespublishing.com

Provides a comprehensive overview of typical & atypical development while explaining key assessment issues and intervention programs. Deals head-on with complex and sensitive subjects such as eligibility for services and NICU ethics. *$44.00*

384 pages Paperback 1997
ISBN 1-55766 -69-X

6401 Infertility and Birth Defects: Is Mercury from Silver Dental Fillings a Hidden Cause?

Bio-Probe
7118 Costello Avenue
Van Nuys, CA 91405 **818-785-1241**

Explains the facts about mercury and lead.

1987

6402 It's All in Your Head

Avery Publishing Group
375 Hudson Street
New York, NY 10014 **212-366-2000**

Dr. Higgins's critique of the use of mercury, a toxic element and environmental hazard, in dentistry. For those suffering mercury poisoning, the book examines a number of conventional and alternative treatments.

6403 Keys to Parenting a Child with a Learning Disability

Barron's Educational Series
250 Wireless Boulevard
Hauppauge, NY 11788 **631-434-3311**
800-645-3476
FAX: 631-434-3723
e-mail: info@barronseduc.com
www.barronseduc.com

Lonny Stein, Director Marketing

The authors discuss the diagnosis and treatment of learning disabilities. They provide a practical course of action for parents who suspect a learning disability is present in their child. They also describe methods of special education, dealing with learning disabled children at home, and integrating them into community activities. *$ 6.95*

208 pages Paperback
ISBN 0-812016-79-3

6404 Kids to the Rescue

Alliance for Parental Involvement in Education
PO Box 59
E Chatham, NY 12060 **518-392-6900**
FAX: 518-392-6900

Parents and children should read this book together. The author offers children the information they need for fourteen emergency situations. *$7.95*

6405 LifeLines

Disabled and Alone
352 Park Avenue S
11th Floor
New York, NY 10010 **212-532-6740**
800-995-0066
FAX: 212-532-3588
e-mail: info@disabledandalone.org
www.disabledandalone.org

Disabled and Alone is a national nonprofit organization whose sole purpose is to assure the well being of disabled individuals, particularly those whose families have died and have engaged Disabled and Alone to provide advocacy and oversight for the lifetime of their disabled children. This newsletter provides information about "future planning" for a person with a disability.

8-16 pages Bi-annual

6406 Making Changes: Family Voices on Living Disabilities

Brookline Books
PO Box 1047
Cambridge, MA
800-666-2665
FAX: 617-868-1772
e-mail: brooklinebks@delphi.com
www.brooklinebooks.com

What are the day to day impacts on the family when a disabled child is born? Or when a child who grows up without a disability becomes disabled through accident or disease? This provocative set of reports illuminates the conditions of those peoples lives, and the way they and those around them adjust to the disabilities. *$16.95*

216 pages Paperback
ISBN 0-91479 -93-

6407 Mobility Training for People with Disabilities

Charles C Thomas
2600 S First Street
Springfield, IL 62704 **217-789-8980**
800-258-8980
FAX: 217-789-9130
e-mail: books@ccthomas.com
www.ccthomas.com

Children and adults with mental, visual, physical and hearing impairments can learn to travel. Also available in cloth. *$ 28.95*

144 pages Paper
ISBN 0-398063-56-7

6408 Mothers Talk About Learning Disabilities

Gallery Bookshop
PO Box 270
Mendocino, CA 95460 **707-937-2665**
FAX: 707-937-3737
e-mail: info@gallerybooks.com
www.gallerybooks.com

In this work, the mother of two learning disabled boys seeks to give mothers in similar circumstances encouragement, support and everyday advice. *$17.95*

157 pages
ISBN 0-13502 -70-1

6409 **New Language of Toys: Teaching Communicati on Skills to Children with Special Needs**

Spina Bifida Association of America
4590 MacArthur Boulevard NW
Suite 250
Washington, DC 20007 **202-944-3285**
800-621-3141
FAX: 202-944-3295
e-mail: sbaa@sbaa.org
www.sbaa.org

A guide for parents and teachers and a reader-friendly resource guide that provides a wealth of information on how play activities affect a child's language development and where to get the toys and materials to use in these activities. *$19.00*

6410 **No More Allergies**

Villiard Books
1540 Braodway
New York, NY 10036 **212-782-9000**
FAX: 212-302-7985

A detailed investigation into the causes of allergies related both to food and the environment, as well as their link to other illnesses, such as asthma, arthritis, chrinic fatigue syndrome, and diabetes. Also outlines testing methods, treatments, and a diet plan to restore immune function.

6411 **No One to Play with: The Social Side of Learning Disabilities**

Special Needs Project
324 State Street
Suite H
Santa Barbara, CA 93101
800-333-6867
FAX: 805-962-5087

Betty Osman

Your child suffers from a learning disability, and you have read reams on how to improve his or her academic skills and now want to address his or her social needs. *$10.00*

188 pages

6412 **No Time for Jello: One Family's Experience**

Brookline Books
PO Box 1046
Cambridge, MA 02238 **617-868-0360**
800-666-2665
FAX: 617-868-1772
e-mail: brooklinebks@delphi.com
www.brooklinebooks.com

One family's story of their attempts to remediate and cure the effects of a cerebral palsied condition the oldest son was born with. The Bratts traveled traditional routes, through distinguished medical centers in Boston, and nontraditional routes in a search for treatments that would help their son. *$17.95*

Softcover
ISBN 0-91479 -56-5

6413 **On the Road to Autonomy: Promoting Self-Competence in Children & Youth with Disabilities**

Brookes Publishing
PO Box 10624
Baltimore, MD 21285 **410-337-9580**
800-638-3775
FAX: 410-337-8539
e-mail: custserv@brookespublishing.com
www.brookespublishing.com

This book provides detailed conceptual, practical, and personal information regarding the promotion of self-esteem, self-determination, and coping skills among children and youth with and without disabilities. *$48.00*

432 pages Paperback
ISBN 1-55766 -35-5

6414 **One-Two-Three Magic: Effective Discipline for Children 2-12**

Child Management
800 Roosevelt Road
Glen Ellyn, IL 60137 **630-469-0484**
800-442-4453
FAX: 800-635-8301

Nancy Roe, Office Manager

Time tested program provides easy-to-follow steps for disciplining children ages 2-12 without arguing, yelling or spanking. Excellent for parents, grandparents and teachers. Available on video ($39.95) audio ($24.95), and book ($12.95) *$12.95*

180 pages Paperback
ISBN 0-96338 -61-9

6415 **Pain Erasure**

M Evans and Company
216 E 49th Street
New York, NY 10017 **212-688-2810**
FAX: 212-486-4544

This book explains Bonnie Prudden's method for pain relief using myotherapy, a method hailed by doctors and patients.

1985
ISBN 0-345331-02-8

6416 **Parent Centers and Independent Living Centers: Collectively We're Stronger**

Independent Living Research Utilization ILRU
2323 S Shepherd Drive
Suite 1000
Houston, TX 77019 **713-520-0232**
FAX: 713-520-5785
www.ilru.org

This article describes several examples of effective working relationships of PTIs and CILs. The examples highlight how parent and consumer organizations have identified complimentary strengths and formed partnerships to better support children with disabilities and their families. These partnerships can also be a very important way of involving youth in the disability movement so they may become leaders of tomorrow.

10 pages

6417 **Parent Survival Manual**

Exceptional Parent Library
120 Sylvan Avenue, Suite 10
PO Box 1807
Englewood Cliffs, NJ 10116
800-535-1910
FAX: 201-947-9376
e-mail: eplibrary@aol.com
www.eplibrary.com

A guide to crises resolution in autism and related developmental disorders. *$39.95*

6418 **Parent-Child Interaction and Developmental Disabilities**

Greenwood Publishing Group
88 Post Road W
Suite 5007
Westport, CT 06880 **203-226-3571**
FAX: 203-222-1502
www.greenwood.com

This volume brings together the original papers by international scholars and practitioners on the question of the effects of parent interaction with developmentally disabled children. $65.00-$69.50.

395 pages Hardcover
ISBN 0-275928-35-7

6419 Parenting

Accent Books & Products
PO Box 700
Bloomington, IL 61702 **309-378-2961**
800-787-8444
FAX: 309-378-4420
e-mail: acmtlvng@aol.com

Raymond C Cheever, Publisher
Betty Garee, Editor

Experienced parents (who are disabled) discuss: raising children from infant to teens, balancing career and motherhood, discipline methods and more when both parents are disabled. *$7.95*

83 pages
ISBN 0-91570 -26-4

6420 Parents and Young Mentally Handicapped Children

Brookline Books
PO Box 1046
Cambridge, MA 02238 **617-868-0360**
800-666-2665
FAX: 617-868-1772
e-mail: brooklinebks@delphi.com
www.brooklinebooks.com

Critically reviews and analyzes the effects of having a developmentally delayed child on the daily life of the family. Examined are the parents' crucial role in their child's development, the part played by other extended family members, parents' attitudes and parents' styles of interaction with their disabled and non-disabled child. *$ 29.95*

Hardcover
ISBN 0-91479 -28-X

6421 Perspectives on a Parent Movement

Brookline Books
PO Box 1046
Cambridge, MA 02238 **617-868-0360**
800-666-2665
FAX: 617-868-1772
e-mail: brooklinebks@delphi.com
www.brooklinebooks.com

This book captures Rosemary Dybwad's truly innovative wisdom and pioneering for people with intellectual limitations in these previously unpublished essays and speeches. *$17.95*

Paperback
ISBN 0-91479 -74-3

6422 Power Dialogues

Option Institute and Fellowship
2080 S Undermountain Road
Sheffield, MA 01257 **413-229-8737**
800-562-7171
FAX: 413-229-8737
e-mail: indigo@option.org
www.optionindigo.com

Kate Wilde

Learn our core system for helping others. This key program teaches participants the simple, yet profound principles and practical skills involved in using the Option Process Dialogue. This process consists of a system of nonjudgmental, non-directive questions that enables people to uncover the beliefs that underlie their feelings and behaviors. *$49.95*

301 pages Paperback
ISBN 1-88725 -06-4

6423 Promoting Communication in Infants and Young Children: 500 Ways to Succeed

Speech Bin
1965 25th Avenue
Vero Beach, FL 32960 **772-770-0007**
800-477-3324
FAX: 772-770-0006
www.speechbin.com

This practical reference for parents, caregivers and professional service providers how to promote communication development in infants and yourn children. Gives down-to-earth information and activities to help your youngest children succeed. It provides step-by-step suggestions for stimulationg children's speech and language skills. Paperback. *$14.95*

6424 Raising Your Child to be Gifted

Brookline Books
PO Box 1047
Cambridge, MA 02238 **617-868-0360**
800-666-2665
FAX: 617-868-1772
e-mail: brooklinebks@delphi.com
www.brooklinebooks.com

Dr. Campbell studied more than 10,000 gifted children in four countries, and found that what they shared most was not IQ, but parents who nurtured their ability and supported their efforts in school. This book explains the underlying principles and strategies these parents used in nurturing their childrens' abilities. *$15.95*

196 pages Paperback
ISBN 1-57129 -00-1

6425 Risk, Resilience, & Prevention: Promoting the Well-Being of All Children

Brookes Publishing
PO Box 10624
Baltimore, MD 21285 **410-337-9580**
800-638-3775
FAX: 410-337-8539
e-mail: custserv@brookespublishing.com
www.brookespublishing.com

This book investigates the implications of a primary prevention agenda for policy, practice, and research. Provides an in-depth examination of the increase in teenage pregnancy, school dropout, neglect and abuse, unintentional injury, depression and mental illness, behavior disorders, sexually transmitted disease, and illiteracy. An essential for health care professionals, educators, and administrators, psychologists, school counselors, policy makers, and child services providers. *$34.00*

384 pages Paperback
ISBN 1-55766 -66-9

6426 Sexuality and the Developmentally Handicapped

Edwin Mellen Press
PO Box 450
Lewiston, NY 14092 **716-754-2266**
FAX: 716-754-4056
e-mail: mellen@wzrd.com

Presents the knowledge, attitudes, and skills pertinent to responding to the sexual problems of developmentally handicapped persons, their families and communities. Details fully documented cases, issues concerning the law, and resource materials available. *$89.95*

245 pages Hardcover
ISBN 0-88946 -32-5

6427 **Shattered Dreams-Lonely Choices: Birth Parents of Babies with Disabilities**

Greenwood Publishing Group
88 Post Road W
Suite 5007
Westport, CT 06880
203-226-3571
FAX: 203-222-1502
www.greenwood.com

Written by a mother who, without warning, gave birth to a boy with Down Syndrome, this book is meant to help parents through the initial shock and the realization that they are not able to care for their child. $29.95-$35.00. *$29.95*

208 pages Hardcover
ISBN 0-897892-86-0

6428 **Sibshops: Workshops for Siblings of Children with Special Needs**

Brookes Publishing
PO Box 10624
Baltimore, MD 21285
410-337-9580
800-638-3775
FAX: 410-337-8539
e-mail: custserv@brookespublishing.com
www.brookespublishing.com

Sibshops is a program that brings together 8-to 13-year-old brothers and sisters of children with special needs. The siblings receive support and information in a recreational setting, so they have fun while they learn. *$32.00*

256 pages Paperback
ISBN 1-55766 -69-3

6429 **Since Owen, A Parent-to-Parent Guide for Care of the Disabled Child**

Special Needs Project
324 State Street
Suite H
Santa Barbara, CA 93101
800-333-6867
FAX: 805-962-5087
www.specialneeds.com

Charles Callahan, Editor

Against the background of his experience as the parent of a severely disabled young man, Callahan writes conscientiously to other parents. *$16.95*

486 pages

6430 **Sleep Better! A Guide to Improving Sleep for Children with Special Needs**

Brookes Publishing
PO Box 10624
Baltimore, MD 21285
410-337-9580
800-638-3775
FAX: 410-337-8539
e-mail: custserv@brookespublishing.com
www.brookespublishing.com

This book offers step-by-step, how to instructions for helping children with disabilities get the rest they need. For problems ranging from bedtime tantrums to night waking, parents and caregivers will find a variety of widely tested and easy-to-implement techniques that have already helped hundreds of children with special needs. *$21.95*

288 pages Paperback 1997
ISBN 1-55766 -15-7

6431 **Slow Motion/Sea Legs**

Aquarius Health Care Videos
5 Powderhouse Lane
PO Box 1159
Sherborn, MA 01770
508-651-2963
FAX: 508-650-4216
e-mail: aqvideos@tiac.net
www.aquariusproductions.com

Leslie Kussmonn, President

Probably the last place you would expect to find a disabled person is flying down a mountain in a bucket...attached to a board. Mario Solis and Carla toll introduce a community where physical limitations need no longer stand in the way of strenuous physical performance... the community of disabled snow skiing *$79.00*

6432 **Something's Wrong with My Child**

Charles C Thomas
2600 S First Street
Springfield, IL 62704
217-789-8980
800-258-8980
FAX: 217-789-9130
e-mail: books@ccthomas.com
www.ccthomas.com

A straight forward presentation to help professionals and parents to better understand themselves in dealing with the emotionally charged subject of disabled children. Also available in cloth. *$26.95*

210 pages Paperback
ISBN 0-398068-99-2

6433 **Sometimes I Get All Scribbly**

Exceptional Parent Library
120 Sylvan Avenue, Suite 10
PO Box 1807
Englewood Cliffs, NJ 07632
800-535-1910
FAX: 201-947-9376
e-mail: eplibrary@aol.com
www.eplibrary.com

Clinical, educational and emotional information from the point of view of a parent. *$16.00*

6434 **Son-Rise: The Miracle Continues**

2080 S Undermountain Road
Sheffield, MA 01257
413-229-2100
800-714-2779
FAX: 413-229-3202
e-mail: sonrise@option.org
www.son-rise.org

Documents Raun Kaufman's astonishing development from a lifeless, autistic, retarded child into a highly verbal, lovable youngster with no traces of his former condition. Details Raun's extraordinary progress from the age of four into young adulthood, also shares moving accounts of five families that successfully used the Son-Rise Program to reach their own special children.

372 pages 1994
ISBN 0-915811-53-7

6435 **Special Parent, Special Child**

Exceptional Parent Library
120 Sylvan Avenue, Suite 10
PO Box 1807
Englewood Cliffs, NJ 07632
800-535-1910
FAX: 201-947-9376
e-mail: eplibrary@aol.com
www.eplibrary.com

Offers information for facing the challenges of being a special parent. *$21.95*

Hardcover

6436 Spoiling Childhood: How Well-Meaning Parents Are Giving Children Too Much...

Guilford Press
72 Spring Street
New York, NY 10012
212-431-9800
800-365-7006
FAX: 212-966-6708
www.guilford.com

$15.95

263 pages Paperback 1999
ISBN 1-572304-50-2

6437 Steps to Independence: Teaching Everyday S kills to Children with Special Needs

Spina Bifida Association of America
4590 MacArthur Boulevard NW
Suite 250
Washington, DC 20007
202-944-3285
800-621-3141
FAX: 202-944-3295
e-mail: sbaa@sbaa.org
www.sbaa.org

A guide to help parents teach life skills to their disabled child. *$28.00*

6438 Strategies for Working with Families of Young Children with Disabilities

Brookes Publishing
PO Box 10624
Baltimore, MD 21285
410-337-9580
800-638-3775
FAX: 410-337-8539
e-mail: custserv@brookespublishing.com
www.brookespublishing.com

This text offers useful techniques for collaborating with and supporting families whose youngest members either have a disability or are at risk for developing a disability. The authors address specific issues such as cultural diversity, transitions to new programs, and disagreements between families and professionals. *$33.00*

272 pages Paperback
ISBN 1-55766 -57-6

6439 Talk with Me

Alexander Graham Bell Association
3417 Volta Place NW
Washington, DC 20007
202-337-5220
FAX: 202-337-8314
e-mail: info@agbell.org
www.agbell.org

This book addresses the urgent need to enlighten parents and professionals responsible for the crucial early decisions that affect the speech, language, social, emotional and intellectual development of children who are deaf and hard of hearing. *$22.95*

222 pages Paperback

6440 That's My Child

Exceptional Parent Library
120 Sylvan Avenue, Suite 10
PO Box 1807
Englewood Cliffs, NJ 07632
800-535-1910
FAX: 201-947-9376
e-mail: eplibrary@aol.com
www.eplibrary.com

Offers information to help parent successfully navigate the maze of resources and services available for children with special needs. *$12.95*

6441 Tips for Teaching Infants & Toddlers

Speech Bin
1965 25th Avenue
Vero Beach, FL 32960
772-770-0007
800-477-3324
FAX: 772-770-0006
www.speechbin.com

A pratical multisensory approach to Early Intervention including a whole year's worth of weekly thematic lessons which give children abundant opportunities to see, hear, feel, manipulate, smell and taste. Lessons cover: early concepts, prespeech and language, body image, directionality, fine and gross motor, categories, early acitons, activities just for fun and attributes. Paperback. *$39.95*

6442 To a Different Drumbeat

Alliance for Parental Involvement in Education
PO Box 59
E Chatham, NY 12060
518-392-6900
FAX: 518-392-6900

Parents of special needs children contributed to this book. *$16.95*

6443 Uncommon Fathers

Woodbine House
6510 Bells Mill Road
Bethesda, MD 20817
301-897-3570
800-843-7323
FAX: 301-897-5838
www.woodbinehouse.com

Nineteen fathers talk about the life-altering experience of having a child with special needs and offer a welcome, seldom-heard perspective on raising kids with disabilities, including autism, cerebral palsy, and Down syndrome. Uncommon Fathers is the first book for fathers by fathers, but it is also helpful to partners, family, friends, and service providers. *$14.95*

206 pages Paperback
ISBN 0-933149-68-9

6444 Vaccination Social Violence and Criminality: Medical Assault on the American Brain

North Atlantic Books
1456 Fourth Street
Berkley, CA
510-559-8277
FAX: 510-559-8279
www.northatlanticbooks.com

The author argues that vaccination has produced a generation of neurologic defectives and changed the tone and atmosphere of modern society.

1990

6445 Vaccinations: Mothering Special Edition

Mothering Magazine
1611 A Paseo De Peralta
Santa Fe, NM 87504
505-984-8116
e-mail: info@mothering.com

Articles and commentary on the pros and cons of vaccinations.

1989

6446 Well Pregnancy Book

Summit Books
1230 Avenue of the Americas
New York, NY 10020
212-698-7000
FAX: 212-698-7099

Information on exercise, nutrition, drugs, sex, and all physical and emotional stages of pregnancy.

Hardcover 1986
ISBN 0-671555-49-9

6447 What Works in Children's Mental Health Services? Uncovering Answers to Critical Questions

Brookes Publishing
PO Box 10624
Baltimore, MD 21285
410-337-9580
800-638-3775
FAX: 410-337-8539
e-mail: custserv@brookespublishing.com
www.brookespublishing.com

Provides a comprehensive overview of research on the effectiveness of eight mental health service components in systems of care for children with emotional and behavioral disabilities. *$30.00*

256 pages Paperback
ISBN 1-55766 -54-1

6448 Why Can't My Child Behave?

Feingold Association of the US
127 E Main Street #106
PO Box 6550
Riverhead, NY 11901
631-369-9340
800-321-3287
FAX: 631-369-2988
e-mail: help@feingold.org
www.feingold.org

$22.00

400 pages

6449 Yeast Connection

Vintage Books
1540 Broadway
New York, NY 10036
212-782-9000
FAX: 212-302-7985
www.randomhouse.com

One of the first and best book giving practicle advice regarding what has come to be known as the candida or yeast problem.

434 pages
ISBN 0-394747-00-3

6450 Your Body's Many Cries for Water

Global Health Solutions
8472 A Tyco Road
Vienna, VA 22182
703-848-2333
800-759-3999
FAX: 703-848-0028
e-mail: shipping@watercure.com
www.watercure.com

Kirstin Swan, Secretary
Joy Barber, Secretary

A fascinating discussion about the importance of water in the body, and how simply increasing the amount of water consumed per day can significantly improve arthritic and other pain conditions. *$14.95*

186 pages 1995
ISBN 0-962994-23-5

6451 Your Child Has a Disability: A Complete So urcebook of Daily and Medical Care

Brookes Publishing
PO Box 10624
Baltimore, MD 21285
410-337-9580
800-638-3775
FAX: 410-337-8539
e-mail: custserv@brookesopublishing.com
www.brookespublishing.com

Offers expert advice on a wide range of issues-from finding the right doctor and investigating the medical aspects of a child's condition to learning care techniques and fulfilling education requirements. *$24.95*

368 pages Paperback 1998
ISBN 1-557663-74-2

6452 Your Defiant Child: Eight Steps to Better Behavior

Guilford Press
72 Spring Street
New York, NY 10012
212-431-9800
800-365-7006
FAX: 212-966-6708
www.guilford.com

Also in cloth at $37.00 (ISBN# 1-57230-405-7) *$15.95*

239 pages Paperback 1998
ISBN 1-572303-21-2

Parenting: Specific Disabilities

6453 AFB Directory of Services for Blind and Visually Impaired Persons in the US and Canada

American Foundation for the Blind/AFB Press
PO Box 1020
Sewickley, PA 15143
412-741-1142
800-232-3044
FAX: 412-741-0609
e-mail: afborders@abdintl.com
www.afb.org

Stephanie Biagioli, Marketing Coordinator

Comprehensive CD-ROM and print resource containing more that 2,500 local, state, regional, and national services throughout the US and Canada for persons who are blind or visually impaired. *$74.95*

624 pages Hardcover/CDROM
ISBN 0-89128 -00-5

6454 Attention Deficit Disorder: Children

Aquarius Health Care Videos
5 Powderhouse Lane
PO Box 1159
Sherborn, MA 01770
508-651-2963
888-440-2963
FAX: 508-650-4216
e-mail: aqvideos@tiac.net
www.aquariusproductions.com

Leslie Kussmann, President/Producer

Everyone has been impulsive or easily distracted for different periods of time, so these symptoms that are hallmarks of Attention Deficit Disorder (ADD) have also led to criticism that too many people are being diagnosed with this biochemical brain disorder. This program examines who is being diagnosed, and what treatments are working. An innovative private school specializing in alternative education is profiled, and tips on structuring the school and home environment are included. *$149.00*

Video

6455 Attention-Deficit/Hyperactivity Disorder, What Every Parent Wants to Know

Brookes Publishing
PO Box 10624
Baltimore, MD 21285
410-337-9580
800-638-3775
FAX: 410-337-8539
e-mail: custserv@brookespublishing.com
www.brookespublishing.com

New easy-to-understand, non-technical edition helps teachers and parents get accessible answers to their ADHD. *$21.95*

304 pages Paperback 1900
ISBN 1-557663-98-X

6456 Bipolar Disorders: A Guide to Helping Children & Adolescents

Patient-Centered Guides
101 Morris Street
Sebastopol, CA 95472
707-829-0515
800-998-9938
FAX: 800-997-9901
e-mail: order@oreilly.com
www.patientcenters.com

Linda Lamb, Editor
Shawnde Paull, Marketing

A million children and adolescents in the U.S. may have childhood-onset bipolar disorder, including an estimated 23 percent of those currently diagnosed with ADHD. Bipolar Disorders helps parents and professionals recognize, treat, and cope with bipolar disorders in children and adolescents. It covers diagnosis, family life, medications, talk therapies, other interventions (improving sleep patterns, diet, preventing seasonal mood swings), insurance, and school. *$24.95*

458 pages Paperback
ISBN 1-565926-56-0

6457 Bowel Continence & Spina Bifida

Spina Bifida Association of America
4590 Macarthur Boulevard NW
Suite 250
Washington, DC 20007
202-944-3285
800-621-3141
FAX: 202-944-3295
e-mail: sbaa@sbaa.org
www.sbaa.org

An excellent book aimed at anyone trying to attain bowel continence with sample menus, bowel tracking charts and glossary of terms. *$8.00*

6458 Can't Your Child See? A Guide for Parents of Visually Impaired Children

Pro-Ed Publications
8700 Shoal Creek Boulevard
Austin, TX 78757
512-451-3246
800-897-3202
FAX: 512-451-8542
e-mail: info@proedinc.com
www.proedinc.com

This second edition offers parents optimistic, practical guidelines for helping visually impaired children reach their full potential. *$26.00*

279 pages Paperback

6459 Cancer Clinical Trials: Experimental Treatments and How They Can Help You

Patient-Centered Guides
101 Morris Street
Sebastopol, CA 95472
707-829-0515
800-998-9938
FAX: 707-829-0104
www.patientcenters.com

Linda Lamb, Editor
Shawnde Paull, Marketing

Most cancer patients face treatment options that are less than ideal, whether because of a risk of recurrence or side effects. Finally, however, basic research on cell biology is leading to promising new treatments. If you are not evaluating potential experimental treatments alongside the standard treatment protocols, you aren't considering all the facts you need. Cancer Clinical Trials guide you through understanding your options and finding and considering experimental treatments. *$14.95*

222 pages Paperback
ISBN 1-565925-66-1

6460 Caring for Children with Cerebral Palsy: A Team Approach

Brookes Publishing
PO Box 10624
Baltimore, MD 21285
410-337-9580
800-638-3775
FAX: 410-337-8539
e-mail: custserv@brookespublishing.com
www.brookespublishing.com

A guide to the interdisciplinary care of children with cerebral palsy. Delivers detailed information on a multitude of issues relevant to treatment and supports. *$38.95*

496 pages Paperback 1998
ISBN 1-55766 -22-X

6461 Childhood Cancer Survivors: A Practical Guide to Your Future

Patient-Centered Guides
101 Morris Street
Sebastopol, CA 95472
707-829-0515
800-998-9938
FAX: 707-829-0104
www.patientcenters.com

Linda Lamb, Editor
Shawnde Paull, Marketing

More than 250,000 people have survived childhood cancer - a cause for celebration. Authors Keene, Hobbie, and Ruccione chart the territory of long-term survivorship: relationships; overcoming employment or insurance discrimination; maximizing health; follow-up schedules; medical late effects. The stories of over sixty survivors - their challenges and triumphs - are told. Includes medical history record-keeper. *$27.95*

510 pages Paperback
ISBN 1-565924-60-6

6462 Childhood Cancer: A Parent's Guide to Solid Tumor Cancers

Patient-Centered Guides
101 Morris Street
Sebastopol, CA 95472
707-829-0515
800-998-9938
FAX: 707-829-0104
www.patientcenters.com

Linda Lamb, Editor
Shawnde Paull, Marketing

Childhood Cancer: A Parent's Guide to Solid Tumor Cancers features a wealth of resources for parents of children with solid tumor cancers, plus many stories of veteran parents. Parents will encounter medical facts simply explained, practical advice to ease their daily lives, and tools to be strong advocates for their child. Includes a passport to record patient's medical history. *$24.95*

537 pages Paperback
ISBN 1-565925-31-9

6463 Childhood Leukemia: A Guide for Families, Friends & Caregivers

Patient-Centered Guides
101 Morris Street
Sebastopol, CA 95472 **707-829-0515**
800-998-9938
FAX: 707-829-0104
www.patientcenters.com

Linda Lamb, Editor
Shawnde Paull, Marketing

The second edition of this comprehensive guide offers detailed and precise medical information for parents that includes day-to-day practical advice on how to cope with procedures, hospitalization, family and friends, school, and social, emotional, and financial issues. It features a wealth of tools for prents and contains significant updates on treatments and procedures. *$24.95*

513 pages Paperback
ISBN 1-565926-32-3

6464 Children with Autism

Woodbine House
6510 Bells Mill Road
Bethesda, MD 20817 **301-897-3657**
800-843-7323
FAX: 301-897-5838
www.woodbinehouse.com

Recommended as the first book parents should read, this volume offers information and a complete introduction to autism, while easing the family's fears and concerns as they adjust and cope with their child's disorder. *$17.95*

368 pages Paperback
ISBN 0-933149-16-6

6465 Helping Your Hyperactive: Attention Deficit Child

Prima Publishing
3000 Lava Ridge Court
PO Box 1260
Rocklin, CA 95677 **916-787-7000**
800-632-8676
FAX: 916-787-7001
e-mail: websupportlife@primapub.com
www.primapublishing.com

$19.95

ISBN 1-559584-23-8

6466 If Your Child Has Diabetes: An Answer Book for Parents

Putnam Publishing Group
200 Madison Avenue
New York, NY 10016 **212-889-6330**

Provides information and recommendations for parents of children with diabetes on subjects such as school, recreation, medical and life insurance and employment as well as general information about diabetes. *$9.95*

6467 If Your Child Stutters: A Guide for Parents

Stuttering Foundation of America
3100 Walnut Grove Road, Suite 603
PO Box 11749
Memphis, TN 38111 **901-452-7343**
800-992-9392
FAX: 901-452-3931
e-mail: stutter@vantek.net
www.stutterhelp.org

A guide that enables parents to provide appropriate help to children who stutter. *$1.00*

6468 Keys to Parenting a Child with Attention Deficit Disorder

Barron's Educational Series
250 Wireless Boulevard
Hauppauge, NY 11788 **631-434-3311**
800-645-3476
FAX: 631-434-3723
e-mail: info@barronseduc.com
www.barronseduc.com

Lonny Stein , Director Marketing

This book shows how to work with the child's school, effectively manage the child's behavior and act as the child's advocate. *$6.95*

160 pages Paperback
ISBN 0-812014-59-6

6469 Keys to Parenting a Child with Cerebral Palsy

Barron's Educational Series
250 Wireless Boulevard
Hauppauge, NY 11788 **631-434-3311**
800-645-3476
FAX: 631-434-3723
e-mail: info@barronsedu.com
www.barronseduc.com

Margaret E Myers, Author

This volume helps parents adjust to the challenge of having a child with cerebral palsy. It stresses the child's potential and encourages independence. Facets of the child's total well-being are discussed, including common health problems, physical, mental and social development, therapy, and new trends in medical management. *$6.95*

Paperback
ISBN 0-764100-91-2

6470 Keys to Parenting a Child with Downs Syndrome

Barron's Educational Series
250 Wireless Boulevard
Hauppauge, NY 11788 **631-434-3311**
800-645-3476
FAX: 631-434-3723
e-mail: info@barronsedu.com
www.barronseduc.com

Lonny Stein, Director Marketing

Down Syndrome poses many challenges for children and their families. This book prepares parents and guardians to raise a child with Down Syndrome by discussing adjustment, advocacy, health and behavior, education and planning for greater independence. *$5.95*

160 pages Paperback
ISBN 0-812014-58-8

6471 **Keys to Parenting the Child with Autism**

Barron's Educational Series
250 Wireless Boulevard
Hauppauge, NY 11788
631-434-3311
800-645-3476
FAX: 631-434-3723
e-mail: barrons@barronseduc.com
www.barronseduc.com

Parents of children with autism will find a solid balance between home and practical information in this book. It explains what autism is and how it is diagnosed, then advises parents on how to adjust to their child and give the best care. *$6.95*

208 pages Paperback
ISBN 0-812016-79-3

6472 **Legislative Handbook for Parents**

NAPVI
PO Box 317
Watertown, MA 02272
617-972-7441
800-562-6265
FAX: 617-972-7444
e-mail: napvi@perkins.org
www.napvi.org

Written by parents for parents in dealing with Legislative Processes that ultimately affect their children's lives. *$5.50*

24 pages Paperback

6473 **Life on Wheels: For the Active Wheelchair User**

Patient-Centered Guides
101 Morris Street
Sebastopol, CA 95472
707-829-0515
800-294-4747
FAX: 800-997-9901
e-mail: order@oreilly.com
www.patientcenters.com

Linda Lamb, Editor
Shawnde Paull, Marketing

For 1.5 million Americans, life includes a wheelchair for mobility. Life on Wheels is for people who want to take charge of their life experience. Author Gary Karp describes medical issues (paralysis, circulation, rehab, cure research); day-to-day living (exercise, skin, bowel and bladder, sexuality, home access, maintaining a wheelchair); and social issues (self-image, adjustment, friends, family, cultural attitudes, activism). *$24.95*

573 pages Paperback
ISBN 1-565922-53-0

6474 **Non-Hodgkin's Lymphomas: Making Sense of Diagnosis, Treatment & Options**

O'Reilly
101 Morris Street
Sebastopol, CA 95472
707-829-0515
800-294-4747
FAX: 800-997-9901
e-mail: order@oreilly.com
www.patientcenters.com

$24.95

580 pages Paperback
ISBN 1-565924-44-4

6475 **Not Deaf Enough: Raising a Child Who is Hard of Hearing**

Alexander Graham Bell Association
3417 Volta Place NW
Washington, DC 20007
202-337-5220
FAX: 202-337-8314
e-mail: info@agbell.org
www.agbell.org

This sensitive book portrays a family's struggle to identify, accept and support their youngest child through his diagnosis of mild to moderate hearing loss. This book provides a much needed overview of this under-diagnosed and under-served disability. *$24.95*

242 pages Paperback

6476 **Obsessive-Compulsive Disorder: Help for Children and Adolescents**

Patient-Centered Guides
101 Morris Street
Sebastopol, CA 95472
707-829-0515
800-998-9938
FAX: 707-829-0104
www.patientcenters.com

Linda Lamb, Editor
Shawnde Paull, Marketing

Obsessive-compulsive disorders (OCD) is one of the most common psychiatric problems faced by children. Childhood OCD can be a truly debilitating disability, not just a minor problem or personality quirk. The good news is that it is very treatable. Obsessive-Compulsive Disorder helps parents secure a diagnosis, manage family life, understand medical interventions, explore therapeutic interventions, get care within their existing healthcare plan, and navigate the special education system. *$24.95*

400 pages Paperback
ISBN 1-565927-58-3

6477 **Parent's Guide to Allergies and Asthma**

National Allergy and Asthma Network
3554 Chain Bridge Road
Suite 200
Fairfax, VA 22030
703-385-4403
FAX: 703-352-4354

A up-to-date, easy-to-read resource offering essential information on asthma and allergies.

6478 **Parent's Guide to Autism**

Autism Society of North Carolina Bookstore
505 Oberlin Road
Suite 230
Raleigh, NC 27605
919-743-0204
800-442-2762
FAX: 919-743-0208
e-mail: dcoffey@autismsociety-nc.org
www.autismsociety-nc.org

Darla Coffey, Bookstore Manager

An essential handbook for anyone facing autism. *$14.00*

6479 Parent's Guide to Down Syndrome: Toward a Brighter Future: 2nd Edition

Brookes Publishing
PO Box 10624
Baltimore, MD 21285 **410-337-9580**
800-638-3775
FAX: 410-337-8539
e-mail: custserv@brookespublishing.com
www.brookespublishing.com

Highlights developmental stages and shows the advances that improve a child's quality of life. Includes discussions on easing the transition from home to school and choosing integration and curricular priorities, as well as guidelines for confronting adolescent and adult issues such as social and sexual needs and independent living and vocational options. *$22.95*

336 pages Paperback
ISBN 1-55766 -60-3

6480 Parents Helping Parents: A Directory of Support Groups for ADD

Novartis Pharmaceuticals Division
Customer Response Literature Dept.
59 Route 10
E Hanover, NJ 07936
800-742-2422

6481 Pervasive Developmental Disorders; Finding a Diagnosis and Getting Help

Patient-Centered Guides
101 Morris Street
Sebastopol, CA 95472 **707-829-0515**
800-998-9938
FAX: 707-829-0104
www.patientcenters.com

Linda Lamb, Editor
Shawnde Paull, Marketing

This unique book encompassess both the practical aspects as well as ther personal stories and emotional facets of living with PDD-NOS, the most common pervasive developmental disorder. Parents of an undiagnosed child may suspect many things, from autism to servere allergies. Pervasive Developmental Disorders is for parents (or newly diagnosed adults) who struggle with this neurological condition that profoundly impacts the life of child and family. *$24.95*

580 pages Paperback
ISBN 1-565925-30-0

6482 Preschool Learning Activities for the Visually Impaired Child

NAPVI
PO Box 317
Watertown, MA 02472 **617-972-7441**
800-562-6265
FAX: 617-972-7444
e-mail: napvi@perkins.org
www.napvi.org

This guide for parents offers games and activities to keep visually impaired children active during the preschool years. *$8.00*

91 pages Paperback

6483 Preventing Secondary Conditions Associated with Spina Bifida or Cerebral Palsy

Spina Bifida Association of America
4590 MacArthur Boulevard NW
Suite 250
Washington, DC 20007 **202-944-3285**
800-621-3141
FAX: 202-944-3295
e-mail: sbaa@sbaa.org
www.sbaa.org

This report is for health professionals, parents and teachers. *$3.00*

6484 Reaching the Autistic Child, 2nd Edition A Parent Training Program

Brookline Books/Lumen Editions
PO Box 1047
Cambridge, MA 02238 **617-868-0360**
800-666-2665
FAX: 617-868-1772
e-mail: brooklinebks@delphi.com

Detailed case studies of social and behavioral change in autistic children and their families show parents how to implement the principles for improved socialization and behavior. *$15.95*

Softcover
ISBN 1-571290-56-7

6485 Retarded Isn't Stupid, Mom! Revised Edition

Brookes Publishing
PO Box 10624
Baltimore, MD 21285 **410-337-9580**
800-638-3775
FAX: 410-337-8539
e-mail: custserv@brookespublishing.com
www.pbrookescom/store/books/kaufman-3785

Sandra Kaufman reveals the feelings of denial, guilt, frustration and eventual acceptance that resulted in a determination to help her daughter, Nicole, live an independent life. This edition, revised on the 10th anniversary of the book's original publication, adds a progress report that updates readers on Nicole's adult years and reflects on the revolutionary changes in society's attitudes toward people with disabilities since Nicole's birth. *$22.95*

272 pages Paperback 1999
ISBN 1-557663-78-5

6486 Show Me How: A Manual for Parents of Preschool Blind Children

American Foundation for the Blind/AFB Press
PO Box 1020
Sewickley, PA 15143 **412-741-1142**
800-232-3044
FAX: 412-741-0609
e-mail: afborders@abdintl.com
www.afb.org

A practical guide for parents, teachers and others who help preschool children attain age-related goals. Covers issues on playing precautions, appropriate toys and facilitating relationships with playmates. Paperback. *$12.95*

56 pages
ISBN 0-891281-13-4

6487 Signing Family: What Every Parent Should Know About Sign Communication

Gallaudet University Press
11030 S Langley Avenue
Chicago, IL 60628
800-621-2736
FAX: 800-621-8476
TTY:800-621-9347
gupress.gallaudet.edu

David A Stewart, Co-Author
Barbara Luetke-Stahlman, Co-Author

This reader-friendly book shows parents how to create a set of goals around the communication needs of their deaf child. Describes in even-handed terms the major signing options available, from American Sign Language to Signed English. *$24.95*

192 pages Softcover

6488 Smart But Stuck: Emotional Aspects of Learning Disabilities and Imprisoned Intelligence

Haworth Press
10 Alice Street
Binghamton, NY 13904
607-722-5857
800-429-6784
FAX: 607-722-6362
e-mail: orders@haworthpress.com
www.haworthpress.com

S Harrington-Miller, Advertising

Elaborates on new research about imprisoned intelligence and the emotional consequences of learning disabilities. It is also for psychoterapists, educators, school social workers, medical personnel, people dealing with prisons, etc. It helps those who struggle with learning disabilities (and people who help them) build self esteem, face LD obstacles, bypass weaknesses, and enhance strenghts. *$34.95*

228 pages Hardcover
ISBN 0-789014-66-1

6489 Social Development and the Person with Spi na Bifida

Spina Bifida Association of America
4590 MacArthur Boulevard NW
Suite 250
Washington, DC 20007
202-944-3285
800-621-3141
FAX: 202-944-3295
e-mail: sbaa@sbaa.org
www.sbaa.org

Examines how spina bifida and hydrocephalus may influence development and learning social skills.

6490 Son-Rise: The Miracle Continues

2080 S Undermountain Road
Sheffield, MA 01257
413-229-2100
800-714-2779
FAX: 413-229-3202
e-mail: sonrise@option.org
www.son-rise.org

Documents Raun Kaufman's astonishing development from a lifeless, autistic, retarded child into a highly verbal, lovable youngster with no traces of his former condition. Details Raun's extraordinary progress from the age of four into young adulthood, also shares moving accounts of five families that successfully used the Son-Rise Program to reach their own special children.

372 pages 1994
ISBN 0-915811-53-7

6491 Special Child

Brookes Publishing
PO Box 10624
Baltimore, MD 21285
410-337-9580
800-638-3775
FAX: 410-337-8539
e-mail: custserv@brookesopublishing.com
www.brookespublishing.com

Patricia S Scola MD MPH, Author
E Weidenman PhD, Author
James C Bernier ACSW, Author

Includes specifics on the detection, prognosis and treatment of various conditions as well as detailed information on education, intervention, advocacy, financial planning and technological advances that may affect the lives of children with special needs. *$ 29.95*

464 pages Paperback 1995
ISBN 1-557661-67-7

6492 Taking Charge of ADHD Complete Authoritative Guide for Parents

Guilford Press
72 Spring Street
New York, NY 10012
212-431-9800
800-365-7006
FAX: 212-966-6708
www.guilford.com

Revised and updated to incorporate the most current information on ADHD and its treatment. Provides parents with the knowledge, guidance and confidence they need to ensure that their child receives the best care possible. Also in cloth at $40.00 (ISBN# 1-57230-600-9 *$18.95*

321 pages Paperback 1900
ISBN 1-572305-60-6

6493 Two Hundred Fifty Tips for Making Life with Arthritis Easier

Arthritis Foundation Distribution Center
PO Box 6996
Alpharetta, GA 30009
800-207-8633
FAX: 770-442-9742
www.arthritis.com

What do aerosol cooking spray and snow-shoveling have in common? Learn the answer to this question, and other clever and handy tips to make your life with-or without-arthritis easier. Plus learn about helpful serviced you didn't know were available through you bank, post office, phone company, grocery store, and other businesses you frequent. *$9.95*

88 pages

6494 Without Reason: A Family Copes with Autism

Books on Special Children
PO Box 305
Congers, NY 10920
845-638-1236
FAX: 845-638-0847
e-mail: irene@boscbooks.com

The author discovers his son has autism. He delves into problems of the autistic person and explains reasons for their actions. *$20.95*

292 pages Hardcover

6495 You and Your ADD Child

Nelson Publications
One Gateway Plaza
Port Chester, NY 10573
914-937-8400
FAX: 914-937-8950

$12.99

252 pages Paperback
ISBN 0-785278-95-8

6496 You and Your Deaf Child: A Self-Help Guide for Parents of Deaf and Hard of Hearing Children

Gallaudet University Press
11030 S Langley Avenue
Chicago, IL 60628
800-621-2736
FAX: 800-621-8476
TTY:800-621-9347
gupress.gallaudet.edu

The classic self-instructional guide has been completely written with more information dealing with feelings, communication and other issues. Includes worksheets and practice exercises. *$19.95*

224 pages Softcover

6497 Your Child in the Hospital: A Practical Guide for Parents

Patient-Centered Guides
101 Morris Street
Sebastopol, CA 95472
707-829-0515
800-998-9938
FAX: 707-829-0104
www.patientcenters.com

Linda Lamb, Editor
Shawnde Paull, Marketing

This book offers advice from dozens of veteran parents on how to cope with a child's hospitalization, relieving anxious parents so they can help dispel their child's fears and concerns. Parents will find easy-to-read tips on preparing their child, handling procedures without trauma, and preventing insurance snafus. The second edition features a journal to help open communication and give the child a measure of control over the experience. *$11.95*

166 pages Paperback
ISBN 1-565925-73-4

Parenting: School

6498 ADHD in Schools: Assessment and Intervention Strategies

Guilford Press
72 Spring Street
New York, NY 10012
212-431-9800
800-365-7006
FAX: 212-966-6708
e-mail: info@guilford.com

This landmark volume emphasizes the need for a team effort among parents, community-based professionals, and educators. Provides practical information for educators that is based on empirical findings. Chapters focus on: how to identify and assess students who might have ADHD; the relationship between ADHD and learning disabilities; how to develop and implement classroom-based programs; communication strategies to assist physicians; and the need for community-based treatments. *$ 36.00*

269 pages Hardcover
ISBN 0-898622-45-X

6499 Adapted Physical Education for Students with Autism

Charles C Thomas
2600 S First Street
Springfield, IL 62704
217-789-8980
800-258-8980
FAX: 217-789-9130
e-mail: books@ccthomas.com
www.ccthomas.com

Focuses on the physical education, needs and curriculum for autistic children. Available in cloth, paperback and hardcover. Also available in cloth. *$23.95*

142 pages Paper
ISBN 0-398060-85-1

6500 Adapting Instruction for the Mainstream: A Sequential Approach to Teaching

McGraw-Hill, School Publishing
220 E Danieldale Road
DeSoto, TX 75115
972-224-1111
800-442-9685
FAX: 972-228-1982
mhschool.com

This text gives both regular and special education teachers everything they need to help mildly handicapped students succeed in the mainstream.

226 pages

6501 Assistive Technology in the Schools: A Guide for Idaho Educators

Idaho Assistive Technology Project
129 W 3rd Street
Moscow, ID 83843
208-885-3559
800-432-8324
FAX: 208-885-3628
e-mail: rseiler@uidaho.edu
www.educ.uidaho.edu/idatech

$15.00

6502 Attention Deficit Disorders: Assessment & Teaching

Brooks/Cole Publishing Company
511 Forest Lodge
Pacific Grove, CA 93950
408-373-0728
FAX: 408-375-6414
e-mail: bc-info@brookscole.com
www.brookscole.com

A handy resource that offers teachers, school psychologists, councelors, social workers, administrators, and parents practical advice for working with children who have attention deficit disorders. *$18.95*

258 pages Paperback
ISBN 0-534250-44-0

6503 Carolina Curriculum for Infants and Toddlers with Special Needs, 2nd Edition

Brookes Publishing
PO Box 10624
Baltimore, MD 21285
410-337-9580
800-638-3775
FAX: 410-337-8539
e-mail: custserv@brookespublishing.com
www.brookespublishing.com

This book includes detailed assessment and intervention sequences, daily routine integration strategies, sensorimotor adaptations, and a sample 24-page Assessment Log that shows readers how to chart a child's individual progress. *$41.95*

384 pages Spiral-bound
ISBN 1-557660-74-3

6504 Carolina Curriculum for Preschoolers with Special Needs

Brookes Publishing
PO Box 10624
Baltimore, MD 21285
410-337-9580
800-638-3775
FAX: 410-337-8539
e-mail: custserv@brookespublishing.com
www.brookespublishing.com

This curriculum provides detailed teaching and assessment techniques, plus a sample 28-page Assessment Log that shows readers how to chart a child's individual progress. This guide is for children between 2 and 5 in their developmental stages who are considered at risk for developmental delay or who exhibit special needs. *$35.95*

352 pages Spiral-bound
ISBN 1-557660-32-8

6505 Children and Youth Assisted by Medical Technology in Educational Settings: 2nd Edition

Brookes Publishing
PO Box 10624
Baltimore, MD 21285
410-337-9580
800-638-3775
FAX: 410-337-8539
e-mail: custserv@brookespublishing.com
www.brookespublishing.com

Guidelines for Care, 2nd Edition. Contains detailed daily care guidelines and emergency-response techniques, including information on working with a range of students who have the HIV infection, that rely on ventilators, that utilize tube feeding, or require catheterization. Also covers every aspect of planning for inclusive classrooms, including information on personnel training, entrance planning and transition, legal requirements, and transportation issues. *$52.00*

432 pages Spiral-bound 1997
ISBN 1-55766 -36-3

6506 Children, Problems and Guidelines: A Resource Book For School & Parents

Slosson Educational Publications
PO Box 280
E Aurora, NY 14052
716-625-0930
888-756-7766
FAX: 800-655-3840
e-mail: slosson@slosson.com
www.slosson.com

Leslie Foote, Office Personnel
Peggy Meyer, Office Personnel

Dr. Casey's book is a professional and responsible resource book which addresses many of the most common problems involving children and their homes or schools. Student achievement is very sensitive to home environments, family structure, emotional state, drugs and alcohol usage, and pressures from a great number of sources. Information relevant to answering questions or concerns is provided for dozens of common but devastating problems such as dicipline, study skills, and school behavior. *$43.00*

99 pages

6507 Choosing Outcomes and Accommodations for Children (COACH) 2nd Edition

Brookes Publishing
PO Box 10624
Baltimore, MD 21285
410-337-9580
800-638-3775
FAX: 410-337-8539
e-mail: custserv@brookespublishing.com
www.brookespublishing.com

A guide to educational planning for students with disabilities, second edition. Focuses on life outcomes such as social relationships and participation in typical home, school, and community activities. *$37.95*

400 pages Spiral bound 1997
ISBN 1-55766 -23-8

6508 Cognitive Strategy Instruction That Really Improves Children's Academic Skills

Brookline Books
PO Box 1046
Cambridge, MA 02238
617-868-0360
800-666-2665
FAX: 617-868-1772
e-mail: brooklinebks@delphi.com
www.brooklinebooks.com

Michael Pressley, Series Editor

A concise and focused work that summarily presents the few procedures for teaching strategies that aid academic subject matter learning: decoding reading comprehension, vocabulary, math, spelling and writing. Learning unrelated facts and science. Completely revised in 1995. *$27.95*

Paperback
ISBN 1-571290-07-9

6509 College Admissions: A Guide for Homeschoolers

Alliance for Parental Involvement in Education
PO Box 59
E Chatham, NY 12060
518-392-6900
FAX: 518-392-6900

The author's son was educated at home through junior and senior high school without much imposed structure. *$7.50*

6510 Complete IEP Guide: How to Advocate for Yo ur Special Ed Child

Spina Bifida Association of America
4590 MacArthur Boulevard NW
Suite 250
Washington, DC 20007
202-944-3285
800-621-3141
FAX: 202-944-3295
e-mail: sbaa@sbaa.org
www.sbaa.org

This all-in-one guide will help you understand special education law, identify your child's needs, prepare for meetings, develop the IEP and resolve disputes. *$28.95*

6511 Exceptional Children in Focus

McGraw-Hill, School Publishing
220 E Danieldale Road
DeSoto, TX 75115
972-224-1111
800-442-9685
FAX: 972-228-1982
mhschool.com

Combines a light, personal look at the problems of special educators experiences with the basic facts of exceptionality.

288 pages

6512 Exceptional Student in the Regular Classroom

McGraw-Hill, School Publishing
220 E Danieldale Road
DeSoto, TX 75115
972-224-1111
800-442-9685
FAX: 972-228-1982
mhschool.com

Offers good, solid information through a practical understandable presentation unencumbered by specialized jargon. Covers topics associated with special learners.

480 pages

6513 Families Writing

Alliance for Parental Involvement in Education
PO Box 59
E Chatham, NY 12060
518-392-6900
FAX: 518-392-6900

This book is full of writing activities and examples of ways writing can be encouraged and enjoyed in the home. *$14.99*

6514 Family Math

Alliance for Parental Involvement in Education
PO Box 59
E Chatham, NY 12060
518-392-6900
FAX: 518-392-6900

Here are dozens of interesting activities to share with your children. *$18.00*

6515 Getting the Best Bite of the Apple

Alliance for Parental Involvement in Education
PO Box 59
E Chatham, NY 12060 **518-392-6900**
FAX: 518-392-6900

This book takes a hard critical look at public school. The author is a parent who is also a former public school classroom teacher, school psychologist and principal. *$11.95*

6516 Home Education Resource Packet for New York State

Longview Publishing
R9 Kinderhook Street
Chatham, NY 12037 **518-392-6900**
FAX: 518-392-6900

For those considering home education in New York State, a packet containing the complete NYS Home Instruction Regulation, the laws referred to in the regulation, how to comply, resource listings, curriculum providers, support groups and more. *$8.00*

Paperback

6517 Homeschooling for Excellence

Alliance for Parental Involvement in Education
PO Box 59
E Chatham, NY 12060 **518-392-6900**
FAX: 518-392-6900

Children will learn if we recognize and respect their different interests and abilities and give them a chance to develop them. *$11.99*

6518 In Their Own Way

Alliance for Parental Involvement in Education
PO Box 59
E Chatham, NY 12060 **518-392-6900**
FAX: 518-392-6900

For the parents whose children are not thriving in school, Armstrong offers insight into individual learning styles. *$11.95*

6519 Inclusive & Heterogeneous Schooling: Assessment, Curriculum, and Instruction

Brookes Publishing
PO Box 10624
Baltimore, MD 21285 **410-337-9580**
800-638-3775
FAX: 410-337-8539
e-mail: custserv@brookespublishing.com
www.brookespublishing.com

Presents methods for successfully restructuring classrooms to enable all students, particularly those with disabilities, to flourish. Provides specific strategies for assessment, collaboration, classroom management, and age-specific instruction. *$34.95*

448 pages Paperback
ISBN 1-557662-02-9

6520 LD Child and the ADHD Child: Ways Parents & Professionals Can Help

1406 Plaza Drive
Winston Salem, NC 27103
800-222-9796
FAX: 336-768-9194
e-mail: blairpub@aol.com
www.blairpub.com

Carolyn Sakowski, President
John F Blair, Publisher

Book about learning disabilities available to parents. Stevens cuts through the jargon and complex theories which usually characterize books on the subject to present effective and practical techniques that parents can employ to help their child succeed at home and at school. New edition adds information about ADHD children. *$12.95*

201 pages Paperback
ISBN 0-895871-42-4

6521 Learning All the Time

Alliance for Parental Involvement in Education
PO Box 59
E Chatham, NY 12060 **518-392-6900**
FAX: 518-392-6900

Writes about how to aid young children in learning and how to allow them to figure things out for themselves, with the same insight and love of children that was apparent in his book. *$12.00*

6522 Magic Feather

Alliance for Parental Involvement in Education
PO Box 59
E Chatham, NY 12060 **518-392-6900**
FAX: 518-392-6900

The Grangers were the victims of the special education system. Their son was mistested, mislabeled and more, but their story has a happy ending. *$9.95*

6523 Mainstreaming: A Practical Approach for Teachers

McGraw-Hill, School Publishing
220 E Danieldale Road
DeSoto, TX 75115 **972-224-1111**
800-442-9685
FAX: 972-228-1982
mhschool.com

Provides teachers, administrators and school psychologists with the background, techniques and strategies they need to offer appropriate services for mildly handicapped students in the mainstream classroom.

6524 Making the Writing Process Work

Brookline Books
PO Box 1047
Cambridge, MA 02238 **617-868-0360**
800-666-2665
FAX: 617-868-1772
e-mail: brooklinebks@delphi.com
www.brooklinebooks.com

Making the Writing Process Work: Strategies for Composition and Self-Regulation is geared toward students who have difficulty organizing their thoughts and developing their writing. The specific strategies teach students how to approach, organize, and produce a final written product. *$24.95*

240 pages Paperback
ISBN 1-57129 -10-9

6525 Negotiating the Special Education Maze: A Guide for Parents and Teachers

Spina Bifida Association of America
4590 MacArthur Boulevard
Suite 250
Washington, DC 20007 **202-944-3285**
800-621-3141
FAX: 202-944-3295
e-mail: sbaa@sbaa.org
www.sbaa.org

An excellent aid for the development of an effective special education program. *$19.00*

6526 **Nurturing Independent Learners Brookline Press**
PO Box 1047
Cambridge, MA 02238
617-868-0360
800-666-2665
FAX: 617-868-1772
e-mail: brooklinebks@delphi.com
www.brooklinebooks.com

Presents programs that effectively improve students' independence—the ability to manage their own learning—and explain how to implement them in the classroom. *$24.95*

256 pages Paperback
ISBN 1-57129 -47-8

6527 **One School at a Time: School Based Management**
Alliance for Parental Involvement in Education
PO Box 59
E Chatham, NY 12060
518-392-6900
FAX: 518-392-6900

School based management is a school-by-school approach to educational reform. Parents, students and other community members work with the principal, teachers and other members of the school staff to shape the schools the community wants. *$8.95*

6528 **Parent Teacher Packet**
Spina Bifida Association of America
4590 MacArthur Boulevard NW
Suite 250
Washington, DC 20007
202-944-3285
800-621-3141
FAX: 202-944-3295
e-mail: sbaa@sbaa.org
www.sbaa.org

Includes educational material, learning disabilities literature, children's book, social development and the person with spina bifida and one copy of each fact sheet. *$14.00*

6529 **Parent's Guide to the Montessori Classroom**
Alliance for Parental Involvement in Education
PO Box 59
E Chatham, NY 12060
518-392-6900
FAX: 518-392-6900

This guide gives a concise explanation of the meaning of Montessori. It describes in detail the Montessori program for children between the ages of three to six. *$5.95*

6530 **Rethinking Attention Deficit Disorder**
Brookline Books
PO Box 1047
Cambridge, MA 02238
617-868-0360
800-666-2665
FAX: 617-868-1772
e-mail: brooklinebks@delphi.com
www.brooklinebooks.com

In contrast to the common focus on behavioral symptoms of attention disorders, this book emphasizes internal factors that make attention regulation difficult. In-depth discussions of social, emotional, and academic consequences and appropriate interventions are provided. *$27.95*

250 pages Paperback
ISBN 1-57129 -37-0

6531 **School Information Packet**
Allergy and Asthma Network/Mothers of Asthmatics
2751 Prosperity Avenue
Suite 150
Fairfax, VA 22031
800-878-4403
FAX: 703-573-7794
www.aanma.org

Practical, medical, and legal information for school administrators and parents of students with asthma. *$7.00*

6532 **Scoffolding Student Learning**
Brookline Books
PO Box 1047
Cambridge, MA 02238
617-495-3682
800-666-2665
FAX: 617-868-1772
e-mail: brooklinebks@delphi.com
www.brooklinebooks.com

Collection of papers on the theory and practice of scoffolding—an interactive style of instructions that helps students develop more powerful thinking tools.. *$21.95*

180 pages Paperback
ISBN 1-571290-36-2

6533 **Sharing Nature with Children**
Alliance for Parental Involvement in Education
PO Box 59
E Chatham, NY 12060
518-392-6900
FAX: 518-392-6900

A book of wonderful games for exploring nature in a natural, comfortable way. *$7.95*

6534 **So Your Child Has a Learning Problem?**
CPPC
605 3rd Avenue
New York, NY 10158
212-476-9000
800-433-8234

Designed for parents of children who are encountering learning problems in the classroom. *$19.95*

160 pages

6535 **Study Power: Study Skills to Improve Your Learning and Your Grades: A Workbook**
Brookline Books
PO Box 1047
Cambridge, MA 02238
617-868-0360
800-666-2665
FAX: 617-868-1772
e-mail: brooklinebks@delphi.com
www.brooklinebooks.com

The techniques in the easy-to-use, self-teaching manual have yielded remarkable success for students from elementary to medical school, at all levels of intelligence and achievement. Key skills covered include: listening, note taking, concentration, summarizing, reading comprehension, memorization, test taking, preparing papers and reports, time management, and more. These abilities are vital to success throughout every stage of learning; the benefits will last a lifetime. 1999.ISBN 157129067X *$15.95*

Paperback 1998
ISBN 1-57129 -46-X

6536 **Symptoms and Treatment of Child's Learning**
Health Publishing Company
PO Box 3805
San Francisco, CA 94119
415-282-8585
FAX: 415-826-1470

Handbook for parents who need to know the symptoms and treatments of a child's learning and academic disorders. *$4.95*

6537 **Taking Charge Through Homeschooling**
Alliance for Parental Involvement in Education
PO Box 59
E Chatham, NY 12060
518-392-6900
FAX: 518-392-6900

While this book offers solid information and suggestions for educating children without school, it also offers concrete suggestions on ways home schoolers can unite to protect their rights and freedoms. *$12.95*

6538 **Teaching Children Self-Discipline**

Alliance for Parental Involvement in Education
PO Box 59
E Chatham, NY 12060
518-392-6900
FAX: 518-392-6900

Mr. Gordon draws on research findings and his experience helping parents and teachers. *$17.95*

6539 **Teaching Students with Learning Problems**

McGraw-Hill, School Publishing
220 E Danieldale Road
DeSoto, TX 75115
972-224-1111
800-442-9685
FAX: 972-228-1982
mhschool.com

Expanded coverage of learning strategies, generalization training, self-monitoring techniques, and techniques for increasing the time students spend on academic tasks.

608 pages

6540 **Teaching Young Children to Read Brookline Books**

PO Box 1047
Cambridge, MA 02238
617-868-0360
800-666-2665
FAX: 617-868-1772
e-mail: brooklinebks@delphi.com
www.brooklinebooks.com

Detailed instructions on teaching reading to preschoolers. Gradually develops full fluency. *$16.95*

192 pages Paperback
ISBN 0-57129 -48-6

6541 **Unlocking Potenial: College and Other Choi ces for People with LD and AD/HD**

Spina Bifida Association of America
4590 MacArthur Boulevard NW
Suite 250
Washington, DC 20007
202-944-3285
800-621-3141
FAX: 202-944-3295
e-mail: sbaa@sbaa.org
www.sbaa.org

An indespensible look for high school students with learning disabilities and AD/HD. Includes comprehensive listing of resources. *$22.95*

6542 **Vermont Interdependent Services Team Approach (VISTA)**

Brookes Publishing
PO Box 10624
Baltimore, MD 21285
410-337-9580
800-638-3775
FAX: 410-337-8539
e-mail: custserv@brookespublishing.com
www.brookespublishing.com

A guide to coordinating educational support services. This manual enables IEP team members to fulfill the related services provisions of IDEA as they make effective support services decisions using a collaborative team approach. *$27.95*

176 pages Spiral bound
ISBN 1-55766 -30-4

6543 **You are Your Child's First Teacher**

Alliance for Parental Involvement in Education
PO Box 59
E Chatham, NY 12060
518-392-6900
FAX: 518-392-6900

Presents principles of Waldorf early education in the home from birth to age six. *$12.95*

6544 **You, Your Child, and Special Education: A Guide to Making the System Work**

Brookes Publishing
PO Box 10624
Baltimore, MD 21285
410-337-9580
800-638-3775
FAX: 410-337-8539
e-mail: custserv@brookespublishing.com
www.brookespublishing.com

This book shows parents how to obtain the educational services their children rightfully deserve. It examines the internal workings of the education system, reveals the challenges that await, lists the services that are available, and discusses the rights that are federally guaranteed. Comes with a resource list, directions for filing a complaint, and explanations of relevant legislation and regulations. *$24.00*

272 pages Paperback
ISBN 1-55766 -15-4

Parenting: Spiritual

6545 **A Miracle to Believe In**

Option Institute and Fellowship
2080 S Undermountain Road
Sheffield, MA 01257
413-229-8737
800-562-7171
FAX: 413-229-8737
e-mail: happiness@option.org
www.option.org

A group of people from all walks of life come together and are transformed as they reach out, under the direction of the Kaufmans, to help a little boy the medical world has given up as hopeless. This heartwarming journey of loving a child back to life will inspire and presents a compelling new way to deal with life's traumas and difficulties. *$7.99*

379 pages Paperback
ISBN 0-44920 -08-2

6546 **After the Tears**

Centering Corporation
1531 N Saddle Creek Road
Omaha, NE 68104
402-553-1200
FAX: 402-533-0507
e-mail: j1200@aol.com
www.centering.org

Offers talk, articles on raising a child with a disability. This one book combines feelings and emotions of parents on the subject of raising their disabled child. *$11.00*

87 pages Paperback
ISBN 0-15602 -00-6

6547 **Before and After Zachariah**

Special Needs Project
324 State Street
Suite H
Santa Barbara, CA 93101
800-333-6867
FAX: 805-962-5087
www.specialneeds.com

This intimate chronicle of one family's life with a severely brain damaged child is recently back in print. *$7.95*

241 pages

6548 Bethy and the Mouse: A Father Remembers His Children with Disabilities

Brookline Books
PO Box 1047
Cambridge, MA 02238
617-868-0360
800-666-2665
FAX: 617-868-1772
e-mail: brooklinebks@delphi.com
www.brooklinebooks.com

A moving collection of poetry, photographs, and prose following a father's experiences with two disabled children—one with Down Syndrome and one with an underdeveloped brain. *$16.95*

184 pages Paperback
ISBN 0-57129 -35-4

6549 Dimensions: Visually Impaired Persons with Multiple Disabilities

American Foundation for the Blind/AFB Press
PO Box 1020
Sewickley, PA 15143
412-741-1142
800-232-3044
FAX: 412-741-0609
e-mail: afborders@abdintl.com
www.afb.org

Stephanie Biagioli, Marketing Coordinator

Twenty-one articles from the Journal of Visual Impairment and Blindness, present a wide range of approaches for working with persons with multiple disabilities. *$24.95*

116 pages Paperback
ISBN 0-89128 -63-0

6550 Disabled God: Toward a Liberatory Theology of Disability

Abingdon Press
201 Eighth Avenue S
S Nashville, TN 37202
615-749-6000
800-251-3320
FAX: 800-836-7802
www.abingdon.org

Dr. Rex Matthews, Senior Editor

Draws on themes of the disability rights movement to identify people with disabilities as members of a socially disadvantaged minority group rather than as individuals who need to adjust. Highlights the history of people with disabilities in the church and society. *$ 13.95*

27 pages Paperback
ISBN 0-68710 -01-2

6551 Dying and Disabled Children: Dealing with Loss and Grief

Haworth Press
10 Alice Street
Binghamton, NY 13904
607-722-5857
800-429-6784
FAX: 607-722-6362
e-mail: orders@haworthpress.com
www.haworthpress.com

Harold M Dick MD, Editor
S Harrington-Miller, Advertising

In this sensitive and compassionate look at terminally ill and disabled children, professionals from the medical community examine the stresses faced by their parents and siblings. They address the crucial element of communication in dealing with a child's serious illness. Ethical decision making, learning to recognize the child's suffering, and talking to children about death are honestly and clearly discussed. *$ 59.95*

153 pages Hardcover
ISBN 0-866567-59-3

6552 Eye-Centered: A Study of Spirituality of Deaf People

NCOD
7202 Buchanan Street
Landover Hills, MD 20784
301-577-1684
FAX: 301-577-1690
e-mail: ncod@erols.com
www.ncod.org

The findings of the five-year De Sales Project conducted by The National Catholic Office for the Deaf. *$12.00*

167 pages

6553 Giant Steps

Option Institute and Fellowship
2080 S Undermountain Road
Sheffield, MA 01257
413-229-8737
800-562-7171
FAX: 413-229-8737
e-mail: indigo@option.org
www.optionindigo.com

Kate Wilde

This book illustrates the powerful, life-changing Option Process Dialogue in action. Barry takes us on a very intimate journey presenting ten uplifting, in-depth portraits of young people engaged in transformative dialogues with him. The reader witnesses moments of extreme crisis involving rape, questions of sexuality, a dying parent, divorce, the prison of drugs as these people learn to break through their pain and triumph in the face of challenge and crisis. *$5.99*

351 pages Paperback
ISBN 0-449215-69-5

6554 Happiness is a Choice

Ballantine Books
2080 S Undermountain Road
Sheffield, MA 01257
413-229-8737
800-562-7171
FAX: 413-229-8737
e-mail: indigo@option.org
www.optionindigo.com

Kate Wilde

Happiness is a Choice represents the cutting edge of Barry Neil Kaufman's evolving teaching, focusing on empowering our moment of change, the moment in which we can make self-acceptance, inner peace, joy and love immediately tangible with these easy-to-use tools. This book takes us step by step on a journey to increase personal power. A book to cherish and to share, a book that will ignite the healing process. *$ 10.95*

284 pages Paperback
ISBN 0-449907-99-6

6555 How to Thrive, Not Just Survive

American Foundation for the Blind/AFB Press
PO Box 1020
Sewickley, PA 15143
412-741-1142
800-232-3044
FAX: 412-741-0609
e-mail: afborders@abdintl.com
www.afb.org

Stephanie Biagioli, Marketing Coordinator

Practical, hands-on guide for parents, teachers, and everyone involved in helping children develop the skills necessary for socialization, orientations and mobility, and leisure and recreational activities. Some of the subjects covered are eating, dressing, personal hygiene, self-esteem and etiquette. *$24.95*

104 pages Paperback
ISBN 0-89128 -48-7

6556 **Hug Just Isn't Enough**

Gallaudet University Bookstore
11030 S Langley Avenue
Chicago, IL 60628 **202-651-5488**
800-621-2736
FAX: 202-651-5489

Offers valuable information for the disabled. *$15.95*

94 pages Hardcover

6557 **In Time and with Love: Caring for the Special Needs Infant and Toddler, Second Edition**

Newmarket Press
18 E 48th Street
New York, NY 10017 **212-832-3575**
FAX: 212-832-3629
e-mail: sales@newmarketpress.com
www.newmarketpress.com

Ellen Simon, Sales Director

For families and caregivers of preteen and handicapped children in their first three years - more than one hundred tips for adjusting and coping. *$15.95*

208 pages
ISBN 1-557044-45-7

6558 **Little Children, Big Needs**

Exceptional Parent Library
120 Sylvan Avenue, Suite 10
PO Box 1807
Englewood Cliffs, NJ 07632
800-535-1910
FAX: 201-947-9376
e-mail: eplibrary@aol.com
www.eplibrary.com

Contains candid interviews with fifty families of children with a wide variety of disabilities. *$12.95*

6559 **Loving & Letting Go**

Centering Corporation
1531 N Saddle Creek Road
Omaha, NE 68104 **402-553-1200**
FAX: 402-533-0507
e-mail: j1200@aol.com
www.centering.org

For parents who decide to turn away from aggressive medical intervention for their critically ill newborn. *$5.95*

48 pages Paperback

6560 **Loving Justice**

Exceptional Parent Library
120 Sylvan Avenue, Suite 10
PO Box 1807
Englewood Cliffs, NJ 07632
800-535-1910
FAX: 201-947-9376
e-mail: eplibrary@aol.com
www.eplibrary.com

How the Americans with Disabilities Act affects religious institutions, including congregations, hospitals, nursing homes, seminaries, universities and more. *$10.00*

6561 **Misunderstood Child**

Gallery Bookshop
PO Box 270
Mendocino, CA 95460 **707-937-2665**
FAX: 707-937-3737
e-mail: info@gallerybooks.com
www.gallerybooks.com

A guide for parents with learning disabled children. *$ 8.95*

224 pages Paperback
ISBN 0-07057 -89-5

6562 **Nobody's Perfect: Living and Growing with Children Who Have Special Needs**

Brookes Publishing
PO Box 10624
Baltimore, MD 21285 **410-337-9580**
800-638-3775
FAX: 410-337-8539
e-mail: custserv@brookespublishing.com
www.brookespublishing.com

This book offers parents who have children with special needs a new and positive perspective on the challenges of family life. This book guides parents through the process of adaptation, describing specific strategies for success in balancing one's own life, developing a parenting partnership, and interacting with children, friends, relatives, professionals, and others. *$21.00*

352 pages Paperback
ISBN 1-55766 -43-X

6563 **Pastoral Care of the Mentally Disabled: Advancing Care of the Whole Person**

Haworth Press
10 Alice Street
Binghamton, NY 13904 **607-722-5857**
800-429-6784
FAX: 607-722-6362
e-mail: orders@haworthpress.com
www.haworthpress.com

S Harrington-Miller, Advertising

The beginning step to encourage a partnership for treating and evaluating patients with mental illness. It addresses the perceived roles of clergy and physicians for hearing the whole person which best occurs when medicine and ministry are linked. *$59.95*

116 pages Hardcover
ISBN 1-560246-65-0

6564 **Place for Everyone: A Guide for Special Education Bible Teaching**

Baptist Sunday School Board
127 Ninth Avenue N
Nashville, TN 37234
800-458-2772
FAX: 615-251-5933
www.bssb.com

Ron Brown, Team Leader
Doug Merritt, Manager

Begin a ministry for exceptional people in your church or strengthen an existing ministry. This resource helps pastors, ministers of education, and Sunday School directors understand educational and developmental issues in meeting special education needs. It will train leaders to minister in specific ways, emphasizing the need to reach disabled persons for Christ and for church membership through life-changing Bible study. *$19.95*

ISBN 0-767318-98-6

6565 **Special Education Bible Study**

LifeWay Christian Resources Southern Baptist Conv.
127 9th Avenue N
Nashville, TN 37234 **615-251-2000**
800-458-2772
FAX: 615-251-5017
e-mail: SpecialEd@lifeway.com
www.lifeway.com

Ellen Beene, Editor

Easy to use Bible study helps for mentally handicapped adults and youth. Features full-color pictures plus an emphasis on applying biblical truth to real-life situations. *$1.50*

48 pages Quarterly

6566 Special Education Teacher Packet

LifeWay Christian Resources Southern Baptist Conv.
127 9th Avenue N
Nashville, TN 37234
615-251-2000
800-458-2772
FAX: 615-251-5017
e-mail: SpecialEd@lifeway.com
www.lifeway.com

Ellen Beene, Editor

Resources to help teachers who lead Sunday School classes for adults and older youth with mental retardation. Includes teaching plans, posters, and one copy of Special Education Bible Study. *$10.00*

Quarterly

6567 Special Kind of Parenting

La Leche League International
PO Box 4079
Schaumburg, IL 60168
847-519-7730
FAX: 847-519-0035
e-mail: LLLI@llli.org
www.lalecheleague.org

Schielany Bautista, Marketing Assistant
Judy Torgus, Publications Director

Disabled children have special needs which challenge their parents' emotional and physical resources. This book guides parents through the problems and helps them discover their disabled child as an individual. The author covers both facts and feelings about handicaps, parents' reactions to the initial diagnosis, the grieving process, and effects on the marriage and the rest of the family. They also provide suggestions for choosing the programs and professionals best suited. *$7.50*

172 pages Softcover
ISBN 0-912500-27-1

6568 That All May Worship

Exceptional Parent Library
120 Sylvan Avenue, Suite 10
PO Box 1807
Englewood Cliffs, NJ 07632
800-535-1910
FAX: 201-947-9376
e-mail: mailto:eplibrary@aol.com
www.eplibrary.com

An interfaith handbook to assist congregations in welcoming people with disabilities to promote acceptance and full participation. *$10.00*

6569 Why Mine?

Centering Corporation
1531 N Saddle Creek Road
Omaha, NE 68104
402-553-1200
FAX: 402-533-0507
e-mail: j1200@aol.com
www.centering.org

Offers quotes from parents all across the country on their fears, feelings, marriage, the ill child and other children. *$3.25*

32 pages Paperback

6570 Worst Loss: How Families Heal from the Death of a Child

Exceptional Parent Library
120 Sylvan Avenue, Suite 10
PO Box 1807
Englewood Cliffs, NJ 07632
800-535-1910
FAX: 201-947-9376
e-mail: mailto:eplibrary@aol.com
www.eplibrary.com

Combines anecdotal case histories and the latest research to help bereaved parents cope with the loss of a child, offering practical and comforting advice on how to overcome the disabling symptoms of grief. *$25.00*

ISBN 0-805032-41-X

Professional

6571 A Practical Guide to Art Therapy Groups

Haworth Press
10 Alice Street
Binghamton, NY 13904
607-722-5857
800-429-6784
FAX: 607-722-6362
e-mail: orders@haworthpress.com
www.haworthpress.com

S Harrington-Miller, Advertising

Unique approaches, materials, and device will inspire you to tap into your own well of creativity to design your own treatment plans. It lays out the ingredients and the skills to get the results you want. *$64.95*

115 pages Hardcover
ISBN 0-789001-36-5

6572 ADHD Report

Guilford Press
72 Spring Street
New York, NY 10012
212-431-9800
800-365-7006
FAX: 212-966-6708
e-mail: info@guilford.com

Presents the most up-to-date information on the evaluation, diagnosis and management of ADHD in children, adolescents and adults. This important newsletter is an invaluable resource for all professionals interested in ADHD. *$49.95*

BiMonthly
ISSN 1065-8025

6573 Aging and Developmental Disability: Current Research, Programming, and Practice

Haworth Press
10 Alice Street
Binghamton, NY 13904
607-722-5857
800-429-6784
FAX: 607-722-6362
e-mail: orders@haworthpress.com
www.haworthpress.com

Joy Hammel PhD, OTR/L, Co-Editor
Susan M Nochajski PhD, OTR, Co-Editor
S Harrington-Miller, Advertising

Explores research findings and their implications for practice in relation to normative and disability-related aging experiences and issues. It discusses the effectiveness of specific intervention targeted toward aging adults with developmental disabilities such as Down's Syndrome, cerebral palsy, autism, and epilepsy, and offers suggestions for practice and future research in this area. *$39.95*

100 pages Hardcover
ISBN 0-789010-39-9

6574 American Association of Spinal Cord Injury Nurses

American Association of Spinal Cord Injury Nurses
7520 Astoria Boulevard
Jackson Heights, NY 11370 **718-397-4181**
FAX: 718-803-0414
www.aascin.org

Sara Lerman MPH, Program Manager

Disseminates information to nurses and others caring for spinal cord injured individuals. Membership in AASCIN represents registered and licensed practical and vocational nurses in the US and Canada who practice in the diverse SCI settings such as intensive care, acute care and long-term care; rehabilitation; home care; and outpatient care. There is a Nursing Research Program which funds research in the area of spinal cord impairment. Annual educational conference.

6575 American Forensic Association Journal

American Forensic Association
University of Wisconsin-River Falls
River Falls, WI 54022 **715-262-3605**
FAX: 715-425-9533
e-mail: james.wpratt@uwrf.edu

Communication disorders newsletter. *$25.00*

6576 American Journal of Art Therapy

Vermont College of Norwich University
Montpelier, VT 05602 **802-828-8540**
FAX: 802-828-8585
e-mail: mzimmerm@norwich.edu

Gladys Agell PhD ATR-BC HLM, Editor

Discusses the graphic and plastic arts as they contribute to human understanding, psycotherapy, rahabilitation and education. *$ 32.00*

35-40 pages Quarterly
ISSN 0007-47 4

6577 American Journal of Orthopsychiatry

American Orthopsychiatric Association
330 7th Avenue
18th Floor
New York, NY 10001 **212-564-5930**
FAX: 212-564-6180
e-mail: amerortho@aol.com

Joan Adler, Managing Editor
Ellen L Bassuk, Editor

Mental health issues from multidisciplinary and interprofessionals perspectives: clinical, research and expository approaches. *$45.00*

160 pages Quarterly

6578 American Journal of Physical Medicine

Lippincott, Williams & Wilkins
PO Box 1551
Hagerstown, MD 21741
800-638-3030
FAX: 301-824-7390
www.lww.com

Journal of the Association of Academic Psychiatrists. Articles covering research and clinical studies and applications of new equipment, procedures and therapeutic advances. *$45.00*

6579 American Journal of Psychiatry

American Psychiatric Publishing
1400 K Street NW
Washington, DC 20005 **202-682-6240**
800-368-5777
FAX: 202-789-2648
e-mail: mailto:accessnumber@psych.org
ajp.psychiatryonline.org

Nancy C Andreasen MD PhD, Editor-In-Chief

Peer-reviewed articles focus on developments in biological psychiatry as well as on treatment innovations and forensic, ethical, economic, and social topics. *$56.00*

Monthly

6580 American Journal of Public Health

American Public Health Association
1015 15th Street NW
Washington, DC 20005 **202-777-2742**
FAX: 202-777-2534
e-mail: comments@msmail.apha.org
www.apna.org

Dr. Mervyn Susser, Editor

Association journal containing professional articles and sections such as Notes from the Field and Association News. Single copies are $15.00. $50.00 per year for special consumer membership.

Monthly
ISSN 0090-00 6

6581 American Journal on Mental Retardation

American Association on Mental Retardation
444 N Capitol Street NW
Washington, DC 20001 **202-387-1968**
800-424-3688
FAX: 202-387-2193
e-mail: aamr@access.digex.net
www.aamr.org

Bruce Appelgen, Director Publications

Articles cover biological, behavioral, and educational research: theory papers; and reviews of research literature on specific aspects of mental retardation. *$142.00*

112 pages BiMonthly

6582 American Rehabilitation

Rehabilitation Services Administration
330 C Street SW
3033 Mes
Washington, DC 20202 **202-205-8296**
FAX: 202-205-9874
e-mail: frank.romano@ed.gov
www.ed.gov/pubs/AmericanRehab

Frank Romano, Editor

Covers medical, social and employment aspects of vocational rehabilitation. *$10.00*

40 pages Quarterly

6583 **Annals of Otology, Rhinology and Larynology**

Annals Publishing Company
4507 Laclede Avenue
Saint Louis, MO 63108 **314-367-4987**
FAX: 314-367-4988
e-mail: manager@annals.com
www.annals.com

Kenneth A Cooper Jr, Business Manager

Original, peer-reviewed articles in the fields of otolaryngology - head and neck medicine and surgery, broncho-esophagology, audiology, speech, pathology, allery, and maxillofacial surgery. Official journal of the American Laryngological Association/American Broncho-Esophagological Association. *$170.00*

112 pages Monthly

6584 **Archives of Neurology**

American Medical Association
515 N State Street
Chicago, IL 60610 **312-464-5000**
FAX: 312-464-4184
e-mail: ama-subs@ama-assn.org
www.archneurol.com

Roger Rosenberg MD, Editor
Nawn Gupta PhD, VP Publishing/Group Publisher
Peter J Murphy, Publishing/Sales/Marketing Dir.

Mission is to publish scientific information primarily important to those physicians caring for people with neurologic disorders, but also for those interested in the structure and function of the normal and diseased nervous system. *$235.00*

198 pages Monthly

6585 **Art Therapy**

American Art Therapy Association
1202 Allanson Road
Mundelein, IL 60060 **847-949-6064**
FAX: 847-556-4580

Nancy Stygar

Publishes articles on the uses of art in the education, enrichment, development and treatment of disabled people. *$10.00*

76+ pages Quarterly
ISSN 0742-16 6

6586 **Careers & the DisABLED Magazine**

Equal Opportunity Publications
445 Broad Hollow Road
Suite 425
Melville, NY 11747 **631-421-9421**
FAX: 631-421-0359
e-mail: jschneider@eop.com
www.eop.com

John R Miller III, President/Publisher
James Schneider, Editorial Director

A career magazine for professional career seekers who have disabilities. Profiles disabled people who have achieved successful careers. Features a career section in Braille, career guide. *$10.00*

64 pages 3X 1987

6587 **Clinician's Practical Guide to Attention-Deficit/Hyperactivity Disorder**

Brookes Publishing
PO Box 10624
Baltimore, MD 21285
800-638-3775
FAX: 410-337-8539
www.brookespublishing.com

Quick reference volume with comprehensive data on psychoeducational and neuropsychological assessment, related symptoms, drug and counseling therapies and critical issues. *$39.95*

368 pages 1999
ISBN 1-557663-58-0

6588 **Colon Health: Key to a Vibrant Life**

Norwalk Press
Prescott, AZ **928-445-5567**
FAX: 928-445-5567

Includes complete glossary of terms and index of referrals.

6589 **Complete Guide to Cancer Prevention**

Harper Collins Publishers/Basic Books
10 E 53rd Street
New York, NY 10022 **212-207-7000**
FAX: 212-207-7901

A comprehensive guide to preventing cancer using nutrition in combination with preventative environmental and psychological measures.

1988

6590 **Connections Newsletter**

Kessler Institute for Rehabilitation
1199 Pleasant Valley Way
W Orange, NJ 07052 **973-731-3600**
888-KES-SLER
FAX: 973-243-6992

Maura Bergen, Editor/Public Relations Coordin.
Maria Anan, Editor/N. NJSCI System Coord.
Karen Hwang, Editor

Quarterly newsletter for individuals with a spinal cord injury. Funded by the Northern New Jersey Spinal Cord Injury System.

Quarterly-Free

6591 **Conquering the Darkness: One Story of Reco vering from a Brain Injury**

Paragon House
2700 University Avenue W
Suite 200
Saint Paul, MN 55114 **651-644-3087**
800-447-3709
FAX: 800-494-0997
e-mail: info@paragonhouse.com
www.paragonhouse.com

Rosemary Yokoi, Publicity Department

The course of recovery from a brain injury by a woman who lived through it. *$15.95*

420 pages 1999
ISBN 1-557787-63-8

6592 **Controlling Asthma**

American Lung Association
61 Broadway
New York, NY 10006
212-315-8700
FAX: 212-315-8870
e-mail: info@lungusa.org
www.lungusa.org

For parents of children with asthma, this news magazine tells how parents can help their child deal with the many problems presented by asthma.

16 pages

6593 **Counseling Parents of Children with Chronic Illness or Disability**

Brookes Publishing
PO Box 10624
Baltimore, MD 21285
410-337-9580
800-638-3775
FAX: 410-337-8539
e-mail: custserv@brookespublishing.com
www.brookespublishing.com

$23.00

144 pages Paperback
ISBN 1-85433 -91-8

6594 **Diabetes Self-Management**

RA Rapaport Publishing
150 W 22nd Street
New York, NY 10011
212-989-0200
FAX: 212-989-4786

James Hazlett, Editor

Publishes practical how-to information, focusing on the day-to-day and long-term aspects of diabetes in a positive and upbeat style. Gives subscribers up-to-date news, facts and advice to help them maintain their wellness and make informed decisions regarding their health. *$18.00*

BiMonthly

6595 **Disability Analysis Handbook**

American Board of Disability Analysts
345 24th Avenue N
Suite 200
Nashville, TN 37203
615-327-2984
FAX: 615-327-9235
e-mail: americanbd@aol.com

Alex Horwitz MD, Executive Officer

Official newsletter of the American Board of Disability Analysts; features Healthnews Headlines, Meeting Calendar, Application Packet and much more. Free to members; $20 per year for non-members. *$60.00*

396 pages
ISBN 0-787226-70-x

6596 **Educating Children with Disabilities A Transdisciplinary Approach, Third Edition**

Brookes Publishing
PO Box 10624
Baltimore, MD 21285
800-638-3775
FAX: 410-337-8539
www.brookespublishing.com

Widely respected textbook presents you with the strategies you need for developing an inclusive curriculum, integrating health care and educational programs and addressing needs and concerns. *$38.00*

512 pages 1996
ISBN 1-557662-46-0

6597 **Education and Training in Mental Retardation and Developmental Disabilities**

Council for Exceptional Children
1110 N Glebe Road
Suite 300
Arlington, VA 22201
703-620-3660
FAX: 703-264-9494
www.cec.sped.org

Janice Burdick, President

A medium for continuing education for teachers and practitioners by providing timely information about the direction, management and accountability of special education programs for individuals with mental retardation and developmental disabilities. Individual, $30; Institution, $75.

Quarterly

6598 **Ethical Conflicts in Management of Home Care**

Springer Publishing Company
536 Broadway
New York, NY 10012
212-431-4370
877-687-7476
FAX: 212-941-7842
e-mail: marketing@springerpub.com
www.springerpub.com

Annette Imperati, Marketing/Sales Director

Offers answers to the questions what is case management and why does it raise ethical issues. *$29.95*

288 pages

6599 **Evaluation of the Association for Children with Learning Disabilities**

National Center for State Courts
300 Newport Avenue
Williamsburg, VA 23185
757-259-7575
800-877-1233
FAX: 757-564-2028
www.ncsconline.org

Final report on children with learning disabilities training institute. *$6.96*

116 pages Manuscript

6600 **Failure to Thrive and Pediatric Undernutrition: A Transdisciplinary Approach**

Brookes Publishing
PO Box 10624
Baltimore, MD 21285
410-337-9580
800-638-3775
FAX: 410-337-8539
e-mail: custserv@brookespublishing.com
www.brookespublishing.com

Offers comprehensive coverage of pediatric undernutrition complete with assessment and intervention techniques. Theoretical as well as practical concerns such as epidemiology, nutrition, medical issues, feeding, families, history, research, and community programs are addressed. A family-centered approach shows practitioners how to enhance treatment by capitalizing on family strengths and acknowledging the impact of larger issues such as culture, social environment, and public policy. *$62.95*

592 pages Hardcover 1998
ISBN 1-55766 -48-3

6601 **Families in Recovery**

Brookes Publishing
PO Box 10624
Baltimore, MD 21285
410-337-9580
800-638-3775
FAX: 410-337-8539
e-mail: custserv@brookespublishing.com
www.brookespublishing.com

This book teaches professionals how to use each families strengths to promote recovery. The authors demonstrate effective, family-focused intervention techniques developed in their combined 35 years of practice. Motivational techniques and stress reducers for counselors are also provided. *$34.00*

352 pages Paperback 1997

ISBN 1-55766 -64-9

6602 **Family and Community Health**

Aspen Publishers
7201 McKinney Circle
Frederick, MD 21704
301-698-7100
800-234-1660
FAX: 301-695-7931
www.aspenpublishers.com

Peer-view journal addressing the information needs of health-care practitioners. *$124.00*

Quarterly

6603 **Health Care Management Review**

Aspen Publishers
7201 McKinney Circle
Frederick, MD 21704
301-698-7100
800-234-1660
FAX: 301-695-7931
www.aspenpublishers.com

Provides health care administrators with useful information on health care management. *$145.00*

6604 **Health Technology Trends**

Emergency Care Research Institute (ECRI)
5200 Butler Pike
Plymouth Meeting, PA 19462
610-825-6000
FAX: 610-834-1275
e-mail: info@ecri.org
www.ecri.org

Damian Carlson, Associate Editor

Provides analysis and information about health care technology to administrators and health care providers. *$275.00*

12 pages Monthly

6605 **Home Health Care Services Quarterly**

Haworth Press
10 Alice Street
Binghamton, NY 13904
607-722-5857
800-429-6784
FAX: 607-722-6362
e-mail: orders@haworthpress.com
www.haworthpress.com

W June Simmons, Editor
S Harrington-Miller, Advertising

Professional journal in book format. *$75.00*

Quarterly

6606 **Immune Deficiency Foundation Newsletter**

Immune Deficiency Foundation
40 W Chesapeake Avenue
Suite 308
Towson, MD 21204
410-321-6647
800-296-4433
FAX: 410-321-9165
e-mail: idf@primaryimmune.org
www.primaryimmune.org

Thomas L Moran, President
Stacy Ledbetter, Office Manager

Offers information on immune deficiencies. How to treat them, what they are and more.

4-6 pages

6607 **Including Students with Severe and Multiple Disabilities in Typical Classrooms**

Brookes Publishing
PO Box 10624
Baltimore, MD 21285
410-337-9580
800-638-3775
FAX: 410-337-8539
e-mail: custserv@brookespublishing.com
www.brookespublishing.com

Straightforward resource gives you the guidance you need to educate learners who have one or more sensory impairments in addition to cognitive and physical disabilities. Offers numerous ideas for modifying the general education curriculum. *$35.00*

244 pages Paperback 1996

ISBN 1-557662-39-8

6608 **Informer**

Simon Foundation
PO Box 835
Wilmette, IL 60091
847-864-3913
800-237-4666
FAX: 847-864-9758
www.simonfoundation.org

Cheryle B Gartley, President

Publishes items of interest to people with bladder or bowel incontinence, including medical articles, helpful devices, publications and a pen pal list. Quarterly newsletter.

6609 **Issues in Law and Medicine**

National Legal Center for the Medically Dependent
3 S Sixth Street
Terre Haute, IN 47807
812-232-0103
FAX: 812-232-0103

James Bopp Jr, Editor-in-Chief
Larry Ligget, Subscriptions

A peer-reviewed journal providing technical and informational assistance to attorneys, health care professionals, educators, and administrators concerned with severely disabled persons of all ages who may be subjected to discrimination in the delivery of medical care. *$89.00*

124 pages 3x Year

ISSN 8756-81 0

6610 **JAMA: The Journal of the American Medical Association**

American Medical Association
515 N State Street
Chicago, IL 60610
312-464-5000
FAX: 312-464-2580
e-mail: ama.jama
jama.ama-assn.org

Roger Rosenberg MD, Editor
Peter Payerli, Publisher

Articles cover all aspects of medical research and clinical medicine. *$66.00*

6611 Journal of Addictions and Offender Counseling

American Counseling Association
5999 Stevenson Avenue
Alexandria, VA 22304
800-347-6647
800-473-2329
FAX: 703-823-6862
www.counseling.org

Jane Carroll, Editor
Carolyn Baker, Publications Director

Contains articles of interest to professionals in the field of addictions and offender counseling and focuses on descriptions of prevention and treatment programs, theoretical and philosophocal rationales for programs with juvenile and adult offenders, and descriptions of research conducted on rehabilitation programs with offenders and public offender counselors. It is also open to literature focusing on the attitudes and behaviors of addictions and offender counselors *$30.00*

64 pages Bi-Annually

6612 Journal of Adolescent Health Care

655 Avenue of the Americas
New York, NY 10010
212-989-5800
FAX: 212-633-3990
www.elsevier.com/locate/jadohea

Micheal Targwwsk, Advertising Representative

Peer-reviewed publication for the multidisciplinary study of adolescent medicine and health care. *$7.00*

6613 Journal of Applied Rehabilitation Counseling

National Rehabilitation Counseling Association
8807 Sudley Road
Suite 102
Manassas, VA 20110
703-361-2077
FAX: 703-361-2489
e-mail: nrcaoffice@aol.com

Debra Harley, Editor
Ellen Fabian, Associate Editor
Hal Cain, Book and Media Review Editor

Articles on counseling history, research and practice of interest in rehabilitation. $20.00 for individuals, $35.00 institutional. *$20.00*

Quarterly

6614 Journal of Children's Communication Development

CEC Div for Childrens' Communication Development
1920 Association Drive
Reston, VA 20191
703-620-3660
FAX: 703-312-9193

Alexander Brice, Editor

Contains scholarly articles pertaining to the many aspects of communication disorders in children, encompassing speech, language, hearing and learning disabilities. *$16.00*

2x Year

6615 Journal of Cognitive Rehabilitation

Neuroscience Publishers
6555 Carrollton Avenue
Indianapolis, IN 46220
317-257-9672
FAX: 317-257-9674
e-mail: nsc@netdirect.net
www.neuroscience.cnter.com

Odie L Bracy III PhD, Editor
Sandra Reichle, Production Manager

Publication for therapists, family and patient, designed to provide information relevant to the rehabilitation of impairment resulting from brain injury. *$40.00*

36-48 pages Quarterly

6616 Journal of Employment Counseling

American Counseling Association
5999 Stevenson Avenue
Alexandria, VA 22304
800-347-6647
800-473-2329
FAX: 703-823-6862
www.counseling.org

Robert Drummond, Editor

$20.00

Quarterly

6617 Journal of Head Trauma Rehabilitation

Aspen Publishers
200 Orchard Ridge Drive
Gaithersburg, MD 20878
301-698-7100
800-234-1660
FAX: 301-695-7931
www.aspenpublishers.com

Scholarly journal designed to provide information on clinical management and rehabilitation of the head-injured for the practicing professional. Published bimonthly. *$119.00*

128 pages

6618 Journal of Humanistic Education and Development

American Counseling Association
5999 Stevenson Avenue
Alexandria, VA 22304
800-347-6647
800-473-2329
FAX: 703-823-6862
www.counseling.org

Richard J Hazler, Editor

$12.00

Quarterly

6619 Journal of Multicultural Counseling and Development

American Counseling Association
5999 Stevenson Avenue
Alexandria, VA 22304
800-347-6647
800-473-2329
FAX: 703-823-6862
www.counseling.org

Frederick D Harper, Editor

$14.00

Quarterly

6620 Journal of Rehabilitation

National Rehabilitation Association (NRA)
633 S Washington Street
Alexandria, VA 22314
703-836-0850
FAX: 703-836-0848
TTY:7038360849
e-mail: info@nationalrehab.org
www.nationalrehab.org

Paul Leung, Editor

This journal offers information on rehabilitation services and programs for the disabled and the professional. *$12.50*

100 pages Quarterly

6621 Journal of Religion, Disability & Health

Haworth Press
10 Alice Street
Binghamton, NY 13904 **607-722-5857**
800-429-6784
FAX: 607-722-6362
e-mail: orders@haworthpress.com
www.haworthpress.com

Wiliam Gaventa MD, Co-Editor
David Coulter MD, Co-Editor
S Harrington-Miller, Advertising/Journal Liaison

This journal aims to inform religious professionals about developments in the field of disability and rehabilitation in order to facilitate greater contributions on the part of pastors, religious educators and pastoral counselors. *$60.00*

Quarterly

6622 Journal of Social Work in Disabilty & Rehabilitation

Haworth Press
10 Alice Street
Binghamton, NY 13904 **607-722-5857**
800-429-6784
FAX: 607-722-6362
e-mail: orders@haworthpress.com
www.haworthpress.com

John T Oardeck PhD, Editor
S Harrington-Miller, Advertising

Presents and explores issues related to disabilities and social policy, practice, research, and theory. Reflecting the broad scope of social work in disabilty practice, this interdisciplinary journal examines vital issues aspects of the field — from innovative practice methods, legal issues, and literature reviews to program descriptions and cuttinf-edge practice research.

Quarterly

6623 Modern Healthcare

Crain Communications
360 N Michigan Avenue
Chicago, IL 60601 **312-649-5200**
FAX: 312-397-5510
www.crain.com

Brenda Stewart, Publishing Director

Business news magazine for healthcare professionals. *$ 7.00*

Weekly

6624 Most Frequently Asked Questions About Lobbying and CILs (Revised 3/98)

Independent Living Research Utilization ILRU
2323 S Shepherd Drive
Suite 1000
Houston, TX 77019 **713-520-0232**
FAX: 713-520-5785
www.ilru.org

This FAQ was written to provide an overview of the federal laws and regulations about lobbying which apply to non-profit organizations. It also covers what constitutes advocacy and what distinguishes it from lobbying. This FAQ is not intended to be a substitute for sound guidance from your organization's attorney and accountant. Consult them before engaging in these activities.

10 pages

6625 National Clearinghouse of Rehabilitation Training Materials

5202 N Richmond Hill Drive
Stillwater, OK 74078 **405-624-7650**
800-223-5219
FAX: 405-624-0695
www.nchrtm.okstate.edu

Judy Seefeld, Director
Carolyn Cash, Information Coordinator

Newsletter produced quarterly to provide information and opportunities to learn more about related fields.

Quarterly

6626 Occupational Therapy in Mental Health

Haworth Press
10 Alice Street
Binghamton, NY 13904 **607-722-5857**
800-429-6784
FAX: 607-722-6362
e-mail: orders@haworthpress.com
www.haworthpress.com

Marie Louise Blount AM BS, Co-Editor
Mary Donohue, Co-Editor
S Harrington-Miller, Advertising/Journal Liaison

An essential journal for all OT's in mental health fields. Provides professionals with a forum in which to discuss challenges. *$ 60.00*

Quarterly

6627 PDP Products

14524 61st Street Ct N
PO Box 2009
Stillwater, MN 55082 **651-439-8865**
FAX: 651-439-0421
e-mail: products@pdppro.com
www.pdppro.com

PDP Products acquires books and therapy materials recommended or developed by therapists and makes those materials available at PDP courses and through mail order.

6628 Parkinsons Report

National Parkinson Foundation
1501 NW 9th Avenue
Bob Hope Road
Miami, FL 33136 **305-547-6666**
800-327-4545
FAX: 305-243-4403
e-mail: mailbox@parkinson.org
www.parkinson.org

Julian Pearson, Administrator

Articles, reports and news on Parkinson's disease and the activities of the National Parkinson Foundation.

32 pages Qarterly

6629 Part B News

United Communications Group
11300 Rockville Pike
Rockville, MD 20852 **301-816-8950**
FAX: 301-816-8945
www.ucg.com

Washington news practical strategies for maximizing Medicare Part B.

6630 Physical & Occupational Therapy in Geriatrics...Current Trends in Geriatrics Rehab

Haworth Press
10 Alice Street
Binghamton, NY 13904
607-722-5857
800-429-6784
FAX: 607-722-6362
e-mail: orders@haworthpress.com
www.haworthpress.com

Ellen Dunievey Taira OTR/L, Editor
Jodi Carison MS, OTR/L, Assistant Editor
S Harrington-Miller, Advertising

Focuses on current practice and emerging issues in the care of the older client, including long-term care in institutional and community settings, crisis intervention, and innovative programming; the entire range of problems experienced by the elderly; and the current skills needed for working with older clients.

Quarterly

6631 Physical Therapy

American Physical Therapy Association
1111 N Fairfax Street
Alexandria, VA 22314
703-684-2782
800-999-2782
FAX: 703-684-7343
TTY:703-683-6748
www.apta.org

Jan Reynolds, Managing Editor

Contains articles on clinical and testing procedures. *$45.00*

Monthly

6632 Professional Report

National Rehabilitation Association (NRA)
633 S Washington Street
Alexandria, VA 22314
703-836-0850
FAX: 703-836-0848
TTY:703-836-0849
e-mail: info@nationalrehab.org
www.nationalrehab.org

Association newsletter containing news, programs and information of interest to the Association and its members.

6633 Provider Magazine

American Health Care Association
1201 L Street NW
Washington, DC 20005
202-842-4444
800-321-0343
FAX: 202-842-3860

Magazine for long-term healthcare professionals. *$48.00*

72 pages Monthly
ISSN 0888-03 2

6634 Psychiatric Rehabilitation Journal

940 Commonwealth Avenue W
Boston, MA 02215
617-353-3549
FAX: 617-353-9209
e-mail: leroys@bu.edu
www.bu.edu/cpr

LeRoy Spaniol PhD, Executive Publisher

Discusses issues, programs and research on psychiatric rehabilitation. Magazine for $55 for individual, $105 for organizations, $10 mailing to Canada, $20 mailing to other countries. Published quarterly.

112 pages Quarterly 1976

6635 Public Health Reports

Oxford Journals
JFK Federal Building
Room 1855
Boston, MA 02203
513-636-0257
FAX: 617-565-4260
e-mail: robert.rinsky@chmcc.org
phr.oupjournals.org

Robert Rinsky PhD, Editor

Scholarly articles on issues that relate to public health and the healthcare system. *$13.00*

BiMonthly

6636 Public Health/State Capitals

Wakeman/Walworth
300 N Washington Street
Alexandria, VA 22314
703-768-9600
800-876-2545
FAX: 703-768-9690
e-mail: newsletters@statecapitals.com
www.statecapitals.com

Keyes Walworth, Publisher
Christine Ryan, Editor

Digest of state and municipal health care financing and legislation, including disease control, medicaid, AIDS, abortion, substance abuse programs, cancer prevention such as smoking restrictions, mental health and disability programs, regulation of hospitals & nursing homes, food safety, medical policies, health insurance for children, home regulation, managerial care, public health issues, pest control, and water quality. Issued weekly-52 issues/year. *$245.00*

10 pages

6637 Ragged Edge Magazine

Advocado Press
PO Box 145
Louisville, KY 40201
502-894-9492
FAX: 502-899-9562
e-mail: circulation@raggededgemagazine.com
www.raggededgemagazine.com

Mary Johnson, Editor

Ragged Edge magazine is the successor to The Disability Rag, and covers disability in America today: rights, culture, ideas and controversy. Here you'll find new voices speaking out about disability culture and lives; you'll get the newest cutting-edge thinking on headlines in the news today on genetic discrimination, assisted suicide, healthcare policy. *$17.50*

40 pages BiMonthly
ISSN 0749-95 6

6638 Rehabilitation Counseling Bulletin

American Counseling Association
5999 Stevenson Avenue
Alexandria, VA 22304
800-347-6647
FAX: 800-473-2329
TTY:7038236862
www.counseling.org

Randall M Parker, Editor

A research journal for professionals in rehabilitation counseling. *$18.00*

64 pages Quarterly

6639 **Rehabilitation Psychology**

Springer Publishing Company
536 Broadway
New York, NY 10012 **212-431-4370**
877-687-7476
FAX: 212-941-7842
e-mail: marketing@springerpub.com
www.springerpub.com

Annette Imperati, Marketing/Sales Director

Publishes articles addressing psychological and behavioral aspects of rehabilitation. *$28.00*

6640 **Reversing Diabetes**

AOL Time Warner Books Groups
1271 Avenue of the Americas
New York, NY 10020 **212-522-7200**
FAX: 212-522-7989
e-mail: publicity@warnerbooks.com
www.twbookmark.com

Dr. Whitaker argues that conventional treatments are unnecessary, even dangerous, and shows how diabetics can naturally control their condition through diet and exercise.

1987

6641 **Saint Anthony's Healthcare Resources Alert**

Saint Anthony Publishing
11410 Isaac Newton Square
Reston,, VA 20190 **703-708-1515**
800-632-0123
FAX: 703-707-5700

Suzanne Vel, Jr Product Manager

News, resources and services for practicing healthcare professionals.

6642 **Sexuality and Disability**

Human Sciences Press
233 Spring Street
New York, NY 10013 **212-620-8000**
800-221-9369
FAX: 212-463-0742
www.wkap.com

A journal devoted to the psychological and medical aspects of sexuality in rehabilitation and community settings. The journal features original scholarly articles that address the psychological and medical aspects of sexuality in the field of rehabilitation, case studies, clinical practice reports, and guidelines for clinical practice. Plenum Publishers is now part of Kluner Academic Publishers. Journal fulfillment in the NYC office as before for HSP and Plenum Journals. *$160.00*

64 pages Quarterly
ISSN 0146-10 4

6643 **Simon Foundation for Continence**

PO Box 835-F
Wilmette, IL 60091 **847-864-3913**
800-237-4666
FAX: 847-864-9758
e-mail: simoninfo@simonfoundation.org
www.simonfoundation.org

Dedicated to providing assistance and support to those suffering incontinence. The work includes aid to those afflicted with incontinence, aid to families of those suffering incontinence, creating public awareness, reviewing relevant legislation and encouraging the medical professions' interest in this long-neglectd area of healthcare.

1983

6644 **Smart But Stuck: Emotional Aspects of Learning Disabilities and Imprisoned Intelligence**

Haworth Press
10 Alice Street
Binghamton, NY 13904 **607-722-5857**
800-429-6784
FAX: 607-722-6362
e-mail: orders@haworthpress.com
www.haworthpress.com

S Harrington-Miller, Advertising

Elaborates on new research about imprisoned intelligence and the emotional consequences of learning disabilities. It is also for psychoterapists, educators, school social workers, medical personnel, people dealing with prisons, etc. It helps those who struggle with learning disabilities (and people who help them) build self esteem, face LD obstacles, bypass weaknesses, and enhance strenghts. *$34.95*

228 pages Hardcover
ISBN 0-789014-66-1

6645 **Socialization Games for Persons with Disabilities**

Charles C Thomas
2600 S First Street
Springfield, IL 62704 **217-789-8980**
800-258-8980
FAX: 217-789-9130
e-mail: books@ccthomas.com
www.ccthomas.com

This text will assist those who want to teach severely multiple disabled students by providing information on: general principles of intervention and classroom organization; managing the behavior of students; physically managing students and using adaptive equipment; teaching eating skills; teaching toileting, dressing , and hygiene skills; teaching cognition, communication, and socialization skills; teaching independent living skills; and teaching infants and preschool students. *$24.95*

140 pages Paperback
ISBN 0-39806 -73-4

6646 **Strategic Health Care Marketing**

Health Care Communications
11 Heritage Lane
Rye, NY 10580 **845-687-2328**

Michele Von Dambrowski, Editor

Marketing strategies for hospitals, medical group practices, home health services, urgent care centers.

12 pages Monthly

6647 **Strategies for Teaching Learners with Special Needs**

McGraw-Hill, School Publishing
220 E Danieldale Road
DeSoto, TX 75115 **972-224-1111**
800-442-9685
FAX: 972-228-1982
mhschool.com

This is a text that helps special educators develop the full range of teaching competencies needed to be effective.

560 pages

6648 **Teaching Adults with Learning Disabilities**

Krieger Publishing Company
PO Box 9542
Melbourne, FL 32902 **321-724-9542**
800-724-0025
FAX: 321-951-3671
e-mail: info@krieger-publishing.com
www.krieger-publishing.com

Designed to teach literacy providers and classroom instructors how to recognize specific learning disability (LD) patterns and block reading, spelling, writing and arithmetic skills in students of all ages. One of the major problems faced by literary providers is keeping low-skill adults involved in basic education programs long enough to increase their literacy skills to the level of success. Shows instructors in adult education how to modify teaching strategies. *$25.50*

160 pages
ISBN 0-894649-10-8

6649 **TeamRehab Report**

23805 Stuart Ranch Road, Suite 235
PO Box 8987
Malibu, CA 90265
800-543-4116
FAX: 310-317-9644

Andria Segedy, Publisher
Kim Pfaff, Managing Editor

A magazine for rehab professionals who prescribe, purchase or recommend assistive technology and related services for clients who are permanently disabled. *$24.00*

48 pages Monthly

6650 **VA Practitioner**

Cahners Publishing Company
275 Washington Street
Newton, MA 02458 **617-964-3030**
FAX: 617-558-4700

The magazine for health care professionals of the Department of Veterans Affairs.

Monthly

6651 **Women with Visible & Invisible Disabilitie es: Multiple Intersections, Issues, Therapies**

Haworth Press
10 Alice Street
Binghamton, NY 13904 **607-722-5857**
800-429-6784
FAX: 607-722-6362
e-mail: orders@haworthpress.com
www.haworthpress.com

Martha E Banks PhD, Co-Editor
Ellyn Kaschak PhD, Co-Editor
S Harrington-Miller, Advertising

Addesses the issues faced by women with disabilities, examines the social construction of disability, and makes suggestions for the development and modification of culturally relevant therapy to meet the needs fo disabled women. *$69.95*

418 pages Hardcover
ISBN 0-789019-36-1

Specific Disabilities

6652 **A Guide to Hydrocephalus**

Spina Bifida Association of America
4590 Macarthur Boulevard NW
Suite 250
Washington, DC 20007 **202-944-3285**
800-621-3141
FAX: 202-944-3295
e-mail: sbaa@sbaa.org
www.sbaa.org

$8.00

1973

6653 **A Miracle to Believe In**

Option Indigo Press
2080 S Undermountain Road
Sheffield, MA 01257 **413-229-2100**
800-714-2779
FAX: 413-229-8931
e-mail: indigo@bcn.net
www.optionindigo.com

A group of people from all walks of life come together and are transformed as they reach out, under the direction of the Kaufmans, to help a little boy the medical world had given up as hopeless. This heartwarming journey of loving a child back to life will not only inspire you, the reader, but presents a compelling new way to deal with life's traumas and difficulties.

379 pages 1981
ISBN 0-449201-08-2

6654 **ADD Challenge: A Practical Guide for Teachers**

Research Press
Department 22W
PO Box 9177
Champaign, IL 61826 **217-352-3273**
800-519-2707
FAX: 217-352-1221
e-mail: rp@researchpress.com
www.researchepress.com/scripts/product.asp?it

$15.95

196 pages
ISBN 0-878223-45-2

6655 **ADD: Helping Your Child**

Warner Books
1271 Avenue of the Americas
New York, NY 10020 **212-522-7200**
FAX: 212-522-7989

$12.95

224 pages Paperback
ISBN 0-446670-13-8

6656 ADHD in the Schools: Assessment and Intervention Strategies

Guilford Press
72 Spring Street
New York, NY 10012
212-431-9800
800-365-7006
FAX: 212-966-6708
e-mail: info@guilford.com
www.guilford.com

The landmark volume emphasizes the need for a team effort among parents, community-based professionals, and educators. Provides practical information for educators that is based on empirical findings. Chapters Focus on how to identify and assess students who might have ADHD, the relationship between ADHD and learning disabilities; how to develop and supplement classroom-based programs. Communication strategies to assist physicians and the need for community-based treatments *$36.00*

269 pages Paperback
ISBN 0-898622-45-X

6657 ADHD: Handbook for Diagnosis & Treatment

Western Psychological Services
12031 Wilshire Boulevard
Los Angeles, CA 90025
310-478-2061
800-648-8857
FAX: 310-478-7838

This second edition helps clinicians diagnose and treat Attention Deficit Hyperactivity Disorder. Written by an internationally recognized authority in the field, it covers the history of ADHD, its primary symptoms, associated conditions, developmental course and outcome, and family context. A workbook companion manual is also available. *$ 68.00*

700 pages

6658 AJAO Newsletter

American Juvenile Arthritis Organization
1330 W Peachtree Street
PO Box 7669
Atlanta, GA 30357
404-872-7100
800-283-7800
FAX: 404-872-9559
e-mail: help@arthritis.org
www.arthritis.org

Janet Austin MEd, Editor

Offers information and updates about the organization's activities and events. Legislative information, medical updates, camp information and more for children living with arthritis.

Quarterly

6659 Activities for Developing Pre-Skill Concepts In Children with Autism

Autism Society of North Carolina Bookstore
505 Oberlin Road
Suite 230
Raleigh, NC 27605
919-743-0204
800-442-2762
FAX: 919-743-0208
e-mail: dcoffey@autismsociety-nc.org
www.autismsociety-nc.org

Darla Coffey, Bookstore Manager

Chapters include auditory development, concept development, social development and visual-motor integration. *$36.00*

6660 Adolescents with Down Syndrome: Toward a More Fulfilling Life

Brookes Publishing
PO Box 10624
Baltimore, MD 21285
410-337-9580
800-638-3775
FAX: 410-337-8539
e-mail: custserv@brookespublishing.com
www.brookespublishing.com

Written for health care professionals, psychologists, other developmental disabilities practitioners, educators, and parents, it covers biomedical concerns; behavioral, psychological, and psychiatric challenges; and education, employment, recreation, community, and legal concerns. *$35.95*

416 pages Paperback 1997
ISBN 1-55766 -81-9

6661 Adult Leukemia: A Comprehensive Guide for Patients and Families

Patients-Centered Guides
101 Morris Street
Sebastopol, CA 95472
707-829-0515
800-998-9938
FAX: 707-829-0104
www.patientcenters.com

Linda Lamb, Editor
Shawnde Paull, Marketing

For the tens of thousands of Americans with adult leukemia, Adult Leukemia: A Comprehensive Guide for Patients and Families addresses diagnosis, medical tests, finding a good oncologist, treatments, side effects, getting emotional and other support, resources for further study, and much more. The book includes real-life stories from those who have battled leukemia themselves. *$29.95*

536 pages Paperback
ISBN 0-596500-01-7

6662 Advanced Breast Cancer: A Guide to Living with Metastic Disease

Patients-Centered Guides
101 Morris Street
Sebastopol, CA 95472
707-829-0515
800-998-9938
FAX: 707-829-0104
www.patientcenters.com

Linda Lamb, Editor
Shawnde Paull, Marketing

This is the only book on breast cancer that deals honestly with the realities of living with metastic disease, yet offers hope and comfort. All aspects of facing the disease are covered, including: coping with the shock of recurrence, seeking information and making treatment decisions, communicating effectively with medical personnel finding support, and handling disease progression and end-of-life issues. A comprehensive guide, it also provides updated resources and treatment developments. *$24.95*

532 pages Paperback
ISBN 1-565925-22-X

6663 Advanced Diagnosis and Treatment for Neck and Back Pain

American Back Society
2647 International Boulevard
Suite 401
Oakland, CA 94601
510-536-9929
FAX: 510-536-1812
e-mail: info@americanbacksoc.org
www.americanbacksoc.org

A membership organization dedicated to relieving the pain and impairment caused by back problems. Sponsors symposia for presenting research findings.

6664 **After School and More**

Resources for Children with Special Needs
116 E 16th Street
5th Floor
New York, NY 10003
212-667-4650
FAX: 212-254-4070
e-mail: info@resourcesnyc.org
www.resourcesnyc.org

Karen Schlesinger, Executive Director
Dianne Littwin, Director Publications

Published every 24-36 months. *$25.00*

240 pages
ISBN 0-967836-55-7

6665 **All About Attention Deficit Disorders, Revised**

Child Management
800 Roosevelt Road
B-309
Glen Ellyn, IL 60137
630-469-0484
FAX: 630-469-4571
www.thomasphelan.com

Nancy Roe, Office Manager

A psychologist and expert on ADD outlines the symptoms, diagnosis and treatment of this neurological disorder. *$12.95*

248 pages Paperback
ISBN 1-889140-11-2

6666 **Alternative Medicine and Multiple Sclerosis**

Demos Medical Publishing
386 Park Avenue S
Suite 201
New Yorok, NY 10016
212-683-0072
800-532-8663
FAX: 212-683-0118
e-mail: orderdep@demospub.com
www.demosmedpub.com

Diana Schneider PhD, President

Offers reliable information on the relevance, safety, and effectiveness of various alternative therapies that are not typically considered in discussions of MS management, yet are in widespread use. *$24.95*

272 pages 2001
ISBN 1-888799-52-8

6667 **American Heart Association Guide to Stroke Treatment, Recovery & Prevention**

Random House
1540 Broadway
New York, NY 10036
212-782-9000
800-726-0600
FAX: 212-302-7985
e-mail: customerservice@randonhouse.com
www.randomhouse.com

From the nation's premier authority on heart disease and stroke, the definitive book on stroke prevention, treatment and recovery. *$29.00*

304 pages

6668 **Amyotrophic Lateral Sclerosis: A Guide for Patients and Families**

Demos Medical Publishing
386 Park Avenue S
Suite 201
New Yorok, NY 10016
212-683-0072
800-532-8663
FAX: 212-683-0118
e-mail: orderdep@demospub.com
www.demosmedpub.com

Diana Schneider PhD, President

This comprehensive guide covers every aspect of the management of ALS. Beginning with discussions of its clinical features of the disease, diagnosis, and an overview of symptom management, major sections deal with medical and rehabilitative management, living with ALS, managing advanced disease and end-of-life issues, and reources that can provide support and assistance. *$34.95*

350 pages 2000
ISBN 1-888799-28-5

6669 **Annals of Dyslexia**

International Dyslexia Association
Chester Building
Suite 382
Baltimore, MD 21286
800-ABC-D123
FAX: 410-296-0232
www.interdys.org

Offers information on auditory discrimination, dyslexia, attitudes, advocacy and more on people with learning disabilities. *$15.00*

Paper

6670 **Answering Your Questions About Spina Bifida**

Spina Bifida Association of America
4590 Macarthur Boulevard NW
Suite 250
Washington, DC 20007
202-944-3285
800-621-3141
FAX: 202-944-3295
e-mail: sbaa@sbaa.org
www.sbaa.org

Provides information to help you understand the basic medical, educational and social issues. Available in Spanish.

1973

6671 **Aphasia: What is It?**

Speech Bin
1965 25th Avenue
Vero Beach, FL 32960
772-770-0007
800-477-3324
FAX: 772-770-0006
www.speechbin.com

Brochures for families and caregivers of persons who have suffered aphasic language disorders secondary to strokes. Set of ten copies. *$14.95*

16 pages Package of 10
ISBN 0-93785 -56-4

6672 **Arthritis 101: Questions You Have Answers You Need**

Arthritis Foundation Distribution Center
PO Box 6996
Alpharetta, GA 30009
800-207-8633
FAX: 770-442-9742
www.arthritis.com

Expert reviewers answer questions about basic arthritis facts, treatments, research, surgery and more. Also, specific information about six common conditions: rheumatoid arthritis, osteoarthritis, osteoporosis, fibromyalgia, lupus and gout. *$11.95*

144 pages

6673 Arthritis Accent

Arthritis Foundation Southern N.E. Chapter
35 Cold Spring Road
Suite 411
Rocky Hill, CT 06067
860-563-1177
800-541-8350
FAX: 860-563-6018
e-mail: inpubne@arthritis.org
www.arthritis.org

Susan Nesci, Program Director - CT

Offers information on chapter events and activities.

Quarterly

6674 Arthritis Foundation of Illinois News

2621 N Knoxville
Peoria, IL 61604
309-682-6600
800-795-9115
FAX: 309-682-6732
e-mail: greaterillinois@arthritis.org

Marilynn J Cason, Chairman

A publication offering information about the activities of the chapter. Program news, legislative information, workshops and resources are also included.

Quarterly

6675 Arthritis Foundation: Greater Southwest Chapter

1313 E Osborn Road
Suite 200
Phoenix, AZ 85014
602-264-7679
800-477-7679
FAX: 602-264-0563
e-mail: info.caz@arthritis.org
www.arthritis.org

Sherry Ladd, Administration

Provides information, programs and services for people affected by arthritis.

Quarterly

6676 Arthritis Helpbook

Addison-Wesley Publishing Company
75 Arlington Street
Suite 300
Boston, MA 02116
617-848-6000
617-848-6034
www.awprofessional.com

A self-care program for coping with arthritis that includes diet, nutrition, exercise, and mind/body techniques such as guided imagery and meditation.

6677 Arthritis Helpbook: A Tested Self-Management Program for Coping

Addison-Wesley Publishing Company
75 Arlington Street
Suite 300
Boston, MA 02116
617-848-6000
800-238-9682
FAX: 617-848-6034
www.awprofessional.com

$13.50

288 pages 4th Edition
ISBN 0-201409-63-1

6678 Arthritis News

Wisconsin Chapter of the Arthritis Foundation
8556 W National Avenue
W Allis, WI 53227
414-321-3933
FAX: 262-872-0457
e-mail: info@wi@arthritis.org
www.arthritis.org

Dana Motley, Public Relations Coordinator

Offers information on activities, events, medical research, information and referrals to persons living in the Wisconsin area that are afflicted with arthritis.

8 pages Quarterly

6679 Arthritis Observer

Rocky Mountain Chapter of the Arthritis Foundation
2280 S Albion
Denver, CO 80222
800-475-6647
e-mail: sturman@arthritis.org

Susan Turman, VP Operations

Offers chapter information and updates on fund-raising events and activities, resources and publications and medical updates for the arthritis community.

Quarterly

6680 Arthritis Relief at Your Fingertips

Warner Books
1271 Avenue of the Americas
New York, NY 10020
212-522-7200
FAX: 212-522-7989
www.twbookmark.com

A self-help guide for relieving arthritis pain through exercise and acupressure massage by a leader in the field.

6681 Arthritis Reporter

New York Chapter of the Arthritis Foundation
122 E 42nd Street
18th Floor
New York, NY 10168
212-984-8700
FAX: 212-878-5960
e-mail: info.ny@arthritis.org
www.arthritis.org

Chapter newsletter offering information on upcoming events, activities and groups for the arthritis community.

Quarterly

6682 Arthritis Self Help Products

Aids for Arthritis
35 Wakefield Drive
Medford, NJ 08055
800-654-0707
FAX: 609-654-8631
e-mail: aidsforar@aol.com
www.aidsforarthritis.com

More than 200 arthritis self-help products for kitchen, resting, dressing, bathroom, driving, therapy and foot care. Available online or through catalog. Low prices, quick shipping, since 1979.

24 pages Quarterly

6683 Arthritis Self-Help Book

Addison-Wesley Publishing Company
75 Arlington Street
Suite 300
Boston, MA 02116
617-848-6000
800-238-9682
FAX: 617-848-6034
www.awprofessional.com

A useful and informative book used in conjunction with the Arthritis Foundation's Self-Help Course. *$12.00*

6684 **Arthritis Today**

Arthritis Foundation
1330 W Peachtree Street
Atlanta, GA 30309
770-253-1300
FAX: 404-872-9559
www.arthritis.org

Magazine for patients, physicians, public authorities and others with an interest in the field of arthritis. (Price noted paid for yearly subscription) *$20.00*

6685 **Arthritis: A Comprehensive Guide**

Addison-Wesley Publishing Company
75 Arlington Street
Suite 300
Boston, MA 02116
617-848-6000
800-238-9682
FAX: 617-848-6034
www.awprofessional.com

Reviews types of arthritis, different aspects of treatment including exercise, medications, surgery, the role of diet and an extensive section on challenges of daily living. *$12.00*

6686 **Arthritis: Stop Suffering, Start Moving**

Walker Publishing Company
435 Hudson Street
New York, NY 10014
212-727-8300
800-289-2553
FAX: 212-727-0984
e-mail: orders@walkerbooks.com
www.walkerbooks.com

$22.95

160 pages
ISBN 0-802713-08-4

6687 **Arthritis: Taking Care of Yourself Health Guide for Understanding Your Arthritis**

Addison-Wesley Publishing Company
75 Arlington Street
Suite 300
Boston, MA 02116
617-848-6000
FAX: 617-848-6034
www.awprofessional.com

$13.50

4th Edition
ISBN 0-201409-17-8

6688 **Arthritis: What Exercises Work**

St. Martin's Press
175 Fifth Avenue
New York, NY 10010
212-674-5151
800-221-7945
FAX: 212-420-9314

$19.95

160 pages
ISBN 0-312097-43-3

6689 **Arthritis: Your Complete Exercise Guide**

Human Kinetics Press
PO Box 5076
Champaign, IL 61825
217-351-5076
FAX: 217-351-2674
e-mail: orders@hkusa.com
www.humankinetics.com

The Cooper Clinic and Research Institute Fitness Series provides an exercise rehabilitation alternative for people with chronic meidcal conditions. *$13.95*

152 pages Paperback
ISBN 0-873223-92-6

6690 **Ask the Doctor: Asthma**

Andrews McMeel Publishing
PO Box 419150
Kansas City, MO 64141
816-932-6700
800-826-4216
FAX: 800-437-8683

$8.95

128 pages Soft Cover
ISBN 0-836270-23-1

6691 **Asthma Challenge**

Asthma and Allergy Foundation of America
1125 15th Street NW
Suite 502
Washington, DC 20005
202-466-7643
FAX: 202-466-8940
e-mail: info@aafa.org
www.aafa.org

Fun and engaging activity to assess asthma knowledge. This custom designed, full colored stand up board comes with two sets of pre-tested question cards and can be used with large or small groups. Players test their knowledge in categories like Sneezes and Wheezes, and Nuts and Bolts. *$50.00*

6692 **Asthma Resource Directory**

National Allergy and Asthma Network
3554 Chain Bridge Road
Suite 200
Fairfax, VA 22030
703-385-4403
FAX: 703-352-4354

Valuable reference tool with over 2,500 listings of resources and products nationwide including suppliers, camps, research centers and support groups.

6693 **Asthma Self-Help Book: How to Live a Normal Life in Spite of Your Condition**

Prima Publishing
3000 Lava Ridge Court
Roseville, CA 95661
916-787-7000
800-632-8676
FAX: 916-787-7001
e-mail: websupportlife@primapub.com
www.primapublishing.com

A through, practical look at asthma that includes information from the National Heart, Lung, and Blood Institute's Asthma Guidelines. *$13.95*

271 pages 1992
ISBN 1-559581-66-2

6694 **Asthma Sourcebook**

Omnigraphics
615 Griswold Street
Detroit, MI 48226
800-234-1340
FAX: 800-875-1340
www.omnigraphics.com

Annemarie S Muth, Editor

Provides information about asthma, including symptoms, remidies and research updates. *$78.00*

650 pages 1900
ISBN 0-780803-81-7

6695 **Asthma and Exercise**

Henry Holt and Company
3554 Chain Bridge Road
Suite 200
Fairfax, VA 22030
703-385-4403
FAX: 703-352-4354

This book offers clear and detailed advice on how adults and children with asthma can participate in exercise and sports activities. *$10.00*

6696 **Asthma in the School: Improving Control with Peak Flow Monitoring**

National Allergy and Asthma Network
3554 Chain Bridge Road
Suite 200
Fairfax, VA 22030
703-385-4403
FAX: 703-352-4354

Comprehensive and practical guide to help the school nurse monitor and assist students with asthma. *$7.00*

6697 **Asthma in the Workplace**

John H Dekker & Sons
2941 Clydon Street SW
Grand Rapids, MI 49509
616-538-5160
FAX: 616-538-0720

$199.00

664 pages
ISBN 0-824787-99-4

6698 **Attention**

Children & Adults with ADHD
8181 Professional Place
Suite 150
Landover, MD 20785
301-306-7070
800-233-4050
FAX: 301-306-6788
www.chadd.org

Clarke Ross, CEO
Karen White, Director Natl Resource Center

A bi-monthly publication from CHADD. Free with membership.

bi-monthly

6699 **Attention Deficit Disorder and Learning Disabilities**

Books on Special Children
PO Box 305
Congers, NY 10920
845-638-1236
FAX: 845-638-0847
e-mail: irene@boscbooks.com

Introduces ADD and learning disabilities. This is an easy reading book. Gives definitions and discusses some effective and controverial medication, dietary, biofeedback, cognitive therapy, and many more issues. *$15.95*

246 pages Softcover
ISBN 0-385469-31-4

6700 **Attention Deficit Disorder in Adults Workbook**

Taylor Publishing Company
1550 W Mockingbird
Dallas, TX 75235
214-819-8100
FAX: 214-819-8580

$17.99

192 pages Paperback
ISBN 0-878338-50-0

6701 **Attention Deficit Disorder: A Different Perception**

Underwood-Miller
708 Westover Drive
Lancaster, PA 17601
717-285-2255
FAX: 717-285-2255

$9.95

180 pages Paperback
ISBN 0-887331-56-4

6702 **Attention-Deficit Hyperactivity Disorder A Handbook for Diagnosis and Treatment**

Guilford Press
72 Spring Street
New York, NY 10012
212-431-9800
800-365-7006
FAX: 212-966-6708
e-mail: info@guilford.com

A second edition that is the handbook on the diagnosis and treatment of ADHD in the 1990s. A companion workbook is also available with forms that may be photocopied. *$55.00*

747 pages Hardcover
ISBN 0-898624-43-6

6703 **Attention-Deficit Hyperactivity Disorder: Symptoms and Suggestons for Treatment**

Slosson Educational Publications
PO Box 280
E Aurora, NY 14052
716-625-0930
FAX: 800-655-3840
e-mail: slosson@slosson.com
www.slosson.com

Leslie Foote, Office Personnel
Peggy Meyer, Office Personnel

An exhaustive review of current research and decades of experience as practicing school-based professionals, as well as being a parent of an ADHD child, have culminated in this brief, to-the-point, and yet informed ADHD package which has recieved tremendous reviews. Well-grounded answers and suggestions which would facillitate behavior, learning, social-emotional functioning, and other factors in preschool and adolesence are discussed. Answers most commonly asked questions about ADHD/ADD. *$60.00*

61 pages

6704 **Augmenting Basic Communciation in Natural Contexts**

Brookes Publishing
PO Box 10624
Baltimore, MD 21285
410-337-9580
800-638-3775
FAX: 410-337-8539
e-mail: custserv@brookespublishing.com
www.brookespublishing.com

Here you will find the techniques needed to establish a basic communication system for people of all ages with cognitive disabilities or motor sensory impairments. *$41.95*

304 pages Paperback
ISBN 1-55766 -43-6

6705 **Autism**

Autism Society of North Carolina Bookstore
505 Oberlin Road
Suite 230
Raleigh, NC 27605
919-743-0204
800-442-2762
FAX: 919-743-0208
e-mail: dcoffey@autismsociety-nc.org
www.autismsociety-nc.org

Darla Coffey, Bookstore Manager

Everything there is to know about autism research book. *$17.95*

6706 Autism Handbook: Understanding & Treating Autism & Prevention Development

Oxford University Press
2001 Evans Road
Cary, NC 27513
212-726-6000
800-451-7556
FAX: 919-677-1303
www.oup-usa.org

$25.00

320 pages
ISBN 0-195076-67-2

6707 Autism Research Institute

4182 Adams Avenue
San Diego, CA 92116
619-281-7165
FAX: 619-563-6840
www.autism.com/ari

Bernard Rimland PhD, Director

Offers information and conducts research on autism and related disorders. Please write for info. *$18.00*

8 pages Qtrly. nwsltr.

6708 Autism Treatment Guide

Autism Society of North Carolina Bookstore
505 Oberlin Road
Suite 230
Raleigh, NC 27605
919-743-0204
800-442-2762
FAX: 919-743-0208
e-mail: dcoffey@autismsociety-nc.org
www.autismsociety-nc.org

Darla Coffey, Bookstore Manager

A comprehensive book covering treatments and methods used to help individuals with autism. *$12.95*

6709 Autism and Asperger Syndrome

Autism Society of North Carolina Bookstore
505 Oberlin Road
Suite 230
Raleigh, NC 27605
919-743-0204
800-442-2762
FAX: 919-743-0208
e-mail: dcoffey@autismsociety-nc.org
www.autismsociety-nc.org

Darla Coffey, Bookstore Manager

Chapters include topics such as the relationship of autism and asperger syndrome, living with the syndrome and asperger syndrome in adulthood. *$23.95*

6710 Autism and Learning

David Fulton Publishers
2 Barbon Close Great Ormond Street
London, WCIN
171-405-5606
FAX: 171-831-4840

This book is about how a cognitive perception on the way in which individuals with autism think and learn may be applied to particular curriculum areas.

160 pages Paperback
ISBN 1-853464-21-X

6711 Autism in Adolescents and Adults

Plenum Publishing Corporation
233 Spring Street
New York, NY 10013
212-620-8000
FAX: 212-463-0742
e-mail: info@plenum.com

$63.00

456 pages
ISBN 0-306410-57-5

6712 Autism...Nature, Diagnosis and Treatment

Autism Society of North Carolina Bookstore
505 Oberlin Road
Suite 230
Raleigh, NC 27605
919-743-0204
800-442-2762
FAX: 919-743-0208
e-mail: dcoffey@autismsociety-nc.org
www.autismsociety-nc.org

Darla Coffey, Bookstore Manager

Covers perspectives, issues, neurobiological issues and new directions in diagnosis and treatment. *$49.00*

6713 Autism: A Strange, Silent World

Filmakers Library
124 E 40th Street
New York, NY 10016
212-808-4980
FAX: 212-808-4983
e-mail: info@filmakers.com
www.filmakers.com

Sue Oscar, Co-President

British educators and medical personnel offer insight into autism's characteristics and treatment approaches through the cameos of three children.

6714 Autism: Explaining the Enigma

Autism Society of North Carolina Bookstore
505 Oberlin Road
Suite 230
Raleigh, NC 27605
919-743-0204
800-442-2762
FAX: 919-743-0208
e-mail: dcoffey@autismsociety-nc.org
www.autismsociety-nc.org

Darla Coffey, Bookstore Manager

Explains the nature of autism. *$27.95*

6715 Autism: From Tragedy to Triumph

Branden Publishing Company
17 Station Street
PO Box 843
Brookline Village, MA 02147
617-734-2045
FAX: 781-790-1056
e-mail: branden@branden.com
www.branden.com

A new book that deals with the Lovaas method and includes a foreward by Dr. Ivar Lovaas. The book is broken down into two parts — the long road to diagnosis and then treatment. *$12.95*

6716 Autism: Identification, Education and Treatment

Autism Society of North Carolina Bookstore
505 Oberlin Road
Suite 230
Raleigh, NC 27605
919-743-0204
800-442-2762
FAX: 919-743-0208
e-mail: dcoffey@autismsociety-nc.org
www.autismsociety-nc.org

Darla Coffey, Bookstore Manager

Chapters include medical treatments, early intervention and communication development in autism. *$36.00*

6717 Autism: The Facts

Oxford University Press
2001 Evans Road
Cary, NC 27513
212-726-6000
800-451-7556
FAX: 919-677-1303
www.oup-usa.org

$19.95

128 pages
ISBN 0-192623-28-1

6718 Autistic Adults at Bittersweet Farms

Haworth Press
10 Alice Street
Binghamton, NY 13904
607-722-5857
800-429-6784
FAX: 607-722-6362
e-mail: orders@haworthpress.com
www.haworthpress.com

Norman Giddan PhD, Editor
Jane Giddan MA, Editor

A touching view of an inspirational residential care program for autistic adolescents and adults. Also available in softcover. *$94.95*

Hardcover
ISBN 1-560240-42-3

6719 Awareness Posters

Spina Bifida Association of America
4590 MacArthur Boulevard NW
Suite 250
Washington, DC 20007
202-944-3285
800-621-3141
FAX: 202-944-3295
e-mail: sbaa@sbaa.org
www.sbaa.org

An aid for building community awareness of Spina Bifida and the need for adequate amounts of folic acid in pregnant women. *$7.00*

6720 Away with Arthritis

Vantage Press
516 W 34th Street
New York, NY 10001
212-736-1767
FAX: 212-736-2273

$12.50

ISBN 0-533108-14-4

6721 BOSC: Directory Facilities for People with Learning Disabilities

Books on Special Children
PO Box 305
Congers, NY 10920
845-638-1236
FAX: 845-638-0847
e-mail: irene@boscbooks.com
www.boscbooks.com

Julius Kliener, Marketing Director

Directory of schools, independent living programs, clinics and centers, colleges and vocational programs, agencies and commercial products. Five sections in special post binder that can be updated annually. Hardcover. *$70.00*

300+ pages Yearly
ISSN 0961-3888

6722 Bell

National Mental Health Association
1021 Prince Street
Alexandria, VA 22314
703-684-7722
800-969-NMHA
FAX: 703-684-5968
TTY:800-433-5959
e-mail: nmhainfo@aol.com
www.nmha.org

Sandy Alexander, Publications Manager
Patrick Cody, Sr Director Media Relations

Targets public and private mental health organizations as well as interested corporations, agencies and individuals. The Bell contains information about a variety of issues pertaining to mental health, including: the effects of managed care on mental health care; the implications of Congressional decisions for mental health; prevention efforts on the local, state and national levels; national anti-stigma efforts and national public education campaigns. *$24.00*

Monthly

6723 Biology of the Autistic Syndromes, 2nd Edition

Autism Society of North Carolina Bookstore
505 Oberlin Road
Suite 230
Raleigh, NC 27605
919-743-0204
800-442-2762
FAX: 919-743-0208
e-mail: dcoffey@autismsociety-nc.org
www.autismsociety-nc.org

Darla Coffey, Bookstore Manager

A revision of the original classic text in the light of new developments and current knowledge. This book covers the epidemiological, genetic, biochemical, immunological and neuropsychological literature on autism. *$74.95*

6724 Blooming Where You're Planted

Meeting Life's Challenges
9042 Aspen Grove Lane
Madison, WI 53717
608-824-0402
FAX: 608-824-0403
e-mail: help@MeetingLifesChallenges.com
www.MeetingLifesChallenges.com

Author Shelley Peterman Schwarz takes you on her journey of self-discovery and change following her diagnosis of multiple sclerosis in 1979. Her personal stories are warm and humorous, and insightful. This 138-page book will motivate and inspire you to rise above life's challenges and live life to its fullest. *$12.95*

138 pages
ISBN 0-891854-01-1

6725 Bone Up on Arthritis

Arthritis Foundation
PO Box 6996
Alpharetta, GA 30009
800-207-8633
FAX: 770-442-9742
www.arthritis.com

A self-help education packet designed for home-study use, this program can improve your pain and function levels by teaching proven self-help techniques. *$19.50*

w/Audio Tapes

6726 Bowel Cancer

Oxford University Press
2001 Evans Road
Cary, NC 27513
212-726-6000
800-451-7556
FAX: 919-677-1303
www.oup-usa.org

Offers information and public awareness on the disease of bowel cancer. *$18.95*

152 pages

6727 Bowel Management: A Manual of Ideas and Techniques

Accent Books & Products
PO Box 700
Bloomington, IL 61702
309-378-2961
800-787-8444
FAX: 309-378-4420
e-mail: acmtlvng@aol.com

Raymond C Cheever, Publisher
Betty Garee, Editor

Paras and quads can gain much greater freedom. Includes considerations as frequency, timing, water intake, exercise and successful programs from three rehab centers. *$3.50*

25 pages Paperback
ISBN 0-91570 -02-7

6728 Breaking the Speech Barrier: Language Develpment Through Augmented Means

Brookes Publishing
PO Box 10624
Baltimore, MD 21285
410-337-9580
800-638-3775
FAX: 410-337-8539
e-mail: custserv@brookespublishing.com
www.brookespublishing.com

This resource describes the creation of the System for Augmenting Language (SAL) for school-age youth with mental retardation and offers important insights into the language development of children who are not learning to communicate typically. *$37.00*

224 pages Paperback
ISBN 1-557663-90-4

6729 Breast Cancer Sourcebook

Omnigraphics
615 Griswold Street
Detroit, MI 48226
800-234-1340
FAX: 800-875-1340
www.omnigraphics.com

Edward J Prucha, Editor

Provides information on the prevention of Breast Cancer, self care, treatment options, alternative therapies and diagnostic methods. *$78.00*

600 pages 1900
ISBN 0-780802-44-6

6730 Breathing Disorders: Your Complete Exercise Guide

Human Kinetics
PO Box 5076
Champaign, IL 61825
217-351-5076
800-747-4457
FAX: 217-351-1549
e-mail: orders@hkusa.com
www.humankinetics.com

$11.95

144 pages Paperback
ISBN 0-873224-26-4

6731 Bronchial Asthma: Principles of Diagnosis and Treatment

Humana Press
999 Riverview Drive
Suite 208
Totowa, NJ 07512
973-256-1165
FAX: 973-256-8341

$125.00

784 pages
ISBN 0-896032-53-1

6732 Building Communicative Competence with Indiv. Who Use Augmentative & Alternative Commun.

Brookes Publishing
PO Box 10624
Baltimore, MD 21285
410-337-9580
800-638-3775
FAX: 410-337-8539
e-mail: custserv@brookespublishing.com
www.brookespublishing.com

This is a hands-on instructional program offering goal-setting, teaching, and coaching methods for improving the communicative skills of people who depend on AAC systems. Appropriate for children, adolescents, and adults at any state of communicative development. *$36.95*

336 pages Spiral-bound 1997
ISBN 1-55766 -24-6

6733 Cancer Industry

Paragon House
2700 University Avenue W
Suite 200
Saint Paul, MN 55114
651-644-3087
800-447-3709
FAX: 800-494-0997
e-mail: info@paragonhouse.com
www.paragonhouse.com

A thorough exploration of the political and economical forces behind the suppression of alternative treatments for cancer.

1989

6734 Cancer Sourcebook for Women, 2nd Edition

Omnigraphics
615 Griswold Street
Detroit, MI 48226
800-234-1340
FAX: 800-875-1340
www.omnigraphics.com

Edward J Prucha, Editor

Provides information on the specific forms of cancer that affect women. *$78.00*

600 pages 1900
ISBN 0-780802-26-8

6735 Cancer Sourcebook, 3rd Edition

Omnigraphics
615 Griswold Street
Detroit, MI 48226
800-234-1340
FAX: 800-875-1340
www.omnigraphics.com

Edward J Prucha, Editor

Includes information on the major forms and stages of cancer. *$78.00*

1100 pages 1900
ISBN 0-780802-27-6

6736 Cancer Victors Journal

International Association for Cancer Victors
5336 Harwood Road
San Jose, CA 95124
408-448-4094
FAX: 408-264-9659
www.cancervictors.org

Published by the volunteer community service organization to inform and support interested persons who want to learn more about natural, nontoxic remedies and practices.

6737 Chadder

Children & Adults with Attention Deficit Disorder
499 NW 70th Avenue
Suite 101
Plantation, FL 33317
954-587-3700
800-233-4050
FAX: 954-587-4599

Quarterly

6738 Charting: The Systematic Approach to Achieving Control

RA Rapaport Publishing
150 W 22nd Street
New York, NY 10011
212-989-0200
FAX: 212-989-4786

One of America's leading diabetes educators shows you, in this book, how to analyze your body's responses to diet, exercises and medication, and how to create a personalized systematic program for total diabetes control. *$3.95*

38 pages Paperback
ISBN 0-96317 -10-

6739 Child Care and the ADA: A Handbook for Inclusive Programs

Brookes Publishing
PO Box 10624
Baltimore, MD 21285
410-337-9580
800-638-3775
FAX: 410-337-8539
e-mail: custserv@brookespublishing.com
www.brookespublishing.com

This book is designed for educators and administrators in child care settings. It offers a straightforward discussion of the Americans with Disabilities Act including children with disabilities in community programs. *$25.95*

240 pages Paperback
ISBN 1-55766 -85-5

6740 Childen with Cerebral Palsy

Woodbine House
6510 Bells Mill Road
Bethesda, MD 20817
301-897-3570
800-843-7323
FAX: 301-897-5838
www.woodbinehouse.com

It provides a complete spectrum of information and compassionate advice about cerebral palsy and its effect on their child's development and education. Covers these areas: diagnosis, medical issues, family life, legal rights, early intervention, coping, therapies, treatment, development, advocacy, special ed., and daily care. *$16.95*

470 pages Paperback
ISBN 0-933149-82-4

6741 Children with Acquired Brain Injury: Education and Supporting Families

Brookes Publishing
PO Box 10624
Baltimore, MD 21285
410-337-9580
800-638-3775
FAX: 410-337-8539
e-mail: custserv@brookespublishing.com
www.brookespublishing.com

Ann Glang PhD, Editor
Janet M Williams MSW, Editor
$28.95

288 pages Paperback 1996
ISBN 1-557662-33-9

6742 Children with Asthma: A Manual for Parents

Allergy Control Products
96 Danbury Road
PO Box 793
Ridgefield, CT 06877
203-438-9580
800-422-3878
FAX: 203-431-8963
www.allergycontrol.com

Known as the asthma bible, this second edition is sprinkled with anecdotes by patients and their parents. *$10.00*

296 pages Paperback

6743 Children with Spina Bifida: A Parents Guide

Spina Bifida Association of America
4590 Macarthur Boulevard NW
Suite 250
Washington, DC 20007
202-944-3285
800-621-3141
FAX: 202-944-3295
e-mail: sbaa@sbaa.org
www.sbaa.org

Provides parents with information, guidance and support to help meet the child's needs through childhood. *$16.95*

6744 Children with Tourette Syndrome

Exceptional Parent Library
120 Sylvan Avenue, Suite 10
PO Box 1807
Englewood Cliffs, NJ 07632
800-535-1910
FAX: 201-947-9376
e-mail: eplibrary@aol.com
www.eplibrary.com

Written by a team of professionals and parents, this book covers medical, educational, legal, family life, daily care, and emotional issues. *$14.95*

6745 Children with Visual Impairments

Woodbine House
6510 Bells Mill Road
Bethesda, MD 20817
301-897-3570
800-843-7323
FAX: 301-897-5838
www.woodbinehouse.com

For families of children with visual impairments ranging from low vision to total blind, this book offers aythoritative and empathetic parental insight on diagnosis and treatment, family adjustment, orientation and mobility, literacy, legal issues, and more. *$16.95*

395 pages Paperback
ISBN 0-933149-36-0

6746 **Cleft Palate-Craniofacial Journal**

104 S Estes Drive
Suite 204
Chapel Hill, NC 27514
919-933-9044
FAX: 919-933-9604
e-mail: info@cleftline.org
www.cleftline.org

Michael P Karnell, President
A Michael Sadove, VP

Publication of the international nonprofit medical society of health care professionals who treat and/or perform research on birth defects of the head and face.

6747 **Clinical Care in the Rheumatic Disease**

Arthritis Foundation Distribution Center
PO Box 6996
Alpharetta, GA 30009
800-207-8633
FAX: 770-442-9742
www.arthritis.com

This book was written for all health professionals caring for people with rheumatic diseases and for students in these disciplines. *$35.00*

224 pages

6748 **Colon & Rectal Cancer: A Comprehensive Guide for Patients & Families**

Patient-Centered Guides
101 Morris Street
Sebastopol, CA 95472
707-829-0515
800-998-9938
FAX: 707-829-0104
www.patientcenters.com

Linda Lamb, Editor
Shawnde Paull, Marketing

The fourth most common cancer, colon and rectal cancer is diagnosed in 130,000 new cases in the United States each year. Patients and families need uo-to-date and in-depth information to participate wisely in treatment decisions (e.g., knowing what sexual and fertility issues to discuss with the doctor before surgery). This book covers coping with tests and treatment side effects, caring for ostomies, finding supportt, and other practical issues. *$24.95*

544 pages Paperback
ISBN 1-565926-33-1

6749 **Come Sign with Us**

Gallaudet University Press
11030 S Langley Avenue
Chicago, IL 60628
800-621-2736
FAX: 800-621-8476
TTY:800-621-9347
gupress.gallaudet.edu

Jan C Hafer, Co-Author
Robert M Wilson, Co-Author

This fun guide for parents and educators on teaching hearing children how to sign has been thoroughly revised with completely new activities that provide contexts for practice. *$29.95*

160 pages Softcover

6750 **Communication Development and Disorders in African American Children**

Brookes Publishing
PO Box 10624
Baltimore, MD 21285
410-337-9580
800-638-3775
FAX: 410-337-8539
e-mail: custserv@brookespublishing.com
www.brookespublishing.com

Research, Assessment, and Intervention. This text presents research on communication disorders and language development in African American children. Also addresses multicultural aspects of service delivery and intervention and discusses issues in assessing, diagnosing, and treating communication disorders. *$39.00*

400 pages Paperback
ISBN 1-55766 -53-3

6751 **Communication Development in Children with Down Syndrome**

Brookes Publishing
PO Box 10624
Baltimore, MD 21285
410-337-9580
800-638-3775
FAX: 410-337-8539
e-mail: custserv@brookespublishing.com
www.brookespublishing.com

This book offers an extensive, detailed explanation of communication development in children with Down syndrome relative to their advancing cognitive skills. It introduces a critical framework for assessing and treating hearing, speech, and language problems and provides explicit intervention methods and tested clinical protocols.

Paperback 1998
ISBN 1-55766 -50-5

6752 **Communication Skills for Visually Impaired Learners**

Charles C Thomas
2600 S First Street
Springfield, IL 62704
217-789-8980
800-258-8980
FAX: 217-789-9130
e-mail: books@ccthomas.com
www.ccthomas.com

Contents of this publication include historical perspectives, reading readiness, approaches to readiness instruction, building word identification skills, assessment of reading skills factors to consider in assessment, identifying visually impaired students with learning problems, teaching techniques for students with learning problems and more. Also available in cloth. *$49.95*

322 pages Softcover
ISBN 0-398066-93-0

6753 **Communication-Based Intervention for Problem Behavior**

Brookes Publishing
PO Box 10624
Baltimore, MD 21285
410-337-9580
800-638-3775
FAX: 410-337-8539
e-mail: custserv@brookespublishing.com
www.brookespublishing.com

A user's guide for producing positive change. This manual details methods for conducting functional assessments, communication-based intervention strategies, procedures for facilitating generalization and maintenance, and crisis management tactics. Useful for handling intense behavior problems. Also included are case studies and checklists of things to do to ensure success. *$38.00*

288 pages Paperback
ISBN 1-557662-46-0

6754 Comprehensive Directory of Programs and Services

Resources for Children with Special Needs
116 E 16th Street
5th Floor
New York, NY 10003
212-667-4650
FAX: 212-254-4070
e-mail: info@resourcesnyc.org
www.resourcesnyc.org

Karen Schlesinger, Executive Director
Dianne Littwin, Director Publications

Published every 24-36 months. *$55.00*

1096 pages
ISBN 0-976836-51-4

6755 Comprehensive Guide to ADD in Adults: Research, Diagnosis & Treatment

Taylor & Francis
7625 Empire Drive
Florence, KY 41042
800-634-7064
FAX: 800-248-4724

$50.95

426 pages
ISBN 0-876307-60-8

6756 Concentration Cockpit: Explaining Attention Deficits

Educators Publishing Service
31 Smith Place
Cambridge, MA 02138
617-367-2700
800-225-5750
FAX: 617-547-0412
www.epsbooks.com

This eight-page pamphlet explains the administration of The Concentration Cockpit, a newly revised poster that helps children with attention deficits gain insight into their problems and monitor their progress in grappling with these problems. *$64.50*

ISBN 0-838820-59-X

6757 Confronting the Challenges of Spina Bifida

Spina Bifida Association of America
4590 Macarthur Boulevard NW
Suite 250
Washington, DC 20007
202-944-3285
800-621-3141
FAX: 202-944-3295
e-mail: sbaa@sbaa.org
www.sbaa.org

A group curriculum addressing self care, self esteem and social skills in eight to 13 year olds. *$19.00*

6758 Coping with ADD/ADHD

Rosen Publishing Group
29 E 21st Street
New York, NY 10010
212-777-3017
800-237-9932
FAX: 888-436-4643
e-mail: rosenpub@tribeca.ios.com

At least 3.5 million American youngsters suffer from attention deficit disorder. This book defines the syndrome and provides specific information about treatment and counseling. *$16.95*

ISBN 0-823920-70-4

6759 Coping with Asthma

Rosen Publishing Group
29 E 21st Street
New York, NY 10010
212-777-3017
800-237-9932
FAX: 888-436-4643
e-mail: rosenpub@tribeca.ios.com

This book prepares students by explaining to them the dangers of asthma, a condition which, when properly treated, is completely manageable. *$16.95*

ISBN 0-823920-69-0

6760 Coping with Cerebral Palsy

Pro-Ed Publications
8700 Shoal Creek Boulevard
Austin, TX 78757
512-451-3246
800-897-3202
FAX: 512-451-8542
e-mail: info@proedinc.com
www.proedinc.com

This second edition book provides parents of children and adults with cerebral palsy the answers to more than 300 questions that have been carefully researched. It represents 40 years of experience by the author and is presented in a highly readable, jargon-free manner. *$26.00*

252 pages

6761 Counseling People with Diabetes

Brookes Publishing
PO Box 10624
Baltimore, MD 21285
410-337-9580
800-638-3775
FAX: 410-337-8539
e-mail: custserv@brookespublishing.com
www.brookespublishing.com

$29.00

158 pages Paperback
ISBN 1-85433 -36-1

6762 Counseling for Heart Disease

Brookes Publishing
PO Box 10624
Baltimore, MD 21285
410-337-9580
800-638-3775
FAX: 410-337-8539
e-mail: custserv@brookespublishing.com
www.brookespublishing.com

$25.00

144 pages Paperback
ISBN 1-85433 -96-9

6763 Counseling in Terminal Care & Bereavement

Brookes Publishing
PO Box 10624
Baltimore, MD 21285
410-337-9580
800-638-3775
FAX: 410-337-8539
e-mail: custserv@brookespublishing.com
www.brookespublishing.com

Provides practical suggestions for addressing the needs of patients and family members who are anticipating or currently dealing with grief and bereavement, such as hospice care, hospitals, or at home care. *$34.00*

210 pages Paperback
ISBN 1-85433 -78-7

6764 Count Us In

Exceptional Parent Library
120 Sylvan Avenue, Suite 10
PO Box 1807
Englewood Cliffs, NJ 07632
800-535-1910
FAX: 201-947-9376
e-mail: eplibrary@aol.com
www.eplibrary.com

Offers information on growing up with Downs Syndrome. *$9.95*

6765 Diabetes 101

Chronimed Publishing
13911 Ridgedale Drive
Minnetonka, MN 55305
952-916-2500
800-848-2793
FAX: 952-513-6170

Sandra A Hintz, Marketing Coord.

A pure and simple guide for people who use insulin. *$ 10.95*

208 pages Paperback
ISBN 1-56561 -24-5

6766 Diagnosis and Treatment of Autism

Autism Society of North Carolina Bookstore
505 Oberlin Road
Suite 230
Raleigh, NC 27605
919-743-0204
800-442-2762
FAX: 919-743-0208
e-mail: dcoffey@autismsociety-nc.org
www.autismsociety-nc.org

Darla Coffey, Bookstore Manager

Various chapters written by professionals working with autistic children and adults. *$150.00*

6767 Dictionary of Congenital Malformations & Disorders

Parthenon Publishing Group
120 Mill Road
Park Ridge, NJ 07656
201-391-6796
800-272-7737
FAX: 800-374-3401
e-mail: orders@crcpress.com
www.crcpress.com

$55.00

193 pages
ISBN 0-850705-77-1

6768 Directions

Families of Spinal Muscular Dystrophy
PO Box 196
Libertyville, IL 60048
847-367-7620
800-886-1762
FAX: 847-367-7623
e-mail: sma@fsma.org
www.fsma.org

Audrey Lewis, Executive Director
Colleen McCarthy

$35.00

60-70 pages Quarterly

6769 Disability Compliance Bulletin

LRP Publications
PO Box 24668
West Palm Beach, FL 33416
215-784-0941
800-341-7874
FAX: 215-784-9639
e-mail: custserve@lrp.com
www.lrp.com

Honora McDowelll, Product Group Manager

This biweekly newsletter gives you timely coverage and insightful analyses of the latest developments in disability law. You'll learn the most recent case law dealing with the Americans with Disabilities Act, the Family and Medical Leave Act and more. Disability Compliance Bulletin will help you understand the laws' obligations and show you emerging legal trends. *$165.00*

24 pages BiWeekly

6770 Disorders of Motor Speech: Assessment, Treatment, and Clinical Characterization

Brookes Publishing
PO Box 10624
Baltimore, MD 21285
410-337-9580
800-638-3775
FAX: 410-337-8539
e-mail: custserv@brookespublishing.com
www.brookespublishing.com

This book provides a probing examination of normal, dysarthric, and apraxic speech. Great for speech-language pathologists, neurologists, physical or occupational therapists, and physiatrists. *$47.00*

400 pages Hardcover
ISBN 1-55766 -23-1

6771 Dressing Tips and Clothing Resources for Making Life Easier

Attainment Company
504 Commerce Parkway
PO Box 930160
Verona, WI 53593
608-845-7880
800-327-4269
FAX: 608-845-8040
e-mail: info@attainmentcompany.com
www.attainmentcompany.com

Don Bastian, President

Learn hundreds of simple tips and techniques to make dressing easier. Learn how to adapt/modify ready-to-wear garments to accommodate your special dressing needs. Find out how to locate more than 100 resources offering specially designed or easy-on/easy-off clothing for men, women, children and/or wheelchair users. You'll find everything you need to look your best. An invaluable resource for people with special dressing needs, people with disabilities, caregivers and healthcare professionals. *$19.00*

144 pages 2000
ISBN 1-578611-19-9

6772 Driven to Distraction

National Alliance for the Mentally Ill
2107 Wilson Boulevard
Suite 300
Arlington, VA 22201
780-524-7600
800-950-6264

A practical book discussing adult as well as child attention deficit disorder (ADD). Non-technical, realistic and optimistic, it is an informative how-to manual for parents and consumers. *$23.00*

6773 **Dyslexia over the Lifespan**

Educators Publishing Service
31 Smith Place
Cambridge, MA 02138
617-367-2700
800-225-5750
FAX: 617-547-0412
www.epsbooks.com

Discusses the educational and career development of 56 dyslexic boys from a private school that was one of the first to have a program to detect and treat developmental language disabilities. *$ 18.00*

224 pages
ISBN 0-838816-70-3

6774 **Eating Disorders Sourcebook**

Omnigraphics
615 Griswold Street
Detroit, MI 48226
800-234-1340
FAX: 800-875-1340
www.omnigraphics.com

Dawn D Mattews, Editor

Provides general imformation, causes and treatments of eating disorders. *$78.00*

600 pages 1900
ISBN 0-780803-35-3

6775 **Effective Teaching Methods for Autistic Children**

Charles C Thomas
2600 S First Street
Springfield, IL 62704
217-789-8980
800-258-8980
FAX: 217-789-9130
e-mail: books@ccthomas.com
www.ccthomas.com

$20.95

124 pages Paper
ISBN 0-398063-09-5

6776 **Encounters with Autistic States**

Jason Aronson
400 Keystone Industrial Park
Dunmore, PA 18512
800-782-0015
FAX: 201-840-7242
www.aronson.com

$50.00

Hardcover
ISBN 0-765700-62-

6777 **Epilepsy: 199 Answers, A Doctor Responds to His Patients Questions**

Demos Medical Publishing
386 Park Avenue S
Suite 201
New Yorok, NY 10016
212-683-0072
800-532-8663
FAX: 212-683-0118
e-mail: orderdep@demospub.com
www.demosmedpub.com

Diana Schneider PhD, President

Clear and concise reference book dealing with the many questions a person with epilepsy or a person who has an interest or connection with epilepsy might want to ask. An essential up-to-date handbook on the subjetc of epilepsy. *$19.95*

144 pages 2002
ISBN 1-888799-70-6

6778 **EpilepsyUSA**

Epilepsy Foundation
4351 Garden City Drive
Landover, MD 20785
301-457-3700
800-332-1000
FAX: 301-577-2684
e-mail: postmaster@efa.org
www.epilepsyfoundation.org

Judith O'Toole, Editor

Magazine reporting on issues of interest to people with epilepsy and their families. *$15.00*

24 pages BiMonthly

6779 **Family Urology**

American Foundation for Urologic Disease
1100 Corporate Boulevard
Linthicum, MD 21090
800-242-2383
FAX: 410-468-1808
e-mail: admin@afud.org
www.afud.org

Jodi L Miller, Director Education

Dedicated to the prevention of urologic diseases through the expansion of patient education, research, public awareness and advocacy. Available with annual membership dues.

Quarterly

6780 **Fetal Alcohol Syndrome**

Brookes Publishing
PO Box 10624
Baltimore, MD 21285
410-337-9580
800-638-3775
FAX: 410-337-8539
e-mail: custserv@brookespublishing.com
www.brookespublishing.com

This text conveys urgent information about medical and social issues surrounding fetal alcohol syndrome (FAS). Explains how to identify the disorder, how to work with children (and adults) who have it, how to talk to parents about it, and how to prevent its occurrence through sensitive education of prospective mothers and society at large. *$ 22.95*

336 pages Paperback 1997
ISBN 1-55766 -83-5

6781 **Fighting for Darla: Challenges for Family Care & Professional Responsibility**

Baker & Taylor, International
1200 US Highway 22 E
Bridgewater, NJ 08807
908-541-7000
FAX: 908-541-7862
e-mail: intsale@bakertaylor.com

Follows the story of Darla, a pregnant adolescent with autism. *$18.95*

176 pages
ISBN 0-807733-56-3

6782 **Focus**

Arthritis Foundation
Central Ohio Chapter
3740 Ridge Mill Drive
Hilliard, OH 43026
614-876-8200
888-382-4673
FAX: 614-876-8363
www.arthritis.org

Offers updated information on arthritis as well as news of the services and activities of the Chapter.

Quarterly

6783 **Focus Newsletter**

Attention Deficit Disorder Association
1788 Second Street
Suite 200
Highland Park, IL 60035 **847-432-2332**
FAX: 847-432-5874
e-mail: michelenovotni@yahoo.com
www.add.org

Michele Novotni, PhD, President/Editor

ADDA's mission is to help people with AD/HD lead happier, more successful lives through education, research and public advocacy. Whether you have AD/HD yourself, someone special in your life does, or you treat, counsel or teach those who do, ADDA is an organization for you. ADDA focuses especially on the needs of AD/HD adults and young adults with AD/HD. Parents of children with AD/HD are also welcome.

6784 **Folic Acid Counseling Kit**

Spina Bifida Association of America
4590 Macarthur Boulevard NW
Suite 250
Washington, DC 20007 **202-944-3285**
800-621-3141
FAX: 202-944-3295
e-mail: sbaa@sbaa.org
www.sbaa.org

Alex Brodrick, Chair
Tim Yoder, Vice Chair

Counseling information for health professionals.

1973

6785 **Folic Acid Counseling Pocket Card**

Spina Bifida Association of America
4590 Macarthur Boulevard NW
Suite 250
Washington, DC 20007 **202-944-3285**
800-621-3141
FAX: 202-944-3295
e-mail: sbaa@sbaa.org
www.sbaa.org

For health care professionals. Quick reference card that fits in the white coat pocket. *$18.00*

6786 **Fourth and Long**

Kent Walderep National Paralysis Foundation
16415 Addison Road
Suite 550
Addison, TX 75001 **972-248-7100**
877-724-2873
FAX: 972-248-7313
e-mail: lkoen@spinalvictory.org
www.spinalvictory.org

Lisa Koen, Office Manager/Media Coordinator
$19.95

207 pages
ISBN 0-824515-08-0

6787 **Fragile Success: Nine Autistic Children, Childhood to Adulthood**

Autism Society of North Carolina Bookstore
505 Oberlin Road
Suite 230
Raleigh, NC 27605 **919-743-0204**
800-442-2762
FAX: 919-743-0208
e-mail: dcoffey@autismsociety-nc.org
www.autismsociety-nc.org

Darla Coffey, Bookstore Manager

A book about the lives of autistic children, whom the author has followed from their early years at the Elizabeth Ives School in New Haven, CT, through to adulthood. *$27.50*

6788 **Frames of Reference for the Assessment of Learning Disabilities**

Brookes Publishing
PO Box 10624
Baltimore, MD 21285 **410-337-9580**
800-638-3775
FAX: 410-337-8539
e-mail: custserv@brookespublishing.com
www.brookespublishing.com

New views on measurement issues. Here you'll find an in=depth look at the fundamental concerns facing those who work with children with learning disabilities - assessment and identification. *$55.00*

672 pages Hardcover
ISBN 1-55766 -38-3

6789 **Freedom from Arthritis Through Nutrition & Help for Allergies Sixth Edition**

Tree of Life Publications
PO Box 126
Joshua Tree, CA 92252 **760-228-9081**
FAX: 760-228-9081

$14.95

256 pages Paperback
ISBN 0-930852-15-X

6790 **Functional Electrical Stimulation for Ambulation by Paraplegics**

Krieger Publishing Company
PO Box 9542
Melbourne, FL 32902 **321-724-9542**
800-724-0025
FAX: 321-951-3671
e-mail: info@krieger-publishing.com
www.krieger-publishing.com

FES is employed to enable spinal cord injury patients who are complete paraplegics to stand and ambulate without bracing. The text covers 12 years of amulation experience. Also available in hardcover, ISBN #0-89464-845-4, selling for $42.50. *$32.50*

210 pages Paper
ISBN 1-575240-28-9

6791 **Going Places, Children Living with Cerebral Palsy**

Gareth Stevens
1555 N River Center Drive
Milwaukee, WI 53212 **414-225-0333**
800-542-2595
FAX: 414-225-0377

Mathias is a charming six-year-old with cerebral palsy. He needs special exercises to help him learn to control his muscles. He is also almost completely deaf. But with the love and encouragement of his family, Mathias is developing an interesting and busy life. Every morning finds him eager to start the day's activities. *$13.95*

48 pages
ISBN 0-836801-99-7

6792 **Growing Up with Epilepsy: A Pratical Guide for Parents**

Demos Medical Publishing
386 Park Avenue S
Suite 201
New Yorok, NY 10016 **212-683-0072**
800-532-8663
FAX: 212-683-0118
e-mail: orderdep@demospub.com
www.demosmedpub.com

Diana Schneider PhD, President

Developed to help parents with the uniques challenges that this disorder presents *$19.95*

156 pages 2003

ISBN 1-888799-74-9

6793 **Handbook of Autism and Pervasive Developmental Disorders**

Autism Society of North Carolina Bookstore
505 Oberlin Road
Suite 230
Raleigh, NC 27605
919-743-0204
800-442-2762
FAX: 919-743-0208
e-mail: dcoffey@autismsociety-nc.org
www.autismsociety-nc.org

Darla Coffey, Bookstore Manager

A list of contributors address such topics as characteristics of autistic syndromes and interventions. *$125.00*

6794 **Health Insurance Resource Manual**

Demos Medical Publishing
386 Park Avenue S
Suite 201
New Yorok, NY 10016
212-683-0072
800-532-8663
FAX: 212-683-0118
e-mail: orderdep@demospub.com
www.demosmedpub.com

Diana Schneider PhD, President

Information about a wide variety of options for individuals who are uninsured, underinsured, or who have questions about insurance and don't know where to begin. *$24.95*

208- pages 2003

ISBN 1-888799-69-2

6795 **Healthcare Guidelines for Spina Bifida and Healthcare Services Throughout Life**

Spina Bifida Association of America
4590 Macarthur Boulevard NW
Suite 250
Washington, DC 20007
202-944-3285
800-621-3141
FAX: 202-944-3295
e-mail: sbaa@sbaa.org
www.sbaa.org

$19.00

6796 **Heart Disease in Persons with Down Syndrome**

Brookes Publishing
PO Box 10624
Baltimore, MD 21285
410-337-9580
800-638-3775
FAX: 410-337-8539
e-mail: custserv@brookespublishing.com
www.brookespublishing.com

Offers access to findings from state-of-the-art research on congenital heart disease in children and adults with Down syndrome. Information on cardiac malformations and anomalies, heart and lung pathology, hemodynamic evaluations, and surgical intervention. *$62.00*

240 pages Hardcover

ISBN 1-55766 -24-X

6797 **Help Yourself Cookbook**

Arthritis Foundation
PO Box 6996
Alpharetta, GA 30009
800-207-0633
FAX: 770-442-9742
www.arthritis.com

$12.95

158 pages

6798 **Help for the Learning Disabled Child: Symptoms and Solutions - Revised**

Slosson Educational Publications
PO Box 280
E Aurora, NY 14052
585-652-0930
800-756-7766
FAX: 800-655-3840
e-mail: slosson@slosson.com
www.slosson.com

Leslie Foote, Office Personnel
Peggy Meyer, Office Personnel

This easy-to-read text describes observable behaviors, offers remediation techniques, materials, and specific tests to assist teachers in further diagnosis. This revision has been updated to include specific information and techniques to use with children who appear to have attention deficit disorders. Teachers and parents gain a better understanding of their child's difficulties in school and at home. *$ 36.00*

48 pages

6799 **Helping People with Autism Manage Their Behavior**

Autism Society of North Carolina Bookstore
505 Oberlin Road
Suite 230
Raleigh, NC 27605
919-743-0204
800-442-2762
FAX: 919-743-0208
e-mail: dcoffey@autismsociety-nc.org
www.autismsociety-nc.org

Darla Coffey, Bookstore Manager

Covers the broad topic of helping people with autism manage their behavior. *$7.00*

6800 **Hidden Child: The Linwood Method for Reaching the Autistic Child**

Woodbine House
6510 Bells Mill Road
Bethesda, MD 20817
301-897-3570
800-843-7323
FAX: 301-897-5838
www.woodbinehouse.com

Chronicle of the Linwood Children's Center's successful treatment program for autistic children. *$17.95*

286 pages Paperback

ISBN 0-933149-06-9

6801 **How to Live with a Spinal Cord Injury**

Accent Books & Products
PO Box 700
Bloomington, IL 61702
309-378-2961
800-787-8444
FAX: 309-378-4420
e-mail: acmtlvng@aol.com

Raymond C Cheever, Publisher
Betty Garee, Editor

A guide packed with realistic information about how this disability affects your life and what you can do about it. Answers lots of questions and gives you positive information providing hope and plenty of encouragement. *$6.95*

58 pages Paperback

ISBN 0-91570 -27-2

6802 How to Teach Autistic & Severely Handicapped Children

Autism Society of North Carolina Bookstore
505 Oberlin Road
Suite 230
Raleigh, NC 27605 **919-743-0204**
800-442-2762
FAX: 919-743-0208
e-mail: dcoffey@autismsociety-nc.org
www.autismsociety-nc.org

Darla Coffey, Bookstore Manager

Book provides procedures for effectively assessing and teaching autistic and other severely handicapped children. *$8.00*

6803 Hydrocephalus: A Guide for Patients, Families & Friends

Patient-Centered Guides
101 Morris Street
Sebastopol, CA 95472 **707-829-0515**
800-998-9938
FAX: 707-829-0104
www.patientcenters.com

Linda Lamb, Editor
Shawnde Paull, Marketing

Hydrocephalus is a life-threatening condition often referred to as, water on the brain, that is treated by surgical placement of a shunt system. Hydrocephalus: A Guide for Patients, Families and Friends educates families so they can select a skilled neurosurgeon, understand treatments, participate in care, know what symptoms need attention, discover where to turn for support, keep records needed for follow-up treatments, and make wise lifestyle choices. *$19.95*

379 pages Paperback

ISBN 1-565924-10-X

6804 Hyperactive Child, Adolescent, and Adult: ADD Through the Lifespan

CACLD
25 Van Zant Street
Suite 15-5
E Norwalk, CT 06855 **203-838-5010**
FAX: 203-866-6108
e-mail: CACLD@optonline.net
www.CACLD.org

Beryl Kaufman, Executive Director

Comprehensive general review. Update on previous research by the author, offering a basic text. Published by Cснnecticut Association for Children & Adults with Learning Disabilities (CACLD). *$8.75*

162 pages

6805 In Control

Arthritis Foundation
1330 W Peachtree Street
PO Box 7669
Atlanta, GA 30309 **404-872-7100**
800-283-7800
FAX: 404-872-9559
e-mail: help@arthritis.org
www.arthritis.org

An excellent at-home program which includes video, audio cassettes and the Arthritis Helpbook. Provides tools to help meet the challenges of arthritis.

6806 Increasing Behaviors of Persons with Severe Retardation and Autism

Research Press
2612 N Mattis Avenue
Champaign, IL 61821 **217-352-3273**
800-519-2707
FAX: 217-352-1221
e-mail: rp@researchpress.com
www.researchpress.com

Russell Pence, VP Marketing

Shows how to increase desirable behaviors by using techniques such as shaping, prompting, fading, modeling, backward chaining, and graduated guidance. Includes exercises, review questions, and numerous examples. *$15.95*

230 pages Paperback

ISBN 0-878222-63-4

6807 Independence Without Sight or Sound

American Foundation for the Blind/AFB Press
PO Box 1020
Sewickley, PA 15143 **412-741-1142**
800-232-3044
FAX: 412-741-0609
e-mail: afborders@abdintl.com
www.afb.org

Stephanie Biagioli, Marketing Coordinator

Written in a personal and informal style, this practical guidebook covers the essential aspects of communicating and working with deaf-blind adults. *$39.95*

193 pages Paperback

ISBN 0-89128 -46-7

6808 Individuals with Arthritis

Mainstream
3 Bethesda Metro Center
Suite 830
Bethesda, MD 20814 **301-951-6122**
800-247-1380
FAX: 301-654-6714
e-mail: info@mainstreaminc.org

Mainstreaming individuals with arthritis into the workplace. *$2.50*

12 pages

6809 Individuals with Cerebral Palsy

Mainstream
3 Bethesda Metro Center
Suite 830
Bethesda, MD 20814 **301-951-6122**
800-247-1380
FAX: 301-654-6714
e-mail: info@mainstreaminc.org

Mainstreaming individuals with cerebral palsy into the workplace. *$2.50*

12 pages

6810 Injured Mind, Shattered Dreams: Brian's Survival from a Severe Head Injury

Brookline Books
PO Box 1046
Cambridge, MA 02238 **617-868-0360**
800-666-2665
FAX: 617-868-1772
e-mail: brooklinebks@delphi.com
www.brooklinebooks.com

Brian, headed for normal adulthood, crashes his car and suffers a severe head injury. This book speaks to the issues in his recovery and the victory a family can achieve through caring advocacy and faith. *$17.95*

Paperback

ISBN 0-91479 -95-6

6811 Inside MS

National Multiple Sclerosis Society
421 New Karner Road
Suite 6
Albany, NY 12205 **518-464-0630**
800-344-4867
FAX: 518-464-1232
e-mail: chapter@msupstateny.org
www.nationalmssociety.org

News and information on research progress, medical treatments, patient services, therapeutic claims and activities.

6812 Insights

Spina Bifida Association of America
4590 Macarthur Boulevard NW
Suite 250
Washington, DC 20007 **202-944-3285**
800-621-3141
FAX: 202-944-3295
e-mail: sbaa@sbaa.org
www.sbaa.org

Alex Brodrick, Chair
Tim Yoder, Vice Chair

Bimonthly newsletter of the nonprofit organization. SBAA's mission is to promote the prevention of spina bifida and to enhance the lives of all affected. Addresses the specific needs of the spina bifida community and serves as the national representative of almost 60 chapters. Toll free 800 information and referral service. Legislative updates.

1973

6813 Insurance Solutions: Plan Well, Live Better

Demos Medical Publishing
386 Park Avenue S
Suite 201
New Yorok, NY 10016 **212-683-0072**
800-532-8663
FAX: 212-683-0118
e-mail: orderdep@demospub.com
www.demosmedpub.com

Diana Schneider PhD, President

Learn how to look at various insurance options from a new perspective — including life, disability, health, and long-term care. Concrete information for dealing with potential problems in your coverage, to secure your financial future. *$24.95*

192 pages 2002

ISBN 1-888799-55-2

6814 Interdisciplinary Clinical Assessment of Young Children with Developmental Disabilities

Brookes Publishing
PO Box 10624
Baltimore, MD 21285 **410-337-9580**
800-638-3775
FAX: 410-337-8539
e-mail: custserv@brookespublishing.com
www.brookespublishing.com

Offers insight from veteran team members on interdisciplinary team assessments. Professionals organizing a team as well as students preparing for practice will find advice on how practitioners gather information, approach assessment, make decisions, and face the challenges of their individual fields. Includes case studies and appendix of photocopiable questionnaires for clinicians and parents. *$42.00*

432 pages Hardcover 1900

ISBN 1-557664-50-1

6815 Introduction to Spina Bifida

Spina Bifida Association of America
4590 Macarthur Boulevard NW
Suite 250
Washington, DC 20007 **202-944-3285**
800-621-3141
FAX: 202-944-3295
e-mail: sbaa@sbaa.org
www.sbaa.org

1973

6816 Is the Child Really Stuttering? Questions & Answers About Disfluency

Speech Bin
1965 25th Avenue
Vero Beach, FL 32960 **772-770-0007**
800-477-3324
FAX: 772-770-0006
www.speechbin.com

In a question and answer format concisely shows differences between normal developmental and abnorlam disfluency and motivates adult listeners to deal with problems speech behaviors in a positive way. Set of ten brochures. *$9.95*

6817 Joslin Guide to Diabetes

Joslin Diabetes Center
1 Joslin Place
Boston, MA 02215 **617-732-2400**
FAX: 617-732-2452
www.joslin.harvard.edu

Discusses the causes of diabetes, the role of diet and exercise, meal planning and complications. Also provide information on drawing blood, mixing and injecting insulin, special challenges, living with diabetes. *$20.00*

352 pages

6818 Key

National Mental Health Consumers' Self-Help
1211 Chestnut Street
Suite 1207
Philadelphia, PA 19107 **215-751-1810**
800-553-4539
FAX: 215-636-6312
e-mail: info@mhselfhelp.org
www.mhselfhelp.org

Tom Leibfried, Editor

12 pages Quarterly

6819 **Labeling the Mentally Retarded**

University of California Press
2120 Berkeley Way
Berkeley, CA 94720 **510-643-7154**
FAX: 510-643-7127
www.ucpress.edu

Clinical and social system perspectives on mental retardation. *$12.95*

333 pages Paper

6820 **Language Disabilities in Children and Adolescents**

McGraw-Hill, School Publishing
220 E Danieldale Road
DeSoto, TX 75115 **972-224-1111**
800-442-9685
FAX: 972-228-1982
mhschool.com

A comprehensive review of research in language disabilities.

6821 **Language-Related Learning Disabilities: Their Nature and Treatment**

Brookes Publishing
PO Box 10624
Baltimore, MD 21285 **410-337-9580**
800-638-3775
FAX: 410-337-8539
e-mail: custserv@brookespublishing.com
www.brookespublishing.com

$47.00

464 pages Paperback
ISBN 1-55766 -53-0

6822 **Lead Poisoning in Childhood**

Brookes Publishing
PO Box 10624
Baltimore, MD 21285 **410-337-9580**
800-638-3775
FAX: 410-337-8539
e-mail: custserv@brookespublishing.com
www.brookespublishing.com

This book examines the epidemiology, etiology, and pathophysiology of lead poisoning - the most prevalent preventable childhood health problem today. Also provides practical prevention strategies that are cost-effective and easy to implement. *$31.95*

256 pages Paperback
ISBN 1-55766 -32-0

6823 **Learning Disabilities, Literacy, and Adult Education**

Brookes Publishing
PO Box 10624
Baltimore, MD 21285 **410-337-9580**
800-638-3775
FAX: 410-337-8539
e-mail: custserv@brookespublishing.com
www.brookespublishing.com

This book focuses on adults with severe learning disabilities and the educators who work with them. Described are the characteristics, demographics, and educational and employment status of adults with LD and the laws that protect them in the workplace and in educational settings.

450 pages Paperback 1998
ISBN 1-55766 -47-5

6824 **Learning Disabilities: Lifelong Issues**

Brookes Publishing
PO Box 10624
Baltimore, MD 21285 **410-337-9580**
800-638-3775
FAX: 410-337-8539
e-mail: custserv@brookespublishing.com
www.brookespublishing.com

Sections of this book are devoted to education, labor, justice, and health and human services offering an overview of research and a critical appraisal of the status of learning disability practices. This book sets forth an agenda for improving the educational and ultimately, the social and economic futures of people with learning disabilities. *$36.00*

352 pages Paperback
ISBN 1-55766 -40-1

6825 **Life Line**

National Hydrocephalus Foundation
12413 Centralia
Lakewood, CA 90715 **562-402-3523**
888-857-3434
888-260-1789
FAX: 562-924-6666
e-mail: debbifields@nhfonline.org
www.nhfonline.org

Debbi Fields, Executive Director

Publication included with membership. *$35.00*

12 pages Quarterly

6826 **Living Well with Asthma**

Guilford Press
72 Spring Street
New York, NY 10012 **212-431-9800**
800-365-7006
FAX: 212-966-6708
www.guilford.com

Cynthia L Divino PhD, Author

$15.95

213 pages Paperback 1998
ISBN 1-572300-51-5

6827 **Living with Rheumatoid Arthritis**

Johns Hopkins University Press
2715 N Charles Street
Baltimore, MD 21218 **410-516-6900**
800-537-5487
FAX: 410-516-6998
www.jhupbooks.com

This book offers practical and usable answers to the questions of everyday life. The authors provide clear explanations of the causes, diagnosis, and treatment of the disease, and why medication, joint protection, physical activity, and good nutrition are essential components of care. *$16.95*

280 pages Paperback
ISBN 0-801851-85-8

6828 **Living with Spina Bifida: A Guide for Fami lies and Professionals**

Spina Bifida Association of America
4590 Macarthur Boulevard NW
Suite 250
Washington, DC 20007 **202-944-3285**
800-621-3141
FAX: 202-944-3295
e-mail: sbaa@sbaa.org
www.sbaa.org

Written for families and professionals who care for children, adolescents and adults with spina bifida. *$19.00*

6829 Lung Cancer: Making Sense of Diagnosis, Treatment, & Option

Patient-Centered Guides
101 Morris Street
Sebastopol, CA 95472
707-829-0515
800-998-9938
FAX: 707-829-0104
www.patientcenters.com

Linda Lamb, Editor
Shawnde Paull, Marketing

Straightforward language and the words of patients and their families are the hallmarks of this book on the number one cancer killer in the US. Written by a widely respected author and patient advocate, Lung Cancer: Making Sense of Diagnosis, Treatment, & Options has been meticulously reviewed by top medical experts and physicians. Readers will find medical facts simply explained, advice to ease their daily life, and tools to be strong advocates for themselves or a family member. *$ 27.95*

530 pages Paperback
ISBN 0-596500-02-5

6830 MSFOCUS Magazine

Multiple Sclerosis Foundation
6350 N Andrews Avenue
Fort Lauderdale, FL 33309
954-776-6805
888-673-6287
FAX: 954-351-0630
e-mail: support@msfocus.org
www.msfocus.org

Kathleen Truax, Case Worker

Contemporary national, nonprofit organization that provides free support services and public education for persons with Multiple Sclerosis, newsletters, toll-free phone support, information, referrals, home care, assitive technology and support groups.

48 pages Quarterly

6831 Management of Autistic Behavior

Pro-Ed
8700 Shoal Creek Boulevard
Austin, TX 78757
512-451-3246
800-897-3202
FAX: 512-451-8542
e-mail: info@proedinc.com
www.proedinc.com

Comprehensive and practical book that tells what works best with specific problems. *$41.00*

450 pages Paperback
ISBN 0-890791-96-1

6832 Managing Attention Disorders in Children: A Guide for Practitioners

Books on Special Children
PO Box 305
Congers, NY 10920
845-638-1236
FAX: 845-638-0847
e-mail: irene@boscbooks.com

Offers information about human personality, structure and dynamics, assessment and adjustment. *$27.50*

214 pages

6833 Managing Post-Polio Syndrome

Polio Connection of America
PO Box 182
Howard Beach, NY 11414
718-835-5536
FAX: 718-738-1509
e-mail: w1066@msn.com
www.geocities.com/w1066w

240 pages

6834 Managing the Symptoms of Multiple Sclerosis

Demos Medical Publishing
386 Park Avenue S
Suite 201
New Yorok, NY 10016
212-683-0072
800-532-8663
FAX: 212-683-0118
e-mail: orderdep@demospub.com
www.demosmedpub.com

Diana Schneider PhD, President

Guide for the management of MS symptoms, providing both up-to-date pathophysiological explanation and carefully weighed clinical advice. *$19.95*

192 pages 2003
ISBN 1-888799-78-1

6835 Meeting the Challenge of Progressive Multiple Sclerosis

Demos Medical Publishing
386 Park Avenue S
Suite 201
New Yorok, NY 10016
212-683-0072
800-532-8663
FAX: 212-683-0118
e-mail: orderdep@demospub.com
www.demosmedpub.com

Diana Schneider PhD, President

A concise, practical and useful overview of worsening MS and the dilemma faced when progression presents its challenges to patients and those who care about them. *$21.95*

136 pages 2001
ISBN 1-888799-46-3

6836 Meniere's Disease

Vestibular Disorders Association
PO Box 4467
Portland, OR 97208
503-229-7705
800-837-8428
FAX: 503-229-8064
e-mail: veda@vestibular.org
www.vestibular.org

Lisa Haven, Editor
Connie Pilcher, Editor

1998

6837 Migraine and the Allergy Connection

Healing Arts Press
1 Park Street
Rochster, VT 05767
802-767-3174
FAX: 802-767-3174
e-mail: info@healartspro.com
www.healartspro.com

Discusses the connection between food, environmental allergies, and migraine headaches.

1990

6838 Migraine: Beating the Odds

Addison-Wesley Publishing Company
75 Arlington Street
Suite 300
Boston, MA 02116
617-848-6000
FAX: 617-848-6034
www.awprofessional.com

Discusses how diet, nutrition, and medicine affect migraine headaches.

1992

6839 Moisture Seekers

Sjogren's Syndrome Foundation
366 N Broadway
Suite PH-W2
Jericho, NY 11753
301-718-0300
800-475-6473
FAX: 301-718-0322
e-mail: ssf@sjogrens.org
www.sjogrens.org

Alexis Stegemann, Executive Director

Newsletter of the organization for lay people and professionals interested in Sjogren's Syndrome. Contains medical news, current research, and essential tips for daily living. *$25.00*

15-16 pages Monthly

6840 Motor Speech Disorders

WB Saunders Company
1810 Creekside Lane
Darien, IL 60561
630-910-0749
FAX: 630-910-5789
www.wbsaunders.com

Professional text on rehabilitation techniques for motor speech disorders. *$74.00*

304 pages

ISBN 0-72162 -78-8

6841 Motor Speech Disorders: Advances in Assessment and Treatment

Brookes Publishing
PO Box 10624
Baltimore, MD 21285
410-337-9580
800-638-3775
FAX: 410-337-8539
e-mail: custserv@brookespublishing.com
www.brookespublishing.com

$38.00

288 pages Paperback

ISBN 1-55766 -37-5

6842 Multiple Sclerosis

Demos Medical Publishing
386 Park Avenue S
Suite 201
New Yorok, NY 10016
212-683-0072
800-532-8663
FAX: 212-683-0118
e-mail: orderdep@demospub.com
www.demosmedpub.com

Diana Schneider PhD, President

Guide for living and coping with multiple sclerosis. *$ 39.95*

615 pages 2000

ISBN 1-888799-43-9

6843 Multiple Sclerosis: A Guide for Patients and Their Families

Lippincott, Williams & Wilkins
227 E Washington Square
Philadelphia, PA 19106
215-238-4200
800-777-2295
FAX: 301-824-7390
www.lpub.com

$16.00

288 pages

6844 Multiple Sclerosis: A Guide for the Newly Diagnosed

Demos Medical Publishing
386 Park Avenue S
Suite 201
New Yorok, NY 10016
212-683-0072
800-532-8663
FAX: 212-683-0118
e-mail: orderdep@demospub.com
www.demosmedpub.com

Diana Schneider PhD, President

A must-have title for anyone who has recently been diagnosed with MS and a good idea for family members and friends. *$ 21.95*

160 pages 2002

ISBN 1-888799-60-9

6845 Muscular Dystrophy and Other Neuromuscular Diseases

Haworth Press
10 Alice Street
Binghamton, NY 13904
607-722-5857
800-429-6784
FAX: 607-722-6362
e-mail: orders@haworthpress.com
www.haworthpress.com

S Harrington-Miller, Advertising

A thoughtful new book from professionals who assist persons afflicted with neuromuscular disorders to help them and their families adapt to lifestyle changes accompanying the onset of these disorders. *$74.95*

250 pages Hardcover

ISBN 1-560240-77-6

6846 NADS News

PO Box 4542
Oak Brook, IL 60522
630-325-9112
FAX: 630-325-8842
www.nads.org

Kim Xidas, Family Support Coordinator

A bi-monthly publication from the National Association for Down Syndrome. Subscription prices: $20 for parents; $25 for professionals.

12 pages Bi-monthly

6847 NHIF Newsletter

National Head Injury Foundation
1776 Massachusetts Avenue NW
Washington, DC 20036
202-452-1999
800-444-6443
FAX: 202-466-4265
www.biausa.org

George Zitnay, President

Contains news and articles for families and professionals concerned with head injury. *$25.00*

6848 Neurobiology of Autism

Johns Hopkins University Press
2715 N Charles Street
Baltimore, MD 21218
410-516-6936
FAX: 410-516-6998

This book discusses recent advances in scientific research that point to a neurobiological basis for autism and examines the clinical implications of this research. *$28.00*

272 pages

ISBN 0-801856-80-9

6849 Neuromotor Speech Disorders: Nature, Assessment, and Management

Brookes Publishing
PO Box 10624
Baltimore, MD 21285
410-337-9580
800-638-3775
FAX: 410-337-8539
e-mail: custserv@brookespublishing.com
www.brookespublishing.com

Topics included in this book are: motor-speech imaging, anatomical structure and function in dysarthria, physiological and acoustic analyses of dysarthria intelligibility, dysphonia, and linguistic considerations in apraxia of speech. *$44.95*

320 pages Hardcover 1998
ISBN 1-55766 -26-2

6850 On the Level

Vestibular Disorders Association
P.O. Box 4467
Portland, OR 97208
503-229-7705
800-837-8428
FAX: 503-229-8064
e-mail: veda@vestibular.org
www.vestibular.org

Lisa Haven, Editor
Connie Pilcher, Outreach Coordinator

Quarterly

6851 Options

PO Box 106273
Washington, DC 20016
301-897-8180
FAX: 202-466-1911
www.polio.org/

Ed Grebenstein, President
Jessica Scheer PhD, Executive Director

Quarterly newsletter of the national not-for-profit voluntary organziation created to provide education resources and support group services to people who had polio and are now experiencing the late effects of polio. Activities include maintenance of a national membership database of polio survivors and health care professionals; sponsorship of major national UPDATE conferences about post-polio issues; and publication of Options, quarterly newsletter.

6852 Options: Revolutionary Ideas in the War on Cancer

People Against Cancer
604 East Street
PO Box 10
Otho, IA 50569
515-972-4444
FAX: 515-972-4415
e-mail: info@PeopleAgainstCancer.net
www.peopleagainstcancer.com

Publication of People Against Cancer, a nonprofit, grassroots public benefit organization dedicated to 'New Directions in the War on Cancer.' We are a democratic organization of people with cancer, their loved ones and citizens working together to protect and enhance medical freedom of choice.

6853 Otitos Media in Young Children: Medical, Developmental, & Educational Considerations

Brookes Publishing
PO Box 10624
Baltimore, MD 21285
410-337-9580
800-638-3775
FAX: 410-337-8539
e-mail: custserv@brookespublishing.com
www.brookespublishing.com

Ina F Wallace PhD, Editor
Frederick W Henderson, Editor

This book reviews the current literature on the epidemiology, diagnosis, and medical management of otitis media; its secondary audiologic and communicative effects; and its impact on children and families. *$48.95*

352 pages Hardcover 1997
ISBN 1-557662-78-9

6854 PDF Newsletter

Parkinson's Disease Foundation
710 W 168th Street
New York, NY 10032
212-923-4700
800-457-6676
FAX: 212-923-4778
e-mail: info@pdf.org
www.pdf.org

Robin Elliott, Executive Director
Patricia Arroyo, Business Administrator

12-16 pages Quarterly

6855 PN/Paraplegia News Magazine

Paralyzed Veterans of America
801 18th Street NW
Washington, DC 20006
202-872-1300
800-424-8200
888-888-2201
e-mail: info@pva.org
www.pva.org

Joseph L Fox Sr, National President
Tom Wheaton, Senior VP
Gene A Crayton, National VP

Publication of the PVA, a congressionally chartered veterans service organization, with unique expertise on a wide variety of issues involving the special needs of our members—veterans of the armed forces who have experienced spinal cord injury or dysfunction.

1946

6856 PSP Advocate

Society for Progressive Supranuclear Palsy
Woodholme Medical Building #515
1838 Greene Tree Road
Baltimore, MD 21208
410-486-3330
800-457-4777
FAX: 410-486-4283
e-mail: spsp@psp.org
www.psp.org

Elizabeth Brisson, President
Stephen Hamer, VP
Kelley Harrison PhD, Secretary

Quarterly newsletter. The society's mission is to promote and fund research into finding the cause and cure for progressive supranuclear palsy (PSP). Provides information, support and advocacy to persons diagnosed with PSP, their families and caregivers. Educates physicians and allied health professionals on PSP and how to improve patient care.

6857 Parenting Preschoolers: Suggestions for Raising Young Blind Children

American Foundation for the Blind/AFB Press
PO Box 1020
Sewickley, PA 15143
412-741-1142
800-232-3044
FAX: 412-741-0609
e-mail: afborders@abdintl.com
www.afb.org

Provides practical answers to questions most frequently asked by parents and gives advice on what to expect, how to adapt to a child's situation and what to look for in early education programs. $50.00/pack of 25.

28 pages
ISBN 0-891289-98-4

6858 Partial Seizure Disorders: Help for Patients and Families

Patient-Centered Guides
101 Morris Street
Sebastopol, CA 95472
707-829-0515
800-998-9938
FAX: 707-829-0104
www.patientcenters.com

Linda Lamb, Editor
Shawnde Paull, Marketing

Partial Seizure Disorders helps patients and families get an accurate diagnosis of this condition, understand medications and their side effects, and learn coping skills and other adjuncts to medication. It walks readers through developmental and school issues for young children; adult issues such as employment and driving; working with an existing health plan; and getting further help through advocacy and support organizations, articles, and online resources. *$19.95*

288 pages Paperback
ISBN 0-596500-03-3

6859 Personal Guide to Living Well with Fibromyalgia

Arthritis Foundation Distribution Center
PO Box 6996
Alpharetta, GA 30009
800-207-8633
FAX: 770-442-9742
www.arthritis.com

With this guide you'll learn the latest information about fibromyalgia, what researchers have uncovered about its causes, and an overview of the best treatment options available. Helpful worksheets and tables allow you to manage your condition and document your progress. *$14.95*

224 pages

6860 Plan Ahead: Do What You Can

Spina Bifida Association of America
4590 Macarthur Boulevard NW
Suite 250
Washington, DC 20007
202-944-3285
800-621-3141
FAX: 202-944-3295
e-mail: sbaa@sbaa.org
www.sbaa.org

Alex Brodrick, Chair
Tim Yoder, Vice Chair

Folic acid information for women at risk for recurrence. Available in Spanish.

1973

6861 Polio Network News

Gazette International Networking Institute
4207 Lindell Boulevard
Suite 110
Saint Louis, MO 63108
314-534-0475
FAX: 314-534-5070
e-mail: gini_intl@msn.com
www.post-polio.org

International newsletter for polio survivors, support groups and health professionals concerned about the late effects of polio. *$20.00*

12 pages Quarterly

6862 Polio Vaccine Coverup Report: The New Polio Deception

Polio Connection of America
PO Box 182
Howard Beach, NY 11414
718-835-5536
FAX: 718-738-1509
e-mail: w1066@msn.com
www.geocities.com/w1066w

57 pages

6863 Post Polio

Accent Books & Products
PO Box 700
Bloomington, IL 61702
309-378-2961
800-787-8444
FAX: 309-378-4420
e-mail: acmtlvng@aol.com

Raymond C Cheever, Publisher
Betty Garee, Editor

What does post-polio syndrome mean? What can make a difference in a persons future mobility? These questions and more are answered in this great guide. *$3.95*

47 pages Paperback
ISBN 0-91570 -21-3

6864 Post-Polio Health

Post-Polio Health International
4207 Lindell Boulevard
Suite 110
Saint Louis, MO 63108
314-534-0475
FAX: 314-534-5070
TTY:800-735-2966
e-mail: info@post-polio.org
www.post-polio.org

To enhance the lives and independence of polio survivors by promoting education, networking, and advocacy among these individuals and healthcare providers. Post-Polio Health supports Post-Polio Health International's educational, research, and advocacy efforts. Offers information about relevant events.

12 pages quarterly

6865 Post-Polio Syndrome Information Book

PO Box 182
Howard Beach, NY 11414
718-835-5536
FAX: 718-738-1509
e-mail: w1066@msn.com
www.geocities.com/w1066w

100 pages

6866 Prader-Willi Alliance of New York Monthly Newsletter

267 Oxford Street
Rochester, NY 14607
716-442-1655
800-442-1655
FAX: 716-271-2782
e-mail: balleregballer@aol.com
www.prader-willi.org

Elinor G Baller, Secretary

The Prader-Willi Foundation is a national, nonprofit public charity that works for the benefit of individuals with Prader-Willi syndrome and their families.

6867 **Pressure Sores**

Accent Books & Products
PO Box 700
Bloomington, IL 61702 **309-378-2961**
800-787-8444
FAX: 309-378-4420
e-mail: acmtlvng@aol.com

Raymond C Cheever, Publisher
Betty Garee, Editor

All it takes is one to put a stop to all of your activities. This book offers ways to be able to be comfortable and worry-free by knowing how to treat, recognize and prevent pressure sores. *$3.50*

29 pages Paperback
ISBN 0-91570 -20-5

6868 **Preventable Brain Damage**

Springer Publishing Company
536 Broadway
New York, NY 10012 **212-431-4370**
877-687-7476
FAX: 212-941-7842
e-mail: marketing@springerpub.com
www.springerpub.com

Annette Imperati, Marketing/Sales Director

Offers information on brain injuries from motor vehicle accidents, contact sports and injuries of children. *$35.95*

256 pages

6869 **Preventing Secondary Conditions Associated with Spina Bifida or Cerebral Palsy**

Spina Bifida Association of America
4590 MacArthur Boulevard NW
Suite 250
Washington, DC 20007 **202-944-3285**
800-621-3141
FAX: 202-944-3295
e-mail: sbaa@sbaa.org
www.sbaa.org

This report is for health professionals, parents and teachers. *$3.00*

6870 **Primer on the Rheumatic Diseases**

Arthritis Foundation
PO Box 6996
Alpharetta, GA 30009
800-207-8633
FAX: 404-872-0457
www.arthritis.com

Written to educate medical students and family physicians, this is the authoritative guide on the rheumatic diseases. *$39.95*

513 pages

6871 **Progress in Research**

Christopher Reeve Paralysis Foundation
500 Morris Avenue
Springfield, NJ 07081 **973-379-6299**
800-225-0292
FAX: 973-912-9433
e-mail: paralysis@aol.com
www.paralysis.org

Summarizes research on paralysis and spinal cord injury, emphasizing neural regeneration.

6872 **Pure Facts**

Feingold Association of the US
127 E Main Street
Suite 106
Riverhead, NY 11901 **631-369-9340**
800-321-3287
FAX: 631-369-2988
e-mail: help@feingold.org
www.feingold.org

Jane Hersey, Editor

Relationship between foods, food additives and behavior/learning problems, including Attention Deficit Disorder (ADD) and hyperactivity. *$38.00*

8 pages 10x Year

6873 **Rasmussen's Syndrome and Hemispherectomy Support Network Newsletter**

8235 Lethbridge Road
Millersville, MD 21108 **410-987-5221**
FAX: 410-987-521
e-mail: rssnlynn@aol.com

Al & Lynn Miller, Founders

National not-for-profit organization dedicated to providing information and support to individuals affected by Rasmussen's Syndrome and Hemispherectomy. Publishes a periodic newsletter and disseminates reprints of medical journal articles concerning Rasmussen's Syndrome and its treatments. Maintains a support network that provides encouragement and information to individuals affected by Rasmussen's Syndrome and their families.

6874 **Reality of Dyslexia**

Brookline Books
PO Box 1047
Cambridge, MA 02238 **617-868-0360**
800-666-2665
FAX: 617-868-1772
e-mail: brooklinebks@delphi.com
www.brooklinebooks.com

An informative and sensitive study of living with dyslexia which affects one in 25. He introduces the reader to the subject by sharing the difficulties of his dyslexic son. He then uses the personal accounts of other children and adult dyslexics, even entire dyslexic families, to illuminate the problems they encounter. *$14.95*

150 pages Paperback
ISBN 1-57129 -17-6

6875 **Record Book for Individuals with Autism**

Autism Society of North Carolina Bookstore
505 Oberlin Road
Suite 230
Raleigh, NC 27605 **919-743-0204**
800-442-2762
FAX: 919-743-0208
e-mail: dcoffey@autismsociety-nc.org
www.autismsociety-nc.org

Darla Coffey, Bookstore Manager

Developed with parent input to provide one place to keep information about an autistic child. *$7.00*

6876 Riddle of Autism: A Psychological Analysis

Jason Aronson
400 Keystone Industrial Park
Dunmore, PA 18512
800-782-0015
FAX: 201-840-7242
www.aronson.com

Dr. Victor examines the myths that cloud an understanding of this disorder and describes the meanings of its specific behavioral symptoms. *$30.00*

356 pages Softcover
ISBN 1-568215-73-8

6877 SCI Psychosocial Process

Amer. Assn. of Spinal Cord Injury Psych./Soc. Wks.
7520 Astoria Boulevard
Jackson Heights, NY 11370
718-803-3782
FAX: 718-803-0414
e-mail: ssofer@epua.org
www.aascipsw.org

E Jason Mask LCSW, Editor

Quarterly newsletter.

6878 SPINabilities: A Young Person's Guide to Spina Bifida

Spina Bifida Association of America
4590 Macarthur Boulevard NW
Suite 250
Washington, DC 20007
202-944-3285
800-621-3141
FAX: 202-944-3295
e-mail: sbaa@sbaa.org
www.sbaa.org

A cool and practical book for young adults becoming independent. *$19.00*

6879 Schools for Children with Autism Spectrum Disorders

Resources for Children with Special Needs
116 E 16th Street
5th Floor
New York, NY 10003
212-667-4650
FAX: 212-254-4070
e-mail: info@resourcesnyc.org
www.resourcesnyc.org

Karen Schlesinger, Executive Director
Dianne Littwin, Director Publications

Published every 24-36 months. *$20.00*

160 pages
ISBN 0-967836-53-0

6880 Self-Therapy for the Stutterer

Stuttering Foundation of America
3100 Walnut Groove Road, Suite 603
PO Box 11749
Memphis, TN 38111
901-452-7343
800-992-9392
FAX: 901-452-3931
e-mail: stutter@vantek.net
www.stutterhelp.org

A guide to help adults who stutter overcome the problem on their own. *$3.00*

191 pages Paperback
ISBN 0-933388-32-2

6881 Sexuality After Spinal Cord Injury: Answers to Your Questions

Brookes Publishing
PO Box 10624
Baltimore, MD 21285
410-337-9580
800-638-3775
FAX: 410-337-8539
e-mail: custserv@brookespublishing.com
www.brookespublishing.com

Anatomy, fertility, sexually transmitted diseases, self-esteem, sexual satisfaction, and parenting are among the many physical and emotional issues discussed in this guide. Question-and-answer format. *$24.95*

272 pages Paperback 1997
ISBN 1-557662-65-7

6882 Sexuality and the Person with Spina Bifida

Spina Bifida Association of America
4590 MacArthur Boulevard NW
Suite 250
Washington, DC 20007
202-944-3285
800-621-3141
FAX: 202-944-3295
e-mail: sbaa@sbaa.org
www.sbaa.org

Dr Sloan foucuses on sexual development, sexual activity and other important issues. *$11.00*

6883 Shoebox Tasks: Work Activities

Autism Society of North Carolina Bookstore
505 Oberlin Road
Suite 230
Raleigh, NC 27605
919-743-0204
800-442-2762
FAX: 919-743-0208
e-mail: dcoffey@autismsociety-nc.org
www.autismsociety-nc.org

Darla Coffey, Bookstore Manager

$250.00

6884 Single-Handed: A Book for Persons with the Use of Only One Hand

Accent Books & Products
PO Box 700
Bloomington, IL 61702
309-378-2961
800-787-8444
FAX: 309-378-4420
e-mail: acmtlvng@aol.com

Raymond C Cheever, Publisher
Betty Garee, Editor

Includes information on devices and aids; special techniques; tips on how-to; illustrations; other helpful publications and more. *$4.25*

25 pages Paperback
ISBN 0-91570 -06-0

6885 Smart But Stuck: Emotional Aspects of Learning Disabilities and Imprisoned Intelligence

Haworth Press
10 Alice Street
Binghamton, NY 13904
607-722-5857
800-429-6784
FAX: 607-722-6362
e-mail: orders@haworthpress.com
www.haworthpress.com

S Harrington-Miller, Advertising

Elaborates on new research about imprisoned intelligence and the emotional consequences of learning disabilities. It is also for psychoterapists, educators, school social workers, medical personnel, people dealing with prisons, etc. It helps those who struggle with learning disabilities (and people who help them) build self esteem, face LD obstacles, bypass weaknesses, and enhance strenghts. *$34.95*

228 pages Hardcover

ISBN 0-789014-66-1

6886 Son-Rise: The Miracle Continues

2080 S Undermountain Road
Sheffield, MA 01257
413-229-2100
800-714-2779
FAX: 413-229-3202
e-mail: sonrise@option.org
www.son-rise.org

Documents Raun Kaufman's astonishing development from a lifeless, autistic, retarded child into a highly verbal, lovable youngster with no traces of his former condition. Details Raun's extraordinary progress from the age of four into young adulthood, also shares moving accounts of five families that successfully used the Son-Rise Program to reach their own special children.

372 pages 1994

ISBN 0-915811-53-7

6887 Soon Will Come the Light

Autism Society of North Carolina Bookstore
505 Oberlin Road
Suite 230
Raleigh, NC 27605
919-743-0204
800-442-2762
FAX: 919-743-0208
e-mail: dcoffey@autismsociety-nc.org
www.autismsociety-nc.org

Darla Coffey, Bookstore Manager

Offers new perspectives on the perplexing disability of autism. *$19.95*

6888 Spectrum

Autism Society of North Carolina
505 Oberlin Road
Suite 230
Raleigh, NC 27605
919-743-0204
800-442-2762
FAX: 919-743-0208
e-mail: dcoffey@autismsociety-nc.org
www.autismsociety-nc.org

David Laxton, Editor

Quarterly publication from the Autism Society of North Carolina. *$30.00*

Quarterly

6889 Spinal Cord Injury Life

National Spinal Cord Injury Association
8701 Georgia Avenue
 # 500
Silver Spring, MD 20910
617-469-0004
800-962-9629
FAX: 301-588-9414
e-mail: nscia2@aol.com
www.spinalcord.org

Thomas H Countee Jr, Executive Director

Includes sections such as Legislative Action, Information Resources and Research Notes. *$30.00*

45-60 pages Quarterly

6890 Spine

JB Lippincott
E Washington Square
Philadelphia, PA 19105
FAX: 215-824-7390

Publishes original papers on theoretical issues and research concerning the spine and spinal cord injuries. *$9.00*

Monthly

6891 Sports n' Spokes Magazine

Paralyzed Veterans of America
801 18th Street NW
Washington, DC 20006
202-872-1300
800-424-8200
888-888-2201
e-mail: info@pva.org
www.pva.org

Joseph L Fox Sr, National President
Tom Wheaton, Senior VP
Gene A Crayton, National VP

Publication of the PVA, a congressionally chartered veterans service organization, with unique expertise on a wide variety of issues involving the special needs of our members—veterans of the armed forces who have experienced spinal cord injury or dysfunction.

1946

6892 Stroke Connection

American Heart Association
7272 Greenville Avenue
Dallas, TX 75231
214-373-6300
800-553-6321
FAX: 214-369-3685

A forum for stroke survivors and their families to share information about coping with stroke. Provides information and referrals, and carries stroke related books, videos and literature available for purchase.

6893 Students with Acquired Brain Injury: The School's Response

Brookes Publishing
PO Box 10624
Baltimore, MD 21285
410-337-9580
800-638-3775
FAX: 410-337-8539
e-mail: custserv@brookespublishing.com
www.brookespublishing.com

This book is designed for school professionals and describes a range of issues that this population faces and presents proven means of addressing them in ways that benefit all students. Included topics are hospital-to-school transitions, effective assessment strategies, model programs in public schools, interventions to assist classroom teachers, and ways to involve family members in the educational program. *$29.95*

424 pages Paperback 1997

ISBN 1-557662-85-1

6894 Stuttering

Federal Government
31 Center Drive MSC2320
Bethesda, MD 20892
800-241-1044
FAX: 301-402-0018
e-mail: nidcdinfo@nidcd.nih.gov
www.nidcd.nih.gov

Marin P Allen PhD, Chief OHCPL

Describes how speech is produced, treatments for stuttering and research supported by the federal government.

6895 TBC Focus

400 S State Street 5 N
Chicago, IL 60605
312-747-4001
800-757-4654
FAX: 312-747-1609
e-mail: mgrady@ch.publib.org

Mamie Grady, Librarian

Published quarterly by the Chicago Public Library Talking Book Center. Free of charge.

4 pages Quarterly

6896 TSA Newsletter

Tourette Syndrome Association
42-40 Bell Boulevard
Bayside, NY 11361
718-224-2999
800-237-0717
FAX: 718-279-9596
e-mail: ts@tsa-usa.org
www.tsa-usa.org

Fred Cook, Editor
Judit Ungar, Editor
Tracy Colletti-Flynn, Editor

Quarterly

6897 Teach and Reach Students with Attention Deficit Disorders

MultiGrowth Resources
12345 Jones Road
Suite 101
Houston, TX 77070
281-890-5334
FAX: 281-894-8611

Handbook adn resource guide for parents and educators of ADD students. *$19.95*

200 pages
ISBN 0-963084-70-4

6898 Teaching Children with Autism: Strategies to Enhance Communication

Autism Society of North Carolina Bookstore
505 Oberlin Road
Suite 230
Raleigh, NC 27605
919-743-0204
800-442-2762
FAX: 919-743-0208
e-mail: dcoffey@autismsociety-nc.org
www.autismsociety-nc.org

Darla Coffey, Bookstore Manager

This valuable new book describes teaching strategies and instructional adaptations which promote communication and socialization in children with autism. *$38.95*

6899 Teaching and Mainstreaming Autistic Children

Love Publishing Company
1777 S Bellaire Street
Denver, CO 80222
303-221-7333
FAX: 303-221-7444
e-mail: lovepublishing@compuserve.com

Dr. Knoblock advocates a highly organized, structured environment for autistic children, with teachers and parents working together. His premise is that the learning and social needs of autistic children must be analyzed and a daily program be designed with interventions that respond to this functional analysis of their behavior. *$24.95*

ISBN 0-891081-11-9

6900 Techniques for Aphasia Rehab: (TARGET) Generating Effective Treatment

Speech Bin
1965 25th Avenue
Vero Beach, FL 32960
772-770-0007
800-477-3324
FAX: 772-770-0006
www.speechbin.com

Practical treatment manual for use by aphasia clinicians. *$45.00*

384 pages
ISBN 0-93785 -50-5

6901 Teenagers with ADD

Woodbine House
6510 Bells Mill Road
Bethesda, MD 20817
301-897-3570
800-843-7323
FAX: 301-897-5838
www.woodbinehouse.com

This best selling guide to understanding and coping with teenagers with attention deficit disorder (ADD) provides complete coverage of the special issues and challenges faced by these teens. Based on current diagnostic criteria and the latest literature and research in the field, the book discusses diagnosis, medical treatment, family and school life, intervention, advocacy, legal rights, and options after high school. Parents find strategies for dealing with their teen's difficult behaviors. *$18.95*

370 pages Paperback
ISBN 0-933149-69-7

6902 Three Hundred Tips for Making Life with Multiple Sclerosis Easier

Demos Medical Publishing
386 Park Avenue S
Suite 201
New Yorok, NY 10016
212-683-0072
800-532-8663
FAX: 212-683-0118
e-mail: orderdep@demosmedpub.com
www.demosmedpub.com

Diana Schneider PhD, President

This latest book in the Making Life Easier series features tip, techniques and shortcuts for conserving time and energy so you can do more of the things you want to do. These tips should help increase the number of good days you have while encouraging you to develop your own techniques for making life easier. *$18.95*

109 pages 1999
ISBN 1-888799-23-4

6903 Tourette Syndrome Association Annual Medical Letter

42-40 Bell Boulevard
Bayside, NY 11361
718-224-2999
800-237-0717
FAX: 718-279-9596
e-mail: ts@tsa-usa.org
www.tsa-usa.org

Fred Cook, Chair
Judit Ungar, President

National, nonprofit membership organization. Mission is to identify the cause of, find the cure for, and control the effects of this disorder. A growing number of local chapters nationwide provide educational materials, seminars, conferences and support groups for over 35,000 members.

6904 Tourette Syndrome Association Newsletter

42-40 Bell Boulevard
Bayside, NY 11361
718-224-2999
800-237-0717
FAX: 718-279-9596
e-mail: ts@tsa-usa.org
www.tsa-usa.org

Fred Cook, Chair
Judit Ungar, President

National, nonprofit membership organization. Mission is to identify the cause of, find the cure for, and control the effects of this disorder. A growing number of local chapters nationwide provide educational materials, seminars, conferences and support groups for over 35,000 members.

Quarterly

6905 Tourette's Syndrome: Finding Answers and Getting Help

Patient-Centered Guides
101 Morris Street
Sebastopol, CA 95472
707-829-0515
800-998-9938
FAX: 707-829-0104
www.patientcenters.com

Linda Lamb, Editor
Shawnde Paull, Marketing

Tourette's Syndrome is a neurological disorder usually diagnosed in childhood and characterized by tics, physical jerks, and involuntary vocalizations. Tourette's can be a devastating disability. The good news is that it's very treatable. Tourette's Syndrome helps you secure a diagnosis, understand medical interventions, get healthcare coverage, and manage Tourette's in family life, school, community, and workplace. *$24.95*

356 pages Paperback
ISBN 0-596500-07-6

6906 Toward Healthy Living: A Wellness Journal

Arthritis Foundation Distribution Center
PO Box 6996
Alpharetta, GA 30009
800-207-8633
FAX: 770-442-9742
www.arthritis.com

This spiral-bound journal has ample pages where you can unleach you thoughts, plus scales to monitor your mook and pain. Throught the book you will also find wisdom from a variety of famous and ordinary people - those who live with chronic ilness, and those whose life lessons can help you gain a more positive outlook on daily living. *$9.95*

144 pages

6907 Transition Matters: from School to Independence

Resources for Children with Special Needs
116 E 16th Street
5th Floor
New York, NY 10003
212-667-4650
FAX: 212-254-4070
e-mail: info@resourcesnyc.org
www.resourcesnyc.org

Karen Schlesinger, Executive Director
Dianne Littwin, Director Publications

Published every 24-36 months. *$35.00*

496 pages
ISBN 0-967836-56-5

6908 Traumatic Brain Injury: Cognitive & Communication Disorders

Federal Government
31 Center Drive MSC2320
Bethesda, MD 20892
800-241-1044
FAX: 301-402-0018
e-mail: nidcdinfo@nidcd.nih.gov
www.nidcd.nih.org

Explains what is traumatic brain injury, who suffer from head trauma, what are the cognitive and communication problems that result from traumatic brain injury, how cognitive and communication probles assessed and how they are treated, and what research is being done for the cognitive and communication prblems caused by traumatic brain injury.

6909 Two Hundred Fifty Tips for Making Life with Arthritis Easier

Longstreet Press
2974 Hardman Court
Atlanta, GA 30305
404-254-0110
FAX: 404-254-0016
e-mail: info@longstreetpress.com
www.longstreetpress.com

Thomas Cogburn, Distribution Director

Is it difficult for you to handle everyday chores because of pregnancy, back problems, or the general effects of aging? If so, you'll find tremendous help in the 250 tips in this book. Discover ways to do everything from adapting your home to completing chores and organizing household activities. Even if your limitations are only minimal, you'll find an abundance of suggestions to help you work smarter, faster and more efficiently. *$9.95*

88 pages 1997
ISBN 1-563523-81-7

6910 Ultimate Stranger, The Autistic Child

Academic Therapy Publications
20 Commercial Boulevard
Novato, CA 94949
800-442-7249
FAX: 415-883-3720
www.bookfinder.com

Anna M Arena, President

Clinical background and theories of rehabilitation for the autistic child. *$15.00*

240 pages Paperback
ISBN 0-878794-46-8

6911 Understanding Asthma: The Blueprint for Breathing

National Allergy and Asthma Network
3554 Chain Bridge Road
Suite 200
Fairfax, VA 22030
703-385-4403
FAX: 703-352-4354

A layman's guide to asthma facts based on a presentation from the first national asthma patient conference.

6912 **Understanding Down Syndrome: An Introduction for Parents**

Brookline Books
PO Box 1046
Cambridge, MA 02238
617-868-0360
800-666-2665
FAX: 617-868-1772
e-mail: brooklinebks@delphi.com
www.brooklinebooks.com

Using positive and readable language, this book helps parents understand Down Syndrome. Medical details are explained in lay terms, and advice is given on working with professionals, obtaining services, and treatment techniques that help the child. Cunningham alerts families to potential problems, the prospects for the child in schooling and the passage to adulthood. Revised 1996. *$14.95*

Softcover
ISBN 1-57129 -09-5

6913 **Understanding Juvenile Rheumatoid Arthritis**

American Juvenile Arthritis Organization
1330 W Peachtree Street
PO Box 7669
Atlanta, GA 30326
404-872-7100
800-283-7800
FAX: 404-872-9559
e-mail: help@arthritis.org
www.arthritis.org

A manual for health professionals to use in teaching children with JRA and their families about disease management and self-care. *$61.20*

372 pages

6914 **Understanding Multiple Sclerosis**

MacMillan Publishing Company
135 S Mount Zion Road
Lebanon, IN 46052
FAX: 800-882-8583

Two psychologists discuss their roles with a member who has multiple sclerosis. Includes chapters on adolescents with multiple sclerosis, employment, and research.

6915 **Understanding and Managing Learning Disabilities in Adults**

Krieger Publishing Company
PO Box 9542
Melbourne, FL 32902
321-724-9542
800-724-0025
FAX: 321-951-3671
e-mail: info@krieger-publishing.com
www.krieger-publishing.com

This book first explains how the brain functions in learning and remembering throughout one's life span. Individual chapters then describe the types of learning disabilities (LD) that exist throughout adulthood: dyslexia, attention deficit disorders, Scotopic Sensitivity syndrome, Nonverbal LD, Social-Emotional LD, and mental health factors that frequently accompany learning disabilities. The discussion is two-fold. First each type of LD is described and explained, then management strategies. *$24.50*

150 pages Hardcover
ISBN 1-575241-08-0

6916 **Understanding the Nature of Autism**

Autism Society of North Carolina Bookstore
505 Oberlin Road
Suite 230
Raleigh, NC 27605
919-743-0204
800-442-2762
FAX: 919-743-0208
e-mail: dcoffey@autismsociety-nc.org
www.autismsociety-nc.org

Darla Coffey, Bookstore Manager

$54.00

6917 **Until Tomorrow: A Family Lives with Autism**

Autism Society of North Carolina Bookstore
505 Oberlin Road
Suite 230
Raleigh, NC 27605
919-743-0204
800-442-2762
FAX: 919-743-0208
e-mail: dcoffey@autismsociety-nc.org
www.autismsociety-nc.org

Darla Coffey, Bookstore Manager

The central theme of this book is an effort to show what it is like to live with a child who cannot communicate. *$10.00*

6918 **Ventilator-Assisted Living**

Post-Polio Health International
4207 Lindell Boulevard
Suite 110
Saint Louis, MO 63108
314-534-0475
FAX: 314-534-5070
TTY:800-735-2966
e-mail: info@post-polio.org
www.post-polio.org

To enhance the lives and independence of ventilator-assisted living by promoting education, networking, and advocacy among these individuals and healthcare providers. Ventilator-Assisted Living supports Post-Polio Health International's educational, research, and advocacy efforts. Offers information about relevant events.

12 pages quarterly

6919 **Victims of Dementia: Services, Support and Care**

Haworth Press
10 Alice Street
Binghamton, NY 13904
607-722-5857
800-429-6784
FAX: 607-722-6362
e-mail: orders@haworthpress.com
www.haworthpress.com

S Harrington-Miller, Advertising

Provides an in-depth look at the concept, construction and operation of Wesley Hall, a special living area at the Chelsea United Methodist retirement home in Michigan. *$74.95*

155 pages Hardcover
ISBN 1-560242-64-7

6920 **Visually Structured Tasks**

Autism Society of North Carolina Bookstore
505 Oberlin Road
Suite 230
Raleigh, NC 27605
919-743-0204
800-442-2762
FAX: 919-743-0208
e-mail: dcoffey@autismsociety-nc.org
www.autismsociety-nc.org

Darla Coffey, Bookstore Manager

Independent activites for students with autism and other visual learners. *$24.95*

6921 **Voice of the Diabetic**

Diabetes Action Network of the NFB
1412 I70 Drive SW
Suite C
Columbia, MO 65203
573-875-8911
FAX: 573-875-8902
e-mail: ebrnant@socvet.net
www.nfb.org/voice.htm

Ed Bryant, Editor

Newsletters containing personal stories and practical guidelines by blind diabetics and medical professionals, medical news, resource column and a recipe corner. We are a support and information network for all diabetics.

28 pages Quarterly

6922 Volunteer Voice

Kentucky Chapter of the Arthritis Foundation
2908 Brownsboro Road
Suite 100
Louisville, KY 40206 **502-585-1866**
FAX: 502-585-1657
www.kecc.org

Newsletter offering information and updates on chapter activities, events, camps, juvenile programs and government/legislative information.

6923 What is Vocal Hoarseness?

Speech Bin
1965 25th Avenue
Vero Beach, FL 32960 **772-770-0007**
800-477-3324
FAX: 772-770-0006
www.speechbin.com

Brochures to teach parents, teachers and individuals with voice disorders about chronic hoarseness and what to do about it. Set of ten copies. *$16.95*

24 pages Package of 10
ISBN 0-93785 -55-6

6924 Winter Blues: Seasonal Affective Disorder: What it is and How to Overcome It

Guilford Press
72 Spring Street
New York, NY 10012 **212-431-9800**
800-365-7006
FAX: 212-966-6708
www.guilford.com

$15.95

355 pages Paperback 1998
ISBN 1-572303-95-6

Visually Impaired

6925 ABC Sign with Me

TJ Publishers
817 Silver Spring Avenue
Suite 206
Silver Spring, MD 20910 **301-585-4440**
800-999-1168
FAX: 301-585-5930
e-mail: TJPubinc@aol.com

Angela K Thames, President
Jerald A Murphy, VP

Offers bright pictures of familiar objects, lower case alphabet and corresponding manual alphabet hand shapes. *$3.95*

32 pages Softcover
ISBN 0-93984 -00-3

6926 AFB News

American Foundation for the Blind/AFB Press
11 Penn Plaza
Suite 300
New York, NY 10001 **212-502-7614**
800-232-3044
FAX: 212-502-7777
e-mail: afborders@abdintl.com
www.afb.org

National newsletter for general readership about blindness and visual impairments featuring people, programs, services and activities.

12 pages Quarterly

6927 Access to Art: A Museum Directory for Blind and Visually Impaired People

American Foundation for the Blind/AFB Press
PO Box 1020
Sewickley, PA 15143 **412-741-1142**
800-232-3044
FAX: 412-741-0609
e-mail: afborders@abdintl.com
www.afb.org

Details the access facilities of over 300 museums, galleries and exhibits in the United States. Also included are organizations offering art-related resources such as, art classes, competitions and traveling exhibits. *$19.95*

144 pages Large Print
ISBN 0-891281-56-8

6928 African Americans in the Profession of Blindness Services

Mississippi State University
PO Box 6189
Mississippi State, MS 39762 **662-325-2001**
800-675-7782
FAX: 662-325-8989
www.blind.msstate.edu

Kelly Schaefer, Dissemination Specialist

This study investigated the level of participation by African Americans in vocational rehab. (VR) services to persons who are visually impaired. Using surveys and interviews with all state VR directors, national Census data and national RSA data, it was found nationally that African Americans are substantially under-represented in the service provider ranks, yet over-represented as clients. *$20.00*

61 pages Paperback

6929 Age-Related Macular Degeneration

National Association for Visually Handicapped
22 W 21st Street
6th Floor
New York, NY 10010 **212-889-2804**
FAX: 212-727-2931
e-mail: staff@navh.org
www.navh.org

Dr Lorraine H Marchi, Founder/CEO
Cesar Gomez, COO

A large booklet offering information and up-to-date research on Macular Degeneration. Also available in Russian. Revised in 2002. *$4.00*

6930 Aging and Vision: Declarations of Independence

American Foundation for the Blind/AFB Press
PO Box 1020
Sewickley, PA 15143 **412-741-1142**
800-232-3044
FAX: 412-741-0609
e-mail: afborders@abdintl.com
www.afb.org

A very personal look at five older people who have successfully coped with visual impairmant and continue to lead active, satisfying lives. Their stories are not only inspirational, but also provide practical, down-to-earth suggestions for adapting to vision loss later in life. 18 minute video tape. Also available in PAL, $52.95, 0-89128-276-9. *$42.95*

VHS
ISBN 0-891282-20-3

6931 American Printing House for the Blind

1839 Frankfort Avenue
PO Box 6085
Louisville, KY 40206 **502-895-2405**
800-223-1839
FAX: 502-899-2274
e-mail: info@aph.org
www.aph.org

Fred Gissoni, Customer Support

Devoted solely to producing products for people who are visually impaired. We manufacture books and magazines in braille, large type and recorded form from over 200 vendors across the U.S. We also make a wide range of educational and daily living aids, such as braille paper and styluses, talking book equipment, and synthetic speech computer products. APH also offers LOUIS, an electronic database that lists accessible books in all formats.

6932 Annual Report/Newsletter

National Accreditation Council for Agencies/Blind
15 E 40th Street
Room 1004
New York, NY 10016 **212-683-5068**
FAX: 212-683-4475

Ruth Westman, Executive Director

Provides standards and a program of accreditation for schools and organizations which serve children and adults who are blind or vision impaired.

6933 Art and Science of Teaching Orientation and Mobility to Persons with Visual Impairments

American Foundation for the Blind/AFB Press
PO Box 1020
Sewickley, PA 15143 **412-741-1142**
800-232-3044
FAX: 412-741-0609
e-mail: afborders@abdintl.com
www.afb.org

Comprehensive decription of the techniques of teaching orientation and mobility, presented along with considerations and strategies for sensitive and effective teaching. Hardcover. Paperback also available. *$48.00*

200 pages
ISBN 0-891282-45-9

6934 Association for Macular Diseases Newsletter

210 E 64th Street
8th Floor
New York, NY 10021 **212-605-3719**
FAX: 212-605-3795
e-mail: association@retinal-research.org
www.macula.org

Nikolai Stevenson, President
Walter Ross, Editor in Chief
Joan Daly, Treasurer

Not-for-profit organization promotes education and research in this scarcely explored field. Acts as a nationwide support group for individuals and their families endeavoring to adjust to the restrictions and changes brought about by macular disease. Offers hotline, educational materials, quarterly newsletter, support groups, referrals and seminars for persons and families affected by macular disease.

1978

6935 Awareness

NAPVI
PO Box 317
Watertown, MA 02472 **617-972-7441**
800-562-6265
FAX: 617-972-7444
e-mail: napvi@perkins.org
www.napvi.org

Susan LaVenture, Executive Director

Newsletter offering regional news, sports and activities, conferences, camps, legislative updates, book reviews, audio reviews, professional question and answer column and more for the visually impaired and their families.

Quarterly

6936 Basic Course in American Sign Language

TJ Publishers
817 Silver Spring Avenue
Suite 206
Silver Spring, MD 20910 **301-585-4440**
800-999-1168
FAX: 301-585-5930
TTY:301-585-4440
e-mail: TJPubinc@aol.com

Angela K Thames, President
Jerald A Murphy, VP

Accompanying videotapes and textbooks include voice translations. Hearing students can analyze sound for initial instruction, or opt to turn off the sound to sharpen visual acuity. Package includes the Basic Course in American Sign Language text, Student Study Guide, the original four 1-hour videotapes plus the ABCASI Vocabulary videotape. *$139.95*

280 pages Video

6937 Beam

1850 W Roosevelt Road
Chicago, IL 60608 **312-666-1331**
FAX: 312-243-8539
www.thechicagolighthouse.org

James Kesteloot, Executive Director
Terrence Longo, Assistant Director

Quarterly newsletter of the organization offering progressive programs for the blind, visually impaired, deaf-blind and multi-disabled children and adults, including vocational programs, computer and office skills training, job placement, independent living skills, orientation and mobility training, counseling and a low vision clinic.

6938 Behavioral Vision Approaches for Persons with Physical Disabilities

Optometric Extension Program Foundation
2912 S Daimler Street
Santa Ana, CA 92705 **949-250-0846**

A discussion of the behavioral vision/neuro-motor approach to providing directions for prescriptive and therapeutic services for the visually handicapped child or adult. *$49.50*

197 pages

6939 Berthold Lowenfeld on Blindness and Blind People

American Foundation for the Blind/AFB Press
PO Box 1020
Sewickley, PA 15143
412-741-1142
800-232-3044
FAX: 412-741-0609
e-mail: afborders@abdintl.com
www.afb.org

These writings of the pioneering educator, author and advocate range over a forty-year period include various ground-breaking papers for the blind educator, a rememberance of Helen Keller and other essays on education, sociology and history. *$21.95*

254 pages Paperback
ISBN 0-891281-01-0

6940 Blind Educator

National Federation of the Blind
1800 Johnson Street
Baltimore, MD 21230
410-659-9314
FAX: 410-685-5653
e-mail: nfb@iamdigex.net
www.nfb.org

Magazine specifically for blind educators.

6941 Blind and Vision-Impaired Individuals

Mainstream
3 Bethesda Metro Center
Suite 830
Bethesda, MD 20814
301-951-6122
800-247-1380
FAX: 301-654-6714
e-mail: info@mainstreaminc.org

Mainstreaming blind individuals into the workplace. *$2.50*

12 pages

6942 Blindness and Early Childhood Development Second Edition

American Foundation for the Blind/AFB Press
PO Box 1020
Sewickley, PA 15143
412-741-1142
800-232-3044
FAX: 412-741-0609
e-mail: afborders@abdintl.com
www.afb.org

A review of current knowledge on motor and locomotor development, perceptual development, language and cognitive processes, and social, emotional and personality development. Paperback. *$34.95*

384 pages
ISBN 0-891281-23-1

6943 Blindness, A Family Matter

American Foundation for the Blind/AFB Press
PO Box 1020
Sewickley, PA 15143
412-741-1142
800-232-3044
FAX: 412-741-0609
e-mail: afborders@abdintl.com
www.afb.org

A frank exploration of the effects of an individual's visual impairment on other members of the family and how those family members can play a positive role in the rehabilitation process. Features interviews with three families whose 'success stories' provide advice and encouragement, as well as interviews with newly blinded adults currently involved in a rehabilitation program. 23 minute video tape. Also available in PAL, $49.95, 0-89128-271-8. *$43.95*

VHS 1986
ISBN 0-891282-22-X

6944 Blindness: What it is, What it Does and How to Live with it

American Foundation for the Blind/AFB Press
PO Box 1020
Sewickley, PA 15143
412-741-1142
800-232-3044
FAX: 412-741-0609
e-mail: afborders@abdintl.com
www.afb.org

A classic work on how blindness affects self-perception and social interaction and what can be done to restore basic skills, mobility, daily living and an appreciation of life's pleasures. *$15.95*

396 pages Paperback
ISBN 0-891282-05-

6945 Braille Book Review

National Library Service for the Blind
1291 Taylor Street NW
Washington, DC 20542
202-707-5100
FAX: 202-707-0712
TTY:202-707-0744
e-mail: nls@loc.gov
www.loc.gov/nls

Robert Fistick, Head Publications/Media Section

New braille books and product news.

30 pages BiMonthly

6946 Braille Documents

Metrolina Association for the Blind
704 Louise Avenue
Charlotte, NC 28204
704-372-3870
800-926-5460
FAX: 704-372-3872

This production shop creates Braille and large-print documents.

6947 Braille Forum

American Council of the Blind
1155 15th Street NW
Suite 1004
Washington, DC 20005
202-467-5081
800-424-8666
FAX: 202-467-5085
e-mail: slovering@acb.org
www.acb.org

Penny Reeder, Editor

Offered in print, braille, cassette, IBM computer disk and e-mail. $25 per format per year for companies and non-US residents.

48 pages Magazine

6948 Braille Monitor

National Federation of the Blind
1800 Johnson Street
Baltimore, MD 21230
410-659-9314
FAX: 410-685-5653
e-mail: nfb@iamdigex.net
www.nfb.org

Leading publication in the blindness field, with a circulation of 30,000, this publication addresses issues of concern to the blind and the philosophy and activities of the National Federation of the Blind.

Monthly

6949 **Building Blocks: Foundations for Learning for Young Blind and Visually Impaired Children**

American Foundation for the Blind/AFB Press
PO Box 1020
Sewickley, PA 15143
412-741-1142
800-232-3044
FAX: 412-741-0609
e-mail: afborders@abdintl.com
www.afb.org

Presents the essential components of a successful early intervnetion program, including collaboration with family members, positive relationships between parents and professionals, public education, and attention to important programming components such as space exploration, braille readiness, orientation and mobility, play, cooking and music. Includes interviews with parents. Available in English or Spanish. 10 minute video tape. Also available in PAL, $33.95, 0-89128-268-8. *$26.95*

VHS
ISBN 0-891282-14-9

6950 **Bulletin**

National Association for Visually Handicapped
22 W 21st Street
New York, NY 10010
212-255-2804
FAX: 212-727-2931
e-mail: staff@navh.org
www.navh.org

Annual report offering information on Association activities and events, conferences, vision aids and resources for the visually impaired.

6951 **Burns Braille Transcription Dictionary**

American Foundation for the Blind/AFB Press
PO Box 1020
Sewickley, PA 15143
412-741-1142
800-232-3044
FAX: 412-741-0609
e-mail: afborders@abdintl.com
www.afb.org

A handy, portable guide that is a quick reference for anyone who needs to check print-to-braille and braille-to-print meanings and symbols. Paperback. *$19.95*

96 pages
ISBN 0-891292-32-7

6952 **Career Perspectives: Interviews with Blind and Visually Impaired Professionals**

American Foundation for the Blind/AFB Press
PO Box 1020
Sewickley, PA 15143
412-741-1142
800-232-3044
FAX: 412-741-0609
e-mail: afborders@abdintl.com
www.afb.org

Profiles of 20 successful archivers who describe in their own words what it takes to pursue and attain professional success in a sighted world. Available in large print, cassette and braille. *$16.95*

96 pages Large Print
ISBN 0-891281-70-3

6953 **Careers in Blindness Rehabilitation Services**

Mississippi State University
PO Box 6189
Mississippi State, MS 39762
662-325-2001
800-675-7782
FAX: 662-325-8989
www.blind.msstate.edu

Kelly Schaefer, Dissemination Specialist

In a follow-up study in a series examining the substantial under-representation of African Americans as professionals in blindness services, researchers questioned college students about their knowledge, opinions and interests in blindness services. *$15.00*

54 pages Paperback

6954 **Cataracts**

National Association for Visually Handicapped
22 W 21st Street
6th Floor
New York, NY 10010
212-889-2804
FAX: 212-727-2931
e-mail: staff@navh.org
www.navh.org

A booklet offering information about Cataracts, diagnosis and treatment of this common condition. *$2.50*

6955 **Characteristics, Services, & Outcomes of Rehab. Consumers who are Blind/Visually Impaired**

Mississippi State University
PO Box 6189
Mississippi State, MS 39762
662-325-2001
800-675-7782
FAX: 662-325-8989
www.blind.msstate.edu

Brenda Cavenaugh, Principal Investigatorst
Steven J Pierce, Graduate Research Assistant
Kelly Schaefer, Dissemination Specialist

Issues regarding the efficacy of separate state agencies providing specialized vocational rehabilitation (VR) services to consumers who are blind have generated spirited discussions within the rehabilitation community throughout the history of the state-federal program. In this monograph, RRTC researches report results of their investigation of services provided to blind consumers in separate and general (combined) rehabilitation agencies. *$20.00*

45 pages Paperback

6956 **Childhood Glaucoma: A Reference Guide for Families**

NAPVI
PO Box 317
Watertown, MA 02472
617-972-7441
800-562-6265
FAX: 617-972-7444
e-mail: napvi@perkins.org
www.napvi.org

6957 **Children with Visual Impairments Wodbine House**

American Foundation for the Blind/AFB Press
11 Penn Plaza
Suite 300
New York, NY 10001
212-502-7600
800-232-3044
FAX: 301-897-5838
e-mail: afborder@abdintl.com
www.afb.org

Written by parents and professional, this book presents a comprehensive overview of the issues that are crucial to the healthy development of children with mild to severe visual impaiments. It also offers insight from parents about coping with the emotional aspects of raising a child with special needs. *$16.95*

416 pages
ISBN 0-933149-36-0

6958 **Choice Magazine Listening**

85 Channel Drive
Port Washington, NY 11050
516-883-8280
888-724-6423
FAX: 516-944-6849
e-mail: choicemag@aol.com
www.choicemagazinelistening.org

Lois Miller, Office Manager

A free audio anthology is available bi-monthly to visually impaired/physically disabled persons nationwide. Playable on the special free 4-track cassette playback equipment which is provided by the Library of Congress through the National Library Service. Each issue features eight hours of unabridged magazine articles, short stories, poetry and media selections from over 100 sources. College level and older. Bimonthly distribution.

Bi-Monthly

6959 **Communication Skills for Visually Impaired Learners**

Charles C Thomas
2600 S First Street
Springfield, IL 62704
217-789-8980
800-258-8980
FAX: 217-789-9130
e-mail: books@ccthomas.com
www.ccthomas.com

This book has been designed to provide a foundation for a better understanding of teaching reading, writing, and listening skills to students with visual impairments from preschool age through adult levels. The plan of the book incorporates the latest research findings with the practical experiences learned in the classroom. *$49.95*

322 pages Paperback 1997
ISBN 0-39806-93-0

6960 **Comprehensive Examination of Barriers to Employment Among Persons who are Blind or Impaired**

Mississippi State University
PO Box 6189
Mississippi State, MS 39762
662-325-2001
800-675-7782
FAX: 662-325-8989
www.blind.msstate.edu

J Elton Moore, Author
Kelly Shaefer, Dissemination Specialist

A multi-phase research project designed to: identify barriers to employment; identify and develop innovative successful strategies to overcome these barriers; develop methods for others to utilize these strategies; disseminate this information to rehabilitation providers; replicate the use of selected strategies in other settings. *$20.00*

90 pages Paperback

6961 **Concept Development for Visually Handicapped Children: A Resource Guide**

American Foundation for the Blind/AFB Press
PO Box 1020
Sewickley, PA 15143
412-741-1142
800-232-3044
FAX: 412-741-0609
e-mail: afborders@abdintl.com
www.afb.org

A program for integrating such concepts as body imagery, gross motor movement, posture and tactile discrimination into the curriculum from kindergarten on. Paperback. *$16.95*

80 pages
ISBN 0-891280-18-9

6962 **Contrasting Characteristics of Blind and Visually Impaired Clients**

Mississippi State University
PO Box 6189
Mississippi State, MS 39762
662-325-2001
800-675-7782
FAX: 662-325-8989
www.blind.msstate.edu

Kelly Schaefer, Publications Manager

This report examines cases in the National Blindness and Low Vision Employment Database to identify and profile environmental and personal characteristics of clients who are blind or visually impaired and who were achieving successful and unsuccessful retention of competitive jobs. A total of 787 cases were analyzed. *$15.00*

44 pages Paperback

6963 **DVH Quarterly**

University of Arkansas at Little Rock
2801 S University Avenue
Little Rock, AR 72204

Bob Brasher, Editor

Offers information on upcoming events, conferences and workshops on and for visual disabilities. Book reviews, information on the newest resources and technology, educational programs, want ads and more.

Quarterly

6964 **Dancing Cheek to Cheek**

Blind Children's Center
4120 Marathon Street
Los Angeles, CA 90029
323-664-2153
800-222-3567
FAX: 323-665-3828
e-mail: info@blindchildrenscenter.org
www.blindchildrenscenter.org

Beginning social, play and language interactions. *$ 10.00*

23 pages

6965 **Data on Blindness and Visual Impairment in the US: A Resource Manual**

American Foundation for the Blind/AFB Press
PO Box 1020
Sewickley, PA 15143
412-741-1142
800-232-3044
FAX: 412-741-0609
e-mail: afborders@abdintl.com
www.afb.org

Provides facts and figures for long-range planning, preparing grant proposals and legislative services. Paperback. *$47.00*

412 pages
ISBN 0-891281-52-5

6966 **Deaf-Blind Perspective**

Teaching Research
345 Monmouth Avenue
Monmouth, OR 97361
800-438-9376
FAX: 503-838-8150
e-mail: dblink@tr.wou.edu
www.tr.wou.edu/dblink

John Reiman PhD, Director

6967 Development of Social Skills by Blind and Visually Impaired Students

American Foundation for the Blind/AFB Press
PO Box 1020
Sewickley, PA 15143
412-741-1142
800-232-3044
FAX: 412-741-0609
e-mail: afborders@abdintl.com
www.afb.org

Offers an examination of the social interactions of blind and visually impaired children in mainstreamed settings and the community that highlights the need to teach social interaction skills to children and provide them with support. Paperback. *$39.95*

232 pages
ISBN 0-891282-17-3

6968 Diabetic Retinopathy

National Association for Visually Handicapped
22 W 21st Street
6th Floor
New York, NY 10010
212-889-2804
FAX: 212-727-2931
e-mail: staff@navh.org
www.navh.org

A booklet offering information about Diabetic Retinopathy.

6969 Dialogue Magazine

Blindskills
PO Box 5181
Salem, OR 97304
800-860-4224
FAX: 503-581-0178
e-mail: blindskl@teleport.com
www.blindskills.com

Carol M McCarl, Editor/Publisher

Publishes quarterly magazine in braille, large-type, cassette and disk of news items, fiction and articles of special interest to visually impaired youth and adults. $40.00 for not blind/legally blind. *$28.00*

Quarterly

6970 Directory of Camps for Blind and Visually Impaired Children & Adults

American Foundation for the Blind/AFB Press
PO Box 1020
Sewickley, PA 15143
412-741-1142
800-232-3044
FAX: 412-741-0609
e-mail: afborders@abdintl.com
www.afb.org

A guide to 200 sleepaway camps and day camps in the United States. Descriptions cover types of campers, age ranges, special activities offered, length of seasons and contact names. *$15.95*

34 pages Papberack
ISBN 0-891281-59-2

6971 Diversity and Visual Impairment: The Influ ence of Race, Gender, Religion and Ethnicity

American Foundation for the Blind
11 Penn Plaza
Suite 300
New York, NY 10001
212-502-7600
800-232-5463
FAX: 212-502-7777
e-mail: afbinfo@afb.net
www.afb.org/store

Carl R Augusto, President/CEO

Cultural, social, ethnic, gender, and religious issues can influence the way an individual perceives and copes with a visual impairment. *$45.95*

480 pages 1901
ISBN 0-891283-83-8

6972 Early Focus: Working with Young Blind and Visually Impaired Children

American Foundation for the Blind/AFB Press
PO Box 1020
Sewickley, PA 15143
412-741-1142
800-232-3044
FAX: 412-741-0609
e-mail: afborders@abdintl.com
www.afb.org

Describes early intervention techniques used with blind and visually impaired children and stresses the benefits of family involvement and transdisciplinary teamwork. Paperback. *$32.95*

176 pages
ISBN 0-891282-15-7

6973 Encyclopedia of Blindness and Vision Impairment Second Edition

Facts on File
132 W 31 Street
17th Floor
New York, NY 10001
212-907-8800
800-322-8755
FAX: 212-967-9196
e-mail: jcchambers@factsonfile.com
www.factsonfile.com

James Chamber, Editor in Chief Arts/Humanities

Designed to provide both laymen and professionals with concise, practical information on the second most common disability in the U.S. *$65.00*

340 pages Hardbound
ISBN 6-810021-53-8

6974 Equals in Partnership: Basic Rights for Families of Children with Blindness

NAPVI
PO Box 317
Watertown, MA 02472
617-972-7441
800-562-6265
FAX: 617-972-7444
e-mail: napvi@perkins.org
www.napvi.org

6975 Eye Research News Briefs

Research to Prevent Blindness
645 Madison Avenue
21st Floor
New York, NY 10022
212-752-4333
800-621-0026
FAX: 212-688-6231
e-mail: info@rpbusa.org
www.rpbusa.org

James V Romano PhD, COO
Thomas Furlong, Director Public Information

Yearly publication from Research to Prevent Blindness. Free.

4 pages Yearly

6976 **Eye and Your Vision**

National Association for Visually Handicapped
22 W 21st Street
6th Floor
New York, NY 10010
212-889-2804
FAX: 212-727-2931
e-mail: staff@navh.org
www.navh.org

A large booklet offering information, with illustrations, on the eye. Includes information on protection of eyesight, how the eye works and vision disorders. Available in Russian and Spanish also. *$ 2.75*

6977 **Fathers: A Common Ground**

Blind Children's Center
4120 Marathon Street
Los Angeles, CA 90029
323-664-2153
800-222-3567
FAX: 323-665-3828
e-mail: info@blindchildrenscenter.org
www.blindchildrenscenter.org

Exploring the concerns and roles of fathers of children with visual impairments. *$10.00*

50 pages

6978 **Fighting Blindness News**

RP Foundation Fighting Blindness
1401 Mt Royal Avenue
4th Floor
Baltimore, MD 21217
410-225-9400
800-683-5555
FAX: 410-225-3936
TTY:410-225-9409

Offers information on medical updates, donor programs, assistive devices, resources and clinical trial information for persons with visual impariments, blindness and retinal degenerative diseases.

2x Year

6979 **First Steps**

Blind Children's Center
4120 Marathon Street
Los Angeles, CA 90029
323-664-2153
800-222-3567
FAX: 323-665-3828
e-mail: info@blindchildrenscenter.org
www.blindchildrenscenter.org

A handbook for teaching young children who are visually impaired. Designed to assist students, professionals and parents working with children who are visually impaired. Visit our website for many publications addressing training very young children who are blind or visually impaired. *$35.00*

203 pages

6980 **Focus**

Visually Impaired Center
725 Mason Street
Flint, MI 48503
313-235-2544

Laurie MacArthur, Executive Director

Newsletter offering information for the visually impaired person in the forms of legislative and law updates, ADA information, support groups, hotlines, and articles on the newest technology in the field.

Quarterly

6981 **Foundations of Orientation and Mobility**

American Foundation for the Blind/AFB Press
PO Box 1020
Sewickley, PA 15143
412-741-1142
800-232-3044
FAX: 412-741-0609
e-mail: afborders@abdintl.com
www.afb.org

This text has been updated and revised and includes current research from a variety of disciplines, an international perspective, and expanded contents on low vision, aging, multiple disabilities, accessibility, program design and adaptive technology from more that 30 eminent subject experts. *$68.95*

775 pages
ISBN 0-891289-46-1

6982 **Foundations of Rehabilitation Counseling with Persons Who Are Blind**

American Foundation for the Blind/AFB Press
PO Box 1020
Sewickley, PA 15143
412-741-1142
800-232-3044
FAX: 412-741-0609
e-mail: afborders@abdintl.com
www.afb.org

Rehabilitation professionals have long recognized that the needs of people who are blind or visually impaired are unique and requie a special knowledge and expertise to provide and corrdinate rehabilitation services. *$59.95*

477 pages
ISBN 0-891289-45-3

6983 **Future Reflections**

Natl. Organization for Parents of Blind Children
1800 Johnson Street
Baltimore, MD 21230
410-659-9314
FAX: 410-685-5653
e-mail: nfb@iamdigex.net

National magazine written specifically for parents and educators of blind children. Each issue addresses various topics important to blind children, their families and to school personnel.

Quarterly

6984 **Get a Wiggle On**

American Alliance for Health, Phys. Ed. & Dance
1900 Association Drive
Reston, VA 20191
703-476-3400
FAX: 703-476-9527
e-mail: aaalf@aahperd.org

Gives teachers and parents practical suggestions for helping blind and visually impaired infants grow and learn like other children. *$5.00*

80 pages
ISBN 0-88314 -77-2

6985 **Gleams Newsletter**

Glaucoma Research Foundation
490 Post Street
Suite 1427
San Francisco, CA 94102
415-986-3162
800-826-6693
FAX: 415-986-3763
e-mail: info@glaucoma.org
www.glaucoma.org

Yuko Madono, Outreach/Public Relations

Offers updated medical & research information on glaucoma. Included are glaucoma treatmant and coping tips, legsilative information, professional articles and book reviews.

6 pages Quarterly 1982

6986 **Guidelines and Games for Teaching Efficient Braille Reading**

American Foundation for the Blind/AFB Press
PO Box 1020
Sewickley, PA 15143 **412-741-1142**
800-232-3044
FAX: 412-741-0609
e-mail: afborders@abdintl.com
www.afb.org

Based on research in the areas of rapid reading and precision teaching, these guidelines represent a unique adaptation of a general reading program to the needs of braille readers. Paperback. *$ 24.95*

116 pages
ISBN 0-891281-05-3

6987 **Guideway**

Guide Dog Foundation for the Blind
371 E Jericho Turnpike
Smithtown, NY 11787 **631-265-2121**
800-548-4337
FAX: 516-361-5192

Offers updates and information on the foundation's activities and guide dog programs. In print form but is also available on cassette.

Monthly

6988 **Handbook for Itinerant and Resource Teachers of Blind Students**

National Federation of the Blind
1800 Johnson Street
Baltimore, MD 21230 **410-659-9314**
e-mail: nfb@iamdigex.net

The Handbook provides help to teachers, school administrators or other school personnel that have experience with blind or visually impaired students. The Handbook devotes 45 pages to Braille and how to teach Braille for parents and teachers. There are other chapters offering information on the law, physical education, fitting in socially, testing and evaluation, home economics, daily living skills and more. *$23.00*

533 pages Softcover
ISBN 0-962412-20-1

6989 **Handbook of Information for Members of the Achromatopsia Network**

PO Box 214
Berkeley, CA 94701 **510-540-4700**
FAX: 510-540-4767
e-mail: futterman@achromat.org
www.achromat.org

6990 **Health Care Professionals Who Are Blind or Visually Impaired**

American Foundation for the Blind
11 Penn Plaza
Suite 300
New York, NY 10001 **212-502-7600**
800-232-5463
FAX: 212-502-7777
e-mail: afbinfo@afb.net
www.afb.org/store

Carl R Augusto, President/CEO

This resource is essential reading for older students and young adults who are blind or visually impaired, their families, and the professionals who work with them. *$21.95*

160 pages 1901
ISBN 0-891283-88-9

6991 **Hearsay**

Int'l Association of Audio Information Services
1102 W International Airport Road
Anchorage, AK 99518 **412-434-6023**
800-280-5325
e-mail: aiblink@ak.net
www.iaais.org

Newsletter for persons interested in radio reading services. *$7.00*

Quarterly

6992 **Heart to Heart**

Blind Children's Center
4120 Marathon Street
Los Angeles, CA 90029 **323-664-2153**
800-222-3567
FAX: 323-665-3828
e-mail: info@blindchildrenscenter.org
www.blindchildrenscenter.org

Parents of children who are blind and partially sighted talk about their feelings. *$10.00*

12 pages

6993 **Helen Keller National Center Newsletter**

111 Middle Neck Road
Sands Point, NY 11050 **516-944-8900**
800-225-0411
FAX: 516-944-7302
e-mail: hkncdir@aol.com
www.helenkeller.org/national

Joseph McNulty, Executive Director

The Center provides evaluation and training in vocational skills, adaptive technology and computer skills, orientation and mobility, independent living, communication, speech-language skills, creative arts, fitness and leisure activities.

6994 **Helen and Teacher: The Story of Helen & Anne Sullivan Macy**

American Foundation for the Blind/AFB Press
PO Box 1020
Sewickley, PA 15143 **412-741-1142**
800-232-3044
FAX: 412-741-0609
e-mail: afborders@abdintl.com
www.afb.org

Stephanie Biagioli, Marketing Coordinator

A pictorial biography emphasizing Hellen Keller's accomplishments in public life over a period of more than 60 years. Traces Anne Sullivan's early years and her meeting with Helen Keller, and goes on to recount the joint events of their lives. A definitive biography. $29.95.

Paperback
ISBN 0-891282-89-0

6995 **Helping the Visually Impaired Child with Developmental Problems**

Teachers College Press
Columbia University
New York, NY 10027
800-575-6566
FAX: 212-678-4149

This book aims to explore the human consequences of severe visual problems combined with other handicaps. The application of child development research to educational interventions, the need for educational and rehabilitative services that serve the human and the special needs of children and their families and the promise of technology in helping to expand communicative possibilities are also discussed. *$18.95*

216 pages Paperback
ISBN 0-807729-02-7

6996 **Hub**

SPOKES Unlimited
415 Main Street
Klamath Falls, OR 97602
541-883-7547
FAX: 541-885-2469
e-mail: spokes@internetcds.com

Wendy Howard, Program Coordinator
Celeste Wolf, Clerical Support Specialist II

Newsletter on rehabilitation, peer counseling, blindness, visual impairments, information and referral.

6997 **If Blindness Comes**

National Federation of the Blind
1800 Johnson Street
Baltimore, MD 21230
410-659-9314
FAX: 410-685-5653
e-mail: nfb@iamdigex.net
www.nfb.org

An introduction to issues relating to vision loss and provides a positive, supportive philosophy about blindness. It is a general information book which includes answers to many common questions about blindness, information about services and programs for the blind and resource listings. Contact the Materials Center.

6998 **If Blindness Strikes Don't Strike Out**

Charles C Thomas
2600 S First Street
Springfield, IL 62704
217-789-8980
800-258-8980
FAX: 217-789-9130
e-mail: books@ccthomas.com
www.ccthomas.com

This book is a storehouse of information on daily life for the visually impaired and those around them. From opticons and laser canes to housekeeping to travel, the author describes how to successfully cope with the problems posed by visual impairment and blindness. Also available in cloth. *$36.95*

316 pages Paperback
ISBN 0-398064-34-2

6999 **Imagining the Possibilities: Creative Approaches to Orientation and Mobility Instruction**

American Foundation for the Blind
11 Penn Plaza
Suite 300
New York, NY 10001
212-502-7600
800-232-5463
FAX: 212-502-7777
e-mail: afbinfo@afb.net
www.afb.org/store

Carl R Augusto, President/CEO

Innovative and varied approaches to O&M techniques and teaching and dynamic suggestions on how to analyze learning styles are just some of the important topics included. *$49.95*

378 pages 1901
ISBN 0-891283-82-X

7000 **Increasing Literacy Levels: Final Report**

Mississippi State University
PO Box 6189
Mississippi State, MS 39762
662-325-2001
800-675-7782
FAX: 662-325-8989
www.blind.msstate.edu

Kelly Schaefer, Dissemination Specialist

This study is composed of three research projects to identify and analyze the appropriate use of and instruction in Braille, optical devices and other technologies as they relate to literacy and employment of individuals who are blind or visually impaired. *$20.00*

148 pages Paperback

7001 **Independence Without Sight and Sound: Suggestions for Practitioners**

American Foundation for the Blind/AFB Press
PO Box 1020
Sewickley, PA 15143
412-741-1142
800-232-3044
FAX: 412-741-0609
e-mail: afborders@abdintl.com
www.afb.org

This practical guidebook covers the essential aspects of communicating and working with deaf-blind persons. Includes useful information on how to talk with deaf-blind people, adapt orientation and mobility techniques for deaf-blind travelers. Paperback. *$39.95*

193 pages
ISBN 0-891282-46-7

7002 **Information Access Project**

National Federation of the Blind
1800 Johnson Street
Baltimore, MD 21230
410-837-6763
FAX: 410-685-5653
e-mail: nfb@iamdigex.net
www.nfb.org

Marc Maurer, President

Assists entities covered by the ADA in finding methods for converting visually displayed information, such as flyers, brochures and pamphlets, to formats accessible to individuals who are visually impaired.

7003 **Inside the Beltway**

DC Regl Lib for the Blind & Physically Handicapped
901 G Street NW
Room 215
Washington, DC 20001
202-727-2142
FAX: 202-727-1129
TTY:202-727-2145
e-mail: lbphb_2000@yahoo.com
www.dclibrary.org

Grace J Lyons, Librarian

Regional library/RPH is network library in the Library of Congress, National Library Services for the Blind and Physically Handicapped.

8 pages Quarterly

7004 Insight

United States Association of Blind Athletes
33 N Institute
Colorado Springs, CO 80903
719-630-0422
FAX: 719-630-0616
e-mail: media@usaba.org
www.usaba.org

Covers news, announcements and activities of the Association.

20 pages Quarterly

7005 International Directory of Libraries for the Disabled

KG Saur/Division of RR Bowker
121 Chanlon Road
New Providence, NJ 07974
212-337-6900
800-521-8110

An essential resource for improving the quality and quantity of materials available to the print-handicapped audience. Featuring talking books, braille books, large print books as well as production centers for these materials. *$46.00*

257 pages
ISBN 3-59821 -81-1

7006 Intervention Practices in the Retention of Competitive Employment

Mississippi State University
PO Box 6189
Mississippi State, MS 39762
662-325-2001
800-675-7782
FAX: 662-325-8989
www.blind.msstate.edu

Kelly Schaefer, Dissemination Specialist

This study investigated the methods by which an individual can retain competitive employment after the onset of a significant vision loss. Interviews were conducted with 89 rehabilitation counselors across the US Strategies that contribute to successful job retention were identified as well as best rehabilitation practices in job retention. *$15.00*

60 pages Paperback

7007 Jewish Braille Review

Jewish Braille Institute of America
110 E 30th Street
New York, NY 10016
212-889-2525
800-433-1531
FAX: 212-689-3692
e-mail: admin@jbilibrary.org
www.jbilibrary.org

Ellen Isler MD, Executive VP
Israel A Taub, Associate Director

The JBI seeks the integration of Jews who are blind, visually impaired and reading disabled into the Jewish community and society in general. More than 20,000 men, women and children in 50 countries receive a broad variety of JBI services.

1931

7008 Jewish Heritage for the Blind

1655 E 24th Street
Brooklyn, NY 11229
718-338-8200

Offers large print traditional prayer books for the High Holy days, festivals, fast days and daily rituals for those finding it difficult or impossible to read small print.

7009 Journal of Visual Impairment and Blindness

Sheridan Press, c/o FB
PO Box 465
Hanover, PA 17331
717-632-3535
800-352-2210
FAX: 717-633-8929
e-mail: pubsvc@tsp.sheridan.com
www.sheridanreprints.com

Sharon Shively, Managing Editor
Jane Erin, Editor-in-Chief

Published in braille, regular print and on ASC II disk and cassette, this journal contains a wide variety of subjects including rehabilitation, psychology, education, legislation, medicine, technology, employment, sensory aids and childhood development as they relate to visual impairments. $130 annual individual subscription, $180 annual institutional subscription.

64 pages Monthly
ISSN 0145-48 x

7010 Kernal Book Series

National Federation of the Blind
1800 Johnson Street
Baltimore, MD 21230
410-659-9314
FAX: 410-685-5653
e-mail: nfb@iamdigex.net
www.nfb.org

A series of books written by the blind themselves. Each book is a collection of articles and stories about the real life experiences of blind persons. These books help educate the blind and the sighted alike about a positive philosophy regarding blindness. Contact the Materials Center.

$5 - $10 each

7011 King James Bible, Large Print

Science Products
Box 888
Southeastern, PA 19399
610-296-2111
800-888-7400
FAX: 610-296-0488

Mary Ann Case, Marketing Director

A hardcover book with 24 point type easily seen with 20/200 acuity. Makes bible reading for children easier too. New Testament ($69.95:

7012 Large Print Loan Library

National Association for Visually Handicapped
22 W 21st Street
New York, NY 10010
212-255-2804
FAX: 212-727-2931
e-mail: staff@navh.org
www.navh.org

A huge large print catalog of all the publications, fiction and non-fiction, cassette tapes, books-on-tape and videos available for the visually impaired from the loan library of the National Association for the Visually Handicapped.

100 pages

7013 Learning to Play

Blind Children's Center
4120 Marathon Street
Los Angeles, CA 90029
323-664-2153
800-222-3567
FAX: 323-665-3828
e-mail: info@blindchildrenscenter.org
www.blindchildrenscenter.org

Presenting play activities to the pre-school child who is visually impaired. *$10.00*

12 pages

7014 Let's Eat

Blind Children's Center
4120 Marathon Street
Los Angeles, CA 90029
323-664-2153
800-222-3567
FAX: 323-665-3828
e-mail: info@blindchildrenscenter.org
www.blindchildrenscenter.org

Feeding a child with visual impairment. *$10.00*

28 pages

7015 Library Resources for the Blind and Physically Handicapped

National Library Service for the Blind
1291 Taylor Street NW
Washington, DC 20542
202-707-5100
FAX: 202-707-0712
TTY:202-707-0744
e-mail: nls@loc.gov
www.loc.gov/nls

NLS administers a national library service that provides braille and recorded books and magazines on free loan to anyone who cannot read standard print because of visual or physical disabilities who are eligible residents of the United States or American citizens living abroad. The directory describes the cooperating libaries. Online at www.loc.gov/reference/directories.html.

83 pages

7016 Library Services for the Blind

South Carolina State University
Miller F Whittaker Library
300 College Street NE
Orangeburg, SC 29117
803-536-8902
FAX: 803-536-8902
e-mail: bagingu@scsu.edu
library.scsu.edu

Mary L Small Dean, Library/Information Services

News and information on developments in library services for readers who are blind and physically disabled.

7017 Library Users of America Newsletter

American Council of the Blind
1155 15th Street NW
Suite 1004
Washington, DC 20005
202-467-5081
800-424-8666
FAX: 202-467-5085
e-mail: info@acb.org
www.acb.org

Sharon Strzalkowski, President

Published twice yearly, the newsletter contains much information about library services of particular interest to blind and visually impaired patrons, and is available in the following formats: Braille, Audiocassette, Large Print and e-mail.

7018 Lifestyles of Employed Legally Blind People

Mississippi State University
PO Box 6189
Mississippi State, MS 39762
662-325-2001
800-675-7782
FAX: 662-325-8989
www.blind.msstate.edu

Lynn W McBroom PhD, Senior Research Scientist

Results from a telephone survey show that visually impaired respondents are involved in a wide variety of activities with little restrictions on their range of activities. Sighted respondents tended to spend more time in child care, obtaining goods and services, attending to self-care activities and engaging in social activities, while visually impaired respondents spent more time in education and passive activities. This report is a study of expenditures and time use. *$10.00*

193 pages Paperback

7019 Light the Way

Blind Children's Center
4120 Marathon Street
Los Angeles, CA 90029
323-664-2153
800-222-3567
FAX: 323-665-3828
e-mail: info@blindchildrenscenter.org
www.blindchildrenscenter.org

Newsletter of the Blind Childrens Center, a family-centered agency which serves children with visual impairments from birth to school-age. The center-based and home-based services help the children to acquire skills and build their independence. The Center utilizes its expertise and experience to serve families and professionals worldwide through support services, education and research.

7020 Lion

Lion's Clubs International
300 22nd Street
Oak Brook, IL 60521
312-571-5466

Publication for the blind.

7021 Living with Achromatopsia

PO Box 214
Berkeley, CA 94701
510-540-4700
FAX: 510-540-4767
e-mail: futterman@achromat.org
www.achromat.org

7022 Long Cane News

American Foundation for the Blind/AFB Press
PO Box 1020
Sewickley, PA 15143
412-741-1142
800-232-3044
FAX: 412-741-0609
e-mail: afborders@abdintl.com
www.afb.org

Liz Greco

SemiAnnual

7023 Low Vision Questions and Answers: Definitions, Devices, Services

American Foundation for the Blind/AFB Press
PO Box 1020
Sewickley, PA 15143
412-741-1142
800-232-3044
FAX: 412-741-0609
e-mail: afborders@abdintl.com
www.afb.org

What does low vision mean? What do low vision services cost? What diseases cause low vision? Answers to these and other questions are presented in a comprehensive format with accompanying photographs. $50.00/pack of 25.

21 pages
ISBN 0-891281-96-7

7024 Low Vision: Reflections of the Past, Issues for the Future

American Foundation for the Blind/AFB Press
PO Box 1020
Sewickley, PA 15143
412-741-1142
800-232-3044
FAX: 412-741-0609
e-mail: afborders@abdintl.com
www.afb.org

Background papers and a strategies section are used to identify the shifting needs of visually impaired persons and the resources that may be needed to address them. Paperback. *$29.95*

ISBN 0-891282-18-1

7025 Mainstreaming and the American Dream

American Foundation for the Blind/AFB Press
PO Box 1020
Sewickley, PA 15143
412-741-1142
800-232-3044
FAX: 412-741-0609
e-mail: afborders@abdintl.com
www.afb.org

Based on in-depth interviews with parents and professionals, this research monograph presents information on the needs and aspirations of parents of blind and visually impaired children. Paperback. *$34.95*

256 pages
ISBN 0-891281-91-6

7026 Mainstreaming the Visually Impaired Child

NAPVI
PO Box 317
Watertown, MA 02472
617-972-7441
800-562-6265
FAX: 617-972-7444
e-mail: napvi@perkins.org
www.napvi.org

A unique, informative guide for teachers and educational professionals that work with the visually impaired. *$10.00*

121 pages Paper

7027 Making Life More Livable

American Foundation for the Blind
11 Penn Plaza
Suite 300
New York, NY 10001
212-502-7600
800-232-5463
FAX: 212-502-7774
e-mail: afborder@abdintl.com
www.afb.org

Shows how simple adaptations in the home and environment can make a big difference in the lives of blind and visually impaired older persons. The suggestions offered are numerous and specific, ranging from how to mark food cans for greater visibility to how to get out of the shower safley. Large print. *$24.95*

128 pages 1901
ISBN 0-891283-87-0

7028 Meeting the Needs of People with Vision Loss: Multidisciplinary Perspective

Resources for Rehabilitation
33 Bedford Street
Suite 19A
Lexington, MA 02420
781-890-6371
FAX: 781-867-7517

Susan Greenblatt

Written by rehabilitation professionals, physicians, and a sociologist, this book discusses how to provide appropriate information and how to serve special populations. Chapters on the role of the family, diabetes and vision loss, special needs of children and adolescents, adults with hearing and vision loss. *$29.95*

ISBN 0-92971 -07-0

7029 More Alike Than Different: Blind and Visually Impaired Children

American Foundation for the Blind/AFB Press
PO Box 1020
Sewickley, PA 15143
412-741-1142
800-232-3044
FAX: 412-741-0609
e-mail: afborders@abdintl.com
www.afb.org

Offers photographs of blind and visually impaired children around the world learning to read and write, travel independently and performing basic living skills. Covers the most recent technological advances and demonstrates the universality of educational needs and goals. Paperback. $100.00/pack of 25.

ISBN 0-891281-69-0

7030 Move With Me

Blind Children's Center
4120 Marathon Street
Los Angeles, CA 90029
323-664-2153
800-222-3567
FAX: 323-665-3828
e-mail: info@blindchildrenscenter.org
www.blindchildrenscenter.org

A parent's guide to movement development for babies who are visually impaired. *$10.00*

12 pages

7031 Musical Mainstream

National Library Service for the Blind
1291 Taylor Street NW
Washington, DC 20542
202-707-5100
FAX: 202-707-0712
e-mail: nls@loc.gov
www.loc.gov/nls

Articles selected from print music magazines.

Quarterly

7032 NLS News

National Library Service for the Blind
1291 Taylor Street NW
Washington, DC 20542
202-707-5100
FAX: 202-707-0712
e-mail: nls@loc.gov
www.loc.gov/nls

Newsletter on current program developments.

Quarterly

7033 NLS Update

National Library Service for the Blind
1291 Taylor Street NW
Washington, DC 20542
202-707-5100
FAX: 202-707-0712
e-mail: nls@loc.gov
www.loc.gov/nls

Newsletter on the services volunteer activities.

Quarterly

7034 **Newsline for the Blind**

National Federation of the Blind
1800 Johnson Street
Baltimore, MD 21230
410-659-9314
FAX: 410-685-5653
e-mail: nfb@iamdigex.net
www.nfb.org

Peggy Chong, Contact

Nation's only digital talking newspaper service for the blind. Allows the blind to read the full text of leading national and local newspapers by using a touch-tone telephone. Service is free of charge and available 24 hours a day, 7 days per week.

7035 **Not Without Sight**

American Foundation for the Blind/AFB Press
PO Box 1020
Sewickley, PA 15143
412-741-1142
800-232-3044
FAX: 412-741-0609
e-mail: afborders@abdintl.com
www.afb.org

This video describes the major types of visual impairment and their causes and effects on vision, while camera simulations approximate what people with each impairmant actually see. Also demonstrates how people with low vision make the best use of the vision they have. 20 minute video tape. Also available in PAL, $52.95, 0-89128-272-6. *$42.95*

VHS 1975
ISBN 0-891282-27-0

7036 **One Two Three Sign with Me**

TJ Publishers
817 Silver Spring Avenue
Suite 206
Silver Spring, MD 20910
301-585-4440
800-999-1168
FAX: 301-585-5930
e-mail: TJPubinc@aol.com

Angela K Thames, President
Jerald A Murphy, VP

Charming full color illustrations include basic shapes and counting. *$3.95*

24 pages Softcover

7037 **Open Windows, Audiocassette**

LifeWay Christian Resources Southern Baptist Conv.
127 9th Avenue N
Nashville, TN 37234
615-251-2000
800-458-2772
FAX: 651-251-5764
e-mail: specialed@lifeway.com
www.lifeway.com

Judy Wooldridge, Product Development Specialist

Guide for personal devotions on audiocassette tape, using Bible references, devotional readings, and prayer calendar of popular Open Windows devotional guide. Available quarterly on three cassette tapes. *$10.70*

Quarterly

7038 **Opportunity**

National Industries for the Blind
1901 N Beauregard Street
Suite 200
Alexandria, VA 22311
703-998-0770
FAX: 703-998-8268
www.nib.org

George J Mertz, President/CEO

Offers information and articles on the newest technology, equipment, services and programs for blind and visually impaired persons.

Quarterly

7039 **Orientation and Mobility Primer for Families and Young Children**

American Foundation for the Blind/AFB Press
PO Box 1020
Sewickley, PA 15143
412-741-1142
800-232-3044
FAX: 412-741-0609
e-mail: afborders@abdintl.com
www.afb.org

Practical information for helping a child learn about his or her environment right from the start. Covers sensory training, concept development and orientation skills. Paperback. *$14.95*

48 pages
ISBN 0-891281-57-6

7040 **Out of Left Field**

American Foundation for the Blind/AFB Press
PO Box 1020
Sewickley, PA 15143
412-741-1142
800-232-3044
FAX: 412-741-0609
e-mail: afborders@abdintl.com
www.afb.org

Illustrates how youngsters who are blind or visually impaired integrated with their sighted peers in a variety of recreational and athletic activities. 17 minute video tape. Also available in PAL, $33.95, 0-89128-270-X. *$26.95*

VHS 1975
ISBN 0-891282-28-9

7041 **Out of the Corner of My Eye Living with Vision Loss in Later Life**

American Foundation for the Blind/AFB Press
PO Box 1020
Sewickley, PA 15143
412-741-1142
800-232-3044
FAX: 412-741-0609
e-mail: afborders@abdintl.com
www.afb.org

Stephanie Biagioli, Marketing Coordinator

A personal account of student's vision loss and subsequent adjustment that is full of practical advice and cheerful encouragement, told by an 87 year old retired college teacher who has maintained her independence and zest for life. Available in paperback or on audio cassette. *$23.95*

120 pages
ISBN 0-891281-82-1

7042 **PB News**

Prevent Blindness America
500 E Remington Road
Schaumburg, IL 60173
847-843-2020
800-331-2020
FAX: 847-843-8458
e-mail: info@preventblindness.org
www.preventblindness.org

Ken West, Director Marketing Comm.
$10.00

Quarterly

7043 **PBA News**

Prevent Blindness America
500 E Remington Road
Schaumburg, IL 60173
847-843-8458
800-331-2020
FAX: 847-843-2020
e-mail: info@preventblindness.org
www.preventblindness.org

Betsy van Die, Media Relations Director
Hugh R Parry, President/CEO
Daniel D Garrett, Senior VP

Publication offered three times yearly.

3 times yearly

7044 **Pediatric Visual Diagnosis Fact Sheets**

Blind Children's Center
4120 Marathon Street
Los Angeles, CA 90029
323-664-2153
800-222-3567
FAX: 323-665-3828
e-mail: info@blindchildrenscenter.org
www.blindchildrenscenter.org

Fact sheets addressing commonly encountered eye conditions, diagnostic tests and materials. *$10.00*

10 pages

7045 **Perkins Activity and Resource Guide: A Handbook for Teachers**

Perkins School for the Blind
175 N Beacon Street
Watertown, MA 02472
617-924-3434
FAX: 781-926-2027
www.perkins.org

This is a comprehensive, two volume guide with over 1,000 pages of activities, resources and instructional strategies for teachers and parents of students with visual and multiple disabilities. *$65.00*

7046 **Personal Reader Update**

Personal Reader Department
9 Centennial Drive
Peabody, MA 01960
978-977-2000
800-343-0311
FAX: 978-977-2409

Offers information on new services, assistive devices and technology for the blind.

7047 **Perspective**

Clovernook Center for Blind & Visually Impaired
7000 Hamilton Avenue
Cincinnati, OH 45231
513-522-3860
888-234-7156
FAX: 513-728-3946
e-mail: clovernook@clovernook.org
www.clovernook.org

Carol Friedman, Editor
Joshua Howard, Editor

8 pages Quarterly

7048 **Picture is Worth a Thousand Words for Blind and Visually Impaired Persons Too!**

American Foundation for the Blind/AFB Press
PO Box 1020
Sewickley, PA 15143
412-741-1142
800-232-3044
FAX: 412-741-0609
e-mail: afborders@abdintl.com
www.afb.org

Audiodescription - the art of describing in words for visually impaired viewers the visual aspects seen in television, film, etc. - is highlighted in this book for the blind and visually impaired person. *$7.95*

32 pages Large Print
ISBN 0-891282-12-2

7049 **Popular Activities and Games for Blind, Visually Impaired & Disabled People**

American Foundation for the Blind/AFB Press
PO Box 1020
Sewickley, PA 15143
412-741-1142
800-232-3044
FAX: 412-741-0609
e-mail: afborders@abdintl.com
www.afb.org

A manual of easy-to-follow instructions for more than 50 games and activities for blind and visually impaired persons of all ages, their families, recreation leaders and health care professionals. Large print. *$19.95*

64 pages
ISBN 0-959974-78-4

7050 **Providing Services for People with Vision Loss: Multidisciplinary Perspective**

Resources for Rehabilitation
33 Bedford Street
Suite 19A
Lexington, MA 02173
781-862-6455
FAX: 781-861-7517
www.nfr.org

A collection of articles by ophthalmologists and rehabilitation professionals, including chapters on operating a low vision service, starting self-help programs, mental health services, aids and techniques that help people with vision loss. *$19.95*

136 pages
ISBN 0-929718-02-0

7051 **Psychoeducational Assessment of Visually Impaired and Blind Students**

Pro-Ed
8700 Shoal Creek Boulevard
Austin, TX 78757
512-451-3246
800-897-3202
FAX: 512-451-8542
e-mail: info@proedinc.com
www.proedinc.com

Professional reference book that addresses the problems specific to assessment of visually impaired and blind children. Of particular value to the practitioner are the extensive reviews of available tests, including ways to adapt those not designed for use with the visually handicapped. *$29.00*

140 pages Paperback
ISBN 0-890791-08-2

7052 **Quarterly Update**

National Association for Visually Handicapped
22 W 21st Street
6th Floor
New York, NY 10010 **212-889-2804**
FAX: 212-727-2931
e-mail: staff@navh.org
www.navh.org

Quarterly newsletter offering information on new products for the visually impaired, advances in medical treatments, new books available in the NAVH large print loan library and any new/updated booklets. Free. *$2.25*

7053 **RP Messenger**

Texas Association of Retinitis Pigmentosa
PO Box 8388
Corpus Christi, TX 78468 **361-852-8515**
FAX: 361-852-8515
e-mail: phstiefel@grande.com.nist

A bi-annual newsletter offering information on Retinitis Pigmentosa. *$15.00*

BiAnnual

7054 **Raised Dot Computing Newsletter**

Raised Dot Computing
408 S Baldwin Street
Madison, WI 53703 **608-257-9595**
e-mail: info@rdcbraille.com

Discusses braille computer techniques and devices for blind persons. *$7.00*

7055 **Reaching, Crawling, Walking....Let's Get Moving**

Blind Children's Center
4120 Marathon Street
Los Angeles, CA 90029 **323-664-2153**
800-222-3567
FAX: 323-665-3828
e-mail: info@blindchildrenscenter.org
www.blindchildrenscenter.org

Orientation and mobility for preschool children who are visually imapired. *$10.00*

24 pages

7056 **Recording for the Blind News**

Recording for the Blind
20 Rosel Road
Princeton, NJ 08540 **609-452-0606**
800-221-4792
FAX: 609-987-8116

A non-profit organization that provides recorded books free of charge to blind and print-handicapped individuals.

3x Year

7057 **Resources for Family Centered Intervention for Infants, Toddlers, and Preschoolers**

Hope
1856 N 1200 E
Logan, UT 84341 **435-245-2888**
FAX: 435-245-2888
e-mail: hope@hopepubl.com
www.hopepubl.com

Susan Watkins, Owner

Describes children with vision impairment in terms of characteristics, needs, and parent concerns. *$98.00*

Two volumes

7058 **SCENE**

Braille Institute
527 N Dale Avenue
Anaheim, CA 92801 **714-821-5000**
800-272-4553
FAX: 714-527-7621
www.brailleinstitute.org

Offers information on the organization, question and answer column, articles on the newest technology and more for visually impaired persons.

7059 **Seeing Eye Guide**

Seeing Eye
Washington Valley Road
PO Box 375
Morristown, NJ 07963 **973-539-4425**
FAX: 973-539-0922
e-mail: info@seeingeye.org
www.seeingeye.org

A quarterly publication from Seeing Eye.

Quarterly

7060 **Selecting a Program**

Blind Children's Center
4120 Marathon Street
Los Angeles, CA 90029 **323-664-2153**
800-222-3567
FAX: 323-665-3828
e-mail: info@blindchildrenscenter.org
www.blindchildrenscenter.org

A guide for parents of infants and preschoolers with visual impairments. *$10.00*

28 pages

7061 **Shared Visions**

PCBVI
2470 El Camino Real
Suite 107
Palo Alto, CA 94306 **650-858-0202**
800-660-2009
FAX: 650-858-0214
e-mail: pbrandin@pcbvi.org
www.pcbvi.org

Pam Brandin, Executive Director

A bi-annual publication from Penninsula Center for the Blind and Visually Impaired.

7062 **Sightings Newsletter**

Schepens Eye Research Institute
20 Staniford Street
Boston, MA 02114 **617-912-0100**
FAX: 617-912-0110
e-mail: geninfo@@vision.eri.harvard.edu
www.eri.harvard.edu/default/htm

J Wayne Streilein MD, President

Prominent center for research on eye, vision, and blinding diseases; dedicated to research that improves the understanding, management, and prevention of eye diseases and visual deficiencies; fosters collaboration among its faculty members; trains young scientists and clinicians from around the world; promotes communication with scientists in allied fields; leader in the worldwide dispersion of basic scientific knowledge of vision.

7063 Smith Kettlewell Rehabilitation Engineering Research Center

Smith-Kettlewell Eye Research Institute
2318 Fillmore Street
San Francisco, CA 94115
415-561-2000
FAX: 415-345-8455
e-mail: rerc@ski.org
www.ski.org

Ruth S Poole, COO

Reports on technology and devices for persons with visual impairments.

7064 Social Maturity Scale for Blind Preschool Children: A Guide to Its Use

American Foundation for the Blind/AFB Press
PO Box 1020
Sewickley, PA 15143
412-741-1142
800-232-3044
FAX: 412-741-0609
e-mail: afborders@abdintl.com
www.afb.org

An adaptation of the Vineland Social Maturity Scale for use with children from infancy to 6 years of age. *$9.95*

57 pages Paperback

ISBN 0-891280-59-6

7065 Specifications for Selecting a Vocabulary and Teaching Method/Braille Readers

American Foundation for the Blind/AFB Press
PO Box 1020
Sewickley, PA 15143
412-741-1142
800-232-3044
FAX: 412-741-0609
e-mail: afborders@abdintl.com
www.afb.org

Specifications for a reading series developing braille developed at the American Printing House For The Blind. Paperback. *$ 12.95*

84 pages

ISBN 0-891280-69-3

7066 Standing On My Own Two Feet

Blind Children's Center
4120 Marathon Street
Los Angeles, CA 90029
323-664-2153
800-222-3567
FAX: 323-665-3828
e-mail: info@blindchildrenscenter.org
www.blindchildrenscenter.org

A guide to constructing mobility devices for children who are visually impaired. *$10.00*

38 pages

7067 Starting Points

Blind Children's Center
4120 Marathon Street
Los Angeles, CA 90029
323-664-2153
800-222-3567
FAX: 323-665-3828
e-mail: info@blindchildrenscenter.org
www.blindchildrenscenter.org

Basic information for the clasroom teacher of 3 to 8 year olds whose multiple disabilities include visual impairment. *$35.00*

157 pages

7068 Step-By-Step Guide to Personal Management for Blind Persons

American Foundation for the Blind/AFB Press
PO Box 1020
Sewickley, PA 15143
412-741-1142
800-232-3044
FAX: 412-741-0609
e-mail: afborders@abdintl.com
www.afb.org

A manual of techniques in the areas of hygiene, grooming, clothing, shopping and child care. *$19.95*

136 pages Spiralbound

ISBN 0-891280-61-8

7069 Student Advocate

National Alliance of Blind Students
1010 Vermont Avenue NW
Suite 1100
Washington, DC 20005
202-393-3666
800-424-8666

A communication forum covering issues of concern to postsecondary students who are blind.

7070 Student Teaching Guide for Blind and Visually Impaired College Students

American Foundation for the Blind/AFB Press
PO Box 1020
Sewickley, PA 15143
412-741-1142
800-232-3044
FAX: 412-741-0609
e-mail: afborders@abdintl.com
www.afb.org

A comprehensive resource designed to enable the student to enter the classroom of a university or college with confidence. Large print. *$14.95*

52 pages

ISBN 0-891281-42-8

7071 Syndicated Columnists Weekly

National Braille Press
88 St Stephen Street
Boston, MA 02115
617-266-6160
800-548-7323
FAX: 617-437-0456
e-mail: orders@nbp.org
www.nhp.org

$24.00

Weekly

7072 Talk to Me

Blind Children's Center
4120 Marathon Street
Los Angeles, CA 90029
323-664-2153
800-222-3567
FAX: 323-665-3828
e-mail: info@blindchildrenscenter.org
www.blindchildrenscenter.org

A language guide for parents of children who are visually impaired. *$10.00*

11 pages

7073 Talk to Me II

Blind Children's Center
4120 Marathon Street
Los Angeles, CA 90029
323-664-2153
800-222-3567
FAX: 323-665-3828
e-mail: info@blindchildrenscenter.org
www.blindchildrenscenter.org

$10.00

15 pages

7074 Talking Book Topics

National Library Services for the Blind
1291 Taylor Street NW
Washington, DC 20542
202-707-5100
FAX: 202-707-0712
e-mail: nls@loc.gov
www.loc.gov/nls

Offers hundreds of listings of books, fiction and nonfiction, for adults and children on cassette. Also offers listings on foreign language books on cassette, talking magazines and reviews.

BiMonthly

7075 Teaching Orientation and Mobility in the Schools: An Instructor's Companion

American Foundation for the Blind
11 Penn Plaza
Suite 300
New York, NY 10001
212-502-7600
800-232-5463
FAX: 212-502-7777
e-mail: afbinfo@afb.net
www.afb.org/store

Carl R Augusto, President/CEO

This book, with its useful forms, checklists, and tips, will help O&M instructors and teachers of visually impaired students master the arts of planning schedules, organizing equipment and work routines, working with school personnel and educational team members, and effectively providing instruction to children with diverse needs. *$ 39.95*

176 pages 1902
ISBN 0-891283-91-1

7076 Teaching Visually Impaired Children

Charles C Thomas
2600 S First Street
Springfield, IL 62704
217-789-8980
800-258-8980
FAX: 217-789-9130
e-mail: books@ccthomas.com
www.ccthomas.com

A comprehensive resource for the classroom teacher who is working with a visually impaired child for the first time, as well as a systematic overview of education for the specialist in visual disabilities. It approaches instructional challenges with clear explanations and practical suggestions, and it addresses common concerns of teachers in a reassuring and positive manner. Also available in cloth. *$35.95*

274 pages Paperback
ISBN 0-398065-96-9

7077 Telephone Pioneer

Telephone Pioneers of America
930 15th Street
12th Floor
Denver, CO 80202
303-571-1200
FAX: 303-571-9292
www.telephonepioneers.org

Quarterly

7078 Textbook Catalog

National Braille Association
3 Townline Circle
Rochester, NY 14623
585-427-8260
e-mail: nbaoffice@compuserve.com
www.nationalbraille.org

Lists hundreds of scholarly, college and professional textbooks offered in large print, braille or on cassette for visually impaired readers.

80 pages

7079 To Love this Life: Quotations by Helen Keller

American Foundation for the Blind/AFB Press
11 Penn Plaza
Suite 300
New York, NY 10001
212-502-7600
800-232-5463
FAX: 212-502-7774
e-mail: afborder@abdintl.com
www.afb.org

Inspirational work that offers the penetrating observations of Helen Keller, the beloved deaf-blind champion of the rights of people with disabilities. Also available on cassette at $21.95 (ISBN# 0-89128-348-X) *$21.95*

144 pages Hardcover 1900
ISBN 0-891283-47-1

7080 Touch the Baby: Blind & Visually Impaired Children As Patients

American Foundation for the Blind/AFB Press
PO Box 1020
Sewickley, PA 15143
412-741-1142
800-232-3044
FAX: 412-741-0609
e-mail: afborders@abdintl.com
www.afb.org

A how-to manual for health care professionals working in hospitals, clinics and doctors' offices. Teaches the special communication and touch-related techniques needed to prevent blind and visually impaired patients from withdrawing from the healthcare workers and the outside world. $25.00/pack of 25.

13 pages
ISBN 0-891281-97-5

7081 Transition Activity Calendar for Students with Visual Impairments

Mississippi State University
PO Box 6189
Mississippi State, MS 39762
662-325-2001
800-675-7782
FAX: 662-325-8989
www.blind.msstate.edu

Kelly Schaefer, Dissemination Specialist

The Transition Activity Calendar guides the student with a visual disability through the maze of college preparation. Beginning in junior high school, clearly written steps are listed for each grade level. Students planning to enter college after high school graduation can check-off their accomplishments each step of the way. The calendar helps students focus on their goals while providing reminders of tasks yet to be completed. It can be used in a self-directed manner or in a group format. *$4.25*

16 pages Paperback

7082 Transition to College for Students with Visual Impairments: Report

Mississippi State University
PO Box 6189
Mississippi State, MS 39762
662-325-2001
800-675-7782
FAX: 662-325-8989
www.blind.msstate.edu

Lynn McBroom PhD, Sr Research Scientist

A report offering results from telephone interviews of college students with visual impairments and mail surveys of college officials which examines the transition experience of successful college students. General domains in the study include demographics, educational history, computers, specialized and adaptive equipment, resources, college preparation, problems adjusting to college and O&M skills. A literature review covers preparing for college, task timelines,and classroom, labs and tests. *$20.00*

151 pages Paperback

7083 **Understanding and Coping with Achromatopsia**

PO Box 214
Berkeley, CA 94701 **510-540-4700**
FAX: 510-540-4767
e-mail: futterman@achromat.org
www.achromat.org

7084 **United States Association of Blind Athletes**

33 N Institute
Colorado Springs, CO 80903 **719-630-0422**
FAX: 719-630-0616
e-mail: media@usaba.org
www.usaba.org

Covers news, announcements and activities of the Association.

20 pages Quarterly

7085 **Unseen Minority: A Social History of Blindness in the United States**

American Foundation for the Blind/AFB Press
PO Box 1020
Sewickley, PA 15143 **412-741-1142**
800-232-3044
FAX: 412-741-0609
e-mail: afborders@abdintl.com
www.afb.org

A lively narrative, peppered with anecdotes, recounts how the blind overcame discrimination to gain full participation in the social, educational, economic and legislative spheres. Hardcover. *$ 40.00*

573 pages
ISBN 0-679505-39-3

7086 **Vision Enhancement**

UN Printing
5707 Brockton Drive
Suite 302
Indianaplis, IN 46220 **317-254-1332**
800-431-1739
FAX: 317-251-6588
e-mail: info@visionww.org
www.visionww.org

Patricia L Price, President/Managing Editor

Sesigned to encourage and support individuals with vision loss, family members, and caregivers. *$25.00*

72-78 pages Quarterly

7087 **Visual Aids and Informational Material**

National Association for Visually Handicapped
22 W 21st Street
6th Floor
New York, NY 10010 **212-889-2804**
FAX: 212-727-2931
e-mail: staff@navh.org
www.navh.org

A complete listing of the visual aids NAVH carries such as magnifiers, talking clocks, large print playing cards, etc. *$2.50*

65 pages

7088 **Visual Handicaps and Learning**

Pro-Ed Publications
8700 Shoal Creek Boulevard
Austin, TX 78757 **512-451-3246**
800-897-3202
FAX: 512-451-8542
e-mail: info@proedinc.com
www.proedinc.com

The major focus of this new third edition is to present a new way of thinking about individuals with visual impairment so that they are viewed as participating members of a seeing world despite their reduced visual functioning. *$28.00*

213 pages

7089 **Visual Impairment: An Overview**

American Foundation for the Blind/AFB Press
PO Box 1020
Sewickley, PA 15143 **412-741-1142**
800-232-3044
FAX: 412-741-0609
e-mail: afborders@abdintl.com
www.afb.org

An overall look at the most common forms of vision loss and their impact on the individual. Includes drawings as well as photographs that stimulate how people with vision loss see. Paperback. *$19.95*

56 pages
ISBN 0-891281-74-6

7090 **Visually Handicapped Child in Your Class**

Brookes Publishing
PO Box 10624
Baltimore, MD 21285
800-638-3775
FAX: 410-337-8539
www.pbrookes.com

This book considers the theory and issues relating to the movement to integrate visually handicapped children into ordinary schools and offers practical suggestions to teachers to help such children participate fully in school life. *$21.50*

192 pages Paper
ISBN 0-304314-00-5

7091 **Viva Vital News**

5016 Silk Oak Drive
Sarasota, FL 34232

Membership service organization offering information for veterans and is an affiliate of the American Council of the Blind.

7092 **Voice of Vision**

GW Micro
725 Airport N Office Park
Fort Wayne, IN 46825 **260-489-3671**
FAX: 260-489-2608
e-mail: sales@gwmicro.com
www.gwmicro.com

Offers product reviews, product announcements, tips for making systems or applications more accessible, or explanations of concepts of interest to any computer user or would-be computer user. This association newsletter is available in braille, in large print, on audio cassette and on 3.5 or 5.25 IBM format diskette.

Quarterly

7093 **Walking Alone and Marching Together**

National Federation of the Blind
1800 Johnson Street
Baltimore, MD 21230
410-659-9314
FAX: 410-685-5653
e-mail: nfb@iamdigex.net
www.nfb.org

The history of the organized blind movement, this book spans more than 50 years of civil rights, social issues, attitudes and experiences of the blind. Published in 1990, it has been read by thousands of blind and sighted persons and is used in colleges, libraries and programs across the country as an important tool in understanding blindness and it's impact on both personal lives and the society at large. Braille $130, 2 track or 4 track cassette $40, Print $33.00. Contact Materials Center.

7094 **We Can Do it Together!**

American Foundation for the Blind/AFB Press
PO Box 1020
Sewickley, PA 15143
412-741-1142
800-232-3044
FAX: 412-741-0609
e-mail: afborders@abdintl.com
www.afb.org

This video illustrates a transdisciplinaty team orientation and mobility program for students with severe visual and multiple impairments, covering both adapted communication systems used to teach mobility skills and basic indoor mobility in the school. For mobility instructors, administrators, teachers of the visually and severely handicapped, occupational, physical and speech therapists and parents. Discussion guide included. 10 minute video tape. Also available in PAL, $33.95, 0-89128-267-X. *$26.95*

VHS
ISBN 0-891282-13-0

7095 **Webster Large Print Thesaurus**

Science Products
Box 888
Southeastern, PA 19399
610-296-2111
800-888-7400
FAX: 610-296-0488

Mary Ann Case, Marketing Director

10 point type, more than 57,000 word entries and illustrations, 14 pt. body copy, 16 pt. heads and 20 pt. page headings. *$22.50*

7096 **What Museum Guides Need to Know: Access for the Blind and Visually Impaired**

American Foundation for the Blind/AFB Press
PO Box 1020
Sewickley, PA 15143
412-741-1142
800-232-3044
FAX: 412-741-0609
e-mail: afborders@abdintl.com
www.afb.org

Explains how blind and visually impaired museum-goers experience art and offers pointers on greeting people, asking if help is needed and teaching about a specific work of art. Contains information on access laws, resources, training guides and guidelines for preparing large print, cassette and braille materials. *$14.95*

64 pages Paperback
ISBN 0-891281-58-4

7097 **When You Have a Visually Impaired Student in Your Classroom: A Guide for Teachers**

American Foundation for the Blind
11 Penn Plaza
Suite 300
New York, NY 10001
212-502-7600
800-232-5463
FAX: 212-502-7777
e-mail: afbinfo@afb.net
www.afb.org/store

Carl R Augusto, President/CEO

This guide provides information on students' abilities and needs, resources and educational team members, federal special education requirements, and technology materials used by students. *$9.95*

84 pages 1901
ISBN 0-891283-93-5

7098 **Witch's Daughter**

JB Lippincott
227 E Washington Square
Philadelphia, PA 19106
215-238-4200
800-777-2295
FAX: 215-824-7390

Perdeta had been scorned by her peers on the small Scottish island where she lived. The island children believed her to be a witch and spent their time chasing and teasing her. When Tim and his blind sister Janey arrived for a vacation, Perdeta had her first opportunity to make friends. Janey and Perdeta enjoyed each other's company immediately, while Tim eventually accepted their new friend.

181 pages Hardcover

7099 **You Seem Like a Regular Kid to Me**

American Foundation for the Blind/AFB Press
PO Box 1020
Sewickley, PA 15143
412-741-1142
800-232-3044
FAX: 412-741-0609
e-mail: afborders@abdintl.com
www.afb.org

An interview with Jane, a blind child, tells other children what it's like to be blind. Jane explains how she gets around, takes care of herself, does her schoolwork, spends her leisure time and even pays for things when she can't see money. Paperback and pamphlet. $25.00/pack of 25. *$25.00*

16 pages Pack of 25
ISBN 0-89128 -21-6

Vocations

7100 **ABC's of Starting a Private School**

Alliance for Parental Involvement in Education
PO Box 59
E Chatham, NY 12060
518-392-6900
FAX: 518-392-6900

Job placement programs, remunerative work services and work adjustment training programs. *$17.95*

7101 **Ability**

George J DePontis
PO Box 370788
Miami, FL 33137

Features articles on living, working, playing and entertainment for the disabled. *$12.00*

7102 **Ability Magazine**

Jobs Information Business Service
1682 Langley Avenue
Irvine, CA 92614 **949-622-1040**
800-453-JOBS

Provides an electronic classified system which allows employers to recruit qualified individuals with disabilities, and people with disabilities to locate employment opportunities.

7103 **Cambridge Career Products Catalog**

Cambridge Educational
PO Box 931
Monmouth Junction, NJ 08852 **304-744-9323**
800-468-4227
FAX: 800-329-6687
e-mail: lisa.schmuclei@films.com
www.cambridgeeducational.com

Lisa Schmuclei, Marketing Director

A full color catalog featuring hundreds of products designed to aid people in career exploration, selecting specific occupations and obtaining these jobs through resume and interview preparation.

64 pages BiAnnual

7104 **Career Development Quarterly**

American Counseling Association
5999 Stevenson Avenue
Alexandria, VA 22304 **800-347-6647**
800-473-2329
FAX: 703-823-6862
www.counseling.org

Mark L Savickas, Editor

$35.00

Quarterly

7105 **Case Management in the Vocational Rehabilitation of Disabled Persons**

Berkeley Planning Associates
440 Grand Avenue
Suite 500
Oakland, CA 94610 **510-465-7884**
FAX: 510-465-7885

Linda Toms Barker

Journal examining the effectiveness of case management services in the context of vocational rehabilitation for persons with psychiatric disabilities.

7106 **Closer Look: The English Program at the Model Secondary School for the Deaf**

Gallaudet University Bookstore
800 Florida Avenue NE
Washington, DC 20002 **202-651-5000**
800-451-1073
FAX: 202-651-5489

Job placement programs, remunerative work services and work adjustment training programs incorporating the whole language philosophy into classroom routines. *$8.50*

67 pages

7107 **College Guide for Students with Learning Disablities**

Riverside Publishing/Wintergreen Orchard House
425 Spring Lake Drive
Itasca, IL 60143 **630-232-7047**
800-323-9540
FAX: 630-467-6194

Tina Tripoli, Marketing/Account Manager

There is a role to play whether you are a teacher, counselor, administrator or parent and this guide explains them all. *$26.95*

372 pages

7108 **Economic Opportunity Report**

Business Publishers
8737 Colesville Road
Suite 1100
Silver Spring, MD 20910
800-274-6737
FAX: 301-587-4530
e-mail: bpinews@bpinews.com
www.bpinews.com

Leonard A Eiserer, Publisher
Lan Wilhelm, Editor

Reports the latest on key poverty programs such as homelessness, housing, welfare reform, job training, early childhood education, health care, adult literacy, and more. *$417.00*

10 pages Newsletter Wkly

7109 **Economics, Industry and Disability**

Paul H Brookes Publishing Company
PO Box 10624
Baltimore, MD 21285
800-638-3775
FAX: 410-337-8539

An analysis of the movement toward nonsheltered employment, this book addresses the expanding opportunities, future challenges and economic changes surrounding efforts to ensure the development of positive and constructive employment for persons with disabilities. *$42.00*

Hardcover

7110 **Employment Standards Administration Department of Labor**

200 Constitution Avenue NW
Washington, DC 20210 **202-219-6666**
877-889-5627
www.dol.gov

Corlis Sellers, Branch Chief

Monitors compliance with sub-minimum wage requirements for handicapped workers in sheltered workshops, competitive industry and hospitals and institutions under Section 14 of the Fair Labor Standards Act of 1938.

7111 **Guide to Developing Language Competence in Handicapped Preschool Children**

Charles C Thomas
2600 S First Street
Springfield, IL 62794 **217-789-8980**
800-258-8980
FAX: 217-789-9130
e-mail: books@ccthomas.com
www.ccthomas.com

Ennio Cipani

Job placement programs, remunerative work services and work adjustment training programs handicaps: teachers, administrators and parents. *$54.95*

268 pages Cloth 1991
ISBN 0-398057-48-6

7112 Handbook for Counseling the Gifted and Talented

American Counseling Association
5999 Stevenson Avenue
Alexandria, VA 22304
800-347-6647
800-473-2329
FAX: 703-823-6862
www.counseling.org

Barbara A Kerr, Editor

Tells how to identify, inspire and nurture gifted and talented students. Effective techniques for making a qualitative and quantitative differentiation of gifted students, conducting a successful search for gifted students, nurturing underachievers and helping multipotential students make career choices. *$32.95*

218 pages
ISBN 1-55620-79-1

7113 Job Placement Digest

National Rehabilitation Association (NRA)
613 S Washington Street
Alexandria, VA 22314
703-548-1502
e-mail: info@nationalrehab.org

Newsletter discussing employment options for persons with disabilities.

7114 Mentally Retarded Individuals

Mainstream
3 Bethesda Metro Center
Suite 830
Bethesda, MD 20814
301-951-6122
800-247-1380
FAX: 301-654-6714
e-mail: info@mainstreaminc.org

Mainstreaming mentally retarded individuals into the workplace. *$2.50*

12 pages

7115 Occupational Outlook Quarterly

US Department of Labor/Bureau of Labor Stats
2 Massachusetts Avenue NE
Washington, DC 20212
202-691-5200
FAX: 202-691-7890

Kathleen Green, Managing Editor

Information on new educational and training opportunities, emerging jobs, prospects for change in the work world, and occupational projections. *$9.50*

40 pages Quarterly

7116 Options

6610 N Clark
Chicago, IL 60660
773-973-7900
FAX: 773-973-5268
e-mail: AskAnixter@Anixter.org
www.anixter.org

Stuart Ferst, President/CEO
Robert Dolgan, Editor

Anixter Center's quarterly publication. Free.

Quarterly

7117 Preparation and Employment of Students

Paul H Brookes Publishing Company
PO Box 10624
Baltimore, MD 21285
800-638-3775
FAX: 410-337-8539

A practical guide on vocational training and employment issues for persons with severe multiple and physical disabilities. *$ 213.00*

224 pages Paper

7118 Principles and a Philosophy for Vocational Education

Center on Education and Training for Employment
Ohio State
1900 Kenny Road
Columbus, OH 43210
614-292-4277
800-848-4815
FAX: 614-292-1260

Att:, Publications Office

Identifies and analyzes underlying principles of vocational education and uses them as a basis for coherent philosophical position for vocational education that reflects human and economic needs, a contemporary knowledge base, and the values inherent in our society. *$15.50*

250 pages

7119 Retaining At-Risk Students: The Role of Career and Vocational Education

Center on Education and Training for Employment
Ohio State - 1900 Kenny Road
Columbus, OH 43210
614-292-1102
800-848-4815
FAX: 614-292-1260

Reviews the causes of at-risk students and their implications for the U.S. Labor force. *$6.00*

48 pages

7120 Social Competence for Workers with Developmental Disabilities

Paul H Brookes Publishing Company
PO Box 10624
Baltimore, MD 21285
800-638-3775
FAX: 410-337-8539

A guide to enhancing employment outcomes in integrated settings. *$35.00*

128 pages Paper 1990

7121 Successful Job Accommodation Strategies

LRP Publications
PO Box 24668
West Palm Beach, FL 33416
215-784-0941
800-341-7874
FAX: 215-784-9639
e-mail: custserve@lrp.com
www.lrp.com

Honora McDowell, Product Group Manager

This monthly newsletter provides you with quick tips, new accommodation ideas and innovative workplace solutions. You learn the outcomes of the latest cases involving workplace accommodations. *$ 140.00*

12 pages Monthly

7122 **Teaching Chemistry to Students with Disabilities**

American Chemical Society
1155 16th Street NW
Washington, DC 20036
202-872-4600
800-227-5558
FAX: 202-776-8299
TTY:202-872-6355
e-mail: cwd@acs.org
membership.acs.org/C/CWD

Dorothy Miner, Editor
Judith Summers-Gates, Chair, CCD
Anne Swanson, Editor

Promotes the full involvement of individuals with physical and learning disabilities in educational and career opportunities in the chemical and allied sciences. CWD members lead the American Chemical Society's efforts to help: individuals with disabilities who seek education or employment in chemical and allied sciences; employers and educators of persons with disabilities; other committees, offices and members of ACS who are interested in the full involvement of persons with disabilities.

148 pages
ISBN 0-841238-16-2

7123 **Transition from School to Work**

Paul H Brookes Publishing Company
PO Box 10624
Baltimore, MD 21285
800-638-3775
FAX: 410-337-8539

A hands-on guide to planning and implementing successful transition programs for adolescents with disabilities. *$25.00*

336 pages Paper 1988

7124 **Transition from School to Work for Persons with Disabilities**

Longman Publishing Group
10 Bank Street
9th Floor
White Plains, NY 10606
914-993-5000
FAX: 914-421-5598

Examines the multidimensional process needed to effectively prepare persons with disabilities for life beyond school and addresses the key issues in the transition process.

251 pages Paper 1989
ISBN 0-801302-28-5

7125 **Vocal Rehabilitation: A Practice Book for Voice Improvement**

Pro-Ed
8700 Shoal Creek Boulevard
Austin, TX 78757
512-451-3246
800-897-3202
FAX: 512-451-8542
e-mail: info@proedinc.com
www.proedinc.com

A complete program that clinicians can use to help clients eliminate vocal misuses or abuse and gain a healthy, proficient voice.

7126 **Vocational Education for Multihandicapped Youth**

Paul H Brookes Publishing Company
PO Box 10624
Baltimore, MD 21285
800-638-3775
FAX: 410-337-8539

The first book with specific vocational teaching strategies, adaptations and rehabilitation guidelines for preteens and young adults with cerebral palsy. *$25.00*

320 pages Paper 1988

7127 **Vocational Evaluation and Traumatic Brain Injury: A Procedural Manual**

Stout Vocational Rehab Institute
University of Wisconsin-Stout
Menomonie, WI 5413G
FAX: 715-232-2356

Ronald R Fry, Manager
Darlene Botterbusch, Program Assistant

This is a written guide for rehabilitation professionals interested in effectively developing new or modifying existing evaluation/assessment services for persons with traumatic brain injury. A practical manual for identifying local support services; creating specific processes, tools and techniques; and formulating meaningful outcome information to facilitate the provision or goal-directed services *$ 14.75*

61 pages Softcover

7128 **Vocational Rehabilitation and Employment**

Books on Special Children
PO Box 305
Congers, NY 10920
845-638-1236
FAX: 845-638-0847
e-mail: irene@boscbooks.com

Defines kinds of work, expectations, goals and programs. Contributions in general issues of supported employment, training and management and community based programs. *$47.00*

372 pages Hardcover

7129 **Vocational Rehabilitation and Supported Employment**

Paul H Brookes Publishing Company
PO Box 10624
Baltimore, MD 21285
800-638-3775
FAX: 410-337-8539

A timely, comprehensive resource on how vocational rehabilitation can play a major role in facilitating and implementing supported employment programs. *$43.00*

384 pages Paper 1988

Pamphlets

7130 **A Guide for People with Disabilities Seeking Employment**

US Department of Justice
950 Pennsylvania Avenue NW DRS-NYAV
Washington, DC 20530
202-307-0663
800-574-0301
FAX: 202-307-1197
www.ada.gov

A 2-page pamplet for people with disabilities providing a general explanation of the employment provisions of the ADA and how to file a complaint with the Equal Employment Opportunity Commission.

7131 **ABC's of Latex Allergy**

Asthma and Allergy Foundation of America
1125 15th Street NW
Suite 502
Washington, DC 20005
202-466-7643
FAX: 202-466-8940
e-mail: info@aafa.org
www.aafa.org

Brochure provides excellent coverage of this topic including symptoms, diagnosis, causes, and treatments.

7132 ADA Business Brief: Restriping Parking Lots

US Department of Justice
950 Pennsylvania Avenue NW DRS-NYAV
Washington, DC 20530
202-307-0663
800-574-0301
FAX: 202-307-1197
www.ada.gov

A 2-page illustrated design guide explaining the number of accessible parking spaces that are required and the restriping requirements for accessible parking spaces for cars and vans.

7133 ADA Business Brief: Service Animals

US Department of Justice
950 Pennsylvania Avenue NW DRS-NYAV
Washington, DC 20530
202-307-0663
800-574-0301
FAX: 202-307-1197
www.ada.gov

A 1-page publication summarizing the ADA rules on service animals.

7134 ADHD

Learning Disabilities Association of America
4156 Library Road
Pittsburgh, PA 15234
412-341-1515
FAX: 412-344-0224
e-mail: info@ldaamerica.org
www.ldaamerica.org

A booklet for parents offering information on Attention Deficit-Hyperactivity Disorders and learning disabilities. *$3.00*

7135 ADHD in the Classroom: Strategies for Teac hers

Guilford Press
72 Spring Street
New York, NY 10012
212-431-9800
800-365-7006
FAX: 212-966-6708
e-mail: info@guilford.com

Designed specifically to help teachers with their ADHD students, thereby providing a better learning environment for the entire class. *$95.00*

ISBN 0-898629-85-3

7136 About Asthma

American Lung Association
61 Broadway
New York, NY 10017
212-315-8700
FAX: 212-315-8870
e-mail: info@lungusa.org
www.lungusa.org

A popular style pamphlet explaining symptoms, treatment and more for persons with asthma.

16 pages

7137 About Attention Disorder

CACLD
25 Van Zant Street
Suite 15-5
E Norwalk, CT 06855
203-838-5010
FAX: 203-866-6108
e-mail: CACLD@optonline.net
www.CACLD.org

Beryl Kaufman, Executive Director

Introduction to ADHD for the child with the disorder, parents, professionals, family and friends. Brief description as well as causes, challenges involved, treatment options, ways for parents and teachers to help and how children can help themselves. Published by Connecticut Association for Children & Adults with Learning Disabilities (CACLD). *$2.00*

14 pages

7138 About Children's Eyes

National Association for Visually Handicapped
22 W 21st Street
6th Floor
New York, NY 10010
212-889-2804
FAX: 212-727-2931
e-mail: staff@navh.org
www.navh.org

How to identify the child with a visual problem.

7139 About Children's Vision: A Guide for Parents

National Association for Visually Handicapped
22 W 21st Street
6th Floor
New York, NY 10010
212-889-2804
FAX: 212-727-2931
e-mail: staff@navh.org
www.navh.org

Offers a better understanding of the normal and possible abnormal development of a child's eyesight. *$.50*

7140 Accessible Stadiums

US Department of Justice
950 Pennsylvania Avenue NW DRS-NYAV
Washington, DC 20530
202-307-0663
800-574-0301
FAX: 202-307-1197
www.ada.gov

A 4-page publication highlighting features that must be accessible in new stadiums including line of sight for wheelchair seating locations.

7141 Agent Orange & Spina Bifida

Spina Bifida Association of America
4590 MacArthur Boulevard NW
Suite 250
Washington, DC 20007
202-944-3285
800-321-6141
FAX: 202-944-3295
e-mail: sbaa@sbaa.org
www.sbaa.org

7142 Ankylosing Spondylitis

Arthritis Foundation
PO Box 7669
Atlanta, GA 30357
404-872-7100
800-283-7800
FAX: 404-872-9559
e-mail: help@arthritis.org
www.arthritis.org

7143 Around the Clock: Parenting the Delayed AD HD Child

Guilford Press
72 Spring Street
New York, NY 10012
212-431-9800
800-365-7006
FAX: 212-966-6708
e-mail: info@guilford.com

This videotape provides both professionals and parents a helpful look at how the difficulties facing parents of ADHD children can be handled. Video. *$150.00*

ISBN 0-898629-68-3

7144 Arthritis Answers: Basic Information About Arthritis

Arthritis Foundation
PO Box 7669
Atlanta, GA 30357
404-872-7100
800-283-7800
FAX: 404-872-9559
e-mail: help@arthritis.org
www.arthritis.org

7145 Arthritis Information: Children

Arthritis Foundation
PO Box 7669
Atlanta, GA 30357
404-872-7100
800-283-7800
FAX: 404-872-9559
e-mail: help@arthritis.org
www.arthritis.org

List of materials for children with arthritis, their families and the health professionals who care for them.

7146 Arthritis and Diet

National Institute of Arthritis
1 AMS Circle
Bethesda, MD 20892
301-495-4484
877-226-4267
FAX: 301-881-2731
e-mail: niamsinfo@mail.nih.gov
www.nih.gov/niams

Offers information on nutrition and diet pertaining to the arthritis community. *$2.00*

16 pages

7147 Arthritis and Employment: You Can Get the Job You Want

Arthritis Foundation
PO Box 7669
Atlanta, GA 30357
404-872-7100
800-283-7800
FAX: 404-872-9559
e-mail: help@arthritis.org
www.arthritis.org

7148 Arthritis and Pregnancy

Arthritis Foundation
PO Box 7669
Atlanta, GA 30357
404-872-7100
800-283-7800
FAX: 404-872-9559
e-mail: help@arthritis.org
www.arthritis.org

How arthritis affects pregnancy, managing pregnancy and a new baby.

7149 Arthritis in Children

National Institute of Arthritis
1 AMS Circle
Bethesda, MD 20892
301-495-4484
877-226-4267
FAX: 301-881-2731
e-mail: niamsinfo@mail.nih.gov
www.nih.gov/niams

7150 Arthritis in Children and La Artritis Infantojuvenil

American Juvenile Arthritis Organization
PO Box 7669
Atlanta, GA 30326
404-872-7100
800-283-7800
FAX: 404-872-9559
e-mail: help@arthritis.org
www.arthritis.org

A medical information booklet about juvenile rheumatoid arthritis. This booklet is written for parents or other adults and includes details about different forms of JRA, medications, therapies and coping issues.

7151 Arthritis in Children: Resources for Children, Parents and Teachers

National Institute of Arthritis
9000 Rockville Pike
Bethesda, MD 20892
301-495-4484
877-226-4267
FAX: 301-881-2731
e-mail: niamsinfo@mail.nih.gov
www.nih.gov/niams

A resource offering information on juvenile arthritis, causes, treatments and prevention.

38 pages

7152 Arthritis on the Job: You Can Work with It

Arthritis Foundation
PO Box 7669
Atlanta, GA 30357
404-872-7100
800-283-7800
FAX: 404-872-9559
e-mail: help@arthritis.org
www.arthritis.org

7153 Arthritis, Rheumatic Diseases and Related Disorders

National Institute of Arthritis
9000 Rockville Pike
Bethesda, MD 20892
301-495-4484
877-226-4267
FAX: 301-881-2731
e-mail: niamsinfo@mail.nih.gov
www.nih.gov/niams

This pamphlet offers information, technical articles and research on arthritis and related disorders. Also included are referral organizations to help patients uncover more information.

7154 Arthritis: Do You Know?

Arthritis Foundation
PO Box 7669
Atlanta, GA 30357
404-872-7100
800-283-7800
FAX: 404-872-9559
e-mail: help@arthritis.org
www.arthritis.org

A brief overview of arthritis and the services of the Arthritis Foundation.

7155 Assistance at Self-Serve Gas Stations

US Department of Justice
950 Pennsylvania Avenue NW DRS-NYAV
Washington, DC 20530
202-307-0663
800-574-0301
FAX: 202-307-1197
www.ada.gov

A 1-page document providing guidance on the ADA and refueling assistance for customers with disabilities at self-serve gas stations.

7156 Asthma & Allergy Medications

Academy of Allergy, Asthma, Immunology
611 E Wells Street
Milwaukee, WI 53202
414-272-6071
800-822-2762
FAX: 414-272-6070
e-mail: info@aaaai.org
www.aaaai.org

$.50

4 pages

7157 **Asthma Alert**

American Lung Association
61 Broadway
New York, NY 10017
212-315-8700
FAX: 212-315-8870
e-mail: info@lungusa.org
www.lungusa.org

Quick reference folders with information on asthma, the symptoms and what to do in an emergency.

7158 **Asthma Handbook**

American Lung Association
61 Broadway
New York, NY 10017
212-315-8700
FAX: 212-315-8870
e-mail: info@lungusa.org
www.lungusa.org

Explains asthma, gives self-care methods for handling it and helps patients work more effectively with their doctor.

28 pages

7159 **Asthma Lifelines**

American Lung Association
61 Broadway
New York, NY 10017
212-315-8700
FAX: 212-315-8700
e-mail: info@lungusa.org
www.lungusa.org

Promotional brochure providing descriptions of ALA asthma education materials.

12 pages

7160 **Asthma and Pregnancy**

Academy of Allergy, Asthma, Immunology
611 E Wells Street
Milwaukee, WI 53202
414-272-6071
800-822-2762
FAX: 414-272-6070
e-mail: info@aaaai.org
www.aaaai.org

$.50

7161 **Attention Deficit-Hyperactivity Disorder: Is it a Learning Disability?**

Georgetown University, School of Medicine
3800 Reservoir Road NW
Washington, DC 20007
202-687-2000

Offers information on learning disabilities and related disorders.

7162 **Avoiding Unfortunate Situations**

Autism Society of North Carolina Bookstore
505 Oberlin Road
Suite 230
Raleigh, NC 27605
919-743-0204
800-442-2762
FAX: 919-743-0208
e-mail: dcoffey@autismsociety-nc.org
www.autismsociety-nc.org

Darla Coffey, Bookstore Manager

A collection of tips and information from and about people with autism and other developmental disabilities. *$5.00*

7163 **BVA Bulletin**

Blinded Veterans Association
477 H Street NW
Washington, DC 20001
202-371-8880
800-669-7079
FAX: 303-914-5832
e-mail: bva@bva.org
www.bva.org

Thomas H Miller, Executive Director
John K Williams, Administrative Director
George E Brummell, Nat'l Dir. Field Service Program

BiMonthly

7164 **Being Close**

National Jewish Center for Immunology
1400 Jackson Street
Denver, CO 80206
303-388-4461
e-mail: allstetterw@njc.org
www.njc.org

William Allstetter, Media Relations Manager

A booklet offering information to patients suffering from a respiratory disorder such as emphysema, asthma or tuberculosis, that discusses sexual problems and feelings.

7165 **Blind and Vision-Impaired Individuals**

Mainstream
1030 5th Street NW
Washington, DC 20005
202-898-1400
e-mail: info@mainstreaminc.org

Mainstreaming blind individuals into the workplace. *$ 2.50*

12 pages

7166 **Books are Fun for Everyone**

National Library Service for the Blind
1291 Taylor Street NW
Washington, DC 20542
202-707-5100
FAX: 202-707-0712
e-mail: nls@loc.gov
www.loc.gov/nls

7167 **Braille: An Extraordinary Volunteer Opportunity**

National Library Service for the Blind
1291 Taylor Street NW
Washington, DC 20542
202-707-5100
FAX: 202-707-0712
e-mail: nls@loc.gov
www.loc.gov/nls

7168 **Bursitis, Tendonitis and Other Soft Tissue Rheumatic Syndromes**

Arthritis Foundation
PO Box 7669
Atlanta, GA 30357
404-872-7100
800-283-7800
FAX: 404-872-9559
e-mail: help@arthritis.org
www.arthritis.org

7169 **Carpal Tunnel Syndrome**

Arthritis Foundation
PO Box 7669
Atlanta, GA 30357
404-872-7100
800-283-7800
FAX: 404-872-9559
e-mail: help@arthritis.org
www.arthritis.org

Offers an introduction to Carpal Tunnel, causes, symptoms, diagnosis and resources.

7170 **Cataracts**

National Eye Institute
Building 31
Room 6A32
Bethesda, MD 20892
301-496-5248
800-869-2020
FAX: 301-402-1065
e-mail: 2020@nei.nih.gov
www.nei.nih.gov

Provides information about this common condition and its treatment.

7171 **Childhood Asthma**

Academy of Allergy, Asthma, Immunology
611 E Wells Street
Milwaukee, WI 53202
414-272-6071
800-822-2762
FAX: 414-272-6070
e-mail: info@aaaai.org
www.aaaai.org

$.50

4 pages

7172 **Childhood Asthma: A Matter of Control**

American Lung Association
61 Broadway
New York, NY 10017
212-315-8700
FAX: 212-315-8700
e-mail: info@lungusa.org
www.lungusa.org

A guide for parents of children with asthma, this booklet covers topics such as identifying asthma signs and symptoms as well as controlling the condition.

28 pages

7173 **Children with ADD: A Shared Responsibility**

Council for Exceptional Children
1110 N Glebe Road
Suite 300
Arlington, VA 22201
703-620-3660
FAX: 703-264-9494
www.cec.sped.org

Janice Burdick, President

This book represents a consensus of what professionals and parents believe ADD is all about and how children with ADD may best be served. Reviews the evaluation process under IDEA and 504 and presents effective classroom strategies.

35 pages
ISBN 0-865862-33-8

7174 **Classification of Impaired Vision**

National Association for Visually Handicapped
22 W 21st Street
6th Floor
New York, NY 10010
212-889-2804
FAX: 212-727-2931
e-mail: staff@navh.org
www.navh.org

Describes various degrees of impaired vision.

7175 **Club Foot & Other Foot Deformities Fact Sheet**

March of Dimes
1275 Mamaroneck Avenue
White Plains, NY 10605
914-428-7100
FAX: 914-997-4763
e-mail: askus@marchofdimes.com
www.marchofdimes.com

Provides information about pregnancy, birth defects, genetics, drug use, environmental hazzards and related topics. The Resource Center's health information specialists provide acccurate and up-to-date information via e-mail and Web site. One copy of this fact sheet can be obtained free of charge by visiting our website.

7176 **Cogrehab**

Life Science Associates
1 Fenimore Road
Bayport, NY 11705
631-472-2111

Divided into six groups for diagnosis and treatment of attention, memory and perceptual disorders to be used by and under the guidance of a professional. $95.-$1,950

7177 **Common ADA Errors and Omissions in New Construction and Alterations**

US Department of Justice
950 Pennsylvania Avenue NW DRS-NYAV
Washington, DC 20530
202-307-0663
800-574-0301
FAX: 202-307-1197
www.ada.gov

This 13-page document lists a sampling of common accessibility errors or omissions that have been identified through the Department of Justice's ongoing enforcement efforts. The significance of the errors is discussed and references are provided to the requirements of the ADA Standards for Accessible Design.

7178 **Common ADA Problems at Newly Constructed Lodging Facilities**

US Department of Justice
950 Pennsylvania Avenue NW DRS-NYAV
Washington, DC 20530
202-307-0663
800-574-0301
FAX: 202-307-1197
www.ada.gov

This 11-page document lists a sampling of common accessibility problems at newly constructed lodging facilities that have been identified through the Department of Justice's ongoing enforcement efforts.

7179 **Commonly Asked Questions About Service Animals in Places of Business**

US Department of Justice
950 Pennsylvania Avenue NW DRS-NYAV
Washington, DC 20530
202-307-0663
800-574-0301
FAX: 202-307-1197
www.ada.gov

A 3-page publication providing information about service animals and ADA requirements.

7180 **Commonly Asked Questions About Title III of the ADA**

US Department of Justice
950 Pennsylvania Avenue NW DRS-NYAV
Washington, DC 20530
202-307-0663
800-574-0301
FAX: 202-307-1197
www.ada.gov

A 6-page publication providing information for state and local governments about ADA requirements for ensuring that people with disabilities receive the same services and benefits as provided to others.

7181 **Communicating with People Who Have Trouble Hearing & Seeing: A Primer**

National Association for Visually Handicapped
22 W 21st Street
6th Floor
New York, NY 10010
212-889-2804
FAX: 212-727-2931
e-mail: staff@navh.org
www.navh.org

Line drawings that depict problems for those with both deficiencies. *$2.00*

7182 **Connect Information Service**

150 S Progress Avenue
Harrisburg, PA 17109
717-657-1798
800-692-7288

Pamphlet offering information on child development, special education programs, resources for parents and local contact persons.

7183 **Department of Justice ADA Mediation Program**

US Department of Justice
950 Pennsylvania Avenue NW DRS-NYAV
Washington, DC 20530
202-307-0663
800-574-0301
FAX: 202-307-1197
www.ada.gov

A 6-page publication describing the Department's ADA mediation program and examples of successful mediation efforts.

7184 **Developing a Functional and Longitudinal Plan**

Autism Society of North Carolina Bookstore
505 Oberlin Road
Suite 230
Raleigh, NC 27605
919-743-0204
800-442-2762
FAX: 919-743-0208
e-mail: dcoffey@autismsociety-nc.org
www.autismsociety-nc.org

Darla Coffey, Bookstore Manager

This booklet examines the importance of planning and possible goals in self-care. *$4.00*

7185 **Diet and Arthritis**

Arthritis Foundation
PO Box 7669
Atlanta, GA 30357
404-872-7100
800-283-7800
FAX: 404-872-9559
e-mail: help@arthritis.org
www.arthritis.org

7186 **Dog Sponsorship Program**

Guide Dog Foundation for the Blind
371 E Jericho Turnpike
Smithtown, NY 11787
631-265-2121
800-548-4337
FAX: 516-361-5192

Offers information to an individual or an organization that wishes to sponsor a guide dog.

7187 **Don't Lose Sight of Cataracts**

National Eye Institute
Building 31
Room 6A32
Bethesda, MD 20892
301-496-5248
800-869-2020
FAX: 301-402-1065
e-mail: 2020@nei.nih.gov
www.nei.nih.gov

7188 **Don't Lose Sight of Glaucoma**

National Eye Institute
Building 31
Room 6A32
Bethesda, MD 20892
301-496-5248
800-869-2020
FAX: 301-402-1065
e-mail: 2020@nei.nih.gov
www.nei.nih.gov

7189 **Easy Access Housing**

Easter Seals
230 W Monroe Street
Suite 1800
Chicago, IL 60606
312-726-6200
FAX: 312-726-1494

Janet D Jamieson, Communications Manager

Booklet with a checklist for finding homes that are already accessible or structurally adaptable to accommodate changes in physical abilities and needs. Includes suggestions for solving common accessibility problems such as narrow doors, high thresholds and round knob fixtures.

12 pages

7190 **Educational Issues Among Children with Spi na Bifida**

Spina Bifida Association of America
4590 Macarthur Boulevard NW
Suite 250
Washington, DC 20007
202-944-3285
800-321-6141
FAX: 202-944-3295
e-mail: sbaa@sbaa.org
www.sbaa.org

7191 **Efficacy of Asthma Education, Selected Abstracts**

American Lung Association
61 Broadway
New York, NY 10017
212-315-8700
FAX: 212-315-8700
e-mail: info@lungusa.org
www.lungusa.org

Abstracts documenting the efficacy of asthma education programs for physicians and other health professionals.

7192 **Enhancing Communication in Individuals with Autism Through Pictures/Words**

Autism Society of North Carolina Bookstore
505 Oberlin Road
Suite 230
Raleigh, NC 27605
919-743-0204
800-442-2762
FAX: 919-743-0208
e-mail: dcoffey@autismsociety-nc.org
www.autismsociety-nc.org

Darla Coffey, Bookstore Manager

Booklet addressing the description and implementation of visually aided communication. *$4.00*

7193 **Exercise and Your Arthritis**

Arthritis Foundation
PO Box 7669
Atlanta, GA 30309
404-872-7100
800-283-7800
FAX: 404-872-9559
e-mail: help@arthritis.org
www.arthritis.org

Types of exercise for people with arthritis and how to do them.

7194 **Exercise-Induced Asthma**

Academy of Allergy, Asthma, Immunology
611 E Wells Street
Milwaukee, WI 53202 **414-272-6071**
800-822-2762
FAX: 414-272-6070
e-mail: info@aaaai.org
www.aaaai.org

This brochure covers testing, treatment, and other advice on how to deal with exercise-induced asthma. *$.50*

7195 **Eye-Q Test**

National Association for Visually Handicapped
22 W 21st Street
6th Floor
New York, NY 10010 **212-889-2804**
FAX: 212-727-2931
e-mail: staff@navh.org
www.navh.org

Five questions and answers to assist in knowing more about vision. Also available in Spanish and Russian.

7196 **Fact Sheet: Attention Deficit-Hyperactivit y Disorder**

Learning Disabilities Association of America
4156 Library Road
Pittsburgh, PA 15234 **412-341-1515**
FAX: 412-344-0224
e-mail: info@ldaamerica.org
www.ldaamerica.org

A pamphlet offering factual information on ADHD.

7197 **Fact Sheet: Autism**

Autism Society of America
7910 Woodmont Avenue
Suite 300
Bethesda, MD 20814 **301-657-0881**
800-3AU-TISM
FAX: 301-657-0869
www.autism-society.org

Offers information on autism. What it is, symptoms, causes, diagnosis, treatments and research.

7198 **Facts About Asthma**

American Lung Association
61 Broadway
New York, NY 10017 **212-315-8700**
FAX: 212-315-8700
e-mail: info@lungusa.org
www.lungusa.org

Primary public information leaflet on asthma.

12 pages

7199 **Facts: Books for Blind and Physically Handicapped Individuals**

National Library Service for the Blind
1291 Taylor Street NW
Washington, DC 20542 **202-707-5100**

e-mail: nls@loc.gov
www.loc.gov/nls

Annual

7200 **Facts: Music for Blind and Physically Handicapped Individuals**

National Library Service for the Blind
1291 Taylor Street NW
Washington, DC 20542 **202-707-5100**

e-mail: nls@loc.gov
www.loc.gov/nls

Annual

7201 **Family Guide to Vision Care**

American Optometric Association
243 N Lindbergh Boulevard
St. Louis, MO 63141 **314-991-4100**
FAX: 314-991-4101
www.aoanet.org

Offers information on the early developmental years of your vision, finding a family optometrist and how to take care of your eyesight through the learning years, the working years and the mature years.

7202 **Family Guide: Growth & Development of the Partially Seeing Child**

National Association for Visually Handicapped
22 W 21st Street
6th Floor
New York, NY 10010 **212-889-2804**
FAX: 212-727-2931
e-mail: staff@navh.org
www.navh.org

Offers information for parents and guidelines in raising a partially seeing child. *$.60*

7203 **Free Information/Membership Kit**

National Association for Visually Handicapped
22 W 21st Street
New York, NY 10010 **212-255-4224**
FAX: 212-727-2931
e-mail: staff@navh.org
www.navh.org

Eva M Cohen, CEO Assistant
Lorraine H Marchi, Founder/CEO

A free packet describing brochures, pamphlets, and flyers available addressing the needs of the partially seeing, their families, friends and professionals who serve them: large print, visual aids, self-help, referrals. Includes information regarding vision dysfunction and coping with vision loss.

Quarterly

7204 **General Facts and Figures on Blindness**

National Society to Prevent Blindness
500 E Remington Road
Schaumberg, IL 60173
800-331-2020

7205 **General Interest Catalog**

National Braille Association
3 Townline Circle
Rochester, NY 14623 **585-427-8260**

e-mail: nbaoffice@compuserve.com
www.nationalbraille.org

Lists hundreds of titles of fiction and nonfiction books offered in large print, braille or on cassette to visually impaired readers.

19 pages

7206 **Genetics and Spina Bifida**

Spina Bifida Association of America
4590 Macarthur Boulevard NW
Suite 250
Washington, DC 20007 **202-944-3285**
800-621-3141
FAX: 202-944-3295
e-mail: sbaa@sbaa.org
www.sbaa.org

7207 **Gift of Sight**

RP Foundation Fighting Blindness
1401 Mt Royal Avenue
Baltimore, MD 21217
410-225-9409
800-683-5555
FAX: 410-225-3936

A pamphlet offering information on the Retina Donor Program, which studies diseased, human retinal tissue in their search for a cure of retinal degenerative diseases.

7208 **Glaucoma**

Glaucoma Research Foundation
490 Post Street
Suite 1427
San Francisco, CA 94102
415-986-3162
800-826-6693
FAX: 415-986-3763
e-mail: info@glaucoma.org
www.glaucoma.org

Yuko Madono, Outreach/Public Relations

Offers information on what glaucoma is, the causes, treatments, types of glaucoma, eye exams and prevention.

7209 **Glaucoma: The Sneak Thief of Sight**

National Association for Visually Handicapped
22 W 21st Street
6th Floor
New York, NY 10010
212-889-2804
FAX: 212-727-2931
e-mail: staff@navh.org
www.navh.org

A pamphlet describing the disease, treatment and medications. Also available in Russian and Spanish. Revised in 1999. *$3.50*

7210 **Guide Dog Foundation Flyer**

Guide Dog Foundation for the Blind
371 E Jericho Turnpike
Smithtown, NY 11787
631-265-2121
800-548-4337
FAX: 516-361-5192

Offers information on the programs and services provided by the Foundation.

7211 **Guidelines for Comprehensive Low Vision Care**

National Association for Visually Handicapped
22 W 21st Street
6th Floor
New York, NY 10010
212-889-2804
FAX: 212-727-2931
e-mail: staff@navh.org
www.navh.org

A description of the proper method to conduct a low vision evaluation. *$.50*

7212 **Guidelines for Helping Deaf-Blind Persons**

Helen Keller National Center
111 Middle Neck Road
Sands Point, NY 11050
516-944-8900
800-225-0411
FAX: 516-944-7302
e-mail: hkncdir@aol.com
www.helenkeller.org

Joseph McNulty, Executive Director

Pamphlet offering information on how persons should interact with deaf-blind individuals. Includes drawings of the one hand manual alphabet.

7213 **Healthy Breathing**

National Jewish Center for Immunology
1400 Jackson Street
Denver, CO 80206
303-388-4461
e-mail: allstetterw@njc.org
www.njc.org

William Allstetter, Media Relations Manager

Offers patients with lung or respiratory disorders information on exercise and healthy breathing.

7214 **Heart to Heart**

Blind Children's Center
4120 Marathon Street
Los Angeles, CA 90029
323-664-2153
800-222-3567
FAX: 323-665-3828
e-mail: info@blindchildrenscenter.org
www.blindchildrenscenter.org

Parents of blind and partially sighted children talk about their feelings. *$10.00*

12 pages

7215 **Heartbreak of Being A Little Bit Blind**

National Association for Visually Handicapped
22 W 21st Street
6th Floor
New York, NY 10010
212-889-2804
FAX: 212-727-2931
e-mail: staff@navh.org
www.navh.org

Summary of what it means to have impaired vision; includes illustrations.

7216 **Helping Others Breathe Easier**

National Allergy and Asthma Network
3554 Chain Bridge Road
Suite 200
Fairfax, VA 22030
703-385-4403
FAX: 703-352-4354

Offers information on educational resources, support groups and the Network for persons afflicted with asthma or allergic disorders.

7217 **Helping Your Child with Attention-Deficit Hyperactivity Disorder**

Learning Disabilities Association of America
4156 Library Road
Pittsburgh, PA 15234
412-341-1515
FAX: 412-344-0224
e-mail: info@ldaamerica.org
www.ldaamerica.org

7218 **Hip Function & Ambulation**

Spina Bifida Association of America
4590 MacArthur Boulevard NW
Suite 250
Washington, DC 20007
202-944-3285
800-621-3141
FAX: 202-944-3295
e-mail: sbaa@sbaa.org
www.sbaa.org

7219 **History and Use of Braille**

American Council of the Blind
1155 15th Street NW
Suite 1004
Washington, DC 20005
202-467-5081
800-424-8666
FAX: 202-467-5085
e-mail: info@acb.org
www.acb.org

7220 **Home Control of Allergies and Asthma**

American Lung Association
61 Broadway
New York, NY 10017 **212-315-8700**
FAX: 212-315-8700
e-mail: info@lungusa.org
www.lungusa.org

Discusses substances in the home that may trigger asthma and allergy problems and offers suggestions for controlling them.

12 pages

7221 **How Does a Blind Person Get Around?**

American Foundation for the Blind/AFB Press
PO Box 1020
Sewickley, PA 15143 **412-741-1142**
800-232-3044
FAX: 412-741-0609
e-mail: afborders@abdintl.com
www.afb.org

Offers information on daily living as a blind person.

7222 **How to Choose an Air Ambulance**

National Air Ambulance
PO Box 22460
Fort Lauderdale, FL 33335 **954-359-9900**
800-327-3710
FAX: 954-359-9500
e-mail: inquiry@nationaljets.com
www.nationalairambulance.com

Alan Altman MD, Medical Director
Thomas E Boy, President
George Martinez, Operations Manager

This booklet was prepared to help inform persons about air ambulance operations and to assist if the need for air ambulance transportation should arise.

15 pages

7223 **How to Find More About Your Child's Birth Defect or Disability**

Birth Defect Research for Children
930 Woodcock Road
Suite 225
Orlando, FL 32803 **407-895-0802**
FAX: 407-895-0824
e-mail: abdc@birthdefects.org
www.birthdefects.org

Betty Mekdeci, Executive Director

An informational fact sheet that encourages parents who have a child with a birth defect or disability to become the expert on the child's disability with some suggestions on how to educate themselves.

7224 **How to Own and Operate an Attention Deficit Disorder**

Learning Disabilities Association of America
4156 Library Road
Pittsburgh, PA 15234 **412-341-1515**
FAX: 412-344-0224
e-mail: info@ldaamerica.org
www.ldaamerica.org

Clear, informative and sensitive introduction to ADHD. Packed with practical things to do at home and school, from a professional and mother of a son with ADHD. *$8.95*

43 pages

7225 **Hyperactivity, Attention Deficits, and School Failure: Better Ways**

Learning Disabilities Association of America
4156 Library Road
Pittsburgh, PA 15234 **412-341-1515**
FAX: 412-344-0224
e-mail: info@ldaamerica.org
www.ldaamerica.org

7226 **Individuals with Arthritis**

Mainstream
1030 5th Street NW
Washington, DC 20005 **202-898-1400**
e-mail: info@mainstreaminc.org

Mainstreaming individuals with arthritis into the workplace. *$2.50*

12 pages

7227 **Indoor Allergens**

Academy of Allergy, Asthma, Immunology
611 E Wells Street
Milwaukee, WI 53202 **414-272-6071**
800-822-2762
FAX: 414-272-6070
e-mail: info@aaaai.org
www.aaaai.org

This brochure covers some good ideas on how to reduce dust in the home. *$.50*

4 pages

7228 **Information on Glaucoma**

Glaucoma Research Foundation
490 Post Street
Suite 1427
San Francisco, CA 94102 **415-986-3162**
800-826-6693
FAX: 415-986-3763
e-mail: info@glaucoma.org
www.glaucoma.org

Yuko Madono, Outreach/Public Releations

7229 **Inhaled Medications for Asthma**

Academy of Allergy, Asthma, Immunology
611 E Wells Street
Milwaukee, WI 53202 **414-272-6071**
800-822-2762
FAX: 414-272-6070
e-mail: info@aaaai.org
www.aaaai.org

This brochure gives helpful information on classes of inhaled medication, types of inhalation devices, spacers and holding chambers, how proper training is necessary. *$.50*

4 pages

7230 **Issues in Independent Living**

Independent Living Research Utilization
2323 S Shepherd
Suite 1000
Houston, TX 77019 **713-520-0232**
FAX: 713-520-5785

Lex Frieden, Program Director

This booklet is a report of the National Study Group on the Implications of Health Care Reform for Americans with Disabilities and Chronic Health Conditions.

30 pages

7231 **It's All Right to be Angry**

National Association for Visually Handicapped
22 W 21st Street
6th Floor
New York, NY 10010
212-889-2804
FAX: 212-727-2931
e-mail: staff@navh.org
www.navh.org

A helpful pamphlet describing reactions to learning to live with vision impairment. Also available in Russian. *$2.25*

7232 **Know Your Eye**

American Council of the Blind
1155 15th Street NW
Suite 1004
Washington, DC 20005
202-467-5081
800-424-8666
FAX: 202-467-5085
e-mail: info@acb.org
www.acb.org

7233 **Large Print Loan Library Catalog**

National Association for Visually Handicapped
22 W 21st Street
6th Floor
New York, NY 10010
212-889-2804
FAX: 212-727-2931
e-mail: staff@navh.org
www.navh.org

Listing of over 7,000 commercially published and NAVH large print books avaiable through NAVH on a loan basis. Includes a limited selection of titles available for purchase. *$5.00*

7234 **Latex Allergy in Spina Bifida Patients**

Spina Bifida Association of America
4590 MacArthur Boulevard NW
Suite 250
Washington, DC 20007
202-944-3285
800-621-3141
FAX: 202-944-3295
e-mail: sbaa@sbaa.org
www.sbaa.org

7235 **Learning Among Children with Spina Bifida**

Spina Bifida Association of America
4590 MacArthur Boulevard NW
Suite 250
Washington, DC 20007
202-944-3285
800-621-3141
FAX: 202-944-3295
e-mail: sbaa@sbaa.org
www.sbaa.org

7236 **Learning to Play**

Blind Children's Center
4120 Marathon Street
Los Angeles, CA 90029
323-664-2153
800-222-3567
FAX: 323-665-3828
e-mail: info@blindchildrenscenter.org
www.blindchildrenscenter.org

Discusses how to present play activities to the visually impaired preschool child. *$10.00*

12 pages

7237 **Ledger**

Mental Health Risk Retention Group
PO Box 206
Cedar Grove, NJ 07009
973-239-9107

Information on the Mental Health Risk Retention Group, a liability insurance company.

7238 **Lipomas & Lipomyelomeningocele**

Spina Bifida Association of America
4590 MacArthur Boulevard NW
Suite 250
Washington, DC 20007
202-944-3285
800-621-3141
FAX: 202-944-3295
e-mail: sbaa@sbaa.org
www.sbaa.org

7239 **Living with Asthma and Allergies Brochure Series**

Asthma and Allergy Foundation of America
1125 15th Street NW
Suite 502
Washington, DC 20005
202-466-7643
FAX: 202-466-8940
e-mail: info@aafa.org
www.aafa.org

Informative series was developed to provide up-to-date, accurate information on common topics. Written in easy to understand language, with helpful illustrations, cover some of the most commonly asked questions about asthma and allergies.

7240 **Mama: Your Guide to a Healthy Pregnancy**

March of Dimes
1275 Mamaroneck Avenue
White Plains, NY 10605
914-428-7100
FAX: 914-997-4763
e-mail: askus@marchofdimes.com
www.marchofdimes.com

The March of Dimes Resource Center provides information about pregnancy, birth defects, genetics, drug use, environmental hazards and related topics. The Resource Center's health information specialists provide accurate, up-to-date information via e-mail and Web site.

7241 **Management of Children and Adolescents with AD-HD**

Learning Disabilities Association of America
4156 Library Road
Pittsburgh, PA 15234
412-341-1515
FAX: 412-344-0224
e-mail: info@ldaamerica.org
www.ldaamerica.org

7242 **Managing Your Activities**

Arthritis Foundation
PO Box 7669
Atlanta, GA 30357
404-872-7100
800-283-7800
FAX: 404-872-9559
e-mail: help@arthritis.org
www.arthritis.org

7243 **Managing Your Fatigue**

Arthritis Foundation
PO Box 7669
Atlanta, GA 30357
404-872-7100
800-283-7800
FAX: 404-872-9559
e-mail: help@arthritis.org
www.arthritis.org

7244 **Managing Your Health Care**

Arthritis Foundation
PO Box 7669
Atlanta, GA 30357
404-872-7100
800-283-7800
FAX: 404-872-9559
e-mail: help@arthritis.org
www.arthritis.org

7245 Managing Your Pain

Arthritis Foundation
PO Box 7669
Atlanta, GA 30357
404-872-7100
800-283-7800
FAX: 404-872-9559
e-mail: help@arthritis.org
www.arthritis.org

7246 Many Faces of Asthma

American Lung Association
61 Broadway
New York, NY 10017
212-315-8700
FAX: 212-315-8700
e-mail: info@lungusa.org
www.lungusa.org

Provides an overview of asthma as a major public health problem, describes what happens during asthma attacks and explains how asthma is treated and managed.

12 pages

7247 Marfan Syndrome Fact Sheet

March of Dimes
1275 Mamaroneck Avenue
White Plains, NY 10605
914-428-7100
FAX: 914-997-4763
e-mail: askus@marchofdimes.com
www.marchofdimes.com

7248 Mental Health Resource Guide

1 Renaissance Boulevard
Oakbrook Terrace, IL 60181
630-792-5000

A small pamphlet listing education programs and publications for community mental health centers, child/adolescent services, adult mental health services and MR/DD services.

7249 Move With Me

Blind Children's Center
4120 Marathon Street
Los Angeles, CA 90029
323-664-2153
800-222-3567
FAX: 323-665-3828
e-mail: info@blindchildrenscenter.org
www.blindchildrenscenter.org

A parent's guide to movement development for visually impaired babies. *$10.00*

12 pages

7250 Myositis

Arthritis Foundation
PO Box 7669
Atlanta, GA 30357
404-872-7100
800-283-7800
FAX: 404-872-9559
e-mail: help@arthritis.org
www.arthritis.org

7251 Myths and Facts

US Department of Justice
950 Pennsylvania Avenue NW DRS-NYAV
Washington, DC 20530
202-307-0663
800-574-0301
FAX: 202-307-1197
www.ada.gov

A 3-page publication dispelling some common misconceptions about the ADA's requirements and implementation.

7252 National Institute of Mental Health: Decade of the Brain

6001 Executive Boulevard
Room 8184 MSC 9663
Bethesda, MD 20892
301-443-4513
FAX: 301-443-4279
www.nimh.nih.gov

A consumer's pamphlet to services for persons with mental illness or retardation.

7253 Nocturnal Asthma

National Jewish Center for Immunology
1400 Jackson Street
Denver, CO 80206
303-388-4461
e-mail: allstetterw@njc.org
www.njc.org

William Allstetter, Media Relations Manager

Offers information to patients about how to understand and manage asthma at night.

7254 Obesity

Spina Bifida Association of America
4590 MacArthur Boulevard NW
Suite 250
Washington, DC 20007
202-944-3285
800-621-3141
FAX: 202-944-3295
e-mail: sbaa@sbaa.org
www.sbaa.org

$8.00

7255 Occulta

Spina Bifida Association of America
4590 MacArthur Boulevard NW
Suite 250
Washington, DC 20007
202-944-3285
800-621-3141
FAX: 202-944-3295
e-mail: sbaa@sbaa.org
www.sbaa.org

$8.00

7256 Occupational Asthma

Academy of Allergy, Asthma, Immunology
611 E Wells Street
Milwaukee, WI 53202
414-272-6071
800-822-2762
FAX: 414-272-6070
e-mail: info@aaaai.org
www.aaaai.org

This brochure also contains a list of most common agents theat cause occupational asthma and who is at risk. *$.50*

4 pages

7257 Occupational Asthma: Lung Hazards on the Job

American Lung Association
61 Broadway
New York, NY 10017
212-315-8700
FAX: 212-315-8700
e-mail: info@lungusa.org
www.lungusa.org

Discusses occupational asthma, a form of asthma in which airways overreact to various irritants in the workplace.

7258 Oral/Facial Clefts Fact Sheet

March of Dimes
1275 Mamaroneck Avenue
White Plains, NY 10605
914-428-7100
FAX: 914-997-4763
e-mail: askus@marchofdimes.com
www.marchofdimes.com

The March of Dimes Resource Center provides information about pregnancy, drug use, environmental hazards and other related topics. The Resource Center's health information specialists provide accurate and up-to-date information via e-mail and Web site.

7259 Osteoarthritis

Arthritis Foundation
PO Box 7669
Atlanta, GA 30357
404-872-7100
800-283-7800
FAX: 404-872-9559
e-mail: help@arthritis.org
www.arthritis.org

Offers introductions, examples, explanations and research pertaining to this type of arthritis.

7260 Out of Darkness

CACLD
25 Van Zant Street
Suite 15-5
E Norwalk, CT 06855
203-838-5010
FAX: 203-866-6108
e-mail: CACLD@optonline.net
www.CACLD.org

Beryl Kaufman, Executive Director

Article by an adult who discovers at age 30 that he has ADD. *$1.00*

4 pages

7261 Overcoming Rheumatoid Arthritis

Arthritis Foundation - Michigan Chapter
17117 W Nine Mile Road
Suite 960
Southfield, MI 48075
248-424-9001
800-968-3030
www.arthritis.org

Provides extensive information about the disease and treatment, with an emphasis on what you can do for yourself. *$5.00*

7262 Parenting Attention Deficit Disordered Teens

CACLD
25 Van Zant Street
Suite 15-5
E Norwalk, CT 06855
203-838-5010
FAX: 203-866-6108
e-mail: CACLD@optonline.net
www.CACLD.org

Beryl Kaufman, Executive Director

Detailed outline of the various problems of adolescents with ADHD. Published by Connecticut Association for Children & Adults with Learning Disabilities (CACLD). *$3.25*

14 pages

7263 Patient's Guide to Visual Aids and Illumination

National Association for Visually Handicapped
22 W 21st Street
New York, NY 10010
212-255-2804
FAX: 212-727-2931
e-mail: staff@navh.org
www.navh.org

A reference booklet offering information on aids for the visually impaired.

7264 Peak Flow Meter: A Thermometer for Asthma

Academy of Allergy, Asthma, Immunology
611 E Wells Street
Milwaukee, WI 53202
414-272-6071
800-822-2762
FAX: 414-272-6070
e-mail: info@aaaai.org
www.aaaai.org

$.50

4 pages

7265 People Against Cancer

604 East Street
PO Box 10
Otho, IA 50569
515-972-4444
FAX: 515-972-4415
e-mail: info@PeopleAgainstCancer.net
www.peopleagainstcancer.com

Publication of People Against Cancer, a nonprofit, grassroots public benefit organization dedicated to 'New Directions in the War on Cancer.' We are a democratic organization of people with cancer, their loved ones and citizens working together to protect and enhance medical freedom of choice.

8 pages

7266 Polymyalgia Rheumatica and Giant Cell Arthritis

Arthritis Foundation
PO Box 7669
Atlanta, GA 30357
404-872-7100
800-283-7800
FAX: 404-872-9559
e-mail: help@arthritis.org
www.arthritis.org

7267 Psoriatic Arthritis

National Institute of Arthritis
1 AMS Circle
Bethesda, MD 20892
301-495-4484
877-226-4267
FAX: 301-881-2731
e-mail: niamsinfo@mail.nih.gov
www.nih.gov/niams/

7268 Raynaud's Phenomenon

Arthritis Foundation
PO Box 7669
Atlanta, GA 30357
404-872-7100
800-283-7800
FAX: 404-872-9559
e-mail: help@arthritis.org
www.arthritis.org

7269 Reaching, Crawling, Walking....Let's Get Moving

Blind Children's Center
4120 Marathon Street
Los Angeles, CA 90029
323-664-2153
800-222-3567
FAX: 323-665-3828
e-mail: info@blindchildrenscenter.org
www.blindchildrenscenter.org

Orientation and mobility for preschool children who are visually imapired. *$10.00*

24 pages

7270 Reading Is for Everyone

National Library Service for the Blind
1291 Taylor Street NW
Washington, DC 20542
202-707-5100
FAX: 202-707-0712
e-mail: nls@loc.gov
www.loc.gov/nls

7271 Reading with Low Vision

National Library Service for the Blind
1291 Taylor Street NW
Washington, DC 20542
202-707-5100
FAX: 202-707-0712
e-mail: nls@loc.gov
www.loc.gov/nls

7272 Reference and Information Services From NLS

National Library Service for the Blind
1291 Taylor Street NW
Washington, DC 20542
202-707-5100
FAX: 202-707-0712
TTY:202-707-0744
e-mail: nls@loc.gov
www.loc.gov/nls

7273 Referring Blind and Low Vision Patients for Rehabilitation Services

American Foundation for the Blind/AFB Press
PO Box 1020
Sewickley, PA 15143
412-741-1142
800-232-3044
FAX: 412-741-0609
e-mail: afborders@abdintl.com
www.afb.org

Clear information on such basic topics as the objectives of low vision services, what's covered in the examinations, what rehabilitation services do and how to locate these services. Available in purchase of bulk quantity only.

ISBN 0-891289-13-5

7274 Reiter's Syndrome

Arthritis Foundation
PO Box 7669
Atlanta, GA 30357
404-872-7100
800-283-7800
FAX: 404-872-9559
e-mail: help@arthritis.org
www.arthritis.org

7275 Resource List for Persons with Low Vision

American Council of the Blind
1155 15th Street NW
Suite 1004
Washington, DC 20005
202-467-5081
800-424-8666
FAX: 202-467-5085
e-mail: info@acb.org
www.acb.org

7276 Rheumatoid Arthritis

National Institute of Arthritis
1 AMS Circle
Bethesda, MD 20892
301-495-4484
877-226-4267
FAX: 301-881-2731
e-mail: niamsinfo@mail.nih.gov
www.nih.gov/niams/

Offers an introduction and definition of Rheumatoid Arthritis, treatments, causes, objectives, daily living, resources and medical information.

7277 School Based Assessment of Attention Deficit Disorders

National Clearinghouse of Rehabilitation Materials
5202 N Richmond Hill Drive
Stillwater, OK 74078
405-624-7650
800-223-5219
FAX: 405-624-0695

Presents an overview of current thoughts concerning ADD from an educational perspective, contrast traditional assessment strategies with an alternative model, and describe phases of evaluation.Paperback *$6.10*

61 pages

7278 Selecting a Program

Blind Children's Center
4120 Marathon Street
Los Angeles, CA 90029
323-664-2153
800-222-3567
FAX: 323-665-3828
e-mail: info@blindchildrenscenter.org
www.blindchildrenscenter.org

A guide for parents of infants and preschoolers with visual impairments. *$10.00*

28 pages

7279 Sex Education: Issues for the Person with Autism

Autism Society of North Carolina Bookstore
505 Oberlin Road
Suite 230
Raleigh, NC 27605
919-743-0204
800-442-2762
FAX: 919-743-0208
e-mail: dcoffey@autismsociety-nc.org
www.autismsociety-nc.org

Darla Coffey, Bookstore Manager

Discusses issues of sexuality and provides methods of instruction for people with autism. *$4.00*

7280 Spina Bifida

Spina Bifida Association of America
4590 MacArthur Boulevard NW
Suite 250
Washington, DC 20007
202-994-3285
800-621-3141
FAX: 202-944-3295
e-mail: sbaa@sbaa.org
www.sbaa.org

7281 Standards for the Diagnosis and Care of Patients with Asthma

American Lung Association
61 Broadway
New York, NY 10017
212-315-8700
FAX: 212-315-8700
e-mail: info@lungusa.org
www.lungusa.org

Standards developed by the American Thoracic Society, the medical section of the ALA. For physicians.

24 pages

7282 Standing On My Own Two Feet

Blind Children's Center
4120 Marathon Street
Los Angeles, CA 90029
323-664-2153
800-222-3567
FAX: 323-665-3828
e-mail: info@blindchildrenscenter.org
www.blindchildrenscenter.org

A step-by-step guide to designing and constructing simple, individually tailored adaptive mobility devices for preschool-age children who are visually impaired. *$10.00*

36 pages

7283 **Surgery: Information to Consider**

Arthritis Foundation
PO Box 7669
Atlanta, GA 30357 **404-872-7100**
800-283-7800
FAX: 404-872-9559
e-mail: help@arthritis.org
www.arthritis.org

7284 **Symptomatic Chiari Malformation**

Spina Bifida Association of America
4590 MacArthur Boulevard NW
Suite 250
Washington, DC 20007 **202-944-3285**
800-621-3141
FAX: 202-944-3295
e-mail: sbaa@sbaa.org
www.sbaa.org

7285 **Talk to Me**

Blind Children's Center
4120 Marathon Street
Los Angeles, CA 90029 **323-664-2153**
800-222-3567
FAX: 323-665-3828
e-mail: info@blindchildrenscenter.org
www.blindchildrenscenter.org

A language guide for parents of deaf children. *$10.00*

11 pages

7286 **Talk to Me II**

Blind Children's Center
4120 Marathon Street
Los Angeles, CA 90029 **323-664-2153**
800-222-3567
FAX: 323-665-3828
e-mail: info@blindchildrenscenter.org
www.blindchildrenscenter.org

A sequel to Talk To Me, available in English and Spanish. *$10.00*

15 pages

7287 **Teaching Social Skills to Youngsters with Disabilities**

Federation for Children with Special Needs
56 Temple Place
Suite 644
Boston, MA 02111 **617-542-7860**
800-537-0446
FAX: 617-542-7832
e-mail: pal@fcsn.org
www.ppal.net

Donna Welles, Director
Lisa Lambert, Assistant Director

Explains the importance of instruction and training to learn appropriate social behavior.

7288 **Teens Talk to Teens about Asthma**

Asthma and Allergy Foundation of America
1125 15th Street NW
Suite 502
Washington, DC 20005 **202-466-7643**
FAX: 202-466-8940
e-mail: info@aafa.org
www.aafa.org

Brochure provides support to a teen you care about. Includes quotes and thoughts from teens that captyure the essence of what it feels like to live with asthma.

7289 **Tethering Cord**

Spina Bifida Association of America
4590 MacArthur Boulevard NW
Suite 250
Washington, DC 20007 **202-944-3285**
800-621-3141
FAX: 202-944-3295
e-mail: sba@sbaa.org
www.sbaa.org

7290 **There are Solutions for the Student with Asthma**

American Lung Association
61 Broadway
New York, NY 10017 **212-315-8700**
FAX: 212-315-8700
e-mail: info@lungusa.org
www.lungusa.org

Leaflet telling how parents and school personnel can work together to make life easier for children with asthma.

4 pages

7291 **Thinking About Tomorrow: A Career Guide for Teens with Arthritis**

Arthritis Foundation
PO Box 7669
Atlanta, GA 30357 **404-872-7100**
800-283-7800
FAX: 404-872-9559
e-mail: help@arthritis.org
www.arthritis.org

7292 **Tips to Remember**

Academy of Allergy, Asthma, Immunology
611 E Wells Street
Milwaukee, WI 53202 **414-272-6071**
e-mail: info@aaaai.org
www.aaaai.org

A set of 23 tip sheets offering information on various topics including allergy and asthma treatments, pregnancy and asthma, animal allergies, sinusitis and more.

7293 **Transition in Adolescence**

Spina Bifida Association of America
4590 MacArthur Boulevard
Suite 250
Washington, DC 20007 **202-944-3285**
800-621-3141
FAX: 202-944-3295
e-mail: sbaa@sbaa.org
www.sbaa.org

7294 **Triggers Management of Asthma**

Academy of Allergy, Asthma, Immunology
611 E Wells Street
Milwaukee, WI 53202 **414-272-6071**
800-822-2762
FAX: 414-272-6070
e-mail: info@aaaai.org
www.aaaai.org

This brochure gives helpful information on what will cause an asthma attack. *$.50*

7295 **Understanding**

Easter Seals
230 W Monroe Street
Suite 1800
Chicago, IL 60606 **312-726-6200**
FAX: 312-726-1494

Janet D Jamieson, Communications Mgr.

A brochure series for use in patient, family and public education programs and in career recruitment and counseling.

10 Brochures

7296 Understanding Asthma

National Jewish Center for Immunology
1400 astackson Street
Denver, CO 80206 **303-388-4461**

e-mail: allstetterw@njc.org
www.njc.org

William Allstetter, Media Relations Manager

Offers a brief introduction to asthma and then goes into the physiology of asthma, the triggers of asthma, and diagnosis and monitoring of asthma.

27 pages

7297 Understanding Learning Disabilities: A Guide for Faculty

CACLD
25 Van Zant Street
Suite 15-5
E Norwalk, CT 06855 **203-838-5010**
FAX: 203-866-6108
e-mail: CACLD@optonline.net
www.CACLD.org

Beryl Kaufman, Executive Director

Written for the faculty at Georgetown to help them identify, understand, teach and advise students in their classes who have learning disabilities. Ideal for any college offering special services to the learning disabled as well as high school guidance counselors and propective college students with LD and their parents. Published by Connecticut Association for Children & Adults with Learning Disabilities (CACLD). *$10.00*

36 pages

7298 Urologic Care of the Child with Spina Bifida

Spina Bifida Association of America
4590 MacArthur Boulevard NW
Suite 250
Washington, DC 20007 **202-944-3285**
800-621-3141
FAX: 202-944-3295
e-mail: sbaa@sbaa.org
www.sbaa.org

7299 What Do You Do When You See a Blind Person - and What Don't You Do?

American Foundation for the Blind/AFB Press
PO Box 1020
Sewickley, PA 15143 **412-741-1142**
800-232-3044
FAX: 412-741-0609
e-mail: afborders@abdintl.com
www.afb.org

Examples of real-life situations that teach sighted persons how to interact effectively with blind persons. Topics covered include how to help someone across the street, how not to distract a guide dog and how to take leave of a blind person.

8 pages
ISBN 0-891281-95-9

7300 What Every Parent Should Know About Learning Diabilities

CACLD
25 Van Zant Street
Suite 15-5
E Norwalk, CT 06855 **203-838-5010**
FAX: 203-866-6108
e-mail: CACLD@optonline.net
www.CACLD.org

Beryl Kaufman, Executive Director

Published by Connecticut Association for Children & Adults with Learning Disabilities (CACLD). *$2.00*

7301 What Everyone Needs to Know About Asthma

National Allergy and Asthma Network
3554 Chain Bridge Road
Suite 200
Fairfax, VA 22030 **703-385-4403**
FAX: 703-352-4354

Offers information and facts on gaining control of asthma, asthma triggers and monitoring asthma disorders.

7302 What is Auditory Processing?

Speech Bin
1965 25th Avenue
Vero Beach, FL 32960 **772-770-0007**
800-477-3324
FAX: 772-770-0006
www.speechbin.com

Jan J Binney, Senior Editor

Booklet for parents and teachers explaining children's difficulties in listening and auditory skills. Set of ten copies. *$ 14.95*

16 pages
ISBN 0-93785 -45-9

7303 What to Do When a Friend is Depressed: Guide for Students

National Institute of Mental Health
5600 Fishers Lane
Government Printing Office
Rockville, MD 20857 **202-512-1800**

This pamphlet provides students with valuable information about depression: how to overcome it and how to help others.

7304 When Your Student Has Arthritis: A Guide for Teachers

Arthritis Foundation
PO Box 7669
Atlanta, GA 30357 **404-872-7100**
800-283-7800
FAX: 404-872-9559
e-mail: help@arthritis.org
www.arthritis.org

A medical information booklet written for teachers or other adults who have arthritis. The booklet describes different forms of juvenile arthritis, how arthritis might affect the child at school, and how to help the child work around these problems.

7305 Without Sight and Sound

Helen Keller National Center
111 Middle Neck Road
Sands Point, NY 11050 **516-944-8900**

e-mail: hkncdir@aol.com
www.helenkeller.org

Joseph McNulty, Executive Director

Pamphlet offering facts, causes, types and descriptions of deaf-blindness.

7306 Your Child and Asthma

National Jewish Center for Immunology
1400 Jackson Street
Denver, CO 80206 **303-388-4461**

e-mail: allstetterw@njc.org
www.njc.org

William Allstetter, Media Relations Manager

A booklet offerring information to parents and family about their child with asthma. Offers information on diagnosis, treatments, triggers and family concerns.

Audio/Visual

7307 A Place for Me

Educational Productions
9000 SW Gemini Drive
Beaverton, OR 97008
503-644-7000
800-950-4949
FAX: 503-350-7000
e-mail: custserve@edpro.com
www.edpro.com

Linda Freedman, President/Co-Owner
Molly Krumm, Marketing Director

In this video, parents discuss the issues they face in planning for their child's future. This program is designed to stimulate discussion of these issues and help increase awareness of the options available in your local community.

7308 ADD, Stepping Out of the Dark

ADD Videos
PO Box 622
New Paltz, NY 12561
845-255-3612
FAX: 845-883-6452

Lenae Madonna, Producer

A powerful, effective video, ideal for health professionals, educators and parents providing a visual montage designed to promote an understanding and awareness of attention deficit disorder. Based on actual accounts of those who have ADD, including a neurologist, an office worker, and parents of children with ADD. The video allows the viewer to feel the frustration and lack of attention that ADD brings to many. *$52.95*

Video

7309 ADHD in Adults

Guilford Press
72 Spring Street
New York, NY 10012
212-431-9800
800-365-7006
FAX: 212-966-6708
e-mail: info@guilford.com
www.guilford.com

This program integrates information on ADHD with the actual experiences of four adults who suffer from the disorder. Representing a range of professions, from a lawyer to a mother working at home, each candidly discusses the impact of ADHD on his or her daily life. These interviews are augmented by comments from family members and other clinicians who treat adults with ADHD. *$95.00*

Video
ISBN 0-898629-86-1

7310 ADHD: What Can We Do?

Guilford Press
72 Spring Street
New York, NY 10012
212-431-9800
800-365-7006
FAX: 212-966-6708
e-mail: info@guilford.com

A video program that introduces teachers and parents to a variety of the most effective technologies for managing ADHD in the classroom, at home, and on family outings. *$95.00*

Video
ISBN 0-898629-72-1

7311 ADHD: What Do We Know?

Guilford Press
72 Spring Street
New York, NY 10012
212-431-9800
800-365-7006
FAX: 212-966-6708
e-mail: info@guilford.com

An introduction for teachers and special education practitioners, school psychologists and parents of ADHD children. Topics outlined in this video include the causes and prevalence of ADHD, ways children with ADHD behave, other conditions that may accompany ADHD and long-term prospects for children with ADHD. *$95.00*

Video
ISBN 0-898629-71-3

7312 Able to Laugh

Fanlight Productions
4196 Washington Street
Suite 2
Boston, MA 02131
617-469-4999
800-937-4113
FAX: 617-469-3379
e-mail: fanlight@fanlight.com
www.fanlight.com

Sandy St Louis, Marketing Director
Kelli English, Publicity Coordinator

An exploration of the world of disability as interpreted by six professional comedians who happen to be disabled. It is also about the awkward ways disabled and able-bodied people relate to one another. *$ 195.00*

ISBN 1-572951-05-2

7313 Access for All: Integrating Deaf, Hard of Hearing and Hearing Preschoolers

Gallaudet University Bookstore
800 Florida Avenue NE
Washington, DC 20002
202-651-5000
800-451-1073
FAX: 202-651-5489

This exciting new 90 minute videotape and manual describes a model program for integrating deaf and hard of hearing children in early education. *$24.95*

150 pages

7314 Activity-Based Intervention: 2nd Edition

Brookes Publishing
PO Box 10624
Baltimore, MD 21285
410-337-9580
800-638-3775
FAX: 410-337-8539
e-mail: custserv@brookespublishing.com
www.brookespublishing.com

This 14 minute video illustrates how activity-based intervention can be used to turn everyday events and natural interactions into opportunities to promote learning in young children who are considered at risk for developmental delays or who have mild to significant disabilities. *$39.00*

ISBN 1-55766 -86-3

7315 All About Attention Deficit Disorders, Revised

Child Management
800 Roosevelt Road
B-309
Glen Ellyn, IL 60137
630-469-0484
FAX: 630-469-4571
www.thomasphelan.com

Nancy Roe, Office Manager

A psychologist and expert on ADD outlines the symptoms, diagnosis and treatment of this neurological disorder. Video ($49.95 - 2 parts) and audio cassette ($24.95).

7316 All of Us: Talking Together, Sex Education for People with Developmental Disabilities

Aquarius Health Care Videos
5 Powderhouse Lane
PO Box 1159
Sherborn, MA 01770 **508-651-2963**
888-440-2963
FAX: 508-650-4216
e-mail: aqvideos@tiac.net
www.aquariusproductions.com

Leslie Kussmann, President/Producer

For parents, caregivers and young people with developmental disabilities often feel isolated and unsure when approaching sex education with their children. In this video, parents of children with developmental disabilities share their difficulties in talking to their children about the social/sexual arena. Real life conversations between parents and their children demonstrate their discomfort, concerns, thoughts and hopes. *$195.00*

Video

7317 All the Way Up There

Britannica Film Company
345 4th Street
San Francisco, CA 94107 **415-777-9876**

This is the story of Bruce Burgess who has Cerebral Palsy but wants to climb a mountain. Bruce makes his dreams come true with the help of Grame Dingle, a New Zealand mountain climber.

Film

7318 Allergic Rhinitis

Academy of Allergy, Asthma, Immunology
611 E Wells Street
Milwaukee, WI 53202 **414-272-6071**
800-822-2762
FAX: 414-272-6070
e-mail: info@aaaai.org
www.aaaai.org

Allergic rhinitis, often called hay fever, affects the quality of life of millions of Americans. This video covers the causes and symptoms of seasonal and chronic allergic rhinitis, as well as controls and treatments. *$25.00*

10-13 Minutes

7319 Anaphylaxis

Academy of Allergy, Asthma, Immunology
611 E Wells Street
Milwaukee, WI 53202 **414-272-6071**
800-822-2762
FAX: 414-272-6070
e-mail: info@aaaai.org
www.aaaai.org

For a few people, allergic reactions can be extremely serios-even life-threatening. This video provides vital information on the symptoms, causes and treatment of those anaphylactic reactions, and how your allergist can help you take precautions to ensure your safety. *$25.00*

10-13 Minutes

7320 As I Am

Fanlight Productions
4196 Washington Street
Suite 2
Boston, MA 02131 **617-469-4999**
800-937-4113
FAX: 617-469-3379
e-mail: fanlight@fanlight.com
www.fanlight.com

Sandy St Louis, Marketing Director

Three young people with developmental disabilities speak for themselves about their lives, the problems they face and their hopes and expectations for the future. *$99.00*

ISBN 1-572950-58-7

7321 Asthma Handbook Slides

American Lung Association
61 Broadway
New York, NY 10017 **212-315-8700**
FAX: 212-315-8700
e-mail: info@lungusa.org
www.lungusa.org

Slides and script based on The Asthma Handbook for asthma patients and others.

Film

7322 Asthma Management

Academy of Allergy, Asthma, Immunology
611 E Wells Street
Milwaukee, WI 53202 **414-272-6071**
800-822-2762
FAX: 414-272-6070
e-mail: info@aaaai.org
www.aaaai.org

Although there is currently no cure for asthma, attacks can be controlled by appropriate asthma management. This video describes what happens during an asthma attack, how your allergists diagnoses asthma, and ways your allergist can help you to manage your condition. *$25.00*

10-13 Minutes

7323 Asthma Triggers

Academy of Allergy, Asthma, Immunology
611 E Wells Street
Milwaukee, WI 53202 **414-272-6071**
800-822-2762
FAX: 414-272-6070
e-mail: info@aaaai.org
www.aaaai.org

In the U.S. alone, over 50 million people suffer from asthma, and the incidence is rising. This video relates how patients with asthma can reduce their risk of an attack by avoiding triggers and practicing appropriate asthma management. *$25.00*

10-13 Minutes

7324 Asthma and the Athlete

Academy of Allergy, Asthma, Immunology
611 E Wells Street
Milwaukee, WI 53202 **414-272-6071**
800-822-2762
FAX: 414-272-6070
e-mail: info@aaaai.org
www.aaaai.org

In the past, people with asthma were sometimes discouraged from exercising. Today we know that everyone, including asthmatics, can benefit from physical actilvity. This video details which exercises are best for those with asthma, and how an allergist can help asthmatic athletes to properly manage and treat their disease. *$25.00*

10-13 Minutes

7325 **Attention Deficit Disorder**

Pro-Ed
8700 Shoal Creek Boulevard
Austin, TX 78757
512-451-3246
800-897-3202
FAX: 512-451-8542
e-mail: info@proedinc.com
www.proedinc.com

A book providing helpful suggestions for both home and classroom management of students with attention deficit disorder.

7326 **Attention Deficit Disorder: Adults**

Aquarius Health Care Videos
5 Powderhouse Lane
PO Box 1159
Sherborn, MA 01770
FAX: 508-650-4216
e-mail: aqvideos@tiac.net
www.aquariusproductions.com

Adults with ADD talk about how the disorder that went undiagnosed for so many years has affected their choice of spouses and work, and what they have found to help them. Biofeedback, which is growing as a treatment, is explained and demonstrated by its founder, Dr. Joel Lubar. Medical treatments like antidepressants and stimulants are also discussed, along with behavioral changes that can help the person with ADD and his or her spouse and family. *$149.00*

Video

7327 **Autism**

Aquarius Health Care Videos
5 Powderhouse Lane
PO Box 1159
Sherborn, MA 01770
FAX: 508-650-4216
e-mail: aqvideos@tiac.net
www.aquariusproductions.com

This video takes you into the lives of autistic people and their families to understand more about autism. What defines autism and how can we help those living with the disability? Children, teens, and adults are also profiled and we begin to see the varying levels of development and new technology to help these people communicate. Preview Available. *$149.00*

Video

7328 **Autism: A World Apart**

Fanlight Productions
4196 Washington Street
Suite 2
Boston, MA 02131
617-469-4999
800-937-4113
FAX: 617-469-3379
e-mail: fanlight@fanlight.com
www.fanlight.com

Karen McMillen, Marketing Director

Autism's cause is unknown. There is no cure, and it strikes each victim differently. In this documentary, three families show us what the textbooks and studies cannot - what it is like to live with autism day after day - to love and raise children who may be withdrawn and violent, and unable to make personal connections with their families. *$195.00*

7329 **Awareness Training**

Landmark Media
3450 Slade Run Drive
Falls Church, VA 22042
703-241-2030
800-342-4336
FAX: 703-536-9540
e-mail: landmarkmed@aol.com
www.landmarkmedia.com

ML Hartogs

Covers disabilities of various types — vision, hearing, speech disorders, loss of limbs, loss of mobility, or mental/emotional limitations and how to integrate such individuals into various business and educational settings. It is a 4-part series designed to identify and enable others to interact effectively with those suffering such disabilities. *$495.00*

Set of 4

7330 **Basic Course in American Sign Language**

Harris Communications
15155 Technology Drive
Eden Prairie, MN 55344
952-906-1180
800-825-6758
FAX: 952-906-1099
e-mail: mail@harriscomm.com
www.harriscomm.com

Bill Williams, National Sales Manager

This series of four one-hour tapes is designed to illustrate the various exercises and dialogues in the text. *$39.95*

Video

7331 **Beginning ASL Video Course**

Harris Communications
15155 Technology Drive
Eden Prairie, MN 55344
952-906-1180
800-825-6758
FAX: 952-906-1099
e-mail: mail@harriscomm.com
www.harriscomm.com

Bill Williams, National Sales Manager

You'll watch a family teach you to learn American Sign Language during funny and touching family situations. A total of 15 tapes in the course. *$49.95*

Video

7332 **Beginning Reading and Sign Language**

Harris Communications
15155 Technology Drive
Eden Prairie, MN 55344
952-906-1180
800-825-6758
FAX: 952-906-1099
e-mail: mail@harriscomm.com
www.harriscomm.com

Bill Williams, National Sales Manager

Features a deaf performer signing more than 120 words while standing in front of the object she is signing. Appropriate for children eighteen months to eight years. *$21.95*

Video

7333 **Beyond the Barriers**

Aquarius Health Care Videos
5 Powderhouse Lane
PO Box 1159
Sherborn, MA 01770
508-651-2963
888-440-2963
FAX: 508-650-4216
e-mail: aqvideos@tiac.net
www.aquariusproductions.com

Leslie Kussmann, Presdient

For too many years, paraplegics, amputees, quadraplegics and the blind have felt trapped by their disabilities. No more! Mark Wellman and other disabled adventurers, rock climb the deser towers of Utah, sail in British Columbia, body-board the big waves of Pipeline and Waimea Bay, scuba dive with sea lions in Mexico and hand glide the California coast. This film delivers the simple message: Don't give up, and never give in. If you can't ever lose, then you can't ever win. Preview option. *$90.00*

Video

7334 **Biology Concepts Through Discovery**

Educational Activities Software
PO Box 754
Baldwin, NY 11510
516-867-7878
800-645-2796
FAX: 516-379-7429
e-mail: achieve@ea-software.com

Alan Stern, Sales

These videos, available in English and Spanish versions, encourage learning by presenting interactive problem solving in an effective VISUAL/AUDITORY style. *$89.00*

Video

7335 **Blindness**

Landmark Media
3450 Slade Run Drive
Falls Church, VA 22042
703-241-2030
800-342-4336
FAX: 703-536-9540

ML Hartogs

Cataracts are the most common cause of blindness in the 42 million people worldwide defined as blind. 90% live in developing countries. Cataracts are the most common cause but now can be treated cheaply and safely. *$250.00*

Video

7336 **Braille Documents**

Metrolina Association for the Blind
704 Louise Avenue
Charlotte, NC 28204
704-372-3870
800-926-5460
FAX: 704-372-3872

This production shop creates Braille and large-print documents.

7337 **Breakthroughs: How to Reach Students with Autism**

Aquarius Health Care Videos
5 Powderhouse Lane
PO Box 1159
Sherborn, MA 01770
508-651-2963
FAX: 508-650-4216
e-mail: aqvideos@tiac.net
www.aquariusproductions.com

A hands-on, how-to program for reaching students with autism, featuring Karen Sewell, Autism Society of America's teacher of the year. Here Sewell demonstrates the successful techniques she's developed over a 20-year career. A separate 250 page manual ($59) is also available which covers math, reading, fine motor, self help, social adaptive, vocational and self help skills as well as providing numerous plan reproducibles and an exhaustive listing of equipment and materials resources. Video. *$99.00*

7338 **Breathe Easy Young People's Guide to Asthma**

Magination Press
2751 Prosperity Avenue
Suite 150
Fairfax, VA 22031
703-385-4403
800-878-4403
FAX: 703-573-7794
www.aanma.org

Practical, personal guide for those up to age 13 with asthma. They will learn how to control their asthma with techniques that will bring increased self-confidence. *$9.95*

Video

7339 **Breathing Lessons: The Life and Work of Mark O'Brien**

Fanlight Productions
4196 Washington Street
Suite 2
Boston, MA 02131
617-469-4999
800-937-4113
FAX: 617-469-3379
e-mail: fanlight@fanlight.com
www.fanlight.com

A new documentary which focuses on poet-journalist Mark O'Brien. Crippled by polio in childhood, and later forced to rely on an iron lung as a result of post-polio syndrome, for more than forty years he has fought against illness and bureaucracy in his determination to lead an independent life. According to Mark O'Brien, the two mythologies of disabled people break down to one: we can't do anything or two; we can do everything. But the truth is we're just human. *$195.00*

35 Minutes

7340 **Bridging the Gap: A National Directory of Services for Women & Girls with Disabilities**

Educational Equity Concepts
114 E 32nd Street
New York, NY 10016
212-686-2531
FAX: 212-725-0947
TTY:212-725-1803
e-mail: infomration@edequity.org
www.edequity.org

Ellen Rubin, Coordinator, Disability Programs
Merle Froschl, Editor

Contains a resource section of publications and videos geared specifically to women and girls with disabilities. Available in print, on cassette, and also in braille. *$24.95*

ISBN 0-931629-16-0

7341 **Bringing Out the Best**

Research Press
PO Box 9177
Champaign, IL 61826
217-352-3273
800-519-2707
FAX: 217-352-1221
e-mail: rp@researchpress.com
www.researchpress.com

Russell Pence, VP Marketing

This video training program introduces teachers, staff and parents to a variety of techniques for teaching expressive communication skills to children with multiple handicaps. The video illustrates how to assess a child's current levels of expressive ability, build on that ability, then gradually work toward more advanced communication. It shows how to use everyday situations to help children move beyond passive understanding to more active, intentional communication. *$150.00*

Video

7342 **Business Enterprise Service: Marketing the Randolph-Sheppard Program**

Mississippi State University
PO Box 6189
Mississippi State, MS 39762
662-325-2001
800-675-7782
FAX: 662-325-8989
www.blind.msstate.edu

Kelly Schaefer, Publications Manager

This 10-minute videotape and Marketing Information Kit are for use by State Licensing Agencies throughout the country. They are designed for use in promoting the BEP with building managers, plant managers, building superintendents and others who might be interested in utilizing the services provided under the Randolph-Sheppard Act. *$ 30.00*

7343 **Business as Usual**

Fanlight Productions
4196 Washington Street
Suite 2
Boston, MA 02131
617-469-4999
800-917-4113
FAX: 617-469-3379
e-mail: fanlight@fanlight.com
www.fanlight.com

Karen McMillen, Marketing Director

An enlightening new documentary, brings a unique international perspective to this struggle. This film examines five innovative programs which create opportunities for people with mental and physical disabilities to own and operate their own businesses. *$145.00*

7344 **Buying Time: The Media Role in Health Care**

Fanlight Productions
4196 Washington Street
Suite 2
Boston, MA 02131
617-469-4999
800-937-4113
FAX: 617-469-3379
e-mail: fanlight@fanlight.com
www.fanlight.com

Karen McMillen, Marketing Director

This video program is a thoughtful and disturbing examination in the role of the media in determining the allocation of health care resources. This program is a powerful tool on ethics, policy, journalism, sociology, medicine and nursing as well as for professional workshops, and continuing education programs. *$99.00*

7345 **Caring for People with Developmental Disabilities**

Research Press
PO Box 9177
Champaign, IL 61826
217-352-3273
FAX: 217-352-1221
e-mail: rp@researchpress.com
www.researchpress.com

Russell Pence, VP Marketing

Respite care is emerging as one of the most frequently requested and rapidly growing services offered to parents of children and young adults with developmental disabilities. Agencies are continually pressed to meet the demand for trained care providers. This video series has been developed to address this critical need. *$495.00*

Video

7346 **Caring for Persons with Developmental Disabilities**

Research Press
2612 N Mattis Avenue
Champaign, IL 61821
217-352-3273
800-519-2707
FAX: 217-352-1221
e-mail: rp@researchpress.com
www.researchpress.com

Russell Pence, VP Marketing

A competency-baced video traning program that teaches the skills needed to care for individuals with a wide range of psysical and mental disabilities. Consists of six videotapes that feature demonstrations of respite care procedures. Provides quizzes in which viewers are asked to respond to on-screen situations. *$495.00*

Video

7347 **Center for Health Research: Eastern Washin gton University**

Showalter 209A
Cheney, WA 99004
509-359-2279
800-221-9369
FAX: 509-359-2778
e-mail: sharon.wilson@mail.ewu.edu
iceberg.ewu.edu

Produces eight videotapes, accompanying printed materials, and a videotaped public services announcement to serve as training and resource materials for use by daycare centers.

7348 **Challenge**

Spina Bifida Association of America
4590 Macarthur Boulevard NW
Suite 250
Washington, DC 20007
202-944-3285
800-621-3141
FAX: 202-944-3295
e-mail: sbaa@sbaa.org
www.sbaa.org

Fourteen minute video tape. An excellent introduction to the physical and social challenges faced by individuals with spina bifida. *$20.00*

7349 **Children's Classics Videotape Sets**

Gallaudet University Bookstore
11030 S Langley Avenue
Chicago, IL 60628
202-651-5488
800-621-2736
FAX: 202-651-5489

Tells fairytales from the Grimm Brothers and Hans Christian Anderson in American Sign Language. Includes The Little Mermaid, Emperor's New Clothes, Fisherman & His Wife, Hansel and Gretal and The Musician's of Bromon. *$29.95*

7350 **Christmas Stories**

Gallaudet University Bookstore
11030 S Langley Avenue
Chicago, IL 60628
202-651-5488
800-621-2736
FAX: 202-651-5489

The unique talents of Bobby Giles and Doris Wilding present these great stories in American Sign Language. *$29.95*

Video

7351 **Clinicians View**

6007 Osuna Road NE
Albuquerque, NM 87109
505-880-0058
FAX: 505-880-0059

Gary J Magrun, President
W Michael Magrun, VP

A video and book publishing catalog dedicated to bringing clinicians (PTs; OTs; SLPs) and parents of children with special needs, the best educational and instructional information available. Paperback and videocassette.

7352 **Clockworks**

Learning Corporation of America
6493 Kaiser Drive
Fremont, CA 94555
510-490-7311

Scotty, who has Down Syndrome, is fascinated by clocks. This film follows him on his adventures of employment in the clock shop.

Film

7353 **Close Encounters of the Disabling Kind**

Mainstream
6930 Carroll Avenue
Suite 204
Takoma Park, MD 20912
301-891-8777
FAX: 301-891-8778
e-mail: info@mainstreaminc.org
www.mainstreaminc.org

Lillie Harrison, Information Programs Clerk
Fritz Rumpel, Editor

A training video that provides a hiring manager with information on how to learn the basics of disability etiquette and, by the end of the video, seems much better prepared and willing to interview qualified individuals with disabilities. Includes trainer and trainee guides. *$99.95*

Video

7354 **Come Back Jack: The Revealing Story of a Child Diagnosed with Autism**

Aquarius Health Care Videos
5 Powderhouse Lane
PO Box 1159
Sherborn, MA 01770
508-651-2963
FAX: 508-650-4216
e-mail: aqvideos@tiac.net
www.aquariusproductions.com

Persistent ear infections, medically misguided over-treatment with antibiotics, and other mysterious physiological factors sent Jack's mind spinning. By the time Jack reached the age of two, his intellectual and emothional development had come to a schreeching halt. Terrified by the prospect of losing their youngest son, Jack's parents began searching for answers. Chronicles the ups and downs. *$ 99.00*

7355 **Concentration Video**

Learning disAbilities Resources
PO Box 716
Bryn Mawr, PA 19010
610-525-8336
800-869-8336
FAX: 610-525-8337

An instructional video which provides a perspective about attention problems, possible causes and solutions. *$19.95*

Video

7356 **Dancing from the Inside Out**

Fanlight Productions
4196 Washington Street
Suite 2
Boston, MA 02131
617-469-4999
800-937-4113
FAX: 617-469-3379
e-mail: fanlight@fanlight.com
www.fanlight.com

Karen McMillen, Marketing Director

This eloquent new video looks at the lives and work of three talented dancers who dance professionally with the acclaimed AXIS Dance Troupe, which includes both disabled and non-disabled dancers. They discuss the process they went through in adapting to their disability and how they came to re-discover physical expression through dance. *$ 195.00*

7357 **Deaf Children Signers**

Harris Communications
15155 Technology Drive
Eden Prairie, MN 55344
952-906-1180
800-825-6758
FAX: 952-906-1099
e-mail: mail@harriscomm.com
www.harriscomm.com

Bill Williams, National Sales Manager

This three-part collection of children signers is great for children, teachers, parents and interpreters. *$39.95*

Video

7358 **Deaf Culture Series**

Harris Communications
15155 Technology Drive
Eden Prairie, MN 55344
952-906-1180
800-825-6758
FAX: 952-906-1099
e-mail: mail@harriscomm.com
www.harriscomm.com

Bill Williams, National Sales Manager

Each video in this five-part series features a topic dealing with the unique culture of deaf people. It is an excellent resource for deaf studies programs, Interpreter Preparation programs and Sign Language programs. *$59.95*

Video

7359 **Deaf Mosaic Series**

Harris Communications
15155 Technology Drive
Eden Prairie, MN 55344
952-906-1180
800-825-6758
FAX: 952-906-1099
e-mail: mail@harriscomm.com
www.harriscomm.com

Bill Williams, National Sales Manager

A national magazine show produced monthly by Gallaudet University, this show has been awarded nine Emmys. As the only nation-wide program about the deaf community, these videotapes are the best of the best from the shows programs. *$29.95*

Video

7360 **Descriptive Video Service**

WGBH Educational Foundation
125 Western Avenue
Boston, MA 02134
617-492-2777
800-333-1203
FAX: 617-300-1011
e-mail: ncam@wgbh.org
www.wgbh.org

Sharon King, Outreach Director
Mary Ann Pack, Assistant Director

A national service that makes PBS television programs, Hollywood movies on video and other visual media accessible to people who are blind or visually impaired. DVS provides narrated descriptions of the key visual elements without interfering with the audio or dialogue of a program or movie. The narration describes visual elements such as actions, settings, body language and graphics.

7361 **Different Heart**

Fanlight Productions
4196 Washington Street
Suite 2
Boston, MA 02131
617-469-4999
800-937-4113
FAX: 617-469-3379
e-mail: fanlight@fanlight.com

Karen McMillen, Marketing Director

Though hundreds of children are born each year with potentially fatal heart disease, their parents may feel isolated from those facing similar crises. This sensitive video profiles three such families. *$99.00*

7362 Do You Hear That?

Alexander Graham Bell Association
3417 Volta Place NW
Washington, DC 20007
202-337-5220
FAX: 202-337-8314
e-mail: info@agbell.org
www.agbell.org

This video shows auditory-verbal therapy sessions of a therapist working individually with 11 children who range in age from 7 months to 7 years old and have hearing aids or cochlear implants.

Video

7363 Doing Things Together

Britannica Film Company
345 4th Street
San Francisco, CA 94107
415-777-9876

Steve went with his parents to an amusement park. He met another boy named Martin who at first was shocked by Steve's prosthetic hand.

Film

7364 Down Syndrome

Aquarius Health Care Videos
5 Powderhouse Lane
PO Box 1159
Sherborn, MA 01770
FAX: 508-650-4216
e-mail: aqvideos@tiac.net
www.aquariusproductions.com

This is an excellent video for families who have just had a baby with Down Syndrome as well as professionals in the field of genetics and nursing. Through honest and open discussion, parents of children with Down Syndrome express the feelings and concerns they had during the early years of their child's life. Preview option available. *$150.00*

Video

7365 Dream Catchers

University of New Hampshire: Inst on Disability
7 Leavitt Lane
Suite 101
Durham, NC 03824
603-862-4320
FAX: 603-862-0555
e-mail: institutedisability@unh.edu
www.iod.unh.edu

Jan Nisbet, Director

This video tells the stories of three young people with disabilities, and how they each pulled together a network of people called the circle of support.

7366 Educating Inattentive Children

Western Psychological Services
12031 Wilshire Boulevard
Los Angeles, CA 90025
800-648-8857
FAX: 310-478-7838

An excellent resources for teachers who encounter inattention and hyperactivity in the classroom. It helps teachers distinguish deliberate misbehavior from the incompetent, nonpurposeful behavior of the inattentive child. *$120.00*

Video

7367 Effective Behavioral Programming

Research Press
PO Box 9177
Champaign, IL 61826
217-352-3273
800-519-2707
FAX: 217-352-1221
e-mail: rp@researchpress.com
www.researchpress.com

Russell Pence, VP Marketing

A comprehensive video-based training program for educators and residential staff who work with people with developmental disabilities. It is presented in clear, nontechnical language and does not require an extensive background in the use of behavioral procedures. The program includes eight instructional videotapes, a leader's guide and a set of five participant's manuals. It is suitable for group training or individual study and has no rigid time line. *$895.00*

Video

7368 Effective Intervention for Self-Feeding Success

Exceptional Parent Library
120 Sylvan Avenue, Suite 10
PO Box 1807
Englewood Cliffs, NJ 07632
800-535-1910
FAX: 201-947-9376
e-mail: eplibrary@aol.com
www.eplibrary.com

An effective and easy to follow video program for parents, which provides the tools needed to be successful in moving your child toward independent self-feeding. *$39.95*

7369 Einstein and Me: Talking About Learning Disabilities

Fanlight Productions
4196 Washington Street
Suite 2
Boston, MA 02131
617-469-4999
800-937-4113
FAX: 617-469-3379
e-mail: fanlight@fanlight.com
www.fanlight.com

Karen McMillen, Marketing Director

In this straightforward and engaging video, panels of teens and younger students speak candidly with Schultz, a Clinical Psychologist, about how they found out about their learning disabilities, the policies and people who have made life difficult, the programs which have helped them cope, their strengths and talents, and their futures. *$99.00*

7370 Emerging Leaders

Mobility International USA
PO Box 10767
Eugene, OR 97440
541-343-1284
FAX: 541-343-6812
e-mail: info@miusa.org
www.miusa.org

Susan Sygall, Executive Director
Pamela Houston, Public Relations Coordinator
Tracy Scharn, Project Assistant

Looks at the emergence of people with disabilities as leaders in the world community this video discusses the value of internation exchange programs in fostering leadership skills. Available in English, Spanish and Russian. *$49.00*

Video

7371 **Emotional Intelligence, Lessons in Conflict and Anger**

Aquarius Health Care Videos
5 Powderhouse Lane
PO Box 1159
Sherborn, MA 01770
508-651-2963
FAX: 508-650-4216
e-mail: aqvideos@tiac.net
www.aquariusproductions.com

Up until recently, most of us expected to learn those kinds of skills, like listening, sharing, being kind, at home, and not find them in any organized class at school. Buth that is changing because of reserach shoing that school age children stay healthier, and learn better, when they know how to handle the ups and downs of growing up. this video profiles classes and programs in the New Have, Conneticut school system and in Highland Park, New Jersey. — Videocassette. *$149.00*

7372 **Endurance & Body Sculpting Exercise Programs**

Seat-A-Robics
PO Box 1253
Jamestown, NC 27282
FAX: 336-454-4615
e-mail: seatarobics@hotmail.com
www.homelife.com/products/1093.asp

Clarice Burns, President

Safe, affordable and medically approved exercise videos developed by a health advisory board in conjunction with a licensed aerobics instructor and paraplegic. These videos are aimed at persons with temporary injuries, permanent disabilities, health professionals and educators. Both programs are available on one tape. *$36.95*

56 Minutes

7373 **Environmental Control Measures**

Academy of Allergy, Asthma, Immunology
611 E Wells Street
Milwaukee, WI 53202
414-272-6071
800-822-2762
FAX: 414-272-6070
e-mail: info@aaaai.org
www.aaaai.org

By conrtolling your environment, you can reduce your exposure to substances called allergens that trigger your allergic symptoms. This program depicts common outdoor and indoor allergens, methods an allergist uses to diagnose which substances you're allergic to, and how to reduce your exposure to allergic triggers. *$25.00*

10-13 Minutes

7374 **Explore the Bible: Adult Audiocassette**

LifeWay Christian Resources Southern Baptist Conv.
127 9th Avenue N
Nashville, TN 37234
615-251-2000
800-458-2772
FAX: 651-251-5764
e-mail: specialed@lifeway.com
www.lifeway.com

Ben Garner, Editor

Full-length recorded bible study lessons as printed in Explore the Bible: Adults. *$12.00*

Quarterly

7375 **Face First**

Fanlight Productions
4196 Washington Street
Suite 2
Boston, MA 02131
617-469-4999
800-937-4113
FAX: 617-469-3379
e-mail: fanlight@fanlight.com
www.fanlight.com

Karen McMillen, Marketing Director
Cynthia Conti, Publicity Coordinator
Mike Grundmann, Producer

In this documentary, the stories told reflect the reality faced by all those who are seen as different. Despite their difficult experiences, the survival of the profiled individuals affords comic relief &, by adulthood, they possess unusual strengths that shape their careers in pediatrics, disability care, public speaking, and journalism. *$ 195.00*

7376 **Fairy Tales & Christmas Stories**

Harris Communications
15155 Technology Drive
Eden Prairie, MN 55344
952-906-1180
800-825-6758
FAX: 952-906-1099
e-mail: mail@harriscomm.com
www.harriscomm.com

Bill Williams, National Sales Manager

A collection of videotapes featuring classic fairytales and Christmas stories signed by deaf storytellers. *$29.95*

Video

7377 **Family Challenges: Parenting with a Disability**

Aquarius Health Care Videos
5 Powderhouse Lane
PO Box 1159
Sherborn, MA 01770
508-651-2963
888-440-2963
FAX: 508-650-4216
e-mail: aqvideos@tiac.net
www.aquariusproductions.com

Leslie Kussmann, President/Producer

When a parent has a disability, everyone in the family is affected. For children, these experiences may profoundly influence their lives and views of the world. In this sensitive film, you will hear about different roles that all the family members take on at varying times. *$195.00*

7378 **Family-Guided Activity-Based Intervention for Toddlers & Infants**

Brookes Publishing
PO Box 10624
Baltimore, MD 21285
410-337-9580
800-638-3775
FAX: 410-337-8539
e-mail: custserv@brookespublishing.com
www.brookespublishing.com

Early childhood professionals will be able to teach parents and other caregivers how to use daily routines and activities to help young children with special needs gain vital skills. Included on the video are activity-based teaching methods that enhance children's development, accommodate families' daily schedules, address children's IFSP goals, and promote family interactions. *$37.00*

20 Minutes

ISBN 1-55766 -19-3

7379 **Fanlight Productions**

4196 Washington Street
Suite 2
Boston, MA 02131
617-469-4999
800-937-4113
FAX: 617-469-3379
e-mail: fanlight@fanlight.com
www.fanlight.com

Sandy St Louis, Marketing Director

Distributor of videos on a wide array of health-related topics. *$195.00*

Video

7380 **Fantastic Series**

Harris Communications
15155 Technology Drive
Eden Prairie, MN 55344
952-906-1180
800-825-6758
FAX: 952-906-1099
e-mail: mail@harriscomm.com
www.harriscomm.com

Bill Williams, National Sales Manager

These videotapes offer a blend of entertainment and information to both deaf and hearing children ages 6-10. A total of eight tapes in the series. *$29.95*

7381 **Fibromyalgia Interval Training**

Arthritis Foundation Distribution Center
PO Box 6996
Alpharetta, GA 30009
800-207-8633
FAX: 770-442-9742
www.arthritis.com

This video was designed for people with fibromyalgia. The video features warm water exercises in shallow and deep water, including warmup, stretching, upper and lower body exercises, aerobics, strengthing, cool-down and relaxation. Designed to help you manage the pain, stiffness and fatigue of fibromyalgia. *$29.99*

7382 **Filmakers Library**

124 E 40th Street
New York, NY 10016
212-808-4980
FAX: 212-808-4983
e-mail: info@filmakers.com
www.filmakers.com

Sue Oscar, Co-President

A distributor of educational, award-winning videotapes and films on issues relating to disabilities for educators, counsellors and organizations. The films and tapes are available for rental or sale to institutions, schools, hospitals and organizations. Among the topics covered in the videotapes are autism, schizophrenia, and physical disabilties.

$100 - $300

7383 **Films & Videos on Aging and Sensory Change**

Lighthouse International
111 E 59 Street
New York, NY 10022
212-821-9737
800-829-0500
FAX: 212-821-9706
e-mail: info@lighthouse.org

Joanna Mellor, VP Information Services

An annotated list of over 80 films and videos dealing with age-related sensory change, divided into sections on vision impairment, hearing impairment, and multiple sensory impairments. *$5.00*

7384 **Fingerspelling: Expressive and Receptive Fluency**

Gallaudet University Bookstore
11030 S Langley Avenue
Chicago, IL 60628
202-651-5488
800-621-2736
FAX: 202-651-5489

Improve your fingerspelling with this new video guide. A 24-page instructional booklet is included with fingerspelling practice suggestions. *$39.95*

120 Minutes

7385 **Foundation Fundamentals for Nonprofit Organizations**

Foundation Center
79 Fifth Avenue
Department ZE
New York, NY 10003
212-421-0771
800-424-9836
FAX: 212-807-3677
www.fdncenter.org

Thomas Buckman, President

This video is designed to give fundraisers a general overview of the foundation funding process and to introduce them to the many resources available through our libraries and cooperating collections. The video gives clear, step-by-step instructions on how to build a fundraising program. *$24.00*

Video

7386 **Foundations: The People and the Money**

Foundation Center
79 Fifth Avenue
Department ZE
New York, NY 10003
212-421-0771
800-424-9836
FAX: 212-807-3677
www.fdncenter.org

Thomas Buckman, President

This award-winning documentary film, introduced by Robert MacNeil, provides a fascinating introduction to the world of American philanthropic foundations. Through interviews with both grant-makers and grantees, this book offers a vivid and human perspective on the work of foundations today. *$5.00*

Video

7387 **Fred's Story**

Aquarius Health Care Videos
5 Powderhouse Lane
PO Box 1159
Sherborn, MA 01770
FAX: 508-650-4216
e-mail: aqvideos@tiac.net
www.aquariusproductions.com

Fred tells about the 40 years he spent inside Mansfield Training School, a Connecticut institution closed in 1990 by the Department of Mental Retardation. The film cuts between Fred's telling of the reality of the institution and black-and-white newsreel footage of state officials describing their visions of and goals for the institution in which Fred lived. Fred's indomitable, lyrical spirit shines throughout. Golden Chris Award, Columbus International Film Festival. Preview option available. *$90.00*

Video

7388 **Free to Breathe**

Allergy and Asthma Network/Mothers of Asthmatics
2751 Prosperity Avenue
Suite 150
Fairfax, VA 22031
800-878-4403
FAX: 703-573-7794
www.aanma.org

Characters rap, joke, and learn different ways to use inhalers. Kids are encouraged to talk to their parents and doctor about their choices. 8 minutes. *$10.00*

Video

7389 **Freedom to Create**

National Institute of Art and Disabilities
551 23rd Street
Richmond, CA 94804
510-620-0290
FAX: 510-620-0326
e-mail: reddot@niadart.org
www.niadart.org

Elias Katz, Author

Presents philosophy and practical experiences enabling teachers to stimulate creativity in the visual arts for students with and without disabilities. Videotape. *$35.00*

7390 **From Mime to Sign Package**

TJ Publishers
817 Silver Spring Avenue
Suite 206
Silver Spring, MD 20910
301-585-4440
800-999-1168
FAX: 301-585-5930
e-mail: TJPubinc@aol.com

Angela K Thames, President
Jerald A Murphy, VP

As a drama professor, television personality, performer and storyteller, multiple Emmy winner Gil Eastman has developed a unique presentation style. Now, he shares his expressive communication approach in a highly illustrated American Sign Language text and videotape series. A text and three videotapes. *$139.95*

183 pages

7391 **Fundamentals of Reading Success**

Educators Publishing Service
31 Smith Place
Cambridge, MA 02138
617-367-2700
800-225-5750
FAX: 617-547-0412
www.epsbooks.com

This video series is designed to help teachers learn a phonics or code-emphasis approach to teaching reading, spelling and handwriting. There is one set for teaching children and one for teaching adults. *$480.00*

Complete Set
ISBN 0-838872-52-2

7392 **Getting Started with Facilitated Communication**

Syracuse University, Institute on Communication
805 S Krouse
Syracuse, NY 13244
315-443-2693

Describes in detail how to help individuals with autism and/or severe communication difficulties to get started with facilitated communication.

Video

7393 **Getting Together: A Head Start/School District Collaboration**

Brookes Publishing
PO Box 10624
Baltimore, MD 21285
410-337-9580
800-638-3775
FAX: 410-337-8539
e-mail: custserv@brookespublishing.com
www.brookespublishing.com

This video describes how to include children with disabilities in the Head Start classrooms. Addresses such issues as leadership, staff support, and policy development. Comes with a 24-page saddle-stitched booklet. *$34.95*

25 Minutes
ISBN 1-55766 -97-5

7394 **Getting in Touch**

Research Press
PO Box 9177
Champaign, IL 61826
217-352-3273
800-519-2707
FAX: 217-352-1221
e-mail: rp@researchpress.com
www.researchpress.com

Russell Pence, VP Marketing

When communicating with a child who is deaf/blind, there are certain basic procedures that can be used to help the child understand. This video introduces these procedures to teachers, staff, parents and others who work with children who have sensory impairments. The video demonstrates techniques that involve the use of two types of tactile cues - Touch Cues (signals made by actually touching the child) and Object Cues (signals made by presenting an object to the child). *$150.00*

19 Minutes

7395 **Going to School with Facilitated Communication**

Syracuse University, School of Education
Educational Resource Center
230 Huntington Hall
Syracuse, NY 13244
315-443-4751

A video in which students with autism and/or severe disabilities illustrate the use of facilitated communication focusing on basic principles fostering facilitated communication.

Video

7396 **Good Weather or Not**

Nat'l Council of Community Mental Health Center
12300 Twinbrook Parkway
Suite 320
Rockville, MD 20852

One of the few resources of its kind, this set will help clinicians present material about parents' mental illness that is generated to young children's levels of thinking. *$290.00*

7397 **Granny Good's Signs of Christmas**

Gallaudet University Bookstore
11030 S Langley Avenue
Chicago, IL 60628
202-651-5488
800-621-2736
FAX: 202-651-5489

Come join the folks at Granny's cottage where Hans Signer, from the silent forest, interprets his favorite story, Twas The Night Before Christmas. *$29.95*

Video

7398 **Harry**

Research Press
PO Box 9177
Champaign, IL 61826
217-352-3273
800-519-2707
FAX: 217-352-1221
e-mail: rp@researchpress.com
www.researchpress.com

Russell Pence, VP Marketing

Harry is one of the most unforgettable documentaries ever produced. It is honest, dramatic, touching and REAL. None of the scenes were staged, actual treatment sessions, conducted by Dr. Richard M. Foxx, were videotaped through a one-way mirror. Harry is the subject of the remarkably successful treatment program. At the time of this taping he was 24 years old and had spent most of his life in institutions wearing various types of physical restraints. 38 minutes. $495.00.

Video

7399 **Hear to Listen & Learn: A Language Approach for Children with Ear Infections**

Brookes Publishing
PO Box 10624
Baltimore, MD 21285
410-337-9580
800-638-3775
FAX: 410-337-8539
e-mail: custserv@brookespublishing.com
www.brookespublishing.com

This video describes the behavioral characteristics that signal when middle ear fluid is causing problems for a child. Also provides professionals with ideas for modifying classrooms and incorporating teaching practices that promote learning opportunities and language acquisition for children with middle ear fluid and associated hearing loss. *$42.00*

20-min VHS
ISBN 1-55766-99-5

7400 **Heart to Heart**

Blind Children's Center
4120 Marathon Street
Los Angeles, CA 90029
323-664-2153
800-222-3567
FAX: 323-665-3828
e-mail: info@blindchildrenscenter.org
www.blindchildrenscenter.org

Parents of blind and partially sighted children talk about their feelings. *$35.00*

Video

7401 **Heart to Heart Video**

Blind Children's Center
4120 Marathon Street
Los Angeles, CA 90029
323-664-2153
800-222-3567
FAX: 323-665-3828
e-mail: info@blindchildrenscenter.org
www.blindchildrenscenter.org

$35.00

7402 **Helping Hands**

Fanlight Productions
4196 Washington Street
Suite 2
Boston, MA 02131
617-469-4999
800-937-4113
FAX: 617-469-3379
e-mail: fanlight@fanlight.com
www.fanlight.com

The ADA mandates equal access and opportunity for the 43 million people with disabilities in the United States. These individuals may have limited speech, sight or mobility; a developmental disability; or a medical condition which limits some life activities. Many, however, are ready, willing and very able to join the workforce. This video demonstrates that many modifications or adaptations can be made simply by using ingenuity or common sense — such as keeping the aisles clear, etc. *$145.00*

37 Minutes

7403 **Helping the Family Understand**

Vestibular Disorders Association
P.O. Box 4467
Portland, OR 97208
503-229-7705
800-837-8428
FAX: 503-229-8064
e-mail: veda@vestibular.org
www.vestibular.org

Lisa Haven, Editor
Connie Pilcher, Editor

1902

7404 **Home is in the Heart: Accommodating People with Disabilities in the Homestay Experience**

Mobility International USA
PO Box 10767
Eugene, OR 97440
541-343-1284
FAX: 541-343-6812
e-mail: info@miusa.org
www.miusa.org

Susan Sygall, Executive Director
Pamela Houston, Public Relations Coordinator
Tracy Scharn, Project Assistant

Provides information and ideas for exchange organizations. Discusses how to recruit homestay families, meet accessibility needs and accommodate international participants with disabilities. *$49.00*

Video

7405 **How Difficult Can This Be ? (Fat City)**

CACLD
25 Van Zant Street
Suite 15-5
E Norwalk, CT 06855
203-838-5010
FAX: 203-866-6108
e-mail: cacld@optonline.net
www.CACLD.org

Beryl Kaufman, Executive Director

This informative and entertaining video allows the viewer to see the world through the eyes of a learning disabled child. It features a unique workshop attended by teacher, psychologists, social workers, parents, siblings and a student with LD They participate in a series of classroom activiteis which cause frustration, anxiety and tension; emotions all too familiar to a student with a learning disability.

7406 **How We Play**

Fanlight Productions
4196 Washington Street
Suite 2
Boston, MA 02131
617-469-4999
800-937-4113
FAX: 617-469-3379
e-mail: fanlight@fanlight.com
www.fanlight.com

Karen McMillen, Marketing Director

Though most of the people in this new, short documentary are in wheelchairs, and one is blind, they are anything but handicapped. Playing tennis, snorkeling, whitewater canoeing, practicing karate - they are living proof that a disability can be a challenge, not an obstacle. *$99.00*

7407 **I Can Do It**

Britannica Film Company
345 4th Street
San Francisco, CA 94107
415-777-9876

Tommy's parents took him shopping. Although he had trouble moving around with his braces he wanted to go shopping alone. In the pet shop he had some trouble moving around, but he was able to solve his problems and even help other customers. A teacher's guide is available with this video.

Film

7408 **I Want My Little Boy Back**

A Britsh Broadcasting Corporation Documentary
2080 S Undermountain Road
Sheffield, MA 01257
413-229-2100
800-714-2779
FAX: 413-229-8931
e-mail: happiness@option.org
www.option.org

A great video for parents and professionals caring for children with special needs. Join one British family and their autistic son before, during and after their journey to America to attend The Son-Rise Program at The Autism Treatment Center of America. This informative, inspirational and deeply moving story not only captures the joy, tears, challenges and triumps of this amazing little boy and his family, but also serves as a powerful introduction to the attitude and principles of the program. *$25.00*

7409 **I'm Not Disabled**

Landmark Media
3450 Slade Run Drive
Falls Church, VA 22042
703-241-2030
800-342-4336
FAX: 703-536-9540

ML Hartogs

Young people talk about their disabilities and the importance of sports in their lives. The afflictions range from blindness and missing limbs to paralysis. Through physical education and therapy they enjoy freedom of movement and participate in sports such as tennis, basketball, kayaking, skiing, and swimming. *$195.00*

Video

7410 **If I Can't Do It**

Fanlight Productions
4196 Washington Street
Suite 2
Boston, MA 02131
617-469-4999
800-937-4113
FAX: 617-469-3379
e-mail: fanlight@fanlight.com
www.fanlight.com

Karen McMillen, Marketing Director
Cynthia Conti, Publicity Coordinator
Walter Brock, Producer

Arthur Campbell, Jr. doesn't want your sympathy, he just wants what most people want: a living wage, a meaningful social life, a few good laughs and the means to get around. This outstanding documentary is an unflinching portrait of one cantankerous and courageous disabled man. *$245.00*

7411 **Imagery Procedures for People with Special Needs**

Research Press
PO Box 9177
Champaign, IL 61826
217-352-3273
800-519-2707
FAX: 217-352-1221
e-mail: rp@researchpress.com
www.researchpress.com

Russell Pence, VP Marketing

This video features numerous training sessions in which clinicians are shown leading individuals through imagery scenes that focus on controlling specific behaviors. *$195.00*

32 Minutes

7412 **In the Middle**

Fanlight Productions
4196 Washington Street
Suite 2
Boston, MA 02131
617-469-4999
800-937-4113
FAX: 617-469-3379
e-mail: fanlight@fanlight.com
www.fanlight.com

Karen McMillen, Marketing Director

Documents the problems and joys shared by Ryanna, who has Spina Bifida, and her parents, teachers and classmates during her first year of being mainstreamed in a Head Start Program. *$99.00*

7413 **In the Mind of the Beholder.... a Video About Newly Blind Adults**

Aquarius Health Care Videos
5 Powderhouse Lane
PO Box 1159
Sherborn, MA 01770
508-651-2963
FAX: 508-650-4216
e-mail: aqvideos@tiac.net

Newly blind adults making the transition to using their non-visual senses. In a society in which most people are terrified of losing their vision- and yet know virtually nothing about vision loss- the blind are wrongly viewed as mysterious, pitiful or courageous. Produced by Karen Brown Davison, this film puts a human face and voice to blindness. By sharing the experience of losing their eyesight and relearning skills they once took for granted, the people in this film: nonvisual clues. *$195.00*

7414 **Include Us**

Exceptional Parent Library
120 Sylvan Avenue, Suite 10
PO Box 1807
Englewood Cliffs, NJ 07632
800-535-1910
FAX: 201-947-9376
e-mail: eplibrary@aol.com
www.eplibrary.com

First children's video to feature a proportionate number of children with disabilities. Inclusion works via eight songs. *$19.95*

7415 Intensive Early Intervention and Beyond School-Based Inclusion Program

Research Press
2612 N Mattis Avenue
Champaign, IL 61821
217-352-3273
800-519-2707
FAX: 217-352-2707
e-mail: rp@researchpress.com
www.researchpress.com

Russell Pence, VP Marketing

Shows the successful application of a school-based inclusion program. The video focuses on the lives of young children with autism who have shown remarkable progress in personal, social, and academic skills. 22 minutes. *$195.00*

Video

7416 Interpretations

Fanlight Productions
4196 Washington Street
Suite 2
Boston, MA 02131
617-469-4999
800-937-4113
FAX: 617-469-3379
e-mail: fanlight@fanlight.com
www.fanlight.com

Karen McMillen, Marketing Director

This new film uses humor and drama to explore the interaction between the deaf and hearing communities. Janice, a freelance photographer who is deaf, has been given her first assignment by an advertising agency. She hires her hearing friend Maureen to interpret for her. When conflicts arise between Janice and the client, Maureen changes Janice words. The film looks at the interplay of dependence and responsibility in the relationship of communicator and interpreter. $145.00.

7417 Invisible Children

Learning Corporation of America
6493 Kaiser Drive
Fremont, CA 94555
510-490-7311

Renaldo was blind, Mandy was deaf, and Mark had Cerebral Palsy and used a wheelchair. These child-size puppet characters interacted with non-handicapped puppets.

Film

7418 Is This Abuse?

YAI: Natl. Institute for People with Disabilities
460 W 34th Street
New York, NY 10001
212-273-6100
FAX: 212-947-7524
www.yai.org

Video clarifies issues of abuse for professionals working with disabled adults. *$145.00*

7419 It's Just Attention Disorder

Western Psychological Services
12031 Wilshire Boulevard
Los Angeles, CA 90025
310-478-2061
800-648-8857
FAX: 310-478-7838

This ground-breaking videotape takes the critical first steps in treating attention-deficit disorder: it enlists the inattentive or hyperactive child as an active participant in his or her treatment. *$99.50*

Video

7420 JBI Voice

Jewish Braille Institute of America
110 E 30th Street
New York, NY 10016
212-889-2525
800-433-1531
FAX: 212-689-3692
e-mail: admin@jbilibrary.org
www.jbilibrary.org

Ellen Isler MD, Executive VP
Israel A Taub, Associate Director

Monthly recorded magazine emphasizing Jewish current events and culture.

1931

7421 Journey

Landmark Media
3450 Slade Run Drive
Falls Church, VA 22042
703-241-2030
800-342-4336
FAX: 703-536-9540

ML Hartogs

A moving portrayal of the extraordinary journey to Japan of 74-year-old Billie Sinclair, who is deaf, blind and mute. He funds his travels by weaving and selling baskets. In Japan he rides a roller coaster, tries judo and visits a deaf and blind acupuncturist. He demonstrates how it is possible to communicate by touch alone. *$195.00*

Video

7422 Juggler

Beacon Press
25 Beacon Street
Boston, MA 02108
617-742-2100
FAX: 617-743-3097

Andre was the young son of a wealthy, early Quebec fur trader. Because he was almost totally blind, he was overly protected by his family, and his movement outside his home was very limited.

Film

7423 Just 4 Kids

Seat-A-Robics
PO Box 1253
Jamestown, BC 27282
336-454-4615
FAX: 336-454-4615
e-mail: seatarobics@hotmail.com
www.seat-a-robics.com

Clarice Burns, President

Seated aerobic exercise program incorporates animation, props and musical themes that children five through adolescent can relate to. Adaptive instruction and safety tips are provided while demonstrating proper form. The warm-up and marching band sections include eight kid instructors as participants. Recommended for ages five through adolescents. *$39.95*

Ages 5-14
ISBN 1-887479-03-1

7424 Keeping the Balance

Fanlight Productions
4196 Washington Street
Suite 2
Boston, MA 02131
617-469-4999
800-937-4113
FAX: 617-469-3379
e-mail: fanlight@fanlight.com
www.fanlight.com

Karen McMillen, Marketing Director

Brothers and sisters of children with serious lung diseases share their experiences of being the normal child. Insightful and articulate, they explore the frequent conflict between their feelings of love and concern, and their resentment over the attention denied to them because of the sibling's illness. *$99.00*

7425 **Key Changes: A Portrait of Lisa Thorson**

Fanlight Productions
4196 Washington Street
Suite 2
Boston, MA 02131
617-469-4999
800-937-4113
FAX: 617-469-3379
e-mail: fanlight@fanlight.com
www.fanlight.com

Karen McMillen, Marketing Director

A documentary profiling Lisa Thorson, a gifted vocalist who uses a wheelchair. Ms. Thorson defines herself as a performer first, a person with a disability second, and this thoughtful portrait respects that distinction. Her work as a jazz singer is at the heart of the film, reflecting her philosophy that the biggest contribution that she can make to the struggle for the rights of people with disabilities is doing her art the best way she can. *$145.00*

7426 **Know Your Diabetes, Know Yourself**

Joslin Diabetes Center
1 Joslin Plaza
Boston, MA 02215
617-732-2400

An hour-long videotape in which Joslin patients talk about daily issues of diabetes management - meal planning, exercise, monitoring, injections, foot and eye care, and managing the disease when sick or traveling. *$3.00*

7427 **Landmark Media**

3450 Slade Run Drive
Falls Church, VA 22042
703-241-2030
800-342-4336
FAX: 703-536-9540
e-mail: landmrkmed@aol.com

Supplier and distributor of educational videocassettes and CD's. $79-$280.00.

7428 **Learning Disabilities and Discipline**

CACLD
25 Van Zant Street
Suite 15-5
E Norwalk, CT 06855
203-838-5010
FAX: 203-866-6108
e-mail: CACLD@optonline.net
www.CACLD.org

Beryl Kaufman, Executive Director

This video comes with a 16 page Program Guide containing information about specific aspects of the learing disabilities profile that can cause misbehavior. Some basic concepts which can be valuable as you develop your own behavior management plans are discussed. Included are dozens of field test techniques and strategies that can be used to monitor, evaluate and manage childrens behavior and more.

7429 **Learning Disabilities and Self Esteem**

CACLD
25 Van Zant Street
Suite 15-5
E Norwalk, CT 06855
203-838-5010
FAX: 203-866-6108
e-mail: CACLD@optonline.net
www.CACLD.org

Beryl Kaufman, Executive Director

The 60 minute Teacher video contains program material for building self-esteem in the classroom. The 60 minute parent video contains program material for building self esteem in the home. A 16 page Program Guide accompanies each video.

7430 **Learning Disabilities and Social Skills**

CACLD
25 Van Zant Street
Suite 15-5
E Norwalk, CT 06855
203-838-5010
FAX: 203-866-6108
e-mail: CACLD@optonline.net
www.CACLD.org

Beryl Kaufman, Executive Director

Noting that LD children do not have the cognitive skills to simply pick up socially correct behavior by watching their parents, like most children do, nationally recognized expert on learning disabilities, Richard Lavoie, gives parents and teachers examples on how to help their LD children succeed in everyday situations where they might normally fail. The program includes an explanation of social autopsies and the techniques Lavoie uses to correct them.

7431 **Let's Eat Video**

Blind Children's Center
4120 Marathon Street
Los Angeles, CA 90029
323-664-2153
800-222-3567
FAX: 323-665-3828
e-mail: info@blindchildrenscenter.org
www.blindchildrenscenter.org

$35.00

7432 **Let's be Friends**

Britannica Film Company
345 4th Street
San Francisco, CA 94107
415-777-9876

The teacher left the room and asked Shelly, a hearing impaired child to be the mother. Margaret, an emotionally disturbed child, became frightened and verbally attacked Shelly. The teacher worked to get them to become friends and understand each other's problems.

Film

7433 **Living with Spinal Cord Injury**

Fanlight Productions
4196 Washington Street
Suite 2
Boston, MA 02131
617-469-4999
800-937-4113
FAX: 617-469-3379
e-mail: fanlight@fanlight.com
www.fanlight.com

Karen McMillen, Marketing Director

A series of three videos produced by an individual who has experienced spinal cord injury himself. Changes; is about the consequences of spinal cord injury and the process of rehabilitation. Outside; emphasizes the life-long aspect of rehabilitation for people with spinal cord injury. Survivors; interviews 23 men and women who have lived at least 24 years with spinal cord injury. *$200.00*

7434 **Look Out for Annie**

Lighthouse International
111 E 59 Street
New York, NY 10022
212-821-9737
800-829-0500
FAX: 212-821-9706
e-mail: info@lighthouse.org

Joanna Mellor, VP Information Services

Depicts an older woman coping with her vision loss. It focuses on the emotional issues surrounding vision loss and conveys the idea that both the person with the vision disorder and their family and friends will need to make adjustments. *$25.00*

Video

7435 Look Who's Laughing

Aquarius Health Care Videos
5 Powderhouse Lane
PO Box 1159
Sherborn, MA 01770
FAX: 508-650-4216
e-mail: aqvideos@tiac.net
www.aquariusproductions.com

This video is packed with laugh-out-loud comedic moments, but is also full of intelligent and inspiring messages. Look Who's Laughing introduces viewers to some of today's funniest comedians - who just happen to be physically disabled. We hear them talk openly and honestly about their limitations as well as their abilities and talents. Helpful for those who work with the disabled and motivational to both the disabled and able-bodied. Preview option available. *$95.00*

Video

7436 Loud, Proud and Passionate

Mobility International USA
PO Box 10767
Eugene, OR 97440
541-343-1284
FAX: 541-343-6812
e-mail: info@miusa.org
www.miusa.org

Susan Sygall, Executive Director
Pamela Houston, Public Relations Coordinator
Tracy Scharn, Project Assistant

Documents MIUSA's Women's Institute on Leadership and Disability. Interviews with participants highlight the vision, determination, challanges and recommendations of women with disabilities who are grassroots leaders in over 25 countries. MIUSA's unique model of international leadership training is illustrated as women with mobility, visual and hearing disabilities are shown in training workshop and team-building activities. Available in English, Spanish and Russian. *$49.00*

Video

7437 Making a Difference: A Wise Approach

Easter Seals
230 W Monroe Street
Chicago, IL 60606
312-726-6200
FAX: 312-726-1494

Janet D Jamieson, Communication Manager

The town of Wise, Virginia, and its leading citizen, Virgil Craft, personify what Making a Difference is all about when a community supports implementing the provisions of the Americans with Disabilities Act. Craft, a person with a disability, has spent his life giving back to the community. The community, in turn, has supported Craft's efforts to improve the environment, education, healthcare and access for disabled persons. A must buy for companies of all sizes, clubs and organizations. *$50.00*

7438 Managed Mental Healthcare Video

Nat'l Council for Community Behavioral Healthcare
12300 Twinbrook Parkway
Suite 320
Rockville, MD 20852
301-984-6200
FAX: 301-881-7159
www.nccbh.org

Get an overview of the managed healthcare climate with this premier strategic planning and training tool.

7439 Manic Depression: Voices of an Illness

Fanlight Productions
4196 Washington Street
Suite 2
Boston, MA 02131
617-469-4999
800-937-4113
FAX: 617-469-3379
e-mail: fanlight@fanlight.com

Karen McMillen, Marketing Director

This audio cassette focuses on the lives of nine people and their families who are living with the pervasive illness. *$29.00*

Audio

7440 Martin Luther Home Society

650 J Street
Suite 305
Lincoln, NE 68508
800-727-8317
FAX: 402-434-3253
e-mail: info@mlhs.com
www.mlhs.com

Faye Colburn, Communications Specialist
David Frye, Communications Director

Video production: public education and public relations programs. Staff training materials. Public Service announcements and script writing services.

7441 More Than Just a Job

Institution on Disability
University of New Hampshire
Morrill Hall, Room 312
Durham, NH 03824

Narrative case studies and interviews with persons with disabilities, their employers, families and experts in the field. *$ 20.00*

7442 My Body is Not Who I Am

Aquarius Health Care Videos
5 Powderhouse Lane
PO Box 1159
Sherborn, MA 01770
508-651-2963
888-440-2963
FAX: 508-650-4216
e-mail: aqvideos@tiac.net
www.aquariusproductions.com

Leslie Kussman, President

This thought-provoking video introduces viewers to people who openly discuss the struggles and triumphs they have experienced living in a body that is physically disabled. They talk honestly about the social stigma of their disability and the problems they face in terms of mobility, health care and family relationships, as well as the challenges of emotional and sexual intimacy. Preview option available. *$195.00*

Video

7443 My Country

Aquarius Health Care Videos
5 Powderhouse Lane
PO Box 1159
Sherborn, MA 01770
508-651-2963
888-440-2963
FAX: 508-650-4216
e-mail: aqvideos@tiac.net
www.aquariusproductions.com

Leslie Kussmann, President

By telling the stories of three people with disabilities and their struggle for equal rights under the law, this film draws a powerful parallel between the efforts of disability rights activists and the civil rights struggle of the 1960s. Great for disability awareness programs, and for discussions of disability rights issues. Should be part of every college curriculum on disabilities. Awarded Best of Show Superfest 98. Preview option available. *$195.00*

Video

7444 Nancy's Special Workout for the Physically Challenged

Laurel Designs
5 Laurel Avenue
Belvedere, CA 94920

FAX: 415-435-1451
e-mail: laureld@ncal.verio.com

Janet Sawyer, Owner
Lynn Montoya, Owner

Aerobic exercise video with syncopated music for seated people with disabilities from minimal to severe. *$42.00*

45 Minutes

7445 Narcolepsy

Fanlight Productions
4196 Washington Street
Suite 2
Boston, MA 02131

617-469-4999
FAX: 617-469-3379
e-mail: fanlight@fanlight.com
www.fanlight.com

Presents the experiences of three individuals who lives and relationships have been disrupted by narcolepsy. Rental $50/day. *$ 195.00*

25 Minutes

7446 No Barriers

Aquarius Health Care Videos
5 Powderhouse Lane
PO Box 1159
Sherborn, MA 01770

FAX: 508-650-4216
e-mail: aqvideos@tiac.net
www.aquariusproductions.com

Everyone faces the world with different abilities and disabilities. But everyone has at least one goal in common...to break through their own barriers says Mark Wellman. Mark, a paraplegic, knows this well. No Barriers takes us into Mark's world where he defies the odds for most able bodied individuals by climbing Yosemite's Half Dome and El Capitan. This video is more than inspiring and fun to watch...it helps one make that paradigm shift from can't do to can do! Preview option available *$90.00*

Video

7447 NoBody's Perfect....Educating Children about Disabilities

Aquarius Health Care Videos
5 Powderhouse Lane
PO Box 1159
Sherborn, MA 01770

508-651-2963
FAX: 508-650-4216
e-mail: aqvideos@tiac.net

An upbeat, inclusion-friendly program for kids that profiles three children with disabilties. Viewers discover that accepting differences is an essential part of growing up. We learn how the kids cope and, in the process, are introduced to signing, prosthetics, and assistive technology and Braille. Videocassette, preview option is available. *$ 99.00*

7448 Nobody is Burning Wheelchairs

Easter Seals
230 W Monroe Street
Chicago, IL 60606

312-726-6200
FAX: 312-726-1494

Janet D Jamieson, Communications Manager

Explains the employment, public accommodations, transportation and telecommunications provisions of the Americans with Disabilities Act and what this law means to people with disabilities and business and industry. The video can be used for training and information seminars, awareness training and for groups interested in learning more about people with disabilities. *$35.00*

7449 Observing Kassandra

Brookes Publishing
PO Box 10624
Baltimore, MD 21285

410-337-9580
800-638-3775
FAX: 410-337-8539
e-mail: custserv@brookespublishing.com
www.brookespublishing.com

Provides professionals with a firsthand opportunity to practice taking notes during a TPBA. Comes with summary forms that can be completed for additional guidance in learning how to use TPBA. Also included is a 28-page saddle-stitched booklet. *$169.00*

50 Minutes
ISBN 1-55766 -66-5

7450 Once Upon a Time...Children's Classics Retold in American Sign Language

Harris Communications
15155 Technology Drive
Eden Prairie, MN 55344

952-906-1180
800-825-6758
FAX: 952-906-1099
e-mail: mail@harriscomm.com
www.harriscomm.com

Bill Williams, National Sales Manager

Children's classics come alive on videotapes. Six tapes are available, each telling a favorite fairy tale. *$29.95*

7451 One to Grow On

Nat'l Council for Community Behavioral Healthcare
12300 Twinbrook Parkway
Suite 320
Rockville, MD 20852

301-984-6200
FAX: 301-881-7159
www.nccbh.org

Provides an important service to clinicians. This video will allow therapists to make in-depth observations of clients' treatment needs and reduce therapist-client mismatches. *$595.00*

7452 Open for Business

Disability Rights Education and Defense Fund
2212 6th Street
Berkeley, CA 94710

510-644-2555
FAX: 510-841-8645
e-mail: dredf@dredf.org
www.dredf.org

Susan Henderson, Managing Director

An award-winning film that depicts the disability and business communities working together in one small town to remove architectural barriers, when readily achievable, as required by the Americans with Disabilities Act. Package includes 15 and 30 minute closed-captioned versions and 15 to 30 minute versions with audio description. *$179.00*

7453 Open to the Public

Aquarius Health Care Videos
5 Powderhouse Lane
PO Box 1159
Sherborn, MA 01770
FAX: 508-650-4216
e-mail: aqvideos@tiac.net
www.aquariusproductions.com

Provides an overview of the Americans with Disabilities Act as it applies to state and local governments. The ADA doesn't provide recommendations for solving common problems, but this film could provide enough information for governments to solve some common problems without turning to high-priced consultants. Preview option available. *$125.00*

Video

7454 PACE II

Arthritis Foundation
PO Box 6996
Alpharetta, GA 30009
800-207-8633
FAX: 770-442-9742
www.arthritis.com

$19.50

7455 Parallels in Time

MN Governor's Council on Development Disabilities
370 Centennial Office Building
658 Cedar Street
St. Paul, MN 55155
651-296-4018
877-348-0505
FAX: 651-297-7200
e-mail: admin.dd@state.mn.us
www.mncdd.org

Colleen Wieck PhD, Executive Director

Parallels in Time traces present attitudes and the treatment of people with disabilities, and supplements the first weekend seesion of Partners in Policymaking. This CD-ROM includes the History of the Parent Movement and the History of the Independent Living Movement, as well as personal stories of self advocates, leaders in the self advocacy movement.

7456 Part of the Team

Easter Seals
230 W Monroe Street
Suite 1800
Chicago, IL 60606
312-726-6200
FAX: 312-726-1494

Janet D Jamieson, Communications Manager

Designed for employers of all sizes, rehabilitation organizations and all others concerned with the employment of people with disabilities. It addresses managers' concerns and questions about supervising persons with disabilities and can be used as a discussion/team-building tool for employees with and without disabilities. The video recognizes people with disabilities as strong contenders for almost any job. *$15.00*

7457 Passion for Justice

Fanlight Productions
4196 Washington Street
Suite 2
Boston, MA 02131
617-469-4999
800-937-4113
FAX: 617-469-3379
e-mail: fanlight@fanlight.com
www.fanlight.com

An engaging portrait of Bob Perske, the author of Unequal Justice and a crusader for the rights of people with developmental disabilities. The tape focuses on cases in which people with developmental disabilities have been convicted of crimes they didn't commit. The tape asks challenging questions about society's responsibility to this population, and about ways to protect their rights to equality and justice. *$99.00*

29 Minutes

7458 Pathways to Better Living

Arthritis Foundation
PO Box 6996
Alpharetta, GA 30009
800-207-8633
FAX: 770-442-9742
www.arthritis.com

$29.95

7459 Paul

Miriam Perrone
440 Park Avenue
Saint Simons Island, GA 31522

How a determined mother carved a semi-independent life for her now-grown Down Syndrome child. *$63.20*

7460 Pharmacologic Therapy of Pediatric Asthma

American Lung Association
61 Broadway
New York, NY 10017
212-315-8700
FAX: 212-315-8700
e-mail: info@lungusa.org
www.lungusa.org

A Learning Resource Program developed by a joint committee of the American Thoracic Society and the ALA.

Film

7461 Pool Exercise Program

Arthritis Foundation Distribution Center
PO Box 6996
Alpharetta, GA 30009
800-207-8633
FAX: 770-442-9742
www.arthritis.com

This video features water exercises that will help you increase and maintain joint flexibility, strengthen and tone muscles, and increase endurance. All exercises are performed in water at chest level. No swimming skills are necessary. *$19.50*

7462 Potty Learning for Children who Experience Delay

Exceptional Parent Library
120 Sylvan Avenue, Suite 10
PO Box 1807
Englewood Cliffs, NJ 07632
800-535-1910
FAX: 201-947-9376
e-mail: eplibrary@aol.com
www.eplibrary.com

This video presents a unique developmental approach to supporting the child in learning independence in the management of bathroom skills. *$39.95*

7463 Raising Kids with Special Needs

Aquarius Health Care Videos
5 Powderhouse Lane
PO Box 1159
Sherborn, MA 01770 **508-651-2963**
FAX: 508-650-4216
e-mail: aqvideos@tiac.net
www.aquariusproductions.com

An intimate look into the lives of parents of three kids with very different disabilities. The objective of this video is an understanding of paprenting a child with special nees. THis outstanding program looks at safety concerns, issues of anger and grief, the importance of a support network and other important issues. Ultimately, this is a narrative about raising and educating a child with disabilities. Preview option is available. *$89.00*

Video

7464 Reasonable Accommodations of the Enabling Kind

Mainstream
3 Bethesda Metro Center
 # 830
Bethesda, MD 20814 **301-654-2400**
e-mail: info@mainstreaminc.org

Lillie Harrison, Information Programs Clerk

In this training video a hiring manager demonstrates the basics of doing a job analysis and is shown using the information in interview sessions to determine the reasonable accommodation needs of three individuals with disabilities. Includes trainer and trainee guide. *$59.95*

7465 Recognizing Children with Special Needs

Aquarius Health Care Videos
5 Powderhouse Lane
PO Box 1159
Sherborn, MA 01770
FAX: 508-650-4216
e-mail: aqvideos@tiac.net
www.aquariusproductions.com

A great overview for caregivers of children on how to recognize special needs. Often-times it is the little things children do everyday to compensate for, or express, a disability that can be observed by their caregiver. All types of disabilities are addressed: emotional, physical, psychological, and chronic illness. A wonderful tool for teachers, childcare staff, and students on how to play a vital role in our children's development. Preview option available. *$125.00*

Video

7466 Regular Kid

American Lung Association
61 Broadway
New York, NY 10017 **212-315-8700**
FAX: 212-315-8700
e-mail: info@lungusa.org
www.lungusa.org

This film shows how families and children cope with asthma problems. Proven asthma management strategies are presented through the experiences of four children with asthma, ranging in age from toddler to teenager.

Film

7467 Relaxation Techniques for People with Special Needs

Research Press
2612 N Mattis Avenue
Champaign, IL 61822 **217-325-3273**
800-519-2707
FAX: 217-352-1221
e-mail: rp@researchpress.com
www.researchpress.com

Gail Salyards, Marketing Services Manager

The developers discuss and demonstrate how to use special relaxation procedures with children and adolescents who have developmental disabilities. They emphasize the need for students to learn relaxation as a means of coping with stress and developing self-control. During the scenes of Dr June Groden conducting relaxation training, viewers will see how to correctly use the training procedures, how to use reinforcement during training and how to use guided imagery. 23 minutes. Includes book. *$195.00*

Video

7468 Right at Home

Aquarius Health Care Videos
5 Powderhouse Lane
PO Box 1159
Sherborn, MA 01770 **508-651-2963**
FAX: 508-650-4216
e-mail: aqvideos@tiac.net
www.aquariusproductions.com

Shows simple solutions for complying with the Fair Hoiusing Act amendments. Emphasizes low-cost, practical solutions, and working with people with disabilities to find the best applicable solution. Ideal for people with disabilities and their families, as well as housing providers, university courses, and disability awareness organizations. Preview option is available. *$99.00*

Video

7469 Say it with Sign Videotape

Harris Communications
15155 Technology Drive
Eden Prairie, MN 55344 **952-906-1180**
800-825-6758
FAX: 952-906-1099
e-mail: mail@harriscomm.com
www.harriscomm.com

Bill Williams, National Sales Manager

Contains both the serious and fun side of signing and provides the basic signs that might be needed in an emergency situation. *$39.95*

Video

7470 Science Accessed for All Students

Center for Accessible Technology
2547 8th Street
Suite 12-A
Berkeley, CA 94710 **510-841-3224**
FAX: 510-841-7956
e-mail: info@cforat.org
www.cforat.org

Lisa Wahl, Director

A 10 minute video that demonstrates inclusive in elementary school science two peer support, adaptation of notifices and assistance technology. *$15.00*

Video

7471 See What I Feel

Britannica Film Company
345 Fourth Street
San Francisco, CA 94107 **415-777-9876**

A blind child tells her friends about her trip to the zoo. Each experience was explained as a blind child would experience it. A teacher's guide comes with this video.

Film

7472 **See What I'm Saying**

Fanlight Productions
4196 Washington Street
Suite 2
Boston, MA 02131 **617-469-4999**
800-937-4113
FAX: 617-469-3379
e-mail: fanlight@fanlight.com
www.fanlight.com

Karen McMillen, Marketing Director

This program illustrates how the acquisition of communication skill, particularly sign language, enhances a child's self esteem and family and peer relationship. The documentary follows Patricia, who is deaf and from a Spanish-speaking family, through her first year at the Kendall Demonstration Elementary School of Gallaudet University. *$195.00*

7473 **See for Yourself**

Lighthouse International
111 E 59 Street
New York, NY 10022 **212-821-9737**
800-829-0500
FAX: 212-821-9706
e-mail: info@lighthouse.org

Joanna Mellor, VP Information Services

This video features older adults with impaired vision who have been helped by vision rehabilitation. *$50.00*

7474 **Shape Up 'n Sign**

Gallaudet University Bookstore
11030 S Langley Avenue
Chicago, IL 60628 **202-651-5488**
800-621-2736
FAX: 202-651-5489

An aerobic exercise tape introducing the basic sign language for deaf and hearing children ages six to ten. *$22.95*

30 Minutes

7475 **Shining Bright: Head Start Inclusion**

Brookes Publishing
PO Box 10624
Baltimore, MD 21285 **410-337-9580**
800-638-3775
FAX: 410-337-8539
e-mail: custserv@brookespublishing.com
www.brookespublishing.com

This documentary depicts the collaborative efforts of a Head Start and a local education agency to include children with severe disabilities in a Head Start program. This video addresses issues such as support for children with severe health impairments, benefits of participating in Head Start, ability of teachers with a general education background to serve children with severe disabilities, and staff relations. Includes a 28-page saddle-stitched booklet. *$45.00*

23 Minutes

ISBN 1-55766 -95-9

7476 **Sight by Touch**

Landmark Media
3450 Slade Run Drive
Falls Church, VA 22042 **703-241-2030**
800-342-4336
FAX: 703-536-9540

ML Hartogs

This video features the life and importance of Louis Braille. Vision-impaired performers and teachers demonstrate how Braille has benefitted their lives, and how improvements are constantly being made. *$195.00*

Video

7477 **Sign of the Times**

Fanlight Productions
4196 Washington Street
Suite 2
Boston, MA 02131 **617-469-4999**
800-937-4113
FAX: 617-469-3379
e-mail: fanlight@fanlight.com
www.fanlight.com

Karen McMillen, Marketing Director

Profiles a public school in the heart of Los Angeles - an American microcosm where over 300 languages are spoken, and where cultures and races collide. Fairfax High, publicized as the site of gang activity and murder, has long been a focus for bad press. But something very right is going on in this school. A Sign of the Times offers a positive example of how the American Dream and American education are still alive *$ 154.00*

7478 **Sleeping Beauty Videotape**

Gallaudet University Bookstore
11030 S Langley Avenue
Chicago, IL 60628 **202-651-5488**
800-621-2736
FAX: 202-651-5489

Presents the entire story of Sleeping Beauty told in American Sign Language. Includes voice over. *$29.95*

30 Minutes

7479 **Small Differences**

Aquarius Health Care Videos
5 Powderhouse Lane
PO Box 1159
Sherborn, MA 01770
FAX: 508-650-4216
e-mail: aqvideos@tiac.net
www.aquariusproductions.com

What happens when you give children with and without disabilities a camera and ask them to produce a video about disabilities? The result is an uplifting, award-winning disability video that both children and adults can relate to. The kids interviewed adults and children with physical and sensory disabilities. A top-quality production that increases understanding and awareness. Winner, Columbus International Film & Video Festival. Winner, National Education Media Network. Preview option availabe *$110.00*

Video

7480 **Social Skills on the Job**

AGS
Publishers Building
PO Box 99
Circle Pines, MN 55014
800-328-2560
FAX: 763-786-9007
www.agsnet.com

Robert Zaske, Market Manager

Gives students a realistic picture of what's expected of them at work and models appropriate behavior on the job through a variety of videos and software. *$259.95*

7481 **Someday's Child**

Educational Productions
9000 SW Gemini Drive
Beaverton, OR 97008 **503-644-7000**
800-950-4949
FAX: 503-350-7000
e-mail: custserv@edpro.com
www.edpro.com

Linda Freedman, President/Co-Owner
Molly Krumm, Marketing Director

This video focuses on three families' search for help and information for their children with disabilities.

7482 Something Magical

Educational Productions
9000 SW Gemini Drive
Beaverton, OR 97008
503-644-7000
800-950-4949
FAX: 503-350-7000
e-mail: custserve@edpro.com
www.edpro.com

Linda Freedman, President/Co-Owner
Molly Krumm, Marketing Director

In 1984 two teachers and one music therapist decided that a collaboration between their two schools would be mutually beneficial. The result is recorded in this heart-warming documentary.

7483 Sound & Fury

Aquarius Health Care Videos
5 Powderhouse Lane
PO Box 1159
Sherborn, MA 01770
508-651-2296
888-440-2963
FAX: 508-650-4216
e-mail: aqvideos@tiac.net
www.aquariusproductions.com

Leslie Kussmann, President/Producer

This film takes viewers inside the seldom seen world of the deaf to witness a painful family struggle over a controversial medical technology called the cochlear implant. Some of the family members celebrate the implant as a long overdue cure for deafness while others fear it will destroy their language and way of life. This documentary explores this seemingly irreconcilable conflict as it illuminates the ongoing struggle for identity among deaf people today. *$195.00*

Video

7484 Sound and Fury

Aquarius Health Care Videos
5 Powderhouse Lane
PO Box 1159
Sherborn, MA 01770
508-651-2963
FAX: 508-650-4216
e-mail: aqvideos@tiac.net
www.aquariusproductions.com

Leslie Kussmonn, President

This film takes viewers inside the seldom seen world of the deaf to witness a painful family struggle over a controversial medical technology called the cochlear implant. Some of the family members celebrate the implant as a long overdue cure for deafness, while others fear it will destroy their language and way of life. This documentary explores this seemingly irreconcilable conflict as it illuminates the ongoing struggle for the identity among deaf people today. Preview option available. *$195.00*

7485 Special Children/Special Solutions

Option Institute and Fellowship
2080 S Undermountain Road
Sheffield, MA 01257
413-229-8727
800-562-7171
FAX: 413-229-8727
e-mail: indigo@option.org
www.optionindigo.com

Kate Wilde

This four-tape audio series presents concrete, down-to-earth, no-nonsense alternatives which are full of love and acceptance for the special child while being wholly supportive of parents, professionals and helpers who want to reach out. The accepting (nonjudgmental) attitude presented is the basis of all Samahria's work and is the foundation for the nurturing teaching process that has encouraged and helped parents, children and others to accomplish more than most would have believed. *$55.00*

Audio

7486 Special Education Cassette Recording

LifeWay Christian Resources Southern Baptist Conv.
127 9th Avenue N
Nashville, TN 37234
615-251-2000
800-458-2772
FAX: 651-251-5764
e-mail: specialed@lifeway.com
www.lifeway.com

Ellen Beene, Editor

This annual audiocassette features the 12 unit songs suggested for a special education Sunday school curriculum. *$15.00*

7487 Stay Tuned

Fanlight Productions
4196 Washington Street
Suite 2
Boston, MA 02131
617-469-4999
800-937-4113
FAX: 617-469-3379
e-mail: fanlight@fanlight.com
www.fanlight.com

Karen McMillen, Marketing Director

This program looks at ways of coping with hearing loss. The program introduces us to one woman who, after suffering a mid-life hearing loss, confronts her situation and regains her ability to function and enjoy her life through taking advantage of hearing aids, speech reading instruction, assistive listening devices and the support of other hearing impaired people. *$99.00*

7488 Stuttering & Your Child: A Videotape for Parents

Stuttering Foundation of America
3100 Walnut Grove Road, Suite 603
PO Box 11749
Memphis, TN 38111
901-452-7343
800-992-9392
FAX: 901-452-3931
e-mail: stutter@vantek.net
www.stutterhelp.org

Anne Edwards, Coordinator

Provides parents withup-to-date information on what stuttering is; what is thought to cause and worsen childhood stuttering; what parents can do to help their child. *$10.00*

7489 TERI

3225 Roymar Road
Oceanside, CA 92054

A private, nonprofit corporation which has been developing and operating programs for individuals with developmental disabilities since 1980. Offers staff training videos, staff training tools and technique manuals.

7490 Teaching People with Developmental Disabilities

Research Press
PO Box 9177
Champaign, IL 61826
217-352-3273
800-519-2707
FAX: 217-352-1221
e-mail: rp@researchpress.com
www.researchpress.com

Russell Pence, VP Marketing

Hands-on video training series designed to help teachers, staff, volunteers, or family members master four behavioral techniques vital to teaching functional living skills. The videotapes which provide clear and simple teaching demonstrations, are designed to be stopped and started frequently to allow time for viewer response. Each tape includes numerous scenes of training sessions in which teachers and staff are shown working with individual students. *$595.00*

Video

7491 Technology for the Disabled

Landmark Media
3450 Slade Run Drive
Falls Church, VA 22042
703-241-2030
800-342-4336
FAX: 703-536-9540

ML Hartogs

Physically disabled people cope with the frustrations of a body they cannot control. The computer age has made many disabled more self-reliant; armless feed themselves, the blind read newspapers and the voiceless speak through marvelous technological breakthroughs. *$195.00*

Video

7492 Telling Stories

Harris Communications
15155 Technology Drive
Eden Prairie, MN 55344
952-906-1180
800-825-6758
FAX: 952-906-1099
e-mail: mail@harriscomm.com
www.harriscomm.com

Bill Williams, National Sales Manager

This international award winning play, now on video, uses the symbols and myths drawn from the struggles between the world of the deaf and the world of the hearing. *$59.95*

Video

7493 Theatre Without Limits

VSA Arts of Maine
PO Box 4002
Portland, ME 04101
207-761-3861
FAX: 207-761-4740
e-mail: me@vsarts.org
vsartsmaine.org

David C Webster, Executive Director

Video demonstrates how to make theatrical performances accessible to people who are blind, deaf, or who have other disabilities.

7494 They Don't Come with Manuals

Fanlight Productions
4196 Washington Street
Suite 2
Boston, MA 02131
617-469-4999
800-937-4113
FAX: 617-469-3379
e-mail: fanlight@fanlight.com
www.fanlight.com

Karen McMillen, Marketing Director

The parents and adoptive parents in this video speak candidly of their day to day experiences caring for children with physical and mental disabilities. *$145.00*

7495 They're Just Kids

Aquarius Health Care Videos
5 Powderhouse Lane
PO Box 1159
Sherborn, MA 01770
508-651-2963
888-440-2963
FAX: 508-650-4216
e-mail: aqvideos@tiac.net
www.aquariusproductions.com

Leslie Kussmann, President/Producer

The importance and value of inclusion, excellent for anyone working with kids with disabilities. The documentary explores the advantages of the inclusion of disabled children in the classroom, cub scouts and other extracurricular activities. *$99.00*

Video

7496 Three R's for Special Education: Rights, Resources, Results

Brookes Publishing
PO Box 10624
Baltimore, MD 21285
410-337-9580
800-638-3775
FAX: 410-337-8539
e-mail: custserv@brookespublishing.com
www.brookespublishing.com

This is a guide for parents, and a tool for educators. Through this video parents learn how to work through the steps of the special education system and work toward securing the best education and services for their children. Reviews the laws to protect children with disabilities in easy to understand language. Also provides a list of national organizations that can offer resources, information and advice to parents. *$49.95*

50 Minutes
ISBN 0-96461 -80-7

7497 Tools for Students

Aquarius Health Care Videos
5 Powderhouse Lane
PO Box 1159
Sherborn, MA 01770
508-651-2963
FAX: 508-650-4216
e-mail: aqvideos@tiac.net
www.aquariusproductions.com

Provides a series of 26 fun occupational therapy sensory processing activities. Designed as an in-home, in-workshop, and in-class exercise leader with students. Activities include: Strenghten the muscles necessary for normal activities, provide the muscles necessary to enhance alertness and concentration, increase the ability to use good posture, help social skills and fitting in and increase coordination; concludes with emphasis on team collaboration between the student, teacher, and parents. *$99.00*

Video

7498 Tools for Teachers: Practical Strategies f or Students with ADD & Learning Disabilities

Aquarius Health Care Videos
5 Powderhouse Lane
PO Box 1159
Sherborn, MA 01770 **508-651-2963**
FAX: 508-650-4216
e-mail: aqvideos@tiac.net
www.aquariusproductions.com

Designed to provide a beneficial overview, Tools for Teachers is ideal for in-service programs, parent education, teacher familiarization, and group discussion. Useful for an adult audience, it explains why students rock in their chairs, why a student may have so much difficulty coordinating hand movements, why untreated sensory integration deficits can bring all kinds of problems in the classroom, how inclusion can be successful, and how OT techniques can help build successful education. *$99.00*

Video

7499 Trackman: Y-Saves (Youth Substance Abuse Video Educational Series)

Michigan Association for Deaf, Hearing and Speech
2929 Covington Center
Lansing, MI 48912 **517-487-0066**
800-YOU-HEAR
e-mail: yourear@msu.edu
www.madhs.org

Katherine Draper, Executive Director
Jody Smith, Program Director

A three part substance abuse educational video program created by the Michigan Association for Deaf, Hearing and Speech services. The program provides a stimulating format for educating youth about drugs and alcohol. This video was written and produced especially for deaf middle and high school students, but is appropriate for all youth as it includes signing, open captioning and voice overs. An extensive guide provides guidance and plenty of ideas for activities and exercises.

7500 Twitch and Shout

Fanlight Productions
4196 Washington Street
Suite 2
Boston, MA 02131 **617-469-4999**
800-937-4113
FAX: 617-469-3379
e-mail: fanlight@fanlight.com
www.fanlight.com

Karen McMillen, Marketing Director
Cynthia Conti, Publicity Coordinator
Laurel Chiten, Producer

This documentary provides an intimate journey into the startling world of Tourette Syndrome (TS), a genetic disorder that can cause a bizarre range of involuntary movements, vocalizations, and compulsions. Through the eyes of a photojournalist with TS, the film introduces viewers to others who have this puzzling disorder. This is an emotionally absorbing, sometimes, unsettling, and finally uplifting program about people who must contend with a society that often sees them as crazy or bad. *$275.00*

7501 Understanding ADHD

Aquarius Health Care Videos
5 Powderhouse Lane
PO Box 1159
Sherborn, MA 01770
FAX: 508-650-4216
e-mail: aqvideos@tiac.net
www.aquariusproductions.com

A look at some of the controversies surrounding Attention Deficit Hyperactivity Disorder. This video shows how the disorder is diagnosed and presents strategies for living with a child with the disorder. Diverse and candid opinions from teachers, social workers, a behavior specialist, a pediatrician and a parent with ADHD twins. Recommended for child development students, social workers, and caregivers. Preview option available. *$120.00*

Video

7502 Understanding Allergic Reactions

Academy of Allergy, Asthma, Immunology
611 E Wells Street
Milwaukee, WI 53202 **414-272-6071**
800-822-2762
FAX: 414-272-6070
e-mail: info@aaaai.org
www.aaaai.org

During an allergic reaction, your body responds to a substance generally considered harmless to most people. This video portrays what happens in you body's immune system during an allergic reaction, how to avoid allergic substances, and methods your allergist uses to treat your allergies. *$25.00*

10-13 Minutes

7503 Understanding Attention Deficit Disorder

CACLD
25 Van Zant Street
Suite 15-5
E Norwalk, CT 06855 **203-838-5010**
FAX: 203-866-6108
e-mail: CACLD@optonline.net
www.CACLD.org

Beryl Kaufman, Executive Director

A video in an interview format for parents and professionals providing the history, symptoms, methods of diagnosis and three approaches used to ease the effects of attention deficit disorder. Published by Connecticut Association for Children & Adults with Learning Disabilities (CACLD). *$20.00*

45 Minutes

7504 Understanding Autism

Fanlight Productions
4196 Washington Street
Suite 2
Boston, MA 02131 **617-469-4999**
800-937-4113
FAX: 617-469-3379
e-mail: fanlight@fanlight.com
www.fanlight.com

Karen McMillen, Marketing Director

This program explores some basic components of a behavioral analysis approach to educating individuals with autism. After giving an introduction to the disability, the program goes on to illustrate the principles of reinforcement, teaching methods and data collection and analysis, as well as outlining the philosophy behind using behavior modification techniques with children with autism. *$195.00*

7505 **Understanding Learning Disabilities**

Aquarius Health Care Videos
5 Powderhouse Lane
PO Box 1159
Sherborn, MA 01770
FAX: 508-650-4216
e-mail: aqvideos@tiac.net
www.aquariusproductions.com

This video explains various learning disabilities that may effect many areas - language, reading, math skills, and behavior. Attention Deficit Disorder is gaining a lot of press these days and here we see the link between it and other disorders. Teaching children new ways to overcome their disability is shown in a how-to method. Preview option available. *$125.00*

Video

7506 **Video Guide to Disability Awareness**

Aquarius Health Care Videos
5 Powderhouse Lane
PO Box 1159
Sherborn, MA 01770
FAX: 508-650-4216
e-mail: aqvideos@tiac.net
www.aquariusproductions.com

President Clinton opens and concludes this informative video about disability awareness. A series of candid interviews with people who have a wide range of disabilities provide personal insights into the issues surrounding visual, hearing, physical and mental disabilities. Video comes with written reference guide and is also available with open or closed captioning. Preview option available. *$195.00*

Video

7507 **Video Intensive Parenting**

Systems Unlimited/LIFE Skills
1556 S 1st Avenue
Iowa City, IA 52240 **319-338-9212**

Ginny Kirschling, Public Information Specialist
Geoffrey Lauer, Program Director

Parents who have children with special needs share their reactions to their child's diagnosis and how they have learned to cope with their feelings. *$69.95*

7508 **Vital Signs: Crip Culture Talks Back**

Fanlight Productions
4196 Washington Street
Suite 2
Boston, MA 02131 **617-469-4999**
800-937-4113
FAX: 617-469-3379
e-mail: fanlight@fanlight.com
www.fanlight.com

Karen McMillen, Marketing Director
Cynthia Conti, Publicity Coordinator

This edgy, raw video documentary explores the politics of disability through the performances, debates and late-night conversations of artists at a recent national conference of disabilities and the art's. Vital Signs conveys the intensity, variety and vitality of disability culture today. *$225.00*

Video

7509 **We're Not Stupid**

Aquarius Health Care Videos
5 Powderhouse Lane
PO Box 1159
Sherborn, MA 01770
FAX: 508-650-4216
e-mail: aqvideos@tiac.net
www.aquariusproductions.com

The U.S. Department of Education has estimated that up to five percent of students have problems in school because of attention deficit disorders. These kids often are impulsive and angry. They hear throughout their schooling what not to do, but not what to do. I know because I was diagnosed in high school with mild dyslexia and ADD. This film is about people discussing what their lives were like having learning problems. $125.00

Video

7510 **What About Me?**

Educational Productions
9000 SW Gemini Drive
Beaverton, OR 97008 **503-644-7000**
800-950-4949
FAX: 503-350-7000
e-mail: custserve@edpro.com
www.edpro.com

Linda Freedman, President/Co-Owner
Molly Krumm, Marketing Director

This video focuses on two siblings of children with disabilities. The siblings (Brian and Julie) share their perspectives, their worries, concerns and victories about living with a sibling with a disability.

7511 **What Can Baby Hear?: Auditory Tests and In terventions for Infants with Multiple Disabilities**

Brookes Publishing
PO Box 10624
Baltimore, MD 21285 **410-337-9580**
800-638-3775
FAX: 410-337-8539
e-mail: custserv@brookespublishing.com
www.brookespublishing.com

This video and accompanying booklet explain the principles and methods of various auditory tests designed for early detection and teach viewers how to assess infants' auditory needs to begin appropriate intervention. *$45.00*

30 Minutes 1997
ISBN 1-557662-88-6

7512 **What School Personnel Should Know About Asthma**

American Lung Association
61 Broadway
New York, NY 10017 **212-315-8700**
FAX: 212-315-8700
e-mail: info@lungusa.org
www.lungusa.org

Professionally produced videotape discussing the triggers, symptoms and management of childhood asthma.

Video

7513 **When Billy Broke His Head...and Other Tales of Wonder**

Fanlight Productions
4196 Washington Street
Suite 2
Boston, MA 02131 **617-469-4999**
800-937-4113
FAX: 617-469-3379
e-mail: info@fanlight.com
www.fanlight.com

Elena Cambio

When Billy Golfus, an award-winning journalist, became brain damaged as the result of a motor scooter accident, he joined the ranks of the 43 million Americans with disabilities, this country's largest and most invisible minority. He helped create this video, which blends humor with politics and individual experience with a chorus of voices, to explain what it is really like to live with a disability in America. #136 *$195.00*

ISBN 1-57295 -36-2

7514 When I Grow Up

Britannica Film Company
345 4th Street
San Francisco, CA 94107 **415-777-9876**

At a costume party each child was to come as what they wanted to be when they grew up. Some of the children had handicaps, and they talked about why their handicaps would not prevent them from fulfilling their desires.

Film

7515 When Parents Can't Fix It

Fanlight Productions
4196 Washington Street
Suite 2
Boston, MA 02131 **617-469-4999**
800-937-4113
FAX: 617-469-3379
e-mail: fanlight@fanlight.com
www.fanlight.com

Karen McMillen, Marketing Director
Cynthia Conti, Publicity Coordinator

This documentary looks at the lives of five families who are raising children with disabilities - the problems they face, how they have learned to cope, and the rewards and stresses of adapting to their child's condition. It explores the medical complexities and financial pressures families encounter, the emotional and physical toll on parents and siblings, and the dangers of child abuse in this population. It offers a very realistic look at different family strengths and coping styles. *$245.00*

7516 When the Brain Goes Wrong

Fanlight Productions
4196 Washington Street
Suite 2
Boston, MA 02131 **617-469-4999**
800-937-4113
FAX: 617-469-3379
e-mail: info@fanlight.com
www.fanlight.com

Elena Cambio, Contact

An extraordinary and provocative series of seven short films which profile individuals with a range of brian dysfunctions. The seven brief segments focus on schizophrenia, manic depression, epilepsy, head injury, headaches and addiction. In addition to the personal stories, the segments include interviews with physicians who speak briefly about what is known about the disorders and treatment. #131 *$245.00*

ISBN 1-572951-31-1

7517 Why My Child

800-313-ABDC
www.birthdefects.org

A 9 1/2 minute video that explores the feelings every parent has when their child is born with a birth defect. Emmy-award-winning producer, Karen Dorsett, has created a compelling video that begins with the parents' question, why my child? Follows through to concerns about links between birth defects and environmental exposures to drugs, pesticides, dioxin, radiation, hazardous wastes, etc. *$25.00*

7518 Why Won't My Child Pay Attention?

Western Psychological Services
12031 Wilshire Boulevard
Los Angeles, CA 90025 **310-478-2061**
800-648-8857
FAX: 310-478-7838

Practical and reassuring videotape, noted child psychologist tells parents about two of the most common and complex problems of childhood: inattention and hyperactivity. *$49.50*

Video

7519 With Standing Ovation

Aquarius Health Care Videos
5 Powderhouse Lane
PO Box 1159
Sherborn, MA 01770 **508-651-2963**
FAX: 508-650-4216
e-mail: aqvideos@tiac.net
www.aquariusproductions.com

Profiles two dynamic young people, Peaches and Daniel, who were born with severe congenital limb deformities; spent much of their time as children in hospitals learning to use mechanical prostheses to aid them in their daily activities. Despite the training however, both shed the devices and mastered active and creative lives with only a minimal reliance on their prostheses. Encourages health care providers to view their occupational therapy and rehabilitation patients as people with abilities. *$195.00*

Video

7520 Without Pity

Aquarius Health Care Videos
5 Powderhouse Lane
PO Box 1159
Sherborn, MA 01770 **508-651-2963**
FAX: 508-650-4216
e-mail: aqvideos@tiac.net
www.aquariusproductions.com

This HBO documentary, narratd by Christopher Reeve, celebrates the eggorts of the disabled to live full, productive lives. We meet a cross section of Americans. A young woman with cerebral palsy cares for her baby, while a man with cerebral palsy lives successfully on his own after forty years in an institution. We go to tschool with a remarkable 6-year-old without arms or legs, visit the workplace of a blind computer expert and meet a professor with polio. Preview option is available. *$129.00*

Video

7521 Work Sight

Lighthouse International
111 E 59 Street
New York, NY 10022 **212-821-9737**
800-829-0500
FAX: 212-821-9706
e-mail: info@lighthouse.org

Joanna Mellor, VP Information Services

Intended for employers and employees who have concerns about vision loss and job performance. *$25.00*

7522 **World Through Their Eyes**

Lighthouse International
111 E 59 Street
New York, NY 10022
212-821-9737
800-829-0500
FAX: 212-821-9706
e-mail: info@lighthouse.org

Joanna Mellor, VP Information Services

Intended to help nursing home staff understand how residents with impaired vision perceive the world. Concrete suggestions help staff provide better care to visually impaired residents. *$25.00*

Web Sites

7523 **Abledata**

disabilities.about.com/health/disabili

Premier source for information on assistive technology.

7524 **Ablewear Aids for Daily Living**

www.ableware.com

Quality products to achieve independence in performing daily living activities.

7525 **Academy for Educational Development**

www.aed.org

Committed to addressing human development needs in the United States and throughout the world.

7526 **Access Unlimited**

e-mail: webmaster@accessunlimited.com
accessunlimited.com

Adaptive transportation and mobility equipment for people with disabilities.

7527 **Ai Squared**

www.aisquared.com

Leaders in low vision software.

7528 **Alternatives in Education for the Hearing Impaired (AEHI)**

www.aehi.org

AEHI fosters literacy and empowers people with hearing impairments to achieve their full potential through unique educational options.

7529 **American Academy of Audiology**

www.audiology.org

7530 **American Association of People with Disabilities**

www.aapd.com

Non-profit, non-partisan, cross-disability, national membership organization whose goals are unity, leadership and impact. AAPD's mission is to advance the economic and political power of all people with disabilities.

7531 **American Botanical Council**

www.herbalgram.org

Conducts research and provides education on the safe, responsible and scientific uses of medicine herbs to the public, healthcare professionals, government, industry, and the media.

7532 **American College of Rheumatology Research and Education Foundation**

e-mail: ref@rheumatology.org
www.rheumatology.org

Arthritis afflictsone in every seven Americans. Your gift supports research, investigates the causes, improves treatment and works toward the prevention and cure of arthritis.

7533 **American Liver Foundation**

www.liverfoundation.org

Is the only national voluntary health organization dedicated to preventing, treating, and curing hepatitis and other liver and gall bladder diseases through research and education.

7534 **American Mobility Personal Mobility Solutions**

e-mail: info@americanmobility.com
www.americanmobility.com

Source of Pride Scooters, Jazzy Power Chairs, personal mobility vehicles, and lift and recline chairs.

7535 **American Speech-Language and Hearing Association**

www.asha.org

Exhibits by companies specializing in alternative and augmentative communications products, publishers, software and hardware compinies, and hearing aid testing equipment manufacturers.

7536 **Americans with Disabilities Act ADA Home Page**

www.usdoj.gov

Provides facts on the Americans with Disabilities Act and other information relating to disability rights.

7537 **Appliance 411**

appliance411.com

A guide to remodeling and appliances for people with disabilities.

7538 Arc of the United States

e-mail: info@thearc.org
www.thearc.org

National organization of and for people with mental retardation anad thier families.

7539 Assist.com

www.assist.com

Assistive technology web resource.

7540 Assistive Technology Disabilities

www.netins.net

Provides information on assistive technology.

7541 Association for the Cure of Cancer of the Prostate

e-mail: hsoule@capcure.org
www.capcure.org.il

CURE is a nonprofit public charity that is dedicated to supporting prostate cancer research and hastening the conversion of research into cures or controls.

7542 Asthma and Allergy Foundation of America

www.aafa.org

Supports research to cure asthma and allergies and helps sufferers through patient education, practical advice, and a nationwide chapter and support group network.

7543 Audiology Foundation of America

www.audfound.org

Commited to fostering the education and training of audiologists to meet the needs of the public, especially those with impaired hearing.

7544 Auditory-Verbal International

www.auditory-verbal.org

7545 Beebe Center

www.beebecenter.org

At the Beebe center our mission is to help hearing-impaired children to listen and talk.

7546 Cancer Biotherapy Research Group

members.aol.com/cancerccsi

Cancer patients receive promising treatments in their communities through a nationwide research network of physicians and hospitals. All contributions are used to fund clinical research.

7547 Cancer Immunology Research Foundation

e-mail: concern@cwix.com
www.cancer-research.org

Immunology research will discover why the immune system fails and cancer develops. Herein lies the cure for cancer, AIDS, and other autoimmune diseases.

7548 Cancer Immunotherapy and Gene Therapy Institute

www.skcc.org

Researches effective, non-toxic therapies for cancer. Accelerates taking promising discoveries from the laboratories to clinics to treat people victimized by cancer. Treatments given at no charge.

7549 Cancer Research Fund of Damon Runyon: Walter Winchell Foundation

e-mail: crfinfo@cancerresearchfund.org
www.cancerresearchfund.org

Goal is to cure cancer. 100% of your gift funds research. With 49 Runyon-Winchell scientists who have won Nobel Prizes, chances are good.

7550 Center on the Social & Emotional Foundations for Early Learning

csefel.uiuc.edu

The center will: focus on promoting the social and emotional developmental of children as a means of preventing challenging behaviors; collaborate with existing T/TA providers for the purpose of ensuring the implementation and sustainability of practices at the local level; provide ongoing identification of training needs and preferred delivery formats of local programs and T/TA providers; disseminate evidence-based practices.

7551 Disability Information and Resources

www.eskimo.com

7552 Disability Mall

www.disabilityproducts.com

Online directory committed to featuring information on disability and medical products, resources and services, with over 2,500 links including over 400 companies for one-stop shopping convenence.

7553 Disability Net

www.bargione.co.uk/disabled.htm

The internet resource for disabled people that offers the latest news and events.

7554 Disability Rights Activist

www.disrights.org

Provides information to enable anyone intersted in the rights of disabled people to work for those rights.

7555 **DisabilityResources.org**

www.disabilityresources.org

Provides information on disability-related material on the Web.

7556 **Discover Technology**

discovertechnology.com

Provides links to websites that are specifically geared toward persons with disabilities who have special interest in adaptive technology.

7557 **Dynamic Living**

www.dynamic-living.com

Kitchen products, bathroom helpers, and unique daily living products that provide a convienient, comfortable, and safe environment for people with disabilities.

7558 **Exploring Autism: A Look at the Genetics of Autism**

www.exploringautism.org

Dedicated to helping families who are living with the challenges of autism stay informed about the exciting breakthroughs involving the genetics of autism. Report and explain new genetic research findings. Explain genetic principles as they relate to autism, provide the latest research news, and seek your imput.

7559 **Federal Resource Center for Special Education**

www.dss.org

7560 **Foundation Fighting Blindness**

www.blindness.org

Largest voluntary, non-government sponsor to cure retinitis pigmentosa (RP), macular degeneration and related inherited disorders—leading causes of blindness and deaf-blindness.

7561 **Freedom Scientific**

www.hj.com

Assistive technology for blind and visually impaired computer users.

7562 **Gallaudet University Press**

www.gallaudet.edu

Kendall Green

Source for titles on deafness and deaf related subjects.

7563 **Glaucoma Research Foundation**

e-mail: info@glaucoma.org
www.glaucoma.org

Yuko Madono, Outreach/Public Relations

Protecting both sight and independence for those with glaucoma, by providing improved treatments and education today and by leading research towards a cure for tomarrow.

7564 **Herb Research Foundation**

e-mail: info@herbs.org
www.herbs.org

Research and public education on the health benefits of medicinal plants. Dedicated to world health through the informed use of herbs.

7565 **Hypokalemic Periodic Paralysis Resource Page**

e-mail: editor@calexplorer.com
www.periodicparalysis.org/PPRC/PP

Provides understandable information on HKPP, dynamia linkage to several additional sources of helpful information on the Internet, and offers several online networking opportunities.

7566 **Innovation Management Group**

e-mail: cs@imgpresents.com
www.imgpresents.com

Jerry Hussong, VP Sales/Marketing

US and international onscreen keyboards, Word Prediction, Switch Scanning, Hover and Dwell, Joystick emulation, and Magnification software programs.

7567 **Interstitial Cystitis Association**

e-mail: icamail@ichelp.org
www.ichelp.com

Providing information, support and assistance to the patients of Interstitial Cystitis, a highly debilitating bladder disease. We'll find a cure by funding and encouraging research.

7568 **LDOnLine**

www.ldonline.org

The interactive guide to learning disabilities for parents, teachers, and children.

7569 **Learning Disabilities Association of America (LDA)**

e-mail: ldanatl@usaor.net
www.ldanatl.org

Our purpose is to advance the education and general welfare of children and adults of normal or potentially normal intelligence who manifest disabilities of a perceptual, conceptual, or coordinative nature.

7570 **Lyme Disease Foundation**

e-mail: lymefnd@aol.com
www.lyme.org

Provides critical information about tick-borne disease prevention, improves healthcare and funds research for solutions. 500,000 children, adults, and professionals assisted 25 countries.

7571 Mainstream Online Magazine of the Able-Disabled

e-mail: webmaster@mainstream-mag.com
www.mainstream-mag.com

The leading news, advocacy and lifestyle magazine for people with disabilities.

7572 Med-Sell

www.kansas.net/~cbaslock/classifi

Helps people buy and sell new and previously owned medical equipment and find accessible housing.

7573 Medem Network Societies American Academy of Opthamology

www.medem.com

Physician web site service empowered by the leading medical specialty societies.

7574 Microsoft Accessibility Technology for Everyone

microsoft.com/enable/

Information about accessibility features and options included in Microsoft products.

7575 MossRehab ResourceNet

www.mossresourcenet.org

Accessible travel, disability fact sheets, ADA, newsgroups, search tools.

7576 Multiple Sclerosis National Research Institute

e-mail: ms-research@ms-national-research.org
www.ms-national-research.org

Conducts research for development of a vaccine to halt progression of mutiple sclerosis. Initial patient trials show promising results. Help us find a cure soon.

7577 National Alliance of the Disabled (NAOTD)

www.naotd.org

Premier source for information on assistive technology.

7578 National Association for Visually Handicapped

www.navh.org

Works with millions of people worldwide in dealing with the difficulties of vision impairment.

7579 National Brain Tumor Foundation

e-mail: nbtf@braintumor.org
www.braintumor.org

Brain tumors strike children and adults in the prime of life. Your support gives help and gives hope by funding research and patient support services.

7580 National Business & Disability Council

www.business-disability.com

Works toward furthering the intersts of business and people with disabilities.

7581 National Organization on Disability

www.nod.org

7582 National Rehabilitation Center

www.naric.com

Serves both professionals and the general public intersted in disability and rehabilitation.

7583 National Women's Health Information Center

www.4women.gov

Provides information for women with disabilities, health professionals, researchers, and caretakers.

7584 NeuroControl Corporation

www.neurocontrol.com

Helps people with spinal cord injuries lead more independent lives.

7585 Osteogenesis Imperfecta Foundation

e-mail: bonelink@oif.org
www.oif.org

Bill Brander, Director Communications/Events

Strives to improve the quality of life for indivduals with this brittle bone disorder through research, education, awareness, and mutual support.

7586 Quantum Technology

www.quantech.com

Provides access to information and tools for independence to serve the visually impaired and those with a learning disability.

7587 Research!America

e-mail: info@researchamerica.org
www.researchamerica.org

Builds active public support for more government and private-industry research to find treatments and cures for both physical and mental disorders.

7588 Skin and Dental Dysfunction Foundation

www.nfed.org

Children left toothless from Ectodermal Dysplasia are provided dentures, support services and education. Established by National Foundation for Ectodermal Dysplasias which searches for a cure.

7589 **Social Security Online**

www.ssa.gov

Official website of the Social Secuirity Administration.

7590 **Special Clothes for Special Children**

www.special-clothes.com

A catalog of adaptive clothing for children with disabilities - helping boys and girls with special needs meet the world with pride and confidence since 1987.

7591 **V Foundation for Cancer Research**

e-mail: info@jimmyv.org
www.jimmyv.org

Named for basketball coach and broadcaster, Jim Valvano. The V Foundation funds critical stage research conducted by young researchers at NCI approved cancer research facilities.

7592 **ValueOptions**

e-mail: info@valueoptions.com
www.valueoptions.com

Serves over 22 million people in behavioral healthcare through publicaly funded, federal, and commercial contracts.

7593 **Wardrobe Wagon The Special Needs Clothing Store**

e-mail: info@wardrobewagon.com
www.wardrobewagon.com

Wearing apparel for individuals with special clothing needs.

7594 **We Magazine**

www.icdri.org/NEWS/WEMagazine.htm

Lifestyle magazine for people with disabilities.

7595 **We Media**

www.wemedia.com

Online network for people with disabilities.

7596 **WebABLE**

www.hisoftware.com/press/webable.html

Provides disability-related internet resources.

7597 **WheelchairNet**

www.wheelchairnet.org

7598 **World Association of Persons with Disabilities**

www.wapd.org

Dedicated to improving the quality of life for those with disabilities.

Associations

7599 Access to Sailing

19744 Beach Boulevard
Suite 340
Huntington Beach, CA 92648 **949-722-5371**
e-mail: dmilne@access2sailing.org
www.access2sailing.org

Duncan Milne, Founder

Sports association.

7600 Achilles Track Club

42 W 38th Street
4th Floor
New York, NY 10018 **212-354-0300**
FAX: 212-354-3978
e-mail: achillestc@aol.com

Leslie Winter, Executive Director

Organization whose goal is to guide disabled athletes into the able-bodied community. Quarterly newsletter has affiliate chapters in various cities overseas.

8 pages

7601 Adaptive Sports Center

PO Box 1639
Crested Butte, CO 81224 **970-349-2296**
866-349-2296
FAX: 970-349-4950
e-mail: info@adaptivesports.org
www.adaptivesports.org

Christopher Hensley, Director
Karen Render, Summer Program Director

Year round adaptive, adventure recreation program located at the base of Crested Butte Mountain Resort, Crested Butte ,CO. The Adaptive Sports Centers provides adaptive downhill and cross country ski lessons, ski rentals and snowboarding lessons in the winter. Offers a variety of wilderness based programs in the summer including multi-day trips into the back country, extensive cycling programs, canoeing, and white water rafting.

7602 American Hearing Impaired Hockey Association

1143 W Lake Street
Chicago, IL 60607 **312-226-5880**
FAX: 312-829-2098
e-mail: ahiha2@aol.com

Cheryl Hager, VP
Stan Mikita, President
Tom Schaffner, Executive Director

Supports hockey for hearing-impaired youths.

7603 American Wheelchair Bowling Association

6264 N Andrews Avenue
Fort Lauderdale, FL 33309 **954-491-2886**
FAX: 954-491-2886

Sports association.

7604 Blind Outdoor Leisure Development

PO Box M
Aspen, CO 81612 **970-923-0578**
800-530-3907
FAX: 970-923-7338
e-mail: possibilities@challengeaspen.com
www.challengeaspen.com

Outdoor recreation for the blind. Winter program of skiing with guides plus numerous summer programs for the visually impaired.

7605 Chesapeake Region Accessible Boating

1525 Grooms Lane
Woodstock, MD 27163 **410-461-8652**
FAX: 410-461-9151
e-mail: crabsailin@aol.com

Michael D Story, Executive Director

CRAB provides opportunities for the disabled and their friends to sail the Chesapeake Bay. Day sails, lessons, organized races. Call for charter information. Sail for free on the fourth Sunday of each month, May through October.

7606 Disabled Watersports Program Mission Bay Aquatic Center

1001 Santa Clara Plaza
San Diego, CA 92109 **858-488-1036**
FAX: 858-488-9625

Peter K Ballantyne, Program Manager
Marci Honstead, Program Coordinator

A cooperative, collegiate waterfront facility which is intended and designed to provide water-oriented programs and equipment and to be a resource center for water oriented sports and activities of all types, instructional and recreational. Since 1980, the center has offered aquatic activities for disabled individuals. This program serves hundreds of people yearly throughout the southwest United States and particularly San Diego, and serves as a model for similar programs.

7607 FORE! Future Opportunity for Recreation and Employment for the Handicapped

Southern California Golfing Association
3740 Cahuenga Boulevard
North Hollywood, CA 91604 **818-980-3630**
FAX: 818-980-1808
e-mail: info@scga.org
www.scga.org

Golfing association for the physically handicapped.

7608 Handicapped Scuba Association International

Handicapped Scuba Association
1104 Prado
San Clemente, CA 92672 **949-498-4540**
FAX: 949-498-6128
e-mail: hsa@hsascuba.com
www.hsascuba.com

Jim Gatacre, President

A nonprofit volunteer organization dedicated to improving the physical and social well being of those with special needs through the exhilarating sport of scuba diving. An educational program for able bodied scuba instructors to learn to teach and certify people with special needs. Accessible travel opportunities. Publishes quarterly newsletter.

7609 ISC: National Organization of People with Physical Disabilities

16 Liberty Street
Larkspur, CA 94939 **415-924-3549**
FAX: 415-927-9556
e-mail: russab@earthlink.net

Russ Bohlke, Executive Secretary

Providing opportunities for the handicapped to participate in accessible community activities is the objective of this service organization which has regional chapters in many states.

7610 **Lakeshore Foundation**

3800 Ridgeway Drive
Birmingham, AL 35209 **205-868-2303**
FAX: 205-868-2069
e-mail: jremick@ikshore.org
www.lakeshore.org

Offers fitness, recreation and competitive sports programs for persons with physical disabilities.

7611 **Leaning Tower YMCA: Conquerors Gym and Swim Program**

Leaning Tower YMCA
6300 W Touhy Avenue
Niles, IL 60714 **847-647-8222**
FAX: 847-647-7736
e-mail: leaningtower@ymcacommunity.net
www.ymcacommunity.net

Jerome Flosch, Assistant Aquatic Director
Nancy Friend, Volunteer Coord./Asst. Coach
Lucy Akers, Head Coach

Mission to support the spiritual, mental and physical well being of inviduals and families in order to improve their quality of life. Provides quality programs to meet the need of the individuals with and without disabilities.

7612 **National Skeet Shooting Association**

5931 Roft Road
San Antonio, TX 78253 **210-688-3371**
800-877-5338
FAX: 210-688-3014
www.nssa-nsca.com

Offers information on sporting clay targets for the disabled hunter.

7613 **Rehabilitation Institute of Chicago's Virginia Wadsworth Sports Program**

710 N Lake Shore Drive
Chicago, IL 60611 **312-908-6000**
FAX: 312-908-1051
e-mail: jjones02@rehabchicago.org
www.richealthfit.org

Jeff Jones, Director
Tom Richey, Sports Coordinator
Mitch Carr, Fitness Coordinator

RIC's Center for Health and Fitness is a full service fitness center for individuals with disablilties and the administrative offices for RIC's Wirtz Sports Program. Eighteen different sport and recreation programs are offered free of charge. The facility is adjacent to RIC's main building and also is the location of a branch of The National Center for Physical Activity and Disability (NCPAD), a joint project operated by the University of Illinois-Chigcago.

7614 **Special Olympics**

1325 G Street NW
Suite 500
Washington, DC 20005 **202-628-3630**
FAX: 202-824-0200
e-mail: soimail@aol.com
www.specialolympics.org

Timothy Shriver, President/CEO
Kim Elliott, COO
J Drake Turrentine, General Counsel

A year-round worldwide program that promotes physical fitness, sports training and athletic competition for children and adults with mental retardation.

7615 **US Hang Gliding Association**

PO Box 1330
Colorado Springs, CO 80903 **719-632-8300**
FAX: 719-632-6417
e-mail: ushga@ushga.org
www.ushga.org

Jayne Defanfilis, CEO

Offers information for the disabled about how they may learn to hang glide or paraglide or try the sports just once with a tandem flight.

7616 **USA Deaf Sports Federation**

3607 Washington Boulevard
 # 4
Ogden, UT 84403
FAX: 801-393-2263
www.usadsf.org

Bobbie Beth Scoggins, President
Valerie G Kinney, Administrative Assistant

Governing body for all deaf sports and recreation in the United States. Sixteen different sports organizations and 20 member clubs are affiliates of USADSF.

7617 **Wheelchair Motorcycle Association**

101 Torrey Street
Brockton, MA 02301 **508-583-8614**

Founded in 1975, after Scott Factor sustained injury resulting in paraplegia, this association offers information on all types of off-road vehicles for use by people with disabilities, also offers a newsletter.

Books

7618 **Adapted Physical Education National Standards**

Human Kinetics
PO Box 5076
Champaign, IL 61825
800-747-4457
FAX: 217-351-2674
e-mail: orders@hkusa.com
www.humankinetics.com

The book presents fifteen broad standards based on the responsibilities and perceived professional needs of practicing physical educators. Each standard is broken down into levels that include content that physical educators who work with individuals with disabilities should know, additional content for adapted physical educators, and sample applications that adapted physical educators should be able to demonstrate. *$28.00*

224 pages Paperback
ISBN 0-873229-62-2

7619 **Adapted Physical Education and Sport, 2nd Edition**

Human Kinetics
PO Box 5076
Champaign, IL 61825
800-747-4457
FAX: 217-351-2674
e-mail: orders@hkusa.com
www.humankinetics.com

Designed as a resource for both present and future physical education leaders, this book is an exceptional book for teaching exceptional children. It emphasizes the physical education of young people with disabilities. *$47.00*

472 pages
ISBN 0-873225-78-1

7620 Bold Tracks: Skiing for the Disabled

Johnson Books: A Cordillera Press Guide
1880 57th Center S
Boulder, CO 80301
800-258-5830
FAX: 303-443-1106
e-mail: books@jpcolorado.com

Richard Croog, Sales/Promotion

The first complete teaching and learning guide to skiing for the disabled. The guide is essential for instructor and student alike. Beginning with the basic American Teaching System and continuing through three-track and four-track methods, the manual covers skiing for the visually and hearing impaired as well as the physically and developmentally disabled. It includes glossaries of skiing and medical terms and tips for skin program development. *$24.95*

160 pages Paperback
ISBN 1-555661-14-9

7621 Conditioning with Physical Disabilities

Human Kinetics
PO Box 5076
Champaign, IL 61825
800-747-4457
FAX: 217-351-2674
e-mail: orders@hkusa.com
www.humankinetics.com

The first practical, authoritative exercise guide for people with all classifications and levels of physical disabilities. The authors share the successful strength and conditioning program they created at the highly regarded Rehabilitation Institute of Chicago - a pioneering program that is now the leading exercise approach for people with physical disabilities. *$22.95*

288 pages
ISBN 0-873226-14-3

7622 Disability and Sport

Human Kinetics
PO Box 5076
Champaign, IL 61825
800-747-4457
FAX: 217-351-2674
e-mail: orders@hkusa.com
www.humankinetics.com

This new book, written by leading experts in adapted physical education and disability sport, is intended to serve as a comprehensive reference about the disability sport world. Topics include adapted equipment, event management, women and disability sport, medical management of disabled athletes and research highlights. This book should serve as a valuable reference for disabled individuals and their families interested in sport, physical educators and medical personnel who work with disabled. *$40.00*

312 pages
ISBN 0-873228-48-0

7623 Exercise Activities for the Elderly

Springer Publishing Company
536 Broadway
New York, NY 10012
212-431-4370
877-687-7476
FAX: 212-941-7842
e-mail: marketing@springerpub.com
www.springerpub.com

Annette Imperati, Marketing/Sales Director

A variety of exercises geared to clients with such conditions as arthritis, diabetes and Parkinson's disease, and others which are designed to build up muscular strength and maintain flexibility. *$39.95*

224 pages Softcover
ISBN 0-826187-03-X

7624 Fitness Programming for Physical Disabilities

Human Kinetics
PO Box 5076
Champaign, IL 61825
800-747-4457
FAX: 217-351-2674
e-mail: orders@hkusa.com
www.humankinetics.com

A book offering information for developing and conducting exercise programs for groups that included people with physical disabilities. A dozen authorities in exercise science and adapted exercise programming explain how to effectively and safely modify existing programs for individuals with physical disabilities. *$32.00*

208 pages
ISBN 0-873224-34-5

7625 Guide to Wheelchair Sports and Recreation

Paralyzed Veterans of America
801 18th Street NW
Washington, DC 20006
202-872-1300
800-424-8200
888-860-7244
FAX: 301-843-0159
e-mail: info@pva.org
www.pva.org

PVA's new booklet has been produced in part through a generous grant from Everest & Jennings, Inc., to serve individuals as a resource guide to sports and recreation activities and equipment suppliers.

28 pages

7626 Inclusive Games

Human Kinetics
PO Box 5076
Champaign, IL 61825
800-747-4457
FAX: 217-351-2674
e-mail: orders@hkusa.com
www.humankinetics.com

Features more than 50 games, helpful illustrations, and hundreds of game variations. The book shows how to adapt games so that children of every ability level can practice, play and improve their movement skills together. The game finder makes it easy to locate an appropriate game according to its name, approximate grade level, difficulty within the grade level, skills required/developed, and number of players. *$14.95*

120 pages Paperback
ISBN 0-873226-39-9

7627 Physical Activity for Individuals with Mental Retardation

Human Kinetics
PO Box 5076
Champaign, IL 61825
800-747-4457
FAX: 217-351-2674
e-mail: orders@hkusa.com
www.humankinetics.com

The first movement-oriented text to cover the life span of people with mental retardation. Readers will discover the characteristics and unique needs of individuals with mental retardation. They will also become familiar with methodologies for facilitating fitness and movement competencies. *$33.00*

480 pages
ISBN 0-873223-61-6

7628 **Physical Fitness Testing of the Disabled**

Human Kinetics
PO Box 5076
Champaign, IL 61825
800-747-4457
FAX: 217-351-2674
e-mail: orders@hkusa.com
www.humankinetics.com

A physical fitness testing manual for selected disabled groups thanks to the research and professional teamwork of the authors. In this manual, they offer practitioners norm-referenced tests of physical fitness for youngsters with cerebral palsy, visual and auditory impairments, and spinoneuro-muscular conditions. *$25.00*

184 pages Spiral bound
ISBN 0-931250-45-7

7629 **Recreation & Sports**

Accent Books & Products
PO Box 700
Bloomington, IL 61702
309-378-2961
800-787-8444
FAX: 309-378-4420
e-mail: acmtlvng@aol.com

Raymond C Cheever, Publisher
Betty Garee, Editor

A guide to fun, excitement and travel offering options for disabled persons. Includes photos and sources of some special products. *$4.95*

65 pages Paperback
ISBN 0-91570-18-3

7630 **Sport Science Review: Adapted Physical Activity**

Human Kinetics
PO Box 5076
Champaign, IL 61825
800-747-4457
FAX: 217-351-2674
e-mail: orders@hkusa.com
www.humankinetics.com

This special issue addresses disability and sport. Researchers from diverse academic backgrounds and parts of the world review the issues and controversies surrounding inclusion in physical education and sport. The papers explore inclusion in school settings, the history of disability sport, psychological and sociological aspects of adapted physical activity, and the need to identify reliable classification systems. *$15.00*

96 pages
ISBN 0-736029-88-5

7631 **Sports & Recreation for the Disabled**

Exceptional Parent Library
120 Sylvan Avenue, Suite 10
PO Box 1807
Englewood Cliffs, NJ 07632
800-535-1910
FAX: 201-947-9376
e-mail: eplibrary@aol.com
www.eplibrary.com

A book designed to make dreams come true. *$32.00*

7632 **Sports and Exercise for Children with Chronic Health Conditions**

Human Kinetics
PO Box 5076
Champaign, IL 61825
800-747-4457
FAX: 217-351-2674
e-mail: orders@hkusa.com
www.humankinetics.com

Written by leading pediatric authorities, the practical guidelines in Sports and Exercise for Children with Chronic Health Conditions address these twenty common medical conditions: spina bifida, epilepsy, childhood progressive neuromuscular disease, cerebral palsy, childhood arthritis, asthma, cystic fibrosis, AIDS, hepatitis, hypertension, congenital heart disease-shunt lesions, congenital obstructive valvular heart disease, carditis, anemia, hemophilia and more. *$49.00*

392 pages Hardcover

7633 **Sports for the Handicapped**

Walker Publishing Company
435 Hudson Street
New York, NY 10014
212-727-8300
800-289-2553
FAX: 212-727-0984
e-mail: orders@walkerbooks.com
www.walkerbooks.com

This text outlines six sports that handicapped individuals may be able to participate in. Skiing, basketball, swimming, track and field, football and horseback riding are each presented. Each of the sports requirements are told by an athlete who is handicapped and who has excelled at the sport. At the end of the text is a good resource/reference guide for organizations that serve handicapped sports enthusiasts.

80 pages Hardcover

7634 **Tennis in a Wheelchair**

United States Tennis Association
707 Alexander Road
Princeton, NJ 08540
609-419-4418
FAX: 985-641-2267

A practical manual of tennis playing techniques for the wheelchair athlete. Included are sections on basic strokes from a wheelchair, wheelchair mobility, singles and doubles strategy, and more. Readers will discover how enjoyable and challenging the game of wheelchair tennis can be. *$3.75*

40 pages Illustrated

Exercise Devices

7635 **Abilitations**

1 Sportime Way
Atlanta, GA 30340
770-449-5700
800-850-8602
FAX: 800-845-1535
e-mail: orders@sportime.com

Ilana Danneman, Marketing Director

Catalog provides products to patients, therapists and parents to assist in maximizing functional levels through movement, cognition, recreation and positioning.

240 pages Quarterly

7636 **CC-M Productions**
8512 Cedar Street
Silver Spring, MD 20910
800-453-6280
FAX: 301-585-2321
e-mail: cc-m@cc-m.com
www.cc-m.com

Jon Abel, Marketing

Armchair Fitness video series. 4 cassettes: Armchair Fitness Aerobic, Armchair Fitness Gentle, Armchair Fitness Strength and Armchair Fitness Yoga. $29.95-$39.95.

$29.95 - $39.95

7637 **Equalizer 1000 Series**
Helm Distributing
1516 Nicholas Road
Dayton, OH 45418
937-268-7415
FAX: 937-268-9525
e-mail: helmdist@infinet.com
http://helm.hypermart.net/

Pruett B Helm, President/Owner

Weight training equipment designed with the wheelchair user in mind. *$7050.00*

7638 **Equalizer 5000 Home Gym**
Helm Distributing
1516 Nicholas Roadad
Dayton, OH 45418
937-268-7415
FAX: 937-268-9525
e-mail: helmdist@infinet.com
http://helm.hypermart.net

Pruett B Helm, President/Owner

Exercise machine for the able-bodied and the disabled, but specifically designed with a wheelchair user in mind. *$4250.00*

7639 **Equalizer Exercise Machines**
Helm Distributing
1516 Nicholas Roadad
Dayton, OH 45418
937-268-7415
FAX: 937-268-9525
e-mail: helmdist@infinet.com
http://helm.hypermart.net

Offers exercise and gym equipment for the disabled.

7640 **Freedom Ryder Handcycles**
Brike International
20589 SW Elk Horn Center
Tualatin, OR 97062
503-692-1029
800-800-5828

Mike Lofgren, President
Brian Stewart, VP

The finest handcycle in the world. The cycles incorporate body, lean steering and the finest bicycle components to make this a three-wheeled vehicle without equal. Suitable for both recreation and competition. *$1995.00*

7641 **Modular QuadDesk**
GPK
535 Floyd Smith Drive
El Cajon, CA 92020
800-468-8679
FAX: 619-593-7514
e-mail: rajesh@gpk.com
www.gpk.com

Rajesh Kanwar, President

Worktable specially dsigned for people in wheelchairs who lack grip strength, or cannot learn or reach. Small or medium.

7642 **Pedal-in-Place Exerciser**
Thoele Manufacturing
475 County Road 100 N
Montrose, IL 62445
217-924-4553
FAX: 217-924-4553

A great in-home exerciser that can benefit quadraplegics, paraplegics, stroke patients or anyone with limited use of their arms and legs.

7643 **Quad Commander**
GPK
535 Floyd Smith Drive
El Cajon, CA 92020
800-468-8679
FAX: 619-593-7514
e-mail: rajesh@gpk.com
www.gpk.com -or- www.quadriplegia.com

Rajesh Kanwar, President

Joystick for people with quadriplegia.

7644 **Seat-A-Robics**
PO Box 630064
Little Neck, NY 11363
800-484-7046
FAX: EXT- 11-30

Daria Alinovi, President

Offers a variety of safe, affordable and medically approved video exercise programs that are listed in our video chapter. In addition the company offers two resources. The first Healthy Eating & Facts For Kids is geared specifically to health professionals and educators that work with disabled children ($39.95). The second is a recreational resource guide that stimulates children to be creative and get involved. It keeps them actively engaged while having fun and getting fit ($29.95).

7645 **Uppertone**
GPK
535 Floyd Smith Drive
El Cajon, CA 92020
800-468-8679
FAX: 619-593-7514
e-mail: rajesh@gpk.com
www.gpk.com -or- www.quadriplegia.com

Rajesh Kanwar, President

Unassisted muscle strengthening and conditioning system for quads. *$2495.00*

7646 **Versatrainer**
PRO-MAX/Division of Bow-Flex of America
2200 NE 65th Avenue
 # C
Vancouver, WA 98661
800-BOW-FLEX
FAX: 360-993-3610
www.boflex.com

One exercise system for the disabled person that does everything. Incorporates full body strength, muscle development, cardiovascular conditioning, gives full muscle movement and balanced muscle development.

Periodicals

7647 **Access to Recreation**

8 Sandra Court
Newbury Park, CA 91320

805-498-7535
800-634-4351
FAX: 805-498-8186
e-mail: dkrebs@accesstr.com
www.accesstr.com

Don Krebs, President

The Access to Recreation catalog is full of recreation and exercise equipment. One can find items such as electric fishing reels and other fishing and hunting equipment for the disabled sportsman. There are also adapted golf clubs, swimming pool lifts, wheelchair gloves and cuffs and bowling equipment. There are devices to help with embroidery, knitting and card playing, videos, books and practical aides such as wheelchair ramps and book.

64 pages Bi-Annually

7648 **Adapted Aquatics: Swimming for Persons with Physical or Mental Impairments**

American Red Cross
2131 K Street NW
Washington, DC 20037

202-728-6400
FAX: 202-728-6647
e-mail: nccteck@usa.redcross.org
www.redcross.org

Magazine for disabled swimmers.

7649 **Outrigger**

National Sports Center for the Disabled
PO Box 1290
Winter Park, CO 80482

970-726-1540
FAX: 970-726-4112
e-mail: info@nscd.org
www.nscd.org

Gigi Doming, Operations Manager

Free newsletter with information and tips for adaptive skiing and other mountain sports for people with disabilities.

6-8 pages Quarterly

7650 **PALAESTRA: Forum of Sport/PE/Recreation for Those with Disabilities**

Challenge Publications, Limited
PO Box 508
Macomb, IL 61455

309-833-1902
FAX: 309-833-1902
e-mail: challpub@macomb.com
www.palaestra.com

Julian Stein, Associate Editor
David Beaver, Editor In Chief

The most comprehensive resource on sport, physical education and recreation for individuals with disabilities, their parents and professionals in the field of adapted physical activity. Published in cooperation with US Paralympics and AAHPERD's Adapted Physical Activity Council. Informative yet entertaining and delivers valuable insights for consumers, families and professionals in the field. Published quarterly.

Skiing

7651 **National Sports Center for the Disabled**

PO Box 1290
Winter Park, CO 80482

970-726-1540
FAX: 970-726-4112
e-mail: info@nscd.org
www.nscd.org

Innovative non-profit organization that provides year-round recreation for children and adults with disabilities. The world's largest adaptive ski program, teaching 25,000 lessons per winter at Winter Park Resort, Colorado. Also snowboarding, ski racing, showshoeing, cross-country skiing. Summer sports: rafting, sailing, camping, hiking, hand cycling, mountain biking, tandem biking, in-line skating, horseback riding, fishing, rock climbing. Sports symposium and clinics.

Products & Programs

7652 **Aerospace Compadre**

Aerospace America
900 Truman Parkway
Suite 189
Bay City, MI 48706

989-684-2121
FAX: 989-684-4173

Murray Sutherland, President

Fully customized golf cart type vehicle for the physically impaired person. Fully equipped with hand controls, wheelchair rack, storage racks, head and tail lights and full safety belts. *$2500.00*

7653 **Basketball: Beeping Foam**

Maxi Aids
42 Executive Boulevard
Suite 3209
Farmingdale, NY 11735

631-752-0521
800-522-6294
FAX: 631-752-0689
TTY:516-752-0738
e-mail: sales@max.aids.com
www.maxiaids.com

Customer Service

This sound making basketball enables the visually impaired to play basketball or other games. *$29.95*

7654 **Bounce Back**

Access to Recreation
8 Sandra Court
Newbury Park, CA 91320

805-498-7535
800-634-4351
FAX: 805-498-8186
e-mail: dkrebs@accesstr.com
www.accesstr.com

Don Krebs, President

7655 **Bowling: Ball Ramp**

Cleo of New York
S Buckout Street
Trent Building
Irvington, NY 10533

800-321-0595

Bowling devices for wheelchair occupants. *$109.00*

7656 Center for Health and Fitness

710 N Lake Shore Drive
Chicago, IL 60671 **312-908-7532**
FAX: 312-908-1051
e-mail: mcsport@megsinet.net

Jeff Jones, Director
Tom Rishey, Sports Coordinator

Provides free sports and programs to individuals with physical disabilities in the greater Chicago area. Programs in 16 different sports including center for health and fitness which provides exercise opportunities seven days a week.

7657 Challenge Golf

Motivation Media
1245 Milwaukee Avenue
Glenview, IL 60025 **847-808-0717**
FAX: 847-297-6829

Dorothy Bauer, Coordinator

A plain-language video, Challenge Golf is packed with information for beginners or veterans. Peter Longo covers 5 handicaps (one-arm, one-leg, in a seated position, blind, and arthritis) clearly and concisely, on how to play golf with a physical disability. In color, complete with special effects, graphs and real handicapped golfers at play. *$38.95*

Home Edition

7658 Disabled Sports USA, Far West

Tahoe Adaptive Ski School
PO Box 9780
Truckee, CA 96162 **530-581-4161**
FAX: 530-581-3127
e-mail: info@dsusafw.org
www.dsusafw.org

Katherine Rodriguez, VP
Haakon Lang-Ree, Program Director
Cindy Smith, Office Manager

Snow ski and snowboard lessons for people with disabilities. December through April. Two and a half hour lesson, adaptive equipment and beginner lift ticket: $50 midweek. Summer programs include: Water Skiing, Whitewater Rafting, Cycling, 4WD Backcountry Access and Kayaking.

7659 EasyStand 6000 Glider

Access to Recreation
8 Sandra Court
Newbury Park, CA 91320 **805-498-7535**
800-634-4351
FAX: 805-498-8186
e-mail: dkrebs@accesstr.com
www.accesstr.com

Don Krebs, President

Provides dynamic leg motion for individuals who are unable to stand upright or walk on their own.

7660 Fairway Spirit Adaptive Golf Car: Model 4852

Fairway Golf Cars
W220 N507 Springdale Road
Suite G
Waukesha, WI 53186 **262-522-0822**
888-320-4850
FAX: 262-542-4258

John Perez, Sales/Marketing Director
Cheryl Tesch, Executive Assistant

Fairway Spirt is designed to allow access to all aspects of the game of golf- even greens and tee. Spirit 4850 features a 48 volt electronic system to provide unsurpassed power, range and speed. Couple the drive system performance with ergonomic features like an adjustable seat with flip up arm rests, 360 degree swivel and an adjustable tilter position.

7661 Golf Xpress

eMotorsports
4275 County Line Road #214
Chalfont, PA 18914 **215-997-9555**
877-494-6532
FAX: 215-997-9560
e-mail: dplabowsky@aol.comm
www.golfxpress.com

Don Labowsky, President

Patented single-rider adaptive golf cart allows you to play golf seated or supported. Hit woods, irons, and putt from the car. Drives onto tees and greens and into traps without damaging the course.

7662 High Adventure Hang Gliding

4231 Sepulveda Avenue
San Bernardino, CA 92404 **909-883-8488**
FAX: 909-883-8488
e-mail: robndi@flytandem.com

Rob McKenzie, Tandem Instructor

Tandem adventures.

7663 National Sports Center for the Disabled

PO Box 1290
Winter Park, CO 80482 **970-726-1540**
FAX: 970-726-4112
e-mail: info@nscd.org
www.nscd.org

Gigi Glass Domingy, Operations Manager

Innovative non-profit organization that provides year-round recreation for children and adults with disabilities. The world's largest adaptive ski program, teaching 25,000 lessons per winter at Winter Park Resort, Colorado. Also snowboarding, ski racing, showshoeing, cross-country skiing. Summer sports: rafting, sailing, camping, hiking, hand cycling, mountain biking, tandem biking, in-line skating, horseback riding, fishing, rock climbing. Sports symposium and clinics.

7664 Rickshaw Exerciser

Access to Recreation
8 Sandra Court
Newbury Park, CA 91320 **805-498-7535**
800-634-4351
FAX: 805-498-8186
e-mail: dkrebs@accesstr.com
www.accesstr.com

Don Krebs, President

This Exerciser develops the muscle used most by those in wheelchairs. It develops the strength you need to lift yourself for pressure relief, doing transfers and pushing your wheelchair.

7665 Sailing Fascination

4010 Park Newport
Apartment 224
Newport Beach, CA 92660 **949-640-1678**
FAX: 949-760-8650
e-mail: bbg2506@webtv.net

Jack W Hester, President
Tom Tolbert, VP

Sailing Fascination provides sailing programs for anyone who is disabled. A non profit educational and charitable California State Corp. with an all volunteer staff, officers, and directors. Year round sailing classes are held on a 24 foot sailboat that is equipped to be accessible to the disabled student sailor.

7666 Wheelchair Roller

Access to Recreation
8 Sandra Court
Newbury Park, CA 91320
805-498-7535
800-634-4351
FAX: 805-498-8186
e-mail: dkrebs@accesstr.com
www.accesstr.com

Don Krebs, President

The McClain Wheelchair Roller allows you to build strength and stamina in the comfort of your own home.

General

7667 AAN's Toll-Free Hotline
National Allergy and Asthma Network
2751 Prosperity Avenue
Suite 150
Fairfax, VA 22031
800-878-4403
FAX: 703-573-7794
www.aanma.org

Offers answers to questions regarding allergies and asthma, provides referrals and support to assist the patient and his or her family.

7668 American SIDS Institute
2480 Windy Hill Road
Suite 380
Marietta, GA 30067
770-612-1030
800-232-7437
FAX: 770-612-8277
www.sids.org

Betty McEntire PhD, Executive Director

Hotline for information on Sudden Infant Death Syndrome. Offers research, clinical services, education and family support/counseling.

7669 American Speech-Language-Hearing Association
10801 Rockville Pike
Rockville, MD 20852
301-897-5700
800-638-8255
FAX: 301-897-7348
e-mail: actioncenter@asha.org
www.asha.org

Joanne Jessen, Publications Director
Frederick T Spahr PhD, Executive Director
John E Bernthal, President

Hotline for the speech and hearing impaired.

7670 Anchor Houses
1212 Monroe Street NW
Washington, DC 20010
202-832-5555
FAX: 202-832-8216

Francis Palilkarambi

Offers support groups and services such as: counseling, case management, advocacy for financial entitlements and more for individuals and families dealing with mental illness.

7671 Arthritis Foundation Information Hotline
PO Box 7669
Atlanta, GA 30357
800-283-7800
FAX: 404-872-9559
e-mail: help@arthritis.org
www.arthritis.org

Offers information and referrals, counseling, physicians information and more to persons living with arthritis.

7672 Aurora of Central New York
518 James Street
Syracuse, NY 13203
315-422-7263
FAX: 315-422-4792
TTY:315422974692
e-mail: auroracny@aol.com

Professional counseling services to assist individuals and their families deal with the trauma of hearing or vision loss.

7673 Autism Society of America
7910 Woodmont Avenue
Suite 300
Bethesda, MD 20814
301-657-0881
800-3AU-TISM
FAX: 301-657-0869
www.autism-society.org

ASA is the largest and oldest grassroots organization within the autism community, with more than 200 chapters and over 20,000 members and supporters nationwide. ASA is the leading source of education, information and referral about autism and has been the leader in advocacy and legislative initiatives for more than three decades.

7674 Braille Institute Orange County Center
527 N Dale Avenue
Anaheim, CA 92801
714-821-5000
800-272-4553
FAX: 714-527-7621
www.brailleinstitute.org

A toll free information and referral service where callers can obtain information about community programs and referrals to organizations serving the blind in their local areas.

7675 Camp New Hope
PO Box 764
Mattoon, IL 61938
217-895-2341
FAX: 217-895-3658
e-mail: cnhinc@rri.net
www.campnewhope.com

Kim Carmack, Executive Director
Terri Taylor, Program Coordinator

Offers advocacy services, social and recreational services and a summer camp for the disabled.

7676 Cancer Information Service
National Cancer Institute
6116 Executive Boulevard
Suite 3036A
Bethesda, MD 20892
800-422-6237
www.nci.nih.gov

A nationwide network of 19 regional field offices supported by the National Cancer Institute which provides accurate, up-to-date information on cancer to patients and their families, health professionals and the general public. The CIS can provide specific information in understandable language about particular types of cancer, as well as information on second opinions and the availability of clinical trials.

7677 Clearinghouse on Disability Information
Office of Special Education & Rehabilitative Svcs
330 C Street SW
Room 3132
Washington, DC 20202
202-205-8241
FAX: 202-401-2608
www.ed.gov/OFFICE/OSERS

Carolyn Corlett, Director

The Clearinghouse provides information to people with disabilities or anyone requesting information, by doing research and providing documents in response to inquiries. The information provided includes areas of federal funding for disability-related programs. Clearinghouse staff is trained to serve as experts in referring requests to other sources of disability-related information, if necessary.

7678 Community Connections
801 Pennsylvania Avenue SE
 # 201
Washington, DC 20003
202-726-2756
FAX: 202-544-5365

Offers support groups and support systems for adults with mental and emotional disabilities.

7679 Community Support Center
13301 Bruce B Downs Boulevard
Tampa, FL 33612
813-228-6724
FAX: 813-250-0941

Cecil Woodside, CSC Division Dir.

Provides an alternative to institutionalization for persons 18 years to 55 years of age, with a mental disability. There are approximately 60 staff members and daily census for clients is about 600.

7680 Community and Support Services
33-R Water Street
Guilford, CT 06437
860-347-4465
FAX: 860-346-6813

Roberta Hurley, Manager

Operate 15 programs at various sites. The services offer development of programs to meet individual needs and to engage in all types of activities which shall promote and foster more normal and independent lives for persons with disabilities.

7681 Compassionate Friends
PO Box 3696
Oak Brook, IL 60522
630-990-0010
877-969-0010
FAX: 630-990-0246
e-mail: nationaloffice@compassionatefriends.org
www.compassionatefriends.org

Patricia Loder, Executive Director

Peer support for bereaved parents, grandparents and siblings, offering 600 chapters in the United States. The organization also offers a quarterly magazine, We Need Not Wake Alone, and TCF resources of booklets, tapes and brochures for the bereaved parent, grandparent and sibling.

7682 Consumer and Patient Information Hotline
Prevent Blindness America
500 E Remington Road
Schaumburg, IL 60173
847-843-8458
800-331-2020
FAX: 847-843-2020
e-mail: info@preventblindness.org
www.preventblindness.org

Betsy van Die, Media Relations Director
Hugh R Parry, President/CEO
Daniel D Garrett, Senior VP

A toll-free line offering free information on a broad range of vision, eye health and safety topics including sports eye safety, diabetic retinopathy, glaucoma, cataracts, children's eye disorders and more.

7683 Cornerstone Services
777 Joyce Road
Joliet, IL 60436
815-741-7602
FAX: 815-723-1177
e-mail: jhogan@cornerstoneservices.org
www.cornerstoneservices.org

James A Hogan, President/CEO
Susan Murphy, Director of Human Resources

Cornerstone Services provides progressive, comprehensive services for people with disabilities, promoting choice, dignity and the opportunity to live and work in the community. Established in 1969, the agency provides developmental, vocational, employment, residential and mental health services at various community-based locations. The nonprofit social service agency helps approximately 750 people each day.

7684 Department of Ophthalmology Information Line
Eye & Ear Infirmary
1855 W Taylor Street
Chicago, IL 60612
773-ITR-AUMA

Offers eye clinic and physician referrals to persons suffering from vision disorders as well as offers emergency information.

7685 Dial-a-Hearing Screening Test
PO Box 1880
Media, PA 19063
610-544-7700
800-222-EARS
FAX: 610-543-2802
e-mail: dahst@aol.com

George Biddle, Executive Director

Hearing help information center. Provides toll free phone number for accurate telephone hearing screening test. Provides referral to audiologist or ear, nose and throat doctor. All services are free. Hours are 9 AM to 5 PM ET Monday to Friday.

7686 Disability Network
3600 S Dort Highway
Suite 54
Flint, MI 48507
810-742-1800
FAX: 810-742-2400
TTY:810-742-7647
e-mail: disnet@tir.com

Mike Zelley, Executive Director

The Disability Network offers the opportunity for everyone in the community to come together as a part of a working and growing system of support for persons with disabilities. This includes Peer Support, Information and Referral of Resources, Advocacy, Planning for Independent Living, and Americans with Disabilities Act Consultations.

7687 Disability and Health, National Center for Birth Defects and Developmental Disabilities
4770 Buford Highway NE
 # F-35
Atlanta, GA 30341
770-488-7080
FAX: 770-488-7075
TTY:770-488-7083
e-mail: ncehinfo@cdc.gov
www.cdc.gov/ncbddd/dh

Lisa Sinclair, Health Policy Analyst

Located within the new CDC, National Center for Birth Defects and Developmental Disabilities, the Disability and Health section, operates a ralatively small program that primarily supports: data collection on the prevalence of people with disabilities & their health status and risk factors for poor health and well-being; research on measures of disability, functioning and health; health promotion intervention studies; and dissemination of health information.

7688 Easter Seals
230 W Monroe Street
Suite 1800
Chicago, IL 60606
312-726-6200
800-221-6827
FAX: 312-726-1494
TTY:312-726-4258
e-mail: info@easter-seals.org
www.easter-seals.org

Joan Fishman, Marketing Manager
James Williams, President/CEO
Rosemary Garza, Resource/Information Specialist

Provides services that help children and adults with disabilities gain greater independence. Primary services medical rehabilitation, job training and employment, child care, adult day services, and camping and recreation benefit more than 1 million individuals and their families families each year through one of 450 center worldwide.

7689 Epilepsy Foundation for the National Capitol Area

4224 6th Street SE
Washington, DC 20032 **202-561-6114**

Sandra Coshner Weinstein

Offers information and referrals, support groups for dually diagnosed persons.

7690 Family Support Project for the Developmentally Disabled

N Central Bronx Hospital
3424 Kossuth Avenue, Room 15A10
Bronx, NY 10467 **718-519-5000**

Monica Sanabria, Project Coordinator

7691 Green Door

1623 16th Street NW
Washington, DC 20009 **202-462-4092**
FAX: 202-462-7562
e-mail: g1admin@aol.com

Judith Johnson, Executive Director
Brenda Randall, Program Director

Green Door is a community program which prepares people with a severe and persistent mental illness to live and work independently. Since 1976, Green Door has provided comprehensive services to mentally ill people-members, including housing, job training, job placement, education, homeless outreach, case management, support for people with substance abuse problems, family support,and specialized help for people who have had repeated hospitalizations.

7692 Head Injury Hotline

PO Box 84151
Seattle, WA 98124 **206-329-1371**
FAX: 206-624-4961
e-mail: brain@headinjury.com
www.headinjury.com

Disseminates head injury information and provides referrals to facilitate adjustment to life following head injury. Organizes seminars for professionals, head injury survivors, and their families.

7693 Headlines Support Group

Center for Community Re-entry
313 N Main Street
Rockford, IL 61101 **815-964-9555**
FAX: 815-962-6113

Pamela Solberg, Office Manageror

A local support group reaching northern Illinois and southern Wisconsin, for survivors and families of brain injury. The group helps survivors and families cope with awareness difficulties, social adjustment, and leisure awareness. The group shares information regarding head injuries and provides updates from the state and national associations. Headlines continually searches for new ideas, information and services which can help survivors fulfill their maximum potential.

7694 Human Policy Press

University Station
PO Box 35127
Syracuse, NY 13235 **315-443-2761**
800-894-0826
FAX: 315-443-4338
e-mail: thechp@sued.syr.edu
soeweb.syr.edu/thechp/HumanPolicyPress

Rachael Zubal-Ruggieri, Information Coordinator

Independent press started by the Center on Human Policy in 1974 to promote positive attitudes towards people with disabilities.

7695 International Braille and Technology Center for the Blind

National Federation of the Blind
1800 Johnson Street
Baltimore, MD 21230 **410-659-9314**
FAX: 410-685-5653
e-mail: nfb@iamdigex.net
www.nfb.org

Richard Ring, Director

World's largest and most complete evaluation and demonstration center of all assistive technology used by the blind from around the world. Includes all Braille, synthetic speech, print-to-speech scanning, internet and portable devices and programs. Available for tours by appointment to blind persons, employers, technology manufacturers, teachers, parents and those working in the assistive technology field.

7696 Job Opportunities for the Blind

National Federation of the Blind
1800 Johnson Street
Baltimore, MD 21230 **410-659-9314**
FAX: 410-685-5653
e-mail: nfb@iamdigex.net
www.nfb.org

Anthony Cobb, Director

A specialized service that provides free support, resources and information to blind persons seeking employment and to employers interested in hiring the blind. A partnership program with the US Department of Labor, this is the most successful program of its kind in helping blind persons find competitive work.

7697 Kaleidoscope Network

1777 NE Loop 410
Suite 300
San Antonio, TX 78217 **210-436-2611**
FAX: 210-829-1388
www.kALIVE.com

Phyllis Nichols, COO
Ron Dixon, President Programming Production

KALEIDOSCOPE Network, inc. (KNI) is a broadband, multimedia health and lifestyle company which produces and distributes television and on-line programming and content emphasizing health and wellness. KNI airs its programming on PAX Television with a reach to 73% of the country or 74 million households. KNI's interactive Web site provides authoritative health content, with links to its more than 240 health and disability-related National Advisory Board organizations.

7698 Kids on the Block Arthritis Programs

Arthritis Foundation
PO Box 7669
Atlanta, GA 30357
404-872-7100
800-283-7800
FAX: 404-872-9559
e-mail: help@arthritis.org
www.arthritis.org

State and local programs that use puppetry to help children understand what it is like for children and adults who have arthritis.

7699 Lighthouse International Information and Resource Service

111 E 59th Street
New York, NY 10022
212-821-9200
800-829-0500
FAX: 212-821-9705
e-mail: info@lighthouse.org
www.lighthouse.org

Provides information about eye diseases, low vision, age-related vision loss, adaptive technology, optical devices, large print and braille publishers, helps people find low vision services, vision rehabilitation services, and support groups across the U.S.; offers large selection of consumer products.

7700 Lung Line Information Service

National Jewish Center for Immunology
1400 Jackson Street
Denver, CO 80206
303-697-5095
800-222-LUNG
www.nationaljewish.org

Lynn Taussig, President

A free information service answering questions, sending literature and giving advice to patients with immunologic or respiratory illnesses. The Line is an educational service and not a substitute for medical care. Diagnosis or suggested treatment will not be provided for a caller's specific condition.

7701 Medic Alert Foundation, International

2323 Colorado Avenue
Turlock, CA 95382
209-668-3333
800-825-3785
FAX: 209-669-2495
e-mail: customer_service@medicalert.org
www.medicalert.org

Tanya Glazebrook, CEO/President

Emergency medallions and bracelets containing emergency medical information and 24-hour emergency information telephone services.

7702 Medicaid Information

7500 Security Boulevard
Baltimore, MD 21244
410-767-1686

Information about eligibility and benefits for needy citizens who require health care is available by contacting the Health Care Financing administration or by contacting the local public welfare office.

7703 Medicare Information

200 Independence Avenue SW
Washington, DC 20201
202-279-6002
www.medicare.gov

Eligibility and benefits for the health care of the older american is available by contacting the health care financing office.

7704 National AIDS Hotline

Centers for Disease Control and Prevention
Mailstop F07
1600 Clifton Road
Atlanta, GA 30333
800-342-2437
www.cdcnac.org

Offers free confidential information and publications on HIV infection and AIDS.

7705 National Association for Home Care

Val J Halomandaris
228 7th Street SE
Washington, DC 20003
202-547-7424
FAX: 202-547-3540
e-mail: subscription@nahc.org
www.nahc.org

This is a non-profit trade association representing various home care, hospice and health aid organizations. Website contains a section with information on how to choose a home care provider and a zip code driven locator for home care and hospice. Publishes monthly newsletter.

7706 National Association for Parents of Children with Visual Impairments (NAPVI)

PO Box 317
Watertown, MA 02472
617-972-7441
800-562-6265
FAX: 617-972-7444
e-mail: napvi@perkins.org
www.napvi.org

Susan LaVenture, Executive Director
Mary Zabelski, President
Lars Anderson, VP

In 1979, a group of parents responding to their own needs founded NAPVI, the National Association for Parents of the Visually Impaired, Inc. Never before was there a self-help organization specific to the needs of families of children with visual impairments. Since that time, NAPVI has grown and helped families across the US and in other countries.

7707 National Autism Hotline

Autism Services Center
605 9th Street
PO Box 507
Huntington, WV 25710
304-525-8014
FAX: 304-525-8026
www.autismservices.com

Ruth C Sullivan PhD, Director

Service agency for individuals with autism and developmental disabilities, and their families. Assists families and agencies attempting to meet the needs of individuals with autism and other developmental disabilities. Makes available technical assistance in designing treatment programs and more. The hotline provides informational packets to callers and assists via telephone when possible.

7708 National Child Safety Council

PO Box 1368
Jackson, MI 49204
517-764-6070
800-222-1464
FAX: 517-764-3069

Hotline.

7709 National Depressive and Manic Depressive Association

730 N Franklin Street
Suite 501
Chicago, IL 60610
312-642-0049
800-826-3632
FAX: 312-642-7243
www.ndmda.org

Lydia Lewis, Executive Director
April Robinson, Program Manager

Mission is to educate patients, families, professionals and the public concerning the nature of depressive and manic-depressive illnesses as treatable medical diseases; to foster self-help for patients and families; to eliminate discrimination and stigma; to improve access to care; and to advocate for research toward the elimination of these illnesses; to improve access to care; and to advocate for research toward the elimination of these illnesses.

7710 National Health Information Center

PO Box 1133
Washington, DC 20013
301-529-7770
800-336-4797
301-468-7394
e-mail: nhicinfo@health.org

Ramona Arnett, Project Director
Alison Telesford, Information Specialist

Identifies health information resources, channels requests for information to these resources and develops publications available for small handling fees.

7711 National Information Center for Health Related Services

University of South Carolina
First Benson
Columbia, SC 29208
803-777-7000
800-922-9236
e-mail: scsis@dccisc.edu

Hotline.

7712 National Institute of Child Health and Human Development

31 Center Drive
Building 31/Room 2A32
Bethesda, MD 20892
800-370-2943
FAX: 301-984-1473
e-mail:
NICHDInformationResourceCenter@mail.nih.gov
www.nichd.nih.gov

Government agency that supports and conducts research on topics related to the health of children, adults, families and communities; offers free materials and information.

7713 National Service Dog Center

Delta Society
580 Naches Avenue SW
Suite 101
Renton, WA 98055
425-226-7357
FAX: 425-235-1076
e-mail: info@deltasociety.org.com
www.deltasociety.org

Linda M Hines, President/CEO
Tamara Whitehall, Program Manager

A service of the Delta Society, provides information about the selection, training, stewardship, and roles of service dogs; referral to service dog training programs and related resources; education to businesses and health care professionals regarding service dog issues; research assistance through a resource library and network of professional experts and advocacy on behalf of people with service dogs.

7714 PALS Support Groups

Parent Professional Advocacy League
56 Temple Place
Suite 664
Boston, MA 02111
617-542-7860
800-537-0446
FAX: 617-542-7832
e-mail: pal@fcsn.org
www.ppal.net

Offers emotional support to parents and families of disabled children.

7715 PXE International

4301 Connecticut Avenue
Suite 404
Washington, DC 20008
202-362-9599
FAX: 202-966-8553
e-mail: info@pxe.org
www.pxe.org

Offers vital services to those with pseudoxanthoma elasticum, a connective tissue disorder causing calcification of connective tissue in various places throughout the body, often affecting the membrane behind the eye.

7716 Parent Assistance Network

Good Samaritan Health Systems
PO Box 1810
Kearney, NE 68848
308-865-2009
FAX: 308-865-2933
e-mail: sheilameyer@catholichealth.net

Sheila Meyer, Parent Assistance Service Coord

Provides information and emotional support to all parents and especially to parents of children with disabilities in the central Nebraska area. Ongoing activities include parent support group meetings, parent-to-parent networking and referrals and Respite Care provider trainings.

7717 Parent Support Network

Independence Square
500 Prospect Street
Pawtucket, RI 02860
401-728-7800
FAX: 401-727-2810
e-mail: mmhra@aol.com

Laure Turn, Director

Offers support groups for parents of children and adolescents with emotional/behavioral disabilities.

7718 Physician Referral and Information Line

Academy of Allergy, Asthma, Immunology
611 E Wells Street
Milwaukee, WI 53202
800-822-2762
FAX: 414-272-6070
e-mail: info@aaaai.org
www.aaaai.org

Referral line offering information on allergy and asthma, referral to an allergy/immunology specialist.

7719 Post-Polio Support Group

Hinsdale Hospital
120 N Oak Street
Hinsdale, IL 60521
630-856-7525
FAX: 630-856-7524
ahsmidwest.org

Information and support for polio patients and their families; meets the fourth Wednesday of each month.

7720 Prevent Child Abuse of Metropolitan Washington
PO Box 57194
Washington, DC 20037
202-223-0020
FAX: 202-296-4046
e-mail: pcamw@juno.com
www.pcamw.org

Kendra Dunn, Executive Director

Through public education, community partnerships and support services, PCAMW helps everyone play a role in prevention. We share information on prevention stategies and effective parenting at community forums and events and advocate for polices and services that keep children safe. We operate PhoneFriend, a telephone support line for children at home without adult supervision and conduct personal safety workshops in schools, camps and libraries. PhoneFriend support line: 202-223-2244.

7721 RET Project: (Rehabilitation Engineering Technology San Francisco State University
1600 Holloway Avenue
San Francisco, CA 94132
415-338-1333
FAX: 415-338-1501
e-mail: rgrott@sfsu.edu

Ray Grott, Director

This program provides assistive technology consultation, assessments, training and custom fabrication.

7722 Recorded Periodicals
Associated Services for the Blind
919 Walnut Street
Philadelphia, PA 19107
215-627-0600
FAX: 215-922-0692

John Corrigan, Manager

A subscription service of Associated Services for the Blind, these periodicals provide 21 magazines through this subscription service. A magazine list can be sent, in both large print and on audio cassette. *$18.00*

7723 Son-Rise Program
2080 S Undermountain Road
Sheffield, MA 01257
413-229-2100
800-714-2779
FAX: 413-229-3202
e-mail: sonrise@option.org
www.son-rise.org

Glenna Klein, Publicist

Internationally renowned and highly effective method for working with children challenged by autism, autism spectrum disorders, PDD and all other developmental difficulties. The program teaches parents, relatives, volunteers and professionals how to design and implement a child-centered, home-based educational program. Modality comprises an innovative and comprehensive system for learning and growth with specific impact in areas including eye contact, speech and communication and more.

7724 Special Children
1306 Wabash Avenue
Belleville, IL 62220
618-234-6876
FAX: 618-234-6150
e-mail: kcullan@peaknet.net
www.specialchildren.net

A nonprofit agency serving children with developmental disabilities ages birth to 21 years old.

7725 Special Education Action Commette
PO Box 161274
Mobile, AL 36616
251-478-1208
800-222-7322
FAX: 251-473-7877
e-mail: seacofmobile@zebra.net
www.dssc.org/frc/TAGuide/pti/al.htm

Carol R Blades, Director

7726 Stuttering Foundation of America
PO Box 11749
Memphis, TN 38111
901-452-7343
800-992-9392
FAX: 901-452-3931
e-mail: stutter@stetteringhelp.org
www.stutteringhelp.org

Jane Fraser, President
Anne Edwards, Coordinator

Toll-free hotline, brochures, books and videotapes on stuttering.

7727 SupportWorks
1018 E Boulevard
Suite 5
Charlotte, NC 28203
704-331-9500
www.supportworks.org

SupportWorks helps people find and form support groups. An 8 page publication Power Tools, clearly walks new group leaders through steps of putting together a healthy self-help group. SupportWorks also has a telephone conference program which allows people with similar diseases or other nonprofit issues to meet by phone conference for free or at very low cost.

7728 Teratogen and Birth Defects Information Project
University of South Dakota
414 E Clark
Vermillion, SD 57069
605-677-5623
FAX: 605-677-5778

For South Dakota residents only.

7729 Toll-Free Information Line
Asthma and Allergy Foundation of America
1125 15th Street
Suite 502
Washington, DC 20005
202-466-7643
800-7AS-THMA
FAX: 202-466-8940
e-mail: info@aafa.org
www.aafa.org

Referral line for questions about asthma and allergies and how to get involved in your local chapter and support groups.

7730 VUE: Vision Use in Employment
Carroll Center for the Blind
770 Centre Street
Newton, MA 02458
617-969-6200
800-852-3131
FAX: 617-969-6204

Dina Rosenbaum, VP Marketing
Robert McGilliuray, Low Vision Administration

Provides engineering solutions plus training to help people keep jobs despite their vision loss.

7731 **Visiting Nurse Association of America**

11 Beacon Street
Suite 9103
Boston, MA 02108
617-523-4042
800-426-2547
FAX: 617-227-4843
www.naa.org

This agency represents independent VNA units across the United States. Each VNA unit may vary in their services, but most provide skilled nursing, physical therapy, occupational therapy, speech therapy, and home health aid services.

7732 **Washington Connection**

American Council of the Blind
1155 15th Street NW
Suite 1004
Washington, DC 20005
202-467-5081
800-424-8666
FAX: 202-467-5085
e-mail: mbrunson@acb.org
www.acb.org

Melanie Brunson, Governmental Affairs Director

Coverage of issues affecting blind people via legislative information, participates in law-making, legislative training seminars and networking of support resources across the US.

General

7733 Age Appropriate Puzzles

7756 Winding Way
Fair Oaks, CA 95628
916-961-3507
FAX: 916-961-0765
e-mail: miltcher@aol.com

Cheryl Meyers, President

These unique puzzles teach numerous concepts: picture, name, color and shape recognition. Each of the two themes (holidays, and clothing) comes with self-adhesive stickers that name each picture in English, Hmong, Russian, Spanish and Vietnamese. A notch at each puzzle piece makes grasping and lifting the pieces easy to use., They are designed for children from 18 months and up. Special needs children, preschool through high school would also benefit. *$9.95*

7734 All-Turn-It Spinner

AbleNet
1081 10th Avenue SE
Minneapolis, MN 55414
800-322-0956
FAX: 612-379-9143
e-mail: customerservice@ablenetinc.com
www.ablenetinc.com

The All-Turn-It Spinner is a random spinner that comes with a dice overlay allowing user's to participate in any commercially-available game that require dice. Activate the spinner with its built-in switch or connect an external switch. Overlays are interchangeable with AbleNet designed spinner games or create your own overlay. A great inclusion tool!. *$89.00*

7735 Anthony Brothers Manufacturing

1945 S Rancho Santa Fe Road
San Marcos, CA 92069
760-744-8299
FAX: 760-744-2994
e-mail: kids@kidtrikes.com
www.kidtrikes.com

Tom Anthony, President
Sue Coffin, VP
Nairne Farner, Executive VP

Manufacture wheeled toys and goods for disabled children.

7736 Automatic Card Shuffler

Maxi Aids
42 Executive Boulevard
Suite 3209
Farmingdale, NY 11735
631-752-0521
800-522-6294
FAX: 631-752-0689
e-mail: sales@maxiaids.com
www.maxiaids.com

Simple to use, the cards are physically challenging for the player with limited hand dexterity. *$14.95*

7737 Backgammon Set: Deluxe

Maxi Aids
42 Executive Boulevard
Suite 3209
Farmingdale, NY 11735
631-752-0521
800-522-6294
FAX: 631-752-0689
e-mail: sales@maxiaids.com
www.maxiaids.com

Completely factual with a felt board, raised white dividers and white braille dice for the blind and visually impaired. *$29.95*

7738 Board Games: Snakes and Ladders

Maxi Aids
42 Executive Boulevard
Suite 3209
Farmingdale, NY 11735
631-752-0521
800-522-6294
FAX: 631-752-0689
e-mail: sales@maxiaids.com
www.maxiaids.com

A dice game for 2 to 6 players. This children's game is also fun for the whole family. Offers recreation, competition and eye/hand coordination skills. *$34.95*

7739 Board Games: Solitaire

Maxi Aids
42 Executive Boulevard
Suite 3209
Farmingdale, NY 11735
631-752-0521
800-522-6294
FAX: 631-752-0689
e-mail: sales@maxiaids.com
www.maxiaids.com

This popular solo board game lends itself to a number of less well-known variations. The board is accompanied by brightly colored pieces that are reversible for the visually impaired player. *$30.95*

7740 Braille Playing Cards: Pinochle

Maxi Aids
42 Executive Boulevard
Suite 3209
Farmingdale, NY 11735
631-752-0521
800-522-6294
FAX: 631-752-0689
e-mail: sales@maxiaids.com
www.maxiaids.com

Cards offer regular print as well as braille on each plastic card for the blind or visually impaired player. *$9.95*

7741 Braille Playing Cards: Plastic

Maxi Aids
42 Executive Boulevard
Suite 3209
Farmingdale, NY 11735
631-752-0521
800-522-6294
FAX: 631-752-0689
e-mail: sales@maxiaids.com
www.maxiaids.com

Playing cards that offer regular print and braille on plastic cards for the blind or visually impaired player. *$9.95*

7742 Braille: Bingo Cards, Boards and Call Numbers

Maxi Aids
42 Executive Boulevard
Suite 3209
Farmingdale, NY 11735
631-752-0521
800-522-6294
FAX: 631-752-0689
e-mail: sales@maxiaids.com
www.maxiaids.com

Bingo products for the visually impaired. Cards, boards and call numbers offer regular print and braille. *$4.99*

7743 Braille: Rook Cards

Maxi Aids
42 Executive Boulevard
Suite 3209
Farmingdale, NY 11735
631-752-0521
800-522-6294
FAX: 631-752-0689
e-mail: sales@maxiaids.com
www.maxiaids.com

This set of cards for Rook, the popular bidding card game with 23 variations, has regular size print and braille print for the blind/visually impaired player. *$13.75*

7744 **Card Holder Deluxe**

Maxi Aids
42 Executive Boulevard
Suite 3209
Farmingdale, NY 11735
800-522-6294
FAX: 631-752-0689
e-mail: sales@maxiaids.com
www.maxiaids.com

A handsome-looking card holder takes the struggle out of holding playing cards in weak or arthritic hands. The two clear plastic tiers hold up to 18 cards. The wooden base has a non-skid bottom to prevent slipping, and is also great for holding recipe cards. *$19.75*

7745 **Cards: Musical**

Sense-Sations
919 Walnut Street
Philadelphia, PA 19107 **215-627-0600**
FAX: 215-922-0692

These cards, for all occasions, play music when they are opened, for the visually impaired and blind persons. *$2.50*

7746 **Cards: UNO**

Maxi Aids
42 Executive Boulevard
Suite 3209
Farmingdale, NY 11735 **631-752-0521**
800-522-6294
FAX: 631-752-0689
e-mail: sales@maxiaids.com
www.maxiaids.com

Traditional card game in Braille for the blind player recreation. *$10.95*

7747 **Checker Set: Deluxe**

Maxi Aids
42 Executive Boulevard
Suite 3209
Farmingdale, NY 11735 **631-752-0521**
800-522-6294
FAX: 631-752-0689
e-mail: sales@maxiaids.com
www.maxiaids.com

A wooden board with sunken playing squares. The squares have drilled holes for inserting the checker, offering help with eye/hand coordination for the physically challenged. *$25.95*

7748 **Chess Set: Deluxe**

Maxi Aids
42 Executive Boulevard
Suite 3209
Farmingdale, NY 11735 **631-752-0521**
800-522-6294
FAX: 631-752-0689
e-mail: sales@maxiaids.com
www.maxiaids.com

Made out of wood material. Boards have raised dark squares and all squares have drilled holes for inserting pegged chessmen, for the physically challenged player with poor eye/hand coordination. *$43.95*

7749 **Dice: Jumbo Size**

New Vision Store
919 Walnut Street
Philadelphia, PA 19107 **215-629-2990**

The large white and black dice are over-sized and have grooved dots to indicate the numbers, for easy reading for the visually handicapped. *$4.95*

7750 **Enabling Devices**

385 Warburton Avenue
Hastings On Hudson, NY 10706 **914-478-0960**
800-832-8697
FAX: 914-479-1369
e-mail: customer_support@enablingdevices.com
www.enablingdevices.com

Elizabeth Bell, Marketing Manager
Karen O'Connor, VP Operations

For more than 25 years, Enabling Devices has been dedicated to providing affordable learning and assistive devices for the physically challenged. Products include Augmentative Communicators, Adapted Toys, Capability Switches, Training and Sensory Devices and Activity Centers. Call for a free catalog.

7751 **Hands-Free Controller**

Nintendo
PO Box 97032
Redmond, WA 98073
800-255-3700

Nintendo controller for the physically disabled.

7752 **One Hundred Board and Pegs**

Maxi Aids
42 Executive Boulevard
Suite 3209
Farmingdale, NY 11735 **631-752-0521**
800-522-6294
FAX: 631-752-0689
e-mail: sales@maxiaids.com
www.maxiaids.com

Cognitive skills and motor stimulation. *$34.95*

7753 **Puzzle Games: Cooking, Eating, Community and Grooming**

Programming Concepts
PO Box 12428
San Antonio, TX 78212
800-594-4263
FAX: 218-248-055

Janie Haugen, Program Director
Jeff McLane, President/CEO

Each game has 63 pieces which are 2 inches in size. The completed full color puzzle is 19 inch x 15 inch. Step 1 - Work the puzzle. Step 2 - Match picture or Word cards to the correct space on the puzzle. These puzzles teach basic life skills. *$19.95*

7754 **Single Switch Latch and Timer**

AbleNet
1081 10th Avenue SE
Minneapolis, MN 55414
800-322-0956
FAX: 612-379-9143
e-mail: customerservice@ablenetinc.com
www.ablenetinc.com

A Single Switch Latch and Timer allows a user to activate a battery-operated toy or appliance in the latch, timed seconds and timed minutes modes of control. Choose for one user and one device at a time. *$63.00*

7755 **Stacking the Deck**

Research Press
PO Box 9177
Champaign, IL 61826 **217-352-3273**
800-519-2707
FAX: 217-352-1221
e-mail: rp@researchpress.com
www.researchpress.com

Russell Pence, VP Marketing

A unique training program designed for use with any table game that involves progressive movement around a game board to home. During the game, players are required to draw cards and react to specific social situations. Training focuses on three areas: general social skills; social/vocational skills; and social/sexual skills. The training package contains 144 situation cards, detailed instructions and reproducible forms for scoring, recording and evaluating progress. *$19.95*

Game

7756 **Take a Chance**

Speech Bin
1965 25th Avenue
Vero Beach, FL 32960
772-770-0007
800-477-3324
FAX: 772-770-0006
www.speechbin.com

Jan J Binney, Senior Editor

Card game for practice of commonly misarticulated speech sounds. *$18.75*

16 pages Book & Cards
ISBN 0-93785 -46-7

7757 **Tic Tac Toe Plus**

Maxi Aids
42 Executive Boulevard
Suite 3209
Farmingdale, NY 11735
631-752-0521
800-522-6294
FAX: 631-752-0689
e-mail: sales@maxiaids.com
www.maxiaids.com

Offers the traditional tic-tac-toe game but with pieces that are 3/4 inch in diameter and 1/4 inch high in black and green, for the visually impaired player. *$5.95*

7758 **Turnabout Game**

Maxi Aids
42 Executive Boulevard
Suite 3209
Farmingdale, NY 11735
631-752-0521
800-522-6294
FAX: 631-752-0689
e-mail: sales@maxiaids.com
www.maxiaids.com

A game of strategy for two, with large playing pieces and a bright gameboard for the visually impaired player. *$7.70*

Newsletters & Books

7759 **A Guide for the Wheelchair Traveler**

Access for Disabled Americans
1475 N Broadway #420
Walnut Creek, CA 94596 **925-932-9001**
FAX: 925-932-9055
e-mail: PSmither@aol.com
www.accessfordisabled.com

All you need to know when traveling in a wheelchair. *$ 30.00*

165 pages Paperback
ISBN 1-928616-00-3

7760 **A World Awaits You**

Mobility International USA
PO Box 10767
Eugene, OR 97440 **541-343-1284**
FAX: 541-343-6812
e-mail: info@miusa.org
www.miusa.org

Susan Sygall, Executive Director
Pamela Houston, Public Relations Coordinator
Tracy Scharn, Project Assistant

A journal of success stories and tips of people with disabilities participating in international exchange programs.

40 pages Yearly

7761 **Access Travel: Airports**

Consumer Information Center
Department 575A
Pueblo, CO 81009 **719-948-3334**
e-mail: catalog.pueblo@gsa.gov

Michael Clark, Public Affairs

Tips and suggestions for easier travel for persons with disabilities and the elderly. Lists designs, facilities, and services at 553 airport terminals worldwide.

7762 **Architectural Barriers Action League**

PO Box 57088
Tucson, AZ 85732 **520-628-8118**

Offers guides to accessible hotels and motels across the country.

7763 **Directory of Accessible Van Rentals**

Disability Bookshop
PO Box 129
Vancouver, WA 98666 **360-694-2462**

Designed to help people with disabilities locate rental vans that are accessible throughout the U.S. *$9.95*

30+ pages
ISBN 0-93326 -09-9

7764 **Directory of Travel Agencies for the Disabled**

Twin Peaks Press
PO Box 129
Vancouver, WA 98666 **360-694-2462**
FAX: 360-696-3210
e-mail: twinpeak@pacifer.com
dmoz.org/Society/Disabled/Travel/Agencies

Directory lists more than 360 travel agents specializing in arrangements for people with disabilities. Handbook provides information about accessibility. *$19.95*

40 pages Paperback
ISBN 0-93326 -04-8

7765 **Elderly Guide to Budget Travel/Europe**

Pilot Books
PO Box 2102
Greenport, NY 11944 **631-477-1094**
FAX: 631-661-4379

Includes a list of over 250 inexpensive hotels in prime tourist areas. Covers special needs of senior citizens including inexpensive accommodations and fares. *$3.95*

7766 **Ideas for Easy Travel**

Accent Books & Products
PO Box 700
Bloomington, IL 61702 **309-378-2961**
800-787-8444
FAX: 309-378-4420
e-mail: acmtlvng@aol.com

Raymond C Cheever, Publisher
Betty Garee, Editor

Ideal for helping the new traveler get started having fun. Points out favorite accessible high-spots as reported by two travel experts (one is disabled), and offers basic ideas to help wherever you go. *$3.25*

55 pages Paperback
ISBN 0-91570 -36-1

7767 **Travel Information Service/Moss Rehab Hospital**

Moss Rehabilitation Hospital
1200 W Tabor Road
Philadelphia, PA 19141 **215-329-5715**

Joan Appel, Manager

Offers information and resources, to telephone callers only, for persons with special traveling/accessibility needs.

7768 **United States Department of the Interior National Park Service**

Superintendent of Documents
1100 Ohio Drive SW
Washington, DC 20024 **202-619-7222**
FAX: 202-619-7302

James Ridenour, Director

Offers an informational packet containing books, guides and tours for the disabled and elderly.

7769 **Wheelin' Around**

Wheelers Accessible Van Rentals
710 N 55th Avenue
Glendale, AZ 85301
800-456-1371
FAX: 602-412-9920
e-mail: wheelens@primenet.com
www.wheelerz.com

Tammy Smith, President

A newsletter for persons with physical disabilities by Wheelers Accessible Van Rentals offering information on automotive assistive devices, van conversions and travel tips for the disabled.

Quarterly

7770 **Where to Stay USA**

Council on International Educational Exchange
633 3rd Avenue
New York, NY 10017 **212-822-2600**
888-COU-NCIL
FAX: 212-822-2649

Priscilla Tovey, Information Services

A guide to low-cost lodging throughout the United States including information on whether the establishment is accessible. *$15.95*

250 pages
ISBN 0-67179 -49-5

Organizations

7771 **Access America**

Northern Cartographic
4050 Williston Road
Suite 131
South Burlington, VT 05403 **802-860-2886**
FAX: 802-865-4912
e-mail: info@ncarto.com
www.ncarto.com

Offers information on 36 national parks, providing detailed information on accessibility.

7772 **Access Wheels**

6614 W Sweetwater Avenue
Glendale, AZ 85304 **623-776-8830**
800-456-1371
FAX: 623-412-9920
e-mail: info@wheelerscanrentals.com
www.wheelersvanrentals.com

Tammy Smith, Manager

Operator of lowered floor mini-vans. Technically advanced engineering features bring a world of independence to the user. Lowered floor modification provided on all GM and Chrysler front wheel drive mini-vans.

7773 **Access Yosemite National Park**

Special Needs Project
324 State Street
Suite H
Santa Barbara, CA 93101
800-333-6867
FAX: 805-962-5087
www.specialneeds.com

Represents unprecedented combinations of intensive information survey data with high quality cartography. *$7.95*

31 pages

7774 **America West Airlines**

4000 E Sky Harbor Boulevard
Phoenix, AZ 85034 **480-693-0800**
FAX: 803-056-2807

Diana Lawson

This airline trains employees to make sure that passengers with disabilities enjoy convenient, safe and comfortable travel.

7775 **American Hotel and Lodging Association**

1201 New York Avenue
Washington, DC 20005 **202-289-3100**
FAX: 202-289-3199
e-mail: comments@ahlaonline.org
www.ahma.com

William Fisher, President/CEO

Will disseminate information, develop and conduct a series of seminars for the hotel and motel industry at state-level association conferences, and develop and distribute an ADA Compliance handbook for use by the lodging industry.

7776 **Amtrak**

60 Massachusetts Avenue NE
Washington, DC 20002 **202-906-2121**
800-USA-RAIL
TTY:800-523-6590
e-mail: access@w0.amtrak.com
www.amtrak.com

Amtrak is committed to making travel for passengers with disabilities more accessible. Anyone interested should contact Amtrak's Special Services Desk at 1-800-USA-RAIL at least 24 hours in advance to arrange for special assistance. The type of equipment and accessibility vary from train to train and station to station.

7777 **Easter Seals Project ACTION**

700 13th Street NW
Suite 200
Washington, DC 20005 **202-347-3066**
800-659-6428
FAX: 202-737-7914
e-mail: project_action@easter-seals.org
www.projectaction.org

Dr Alan Abeson, Director
Liz Moore, Communications Manager

A national technical assistance program designed to improve access to transportation services for people with disabilities and assist transit providers in implementing the Americans with Disabilities Act. Publishes quarterly newsletter.

7778 **Easy Access to National Parks: The Sierra Club Guide for the Disabled**

Sierra Club Books
2530 San Pablo Avenue
Suite Ior
Berkeley, CA 94702 **510-848-0800**
FAX: 510-848-3383
e-mail: san-francisco-bay.chapter@sierraclub.org
sanfranciscobay.sierraclub.org/leadership.asp

Includes practical information on planning safe trips to 50 national parks that are designated as best visits for their accessibility. *$16.00*

432 pages
ISBN 0-87156 -20-6

7779 **General Motors Mobility Program for Persons with Disabilities**

GM Mobility Program
PO Box 9011
Detroit, MI 48202
800-323-9935

Mary Anne Meade, Manager GM Mobility

GM Mobility Program provides up to $1000 reimbursement toward mobility adaptations for drivers or passengers and/or vehicle alerting devices for drivers who are deaf or hard of hearing. Provided on eligible new Chevrolet, Pontiac, Oldsmobile, Buick, Cadillac, and GMC vehicles. Complete GMC financing available. GM Mobility also offers free resource information, including list of area adaptive equipment installers, plus free resource video.

7780 **Kenny Foundation**
21700 Northwestern Highway
Suite 730
Southfield, MI 48075 **248-552-0202**
800-237-3422
FAX: 248-552-0275
www.comnet.org/kenny

Susan Burstein, Executive Director

Provides education, advocacy & direct services to people with mobility impairments throughout Michigan. Services include Equipment Connection, a database, available online, that connects buyers & sellers of used adaptive equipment; Attitudes is a disability awareness program for 1st & 2nd graders; Information & Referral services; and Accessbility, a program that uses volunteer labor and donated materials to buid ramps for people who can't afford them.

7781 **Melwood Access Adventures**
9035 Ironsides Road
Nanjemoy, MD 20662 **301-870-3226**
FAX: 301-870-2620
e-mail: accessadventures@erols.com

Heidi Aldous, Director
Ann Davis, Office Manager

A year round recreation facility that serves mentally and physically disabled individuals, offers a variety of vacations, outdoor recreation, travel and respite care.

7782 **Nantahala Outdoor Center**
13077 Highway 19 W
Bryson City, NC 28713 **828-488-2175**
800-232-7238
FAX: 828-488-2498
e-mail: rafting@noc.com
www.noc.com

Jennifer Petos, Marketing Department

Nantahala Outdoor Center, the leader in outdoor recreation and education for over 30 years, strongly encourages and supports participants with disabilities. We offer whitewater rafting adventures on six rivers in the Southeast for all skill and thrill levels, also kayak and canoe adaptive instruction. NOC will tailor a whitewater program to your skill and ability level, modify the gear, and pace instruction for you. We also offer a Ropes Challenge Course and team building programs.

7783 **Paralysis Society of America**
Paralyzed Veterans of America
801 18th Street NW
Washington, DC 20006 **202-872-1300**
800-424-8200
FAX: 202-973-8421
e-mail: info@pva.org
www.pva.org

Michelle Mearham, Communications Coordinator

A national organization whose members are people with spinal cord injury or disease, their family members and caregivers, health-care professionals, and others with an interest in the disciplines of spinal cord medicine and paralsis. One year membership includes NewsWheels, a quarterly newsletter. *$10.00*

7784 **Professional Respite Care**
Act for Health
1385 S Colorado Boulevard
Denver, CO 80222 **303-757-4808**
FAX: 303-757-3821

Pamela Erickson, RN

Offers travel accompaniment services for disabled persons or senior citizens.

7785 **Rodeway Inns Airport**
124 S 24th Street
Phoenix, AZ 85034 **602-220-0044**
FAX: 602-244-0174
e-mail: jimp124@juno.com

Jaeques Pichardie, General Manager
Rita Reyes, Assistant Manager

This organization has a limited number of rooms for the handicapped with extra wide doors and special bathroom assist bars.

7786 **Shilo Inn Hotel: Gresham**
2752 NE Hogan
Gresham, OR 97030 **503-907-1777**
800-222-2244
FAX: 503-674-5985
e-mail: gresham@shiloinns.com
www.shiloinns.com

Tim VanHouten, General Manager

Full-Service hotel conveniently located to Mt. Hood and the Columbia River Gorge. Special Assist rooms have wheelchair access, include larger sized bathrooms with roll in shower and shower seat and assist bar around toilet and bathtub. Pets welcome with fee. Check out our website www.shiloinns.com to view property and amenities. Call 1-800-222-2244 for more details and to make reservations.

7787 **Shilo Inn Hotel: Portland Beaverton**
9900 SW Canyon Road
Portland, OR 97225 **503-297-2551**
800-222-2244
FAX: 503-297-7708
e-mail: beaverton@shiloinns.com
www.shiloinns.com

Naeem Khan, General Manager

Full-Service hotel conveniently located to local attractions, shopping and Downtown Portland. Special Assist rooms are located on the first floor and have interior entry. Bathrooms have wheelchair access. Special assist dogs are welcome free of charge. Check out out website www.shiloinns.com to view property and amenities. Call 1-800-222-2244 for more details and to make reservations.

7788 **Shilo Inn Hotel: Richland**
50 Comstock Street
Richland, WA 99352 **509-946-4661**
800-222-2244
FAX: 509-943-6741
e-mail: richland@shiloinns.com
www.shiloinns.com

Joyce Bennet, General Manager

Full-Service hotel overlooking the Columbia River. Special Assit rooms have wheelchair access and include larger sized bathrooms with assist bar around toilet and bathtub and hand held shower available. Special assist dogs are welcome free of charge. Check out our website www.shiloinns.com to view property and amenities. Call 1-800-222-2244 for more details and to make reservations.

7789 **Shilo Inn Hotel: Salt Lake City**
206 SW Temple
Slat Lake City, UT 84101 **801-521-9500**
800-222-2244
FAX: 801-359-6527
e-mail: saltlakecity@shiloinns.com
www.shiloinns.com

Del Brewster, General Manager

Full-Service hotel located in downtown Salt Lake City. Special Assist rooms have wheelchair access and include larger sized bathrooms with assist bar around toilet and bathtub and bench/stool. Special assist dogs are welcome free of charge. Check out our website www.shiloinns.com to view property and amenities. Call 1-800-222-2244 for more details and to make reservations.

7790 **Shilo Inn Hotel: Spokane**

E 923 Third Avenue
Spokane, WA 99202
509-535-9000
800-222-2244
FAX: 509-535-5740
e-mail: spokane@shiloinns.com
www.shiloinns.com

Ken Anderson, General Manager

Full-Service hotel conveniently located near downtown off I-90. Special Assist rooms have wheelchair access and include larger sized bathrooms with assist bar around toilet and bathtub, shower seat and hand held shower. Hearing impaired kits available. Special assist dogs are welcome free of charge. Check out our website www.shiloinns.com to view property and amenities. Call 1-800-222-2244 for more details and to make reservations.

7791 **Shilo Inn Hotel: Yuma**

1550 S Castle Dome Avenue
Yuma, AZ 85365
928-782-9511
800-222-2244
FAX: 928-783-1538
e-mail: yuma@shiloinns.com
www.shiloinns.com

Sandy Potter, General Manager

Full-Service hotel is located in the heart of the"American Sahara. Special Assist rooms have wheelchair access and include larger sized bathrooms with assist bar around toilet and bathtub; hand held shower and shower seat available. Special assist dogs are welcome free of charge. Check out our website www.shiloinns.com to view property and amenities. Call 1-800-222-2244 for more details and to make reservations.

7792 **Shilo Inn Suite: Elko**

2401 Mountain City Highway
Elko, NV 89801
775-738-5522
800-222-2244
FAX: 775-738-6247
e-mail: elko@shiloinns.com
www.shiloinns.com

Dorothy Kirkwood, General Manager

Conveniently located 2-3 miles from Convention Center and Casinos. Special Assist rooms have wheelchair access, include larger sized bathrooms with assist bar around toilet and bathtub and hand held shower. Special assist dogs are welcome free of charge. Check out our website www.shiloinns.com to view property and amenities. Cal 1-800-222-2244 for more details and to make reservations.

7793 **Shilo Inn Suite: Eugene/Springfield**

3350 Gateway
Springfield, OR 97477
541-747-0332
800-222-2244
FAX: 541-726-0587
e-mail: eugene@shiloinns.com
www.shiloinns.com

Bruce Pedersen, General Manager

Full-Service hotel conveniently located off I-5. Special Assit rooms have wheelchair access, include larger sized bathrooms with assist bar around toilet and bathtub and hand held shower. Special assist dogs welcome free of charge. Check out our website www.shiloinns.com to view property and amenities. cal 1-800-222-2244 for more details and to make reservations.

7794 **Shilo Inn Suite: Salem**

3304 Market Street NE
Salem, OR 97301
503-581-4001
800-222-2244
FAX: 503-399-9385
e-mail: salem@shiloinns.com
www.shiloinns.com

Kathy Sharp, General Manager

Located right off I-5 and near Oregon State Fairgrounds and shopping. Special Assit rooms have wheelchair access and include larger sized bathrooms with assist bar around toilet and bathtub, shower seat and hand held shower. Special assist dogs are welcome free of charge. Check out our website www.shiloinns.com to view property and amenities. Call 1-800-222-2244 for more details and to make reservations.

7795 **Shilo Inn Suites Hotel-Bend Oregon**

3105 OB Riley Road
Bend, OR 97701
584-138-9960
800-222-2244
FAX: 541-382-4310
e-mail: bend@shiloinns.com
www.shiloinns.com

Mike Shirley, General Manager
Donnis Shirley, General Manager

Full-Service Hotel located on the banks of the Deschutes River. Special Assist rooms have wheelchair access, include larger sized bathrooms with assit bar around toilet and bathtub and a hand held shower. Some rooms available with in-room spa. Pets are welcome with a fee. Check out our website www.shiloinns.com to view property and amenities. Call 1-800-222-2244 for more details and to make reservations.

7796 **Shilo Inn Suites Hotel: Portland Airport**

11707 NE Airport Way
Portland, OR 97220
503-252-7500
800-222-2244
FAX: 503-254-0794
e-mail: portland205@shiloinns.com
www.shiloinns.com

Maureen Buscio, General Manager

Full-Service hotel near Portland International Airport. Special Assist room ahve wheelchair access and include a larger bathroom with assist bar around toilet and bathtub and hand held shower. Special assist dogs are welcome free of charge. Check out our website www.shiloinns.com to view property and amenities. Call 1-800-222-2244 for more detailsand to make reservations.

7797 **Shilo Inn Suites: Boise Airport**

4111 Broadway Avenue
Boise, ID 83705
208-343-7662
800-222-2244
FAX: 208-344-0318
e-mail: boiseairport@shiloinns.com
www.shiloinns.com

Hakan Kalinov, General Manager

Located 1 mile from Boise International Airport. Special Assist rooms have wheelchair access, include larger sized bathrooms with roll in shower, assist bar around toilet and bathtub and a hand held shower. Special assist dogs are welcome free of charge. Check out our wesite www.shiloinns.com to view property and amenities. Cal 1-800-222-2244 for more details and to make reservations.

7798 **Shilo Inn Suites: Coeur D'Alene**

702 W Appleway
Coeur D'Alene, ID 83814 **208-664-2300**
800-222-2244
FAX: 208-667-2863
e-mail: coeurdalene@shiloinns.com
www.shiloinns.com

Dick Scheets, General Manager

Conveniently located near local attractions, shopping and convention centers. Special Assist rooms have wheelchair access, include larger sized bathrooms with assist bar around toilet and bathtub and hand held shower. Special assist dogs are welcome free of charge. Check out our website www.shiloinns.com to view property and amenities. Call 1-800-222-2244 for more details and to make reservations.

7799 **Shilo Inn Suites: Corning**

3350 Sunrise Way
Corning, CA 96021 **530-824-2940**
800-222-2244
FAX: 530-824-2983
e-mail: corning@shiloinns.com
www.shiloinns.com

Lisa Dowd, General Manager

Located across I-5 from newly opened Rolling Hills casino. Special Assist rooms have wheelchair access include larger sized bathrooms with assit bar around toilet and bathtub and hand held shower. Special assist dogs welcome free of charge. Check out our website www.shiloinns.com to view property and amenities. Call 1-800-222-2244 for more details and to make reservations.

7800 **Shilo Inn Suites: Idaho Falls**

780 Lindsay Boulevard
Idaho Falls, ID 83402 **208-523-0088**
800-222-2244
FAX: 208-522-7420
e-mail: idahofalls@shiloinns.com
www.shiloinns.com

Stacey Mason, General Manager

Full-Service hotel overlooking the Snake River near the falls. Special Assit rooms have wheelchair access, include larger sized bathrooms with assist bar around toilet, hand held shower and shower seat. Special assist dogs are welcome free of charge. Check out our website www.shiloinns.com to view property and amenities. Call 1-800-222-2244 for more details and to make reservations.

7801 **Shilo Inn Suites: Kanab**

296 W 100 N
Kanab, UT 84741 **435-644-2562**
800-222-2244
FAX: 435-644-5333
e-mail: kanab@shiloinns.com
www.shiloinns.com

Linda Clark, General Manager

Located within an easy drive to six national parks and monuments, including Grand Canyon. Special Assist rooms have wheelchair access, include larger sized bathrooms with assist bar around bathtub, hand held shower available. Special assist dogs are welcome free of charge. Check out our website www.shiloinns.com to view property and amenities. Call 1-800-222-2244 for more details and to make reservations.

7802 **Shilo Inn Suites: Klamath Falls**

2500 Almond Street
Klamath Falls, OR 97601 **541-885-7980**
800-222-2244
FAX: 541-885-7959
e-mail: klamathfalls@shiloinns.com
www.shiloinns.com

Judy Weitzel, General Manager

Full-Service hotel overlooking Klamath Lake and Cascade Mountain Range and within driving distance to Carter Lake. Special Assist rooms have wheelchair access and lake view; include larger bathrooms with assist bar around toilet and bathtub, hand held shower. Special assist dogs are welcome free of charge. Check out our website www.shiloinns.com to view property and amenities. Call 1-800-222-2244 for more details and to make reservations.

7803 **Shilo Inn Suites: Mammoth Lakes**

2963 Main Street
PO Box 2179
Mammoth Lakes, CA 93546 **760-934-4500**
800-222-2244
FAX: 760-934-7594
e-mail: mammothlakes@shiloinns.com
www.shiloinns.com

Joan Coleman, General Manager

Year-round resort located in city center and adjacent to California's largest ski area. Special Assist rooms have wheelchair access include larger sized bathrooms with assist bar around toilet and bathtub, hand held shower and shower seat. Special assist dogs are welcome free of charge. Check out our website www.shiloinns.com to view property and amenities. Call 1-800-222-2244 for more details and to make reservations.

7804 **Shilo Inn Suites: Moses Lake**

1819 E Kittleson
Moses Lake, WA 98837 **509-765-9317**
800-222-2244
FAX: 509-765-5058
e-mail: moseslake@shiloinns.com
www.shiloinns.com

Terry Ziegelman, General Manager
Claudia Ziegelman, General Manager

Located near outdoor recreational oasis in the Columbia Basin. Specail Assist rooms have wheelchair access include larger sized bathrooms with assist bar around toilet and bathtub and hand held shower. Special assist dogs welcome free of charge. Check out our website www.shiloinns.com to view property and amenities. Call 1-800-222-2244 for more details and to make reservations.

7805 **Shilo Inn Suites: Newberg**

501 Sitka Avenue
Newberg, OR 97132 **503-537-0303**
800-222-2244
FAX: 503-537-0442
e-mail: newberg@shiloinns.com
www.shiloinns.com

Sean O'Hara, General Manager

Newberg is located in the heart of the Willamette Valley and the local wineries that were voted Most Romantic Destination in the World by Fodor's. Special Assistn rooms have wheelchair access and include larger sized bathrooms with assist bar around toilet and bathtub and hand held shower. Special assist dogs are welcome free of charge. Check out our website www.shiloinns.com to view property and amenities. Call 1-800-222-2244 for more details and to make reservations.

7806 **Shilo Inn Suites: Oakhurst/Yosemite**

40644 Highway 41
Oakhurst, CA 93644 **559-683-3555**
800-222-2244
FAX: 559-683-3386
e-mail: oakhurst@shiloinns.com
www.shiloinns.com

Lois Bergeron, General Manager

Oakhurst is located just 15 miles form the south entrance to Yosemite Park. Special Assist rooms have wheelchair access and include larger sized bathrooms with assist bar around toilet and bathtub and hand held shower, shower seat available. Special assist dogs are welcome free of charge. Check out our website www.shiloinns.com to view property and amenities. Call 1-800-222-2244 for more details and to make reservations.

7807 **Shilo Inn Suites: Palm Springs**

1875 N Plam Canyon Drive
Plam Springs, CA 92262 **760-320-7676**
800-222-2244
FAX: 760-320-9543
e-mail: plamsprings@shiloinns.com
www.shiloinns.com

David Herring, General Manager

Plam Springs features local attractions, shopping and Aerial Tramway nearby. Special Assist rooms have wheelchair access and include larger sized bathrooms with assist bar around toilet and bathtub and hand held shower. Special assist dogs are welcome free of charge. Check out our website www.shiloinns.com to view property and amenities. Call 1-800-222-2244 for more details and to make rservations.

7808 **Shilo Inn Suites: Seaside East**

900 S Holladay
Seaside, OR 97138 **503-738-0549**
800-222-2244
FAX: 503-738-0532
e-mail: seasideeast@shiloinns.com
www.shiloinns.com

Val Perry, General Manager

Seaside is conveniently located within walking distance to the beach. Special Assist rooms have wheelchair access and include larger sized bathrooms with assist bar around toilet and bathtub and hand held shower. Special assist dogs are welcome free of charge. Check out our website www.shiloinns.com to view property and amenities. Call 1-800-222-2244 for more details and to make reservations.

7809 **Shilo Inn Suites: Tillamook**

2515 N Main
Tillamook, OR 97141 **503-842-7971**
800-222-2244
FAX: 503-842-7960
e-mail: tillamook@shiloinns.com
www.shiloinns.com

David Sutton, General Manager

Being located on the Wilson River makes this a perfect getaway for the avid fishing enthusiast. Special Assist rooms have wheelchair access and include larger sized bathrooms with assist bar around toilet and bathtub and hand held shower. Special assist dogs are welcome free of charge. Check out our website www.shiloinns.com to view property and amenities. Call 1-800-222-2244 for more details and to make reservations.

7810 **Shilo Inn Suites: Twin Falls**

1586 Blues Lakes Boulevard
Twin Falls, ID 83301 **208-733-7545**
800-222-2244
FAX: 208-736-2019
e-mail: twinfalls@shiloinns.com
www.shiloinns.com

Jim Harris, General Manager
Florine Harris, General Manager

Located in the heart of Southern Idaho near Snake River Canyon and Shoshone Falls. Special Assist rooms have wheelchair access and include larger sized bathrooms with assist bar around toilet and bathtub and hand held shower. Special assist dogs are welcome free of charge. Check out our website www.shiloinns.com to view property and amenities. Call 1-800-222-2244 for more details and to make reservations.

7811 **Shilo Inn Suites: Warrenton/Astoria**

1609 W Harbor Drive
Warrenton, OR 97146 **503-861-2181**
800-222-2244
FAX: 503-861-2980
e-mail: warrenton@shiloinns.com
www.shiloinns.com

Elsbeth Kenoyer, General Manager

Full-Service hotel a short distance to the Pacific Ocean. Special Assist rooms have wheelchair access and include larger sized bathrooms with assist bar around toilet and bathtub and hand held shower. Special assist dogs are welcome free of charge. Check out our website www.shiloinns.com to view property and amenities. Call 1-800-222-2244 for more details and to make reservations.

7812 **Shilo Inn: Casper**

I25 & Curtis Road
PO Box 246
Evansville, WY 82636 **307-237-1335**
800-222-2244
FAX: 307-577-7429
e-mail: casper@shiloinns.com
www.shiloinns.com

Monty Blare, General Manager

Full-Service hotel located at I-25 and Curtis Road. Special Assist rooms have wheelchair access, include lager sized bathrooms with assist bar around bathtub. Special assist dogs are welcome free of charge. Check out our website www.shiloinns.com to view property and amenities. Call 1-800-222-2244 for more details and to make reservations.

7813 **Shilo Inn: Dalles**

3223 Bret Clodfelter Way
The Dalles, OR 97058 **541-298-5502**
800-222-2244
FAX: 541-298-4673
e-mail: thedalles@shiloinns.com
www.shiloinns.com

Laura Comini, General Manager

The Dalles is locted on the Cloumbia River off I-84, overlooking the Lone Pine Indian Village and The Dalles Dam. Special Assist rooms have wheelchair access and include larger bathrooms with assist bar around toilet and bathtub and hand held shower. Special assist dogs are welcome free of charge. Check out our website www.shiloinns.com to view property and amenities. Call 1-800-222-2244 for more details and to make reservations.

7814 **Shilo Inn: Grants Pass**

1880 NW Sixth Street
Grants Pass, OR 97526
541-479-8391
800-222-2244
FAX: 541-474-7344
e-mail: grantspass@shiloinns.com
www.shiloinns.com

Sarah Ainsworth, General Manager

Conveniently located off I-5, just 2 miles from city center. Special Assist rooms have wheelchair access, include larger sized bathrooms with assist bar around bathtub and shower seat is available upon request. Special Assist dogs are welcome free of charge. Hearing impaired kits available at front desk. Checkout our website www.shiloinns.com to view property and amenities. Call 1-800-222-2244 for more details and to make reservations.

7815 **Shilo Inn: Helena**

2020 Prospect Avenue
Helena, MT 59601
406-442-0320
800-222-2244
FAX: 406-449-4426
e-mail: helena@shiloinns.com
www.shiloinns.com

Kathy Cox, General Manager

Conveniently located between Yellowstone and Galcier National Parks. Special Assist rooms have wheelchair access, include larger sized bathrooms with assist around bathtub. Special assist dogs are welcome free of charge. Check out our website www.shiloinns.com to view property and amenities. Call 1-800-222-2244 for more details and to make reservations.

7816 **Shilo Inn: Lincoln City Oceanfront Resort**

1501 NW 40th Place
Lincoln City, OR 97367
541-994-3655
800-222-2244
FAX: 541-994-2199
e-mail: lincolncity@shiloinns.com
www.shiloinns.com

Scott Mason, General Manager

Full-Service resort with low beach access; overlooking Pacific Ocean and located adjacent to Gaming Center. Special Assist rooms have wheelchair access include larger sized bathrooms with assist bar around toilet and bathtub, hand held shower. Special Assist dogs are welcome free of charge. Check out our website www.shiloinns.com to view property and amenities. Call 1-800-222-2244 for more details and to make reservations.

7817 **Shilo Inn: Medford**

2111 Biddle Road
Medford, OR 97504
541-770-5151
800-222-2244
FAX: 541-776-0417
e-mail: medford@shiloinns.com
www.shiloinns.com

Randy Butts, General Manager

Conveniently located off I-5, approximately 77 miles form Carter Lake. Special Assist rooms have wheelchair access include larger sized bathrooms with assist bar around bathtub and hand held shower. Pets are welcome with fee. Check out website www.shiloinns.com to view property and amenities. Call 1-800-222-2244 for more details and to make reservations.

7818 **Shilo Inn: Nampa Suites**

1401 Shilo Drive
Nampa, ID 83687
208-465-3250
800-222-2244
FAX: 208-465-5929
e-mail: nampasuites@shiloinns.com
www.shiloinns.com

Shelley Quintana, General Manager

Full-Sevice hotel located 5 miles from city center and within easy distance of local wineries. Special Assist rooms have wheelchair access and include larger sized bathrooms with assist bar around toilet and bathtub and hand held shower. Special assist dogs are welcome free of charge. Check out our website www.shiloinns.com to view property and amenities. Call 1-800-222-2244 for more details and to make reservations.

7819 **Shilo Inn: Newport Oceanfront Resort**

536 SW Elizabeth
Newport, OR 97365
541-265-7701
800-222-2244
FAX: 541-265-5687
e-mail: newport@shiloinns.com
www.shiloinns.com

Karen Anderson, General Manager

Full-Service resort located right on the ocean's edge and all guest rooms have ocean view. Special Assist rooms have wheelchair access and include larger sized bathrooms with assist bar around toilet and bathtub and shower seat, hand held shower available. Special assist dogs are welcome free of charge. Check out our website www.shiloinns.com to view property and amenities. Call 1-800-222-2244 for more details and to make reservations.

7820 **Shilo Inn: Ocean Shores Beach Front Resort**

707 Ocean Shores Boulevard NW
Ocean Shores, WA 98569
360-289-4600
800-222-2244
FAX: 360-289-0355
e-mail: oceanshores@shiloinns.com
www.shiloinns.com

Bob Hugo, General Manager

Full-Service resort located right on the beach. Special Assist rooms have wheelchair access and include larger sized bathrooms with assist bar around toilet and bathtub, hand held shower and 2 shower seats. Special assist dogs are welcome free of charge. Check out our website www.shiloinns.com to view property and amenities. Call 1-800-222-2244 for more details and to make reservations

7821 **Shilo Inn: Pomona Hilltop Suites**

3101 Temple Avenue
Pomona, CA 91768
909-598-7666
800-222-2244
FAX: 909-598-5654
e-mail: pomonahilltop@shiloinns.com
www.shiloinns.com

Heinz Gehner, General Manager

Full-Sevice hotel with view of San Gabriel Mountains and valley. Special Assist rooms have wheelchair access and include larger sized bathrooms with assist bar around toilet and bathtub and hand held shower, shower seat available. Special assist dogs are welcome free of charge. Check out our website www.shiloinns.com to view property and amenities. Call 1-800-222-2244 for more details and to make reservations.

7822 **Shilo Inn: Pomona Hotel**

3200 Temple Avenue
Pomona, CA 91768 **909-598-0073**
800-222-2244
FAX: 909-594-5862
e-mail: pomona@shiloinns.com
www.shiloinns.com

Heinz Gehner, General Manager

Located conveniently of Southern California sights and attractions and right across the street from Shilo Inn Pomona Hilltop. Special Assist rooms have wheelchair access and include larger sized bathrooms with assist bar around toilet and bathtub and hand held shower, shower seat available. Special assist dogs are welcome free of charge. Check out our website www.shiloinns.com to view property and amenities. Call 1-800-222-2244 for more details and to make reservations.

7823 **Shilo Inn: Portland**

7300 Hazelfern Road
Tigard, OR 97224 **503-639-2226**
800-222-2244
FAX: 503-639-9130
e-mail: i5south@shiloinns.com
www.shiloinns.com

Shahab Shahbazzadeh, General Manager

Located directly off I-5 just south of Portland. Special Assist rooms have wheelchair access and include larger sized bathrooms. Special assist dogs are welcome free of charge. Check out our website www.shiolinns.com to view property and amenities. Call 1-800-222-2244 for more detials and to make reservations.

7824 **Shilo Inn: Seaside Oceanfront Resort**

30 N Prom
Seaside, OR 97138 **503-738-9571**
800-222-2244
FAX: 503-738-0674
e-mail: seasideoceanfront@shiloinns.com
www.shiloinns.com

Val Perry, General Manager

Full-Service resort located on the oceanfront. Special Assist rooms have wheelchair access and include larger sized bathrooms with assist bar around toilet and bathtub and hand held shower. Special assist dogs are welcome free of charge. Check out our website www.shiloinns.com to view property and amenities. Call 1-800-222-2244 for more details and to make reservations.

7825 **Shilo Inn: Tacoma**

7414 S Hosmer
Tacoma, WA 98408 **253-475-4020**
800-222-2244
FAX: 253-475-1236
e-mail: tacoma@shiloinns.com
www.shiloinns.com

Alan Harrison, General Manager

Conveniently located off I-5, near McChord Air Force Base and Ft. Lewis Army Base. Special Assist rooms have wheelchair access and include larger sized bathrooms with assist bar around toilet and bathtub. Special assist dogs are welcome free of charge. Check out our website www.shiloinns.com to view property and amenities. Call 1-800-222-2244 for more details and to make reservations.

7826 **Shilo Inn: Vancouver**

401 E 13th Street
Vancouver, WA 98660 **360-696-0411**
800-222-2244
FAX: 360-750-0933
e-mail: vancouuver@shiloinns.com
www.shiloinns.com

Erik Seaburg, General Manager

Located in downtown Vancouver and a short distance to local attractions and shopping. Special Assist rooms have wheelchair access and include larger sized bathrooms with assist bar around toilet and bathtub; some units have hand held shower. Special assist dogs are welcome free of charge. Check out our website www.shiloinns.com to view property and amenities. Call 1-800-222-2244 for more details and to make reservations.

7827 **Shilo Inn: Washington Square**

10830 SW Greenburg Road
Tigard, OR 97223 **503-620-4320**
800-222-2244
FAX: 503-620-8277
e-mail: washingtonsquare@shiloinns.com
www.shiloinns.com

Naeem Khan, General Manager

Conveniently located across freeway from Washington Square shopping mall. Special Assist rooms have wheelchair access and include larger sized bathrooms with assist bar around toilet, all rooms have showers and hand held shower available. Special assist dogs are welcome free of charge. Check out our website www.shiloinns.com to view property and amenities. Call 1-800-222-2244 for more deatils and to make reservations.

7828 **Shilo Inns & Resorts**

11600 SW Shilo Lane
Portland, OR 97225 **503-641-6565**
800-222-2244
FAX: 503-644-0868
www.shiloinns.com

Ivan McAffee, National Sales/Marketing Dir.

Shilo Inns offers Affordable Excellence with Special Assist rooms at many of our locations. These rooms include larger sized bathrooms equipped with assistance railings and wheelchair access. Special assist dogs are welcome free of charge ar most Shilo Inns. Call 1-800-222-2244 for details or make reservations or check out www.shiloinns.com

7829 **Special Assistance Services (SAS)**

3 High Street
Helmetta, NJ 08828
FAX: 732-521-9333

James J Muzikowski, President
Steve Rosenel, Assistant Travel Coordinator

The mission of this organization is to empower the quest to travel. They supply this by offering flexible plans and personal assistance. S.A.S. is dedicated to providing various types of assistance to persons with disabilities. The organization serves guests with a variety of special needs, including but not limited to persons with visual and hearing impairments, physical and development disabilities, and the mentally challenged.

7830 **Ticket Counter**

6900 Wisconsin Avenue
Suite 706
Chevy Chase, MD 20815 **301-986-0790**
FAX: 301-913-0166

Tracey Bullan Rattner

Offers airlines, train, vacation and honeymoon packages, leisure and business, cruises, skiing, horseback riding and other interest tickets to persons with or without disabilities.

7831 Travelers Aid Society
1612 K Street NW
Washington, DC 20006 **202-546-1127**
FAX: 202-546-1625

Pauline Dunn

Provides crisis intervention and casework services, limited financial assistance, protective travel assistance and information and referrals for travelers, transients and newcomers.

7832 US Servas
11 John Street
Room 505
New York, NY 10038 **212-267-0252**
FAX: 212-267-0292
e-mail: info@usservas.org
www.usservas.org

Lara Fisher, Administrator
Julieie Schumacher, Assistant Administrator

International network that links travelers with hosts in 130+ countries with the hope of building world peace through understanding and friendship.

Quarterly

7833 Westin Hotels and Resorts
PO Box 141609
Austin, TX 78714
FAX: 512-835-4417
www.westin.com

Westin Hotels include special parking stalls, wheelchair ramps, wide doors, wheelchairs, braille elevator buttons, recreational facilities for people with disabilities, restaurants and restrooms.

7834 Wilderness Inquiry
1313 5th Street SE
Minneapolis, MN 55414 **612-379-3854**
800-728-0179
FAX: 612-379-5972

Greg Lais, Executive Director
Tracy Fredin, Outreach Director

Allows people of all ages and abilities to share the adventure of wilderness travel. This nonprofit organization was formed in 1978 and conducts tours to some of the most beautiful and remote parts of the world.

Tours

7835 Accessible Journeys
35 W Sellers Avenue
Ridley Park, PA 19078 **610-521-0339**
800-846-4537
FAX: 610-521-6959
e-mail: sales@disabilitytravel.com
www.disabilitytravel.com

Howard Mccoy III, Director
Deborah Richards, Associate Director

Tour operator for slow walker and wheelchair travelers their families and their friends offering tours to culturally intriguing destinations like Africa, China, Brazil, Alaska and Hawaii. Also offers a quarterly newsletter.

7836 Anglo California Travel Service
4250 Williams Road
San Jose, CA 95129 **408-257-2257**
FAX: 408-257-2664

Helen Jones

Plans for one and two week accessible tours.

7837 Bill Dvorak, Kayak and Rafting Expeditions
17921 US Highway 285
Nathrop, CO 81236 **719-539-6851**
800-824-3795
FAX: 719-539-3378
e-mail: dvorakex@amigo.net
www.dvorakexpeditions.com

Bill Dvorak, President
Jaci Dvorak, VP

This organization does river trips for people who are deaf, visually impaired, physically or mentally disabled. Rafting trips with groups and families and whitewater instruction.

7838 Cunard Line
6100 Blue Lagoon Drive
Miami, FL 33126 **305-463-3000**
800-528-6273
FAX: 305-463-3010
www.cunard.co.uk

Cunard Line, one of the world's most recognized brand names with a classic British heritage, operated by Cunard Line Limited, has provided the ultimate in deluxe ocean travel experience for the past 158 years. The fleet consists of famed liner Queen Elizabeth 2 and the Caronia, a classic ship formerly identified as Vistafjord. The Cunard Line brand, the epitome of British essence, focuses on recalling the golden age of sea travel for those who missed the first.

7839 Dell Rapids Sportsmen's Club
714 E 9th Street
PO Box 126
Dell Rapids, SD 57022 **605-428-5501**
FAX: 605-428-5502
e-mail: ezhealth@sd.cybernex.net
www.rodandgunclub.com

A club offering education and experience in planning, designing or using accessible shooting or gun club.

7840 Diabetic Cruise Desk
Hartford Holiday Travel
PO Box 536
Williston Park, NY 11596 **516-746-6670**
800-645-2120

Offers a seven-day cruise to Alaska for people with diabetes. Includes seminars on diabetes, self management, planning, special guidance for exercise classes and individual dietary advice.

7841 Dialysis at Sea Cruises
107 13th Avenue
 # 218
Indian Rocks Beach, FL 33785 **727-518-7311**
800-544-7604
FAX: 727-518-7332
e-mail: dasc@dialysis-at-sea.com
dialysisatsea.com

Andrew Carrabus, President

Been in the business of providing travel opportunities for persons on hemodialysis and CAPD since 1977. Handle all aspects of their travel and medical requirements. Not Sold Through Travel Agents! Make all reservations and coordinates the total set-up and operation of an onboard ship mobile dialysis clinic. Cruises run from seven days to three weeks and have departures from cities around the world on a variety of cruise lines.

7842 Directions Unlimited Acccessible Tours

123 Green Lane
Bedford Hills, NY 10507 **914-241-4477**
800-533-5343
FAX: 914-241-0243

Lois Bonanni, Director

Arrange vacations throughout the world for all disabilities including accessible cruises, African safari, rafting and scuba diving, European and Caribbean vacations.

7843 Environmental Traveling Companions

Fort Mason Center Building C
San Francisco, CA 94123 **415-474-7662**
FAX: 415-474-7662
www.etctrips.org

Diane Poslosky

Aids travelers regardless of physical or financial limitations to experience the beauty and challenge of the wilderness.

7844 Flying Wheels Travel

143 W Bridge Street
PO Box 382
Owatonna, MN 55060 **507-451-5005**
FAX: 507-451-1685
e-mail: thq@ll.net
www.flyingwheelstravel.com

Barbara Jacobson, President

Arranges escorted group and individual cruise trips to the Caribbean, Panama Canal and Europe. People traveling in wheelchairs will need to be able to push themselves and take care of personal needs or bring along an attendant.

7845 Golden Eagle Passport

US Dept. of the Interior, National Park Service
1849 C Street NW
Washington, DC 20240 **202-208-6843**

www.natlforests.org/2003/passport/passport_go

A free lifetime passport to federally operated parks, monuments, historic sites, recreation areas and wildlife refuges for persons who are blind or permanently disabled.

7846 Guide Service of Washington

733 15th Street NW
Washington, DC 20005 **202-628-2842**
FAX: 202-638-2812

Renee Price, Resident

A guide service offering tours of Washington DC and vicinity.

7847 Guided Tour for Persons 17 & Over with Developmental and Physical Challenges

7900 Old York Road
Suite 114B
Elkins Park, PA 19027 **215-782-1370**
FAX: 215-635-2637
e-mail: gtour400@aol.com
www.guidetour.com

Irv Segal DCSW LSW, Director
Ari Segal LSW, Assistant Director
Doron Segal, Coodinator

Offers unique travel and vacation programs for individuals with mild to moderate developmental disabilities. We publish a free Rates & Dates brochure twice a year.

7848 Hostelling North America Hostelling International: American Youth Hostels

733 15th Street NW
Suite 840
Washington, DC 20005 **202-783-6161**
FAX: 202-783-6171
e-mail: hiayhserv@hiayh.org
www.hiayh.org

Ms. Toby Pyle, PR Manager

Hostels are very inexpensive accommodations for travelers of all ages. They provide dorm-style sleeping rooms with separate quarters for males and females, fully equipped self-service kitchens, dining areas and common rooms for relaxing and socializing. HI-AYH has hostels in major cities, in national and state parks, near beaches and in the mountains. Send for a copy of Hostelling North America, a directory of hostels in U.S. and Canada, which lists hostels that are handicap accessible. *$ 3.00*

400 pages Yearly

7849 New Courier Travel

532 Duane Street
Glen Ellyn, IL 60137 **630-469-7349**
FAX: 630-469-7390

Janice Perkins, Travel Consultant

Offers specialized assistance for independent travel or tours for persons with disabilities including cruises and travel in the USA and abroad. Fee charged for out-of-state clients, long-distance calls and clients who have free air.

7850 New Directions

5276 Hollister Avenue
Suite 207
Santa Barbara, CA 93111 **805-967-2841**
888-967-2841
FAX: 805-964-7344
e-mail: info@newdirectionstravel.com
www.newdirectionstravel.com

Dee Duncan, Executive Director

New Directions is a 501 (c) non-profit organization providing vacation travel and special educational exchange programs for people with developmental disabilities. The purpose of the program is to promote understanding, acceptance, and appreciation of people with disabilities as important and contributing members of society.

7851 Norwegian Cruise Line

7665 NW 19th Street
Miami, FL 33126 **305-436-4652**
800-327-7030
FAX: 305-436-4117
www.ncl.com

Has accessible cabins but urges mobility impaired passengers to travel in the same cabin with a person who is not mobility impaired. Cruise fares vary.

7852 People and Places

3909 Genesee Street
Cheektowaga, NY 14225 **585-937-1813**

Joie Budington, Director
Patty Brown Schieder, Assistant Director

Nonprofit organization that provides escorted small group vacation opportunities and outdoor experiences throughout the world for persons with developmental disabilities. Brochure available.

7853 **River Odysseys West: ROW**

PO Box 579-DI
Coeur D'Alene, ID 83816 **208-667-1835**
800-451-6034
FAX: 208-667-6506
e-mail: info@rowinc.com
www.rowinc.com

Offers one to six day rafting trips to physically disadvantaged people. Designs custom itineraries, or trips with a special focus for small groups. For those with special dietary needs, they prepare special meals. So come ride the rapids and enjoy life. They also offer canoe trips aboard 34' voyager canoes along the trail of Lewis and Clark on Montana's upper Missouri River. Free brochure upon request.

7854 **Search Beyond Adventures**

4603 Bloomington Avenue
Minneapolis, MN 55407 **612-721-2800**
800-800-9979
FAX: 612-721-3409
e-mail: travel@searchbeyond.com
www.searchbeyond.com

Operates a wide variety of tours for adults with mental retardation. Programs vary from 2 to 16 days throughout North America, the Caribbean and Europe. Offices in Minneapolis, Chicago, Denver, Boston and Phoenix areas. Camping and accommodation tours are also offered. Catalog of over 135 tours are available.

7855 **Sundial Special Vacations**

Sundial Tours
2609 Highway 101 N
Seaside, OR 97138 **503-738-9491**
800-547-9198
FAX: 503-738-3369
e-mail: patsy@sundial-travel.com

Bruce Conner, Tour Operations Dir/Owner
Patsy Conner, Owner

Provides special vacations for developmentally disabled persons. Provides quality vacations for persons with developmental disabilities. Ratio is 1 for 7 or 1 for 5 depending on tour. Only two people to a room. Exciting destinations. 3 to 4 star properties. Great fun.

7856 **Ventures Travel**

Friendship Ventures
10509 108th Street NW
Annandale, MN 55302 **952-852-0101**
800-450-8376
FAX: 952-852-0123
e-mail: fv@friendshipventures.org
www.friendshipventures.org

Ventures Travel is a service of Friendship Ventures-a non-profit organization that has been enriching the lives of people with mental retardation and related developmental disabilities since 1964. Contact us to learn about our other programs, employment information, volunteer openings or donor opportunities.

7857 **Wheelchair Express**

PO Box 700637
Saint Cloud, FL 34770
FAX: 407-957-2043

Robert Mann, President

Transports individuals, families or groups, with disabilities in Central Florida. All attractions, plus a Florida tour.

7858 **Wheelchair Getaways**

Nationwide Locations
PO Box 605
Versailles, KY 40383 **859-873-4973**
800-642-2042
FAX: 859-873-8039
e-mail: corporate@wheelchairgetaways.com
www.wheelchairgetaways.com

Wheelchair Getaways, the largest wheelchair/scooter accessible van rental company in the US, has 50 franchise locations serving major cities and airports throughout the continental US and Hawaii. Rentals by the day, week, month or longer. Delivery/pickup available.

Vehicle Rentals

7859 **ABC Union, ACE, ANLV, Vegas Western Cab**

5010 S Valley View Boulevard
Las Vegas, NV 89118 **702-643-1041**
FAX: 702-736-8813

Art McGill, Manager

Taxi service in Las Vegas that uses vans with wheelchair lifts at regular taxi rates.

7860 **Avis Rent-A-Car**

900 Old Country Road
Garden City, NY 11530 **516-222-3000**
800-331-1212
FAX: 918-621-4819
e-mail: custserv@avis.com
www.avis.com

James A Keyes, VP Human Resourses
Richard A Fuller, VP Media Relations

Requires 24-hour notice for hand control vehicles, available in any location across the US.

7861 **CEH**

4457 63rd Circle
Pinellas Park, FL 33781 **727-522-0364**
800-677-0364
FAX: 727-522-9024

Phillip G Faas, President

New vans, used vans, rental vans; specializing in quad conversions, all types of handicap equipment. Celebrating 28 years in business.

7862 **Mobile Care**

6201 Riverdale Road
Suite 101
Riverdale, MD 20737 **301-649-0564**
FAX: 301-699-1865
e-mail: jaklimo@aol.com

Jeffery A Koch, President

Specializing in non-emergency wheelchair service for the elderly and physically challenged.

7863 **National Car Rental System**

1795 Perimeter Roadvenue
Dania, FL 33004 **954-359-8303**
800-CAR-RENT
FAX: 954-359-8313
www.nationalcar.com

Accommodates special requests subject to availability. Offers hand controls, bench seats, extra mirrors and vans with lifts at many major locations.

7864 Northwest Limousine Service

9950 W Lawrence Avenue
Schiller Park, IL 60176
847-671-5444
800-376-5466
FAX: 847-671-5482

Kathleen Maloney, Manager
Ann Walsh, Office Reservations

Offers wheelchair accessible mini vans, sedans, stretch and super stretch limousines for hourly or daily rental.

7865 Over the Rainbow Disabled Travel Services & Wheelers' Accessible Van Rentals

186 Mehani Circle
Kihei, HI 96753
808-879-5521
FAX: 808-871-7533

David McKown, VP/Director

Offers the disabled traveler Hawaii airport arrangements and ticketing accessible accommodations, hotels and condos including roll-in showers, Wheelers' Accessible Van Rentals on Maui and Honolulu or cars with hand controls, personal care attendants, medical or recreational equipment rentals and activities such as: helicopter rides, luau's, whalewatching, boating and more. Airfare varies from departure points and time of the year.

7866 Rehabiliation Engineering Center for Personal Licensed Transportation

University of Virginia School of Engineering
PO Box 9003
Charlottesville, VA 22906
434-924-0311
FAX: 434- -

7867 Wheelchair Getaways Wheelchair/Scooter Accessible Van Rentals

Nationwide Locations
PO Box 605
Versailles, KY 40383
859-873-4973
800-642-2042
FAX: 859-873-8039
e-mail: corporate@wheelchairgetaways.com
www.wheelchairgetaways.com

Rents wheelchair/scooter accessible vans by the day, week, month or longer and offers delivery to major airports and other convenient locations in more than 200 cities in 42 states and Puerto Rico. Also offers full size and mini vans with automatic lifts and ramps. Some vans are equipped with hand controls, six-way power seats and remote controls for powered door operation and lifts.

7868 Wheelers

7101 N 55th Avenue
Glendale, AZ 85301
800-456-1371
FAX: 623-435-9989

Offers delivery to airports in 29 states and Washington, D.C. In about 40 cities, Wheelers works directly with Avis Rent-a-Car. Wheelers offers a variety of van configurations with capacity for up to three wheelchairs, automatic ramps or lifts and nylon tie-downs, hand controls or other modifications.

7869 Wheelers Accessible Van Rentals

7101 N 55th Avenue
Glendale, AZ 85301
602-931-7474
800-456-1371
FAX: 623-435-1518

Tammy Smith, President

National Administrations

7870 DAV National Service Headquarters

807 Maine Avenue SW
Washington, DC 20024 **202-554-3501**
FAX: 202-554-3581
e-mail: feedback@davmail.org
www.dav.org

Arthur H Wilson, National Adjutant
David W Gorman, Executive Director

Serves America's disabled veterans and their families. Direct services include legislative advocacy; professional counseling about compensation, pension, educational and job training programs and VA health care; and assistance in applying for those entitlements.

7871 Department of Medicine and Surgery Veterans Administration

810 Vermont Avenue NW
Washington, DC 20420 **202-273-8504**
FAX: 202-273-9108

Gerald McDonald MD, Senior Consultant

Provides hospital and outpatient treatment as well as nursing home care for eligible veterans in Veterans Administration facilities. Services elsewhere provided on a contract basis in the United States and its territories. Provides non-vocational inpatient residential rehabilitation services to eligible legally blinded veterans of the armed forces of the United States.

7872 Department of Veterans Affairs Regional Office - Vocational Rehab Division

380 Westminster Street
Providence, RI 02903 **401-528-4580**
800-827-1000
FAX: 401-528-4894

Gerald E Allen, Counseling Officer

Vocational rehabilitation is a program of services administered by the Department of Veterans Affairs for service members and veterans with service-connected physical or mental disabilities. If persons are compensibly disabled and are found in need of rehabilitation services because they have an employment handicap, this program can prepare them for a suitable job; get and keep that job; assist persons to become fully productive and independent.

7873 Department of Veterans Benefits

810 Vermont Avenue NW
Washington, DC 20420
800-827-1000

Raymond Vogel, Chief Benefits

Furnishes compensation and pensions for disability and death to veterans and their dependents. Provides vocational rehabilitation services, including counseling, training, assistance and more towards employment, to blinded veterans disabled as a result of service in the armed forces during World War II, Korea and the Vietnam era; also provides rehabilitation services to certain peace-time veterans.

7874 Disabled American Veterans

PO Box 14301
Cincinnati, OH 45250 **859-441-7300**
FAX: 859-441-1416
www.dav.org

Advises veterans of their rights and employers of their obligations, under the Rehabilitation Act, the Americans with Disabilities Act, and legislation governing the employment and training of Vietnam era veterans with disabilities.

7875 Federal Benefits for Veterans and Dependents

Government Printing Office
Washington, DC 20402 **202-512-1067**
800-827-1000

Offers information on benefits for veterans and their families.

93 pages
ISBN 0-16048 -58-

7876 Hospitalized Veterans Writing Project

5920 Nall Avenue
Suite 105
Mission, KS 66202 **913-432-1214**

Charlotte Black, Secretary

Individuals and organizations united to encourage hospitalized veterans to write for pleasure and rehabilitation during the hospital stay. Maintains speakers' bureau and audio tape version for the blind. Bestows numerous monetary awards in six areas: article; book review; cartoon and drawing; light verse; poetry and short story. *$ 15.00*

64 pages Magazine
ISSN 0504-07 9

7877 US Department of Veterans Affairs National Headquarters

1120 Vermont Avenue NW
Washington, DC 20420 **202-273-5400**
800-827-1000
e-mail: washingtondc.query@vba.va.gov
www.va.gov

Togo D West Jr, Secretary of Veterans Affairs
Hershel W Gober, Deputy Secretary of Vet. Affairs

Administers the laws providing benefits and other services to veterans, their dependents, and their beneficiaries. Acts as their principal advocate in ensuring that they recieve medical care, benefits, social support, and lasting memorials promoting the health, welfare, and dignity of all veterans in recognition of their service to this nation. As the DVA heads into the 21st century, they will strive to meet the needs of the Nation's veterans today and tomorrow.

7878 US Veteran's Administration

810 Vermont Avenue NW
Washington, DC 20420 **202-273-5400**

Provides a wide range of services for those who have been in the military and their dependents, as well as offering information on driver assessment and education programs.

Alabama

7879 Alabama VA Regional Office

Veterans Benefits Administration, US Dept. of VA
345 Perry Hill Road
Montgomery, AL 36109
800-827-1000
e-mail: montgomery.query@vba.va.gov
www.va.gov

7880 Birmingham VA Medical Center

Veterans Health Administration, US Dept. of VA
700 S 19th Street
Birmingham, AL 35233 **205-933-8101**
800-827-1000
e-mail: g.vhacss@forum.va.gov
www.va.gov

7881 **Central Alabama Veterans Healthcare System**
Veterans Health Administration, US Dept. of VA
West Campus
215 Perry Hill Road
Montgomery, AL 36109
334-272-4670
800-827-1000
e-mail: g.vhacss@forum.va.gov
www.va.gov

7882 **Tuscaloosa VA Medical Center**
Veterans Health Administration, US Dept. of VA
3701 Loop Road, E
Tuscaloosa, AL 35404
205-554-2000
FAX: 205-554-2845
www.va.gov

Donna Channell, Director Public Affairs

Alaska

7883 **Anchorage Regional Office**
Veterans Benefits Administration, US Dept. of VA
2925 DeBarr Road
Anchorage, AK 99508
907-257-4700
800-827-1000
e-mail: anchorage.query@vba.va.gov
www.va.gov

7884 **DAV Department of Alaska**
2925 DeBarr Road
Room 3101
Anchorage, AK 99508
907-276-2842
FAX: 907-258-9828

George Hausermann, Treasurer

Arizona

7885 **Carl T Hayden VA Medical Center**
Veterans Health Administration, US Dept. of VA
650 E Indian School Road
Phoenix, AZ 85012
602-277-5551
800-827-1000
e-mail: g.vhacss@forum.va.gov
www.va.gov

Carl Hayden

7886 **Northern Arizona VA Health Center**
Veterans Health Administration, US Dept. of VA
500 N Highway 89
Prescott, AZ 86313
928-445-4860
800-827-1000
FAX: 928-768-6076
e-mail: g.vhacss@forum.va.gov
www.va.gov

7887 **Phoenix Regional Office**
Veterans Benefits Administration, US Dept. of VA
3225 N Central Avenue
Phoenix, AZ 85012
800-827-1000
e-mail: phoenix.query@vba.va.gov
www.va.gov

7888 **Southern Arizona VA Healthcare System**
Veterans Health Administration, US Dept. of VA
3601 S 6th Avenue
Tucson, AZ 85723
520-792-1450
800-827-1000
e-mail: g.vhacss@forum.va.gov
www.va.gov

Arkansas

7889 **Eugene J Towbin Healthcare Center**
Veterans Health Administration, US Dept. of VA
2200 Fort Roots Drive
North Little Rock, AR 72114
501-396-4444
800-827-1000
e-mail: g.vhacss@forum.va.gov
www.va.gov

7890 **Fayetteville VA Medical Center**
Veterans Health Administration, US Dept. of VA
1100 N College Avenue
Fayetteville, AR 72703
479-444-4301
800-827-1000
e-mail: g.vhacss@forum.va.gov
www.va.gov

7891 **John L McClellan Memorial Hospital**
Veterans Health Administration, US Dept. of VA
4300 W 7th Street
Little Rock, AR 72205
501-257-1000
800-827-1000
e-mail: g.vhacss@forum.va.gov
www.va.gov

7892 **North Little Rock Regional Office**
Veterans Benefits Administration, US Dept. of VA
Building 65, Fort Roots
PO Box 1280
Little Rock, AR 72115
800-827-1000
e-mail: littlerock.query@vba.va.gov
www.va.gov

California

7893 **Jerry L Pettis Memorial VA Medical Center**
Veterans Health Administration, US Dept. of VA
11201 Benton Street
Loma Linda, CA 92357
909-825-7084
800-827-1000
e-mail: g.vhacss@forum.va.gov
www.va.gov

7894 **Long Beach VA Medical Center**
Veterans Health Administration, US Dept. of VA
5901 E 7th Street
Long Beach, CA 90822
562-597-3592
800-827-1000
e-mail: g.vhacss@forum.va.gov
www.va.gov

7895 **Los Angeles Regional Office**
Veterans Benefits Administration, US Dept. of VA
Federal Building
11000 Wilshire Boulevard
Los Angeles, CA 90024
800-827-1000
e-mail: losangeles.query@vba.va.gov
www.va.gov

7896 **Martinez Center for Rehab & Extended Care**
Veterans Health Administration, US Dept. of VA
150 Muir Road
Martinez, CA 94553
925-372-2665
800-827-1000
e-mail: g.vhacss@forum.va.gov
www.va.gov

7897 **Oakland VA Regional Office**
Veterans Benefits Administration, US Dept. of VA
1301 Clay Street
Suite 1300N
Oakland, CA 94612
800-827-1000
e-mail: oakland.query@vba.va.gov
www.va.gov

7898 **Rehabilitation Research and Development Center**
Dept of Veteran's Affairs
3801 Miranda Avenue
MS-153
Palo Alto, CA 94304 **650-493-5000**
e-mail: jaffe@roses.stanford.edu
http://guide.stanford.edu

Christopher Jacobs PhD, Director
Nicholas J Giori MD PhD, Medical Director
David L Jaffe MS, Research Biomedical Engineer

The VA Center of Excellence on Mobility in Palo Alto, CA is dedicated to developing innovative clinical treatments and assistive devices for veterans with physical disabilities to increase their independence and improve their quality of life. The clinical emphasis of the Center is to improve mobility, either ambulation or manipulation, in individuals with Neurologic Impairments or Orthopaedic Impairments. We do not publish any printed books, journals or periodicals.

7899 **Sacramento Medical Center**
Veterans Health Administration, US Dept. of VA
10535 Hospital Way
Sacramento, CA 95655 **916-366-5470**
800-827-1000
e-mail: g.vhacss@forum.va.gov
www.va.gov

7900 **San Diego VA Regional Office**
Veterans Benefits Administration, US Dept. of VA
8810 Rio San Diego Drive
San Diego, CA 92108
800-827-1000
e-mail: oakland.query@vba.va.gov
www.va.gov

7901 **San Francisco VA Medical Center**
Veterans Health Administration, US Dept. of VA
4150 Clement Street
San Francisco, CA 94121 **415-221-4810**
877-487-2838
FAX: 415-750-2185
www.sf.med.va.gov

Gene Gibson, Public Affairs Officer

The San Francisco VA Medical Center (SFVAMC) serves as a major tertiary care referral center for veterans throughout Northern California. The facility has 124 acute care hospital beds. It is a high acuity medical center with over a third of bed days of care being in intensive care or monitored beds. Long term care programs include a 120 bed nursing home care unit at the San Francisco site and a home-based primary care program.

7902 **VA Central California Health Care Syste**
Veterans Health Administration, US Dept. of VA
2615 E Clinton Avenue
Fresno, CA 93703 **559-225-6100**
FAX: 559-268-6911
e-mail: g.vhacss@forum.va.gov
www.va.gov

7903 **VA Greater Los Angeles Healthcare System**
Veterans Health Administration, US Dept. of VA
11301 Willchire Boulevard
Los Angeles, CA 90073 **310-478-3711**
800-827-1000
FAX: 310-268-4848
e-mail: g.vhacss@forum.va.gov
www.va.gov

7904 **VA Northern California Healthcare System**
Veterans Health Administration, US Dept. of VA
150 Muir Road
Martinez, CA 94553 **925-372-2179**
800-827-1000
FAX: 925-372-2020
e-mail: g.vhacss@forum.va.gov
www.va.gov

7905 **VA San Diego Healthcare System**
Veterans Health Administration, US Dept. of VA
3350 La Jolla Village Drive
San Diego, CA 92161 **858-552-8585**
800-827-1000
e-mail: g.vhacss@forum.va.gov
www.va.gov

Colorado

7906 **Boulder Vet Center**
2336 Canyon Boulevard
Suite 103
Boulder, CO 80302 **303-440-7306**
FAX: 303-449-3907

Stew Brown PhD, Team Leader

Offers trauma and readjustment from military and civilian life counseling and assistance with disability claims, military benefits and employment are provided.

7907 **Colorado/Wyoming VA Medical Center**
Veterans Benefits Administration, US Dept. of VA
155 Van Gordon Street
Lakewood, CO 80228
800-827-1000
e-mail: denver.query@vba.va.gov
www.va.gov

7908 **Denver VA Medical Center**
Veterans Health Administration, US Dept. of VA
1055 Clermont Street
Denver, CO 80220 **303-399-8020**
800-827-1000
e-mail: g.vhacss@forum.va.gov
www.va.gov

7909 **Grand Junction VA Medical Center**
Veterans Health Administration, US Dept. of VA
2121 N Avenue
Grand Junction, CO 81501 **970-242-0731**
800-827-1000
FAX: 970-244-1300
e-mail: g.vhacss@forum.va.gov
www.va.gov

7910 **National Veterans Training Institute**
University of Colorado at Denver
1100 Stout Street
Suite 300
Denver, CO 80204 **303-871-2000**
800-331-0562
FAX: 303-825-0977

Training for specialists who serve veterans with disabilities.

7911 **Southern Colorado Healthcare System System**
Veterans Health Administration, US Dept. of VA
1339 S Pueblo Boulevard
Pueblo, CO 81005
719-566-6193
888-544-6724
FAX: 719-560-1806
e-mail: g.vhacss@forum.va.gov
www.va.gov

Connecticut

7912 **Disabled American Veterans: Connecticut**
35 Cold Spring Road
Suite 315
Rocky Hill, CT 06067
203-639-8387
www.davct.org/pages/youcanhelp.html

7913 **Hartford Regional Office**
Veterans Benefits Administration, US Dept. of VA
450 Main Street
Hartford, CT 06103
800-827-1000
e-mail: hartford.query@vba.va.gov
www.va.gov

7914 **VA Connecticut Healthcare System: Newington Division**
Veterans Health Administration, US Dept. of VA
555 Willard Avenue
Newington, CT 06111
860-666-6951
800-827-1000
FAX: 860-667-6764
e-mail: g.vhacss@forum.va.gov
www.va.gov

The mission of VA Connecticut Healthcare Systems is to fulfill a nation's commitment to its veterans by providing quality healthcare, promoting health through prevention and maintaining excellence in teaching and research. Provides primary, secondary and tertiary care in medicine, geriatrics, neurology, psychiatry and surgery with an operating capacity of 211 hospital beds.

7915 **VA Connecticut Healthcare System: West Haven**
Veterans Health Administration, US Dept. of VA
950 Campbell Avenue
W Haven, CT 06516
203-932-5711
FAX: 203-937-3868
e-mail: g.vhacss@forum.va.gov
www.va.gov

Delaware

7916 **Delaware Commission of Veterans Affairs**
Robbins Building
802 Silver Lake Boulevard,Suite 100
Dover, DE 19904
302-739-2792
800-344-9900
FAX: 302-739-2794
e-mail: adavila@state.de.us
www.state.de.us/veteran/index.htm

Antonio Davila, Executive Director

To assist, advise, and represent Delaware's military veterans and their families regarding programs and benefits available to them under federal and state laws.

7917 **Delaware VA Regional Office**
Veterans Benefits Administration, US Dept. of VA
1601 Kirkwood Highway
Wilmington, DE 19805
800-827-1000
e-mail: wilmington.query@vba.va.gov
www.va.gov

7918 **Wilmington VA Medical**
Veterans Health Administration, US Dept. of VA
1601 Kirkwood Highway
Wilmington, DE 19805
302-994-2511
800-827-1000
FAX: 302-633-5516
e-mail: g.vhacss@forum.va.gov
www.va.gov

District of Columbia

7919 **Disabled American Veterans, National Service & Legislative Headquarters**
807 Maine Avenue SW
Washington, DC 20024
202-554-3501
www.dav.org/nsf/awards.html

7920 **PVA Sports and Recreation Program**
Paralyzed Veterans of America
801 18th Street NW
Washington, DC 20006
202-273-8479
800-424-8200
FAX: 202-416-7639
e-mail: info@pva.org
www.pva.org

Andy Krieger, Director, Sports and Recreation

7921 **VA Medical Center, Washington DC**
50 Irving Street NW
Washington, DC 20422
202-273-5400
888-553-0242
www.washington.med.va.gov

Acute general and specialized services in medicine, surgery, neurology, and psychiatry.

7922 **Washington DC VA Medical Center**
Veterans Health Administration, US Dept. of VA
50 Irving Street NW
Washington, DC 20422
202-745-8000
800-827-1000
FAX: 202-754-8530
e-mail: g.vhacss@forum.va.gov
www.va.gov

Florida

7923 **Bay Pines VA Medical Center**
Veterans Health Administration, US Dept. of VA
10000 Bay Pines Boulevard
Bay Pines, FL 33744
727-398-6661
800-827-1000
e-mail: g.vhacss@forum.va.gov
www.va.gov

7924 **Gainesville Division, North Florida/South Georgia Veterans Healthcare System**

Veterans Health Administration, US Dept. of VA
1601 SW Archer Road
Room 165A
Gainesville, FL 32608
352-376-1611
800-324-8387
FAX: 352-379-7445
e-mail: g.vhacss@forum.va.gov
www.va.gov

Donald Holcomb, Disabled American Veterans Svc.

7925 **James A Haley VA Medical Center**

Veterans Health Administration, US Dept. of VA
13000 Bruce B Downs Boulevard
Tampa, FL 33612
813-972-2000
800-827-1000
e-mail: g.vhacss@forum.va.gov
www.va.gov

7926 **Lake City Division, North Florida/South Georgia Veterans Healthcare System**

Veterans Health Administration, US Dept. of VA
801 S Marion Street
Lake City, FL 32025
386-755-3016
800-827-1000
FAX: 386-758-3209
e-mail: g.vhacss@forum.va.gov
www.va.gov

7927 **Miami VA Medical Center**

Veterans Health Administration, US Dept. of VA
1201 NW 16th Street
Miami, FL 33125
305-324-4455
800-827-1000
e-mail: g.vhacss@forum.va.gov
www.va.gov

7928 **St. Petersburg Regional Office**

Veterans Benefits Administration, US Dept. of VA
9500 Ba Pines Boulevard
St. Petersburg, FL 33744
800-827-1000
e-mail: stpete.query@vba.va.gov
www.va.gov

7929 **West Palm Beach VA Medical Center**

Veterans Health Administration, US Dept. of VA
7305 N Military Trail
W Palm Beach, FL 33410
561-882-8262
800-827-1000
FAX: 561-882-6707
e-mail: g.vhacss@forum.va.gov
www.va.gov

Georgia

7930 **Atlanta Regional Office**

Veterans Benefits Administration, US Dept. of VA
730 Peachtree Street NE
Atlanta, GA 30365
800-827-1000
e-mail: atlanta.query@vba.va.gov
www.va.gov

7931 **Atlanta VA Medical Center**

Veterans Health Administration, US Dept. of VA
1670 Clairmont Road
Decatur, GA 30033
404-321-6111
800-827-1000
FAX: 404-728-7734
e-mail: g.vhacss@forum.va.gov
www.va.gov

7932 **Augusta VA Medical Center**

Veterans Health Administration, US Dept. of VA
One Freedom Way
Augusta, GA 30904
706-733-0188
800-827-1000
FAX: 706-823-3934
e-mail: g.vhacss@forum.va.gov
www.va.gov

7933 **Carl Vinson VA Medical Center**

Veterans Health Administration, US Dept. of VA
1826 Veterans Boulevard
Dublin, GA 31021
478-272-1210
FAX: 478-277-2717
e-mail: dana.doles@med.va.gov
www.va.gov

Dana F Doles, Public Affairs Officer

7934 **Georgia Veterans Centers**

922 W Peachtree Street NW
Atlanta, GA 30309
FAX: 404-347-7274

Veterans medical clinic offering disabled veterans medical treatments.

Hawaii

7935 **Hawaii Veterans Centers**

Keewe Street
Suite 201
Hilo, HI 96720
808-969-3833
FAX: 808-969-2025

Veterans medical clinic offering disabled veterans medical treatments.

7936 **Honolulu VBA Regional Office**

Veterans Benefits Administration, US Dept. of VA
300 Ala Moana Boulevard
Room 1004
Honolulu, HI 96850
808-541-2570
800-827-1000
e-mail: honolulu.query@vba.va.gov
www.va.gov

7937 **Spark M Matsunaga VA Medical Center & Regional Office**

Veterans Health Administration, US Dept. of VA
459 Patterson Road
Honolulu, HI 96819
808-433-1000
800-827-1000
FAX: 808-433-0390
e-mail: g.vhacss@forum.va.gov
www.va.gov

Idaho

7938 **Boise Regional Office**

Veterans Benefits Administration, US Dept. of VA
805 W Franklin Street
Boise, ID 83702
800-827-1000
e-mail: boise.query@vba.va.gov
www.va.gov

7939 **Boise VA Medical Center**
Veterans Health Administration, US Dept. of VA
500 W Fort Street
Boise, ID 83702
208-422-1000
800-827-1000
FAX: 208-422-1326
e-mail: g.vhacss@forum.va.gov
www.va.gov

7940 **Idaho Division of Veterans' Services**
320 Collins Road
Boise, ID 83702
208-334-3513
FAX: 208-334-2627
www.idvs.state.id.us

Richard W Jones, Administrator
Bonnie Dodson, Administrative Assistant

Illinois

7941 **Chicago-Lakeside VA Medical Center**
Veterans Health Administration, US Dept. of VA
333 E Huron Street
Chicago, IL 60611
312-943-6600
800-827-1000
FAX: 312-640-2248
e-mail: g.vhacss@forum.va.gov
vagreatlakes.org/fac/facmedcenter.asp?id=537a

7942 **Chicago-West Side VA Medical Center**
Veterans Health Administration, US Dept. of VA
820 S Damen Avenue
Chicago, IL 60612
312-666-6500
800-827-1000
e-mail: g.vhacss@forum.va.gov
www.va.gov

Thomas Stelmack OD, Director

Interdisciplinary team of optometry, ophthalmology, low vision training specialists, psychology, social work and audiology provide comprehensive low vision rehabilitation services for the partially sighted.

7943 **Edward Hines Jr Hospital**
Veterans Health Administration, US Dept. of VA
Fifth Avenue & Roosevelt Road
Hines, IL 60141
708-202-8387
800-827-1000
FAX: 708-202-2506
e-mail: g.vhacss@forum.va.gov
www.va.gov/sta/guide/facility.asp?ID=58

7944 **Illinois VA Regional Office Center**
Veterans Benefits Administration, US Dept. of VA
536 S Clark Street
Chicago, IL 60605
800-827-1000
e-mail: chicago.query@vba.va.gov
www.va.gov

7945 **Marion VA Medical Center**
Veterans Health Administration, US Dept. of VA
2401 W Main Street
Marion, IL 62959
618-997-5311
800-827-1000
e-mail: g.vhacss@forum.va.gov
www.va.gov

7946 **North Chicago VA Medical Center**
Veterans Health Administration, US Dept. of VA
3001 Green Bay Road
North Chicago, IL 60064
847-688-1900
800-827-1000
e-mail: g.vhacss@forum.va.gov
www.va.gov

7947 **VA Illiana Health Care System**
Veterans Health Administration, US Dept. of VA
1900 E Main Street
Danville, IL 61832
217-442-8000
800-827-1000
FAX: 217-554-4552
e-mail: g.vhacss@forum.va.gov
www.va.gov

Indiana

7948 **Indianapolis Regional Office**
Veterans Benefits Administration, US Dept. of VA
575 N Pennsylvania Street
Indianapolis, IN 46204
317-226-7860
800-827-1000
e-mail: indianapolis.query@vba.va.gov
www.va.gov

7949 **Richard L Roudebush VA Medical Center**
Veterans Health Administration, US Dept. of VA
1481 W 10th Street
Indianapolis, IN 46202
317-554-0000
800-827-1000
FAX: 317-554-0127
e-mail: g.vhacss@forum.va.gov
www.va.gov

7950 **VA North Indiana Health Care System: Marion Campus**
Veterans Health Administration, US Dept. of VA
1700 E 38th Street
Marion, IN 46953
765-674-3321
800-827-1000
e-mail: g.vhacss@forum.va.gov
www.va.gov

7951 **VA North Indiana Health Care System: Fort Wayne Campus**
Veterans Health Administration, US Dept. of VA
2121 Lake Avenue
Fort Wayne, IN 46805
260-426-5431
800-827-1000
FAX: 260-460-1336
e-mail: g.vhacss@forum.va.gov
www.va.gov

Iowa

7952 **Des Moines VA Medical Center**
Veterans Health Administration, US Dept. of VA
3600 30th Street
Des Moines, IA 50310
515-699-5850
800-827-1000
FAX: 515-699-5862
e-mail: g.vhacss@forum.va.gov
www.va.gov

7953 **Des Moines VA Regional Office**
Veterans Benefits Administration, US Dept. of VA
210 Walnut Street
Des Moines, IA 50309
800-827-1000
e-mail: desmoines.query@vba.va.gov
www.va.gov

7954 **Iowa City VA Medical Center**
Veterans Health Administration, US Dept. of VA
Highway 6 W
Iowa City, IA 52246
319-338-0581
800-827-1000
e-mail: g.vhacss@forum.va.gov
www.va.gov

Kirt A Sickels, Public Affairs Officer

Tertiary care facility, affiliated teaching hospital, and research center seving an aging veteran populatiaon in eastern Iowa and western Illinois. Satellite clinics are located in Bettendord, Dubuque, and Waterloo, Iowa and in Quincy and Galesburg, Illinois.

7955 **Knoxville VA Medical Center**
Veterans Health Administration, US Dept. of VA
1515 Pleasant Street
Knoxville, IA 50138
641-828-5000
800-827-1000
FAX: 641-828-5124
e-mail: g.vhacss@forum.va.gov
www.va.gov

7956 **VA Central Iowa Health Care System**
3600 30th Street
Des Moines, IA 50130
515-699-5999
FAX: 515-699-5214

Elaine Brewster, EEO Program Manager

Fulfilling the promise is our primary mission.

Kansas

7957 **Colmery-O'Neil VA Medical Center**
Veterans Health Administration, US Dept. of VA
2200 Gage Boulevard
Topeka, KS 66622
785-350-3111
800-827-1000
e-mail: g.vhacss@forum.va.gov
www.va.gov

7958 **Dwight D Eisenhower VA Medical Center**
Veterans Health Administration, US Dept. of VA
4101 S 4th Street
Leavenworth, KS 66048
913-682-2000
800-827-1000
e-mail: g.vhacss@forum.va.gov
www.va.gov

7959 **Kansas VA Regional Office**
Veterans Benefits Administration, US Dept. of VA
5500 E Kellogg
Wichita, KS 67218
800-827-1000
e-mail: wichita.query@vba.va.gov
www.va.gov

7960 **Wichita VA Medical Center**
Veterans Health Administration, US Dept. of VA
5500 E Kellogg Drive
Wichita, KS 67218
316-685-2221
800-827-1000
e-mail: g.vhacss@forum.va.gov
www.va.gov

Kentucky

7961 **Lexington VA Medical Center**
Veterans Health Administration, US Dept. of VA
Lexington, KY 40511
859-233-4511
800-352-4000
e-mail: g.vhacss@forum.va.gov
www.va.gov/sta/guide/facility.asp?ID=72

7962 **Louisville VA Medical Center**
Veterans Health Administration, US Dept. of VA
800 Zorn Avenue
Louisville, KY 40206
502-895-3401
800-827-1000
e-mail: g.vhacss@forum.va.gov
www.va.gov

7963 **Louisville VA Regional Office**
Veterans Benefits Administration, US Dept. of VA
545 S 3rd Street
Louisville, KY 40202
800-827-1000
e-mail: louisville.query@vba.va.gov
www.va.gov

Louisiana

7964 **Alexandria VA Medical Center**
Veterans Health Administration, US Dept. of VA
2495 Highway 71 N
Alexandria, LA 71301
318-473-0010
800-827-1000
FAX: 318-483-5029
e-mail: g.vhacss@forum.va.gov
www.va.gov

7965 **New Orleans VA Medical Center**
Veterans Health Administration, US Dept. of VA
1601 Perdido Street
New Orleans, LA 70112
504-568-0811
800-935-8387
FAX: 504-589-5210
e-mail: Stacie.Rivera@med.va.gov
www.va.gov

John D Church, Jr, Medical Center Director
Fernando Rivera, Assoc Medical Center Director
Sam Lucero, Special Assistant to Director

A teaching hospital, providing a full range of patient care services, with state-of-the-art technology as well as education and research. Comprehensive health care is provided through primary care, tetiary care, and long-term care in areas of medicine, surgery, psychiatry, physical medicine and rehabilitation, neurology, oncology, dentistry, geriatrics, and extended care.

7966 **Shreveport VA Medical Center**
Veterans Health Administration, US Dept. of VA
510 E Stoner Avenue
Shreveport, LA 71101
318-221-8411
800-827-1000
FAX: 318-424-6156
e-mail: g.vhacss@forum.va.gov
www.va.gov

Maine

7967 **Chapter 15 Disabled American Veterans**
PO Box 544
Brunswick, ME 04011 207-677-6033
e-mail: re.nee@verizon.net

Cliff Workman, Commander

7968 **Disabled American Veterans: Maine**
PO Box 3151
Togus, ME 04330 207-623-5725
e-mail: dav@mint.net
www.dav.org

7969 **Maine VA Regional Office**
Veterans Benefits Administration, US Dept. of VA
One VA Center
Togus, ME 04330
800-827-1000
e-mail: togus.query@vba.va.gov
www.va.gov

7970 **Togus VA Medical Center**
Veterans Health Administration, US Dept. of VA
1 VA Center
Togus, ME 04330 207-623-8411
800-827-1000
e-mail: g.vhacss@forum.va.gov
www.va.gov

Maryland

7971 **Baltimore Regional Office**
Veterans Benefits Administration, US Dept. of VA
31 Hopkins Plaza Federal Building
Baltimore, MD 21201
800-827-1000
e-mail: baltimore.query@vba.va.gov
www.va.gov

7972 **Baltimore VA Medical Center**
Veterans Health Administration, US Dept. of VA
10 N Greene Street
Baltimore, MD 21201 410-605-7000
800-463-6295
e-mail: g.vhacss@forum.va.gov
www.vamhcs.med.va.gov/balto/baltimor.htm

7973 **Fort Howard VA Medical Center**
Veterans Health Administration, US Dept. of VA
9600 N Point Road
Fort Howard, MD 21052 410-477-1800
800-827-1000
e-mail: g.vhacss@forum.va.gov
www.va.gov

7974 **Maryland Veterans Centers**
6666 Security Boulevard
Suite 2
Gwynn Oak, MD 21207 410-277-3600
FAX: 410-277-3605

Veterans medical clinic offering disabled veterans medical treatments.

7975 **Perry Point VA Medical Center**
Veterans Health Administration, US Dept. of VA
Perry Point, MD 21902 410-642-2411
800-827-1000
e-mail: g.vhacss@forum.va.gov
www.va.gov

7976 **VA Maryland Health Care System**
10 N Greene Street
Baltimore, MD 21201 410-605-7000
800-827-1000
FAX: 410-605-7900
www.vamhcs.med.va.gov

R Daved Edwards, Chief Public/Community Relations
Monica A Smith, Public Affairs Specialist

A dynamic and exciting health care organization that is dedicated to providing quality, compassionate and accessible care and service to Maryland's veterans. As a part of one of the largest health care systems in the United States, the VAMHCS has a reputation as a leader in veterans' health care, reserch and education. Provides comprehensive service to veterans including medical, surgical, rehabilitative, nurological and mental health care on both an inpatient and outpatient basis.

Massachusetts

7977 **Boston VA Regional Office**
Veterans Benefits Administration, US Dept. of VA
JFK Federal Building
Government Center
Boston, MA 02114
800-827-1000
e-mail: boston.query@vba.va.gov
www.va.gov

7978 **Edith Nourse Rogers Memorial Veterans Hospital**
Veterans Health Administration, US Dept. of VA
200 Springs Road
Bedford, MA 01730
800-827-1000
e-mail: g.vhacss@forum.va.gov
www.va.gov

7979 **Northampton VA Medical Center**
Veterans Health Administration, US Dept. of VA
421 N Main Street
Leeds, MA 01053 413-584-4040
800-827-1000
FAX: 413-582-3121
e-mail: g.vhacss@forum.va.gov
www.va.gov

7980 **VA Boston Healthcare System: Brockton Division**
Veterans Health Administration, US Dept. of VA
940 Belmont Street
Brockton, MA 02310 508-583-4500
800-827-1000
FAX: 617-323-7700
e-mail: g.vhacss@forum.va.gov
www.va.gov

7981 **VA Boston Healthcare System: Jamaica Plain Campus**
Veterans Health Administration, US Dept. of VA
150 S Huntington Avenue
Boston, MA 02130 617-232-9500
800-827-1000
FAX: 617-278-4549
e-mail: g.vhacss@forum.va.gov
www.va.gov

7982 **VA Boston Healthcare System: West Roxbury Division**

Veterans Health Administration, US Dept. of VA
1400 VFW Parkway
W Roxbury, MA 02132
413-584-4040
800-827-1000
FAX: 413-582-3121
e-mail: g.vhacss@forum.va.gov
www.va.gov

Providing a broad range of counseling outreach and referral services to eligible veterans in order to help make readjustments to cilvilian life.

Michigan

7983 **Aleda E Lutz VA Medical Center**

Veterans Health Administration, US Dept. of VA
1500 Weiss Street
Saginaw, MI 48602
989-497-2500
800-827-1000
FAX: 989-791-2428
e-mail: g.vhacss@forum.va.gov
www.va.gov

7984 **Battle Creek VA Medical Center**

Veterans Health Administration, US Dept. of VA
5500 Armstrong Road
Battle Creek, MI 49016
269-966-5600
800-827-1000
FAX: 269-966-5483
e-mail: g.vhacss@forum.va.gov
www.va.gov

7985 **Iron Mountain VA Medical Center**

Veterans Health Administration, US Dept. of VA
325 E H Street
Iron Mountain, MI 49801
906-774-3300
800-827-1000
FAX: 906-779-3114
e-mail: g.vhacss@forum.va.gov
www.va.gov

7986 **John D Dingell VA Medical Center**

Veterans Health Administration, US Dept. of VA
4646 John R
Detroit, MI 48201
313-576-1000
800-827-1000
FAX: 313-576-1025
e-mail: g.vhacss@forum.va.gov
www.va.gov

7987 **Michigan VA Regional Office**

Veterans Benefits Administration, US Dept. of VA
Patrick V McNamara Federal Building
477 Michigan Avenue, Room 1400
Detroit, MI 48226
800-827-1000
e-mail: detroit.query@vba.va.gov
www.va.gov

7988 **VA Ann Arbor Healthcare System**

Veterans Health Administration, US Dept. of VA
2215 Fuller Road
Ann Arbor, MI 48105
734-769-7100
FAX: 734-761-7870
e-mail: g.vhacss@forum.va.gov
www.va.gov

Accepting eligible veterans.

7989 **Vet Center Readjustment Counseling Service**

1940 Eastern Avenue SE
Grand Rapids, MI 49507
616-243-0385
FAX: 616-243-5390

William Busby PhD, Team Leader
Lynn Hall PhD, Clinical Coordinator

Minnesota

7990 **Minneapolis VA Medical Center**

Veterans Health Administration, US Dept. of VA
One Veterans Drive
Minneapolis, MN 55417
612-725-2000
800-827-1000
FAX: 612-725-2049
e-mail: g.vhacss@forum.va.gov
www.va.gov

7991 **St. Cloud VA Medical Center**

Veterans Health Administration, US Dept. of VA
4801 8th Street N
St. Cloud, MN 56303
320-252-1670
800-827-1000
FAX: 320-255-6494
e-mail: g.vhacss@forum.va.gov
www.va.gov

7992 **St. Paul Regional Office**

Veterans Benefits Administration, US Dept. of VA
One Federal Drive
Fort Snelling
St. Paul, MN 55111
800-827-1000
e-mail: stpaul.query@vba.va.gov
www.va.gov

7993 **Vet Center**

405 E Superior Street
Duluth, MN 55802
218-722-8654
FAX: 218-723-8212

Cynthia Macaulay MEd, Counselor
Rob Evanson, Counselor
Debbie Burt, Office Manager

Counseling, social services and benefits assistance for combat veterans and those sexually traumatized in the military.

Mississippi

7994 **Biloxi/Gulfport VA Medical Center**

Veterans Health Administration, US Dept. of VA
400 Veterans Avenue
Biloxi, MS 39531
228-523-5000
800-827-1000
e-mail: g.vhacss@forum.va.gov
www.va.gov

7995 **Jackson Regional Office**

Veterans Benefits Administration, US Dept. of VA
1600 E Woodrow Wilson Avenue
Jackson, MS 39216
800-827-1000
e-mail: jackson.query@vba.va.gov
www.va.gov

7996 **Jackson VA Medical Center**

Veterans Health Administration, US Dept. of VA
1500 E Woodrow Wilson Drive
Jackson, MS 39216
601-362-4471
800-362-1000
FAX: 601-364-1359
e-mail: g.vhacss@forum.va.gov
www.va.gov

Missouri

7997 Harry S Truman Memorial Veterans' Hospital
Veterans Health Administration, US Dept. of VA
800 Hospital Drive
Columbia, MO 65201
573-814-6000
800-349-8220
FAX: 573-814-6600
e-mail: g.vhacss@forum.va.gov
www.va.gov

7998 John J Pershing VA Medical Center
Veterans Health Administration, US Dept. of VA
1500 N Westwood Boulevard
Poplar Bluff, MO 63901
573-686-4151
800-827-1000
e-mail: g.vhacss@forum.va.gov
www.va.gov

7999 Kansas City VA Medical Center
Veterans Health Administration, US Dept. of VA
4801 Linwood Boulevard
Kansas City, MO 64128
816-861-4700
800-827-1000
e-mail: g.vhacss@forum.va.gov
www.va.gov

Juliette Leach, EEO Manager
Thirza Thompson, SEPM Manager

The Kansas City VA Medical Center is a modern, well-equipped teriary care inpatient and outpatient center. As the third largest teaching hospital in the metropolitan area, it maintains educational affiliations with the University of Kansas School of Medicine.

8000 Missouri Veterans Centers
3931 Main Street
Kansas City, MO 64111
816-753-1866
FAX: 816-753-2328

Veterans medical clinic offering disabled veterans medical treatments.

8001 St. Louis Regional Office
Veterans Benefits Administration, US Dept. of VA
Federal Building
400 S 18th Street
St. Louis, MO 63103
800-827-1000
e-mail: stlouis.query@vba.va.gov
www.va.gov

8002 St. Louis VA Medical Center
Veterans Health Administration, US Dept. of VA
Jefferson Barracks Division #1
Jefferson Barracks Drive
St. Louis, MO 63125
314-652-4100
800-827-1000
e-mail: g.vhacss@forum.va.gov
www.va.gov

Montana

8003 Montana VA Regional Office
Veterans Benefits Administration, US Dept. of VA
Williams Street
Fort Harrison, MT 59636
800-827-1000
e-mail: ftharrison.query@vba.va.gov
www.va.gov

8004 VA Montana Healthcare System
Veterans Health Administration, US Dept. of VA
William Street
Fort Harrison, MT 59636
406-442-6410
800-827-1000
FAX: 406-447-7965
e-mail: g.vhacss@forum.va.gov
www.va.gov

8005 Vet Center
1234 Avenue C
Billings, MT 59102
406-657-6071
FAX: 406-657-6603

Bob Phillips MSW, Team Leader
Luanne Oakland MS, Office Manager
Barry Osgard MS, Counselor

Readjustment counseling service for counseling veterans who are having difficulty adjusting from military service especially those diagnosed with PTSD.

Nebraska

8006 Grand Island VA Medical System
Veterans Health Administration, US Dept. of VA
2201 N Brodwell Avenue
Grand Island, NE 68803
308-382-3660
800-827-1000
e-mail: g.vhacss@forum.va.gov
www.va.gov

8007 Lincoln Regional Office
Veterans Benefits Administration, US Dept. of VA
5631 S 48th Street
Lincoln, NE 68516
800-827-1000
e-mail: lincoln.query@vba.va.gov
www.va.gov

8008 Lincoln VA Medical Center
Veterans Health Administration, US Dept. of VA
600 S 70th Street
Lincoln, NE 68510
402-489-3802
800-827-1000
FAX: 402-486-7840
e-mail: g.vhacss@forum.va.gov
www.va.gov

8009 VA Nebraska-Western Iowa Health Care System
Veterans Health Administration, US Dept. of VA
4101 Woolworth Avenue
Omaha, NE 68105
402-346-8800
FAX: 402-449-0684
www.va.gov

Sharon King, People with Disabilities Chair
Cheri DeWispelare, EEO Manager

Nevada

8010 Las Vegas Veterans Center
1040 E Sahara Avenue
Suite 102
Las Vegas, NV 89104
702-388-6369
FAX: 702-388-6664

Gerald Eusf, Clinical Coordinator, LCSW
Daryl Harding, Resident Counselor LCSW
Matt Watson, Team Leader MSW

Veterans clinical counseling center for veterans and their dependent individual and group counseling, marital and family counseling, alcohol and drug assessment referral or treatment. Community education and consultation, employment counseling.

8011 Reno Regional Office
Veterans Benefits Administration, US Dept. of VA
1201 Terminal Way
Reno, NV 89520
800-827-1000
e-mail: reno.query@vba.va.gov
www.va.gov

8012 VA Sierra Nevada Healthcare System
Veterans Health Administration, US Dept. of VA
1000 Locust Street
Reno, NV 89502
775-786-7200
888-838-6256
FAX: 775-328-1464
www.va.gov

Lisa Howard, Office of the Director

8013 VA Southern Nevada Healthcare System
Veterans Health Administration, US Dept. of VA
1700 Vegas Drive
Las Vegas, NV 89106
702-636-3000
800-827-1000
FAX: 707-636-4000
e-mail: g.vhacss@forum.va.gov
www.va.gov

New Hampshire

8014 Manchester Regional Office
Veterans Benefits Administration, US Dept. of VA
Norris Cotton Federal Building
275 Chestnut Street
Manchester, NH 03101
800-827-1000
e-mail: manchester.query@vba.va.gov
www.va.gov

8015 Manchester VA Medical Center
Veterans Health Administration, US Dept. of VA
718 Smyth Road
Manchester, NH 03104
603-624-4366
800-827-1000
e-mail: g.vhacss@forum.va.gov
www.va.gov

8016 New Hampshire Veterans Centers
103 Liberty Street
Manchester, NH 03104
603-668-7060
FAX: 603-666-7404

Caryl Ahern MSW, Team Leader
Paulette Landry, Office Manager

Veterans clinic offering combat veterans outpatient counseling

New Jersey

8017 Disabled American Veterans, New Jersey Northern Valley Chapter 32
PO Box 505
8 Veterans Plaza
Bergenfield, NJ 07621
201-384-0001
e-mail: DAV32GIN@aol.com
www.davnj.org

Virginia McAleer-Hujber, Adjutant

8018 Disabled American Veterans: Ocean County
PO Box 1806
Toms River, NJ 08754
732-929-0907
e-mail: bvenga@thecore.com
http://community.nj.com/cc/dav24

Mary Bencivenga, Contact

8019 East Orange Campus of the VA New Jersey Healthcare System
Veterans Health Administration, US Dept. of VA
385 Tremont Avenue
E Orange, NJ 07018
973-676-1000
800-827-1000
FAX: 973-676-4226
e-mail: g.vhacss@forum.va.gov
www.va.gov

8020 Lyons Campus of the VA New Jersey Healthcare System
Veterans Health Administration, US Dept. of VA
151 Knollcroft Road
Lyons, NJ 07939
908-647-0180
800-827-1000
FAX: 908-647-3452
e-mail: g.vhacss@forum.va.gov
www.va.gov

8021 Newark Regional Office
Veterans Benefits Administration, US Dept. of VA
20 Washington Place
Newark, NJ 07102
800-827-1000
e-mail: newark.query@vba.va.gov
www.va.gov

New Mexico

8022 Albuquerque Regional Office
Veterans Benefits Administration, US Dept. of VA
Danis Chevez Federal Building
500 Gold Avenue SW
Albuquerque, NM 87102
800-827-1000
e-mail: albuquerque.query@vba.va.gov
www.va.gov

8023 New Mexico VA Healthcare System
Veterans Health Administration, US Dept. of VA
1501 San Pedro Drive SE
Albuquerque, NM 87108
505-265-1711
800-827-1000
FAX: 505-256-2855
e-mail: g.vhacss@forum.va.gov
www.va.gov

8024 **New Mexico Veterans Centers**
PO Box 927
TRC, NM 87901 **505-894-4200**

Veterans medical clinic offering disabled veterans medical treatments.

New York

8025 **Albany VA Medical Center: Samuel S Stratton**
Veterans Health Administration, US Dept. of VA
113 Holland Avenue
Albany, NY 12208 **518-626-5000**
800-827-1000
FAX: 518-626-5500
e-mail: g.vhacss@forum.va.gov
www.va.gov

Linda Blumenstock, Marketing Director

8026 **Albany Vet Center**
875 Central Avenue
Albany, NY 12206 **518-438-2505**
FAX: 518-458-8613

Maureen Chauvin, Office Manager

Provides readjustment counseling for combat veterans and also provides benefits and job counseling.

8027 **Bath VA Medical Center**
Veterans Health Administration, US Dept. of VA
76 Veterans Medical Center
Bath, NY 14810 **607-664-4000**
800-827-1000
FAX: 607-664-4000
e-mail: g.vhacss@forum.va.gov
www.va.gov

8028 **Bronx VA Medical Center**
Veterans Health Administration, US Dept. of VA
130 W Kingsbridge Road
Bronx, NY 10468 **718-584-9000**
800-827-1000
e-mail: g.vhacss@forum.va.gov
www.va.gov

8029 **Brooklyn Campus of the VA NY Harbor Healthcare System**
Veterans Health Administration, US Dept. of VA
800 Poly Place
Brooklyn, NY 11209 **718-836-6600**
800-827-1000
e-mail: g.vhacss@forum.va.gov
www.va.gov

8030 **Buffalo Regional Office**
Veterans Benefits Administration, US Dept. of VA
Federal Building
111 W Huron Street
Buffalo, NY 14202
800-827-1000
e-mail: buffalo.query@vba.va.gov
www.va.gov

8031 **Canandiagua VA Medical Center**
Veterans Health Administration, US Dept. of VA
400 Fort Hill Avenue
Canandaigua, NY 14424 **585-394-2000**
800-827-1000
e-mail: g.vhacss@forum.va.gov
www.va.gov

8032 **Castle Point Campus of the VA Hudson Valley Healthcare System**
Veterans Health Administration, US Dept. of VA
Castle Point, NY 12511 **914-831-2000**
800-827-1000
e-mail: g.vhacss@forum.va.gov
www.va.gov

8033 **New York City Campus of the VA NY Harbor Healthcare System**
Veterans Health Administration, US Dept. of VA
423 E 23rd Street
New York, NY 10010 **212-686-7500**
800-827-1000
FAX: 212-951-3487
e-mail: g.vhacss@forum.va.gov
www.va.gov

8034 **New York Regional Office**
Veterans Benefits Administration, US Dept. of VA
245 W Houston Street
New York, NY 10014
800-827-1000
e-mail: newyork.query@vba.va.gov
www.va.gov

8035 **Northport VA Medical Center**
Veterans Health Administration, US Dept. of VA
79 Middlevale Road
Northport, NY 11768 **631-261-4400**
800-827-1000
e-mail: g.vhacss@forum.va.gov
www.va.gov

8036 **Syracuse VA Medical Center**
Veterans Health Administration, US Dept. of VA
800 Irving Avenue
Syracuse, NY 13210 **315-476-7461**
800-827-1000
e-mail: g.vhacss@forum.va.gov
www.va.gov

8037 **Torah Alliance of Families of Kids with Disabilities**
TAFKID
1433 Coney Island Avenue
Brooklyn, NY 11230 **718-252-2236**
FAX: 718-252-2216
e-mail: tafkid@worldnet.att.net
www.tafkid.org

Juby Shapiro, President/Program Director

Serves over 1k families whose children have a variety of disabilities and special needs. Many of these families are large families in the low socioeconomic level. Offers monthly meetings, guest lectures, parent matching, information of new developments in software, technology and techniques, sibling support groups, pen pal lists, audio and video library, alternative medicine and nutrition information and education on legal awareness and rights of disabled citizens.

8038 **VA Hudson Valley Health Care System**
PO Box 100
Montrose, NY 10548 **845-737-4400**
FAX: 845-788-4244

8039 **VA Western NY Healthcare System, Batavia**
Veterans Health Administration, US Dept. of VA
222 Richmond Avenue
Batavia, NY 14020 **585-343-7500**
800-827-1000
e-mail: g.vhacss@forum.va.gov
www.va.gov

8040 VA Western NY Healthcare System, Buffalo
Veterans Health Administration, US Dept. of VA
3495 Bailey Avenue
Buffalo, NY 14215
716-834-9200
800-827-1000
e-mail: g.vhacss@forum.va.gov
www.va.gov

North Carolina

8041 Asheville VA Medical Center
Veterans Health Administration, US Dept. of VA
1100 Tunnel Road
Asheville, NC 28805
828-298-7911
800-827-1000
FAX: 828-299-2502
e-mail: g.vhacss@forum.va.gov
www.va.gov

8042 Charlotte Vet Center
223 S Brevard Street
Suite 103
Charlotte, NC 28202
704-333-6107
FAX: 704-344-6470

Loretta Deaton, Team Leader

Preadjustment Counseling for Combat Veterans with Post Traumatic Stress Disorder (PTSD).

8043 Durham VA Medical Center
Veterans Health Administration, US Dept. of VA
508 Fulton Street
Durham, NC 27705
919-286-0411
800-827-1000
FAX: 919-286-6825
e-mail: g.vhacss@forum.va.gov
www.va.gov

8044 Fayetteville VA Medical Center
Veterans Health Administration, US Dept. of VA
2300 Ramsey Street
Fayetteville, NC 28301
910-488-2120
800-827-1000
FAX: 910-822-7927
e-mail: g.vhacss@forum.va.gov
www.va.gov

8045 Franklin Delano Roosevelt Campus of the VA Hudson Valley Healthcare System
Veterans Health Administration, US Dept. of VA
Route 9A, 622 Albany Post Road
PO Box 100
Montrose, NC 10548
845-737-4400
800-887-2001
FAX: 914-788-4244
e-mail: g.vhacss@forum.va.gov
www.va.gov

8046 WG Hefner VA Medical Center
Veterans Health Administration, US Dept. of VA
1601 Brenner Avenue
Salisbury, NC 28301
704-638-9000
800-827-1000
FAX: 704-638-3395
e-mail: g.vhacss@forum.va.gov
www.va.gov

8047 Winston-Salem Regional Office
Veterans Benefits Administration, US Dept. of VA
Federal Building
251 N Main Street
Winston-Salem, NC 27155
800-827-1000
e-mail: winsalem.query@vba.va.gov
www.va.gov

North Dakota

8048 Fargo VA Medical Center
Veterans Health Administration, US Dept. of VA
2101 Elm Street
Fargo, ND 58102
800-827-1000
e-mail: g.vhacss@forum.va.gov
www.va.gov

8049 North Dakota Department of Veterans' Affairs
PO Box 9003
1411 32nd Street S
Fargo, ND 58106
701-239-7165
FAX: 701-239-7166
www.nasdva.com/northdakota.html

Ray Harkema, Commissioner

8050 North Dakota VA Regional Office
Veterans Benefits Administration, US Dept. of VA
2101 Elm Street
Fargo, ND 58102
800-827-1000
e-mail: fargo.query@vba.va.gov
www.va.gov

Ohio

8051 Chillicothe VA Medical Center
Veterans Health Administration, US Dept. of VA
17273 State Route 104
Chillicothe, OH 45601
740-773-1141
800-827-1000
FAX: 740-772-7023
e-mail: g.vhacss@forum.va.gov
www.va.gov

8052 Cincinnati VA Medical Center
Veterans Health Administration, US Dept. of VA
3200 Vine Street
Cincinnati, OH 45220
513-861-3100
800-827-1000
FAX: 513-475-6500
e-mail: g.vhacss@forum.va.gov
www.va.gov

8053 Cincinnati Veterans Centers
801B W 8th Street
Suite 126
Cincinnati, OH 45203
513-741-5600
FAX: 513-763-3505

Veterans medical clinic offering disabled veterans medical treatments.

8054 Cleveland Regional Office
Veterans Benefits Administration, US Dept. of VA
AJ Celebrezze Federal Building
1240 E 9th Street
Cleveland, OH 44199
800-827-1000
e-mail: cleveland.query@vba.va.gov
www.va.gov

8055 Dayton VA Medical Center
Veterans Health Administration, US Dept. of VA
4100 W 3rd Street
Dayton, OH 45428
937-268-6511
800-827-1000
FAX: 937-262-2179
e-mail: g.vhacss@forum.va.gov
www.va.gov

8056 Louis Stokes VA Medical Center
Veterans Health Administration, US Dept. of VA
10701 E Boulevard
Cleveland, OH 44106
440-526-3030
800-827-1000
FAX: 440-838-6017
e-mail: g.vhacss@forum.va.gov
www.va.gov

Oklahoma

8057 Muskogee VA Medical Center
Veterans Benefits Administration, US Dept. of VA
1011 Honor Heights Drive
Muskogee, OK 74401
918-683-3261
800-827-1000
e-mail: muskogee.query@vba.va.gov
www.va.gov

8058 Oklahoma City VA Medical Center
Veterans Health Administration, US Dept. of VA
921 NE 13th Street
Oklahoma City, OK 73104
405-270-0501
800-827-1000
FAX: 405-270-5132
e-mail: g.vhacss@forum.va.gov
www.va.gov

Steven J Gentling, Director
Kathleen Fogarty, Associate Director
D Robert McCaffree MD, Chief of Staff

8059 Oklahoma Veterans Centers Vet Center
3033 N Walnut Avenue
Suite W101
Oklahoma City, OK 73105
405-528-5583
FAX: 405-270-5125

Peter Sharp, Team Leader

PTSP Counseling for all combat Veterans and victims of sexual trauma/sexual harassment.

Oregon

8060 Oregon Health Sciences University
3181 SW Sam Jackson Park Road
Portland, OR 97201
503-418-4016

Thomas Talboe

Offers services for the totally blind, legally blind, visually impaired, mentally retarded blind and more with health, counseling, educational, recreational, rehabilitation, computer training and professional training services.

8061 Portland Regional Office
Veterans Benefits Administration, US Dept. of VA
1220 SW 3rd Avenue
Portland, OR 97204
800-827-1000
e-mail: portland.query@vba.va.gov
www.va.gov

8062 Portland VA Medical Center
Veterans Health Administration, US Dept. of VA
3710 SW US Veterans Hospital Road
PO Box 1034
Portland, OR 97201
503-220-8262
800-827-1000
FAX: 503-273-5319
e-mail: g.vhacss@forum.va.gov
www.va.gov

8063 Roseburg VA Medical Center
Veterans Health Administration, US Dept. of VA
913 NW Garden Valley Boulevard
Roseburg, OR 97470
541-440-1000
800-827-1000
FAX: 541-440-1225
e-mail: g.vhacss@forum.va.gov
www.va.gov

8064 White City VA Domiciliary
Veterans Health Administration, US Dept. of VA
8495 Crater Lake Highway
White City, OR 97503
541-826-2111
800-827-1000
e-mail: g.vhacss@forum.va.gov
www.va.gov

Pennsylvania

8065 Butler VA Medical Center
Veterans Health Administration, US Dept. of VA
325 New Castle Road
Butler, PA 16001
724-287-4781
800-827-1000
FAX: 724-282-4408
e-mail: g.vhacss@forum.va.gov
www.va.gov

8066 Coatesville VA Medical Center
Veterans Health Administration, US Dept. of VA
1400 Black Horse Hill Road
Coatesville, PA 19320
610-384-7711
800-827-1000
e-mail: g.vhacss@forum.va.gov
www.va.gov

8067 Erie VA Medical Center
Veterans Health Administration, US Dept. of VA
135 E 38th Street
Erie, PA 16504
814-868-8661
800-827-1000
e-mail: g.vhacss@forum.va.gov
www.va.gov

8068 **James E Van Zandt VA Medical Center**
Veterans Health Administration, US Dept. of VA
2907 Pleasant Valley Boulevard
Altoona, PA 16602
814-943-8164
800-827-1000
FAX: 814-940-7898
e-mail: g.vhacss@forum.va.gov
www.va.gov

8069 **Lebanon VA Medical Center**
Veterans Health Administration, US Dept. of VA
1700 S Lincoln Avenue
Lebanon, PA 17042
717-272-6621
800-409-8771
FAX: 717-228-5907
e-mail: g.vhacss@forum.va.gov
www.va.gov

8070 **Pennsylvania Veterans Centers**
G Daniel Baldwin Building
1000 State Street
Suite 2
Erie, PA 16501
FAX: 814-456-5464

Veterans medical clinic offering disabled veterans medical treatments.

8071 **Philadelphia Regional Office and Insurance Center**
Veterans Benefits Administration, US Dept. of VA
5000 Wissahickon Avenue
Philadelphia, PA 19101
800-827-1000
e-mail: phillyro.query@vba.va.gov
www.va.gov

8072 **Philadelphia VA Medical Center**
Veterans Health Administration, US Dept. of VA
University and Woodland Avenues
Philadelphia, PA 19104
215-823-5800
800-827-1000
e-mail: g.vhacss@forum.va.gov
www.va.gov

8073 **Pittsburgh Regional Office**
Veterans Benefits Administration, US Dept. of VA
1000 Liberty Avenue
Pittsburgh, PA 15222
800-827-1000
e-mail: pittsburgh.query@vba.va.gov
www.va.gov

8074 **VA Pittsburgh Healthcare System, University Drive Division**
Veterans Health Administration, US Dept. of VA
University Drive
Pittsburgh, PA 15240
412-688-6000
800-827-1000
FAX: 412-688-6901
e-mail: g.vhacss@forum.va.gov
www.va.gov

8075 **VA Pittsburgh Healthcare System, Highland Drive Division**
Veterans Health Administration, US Dept. of VA
7180 Highland Drive
Pittsburgh, PA 15206
412-365-4900
800-827-1000
e-mail: g.vhacss@forum.va.gov
www.va.gov

8076 **Wilkes-Barre VA Medical Center**
Veterans Health Administration, US Dept. of VA
1111 E End Boulevard
Wilkes-Barre, PA 18711
570-824-3521
800-827-1000
e-mail: g.vhacss@forum.va.gov
www.va.gov

Rhode Island

8077 **Providence Regional Office**
Veterans Benefits Administration, US Dept. of VA
380 Westminister Hall
Providence, RI 02903
800-827-1000
e-mail: providence.query@vba.va.gov
www.va.gov

8078 **Providence VA Medical Center**
Veterans Health Administration, US Dept. of VA
830 Chalkstone Avenue
Providence, RI 02908
401-273-7100
800-827-1000
FAX: 401-457-3370
e-mail: g.vhacss@forum.va.gov
www.va.gov

Alan Kordlenko, Human Resources Mgmt Service
Benson Werthan, EED Manager

8079 **Rhode Island Veterans Center**
789 Park Avenue
Cranston, RI 02910
401-467-2046
FAX: 401-528-5253

Veterans medical clinic offering disabled veterans medical treatments.

South Carolina

8080 **Columbia Regional Office**
Veterans Benefits Administration, US Dept. of VA
1801 Assembly Street
Columbia, SC 29201
803-734-0200
800-827-1000
e-mail: columbia.query@vba.va.gov
www.va.gov

8081 **Ralph H Johnson VA Medical Center**
Veterans Health Administration, US Dept. of VA
109 Bee Street
Charleston, SC 29401
843-937-5011
800-827-1000
FAX: 843-937-6100
e-mail: g.vhacss@forum.va.gov
www.va.gov

8082 **William Jennings Bryan Dorn VA Medical Center**
Veterans Health Administration, US Dept. of VA
6439 Garners Ferry Road
Columbia, SC 29209
803-776-4000
800-827-1000
FAX: 803-695-6739
e-mail: g.vhacss@forum.va.gov
www.va.gov

South Dakota

8083 **Sioux Falls VA Medical Center**
Veterans Health Administration, US Dept. of VA
2501 W 22nd Street
PO Box 5046
Sioux Falls, SD 57117
605-336-3230
800-827-1000
FAX: 605-333-6878
e-mail: g.vhacss@forum.va.gov
www.va.gov

8084 **South Dakota VA Regional Office**
Veterans Benefits Administration, US Dept. of VA
PO Box 5046
Sioux Falls, SD 57117
800-827-1000
e-mail: siouxfalls.query@vba.va.gov
www.va.gov

8085 **South Dakota Veterans Centers**
610 Kansas City Street
Rapid City, SD 57701
605-348-0077
FAX: 605-348-0878

Veterans medical clinic offering disabled veterans medical treatments.

Tennessee

8086 **Alvin C York VA Medical Center**
Veterans Health Administration, US Dept. of VA
3400 Lebanon Road
Murfreesboro, TN 37129
615-893-1360
800-827-1000
FAX: 615-867-5802
e-mail: g.vhacss@forum.va.gov
www.va.gov

8087 **Memphis VA Medical Center**
Veterans Health Administration, US Dept. of VA
1030 Jefferson Avenue
Memphis, TN 38104
901-523-8990
800-827-1000
e-mail: g.vhacss@forum.va.gov
www.va.gov

8088 **Mountain Home VA Medical Center**
Veterans Health Administration, US Dept. of VA
Mountain Home, TN 37684
423-926-1171
800-827-1000
e-mail: g.vhacss@forum.va.gov
www.va.gov

8089 **Nasheville Regional Office**
Veterans Benefits Administration, US Dept. of VA
110 9th Avenue S
Nashville, TN 37203
800-827-1000
e-mail: nashville.query@vba.va.gov
www.va.gov

8090 **Nashville VA Medical Center**
Veterans Health Administration, US Dept. of VA
1310 24th Avenue S
Nashville, TN 37212
615-327-4751
800-827-1000
FAX: 615-321-6350
e-mail: g.vhacss@forum.va.gov
www.va.gov

Texas

8091 **Amarillo VA Healthcare System**
Veterans Health Administration, US Dept. of VA
Amarillo, TX 79106
806-355-9703
800-827-1000
FAX: 806-354-7869
e-mail: g.vhacss@forum.va.gov
www.va.gov

8092 **Amarillo Vet Center**
Department of Veterans Affairs
3414 Olsen Boulevard
Suite E
Amarillo, TX 79109
806-354-9779
FAX: 806-354-7869
e-mail: info@roses.stanford.edu

Pedro Garcia Jr, Team Leader
Mary J Williams, Program Assistant

Provides individual, group and family counseling to veterans who served in combat theaters of World War II and Korea, Veterans of the Vietnam Era, and veterans of conflicts zones in Lebanon, Grenada, Panama, the Persian Guld and Somalia.

8093 **El Paso VA Healthcare Center**
Veterans Health Administration, US Dept. of VA
5001 N Piedras Street
El Paso, TX 79930
915-564-6100
800-827-1000
FAX: 915-564-7920
e-mail: g.vhacss@forum.va.gov
www.va.gov

8094 **Houston Regional Office**
Veterans Benefits Administration, US Dept. of VA
6900 Almeda Road
Houston, TX 77030
713-791-1414
800-827-1000
e-mail: houston.query@vba.va.gov
www.va.gov

8095 **Houston VA Medical Center**
Veterans Health Administration, US Dept. of VA
2002 Holcombe Boulevard
Houston, TX 77030
713-791-1414
800-827-1000
e-mail: g.vhacss@forum.va.gov
www.va.gov

8096 **South Texas Veterans Healthcare System**
Veterans Health Administration, US Dept. of VA
7400 Merton Minter Boulevard
San Antonio, TX 78284
210-617-5300
800-827-1000
e-mail: g.vhacss@forum.va.gov
www.va.gov

8097 **VA North Texas Health Care System: Sam Rayburn Memorial Veterans Center**
Veterans Health Administration, US Dept. of VA
1201 E 9th Street
Bonham, TX 75418
800-924-8387
FAX: 903-583-6688
e-mail: g.vhacss@forum.va.gov
www.va.gov

Lenore Sanders, Social Worker

8098 VA North Texas Health Veterans Affairs Car e System: Dallas VA Medical Center
Veterans Health Administration, US Dept. of VA
4500 S Lancaster Road
Dallas, TX 75216
214-742-8387
800-849-3597
FAX: 214-857-1171
www.va.gov

Alan G Harper, Director
William E Cox, Associate Director
Daniel K Heers, Assistant Director

Health care system which serves veterans with medical care and rehabilitation services including spinal cord injury center. For VA benefit inquiries contact 1-800-827-1000. This system has locations in Bonham, Dallas, and Fort Worth.

8099 Waco Regional Office
Veterans Benefits Administration, US Dept. of VA
1 Veterans Plaza
701 Clay Avenue
Waco, TX 76799
800-827-1000
e-mail: waco.query@vba.va.gov
www.va.gov

8100 West Texas VA Healthcare System
Veterans Health Administration, US Dept. of VA
300 Veterans Boulevard
Big Spring, TX 79720
915-263-7361
800-728-7000
FAX: 915-264-4834
e-mail: g.vhacss@forum.va.gov
www.va.gov

Utah

8101 Disabled American Veterans Department of Utah
272 E 800 S
Salt Lake City, UT 84111
801-359-8168
FAX: 801-328-3442
e-mail: utdav.juno.com
www.utdav.org/

8102 Salt Lake City Regional Office
Veterans Benefits Administration, US Dept. of VA
125 S State Street
Salt Lake City, UT 84147
800-827-1000
e-mail: saltlake.query@vba.va.gov
www.va.gov

8103 VA Salt Lake City Healthcare System
Veterans Health Administration, US Dept. of VA
500 Foothill Drive
Salt Lake City, UT 84148
801-582-1565
800-827-1000
FAX: 801-584-1289
e-mail: g.vhacss@forum.va.gov
www.va.gov

Vermont

8104 Vermont VA Regional Office Center
Veterans Benefits Administration, US Dept. of VA
215 N Main Street
White River Junction, VT 05009
800-827-1000
e-mail: whiteriver.query@vba.va.gov
www.va.gov

8105 Vermont Veterans Centers
359 Dorset Street
South Burlington, VT 05403
802-862-1806

Veterans medical clinic offering disabled veterans medical treatments.

8106 White River Junction VA Medical
Veterans Health Administration, US Dept. of VA
215 N Main Street
White River Junction, VT 05009
802-295-9363
800-827-1000
e-mail: g.vhacss@forum.va.gov
www.va.gov

Virginia

8107 Hampton VA Medical Center
Veterans Health Administration, US Dept. of VA
100 Emancipation Drive
Hampton, VA 23667
757-722-9961
800-827-1000
FAX: 757-723-6620
e-mail: mike.eisenberg@med.va.gov
www.va.gov/sta/guide/facility.asp?ID=57

Jenny Tankersly, Public Affairs Officer
Mike Eisenberg PhD, Chief Psychology Services

8108 Hunter Holmes McGuire VA Medical Center
Veterans Health Administration, US Dept. of VA
1201 Broad Rock Boulevard
Richmond, VA 23249
804-675-5000
800-827-1000
FAX: 804-675-5585
e-mail: g.vhacss@forum.va.gov
www.va.gov

8109 Roanoke Regional Office
Veterans Benefits Administration, US Dept. of VA
210 Franklin Road, SW
Roanoke, VA 24011
540-857-7104
800-827-1000
e-mail: roanoke.query@vba.va.gov
www.va.gov

8110 Salem VA Medical Center
Veterans Health Administration, US Dept. of VA
1970 Roanoke Boulevard
Salem, VA 24153
540-982-2463
800-827-1000
FAX: 540-983-1096
e-mail: g.vhacss@forum.va.gov
www.va.gov

Washington

8111 Jonathan M Wainwright Memorial VA Medical Center
Veterans Health Administration, US Dept. of VA
77 Wainwright Drive
Walla Walla, WA 99362
509-525-5200
888-687-8863
FAX: 509-527-3452
www.va.gov

Bruce E Stewart, Deputy Director

8112 **Seattle Regional Office**
Veterans Benefits Administration, US Dept. of VA
Federal Building
915 2nd Avenue
Seattle, WA 98174
800-827-1000
e-mail: seattle.query@vba.va.gov
www.va.gov

8113 **Spokane VA Medical Center**
Veterans Health Administration, US Dept. of VA
4815 N Assembly
Spokane, WA 99205
509-434-7000
800-827-1000
FAX: 509-434-7119
e-mail: g.vhacss@forum.va.gov
www.va.gov

8114 **VA Puget Sound Health Care System**
Veterans Health Administration, US Dept. of VA
1660 S Columbian Way
Seattle, WA 98108
206-762-1010
800-827-1000
e-mail: g.vhacss@forum.va.gov
www.va.gov

West Virginia

8115 **Beckley VA Medical Center**
Veterans Health Administration, US Dept. of VA
200 Veterans Avenue
Clarksburg, WV 25801
304-255-2121
800-827-1000
FAX: 304-255-2431
e-mail: g.vhacss@forum.va.gov
www.va.gov

8116 **Huntington Regional Office**
Veterans Benefits Administration, US Dept. of VA
640 Fourth Avenue
Huntington, WV 25701
800-827-1000
e-mail: huntington.query@vba.va.gov
www.va.gov

8117 **Huntington VA Medical Center**
Veterans Health Administration, US Dept. of VA
1540 Spring Valley Drive
Huntington, WV 25704
304-623-3461
800-827-1000
e-mail: g.vhacss@forum.va.gov
www.va.gov

8118 **Louis A Johnson VA Medical Center**
Veterans Health Administration, US Dept. of VA
One Medical Center Drive
Clarksburg, WV 26301
304-623-3461
800-827-1000
e-mail: g.vhacss@forum.va.gov
www.va.gov

8119 **Martinsburg VA Medical Center**
Veterans Health Administration, US Dept. of VA
Route 9
Martinsburg, WV 25401
304-263-0811
800-827-1000
FAX: 304-262-7433
e-mail: g.vhacss@forum.va.gov
www.va.gov

Marilyn La Freniere, Sci Coordinator

8120 **US Department Veterans Affairs Beckley Vet Center**
101 Ellison Avenue
Beckley, WV 25801
304-252-8220
FAX: 304-254-8711

Vet Center services includes individual and group readjustment counseling, referral for benefits assistance, liason with community agencies, marital and family counseling, substance abuse counseling, job counseling and referral, sexual trauma counseling, and community education.

Wisconsin

8121 **Clement J Zablocki VA Medical Center**
Veterans Health Administration, US Dept. of VA
5000 W National Avenue
Milwaukee, WI 53295
414-384-2000
800-827-1000
FAX: 414-382-5319
e-mail: g.vhacss@forum.va.gov
www.va.gov

8122 **Tomah VA Medical Center**
Veterans Health Administration, US Dept. of VA
500 E Veterans Street
Tomah, WI 54660
608-372-3971
800-827-1000
e-mail: g.vhacss@forum.va.gov
www.va.gov

8123 **William S Middleton Memorial VA Medical Center**
Veterans Health Administration, US Dept. of VA
2500 Overlook Terrace
Madison, WI 53705
608-256-1901
800-827-1000
e-mail: g.vhacss@forum.va.gov
www.va.gov

8124 **Wisconsin VA Regional Office**
Veterans Benefits Administration, US Dept. of VA
5000 W National Avenue
Building 6
Milwaukee, WI 53295
800-827-1000
e-mail: milwaukee.query@vba.va.gov
www.va.gov

Wyoming

8125 **Cheyenne VA Medical Center**
Veterans Health Administration, US Dept. of VA
2360 E Pershing Boulevard
Cheyenne, WY 82001
800-827-1000
e-mail: g.vhacss@forum.va.gov
www.va.gov

8126 **Sheridan VA Medical Center**
Veterans Health Administration, US Dept. of VA
1898 Fort Road
Sheridan, WY 82801
307-672-1639
800-827-1000
FAX: 307-672-1900
e-mail: g.vhacss@forum.va.gov
www.va.gov

8127 **Wyoming Veterans Centers**

111 S Jefferson Street
Casper, WY 82601
307-266-3633
FAX: 307-261-5439

Veterans medical clinic offering disabled veterans medical treatments.

8128 **Wyoming/Colorado VA Regional Office**

Veterans Benefits Administration, US Dept. of VA
155 Van Gordon Street
Lakewood, CO 80228
800-827-1000
e-mail: denver.query@vba.va.gov
www.va.gov

Alabama

8129 **Coffee County Training Center**
801 Aviation Boulevard
PO Box 311343
Enterprise, AL 36330 **334-347-1732**
FAX: 334-347-0252

Vickie Florence, Director

Clients 21 years and up receive training in Independent Living Skills, Self-Care, Language Skills, Learning, Self-Direction and Economic Self-Sufficiency. Transportation is also provided to clients of the center.

8130 **Easter Seal: Achievement Center**
510 W Thomason Circle
Opelika, AL 36801 **334-745-3501**
FAX: 334-749-5808
e-mail: info@achievement-center.org
www.achievement-center.org

Willie Huff, CEO
Elizabeth Griffin, Administratives Services

Job placement programs, remunerative work services and work adjustment training programs. Clients must be at least 16 years old.

8131 **Easter Seal: Opportunity Center**
PO Box 2247
Anniston, AL 36202 **256-237-0381**

Mike Almaroad

Work adjustment and remunerative work programs.

8132 **Employment Service Division: Alabama**
Department of Industrial Relations
649 Monroe Street
Room 2813
Montgomery, AL 36131 **334-242-8003**
FAX: 334-242-8012
e-mail: shorton@dir.state.al.us
www.dir.state.al.us/es

Stephen A Horton, ES Programs Manager

8133 **Fort Payne-Dekalb Rehab Center**
311 Gault Avenue N
Fort Payne, AL 35967 **256-845-9367**
FAX: 256-547-5761

Kenny Maness, Work Adjustment

Offers work adjustment, evaluation and job readiness skills for people with disabilities.

8134 **Lakeshore Rehabilitation Facility**
3830 Ridgeway Drive
PO Box 59127
Birmingham, AL 35259 **205-870-5999**
800-441-7609
FAX: 205-879-2685

8135 **Montezuma Training Center**
Academy Drive
Andalusia, AL 36420 **334-222-2525**

Lillian Dixon, Director

Individuals served in this program must be at least 21 years of age and have a primary diagnosis of mental retardation. Clients receive training in Independent Living Skills, Learning, Self-Direction and Economic Self-Sufficiency. Special Olympic activities are also emphasized.

8136 **Thomasville Rehabilitation Center**
Adams Building, Bashi Road
PO Box 1006
Thomasville, AL 36784 **334-636-5421**
800-335-3237
FAX: 334-636-5421
www.rehab.state.al.us

8137 **Vocational Rehabilitation Service Opelika**
520 W Thomason Circle
Opelika, AL 36801 **334-749-1259**
800-671-6835
FAX: 334-749-8753
www.rehab.state.al.us

8138 **Vocational Rehabilitation Service: Scottsboro**
203 S Market Street
PO Box 296
Scottsboro, AL 35768 **256-574-5813**
800-418-8823
FAX: 256-574-6033
www.rehab.state.al.us

8139 **Vocational Rehabilitation Service: Dothan**
795 Ross Clark Circle NE
Dothan, AL 36303 **334-792-0022**
800-275-0132
FAX: 334-792-1783
www.rehab.state.al.us

8140 **Vocational Rehabilitation Service: Gadsden**
1100 George Wallace Drive
Gadsden, AL 35903 **256-547-6974**
800-671-6839
FAX: 256-543-1784
www.rehab.state.al.us

8141 **Vocational Rehabilitation Service: Homewoo d**
236 Goodwin Crest Drive
PO Box 19888
Homewood, AL 35219 **205-290-4400**
800-671-6837
FAX: 205-290-0486
www.rehab.state.al.us

8142 **Vocational Rehabilitation Service: Huntsvi lle**
2939 Johnson Road SW
Huntsville, AL 35805 **256-650-8219**
800-671-6840
FAX: 256-650-8250
www.rehab.state.al.us

8143 **Vocational Rehabilitation Service: Jackson**
1401 Forest Avenue
PO Box 1005
Jackson, AL 36545 **251-246-5708**
800-671-6836
FAX: 251-246-5224
www.rehab.state.al.us

8144 **Vocational Rehabilitation Service: Jasper**
301 N Walston Bridge Road
Suite 116
Jasper, AL 35504 **205-221-7840**
800-671-6841
FAX: 205-221-1062
www.rehab.state.al.us

8145 **Vocational Rehabilitation Service: Mobile**
2419 Gordon Smith Drive
Mobile, AL 36617 **251-479-8611**
800-671-6842
FAX: 251-478-2197
www.rehab.state.al.us

8146 **Vocational Rehabilitation Service: Muscle Shoals**
1450 E Avalon Avenue
Muscle Shoals, AL 35662 **256-381-1110**
800-275-0166
FAX: 256-389-3149
www.rehab.state.al.us

8147 **Vocational Rehabilitation Service: Selma**
2906 Citizens Parkway
Selma, AL 36701 **334-872-8422**
888-761-5995
FAX: 334-877-3796
www.rehab.state.al.us

8148 **Vocational Rehabilitation Service: Tallade ga**
4 Medical Office Park
Talladega, AL 35160 **256-362-1300**
800-441-7592
FAX: 256-362-6387
www.rehab.state.al.us

8149 **Vocational Rehabilitation Service: Troy**
518 S Brundidge Street
Troy, AL 36081 **334-566-2491**
800-441-7608
FAX: 334-566-9415
www.rehab.state.al.us

8150 **Vocational Rehabilitation Service: Tuscalo osa**
1305 37th Street E
PO Drawer 1610
Tuscaloosa, AL 35405 **205-554-1300**
800-331-5562
FAX: 205-554-1369
www.rehab.state.al.us

8151 **Vocational Rehabilitation Services: Andalu sa**
580 W Bypass
Andalusa, AL 36420 **334-222-4114**
800-671-6833
FAX: 334-427-1216
www.rehab.state.al.us

8152 **Vocational Rehabilitation Services: Annist on**
1105 Woodstock Avenue
Anniston, AL 36207 **256-238-9300**
800-671-6834
FAX: 256-231-4852
www.rehab.state.al.us

8153 **Vocational and Rehabilitation Agency**
2129 E S Boulevard
PO Box 11586
Montgomery, AL 36111 **334-281-8780**
800-441-7607
FAX: 334-281-1973
TTY:888-737-2032
e-mail: sshivers@rehab.state.al.us
www.rehab.state.al.us

8154 **Vocational and Rehabilitation Service Columbiana**
Community Service Building
PO Box 856
Columbiana, AL 35051 **205-669-3829**
FAX: 205-669-0605
www.rehab.state.al.us

8155 **Vocational and Rehabilitation Service: Dec atur**
621 Cherry Street NE
PO Box 1686
Decatur, AL 35601 **256-353-2754**
800-671-6838
FAX: 256-351-2476
www.rehab.state.al.us

8156 **Wiregrass Rehabilitation Center**
805 Ross Clark Circle
Dothan, AL 36303 **334-792-0022**

Dorothy Morris, Administrator
Provides remunerative work.

8157 **Workshops**
4244 3rd Avenue S
Birmingham, AL 35222 **205-592-9683**
FAX: 205-592-9687
e-mail: mail@workshopsinc.com
www.workshopsinc.com

JE Crim, Executive Director
Shan Amerman, Director Client Services
Provides vocational training, sheltered employment and other support services to people with disabilities in central Alabama.

Alaska

8158 **Anchorage Job Training Center**
235 E 8th Avenue
Anchorage, AK 99501 **907-334-2281**
FAX: 907-334-2286
www.ci.anchorage.ak.us

8159 **Employment Service: Alaska**
Alaska Department of Labor
PO Box 25509
Juneau, AK 99802 **907-465-2723**

8160 **Fair Employment Practice Agency**
Alaska State Commission for Human Rights
800 A Street
Anchorage, AK 99501 **907-276-6563**

8161 **Vocational and Rehabilitation Agency**
801 W 10th Street
Suite A
Juneau, AK 99801 **907-465-2814**
800-478-2815
FAX: 907-465-2856
TTY:907-465-2856
e-mail: duane_french@labor.state.ak.us
www.labor.state.ak.us

Duane French, Director

Arizona

8162 **Downtown Neighborhood Learning Center**

1001 W Jefferson Street
Phoenix, AZ 85007 **602-256-0784**
800-869-8521
FAX: 602-256-2524
e-mail: marcian@first.inter.net

Marcia R Newman, Executive Director
Mattie Johnson, Receptionist
Peg Osinski, El Mirage Learning Lab

Adult education agency providing basic skills, GED, ESOL, life skills, computer skills, resume assistance and career testing.

8163 **Employment Service: Arizona**

Department of Economic Security
PO Box 6160
Phoenix, AZ 85005 **602-254-7213**
FAX: 602-271-4128
www.de.state.az.us/tp/portal.asp

Bill Hernandez, Assistant Director

8164 **Fair Employment Practice Agency: Arizona**

Arizona Civil Rights Division
1275 W Washington Street
Phoenix, AZ 85007 **602-542-5263**

8165 **JOBS Administration Job Opportunities & Basic Skills**

1717 W Jefferson Street
Phoenix, AZ 85007 **602-542-9596**
FAX: 602-542-5171

Gretchen Evans, Program Administrator

Assist applicants and recipients of temporary assistance to needy families to obtain job training and employment that will lead to economic independence.

8166 **Job Training Program Liaison: Arizona**

Department of Economic Security
PO Box 6160
Phoenix, AZ 85005 **602-254-7213**
FAX: 602-271-4128
www.utilitytraderaz.com

Gretchen Evans, Program Administrator

The Job Opportunities and Basic Skills Administration assists applicants and recipients of Temporary Assistance to needy families to obtain training and employment.

8167 **TETRA Corporation**

308 W Glenn Street
Tucson, AZ 85705 **520-622-4874**

Steven King

Work hardening and disciplinary programs.

8168 **Vocational and Rehabilitation Agency Rehabilitation Services Administrations**

Division of Employment & Rehabilitation Services
Department of Economic Security
1789 W Jefferson Street
Phoenix, AZ 85007 **602-542-3332**
800-563-1221
FAX: 602-542-3778
TTY:602-542-6049
e-mail: azrsa@rehabnetwork.org
www.de.state.az.us/rsa/

Jozef de Groot, Manager Program Services
Skip Bingham, Administrator

This program serves individuals with disabilities seeking jobs and job training.

8169 **Yavapal Rehabilitation Center**

436 N Washington Avenue
Prescott, AZ 86301 **928-445-0991**

Bradley Newman

Provides remunerative work.

Arkansas

8170 **Arkansas Employment Service Agency and Job Training Program**

Arkansas Employment Security Department
PO Box 2981
Little Rock, AR 72203 **501-682-2121**

8171 **Easter Seal Work Center**

11801 Fairview Road
Little Rock, AR 72212 **501-223-8077**

Renee Hubbard

Work hardening and disciplinary programs.

8172 **VCT/A Job Retention Skill Training Program**

Hot Springs Rehabilitation Center
PO Box 1358
Hot Springs, AR 71902 **501-624-4411**
FAX: 501-624-0019

A training program designed for use in rehabilitation and educational settings. Using a social skill training strategy, VCT helps participants learn how to solve on-the-job problems and cope with common supervisory demands.

8173 **Vocational and Rehabilitation Agency Division of Services for the Blind**

700 Main Street
Little Rock, AR 72203 **501-682-5463**
800-960-9270
FAX: 501-682-0366
TTY:501-682-0093
e-mail: jim.hudson@mail.state.ar.us
www.state.ar.us

Lyndel Lybarger, Field Adminstrator

8174 **Vocational and Rehabilitation Agency for Persons Who Are Visually Impaired**
Arkansas Department of Human Services
PO Box 3237
Little Rock, AR 72203 **501-682-5463**
800-960-9270
TTY:501-324-9271
e-mail: arkblind@edu.gte.net

James C Hudson, Director

California

8175 **ARC-Adult Vocational Program**
657 Harrison Street
San Francisco, CA 94107 **415-626-5710**

Patricia Kemerling

Job placement programs, remunerative work services and work adjustment training programs.

8176 **Ability First**
3770 E Willow Street
Long Beach, CA 90815 **562-426-6161**
FAX: 562-426-6148

Michael Lande

Job placement programs, remunerative work services and work adjustment training programs.

8177 **Bakersfield Association for Retarded Citizens**
BARC
2240 S Union Avenue
Bakersfield, CA 93307 **661-834-2272**
FAX: 661-834-9813
e-mail: barc@lightspeed.net

Skip Covell, Executive Director

Employment training & placement.

8178 **California Department of Fair Employment & Housing**
2014 T Street
Suite 210
Sacramento, CA 95814 **916-227-2873**
800-884-1684
FAX: 916-227-2870
www.dfeh.ca.gov

Dia S Poole, Deputy Director Public Affairs

8179 **Career Connection Transition Program**
Whittier High School District
9401 Painter Avenue
Whittier, CA 90605 **562-698-8121**
FAX: 562-693-4414
e-mail: Richard.Rosenberg@wuhsd.k12.co.us
www.wehsd.k12.co.us

Richard L Rosenberg PhD, Vocational Coordinator

Job placement programs, remunerative work services and work adjustment training programs. Transition services.

8180 **Career Development Program (CDP)**
260 W Grand Avenue
Escondido, CA 92025 **760-738-0277**
FAX: 760-741-9452

Dr. Richard Brady
Wendy Hope, Supported Employment
Jill Hennessy, Independent Living

Work hardening and disciplinary programs.

8181 **Center for Rehabilitation Engineering and Appropriate Technology Education**
1600 Holloway Avenue
San Francisco, CA 94132 **415-338-1001**

Offers federally funded education programs leading to a master's degree in several areas.

8182 **Community Outpatient Rehabilitation Center**
1925 E Dakota Avenue
Suite 120A
Fresno, CA 93726 **559-459-1842**
FAX: 559-459-1004

Tracie Rawson, Case Manager
Jan Erik Paris, Service Coordinator

Physical occupation and speech Therapy, Neuropsychology services available for orthopedic and neurological diagnosis. Lymphedema program.

8183 **Cry-Rop: Colton-Redlands-Yucaipa Rop**
1214 Indiana Court
Redlands, CA 92374 **909-793-3115**
FAX: 909-793-6901
www.cryrop.kla.ca.us

Stephanie Houston, Manager of Grants/Adult Service

Provides quality hands-on training programs in over 40 high demand career fields to assist high school students and adults in acquiring marketable job skills. Works in cooperation with local high schools, adult education colleges, and employers providing a collaborative team of academic and ROP occupational teachers who integrate academic and vocational competencies to provide sequenced paths within career majors. Support services, career guidance and services are provided to disabled people.

8184 **Desert Haven Training Center**
PO Box 2119
Lancaster, CA 93539 **661-948-8402**

Roy Williams

Work adjustment and remunerative work programs.

8185 **Do-It-Leisure: Work Training Center**
621 1/2 Mangrove Avenue
Chico, CA 95926 **530-343-6055**
FAX: 530-343-4619
e-mail: doitl@ewrc.org

Ken Steidley, Program Manager
Carl Ochsner, Executive Director

Therapeutic recreation programs providing a wide variety of services designed to meet individual needs with specialized, transitional or integrated activities.

8186 **ESS Work Center**
858 Stanton Road
Burlingame, CA 94010 **650-692-3377**

Jerry Martin, Executive Director

8187 **Employment Service: California**
Employment Development Department
PO Box 826880
Sacramento, CA 94280 **916-654-9072**

8188 Feather River Industries
1811 Kusel Road
Oroville, CA 95966 **530-534-4112**
FAX: 530-534-3137

Amy Brown, Rehabilitation Coordinator

Vocational training for persons with developmental disabilities provided through wood products fabrication and assembly tasks. Instructor to trainer rating ranging from 1 to 12, 1 to 8, 1 to 6, and 1 to 4 depending on individual needs and complexity of tasks.

8189 Fit to Work
3581 Palmer Drive
Suite 401
Cameron Park, CA 95682 **530-676-7485**
FAX: 530-676-9114

Jennifer Roach

Provides remunerative work.

8190 Fresno City College: Disabled Students Programs and Services
1101 E University Avenue
Fresno, CA 93741 **559-442-8237**
FAX: 559-485-7304
www.fresnocitycollege.com

Dr Ned Doffoney, President
Dr Janice Emerzian, Director

This program offers services to students with physical, learning and/or psychological disabilities beyond those provided by conventional Fresno City College Programs and enables students to successfully persue their individual educational, vocational and personal goals.

8191 Heartland Opportunity Center
323 N E Street
Madera, CA 93638 **559-674-8828**
FAX: 559-674-8857

Robert J Hand, Director

Job placement programs, remunerative work services and work adjustment training programs.

8192 Hollister Workshop
Hope Rehabilitation Services
2300 Technology Parkway
Suite 7
Hollister, CA 95023 **831-637-8283**
FAX: 831-637-8726

Work adjustment and remunerative work programs.

8193 Job Training Program Liaison: California
Employment Development Department
800 Capitol Mall MIC83
Sacramento, CA 95814 **916-654-9072**

8194 King's Rehabilitation Center
490 E Hanford Armona Road
Hanford, CA 93230 **559-582-9234**
FAX: 559-582-1182

Carol A Rogers, Executive Director

8195 Konocti Industries: People Services
4195 Lakeshore Boulevard
Lakeport, CA 95453 **707-263-3811**
FAX: 707-263-0552

Hank Montgomery

Work hardening and disciplinary programs.

8196 Morongo Basin Work Activity Center
74325 Joe Davis Drive
Twentynine Palms, CA 92277 **760-366-8474**

Sheree Fraser

Job placement programs, remunerative work services and work adjustment training programs.

8197 Mother Lode Rehabilitation Enterprises
399 Placerville Drive
Placerville, CA 95667 **530-622-4848**

Jerry Demarest

Job placement programs, remunerative work services and work adjustment training programs.

8198 NCI Affiliates
1434 Chestnut Street
Paso Robles, CA 93446 **805-238-6630**

Laura Simpson, Executive Director
Judy Jacobson, Services Director

Provides independent living skills and vocational training to people with disabilities.

8199 Napa Valley PSI
651 Trabajo Lane
PO Box 600
Napa, CA 94559 **707-255-0177**
FAX: 707-255-0802

Jeanne Fauquet, Executive Director

Work adjustment, work training and educational services for developmentally disabled adults. Emphasis is on manufacture of quality wood products, primarily wooden office furniture.

8200 New Opportunity Workshops
PO Box 91476
Pasadena, CA 91109

Ron Johnston, Rehabilitation Mgr.

Offers a work services program, vocational rehabilitation, work activity programs and supported employment programs.

8201 Oakland Work Activity Area
6315 San Leandro Street
Oakland, CA 94621 **510-639-9350**

Greg Whalley

Job placement programs, remunerative work services and work adjustment training programs.

8202 Opportunities for the Handicapped
3340 Marysville Boulevard
Sacramento, CA 95838 **916-925-3522**

Kathy Dodd

Work adjustment and remunerative work programs.

8203 **Orange County ARC**
225 W Carl Karcher Way
Anaheim, CA 92801 **714-444-5301**
FAX: 714-744-5312

Joyce Hearn, Chief Executive Officer
Provides remunerative work through both site and community placements.

8204 **PRIDE Industries**
10030 Foothills Boulevard
Roseville, CA 95747 **916-788-2100**
800-550-6005
FAX: 916-788-2560
e-mail: info@prideindustries.com
www.prideindustries.com

Michael Ziegler, President
Rosemary Elston, Director of Rehabilitation
Roxanne Snyder, Employment Services Manager
Vocational rehabilitation and employment services creating jobs for people with disabilites; services include career counseling, vocational assessment, work adjustment, work services, job seeking skills, job development, job placement, on-the-job support (coaching), mentoring, independent living skills, transition services and case management.

8205 **Pomona Valley Workshop**
4650 Brooks Street
Montclair, CA 91763 **909-624-3555**
FAX: 909-624-5675
e-mail: pvwkaren@juno.com

Karen Jones, Executive Director
Assisting adults with disabilities reach their potential in vocational and socialization skills in order that they may achieve their highest level of employment and comminity integration in Work Program, Supported Employment Services, Adult Dev. Center and Senior Services.

8206 **Porterville Sheltered Workshop**
187 W Olive Avenue
Porterville, CA 93257 **559-784-1399**
FAX: 559-781-5651

Nick Brown
Work adjustment and remunerative work programs.

8207 **Project Independence Supported Employment**
3505 Cadillac P 101
Costa Mesa, CA 92626 **714-549-3464**
FAX: 714-549-3559
P-I.org

Andrea Erickson
Provides remunerative work.

8208 **Ramona Training Center**
2138 San Vicente Road
Ramona, CA 92065 **760-789-6018**

Charlene Wutthe
Job placement programs, remunerative work services and work adjustment training programs.

8209 **Sacramento Vocational Services**
6950 21st Avenue
Sacramento, CA 95820 **916-484-0550**

Diane De Rodeff, Director
Work hardening and disciplinary programs.

8210 **Salinas Valley Training Center**
PO Box 453
Salinas, CA 93902 **831-758-8270**

Rosemary Anderson, Day Activity Manager

8211 **San Francisco Vocational Services**
814 Mission Street
Suite 600
San Francisco, CA 94103 **415-512-9500**
FAX: 415-512-9507
www.sfvocationalservices.org

Craig King, Executive Director
Jeffrey Faircloth, Manager Case Management
Comprehensive vocational rehabilitation center offering vocational evaluation, rehabilitative counseling, business office training, work experience, and job placement.

8212 **Shasta County Opportunity Center**
1265 Redwood Boulevard
Redding, CA 96003 **530-225-5000**

Carol Keating, Executive Director

8213 **Social Vocational Services**
350 S Crenshaw
Suite A104
Torrance, CA 90503 **310-787-4740**

Dr. Dale Dutton, Executive Director

8214 **South Bay Vocational Center**
1526 240th Street
Harbor City, CA 90710 **310-784-2032**
FAX: 310-539-6342

Corey Sylve, President/CEO
Clare Grey, Director Programs

8215 **Tri-County Independent Living Center**
955 Myrtle Avenue
Eureka, CA 95501 **707-445-8404**
877-576-5000
FAX: 707-445-9751

Gay Larsen, Executive Director
To provide programs, services and information for people with disabilities living in Humboldt, Del Norte and Trinity Counties in northern California in an effort to allow choices for individuals to optimize their independence.

8216 **Tulare County Training Center Able Industries**
2525 S K Street
Tulare, CA 93274 **559-686-8506**

Robert Stephenson
Provides remunerative work.

8217 **Tulare Workcenter Able Industries**
2325 S K Street
Tulare, CA 93274

Gary Horton, Executive Director

8218 **Unyeway**
2330 Main Street
Suite E
Ramona, CA 92065

Hank Newman, Director
Job placement programs, remunerative work services and work adjustment training programs.

8219 **V-Bar Enterprises**
720 Gordon Circle
Suisun City, CA 94585 **707-864-1334**

Lu Brunet
Job placement programs, remunerative work services and work adjustment training programs.

8220 **Valley Light Industries**
822 N Grand Avenue
Covina, CA 91724 **626-331-9966**

Gary Miller
Provides remunerative work.

8221 **Visalia Workshop**
2544 E Valley Oaks Drive
Visalia, CA 93292 **559-734-1964**

Hortensia Venegas
Work hardening and disciplinary programs.

8222 **Vocational Services**
Parents & Friends
350 Cypress Street
Fort Bragg, CA 95437 **707-964-4940**
FAX: 707-964-2701
e-mail: friends@mcn.org

Russ Pals, Director
Vocational Services provides opportunities for persons with developmental challenges and similar needs to participate fully in our community.

8223 **Westside Opportunity Workshop**
9503 Jefferson Boulevard
Culver City, CA 90232 **310-838-0521**

Edward Oritz
Job placement programs, remunerative work services and work adjustment training programs.

8224 **Work Training Center for the Handicapped**
2255 Fair Street
Chico, CA 95928 **530-343-3107**

Barrie Dyer
Work hardening and disciplinary programs.

8225 **Work Training Programs**
20931 Nordhoff Street
Chatsworth, CA 91311 **818-773-9000**

Stephen Miller
Work hardening and disciplinary programs.

Colorado

8226 **Cheyenne Village**
6275 Lehman Drive
Colorado Springs, CO 80918 **719-592-0200**
FAX: 719-548-9947

Carol Glaze, Co-Director
Ann Turner, Co-Director
Residential and employment programs for adults with developmental disabilities.

8227 **Colorado Civil Rights Divsion**
1560 Broadway
Suite 1050
Denver, CO 80202 **303-894-2997**
800-262-4845
FAX: 303-894-7830
e-mail: ccrd@dora.state.co.us
www.dora.state.co.us

Wendell Pryer, Division Director
Faye Thompson, Compliance Manager
Nancy Snow, Housing Specialist
Fair employment practices agency for Colorado. Accepts and investigates charges of discrimination. Doles outreach, alternative dipute resolution and free technical training in discrimination laws.

8228 **Colorado Employment Service**
Department of Labor and Employment
600 Grant Street
Suite 900
Denver, CO 80203 **303-676-7461**

8229 **Developmental Training Services**
1401 Oak Creek Grade Road
Canon City, CO 81212 **719-275-4504**

Roger Jensen, President

8230 **Dynamic Dimensions**
1778 Martin Avenue
Burlington, CO 80807 **719-346-5367**
FAX: 719-346-6010

Cheryl Reese, Executive Director
Vocational, evaluation and assessment, training and placement for most disabilities.

8231 **Gray Street Workcenter**
5685 Gray Street
Arvada, CO 80002 **303-422-1305**
FAX: 303-467-2793

Shelley Richardson, Executive Director

8232 **Hope Center**
3400 Elizabeth Street
Denver, CO 80205 **303-388-4801**
FAX: 303-388-0249

George Brantley
Work adjustment and remunerative work programs.

8233 **Imagine: Innovative Resources for Cognitive & Physical Challenges**

1400 Dixon Avenue
Lafayette, CO 80026 **303-665-7789**
FAX: 303-665-2648
e-mail: caroline@imaginecolorado.org
www.imaginecolorado.org

John Taylor, Executive Director
Caroline Siegfried, Executive Assistant

Creating and offering innovative supports to people of all ages with cognitive, developmental, physical and health related needs, so they may live lives of independence and quality in their homes and communities.

8234 **Las Animas County Rehabilitation Center**

1205 Congress Drive
Trinidad, CO 81082 **719-846-3388**
FAX: 719-846-4543

Duane Roy

Job placement programs, remunerative work services and work adjustment training programs.

8235 **NORESCO Workshop**

903 E Burlington Avenue
Fort Morgan, CO 80701

Robert Duffield

Provides remunerative work.

8236 **Regional Assessment and Training Center**

3520 W Oxford Avenue
Denver, CO 80236 **303-866-7253**

Russell Porter, Executive Director

8237 **Sedgwick County Workshop**

113 Elm Street
Julesburg, CO 80737 **970-474-3504**

Robert Christiansen

Provides remunerative work.

8238 **Valley Industries**

330 State Avenue
Alamosa, CO 81101

Tim Johnson

Provides remunerative work.

8239 **Vocational and Rehabilitation Agency**

2211 W Evans
Building B
Denver, CO 80223 **720-884-1234**
FAX: 720-884-1213
TTY:720-884-1234
e-mail: diana.huerta@state.co.us
www.cdhs.state.co.us

8240 **Yuma County Workshop**

710 E 2nd Avenue
Yuma, CO 80759 **970-848-3011**

Robert Stephens

Provides remunerative work.

Connecticut

8241 **Area Cooperative Educational Services (ACES)**

350 State Street
North Haven, CT 06473 **203-498-6800**
FAX: 203-498-6890
e-mail: acesinfo@aces.k12.ct.us
www.aces.k12.ct.us

Patricia Krakowski, Assistant Executive Director
Joseph Sullivan, Director of Pupil Services
Vanessa Taragowski, Supervisor of Special Education

Regional Educational Service Center providing high quality educational services in the south central Connecticut region.

8242 **CCARC**

1 Hartford Square
New Britain, CT 06052 **860-224-6993**

Julie Erickson, Day Service Director

Supported employment, work services, habilitation services, advocacy, recreation and residential services.

8243 **Cheshire Occupational and Career Center**

615 W Johnson Avenue
Suite 3
Cheshire, CT 06410 **203-272-5607**
FAX: 203-272-4284

Peter Mason

Work adjustment and remunerative work programs.

8244 **Community Enterprises**

41 Mechanic Street
PO Box 176
Windsor, CT 06095 **860-688-7918**
FAX: 860-688-5599
e-mail: cehftd@aol.com
www.communityenterprises.com

Susan Cauley, VP CT Operations

Provide supported Education services in a community college setting; supported employment including job training, placement and follow-up; transitional services from group homes and other settings to supported living within the community.

8245 **Connecticut Governor's Committee on Employment of Disabled Persons**

200 Folly Brook Boulevard
Wethersfield, CT 06109 **860-566-5505**

8246 **Constructive Workshops**

24 Willow Street
E Hartford, CT 06118 **860-549-1410**
FAX: 860-895-1168

Sandie Lavoy, Coordinator

8247 **Fotheringhay Farms**

84 Waterhole Road
Colchester, CT 06415 **860-267-4463**
FAX: 860-267-7628

Dr. Wesley Martins

Job placement programs, remunerative work services and work adjustment training programs.

8248 George Hegyi Industrial Training Center
5 Coon Hollow Road
Derby, CT 06418 **203-735-8727**

Joan Bucci
Work adjustment and remunerative work programs.

8249 Greater Enfield Association of Retarded Citizens
3 Pearson Way
Enfield, CT 06082 **860-763-0192**

Dean Wem
Work hardening and disciplinary programs.

8250 Hartford Vet Center
30 Jordan Lane
Wethersfield, CT 06109 **860-563-2320**
FAX: 860-563-7246
e-mail: donna.hryb@med.va.gov

Donna Dube Hryb LCSW, Team Leader
Urania Petit BA, Office Manager
A U.S. Department of Veterans Affairs counseling center offering counseling to Vietnam era and combat veterans. Sexual trauma/harassment counseling, medical screening and benefit referral is available to all veterans.

8251 Kennedy Center
2440 Reservoir Avenue
Trumbull, CT 06611 **203-365-8522**
FAX: 203-365-8533
e-mail: mschwartz@kennedyctr.org
www.kennedyctr.org

Martin D Schwartz, President/CEO
Provides vocational rehabilitation, job training and job placement services to 1,000 adults with disabilities including mental retardation, traumatic brain injury, psychiatric disabilities and more. Residential services, well integrated within the community, serve 97 individuals on a daily basis. Children's programs provide support to 85 children age birth to three, in addition to after hours and recreation programs to appromxately 100 school age children. Staff size is presently 400 employees.

8252 Quaezar
2480 Black Rock Turnpike
Suite 8
Fairfield, CT 06432 **203-339-3476**
FAX: 203-377-6144

William J Sedarweck, President
Agency for adult mentally retarded/autistic people providing residential care in a group home or apartment setting. Also provides placement in community employment.

8253 TEAM Vocational Program
227 Elm Street
W Haven, CT 06516 **203-934-5221**

Peter Schwartz, Executive Director
Hannah Carlson, DD Director
Provides remunerative work, vocational training, supported employment, and supportive services. Residential program including group living and supervised apartment, social club.

8254 Valley Memorial Health Center
435 E Main Street
Ansonia, CT 06401

Marilyn Cormack, Director
Provides remunerative work.

8255 Vocational and Rehabilitation Agency
184 Windsor Avenue
Windsor, CT 06095 **860-602-4000**
800-842-4570
FAX: 860-602-4030
e-mail: Brian.Sigman@po.state.ct.us
www.besb.state.ct.us

Dr. Donna Balaski, Executive Director
Carole Donagher, Finance Director

8256 Vocational and Rehabilitation Agency: State Department of Social Services
25 Sigourney Street
Hartford, CT 06106 **860-424-4844**
800-537-2549
FAX: 860-424-4850
TTY:8004244839
e-mail: brs.dss@po.state.ct.us
www.dss.state.ct.us

Delaware

8257 Delaware Division of Vocational Rehabilitation-Department of Labor
4425 N Market Street
PO Box 9969
Wilmington, DE 19809 **302-761-8275**
FAX: 302-761-6611
www.delawareworks.com/divisions/dvr/welcome.h

Andrea Guest, Director
Cynthia Fairwell, Program Specialist
Provides opportunities and resources to eligible individuals with disabilities leading to success in employment and independent living.

8258 Delaware Fair Employment Practice Agency
Delaware Department of Labor
820 N French Street
6th Floor
Wilmington, DE 19801 **302-577-3970**

8259 Delaware Job Training Program Liaison
Division of Employment & Training
PO Box 9828
Wilmington, DE 19809 **302-761-8127**

8260 Opportunity Center
3030 Bowers Street
Wilmington, DE 19802 **302-762-0300**
FAX: 302-762-8797
e-mail: blennon@oppctr.com
www.oppctr.com

Bob Lennon, VP Community Development
Cindy Sterling, VP Employment Services
Cathie Field Lloyd, President/CEO
Work adjustment and remunerative work programs. Also offers career guidance, supported employment, work readiness and job placement.

8261 Wilmington Vet Center
1601 Kirkwood Highway
Wilmington, DE 19805 **302-998-9448**
FAX: 302-633-5250

Mark A Kaufki EdD, Team Leader

Veterans counseling program offering individual counseling services, advocacy services and group counseling. The focus is the counseling of all veterans coping with the aftermath of war, sexual abuse/harassment in the military and all veterans of the Vietnam era. The center also has an active outreach program to seek veterans needing services. Hours of operation are between 8:00 AM - 4:30 PM, Monday - Friday and other times by appointment only. Services are free.

District of Columbia

8262 Davis Memorial Goodwill Industries
2200 S Dakota Avenue NE
Washington, DC 20018 **202-636-4225**
FAX: 202-526-3994

David Becker, President

Offers vocational training, job training, sheltered employment and work experience.

8263 District of Columbia Department of Employment Services
500 C Street NW
Room 600
Washington, DC 20001 **877-319-7346**
877-319-7346
FAX: 202-724-7112
e-mail: des15@erols.com
does.ci.washington.dc.us

Diana C Johnson, Public Information Officer
Marianna Lourenco, Specialist/ADA Coordinator

To foster economic development and growth in the District of Columbia by providing workforce training, bringing together job seekers and employers, compensating unemployed and injured workers and promoting safe and healthy workplaces.

8264 District of Columbia Dept. of Employment Services: Office of Workforce Development
500 C Street NW
Washington, DC 20001 **877-319-7346**
877-319-7346
FAX: 202-724-7112
e-mail: des15@erols.com
does.ci.washington.dc.us

Diana C Johnson, Public Information Officer
Marianna Lourenco, Specialist/ADA Coordinator

To foster economic development and growth in the District of Columbia by providing workforce training, bringing together job seekers and employers, compensating unemployed and injured workers and promoting safe and healthy workplaces.

8265 District of Columbia Fair Employment Practice Agencies
DC Office of Human Rights
2000 14th Street NW
Suite 3
Washington, DC 20009 **202-727-3071**

8266 Green Door
1623 16th Street NW
Washington, DC 20009 **202-462-4092**
FAX: 202-462-7562
e-mail: gdiadmin@aol.com

Judith Johnson, Director

Green Door is a community program which prepares people with a severe and persistent mental illness to live and work independently. Since 1976, Green Door has provided comprehensive services to mentally ill people, including housing, job training, job placement, education, homeless outreach, case management, support for people with substance abuse problems, family support,and specialized help for people who have had repeated hospitalizations.

8267 Operation Job Match
2021 K Street NW
Suite 715
Washington, DC 20006 **202-887-0136**
FAX: 202-296-3425

Diane Afes, Program Director
Steve Nissen, Program Supervisor

Job readiness program for individuals with adult-onset physical disabilities.

8268 President's Committee on Employment of People with Disabilities
1331 F Street NW
Washington, DC 20004 **202-693-7880**
FAX: 202-693-7888
e-mail: info@pcepd.gov
www.ada-ohio.org/default.htm

An independent federal agency whose mission is to facilitate the communication, coordination and promotion of public and private efforts to enhance the employment of people with disabilities. The Committee provides information, training and technical assistance to America's business leaders, organized labor, rehabilitation and service providers, advocacy organizations, families and individuals with disabilities.

8269 Vocational and Rehabilitation Agency
810 1st Street NE
10th Floor
Washington, DC 20002 **202-442-8400**
FAX: 202-442-8742

Elizabeth Parker, Administrator

State Rehabilitation Agency providing services to eligible persons with disabilities.

8270 WAVE Work, Achievement, Value, & Education
525 School Street SW
Suite 500
Washington, DC 20024 **202-484-0103**
800-274-2005
FAX: 202-488-7595
e-mail: wave4kids@aol.com
www.waveinc.org

Job placement programs, remunerative work services and work adjustment training programs for 18 and 21 years of age in many cities across the country including Drop-Out Recovery Programs and Drop-Out Prevention Programs. Programs also available for youth ages 12-18. Youth Professionals Development and Training and key aspects of WAVE services, as well.

Florida

8271 Abilities of Florida: An Affiliate of Service Source

2735 Whitney Road
Clearwater, FL 33760 **727-538-7370**
FAX: 727-538-7387
e-mail: rabbott@ourpeoplework.org
www.ourpeoplework.org

Rhonda Abbott, VP Rehabilitation Services

Provides a full range of employment services including work evaulation, training, job coaching, job placement, advocacy and education. Also provides housing assistance and specialized to adults with cystic fibrosis.

8272 Adult Day Training

Goodwill Industries-Suncoast
10596 Gandy Boulevard N
St Petersburg, FL 33702 **727-523-1512**
888-279-1988
FAX: 727-563-9300
www.goodwill-suncoast.org

An innovative program which uses job skills to teach self-help, daliy living, communication, mobility, travel, decision-making, behavioral and social skills. This focus provides concrete, transferable experiences to help prepare individuals for greater community inclusion by achieving the highest possible degree of independence in their daily life, increasing their confidence and supporting their successful transitions to less structured, self-sufficient environments.

8273 Career Assessment & Planning Services

Goodwill Industries-Suncoast
10596 Gandy Boulevard N
St Petersburg, FL 33702 **727-523-1512**
888-279-1988
FAX: 727-563-9300
www.goodwill-suncoast.org

Provides comprehensive assessment, which can predict current and future employment and potential adjustment factors for physically, emotionally or developmentally disabled persons who may be unemployed or underemployed. Assessment evaluate interests, aptitudes, academic acheivements and physical abilities through coordinated testing, interviewing and behavioral observations.

8274 Center for Independence, Training and Education

215 E New Hampshire Street
Orlando, FL 32804 **407-896-3177**
FAX: 407-895-5255

Mara Schlosser, Program Director

Offers services for the totally blind, legally blind, visually impaired, mentally retarded blind and more with health, counseling, educational, recreational, rehabilitation, computer training and professional training services.

8275 Choices for Work Program

Goodwill Industries-Suncoast
10596 Gandy Boulevard N
St Petersburg, FL 33702 **727-523-1512**
888-279-1988
FAX: 727-563-9300
www.goodwill-suncoast.org

Assisting individuals currently eligible for Workman's Compensation, this program allows those recovering from injury on the job to prepare to return to independent employment, either through increasing ability and confidence in using adaptive behaviors and/or equipment to return to related employment, or adjusting to a more compatible employment environment.

8276 Florida Division of Vocational Rehabilitation

4221 N Himes Avenue
Tampa, FL 33607 **813-871-7300**
FAX: 813-873-4773

Renee Dominic, Librarian

Rehabilitation services are important when a physical or mental handicap interferes with your ability to work. Our purpose is to help prepare for, and return to, gainful employment.

8277 Florida Fair Employment Practice Agency

Florida Commission on Human Relations
325 John Knox Road
Building F
Tallahassee, FL 32303 **850-297-1386**

8278 Florida Vocational Rehabilitation for Persons Who Are Visually Impaired

2540 W Executive Center Circle
Tallahassee, FL 32399

8279 Florida's Governor's Alliance of Citizens with Disabilities

106 E College Avenue
Suite 820
Tallahassee, FL 32301 **850-224-4493**
888-838-2253
FAX: 850-224-4496
e-mail: info@abletrust.org
www.abletrust.org

Sharon Griffith, President/CEO
Kristen Knapp, VP Public Relations
Guenevere Crum, Grants Director

Provides grant funds purchasing equipment for current employment for people with disabilities and employment-related programs for nonprofit agencies in Florida. Assists families, individuals and agencies through educational conferences, and youth training programs. Provides businesses free resources for hiring people with disabilities.

8280 Goodwill Temporary Services

Goodwill Industries-Suncoast
10596 Gandy Boulevard N
St Petersburg, FL 33702 **727-523-1512**
888-279-1988
FAX: 727-563-9300
www.goodwill-suncoast.org

Provides employment links from potential employees, both disabled and non-disabled alike to employers with immediate employment opportunities seeking qualified candidates. Pre-screening on all applicants include: Employment history, personal references, law enforcement background checks and substance screening.

8281 Impact: Ocala Vocational Services

Goodwill Industries-Suncoast
10596 Gandy Boulevard N
St Petersburg, FL 33702 **727-523-1512**
888-279-1988
FAX: 727-563-9300
www.goodwill-suncoast.org

Designed to enable individuals with disabilities to work in integrated settings in the community, receiving wages and benefits matching those of non-handicapped workers.

8282 Job Works NISH Food Service

Goodwill Industries-Suncoast
10596 Gandy Boulevard N
St Petersburg, FL 33702 **727-523-1512**
888-279-1988
FAX: 727-563-9300
www.goodwill-suncoast.org

An enclave style (or group) supported employment program designed to give consumers additional supports that allow and encourage increasingly independent employment opportunities within a food services environment.

8283 Job Works NISH Postal Service

Goodwill Industries-Suncoast
10596 Gandy Boulevard N
St Petersburg, FL 33702 **727-523-1512**
888-279-1988
FAX: 727-563-9300
www.goodwill-suncoast.org

An enclave style (or group) supported employment program designed to give consumers additional supports that allow and encourage increasingly independent employment opportunities within a mailroom environment.

8284 MAClown Vocational Rehabilitation Workshop

6390 NE 2nd Avenue
Miami, FL 33138 **305-754-5015**

Pat Chavis

Provides remunerative work.

8285 One-Stop Service

Goodwill Industries-Suncoast
10596 Gandy Boulevard N
St Petersburg, FL 33702 **727-523-1512**
888-279-1988
FAX: 727-563-9300
www.goodwill-suncoast.org

Provides universal job search and placement related services are available to any person entering the service center. Each One-Stop Services Center provides on-site representation from a variety of employment-related service providers. All One-Stops host and/or facilitate local employment fairs and provides access to computerized job-postings.

8286 Palm Beach Habilitation Center

4522 S Congress Avenue
Lake Worth, FL 33461 **561-965-8500**

Tina Philips, President/CEO

Providing work evaluation, work adjustment, job placement, employment, residential and retirement services for mentally, emotionally and physically disabled adults.

8287 Primrose Supported Employment Programs

2733 S Ferncreek Avenue
Orlando, FL 32806 **407-898-7201**

Terry Provancha

Provides remunerative work.

8288 SCARC

213 W McCollum Avenue
Bushnell, FL 33513 **352-793-5156**

Marsha Woodard Perkins, Executive Director

Training and employment program for adults with disabilities. SCARC offers vocational evaluation, training, work services, transportation, supported independent living and community based training.

8289 Seagull Industries for the Disabled

3879 W Industrial Way
Riviera Beach, FL 33404 **561-842-5814**
FAX: 561-881-3554
e-mail: main@seagull.org
www.seagull.org

Alfred Elsinger, Executive Director

Dedicated to improving the quality of life of mentally, physically and emotionally challenged adults in Palm Beach County, Florida through advocacy and the provision of a variety of social service, vocational training and residential programs designed to encourage self reliance and independence.

8290 Supported Employment Program

Goodwill Industries-Suncoast
10596 Gandy Boulevard N
St Petersburg, FL 33702 **727-523-1512**
888-279-1988
FAX: 727-563-9300
www.goodwill-suncoast.org

Provides an employment option that enables individuals with severe disabilities to work in integrated settings in the community, receiving wages and benefits matching those of their non-disabled counterparts. The individual is provided with intensive, on-the-job training at job sites that have been carefully analyzed to be suitable for each individual.

8291 Vocational and Rehabilitation Agency Department of Education

2002 Old Saint Augustin Road
Building A
Tallahassee, FL 32399 **850-488-6925**
800-451-4327
FAX: 850-488-8062
TTY:850-488-0867
www.2myflorida.com

8292 Vocational and Rehabilitation Agency: Division of Blind Services

2551 Executive Center Circle W
Lafayette Building, Suite 200
Tallahassee, FL 32399 **850-488-1330**
800-342-1828
FAX: 850-487-1804
e-mail: craig_kiser@dbe.doe.state.fl.us
www.state.fl.us/dbs

Craig Kiser, Director

8293 Work Exploration Center

3000 NW 83rd Street I40
Gainesville, FL 32606 **352-395-5265**
FAX: 352-395-5271

Patsy Frenchman, Coordinator
Karla Wooten, Employment Specialist
Rosalyn Burgman, Vocation Evaluator

The Work Exploration Center embraces a holistic approach to Comprehensive Vocational Evaluation and Community Employment services, encouraging individual understanding, hope and growth for a productive and fulfilling future.

Georgia

8294 Employment and Training Division, Region B

Goodwill Industries of North Georgia
PO Box 447
Ellijay, GA 30540
706-276-4722
888-514-8112
FAX: 706-276-4732
e-mail: vti@ellijay.com

Linda Rau, Director Programs/Services

Employment training, assessment and job placement for people who have disabilities and/or are disadvantaged. Serving 15 counties in Northern Georgia.

8295 Fair Housing and Fair Employment

Georgia Commission on Equal Opportunity
229 Peachtree Street NE
710 Int Tower
Atlanta, GA 30303
404-656-1736
FAX: 404-656-4399
e-mail: gceo@gceo.state.ga.us
www.gceo.state.ga.us

Judith A Harris, Acting Fair Housing Manager
Stephanie Randolph, Intake Coordinator/Housing
Lisa Burroughs, Equal Employment Manager

8296 Griffin Area Resource Center Griffin Community Workshop Division

511 Hamilton Boulevard
 # 847
Griffin, GA 30223
770-228-3766
FAX: 770-228-3448
e-mail: griffincomwrkshp@aol.com

Lynn H Leaptrot, Workshop Director
Charles Cary Grubbs, GARC Executive Director

A CARF (The Rehabilitation Accreditation Commission) accredited Employment and Community Support organization providing daily services to participants with disabilities from 16 years of age and up in a 5 county area.

8297 IBM National Support Center

Special Needs Systems
PO Box 2150
Atlanta, GA 30301
404-238-3000
800-228-0752
FAX: 561-982-6059

Serves to help health care leaders, agency directors, policy makers, employers, educators, public officials and individuals learn how computers can enhance the quality of life for the disabled person in the school, home and workplace. Also provide information and resource guides on disabilities affecting hearing, learning, speech and language, mobility and vision.

8298 Kelley Diversified

265 Newton Bridge Road
PO Box 967
Athens, GA 30603
706-549-4398
FAX: 706-549-4479

Mary Patton, Executive Director
Sherry Burns, Rehabilitation Services Director
Jenny Taylor, Business Operations Manager

Work adjustment and remunerative work programs.

8299 New Ventures

304 Fort Drive
LaGrange, GA 30240
706-882-7723

Dave Miller, Executive Director

A rehabilitation and work training facility for individuals with barriers to employability. The program utilizes community based industrial work of varying levels of difficulty. A return to work conditioning program for the industrially injured is offered which features: first-day contact, workers compensation rehabilitation team management, and light-duty work conditioning. A training stipend is paid to defray costs associated with training.

Hawaii

8300 ASSETS School

1 Ohana Nui Way
Honolulu, HI 96818
808-423-1356
FAX: 808-422-1920
e-mail: info@assets-school.net
assets-school.net

Lou Salza, Head of School
Ron Yoshmoto, Principal K-8
Patti Jenks, Principal, High School

ASSETS is an independent school for gifted and or dyslexic children that provides an individualized, integrated learning enviroment. ASSETS' enviroment empowers these children to maximize their potential and to find their place as lifelong learners in school and society.

8301 Hawaii Fair Employment Practice Agency

888 Mililani Street Ph 2
Honolulu, HI 96813
808-599-5449
800-586-8800

8302 Hawaii Vocational Rehabilitation Division

601 Kamokila Boulevard
Room 515
Kapolei, HI 96707
808-692-7715
FAX: 808-692-7727

8303 Lanakila Rehabilitation Center

1809 Bachelot Street
Honolulu, HI 96817
808-531-0555
FAX: 808-533-7264
e-mail: lanakila@lanakilahawaii.org
www.lanakilahawaii.org

Laura K M Colbert, President
Debbie Kim Morikawa, VP Programs

Lanakila is a private nonprofit organization whose mission is to provide services and supports that assist individuals with physical, mental, or age-related challenges to live as independently as possible within our community. A broad range of services are offered which include meal/senior services, community based adult day programming for individuals with disabilities, work training opportunities, and extended/supported employment for individuals with special needs.

8304 Vocational and Rehabilitation Agency

Services for the Blind
PO Box 339
Honolulu, HI 96707
808-692-7715
FAX: 808-692-7727
e-mail: nshim@dhs.state.hi.us

8305 Wahiawa Family

330 Walker Avenue
Wahiawa, HI 96786
808-621-7407

Leslie Chinna

Work adjustment and remunerative work programs.

Idaho

8306 **High Reachers Employment and Training**
245 E 6th S
Mountain Home, ID 83647 **208-587-5804**

Joe McNeal, Executive Director

8307 **Idaho Employment Service and Job Training Program Liaison**
Idaho Department of Employment
317 Main Street
Boise, ID 83735 **208-334-4200**

8308 **Idaho Fair Employment Practice Agency**
Idaho Human Rights Commission
450 W State Street
Boise, ID 83702 **208-334-5747**

8309 **Idaho Governor's Committee on Employment of People with Disabilities**
317 Main Street
Boise, ID 83735

8310 **Idaho Vocational Rehabilitation Agency**
650 W State Street
Boise, ID 83702

8311 **Vocational and Rehabilitation Agency**
Idaho Commission for the Blind and Visually Impaired, PO Box 83720
Boise, ID 83702 **208-334-3220**
800-542-8688
FAX: 208-334-2963
e-mail: mgraham@icbvi.state.id.us
www.icbvi.state.id.us

Michael Graham, Administrator
Mike Blackaller, Rehab Services Chief
Maggie Starkovich, Administrative Assistant

Vocational rehabilitation, independent living training, medical intervention, adaptive technology and devices and employer advocacy.

Illinois

8312 **Ada S McKinley Vocational Services**
725 S Wells Street
Chicago, IL 60607 **312-554-0600**
FAX: 312-554-0292
TTY:312-697-9794
e-mail: ksmith@adasmckinley.org
www.adasmckinley.org

Aberra Zewdie, Division Director
Kent Smith, Chief Development Officer

8313 **Anixter Center**
6610 N Clark
Chicago, IL 60660 **773-973-7900**
FAX: 773-973-5268
e-mail: AskAnixter@anixter.org
www.anixter.org

Stuart Ferst, President/CEO

A Chicago-based human services agency that assists people with disabilities to live and work successfully in the community. Anixter Center provides vocational training, employment services, residences, special education, prevention programs, community services and health care. In addition, Anixter Center offers Illinois' only substance abuse treatment programs specifically for people with disabilities including Addiction Recovery of the Deaf.

8314 **C-4 Work Center**
5710 N Broadway
Chicago, IL 60660 **773-728-1000**
FAX: 773-728-6517

Gino Balbuena, Production Manager
Anthony A Kopera, CEO
Mark T Hicks, Program Director

Aftercare, case finding, information and referrals, vocational training and work activities offered to mentally ill persons.

8315 **Cornerstone Services**
777 Joyce Road
Joliet, IL 60436 **815-741-7602**
FAX: 815-723-1177
e-mail: jhogan@cornerstoneservices.org
www.cornerstoneservices.org

James A Hogan, President/CEO
Susan Murphy, Coordinator of PR

Cornerstone Services provides progressive, comprehensive services for people with disabilities, promoting choice, dignity and the opportunity to live and work in the community. Established in 1969, the agency provides developmental, vocational, employment, residential and mental health services at various community-based locations. The nonprofit social service agency helps approximately 750 people each day.

8316 **Crystal Lake Vocational Rehabilitation Center**
Pioneer Center
3941 W Dayton Street
McHenry, IL 60050 **815-344-1230**

Thomas Gollan, Executive Director

8317 **Fulton County Rehab Center**
500 N Main Street
Canton, IL 61520 **309-649-1000**
FAX: 309-649-1047

Rex Lewis

Work adjustment and remunerative work programs.

8318 **Glenkirk**
3504 Commercial Avenue
Northbrook, IL 60062 **847-272-5111**
FAX: 847-272-7350

Alan Spector, Executive Director

Helps infants, children and adults with developmental disabilities reach higher levels of independence. A non-profit organization serving people in north and northwest Chicago suburbs. Glenkirk's residential, vocational, educational and support programs include services which provide individual evaluation, therapeutic treatment and training.

8319 **Illinois Employment Service**
Department of Employment Security
401 S State Street
Room 615
Chicago, IL 60605 **312-353-5133**

8320 **Jewish Vocational Services**
1 S Franklin Street
Chicago, IL 60606 **312-357-4500**
FAX: 312-855-3282

Occupational training and job placement for handicapped persons of all religions.

8321 **JoDavies Workshop**
706 S W Street
Galena, IL 61036

Intake and referral, early intervention for children only, vocational evaluation and work adjustment training services offered.

8322 **Kennedy Job Training Center**
7361 S Meade
Bedford Park, IL 60638 **708-594-7155**
FAX: 708-594-7156

Robin Mertes, Placement Manager
Kandy Stamer, QMRP/Intake Coordinator

Offers vocational evaluation, vocational training work adjustment training, and job placement services for developmentally disabled and hearing impaired persons.

8323 **Knox County Council for Developmental Disabilities**
2015 Windish Drive
Galesburg, IL 61401 **309-344-2600**
FAX: 309-344-1754
e-mail: kccdd@galesburg.net

Ned Hippensteel, Executive Director

Developmental training, vocational evaluation, work adjustment training, extended training, placement, supported employment, and CILA.

8324 **Kreider Services**
500 Anchor Road
Dixon, IL 61021 **815-453-2074**
FAX: 815-288-1636

Arlan McClain, Executive Director

Offers day service programs, vocational training programs, job placement, supported employment, respite care, residential and family support for ages birth to three years.

8325 **Lambs Farm**
PO Box 520
14245 W Rockland Road
Libertyville, IL 60048 **847-362-4636**
FAX: 847-362-0742
e-mail: info@lambsfarm.org
www.lambsfarm.org

Dianne Yacanetti, President/CEO
Marty Buckley, Director Program Services
Jim Hutson, Asst Dir Vocational Services

Person-centered, comprehensive program of residential, vocational and social support service for adults with developmental disabilities.

8326 **Land of Lincoln Goodwill Industries**
800 N 10th Street
PO Box 8528
Springfield, IL 62703 **217-789-0400**
FAX: 217-789-0540

Larry Hupp, Executive Director

Offers a developmental training and community employment programs for persons with disabilities.

8327 **Orchard Association for the Retarded**
7670 Marmora Avenue
Skokie, IL 60077 **847-967-1800**

Vocational program and counseling, respite services and community living facility for the retarded.

8328 **Owens Vocational Training Center**
2639 N Kildare Avenue
Chicago, IL 60639

Janie Nelson, Executive Director

8329 **President's Committee on Employment of Employment of the Disabled**
623 E Adams Street
Springfield, IL 62701 **217-785-0218**
800-ASK-DORI
TTY:217-782-5734

Audrey McCrimon, Director

8330 **Sertoma Centre**
4343 W 123rd Street
Alsip, IL 60803 **708-371-9700**

Gus van den Brink, Executive Director

Offers vocational services to promote independence and community integration; day training and residential services provided to individuals. Programs include: vocational evaluation, work adjustment training, janitorial training, job placement, sheltered work, supported employment, developmental training, respite care, residential services.

8331 **Shore Training Center**
8035 Austin Avenue
Morton Grove, IL 60053 **847-581-0200**

Mark Robinson

Provides remunerative work.

8332 **Skills**
1122 5th Avenue
Moline, IL 61265 **309-797-3586**
FAX: 309-797-4914

Stuart Olson, President
William Taylor, Transitional Service

Accredited through the Commission on Accreditation of Rehabilitation Facilities; offers job training partnership act and vocational evaluation services offered.

8333 **Thresholds AMISS**
12145 Western Avenue
Blue Island, IL 60406 **708-597-7997**
FAX: 708-597-8073

Julia Rupp, Executive Director
Camille Rucks, Team Leader

Services offered include psychosocial, vocational and residential programs for ages 18 or older with a primary diagnosis of mental illness. Facility is wheelchair accessible.

8334 **Vocational and Rehabilitation Agency**
623 E Adams Street
PO Box 19429
Springfield, IL 62794 **217-785-0218**
800-843-6154
FAX: 217-785-5733
TTY:217-782-5734
e-mail: dhsbr@dhs.state.il.us
www.state.il.us

8335 **Washington County Vocational Workshop**
PO Box 273
Nashville, IL 62263 **618-327-4461**

Keith Currin, Executive Director

8336 **Westside Parents Work Activity Center**
3765 W Odgen Avenue
Chicago, IL 60623 **773-522-1200**

Offers developmental training programs providing basic skills in self care for multiply and physically handicapped persons.

Indiana

8337 **ADEC Resources for Independence**
19607 State Road 120
Boonville, IN 46507 **574-293-9597**

Matt Leachman, Contact

Serves Elkhart County and surrounding area.

8338 **ARC of Allen County**
2542 Thompson Avenue
Fort Wayne, IN 46807 **260-456-4534**
FAX: 260-745-5200

Dan Winkle, Contact

8339 **BI-County Services**
425 E Harrison Road
Bluffton, IN 46714 **260-824-1253**
FAX: 260-824-1892
e-mail: jbussard@adifferentlight.com

Joyce Bussard, Program Director

Serves Wells and Adam Counties. Infant services, Medicaid waivers, music therapy, ICF, MR, group homes, sheltered employment, pay program and supported employment services available.

8340 **Balance Centers of America**
521 E 86th Avenue
Suite H
Merrillville, IN 46410 **219-736-2930**

Jane Labar, Contact

8341 **Bridgepointe Goodwill Industries and Easter Seal Society**
1329 Applegate Lane
PO Box 2117
Clarksville, IN 47129 **812-283-7908**
FAX: 812-283-6248

Terry Richards, Contact

8342 **Carey Services**
2724 S Carey Street
Marion, IN 46795 **765-668-8961**
FAX: 765-664-6747

Grant Black, Contact

8343 **Evansville Association for the Blind**
500 Second Avenuke
PO Box 6445
Evansville, IN 47719 **812-422-1181**
FAX: 812-424-3154
www2.evansville.edu/ebaweb

Karla Horrell, Director Rehabilitation
Diane Hagler, Vocational Specialist
Krysti Kite, Orientation/Mobility

An community rehabilitation facility untilizing individual goals to assist persons with disabilities achieve or maintain potenial

8344 **Four Rivers Resource Services**
PO Box 249
Linton, IN 47441 **812-847-2231**
FAX: 812-847-8836
e-mail: fourrivers@frrs.org
www.frrs.org

Stephen Sacksteder, CEO
Lyna Landis, Marketing Coordinator

Employment, community living, connections, follow-along, early intervention, preschool, healthy families, child care resource and referral and child care voucher program, impact, and transpotation services.

8345 **Gateway Services/JCARC**
PO Box 216
Franklin, IN 46131 **317-738-5500**
FAX: 317-738-5522

Beth Hurst, Contact

8346 **Goodwill Industries of Central Indiana**
1635 W Michigan Street
Indianapolis, IN 46222 **317-264-1313**
FAX: 317-264-1336

Irene McClesky, Contact

8347 **Indiana Employment Services and Job Training Program Liaison**
10 N Senate Avenue
Indianapolis, IN 46204 **317-232-6702**
FAX: 317-233-5499

8348 **Indiana Fair Employment Practice Agency**
32 E Washington Street
Suite 900
Indianapolis, IN 46204 **317-872-9991**

8349 **LCAR**
2650 W 35th Street
Gary, IN 46408 **219-884-1138**

Brian Davis, Contact

8350 **LaPorte County Sheltered Workshop**
4315 E Michigan Boulevard
Michigan City, IN 46360 **219-874-4288**
FAX: 219-879-2139

Vocational training center for persons 16 and older with disabilities.

8351 **New Hope Services**
725 Wall Street
Jeffersonville, IN 47130
812-288-8248
FAX: 812-228-1206

Lynn Snow, Contact

8352 **New Horizons Rehabilitation**
237 Six Pine Ranch Road
PO Box 98
Batesville, IN 47006
812-934-4528

Greg Tow, Contact

Serves Ripley, Franklin, Ohio, Switzerland Dearborn, and Decatur.

8353 **Noble Centers**
2400 N Tibbs Avenue
Indianapolis, IN 46222
317-264-1510
FAX: 317-264-5300

Tom Cain, Contact

8354 **Putnam County Comprehensive Services**
630 Tennessee Street
Greencastle, IN 46135
765-653-9753
FAX: 765-653-7646

Tammy Amore

8355 **Southern Indiana Resource Solutions**
1579 S Folsomville Road
Boonville, IN 47601
812-897-4840
FAX: 812-897-0123
e-mail: jward@sirs.org
www.sirs.org

Kris Lasher, Marketing Director

8356 **Sycamore Rehabilitation Services**
1001 Sycamore Lane
Danville, IN 46122
317-745-4715
FAX: 317-745-8271

Patrick Cockrum, Contact

8357 **Vocational and Rehabilitation Agency**
402 W Washington Street, Room W-451
PO Box 7083
Indianapolis, IN 46207
317-232-1147
800-545-6776
FAX: 317-232-1240
e-mail: mschultz@fssa.state.in.us

Jeff Hendrickson, Contact

8358 **Wabash/Employability Center**
SC6395 Earl Avenue
Suite 2
Lafayette, IN 47903
765-447-0300
FAX: 765-447-6456

Bill Carmichael, Contact

Serves Tippecanoe County.

Iowa

8359 **ACT Assessment Test Preparation Reference Manual**
American College Testing Program
2201 Dodge
168
Iowa City, IA 52243
319-337-1000
FAX: 319-337-1771

This reference manual was developed as a resource for high school teachers and counselors in assisting students with test preparation.

8360 **ACT Asset Technical Manual**
American College Testing Program
2201 Dodge
Suite 168
Iowa City, IA 52243
319-337-1000
FAX: 319-337-1771

Provides a technical description of the ASSET program to guide users in working with the program and interpreting test results.

8361 **Franklin County Work Activity Center**
20 5th Street NW
Hampton, IA 50441
641-456-5293

Steven Paul Woods, Executive Director

Nonprofit organization providing residential and vocational services in Franklin and Hardin counties in the state of Iowa. Residential Services include RCF/MR services, Supported Community Living Services and Community Supervised Apartment Living Arrangement Services. Vocational Services include Work Services and Supported Employment Services. Accredited by the Commission on Accreditation of rehabilitation Facilities since 1984, and serves individuals with a wide range of needs.

8362 **Innovative Industries**
405 E Madison Street
Winterset, IA 50273
515-462-2926
FAX: 515-462-2870
e-mail: winnind@iowalink.com

Sandi Smith, Secretary
Connie Bailey, Program Manager

8363 **Iowa Civil Rights Commission**
400 E 14th Street
Des Moines, IA 50319
515-281-4121
FAX: 515-242-5840
www.state.ia.us/government/crc

8364 **Iowa Employment Service**
1000 E Grand Avenue
Des Moines, IA 50319
515-281-6647

8365 **Iowa Job Training Program Liaison**
Iowa Department of Economic Development
200 E Grand Avenue
Des Moines, IA 50309
515-242-4827

8366 **Iowa Valley Community College**
3702 S Center Street
Marshalltown, IA 50158
641-752-4643
FAX: 641-752-5909

Bill Martin, Career Development

Offers two levels of specialized vocational preparatory programming for adults with disabilities. The Career Development Center serves dependent adults. The goal of the program is to maintain or improve skills to enable persons served to enter sheltered or supported employment. The IRP/CBVT programs are non-credit specialized vocational programs for independent adults served by Vocational Rehabilitation and our programs. The goals are for competitive placements in jobs. CARF accredited.

8367 **Iowa Vocational Rehabilitation Agency**

510 E 12th Street
Des Moines, IA 50309 **515-281-4311**
FAX: 515-281-7643

8368 **New Focus**

102 W Washington
Centerville, IA 52544 **641-437-1722**

Keith Lindley, Executive Director
Peggy Oden, Director Rehabilitation

Provides vocational services for adults with disabilities. Includes work activity, supported employment and supported community living.

8369 **Second Time Around**

110 W Jackson Street
Centerville, IA 52544 **641-437-7355**

Keith Lindley, Executive Director
Debbie Steen, Store Supervisor

Work training site for adults with disabilities.

8370 **Vocational and Rehabilitation Agency**

510 E 12th Street
Des Moines, IA 50319 **515-281-4311**
FAX: 515-281-7645
TTY:515-281-4311
e-mail: dcarlson@dvrs.state.ia.us
www.dvrs.state.ia.us

John Larson, Assistant Chief

Kansas

8371 **Clay Center Adult Training Center**

701 4th Street
Clay Center, KS 67432 **785-632-5357**
FAX: 785-632-5371

Lillian Bosch, Executive Director

8372 **Kansas Fair Employment Practice Agency**

900 SW Jackson Street
Topeka, KS 66612 **785-296-1500**

8373 **Kansas Vocational Rehabilitation Agency**

300 SW Oakley Avenue
Biddle Building, 1st Floor
Topeka, KS 66606 **785-296-3911**
TTY:913-296-7029
e-mail: jac@srkspo.wpo.state.ks.us

Joyce Cussimanio, Director

Kentucky

8374 **Kentucky Committee on Employment of People with Disabilities**

600 W Cedar Street
Louisville, KY 40202 **502-595-4165**

8375 **Kentucky Department for Employment Service and Job Training Program Liaison**

275 E Main Street 2-W
Frankfort, KY 40621 **502-564-2367**
FAX: 502-564-7799
www.desky.org

8376 **Kentucky Department for the Blind**

209 St Clair Street
PO Box 757
Frankfort, KY 40601 **502-695-6350**
800-321-6661
TTY:502-564-2929
e-mail: dbohannon@state.ky.us.dfblind
www.state.ky.us/agencies/wforce

Denise Placido, Commissioner (Acting)

Provides career services and assistance to adults with severe visual handicaps who want to become productive in the home or work force. Also provides the Client Assistance Program established to provide advice, assistance and information available from rehabilitation programs to persons with handicaps.

8377 **Kentucky Vocational Rehabilitation Agency**

500 Mero Street
Frankfort, KY 40601 **502-564-4896**

8378 **Pioneer Vocational/Industrial Services**

590 Stanford Road
Danville, KY 40422

Jack Goodbey, Executive Director

8379 **Vocational and Rehabilitation Agency**

209 Saint Clair
PO Box 757
Frankfort, KY 40601 **502-564-4440**
800-372-7172
FAX: 502-564-6745
TTY:502-564-6817
e-mail: wfd.vocrehab@mail.state.ky.us
kydvr.state.ky.us

8380 **Work Enhancement Center of Western Kentucky**

803 Poplar Street
Murray, KY 42071 **502-762-1100**
FAX: 502-767-3600

Steve Passmore, Director

The center has been established in order to service industry in the three state area surrounding Kentucky. This service includes job/skill evaluation, job design consultation, pre-employment employee evaluations and economic evaluation.

Louisiana

8381 Community Opportunities of East Ascension
1122 E Ascension Complex Boulevard
Gonzales, LA 70737 **225-621-2000**
FAX: 225-621-2022

Mark Thomas, Director

Committed to affording individuals the opportunities that reflect and support choices, dignity, individuality, self-determination, community, coherency and commen sense. Programs incloude Respite, Personal Care Attendant, Support Living, Support Environment, Adult Day Training, and Elderly/Adult Waiver Services.

8382 Louisiana Employment Service and Job Training Program Liaison
PO Box 94094
Baton Rouge, LA 70804 **225-342-3111**
FAX: 225-342-3030

8383 Louisiana Vocational Rehabilitation Agency
4051 Veterans Boulevard
Suite 408
Metairieuge, LA 70002 **504-838-5180**
FAX: 504-838-5413

8384 St. James Association for Retarded Citizens
29150 Health Unit Street
Vacherie, LA 70090 **225-265-7910**

A private sheltered work program for mentally retarded and developmentally disabled adults.

8385 Westbank Sheltered Workshop
1728 Hermosa Street
New Orleans, LA 70114 **504-362-1311**

A private non-residential facility serving severely disabled individuals referred through Louisiana Rehabilitation Services.

Maine

8386 Addison Point Specialized Services
PO Box 207
Addison, ME 04606 **207-483-2817**
FAX: 207-483-2817

Paula Chartrand, Executive Officer

Provides services to individuals who are deaf/blind, mentally retarded, autistic, behaviorally challenged and/or dual diagnosed. Training services to place these individuals in community employment.

8387 Bangor Veteran Center: Veterans Outreach Center
352 Harlow Street
Bangor, ME 04401 **207-947-3391**
FAX: 207-941-8195
e-mail: bangorvc@aol.com
http://www.hud.gov/offices/cpd/about/hudvet/

Joseph A DeGrasse, Team Leader
Robert L Daisey MSW, Clinical Coordinator

Readjustment counseling services for veterans of Vietnam, Vietnam Era, Persian Gulf, Panama, Grenada, Lebanon, Somalia, WWII and Korean conflicts.

8388 Creative Work Systems
443 Congress Street
Portland, ME 04101 **207-879-1140**
FAX: 207-879-1146
e-mail: cws@gwi.net
www.creativesystems.com

Susan Percy, Executive Director

Provides residential, day habilitation and supported emploment in Central and Southern Maine.

8389 Maine Employment Service
20 Union Street
Augusta, ME 04330 **207-287-3788**

8390 Maine Fair Employment Practice Agency
Maine Human Rights Commission
51 State House Station
Augusta, ME 04333 **207-624-6050**
FAX: 207-624-6063
www.state.me.us/mhrc

State agency with the responsibility of enforcing Maine's anti-discrimination laws. The commission investigates complaints of unlawful discrimination in employment, housing, education, access to public accommodations, extension of credit and offensive names.

8391 Maine Governor's Committee on Employment of the Disabled
35 Anthony Avenue
Augusta, ME 04330 **207-624-5335**

8392 Northeast Occupational Exchange
248 Center Street
Bangor, ME 04401 **207-942-3816**

Dr. Charles Tingley, Executive Director

8393 Vocational and Rehabilitation Agency
Division for the Blind
2 Anthony Avenue, 150 SHS
Augusta, ME 04333 **207-624-5959**
800-698-4440
FAX: 207-624-5980
TTY:207-624-5955
e-mail: paul.e.cote@state.me.us

Maryland

8394 Ardmore Developmental Center
3000 Lottsford Vista Road
Bowie, MD 20721
FAX: 301-731-4551

Donalda Lovelace, Chief Executive Officer

Offers supported employment programs and vocational education for persons who are mentally retarded as well as residential services and Emergency Respite Care.

8395 Job Opportunities for the Blind
National Federation of the Blind
1800 Johnson Street
Baltimore, MD 21230 **410-837-6763**
FAX: 410-685-5653
e-mail: nfb@iamdigex.net
www.nfb.org

James Geshel , Director Governmental Affairs
Anthony Cobb, Director Job Opportinities for

This free service allows individuals touch-tone telephone access to the thousands of jobs listed in America's Job Bank, and internet service run by the Department of Labor. Any person registered with either a state rehabilitation agency or a state employment service can search across the country for jobs by either type of work or location.

8396 **Mainstream**

3 Bethesda Metro Center
Suite 830
Bethesda, MD 20814 **301-891-8777**
FAX: 301-891-8778
e-mail: mainstrm@aol.com

Patricia M Jackson, Executive Director

Nonprofit organization dedicated to improving competitive employment opportunities for persons with disabilities. Provides specialized services and acts as a bridge that links service providers, employers and persons with disabilties. Provides training, educational publications, and videos on disablityemployment issues. Educationa materials include a magazine, brochures, and audio-visual aids.

8397 **Maryland Employment Services and Job Training Program Liaison**

1100 N Eutaw Street
Room 600
Baltimore, MD 21201 **410-767-2173**

8398 **Maryland Fair Employment Practice Agency**

400 Washington Avenue
Room 124
Towson, MD 21204 **410-887-5557**
FAX: 410-769-8914

8399 **Maryland State Department of Education**

Division of Rehabilitation Services (DIRS)
2301 Argonne Drive
Baltimore, MD 21218 **410-554-9385**

Robert Burns, Asst. State Super.

The Vocational Rehabilitation Program delivers to eligible individuals with physical and/or mental disabilities to enable them to become employed. The Independent Living Program's goal is to assist people in remaining in their homes and communities. The Division operates the Maryland Rehabilitation Center, a comprehensive evaluation and training center that has dormitory space. There are field offices located statewide with counselors to advise and manage the provision of services offered.

8400 **PWI Profile**

Projects W/Industry, Goodwill Industries of Amer.
9200 Wisconsin Avenue
Bethesda, MD 20814

Newsletter on employment of persons with disabilities.

8401 **Project LINK**

Mainstream
3 Bethesda Metro Center
Suite 830
Bethesda, MD 20814 **301-891-8777**
800-247-1380
FAX: 301-891-8778
e-mail: info@mainstreaminc.org
www.mainstreaminc.org

Provides job development and placement in services to dislocated workers with disabilities in the Washington, DC and Dallas, TX areas.

8402 **Treatment and Learning Centers (TLC)**

9975 Medical Center Drive
Rockville, MD 20850 **301-738-1415**

Richard Pavlin, Executive Director

Helps parents, children and teachers understand and overcome educational difficulties. They offer interdisciplinary diagnostic testing individually tailored to pinpoint the specific strengths and needs of students who may have learning disabilities, Dyslexia or other learning problems.

Massachusetts

8403 **Division of Employment & Training**

State of Massachusetts
19 Staniford Street
3rd Floor
Boston, MA 02114 **617-626-6560**

8404 **Gateway Arts Program, Crafts Store & Gallery**

62 Harvard Street
Brookline, MA 02445 **617-734-1577**
FAX: 617-734-3199
e-mail: gateway@vinfen.org
www.gatewayarts.org

Rae T Edelson, Program Director
Ted Lampe, Assistant Program Director
Mona Thaler, Marketing Director

An arts-based vocational service for adults with developmental and other disabilities including mental illness, autism and head injury who can pursue paid work in fine art and crafts with the aid of professional artists/teachers, a professional marketer and a Crafts Store and Gallery. A service of Vinfen.

8405 **Massachusetts Fair Employment Practice Agency**

1 Ashburton Place
Room 601
Boston, MA 02108 **617-727-8900**

8406 **Massachusetts Governor's Commission on Employment of Disabled Persons**

19 Standiford Street
3rd Floor
Boston, MA 02114 **617-864-2000**

8407 **Vocational Rehabilitation Agency**

27-43 Wormwood Street
Boston, MA 02210 **617-204-3604**
800-642-0249
FAX: 617-727-1354
TTY:800-764-0200
e-mail: elmer.bartels@mrc.state.ma.us
www.state.ma.us

8408 **Vocational and Rehabilitation Agency Massachusetts Commission for the Blind**

88 Kingston Street
Boston, MA 02111 **617-727-5550**
800-392-6450
TTY:800-392-6556
e-mail: poliver@state.ma.us
www.state.ma.us

8409 **Work**
3 Arlington Street
North Quincy, MA 02171 **617-328-0300**

Dr. William Wolk, Executive Director

Michigan

8410 **Disability Community Small Business Development Center**
Ann Arbor Center for Independent Living
2568 Packard
Ann Arbor, MI 48104 **734-484-5310**
FAX: 734-971-0826

Roseanne Herzog, Director

Offers small business counseling and training to individuals with disabilities in the state of Michigan.

8411 **Lamplighter's Work Center**
1320 W State Street
Cheboygan, MI 49721 **906-274-5456**

Robert Spinella, Executive Director

8412 **Michigan Employment Service**
7310 Woodward Avenue
Detroit, MI 48202 **313-876-5217**

8413 **Michigan Fair Employment Practice Agency**
1200 Sixth Avenue, N Tower
6th Floor
Detroit, MI 48226 **313-256-2202**
FAX: 313-256-2167

8414 **Vocational and Rehabilitation Agency**
201 N Washington Square
PO Box 30652
Lansing, MI 48909 **517-373-2062**
800-292-4200
FAX: 517-335-5140
TTY:5173734025
e-mail: kreinerc@state.mi.us
www.mfia.state.mi.us

8415 **Vocational and Rehabilitation Agency: Michigan Department of Career Development**
PO Box 30010
Lansing, MI 48909 **517-373-3390**
800-605-6722
FAX: 517-335-7277
e-mail: davisr1@state.mi.us
www.michigan.gov

Minnesota

8416 **Jewish Vocational Service of Jewish Family and Children's Services**
1500 Lilac Drive S
Suite 311
Minneapolis, MN 55416 **612-546-0616**
FAX: 612-593-1778

Jeremy Waldman, Executive Director

8417 **Minnesota Employment Practice Agency**
Laura Sengil, Dept. of Human Rights
190 E 5th Street
Suite 700
St. Paul, MN 55101 **651-296-9044**

8418 **PWI Forum**
Multi Resource Centers
1900 Chicago Avenue
Minneapolis, MN 55404 **612-871-2402**

Newsletter for business, community and government leaders. Focuses on employment of persons with disabilities.

8419 **Vocational Rehabilitation Agency**
Rehabilitation Services Branch
390 N Robert Street
Saint Paul, MN 55101 **651-296-9981**
800-328-9095
FAX: 651-297-5159
TTY:800-657-3973
e-mail: Paul.Bridges@state.mn.us
www.MNWorkForceCenter.org

Paul Bridges, Contact

8420 **Vocational and Rehabilitation Agency**
21200 University Avenue W
Suite 240
Saint Paul, MN 55114 **612-642-0500**
800-652-9000
FAX: 651-284-3307
TTY:612-642-0506
e-mail: info@ngwmail.des.state.mn.us
www.mnwfc.org

Mississippi

8421 **Allied Enterprises of Tupelo**
613 Pegram Drive
Tupelo, MS 38801 **662-287-1461**
FAX: 662-287-1463

J Barry Bray, Facility Manager

Vocational evaluation, work adjustment and job placement of disabled persons in a rehabilitation workshop.

8422 **Mississippi Department of Rehabilitation Services**
PO Box 1698
Jackson, MS 39215 **601-853-5100**
800-443-1000
FAX: 601-853-5158
TTY:800-443-1000
e-mail: bmcmillan@mdrs.state.ms.us
www.mdrs.state.ms.us

Offers low vision aids and appliances, counseling, social work, educational and professional training, residential services, recreational services, computer training and employment opportunities for the handicapped.

8423 **Mississippi Employment Secutity Commission**
PO Box 1669
Jackson, MS 39215 **601-961-7501**
FAX: 601-961-7405
www.mesc.state.ms.us

8424 **Vocational and Rehabilitation Agency Department of Rehabilitation Services**
1281 Highway 51
PO Box 1698
Jackson, MS 39215
601-853-5230
800-443-1000
FAX: 601-853-5205
e-mail: gneely@mdrs.state.ms.us

8425 **Worksight**
Mississippi State University
PO Box 6189
Mississippi State, MS 39762
662-325-2001
800-675-7782
FAX: 662-325-8989
www.blind.msstate.edu

Discusses news, activities, research projects and training programs of the Center.

Missouri

8426 **Missouri Fair Employment Practice Agency**
3315 W Truman Boulevard
Jefferson City, MO 65102
573-751-4091
www.dolir.state.mo.us

Renell Wynn, Director

8427 **Missouri Governor's Council on Disability**
PO Box 1668
Jefferson City, MO 65102
573-751-2600
800-877-8249
FAX: 573-526-4109
TTY:573-751-2600
e-mail: gcd@dolir.state.mo.us
www.dolir.mo.gov/gcd

Robert Honan, Executive Director

Advocate training, civil rights, community education services, community resource referral, conferences, consumer education, disability awareness program, educational information and resources, information and education services, information and referral, newsletter, policy issues and services, publications, resource directory, seminars, technical assistance, training and seminars.

8428 **Missouri Job Training Program Liaison**
221 Metro Drive
Jefferson City, MO 65109
573-634-2321

8429 **Missouri Vocational Rehabilitation Agency**
3024 W Truman Boulevard
Jefferson Cty, MO 65109
573-751-3251
FAX: 573-741-1441
TTY:573-751-3251

Don Glann, Assistant Commissioner

8430 **Vocational and Rehabilitation Agency**
3024 Dupont Circle
Jefferson City, MO 65109
573-751-3251
877-222-8963
FAX: 573-751-1441
TTY:573-751-0881
www.vr.dese.state.mo.us

8431 **WX: Work Capacities**
17331 E 40th Highway
Suite 103
Independence, MO 64055

Carol Lett, Executive Director

Montana

8432 **Montana Employment Services and Job Training Programs Liaison**
PO Box 1728
Helena, MT 59624
406-444-3697

8433 **Montana Fair Employment Practice Agency**
PO Box 1728
Helena, MT 59624
406-444-3697
800-542-0807

8434 **Montana Governor's Committee on Employment of Disabled People**
Mitchell Building
Room 130
Helena, MT 59620

Nebraska

8435 **Nebraska Employment Services**
Department of Labor
550 S 16th Street
Lincoln, NE 68508
816-426-5481

8436 **Nebraska Fair Employment Practice Agency**
301 Centennial Mall S
Lincoln, NE 68508
402-471-4997

8437 **Nebraska Governor's Committee on the Employment of the Handicapped**
550 S 16th Street
Lincoln, NE 68508
402-472-1415

8438 **Nebraska Vocational Rehabilitation Agency**
301 Centennial Mall S
Lincoln, NE 68509
402-471-3644
877-637-3422
FAX: 402-471-0788
e-mail: vr_stateoffice@vocrehab.state.ne.us

Services for individuals with disabilities who want to become employed. Services are free to those who qualify.

8439 **Nebraska Work Force Development**
550 S 16th Street
Lincoln, NE 68509
402-471-9792
FAX: 402-471-2318

Fernando Lecuona III, Commissioner

8440 **Vocational and Rehabilitation Agency**
State Department of Education
PO Box 94987
Lincoln, NE 68509
402-471-3649
877-637-3422
FAX: 402-471-0788
TTY:402-471-3659
e-mail: vr_stateoffice@vocrehab.state.ne.us
www.vocrehab.state.ne.us

Nevada

8441 **Nevada Fair Employment Practice Agency**
1515 E Tropicana Avenue
Suite 590
Las Vegas, NV 89119

8442 **Nevada Governor's Committee on Employment of Persons with Disabilities**
3100 Mill Street
Suite 115
Reno, NV 89502

8443 **Nevada Job Training Program Liaison**
400 Capitol
Carson City, NV 89710

8444 **Vocational and Rehabilitation Agency**
505 E King Street
Suite 502
Carson City, NV 89701
775-684-4040
FAX: 775-684-4184
e-mail: mryasmer@nvdetr.org
detr.state.nv.us

Maynard Yasmer, Administrator
Peter Singleton, Rehab. Program Supervisor
Bob Nichols, Rehabilitation Manager

The Rehabilitation Division is comprised of four bureaus and the community-based services unit to address prevention, assessment, training, treatment and job placement for Nevadans with functional disabilities. The division places primary emphasis on providing necessary services to help clients work and live independently and substance-free. The division administrator, based in Carson City, oversees programs offered in offices throughout the state.

New Hampshire

8445 **Fit for Work at Exeter Hospital**
10 Buzell Avenue
Exeter, NH 03833
603-778-7311
FAX: 603-778-6671

Staffed by a team of allied health professionals, our outpatient rehabilitation program offers functional restoration, work therapy, diagnostic testing and physical therapy.

8446 **New Hampshire Employment Security**
32 S Main Street
Concord, NH 03301
603-224-3311
800-852-3400
FAX: 603-228-4145
TTY:800-735-2964
www.nhes.state.nh.us

Sandy Smith Dupree, Public Information Officer

Operates a free public employment service and provides assisted and self directed employment and career related services and labor market information for employers and the general public.

8447 **New Hampshire Fair Employment Practice Agency**
2 Chenell Drive
Concord, NH 03301
603-225-3699
FAX: 603-271-6339

8448 **New Hampshire Job Training Program Liaison**
64 Old Suncook Road
Concord, NH 03301
603-228-3349

8449 **Vocational and Rehabilitation Agency**
78 Regional Drive
Building 2
Concord, NH 03301
603-271-3471
800-299-1647
FAX: 603-271-7095
TTY:603-271-3471
e-mail: pleather@ed.state.nh.us
www.ed.state.nh.us

Paul Leather, Director

Offers services for the totally blind, legally blind, visually impaired, mentally retarded blind and more with health, counseling, educational, recreational, rehabilitation, computer training and professional training services.

New Jersey

8450 **ARC of Gloucester County**
1555 Gateway Boulevard
Woodbury, NJ 08096
856-848-8648
FAX: 856-848-7753
www.thearcgloucester.org

Mike Carlin, Contact

8451 **ARC of Hunterdon County**
1322 State Route 31
Suite 5
Annandale, NJ 08801
980-730-7827
FAX: 980-730-7726

Barbara Gustassen, Contact

Serves Hunterdon County.

8452 **ARC of Mercer County**
180 Ewingville Road
Ewing, NJ 08638
609-406-0181
FAX: 609-406-9258
www.arcmercer.org

Joseph Gousie, Executive Director

8453 **ARC of Monmouth**
1158 Wayside Road
Tinton Falls, NJ 07712
732-493-1919
FAX: 732-493-3604
e-mail: info@arcofmonmouth.org
www.arcofmonmouth.org

Jacqueline Moskowitz, Director, Social Services

8454 **Abilities Center of New Jersey**
790 N Delsea Drive
Westville, NJ 08093
856-848-1025
FAX: 856-848-8429

Susan Buchaman, Contact

8455 **Abilities of Northwest New Jersey**
264 Route 31 N
PO Box 251
Washington, NJ 07882
908-689-1118
FAX: 908-689-6363

Denny Senke, Contact

Serves northwestern New Jersey.

8456 **Alliance for Disabled in Action New Jersey**
629 Amboy Avenue
Suite LL
Edison, NJ 08837
732-738-4388
FAX: 732-738-4416
TTY:732-738-9644
e-mail: adacil@adacil.org
www.adacil.org

Richard Ringhof, Executive Director

Serves Somerset, Union and Middlesex Counties in New Jersey.

8457 **Alternatives for Growth: New Jersey**
16-00 208 S
Fair Lawn, NJ 07410
201-797-8330
FAX: 201-797-3586

Donna Flannery, Contact

Serves all New Jersey.

8458 **Arc of Bergen and Passaic Counties**
223 Moore Street
Hackensack, NJ 07601
201-343-0322
FAX: 201-343-0401
e-mail: arcbp@aol.com
www.arcbergenpassaic.org

Alice Siegel, Community Residential Serv. Dir.
Kathy Walsh, Senior VP Program Services
Anne Gallucci, Vocational Services Director

Serving persons with mental retardation and disabilities and their families in Bergen and Passaic Counties, NJ.

8459 **Career Opportunity Development of New Jersey**
901 Atlantic Avenue
Egg Harbor, NJ 08215
732-756-5575

Jenine Emil, Contact

Serves Bergen and Passaic Counties.

8460 **Center for Educational Advancement New Jersey**
11 Minneakoning Road
Flemington, NJ 08822
908-782-1480
FAX: 908-782-5370
e-mail: jkunz@ceaemployment.com
www.ceaemployment.com

Joanne Kunz, Sr Director, Employment Services

Serves Summerset and Mercer Counties. Skills training in office technology and food service. Job placement and job coaching services are available. Employer Network for Ticket to Work.

8461 **Cerebral Palsy Association of Middlesex County**
Roosevelt Park
Oak Drive
Edison, NJ 08837
201-549-5580
FAX: 201-603-0284

Dominic Ursino, Contact

Serves Central New Jersey.

8462 **Easter Seal Hackensack**
171 Atlantic Street
Hackensack, NJ 07601
201-342-5739
FAX: 201-342-4480

Denise Sredeen, Contact

Serves Hackensack.

8463 **Easter Seal Society of New Jersey Highlands Workshop**
133 Main Street
Franklin, NJ 07416
973-827-9066
FAX: 973-827-3828

Dave Shickle, Contact

Serves all New Jersey.

8464 **Easter Seal of Ocean County**
150 Oberlin Avenue
Lakewood, NJ 08701
732-363-6621
FAX: 732-363-7540

Greg Makely, Contact

8465 **Easter Seals New Jersey**
1 Kimberly Road
E Brunswick, NJ 08815
732-257-6662

Wilma Rosa, Contact

Serves all New Jersey.

8466 **Eden WERCS**
1 Eden Way
Princeton, NJ 08540
609-987-0099
FAX: 609-734-0069

Peter Gerhardt, Contact

8467 **Edison Sheltered Workshop**
328 Plainfield Avenue
Edison, NJ 08817
732-985-3844
FAX: 732-985-2216

Ann Marie Stone, Vocational Rehab. Counselor

Serves Middlesex County. Vocational training and job placement services.

8468 **First Occupational Center of New Jersey**
391 Lakeside Avenue
Orange, NJ 07050
973-672-5800
800-894-6265
FAX: 973-672-0065
e-mail: ocnj@idt.net
www.focnj.com or www.dcnj.org

Rocco J Meola, President/CEO
Tina Blakely, Assistant Director Prof Services
Kathy Brown, Manager Employment Services

A private, nonprofit multi-service community rehabilitation program. Services are offered to all people, such as developmentally disabled, visually impaired, hearing impaired and welfare recipients. Services include vocational evaluation and training, respite care, basic and remedial education and job placement and community support services.

8469 **Goodwill Industries of Southern New Jersey**

2835 Route 735
Maple Shades, NJ 08052 **856-665-7270**

Dan Hanson, Contact

8470 **Hausmann Industries**

130 Union Street
Northvale, NJ 07647 **201-767-0255**
FAX: 201-767-1369
e-mail: sales@hausmann.com
www.hausmann.com

George Batchelor, Director Sales/Marketing

Wheelchair acessible exam tables, treatment tables and mat platforms.

8471 **Jersey Cape Diagnostic Training & Opportunity Center**

152 Crest Haven Road
Cape May Court House, NJ 08210 **609-465-4117**
FAX: 609-465-3899

George Plewa, Contact

Serves Cape May County.

8472 **New Jersey Commission for the Blind and Visually Impaired**

153 Halsey Street, 6th Floor
PO Box 47017
Newark, NJ 07102 **973-648-2324**
877-685-8878
FAX: 973-648-7364
e-mail: Vito.DeSantis@dhs.state.nj.us
www.state.nj.us/humanservices/cbvi

Vito J DeSantis, Executive Director
Pamela Gaston, Executive Assistant
Khmbrly Howard PhD, Deputy Executive Director

Offers services for the totally blind, legally blind, visually impaired, deaf blind and more with eye health, counseling, educational, recreational, rehabilitation, computer training and vocational services.

8473 **New Jersey Employment Service and Job Training Program Services**

Department of Labor
Trenton, NJ 08625 **609-292-1040**

8474 **Occupational Center of Hudson County**

780 Montgomery Street
Jersey City, NJ 07306 **201-432-5959**
FAX: 201-432-6227

Christine Romier, Contact

Serves Hudson County.

8475 **Occupational Center of Union County**

301 Cox Street
Roselle, NJ 07203 **908-241-7200**
FAX: 908-241-2025
e-mail: OCUC@OCUCNJ.com

Michele Ford, VP

Provides vocational rehabilitation and mental health service.

8476 **Occupational Training Center of Burlington County**

130 Hancock Lane
Mount Holly, NJ 08060 **609-267-6677**
FAX: 609-265-8418

Karen Elliott, Contact

8477 **Occuptational Training Center of Camden County, New Jersey**

215 W White Horse Pike
Berlin, NJ 08009 **856-768-0845**
FAX: 856-767-1378

Peggy Engelburt, Contact

Serves Camden County.

8478 **Pathway to Independence**

450 Schuyler Avenue
Kearny, NJ 07306 **201-997-6155**
FAX: 201-997-7070

Lisa Johnson, Contact

Serves Hudson and Bergen Counties.

8479 **Somerset Training and Employment Program**

36 4th Street
Somerville, NJ 08876 **732-846-2734**

Laurie Falka, Executive Director

8480 **St. John of God Community Services Vocational Rehabilitation**

1145 Delsea Drive
Westville Grove, NJ 08093 **856-848-4700**
FAX: 856-848-1512

Carol Stark, Contact

Serves Gloucester and Camden Counties.

8481 **United Cerebral Palsy Associations of New Jersey**

354 S Broad Street
Trenton, NJ 08608 **609-392-4004**
FAX: 609-392-3505

Jacqueline Stroman, Contact

8482 **Vocational and Rehabilitation Agency**

135 E State Street
PO Box 398
Trenton, NJ 08625 **609-292-5987**
FAX: 609-292-8347
TTY:609-292-2919
e-mail: tjennings@dol.state.nj.us
www.state.nj.us

Thomas G Jennings, Director

8483 **West Essex Rehab Center**

83 Walnut Street
Montclair, NJ 07042 **201-744-7733**
FAX: 201-744-3744

Ben Viearisi, Contact
Shannon Williams, Contact

New Mexico

8484 **Adelante Development Center**
4906-A Jefferson, NE
Albuquerque, NM 88310 **505-341-2000**

Reina Chavez, Contact
Serves Albuquerque and Belin.

8485 **Goodwill Industries of New Mexico**
5000 San Mateo Boulevard NE
Albuquerque, NM 87109 **505-881-6401**
FAX: 505-884-3157
www.goodwillnm.org

Maria A Prindle, Marketing Director
Serves Albuquerque, Santa Fe and Rio Rancho.

8486 **New Mexico Employment Services and Job Training Liaison**
PO Box 1928
Albuquerque, NM 87103 **505-827-6827**
FAX: 505-827-6860
e-mail: djones2@state.nm.us

8487 **Opportunity Center: New Mexico**
873 Wright Avenue
Alamogordo, NM 88310 **505-437-0919**
FAX: 505-437-1135

Larry Weber, Contact
Serves Alamogorda area.

8488 **RCI**
1023 Stanford Drive NE
Albuquerque, NM 87106 **505-255-5501**
FAX: 505-255-9971

Elizabeth Domzalski, Contact
Serves Bernalillo County.

8489 **Tohatchi Area of Opportunity & Services**
PO Box 49
Tohatchi, NM 87325 **505-733-2200**
FAX: 505-733-2678

Patrick Keptner, Executive Director
Marcella Franklin, Program Director
Daric Kalleco, Community Living Coordinator
Serves McKinley County, San Jose County and the Havanjo Nation.

8490 **Vocational Rehabilitation Agency**
435 Saint Michaels Drive
Building D
Santa Fe, NM 87505 **505-954-8511**
800-224-7005
FAX: 505-954-8562
TTY:8779548583
e-mail: dvris@state.nm.us
www.dvrgetsjobs.com

8491 **Vocational and Rehabilitation Agency**
2905 Rodeo Park Drive E
Building 4, Suite 100
Santa Fe, NM 87505 **505-476-4479**
888-513-7968
FAX: 505-476-4475
e-mail: greg.trapp@state.nm.us
www.state.nm.us

Greg Trapp, Executive Director
James Salas, Deputy Director-VR
Adelmo Vigil, Deputy Director-IL/OB

New York

8492 **JOBS V and SAGE**
PESCO International
21 Paulding Street
Pleasantville, NY 10570 **914-769-4266**
800-431-2016
FAX: 914-769-2970
e-mail: pesco@pesco.org
www.pesco.org

Charles Kass, VP
A computerized matching system matching people to occupations, training, local jobs, local employers and giving job outlooks for the year 2005. Sage 2010 is online computerized testing with the ability for system to read all questions, and job descriptions. Sage is a hands on-computer scored test battery with various adaptation. Braille, large print, bi-lingual and special devices.

8493 **Just One Break (JOBS)**
120 Wall Street
Floor 20
New York, NY 10005 **212-785-7300**
FAX: 212-785-4513
e-mail: justonebreak@interactive.net
www.justonebreak.com

8494 **New York State Department of Labor**
State Office Campus
Building 12
Albany, NY 12240 **518-432-9000**
e-mail: nysdol@labor.state.ny.us
www.labor.state.ny.us

James J McGowan, Commissioner
Fredda Peritz, Employment Servic. Div. Dir.
Thomas Malone, Unemployment Insur. Div. Dir.
The missin of the New York State Department of Labor is to help New York work by preparing individuals for the jobs of today and tomorrow. Provides direct job search and counseling services to job seekers, and can refer people who have disabilities for training opportunities. Provides unemployment insurance for those out of work through no fault of their own.

8495 **Rational Effectiveness Training Systems**
IRET Corporate Services Division
45 E 65th Street
New York, NY 10021 **212-570-2868**

Dr. Dominic DiMattie, Director
Offers advanced training for employee assistance professionals, full service outpatient counseling, consulting services and on-site workshops for the disabled.

8496 Special Education and Vocational Rehabilitation Agency: New York

VESID
One Commerce Plaza, Room 1606
Albany, NY 12234
518-474-2714
800-222-5662
FAX: 518-474-8802
TTY:518-474-5652
www.vesid.nysed.gov

North Carolina

8497 Division of Employment & Training

4111 N Harrington Street
Raliegh, NC 27603
919-715-6500

8498 Iredell Vocational Workshop

PO Box 8
Troutman, NC 28166
704-873-5646
FAX: 704-871-9881

Ben Garrison, Director

8499 North Carolina Division of Services for the Blind

2601 Mail Service Center
Raleigh, NC 27699
919-733-9822
FAX: 919-733-9769
TTY:919-733-9700
e-mail: john.deluca@ncmail.net
www.dhhs.state.nc.us/dsb

John Deluca, Director

8500 Rowan County Vocational Workshop

2728 Old Concord Road
Salisbury, NC 28146
704-633-6223
FAX: 704-633-6224

Terry Osborne, Executive Director

Offers vocational assessment and training, adult developmental activities.

8501 Rutherford Vocational Workshop

200 Fairground Road
Spindale, NC 28160
828-287-9302

Judith Toney, Executive Director

8502 Transylvania Vocational Services

PO Box 1115
Brevard, NC 28712
828-884-3195
FAX: 828-884-3102

Nancy Stricker, Executive Director

8503 Vocational and Rehabilitation Agency

309 Ashe Avenue
2601 Mail Service Center
Raleigh, NC 27699
919-733-9822
FAX: 919-733-9769
TTY:919-733-9700
e-mail: John.DeLuca@ncmail.net
www.dhhs.state.nc.us

Bob Philbeck, Director

Offers services for the totally blind, legally blind, visually impaired, mentally retarded blind and more with health, counseling, educational, recreational, rehabilitation, computer training and professional training services.

8504 Vocational and Rehabilitation Agency: Department of Health and Human Services

2801 Mail Service Center
Raleigh, NC 27699
919-733-3364
FAX: 919-733-7968
TTY:919-733-5924
e-mail: bob.philbeck@ncmail.net
dvr.dhhs.state.nc.us

8505 Webster Enterprises of Jackson County

PO Box 220
Webster, NC 28788
828-586-8981
FAX: 828-586-8125

Arlene C Stewart, Executive Director
Doug Lamb, Director Operations

A community based employment and training program for people with disabilities. A full service program which includes a youth transitional program for life beyond high school, job coaching, vocational assessment and job placement.

8506 Western Regional Vocational Rehabilitation Facility Clifford File, Jr.

PO Box 1443
Morganton, NC 28680

Clifford File Jr, Executive Director

Vocational Evaluation, Work Adjustment, Job Placement, On-site Work Services Program. Serves most disability groups including CMI, DD, Deaf and Physically impaired.

North Dakota

8507 North Dakota Department of Labor, Equal Employment Opportunity Division

600 E Boulevard Avenue
Dept 406
Bismarck, ND 58505
701-328-2660
800-582-8032
FAX: 701-328-2031
e-mail: labor@state.nd.us
www.state.nd.us/labor

Through a work-sharing agreement with the Equal Employment Opportunity Commission (EEOC), the North Dakota Department of Labor enforces the Americans with Disabilities Act (ADA) as related to employment discrimination.

8508 North Dakota Employment Service and Job Training Program Liaison

Job Service North Dakota
PO Box 1537
Bismarck, ND 58502
701-258-6353

8509 North Dakota Governor's Committee on Employment of Disabled Persons

600 S 2nd Street
Suite 1B
Bismarck, ND 58501
701-328-8953
FAX: 701-328-8969

8510 North Dakota Vocational Rehabilitation Agency

Department of Human Services
600 S Second Street, Suite 1B
Bismarck, ND 58504
701-328-8950
800-755-2745
FAX: 701-328-8969
TTY:701-328-8968
e-mail: sohysg@state.nd.us
lnotes.state.nd.us

Gene Hysjulien, Director

Offers services for the totally blind, legally blind, visually impaired, mentally retarded blind and more with health, counseling, educational, recreational, rehabilitation, computer training and professional training services.

Ohio

8511 Cornucopia

18120 Sloane Avenue
Lakewood, OH 44107
216-521-4600
FAX: 216-521-9460
www.lkwdpl.org/paths/healingarts/#Nature's

Chris Yurick, Program Manager

Provides work adjustment training for people with and developmental disabilities in a unique community based setting; Nature's Bin, a natural fresh foods market. Consumers learn through participation in retail operations in produce, grocery, bakery, deli, maintenance and customer service areas. Retail revenues help offset the cost of the program. Job search skills training and placement assistance available to program graduates.

8512 Great Oaks Joint Vocational School

3254 E Kemper Road
Cincinnati, OH 45241
513-772-4603

Dr. Harold Carr, Executive Director

8513 Hearth Day Treatment and Vocational Services

8301 Detroit Avenue
Cleveland, OH 44102
216-281-2660

Ralph Fee, Executive Director

8514 Highland Unlimited Business Enterprises of CRI

1322 E McMillan Street
Cincinnati, OH 45206
513-569-4730
FAX: 513-751-2938
e-mail: ddutton@cricincy.com
www.cricincy.com

Debbie Dutton Lambert, Director Employment Programs

8515 Ohio Civil Rights Commission

1111 E Broad Street
 # 301
Columbus, OH 43205
614-466-5928
FAX: 614-644-8776

8516 Ohio Employment Services and Job Training

145 S Front Street
Columbus, OH 43215
614-466-4000
FAX: 614-752-9049

8517 Vocational and Rehabilitation Agency

400 E Campus View Boulevard
Columbus, OH 43235
614-438-1210
800-282-4536
FAX: 614-785-5012
TTY:614-438-1334
e-mail: john.connellyu@rsc.state.oh.us
www.state.oh.us

Oklahoma

8518 Oklahoma Department of Rehabilitation Services (DRS)

3535 NW 58 Avenue
Suite 500
Oklahoma City, OK 73112
405-951-3400
800-845-8476
FAX: 405-951-3529
e-mail: jprice@drs.state.ok.us
www.okrehab.org

Jody Harlem, Public Information Administrator

8519 Oklahoma Employment Services and Job Training Program Liaison

2401 N Lincoln Boulevard
Oklahoma City, OK 73105
405-557-7211
FAX: 405-557-5368

8520 Oklahoma Governor's Committee on Employment of People with Disabilities

2712 Villa Prom
Oklahoma City, OK 73107
405-424-8378
FAX: 405-943-7550

Orgon

8521 Bend Work Activity Center

275 NE 2nd
Bend, OR 97701
541-389-0129
FAX: 541-389-2084

Bob Weeber, Executive Director

8522 Oregon Fair Employment Practice Agency

Oregon Bureau of Labor & Industry
PO Box 800
Portland, OR 97207
503-229-6601

8523 Oregon Vocational Rehabilitation Agency

1768 Auburn Avenue
Baker City, OR 97814
541-523-3648
866-752-5235
FAX: 541-523-9743

Wendy Wall, Counselor Assistant
Emmy Whitman, VR Counselor
Mary Tomlinson, Branch Manager

8524 Vocational and Rehabilitation Agency

Department of Human Services
500 Summer Street NE
Salem, OR 97301
503-945-5880
877-277-0513
FAX: 503-947-5025
TTY:503-945-5894
e-mail: bobby.c.simpson@state.or.us
vrdweb.hr.state.or.us

8525 **Vocational and Rehabilitation Agency: Commision for the Blind**
535 SE 12th Avenue
Portland, OR 97214
503-731-3221
FAX: 503-731-3230
e-mail: linda.mock@state.or.us
www.cfb.state.or.us

Linda Mock, Administrator

Pennsylvania

8526 **AC-ACLD/An Association for Children and Adults with Learning Disabilities**
4900 Girard Road
Pittsburgh, PA 15227
412-881-2253
FAX: 412-881-2263
e-mail: info@acldnline.org

Thomas Fogarty, President

Offers services to children, adolescents and adults with specific learning disabilities.

8527 **Office of Vocational Rehabilitation**
7th and Forester Street
Harrisburg, PA 17120
717-787-4746
FAX: 717-783-5221

Barry Brandt, Rehab. Specialist

Information in vocational counseling and the governor's committee on Employment of People with Disabilities. Also serves persons with disabilities that present a substantial handicap to employment and independence. Services are provided when there is a reasonable expectation that employment is possible as a result of those services.

8528 **Pennsylvania Employment Services and Job Training**
Labor & Industry Building
Room 1708
Harrisburg, PA 17120
717-787-5279
FAX: 717-787-8826

8529 **Pennsylvania Governor's Committee on Employment of Disabled Persons**
7th and Forester Street
Harrisburg, PA 17120
717-787-4746

8530 **Pennsylvania Human Relations Commission Agency**
301 Chestnut Street
Suite 300
Harrisburg, PA 17101
717-787-4410
FAX: 717-787-0420
www.phrc.state.pa.us

8531 **US Healthworks**
1114 Commons Boulevard
Reading, PA 19605
611-926-0960
FAX: 610-926-6225

Helps injured workers overcome injuries or disabilities and return to their jobs.

8532 **Vocational and Rehabilitation Agency**
Office of Vocational Rehabilitation
909 Green Street
Harrisburg, PA 17102
717-787-5244
800-442-6351
FAX: 717-787-3210
TTY:717-787-5244
e-mail: ovr@dli.state.pa.us
www.dli.state.pa.us

8533 **Vocational and Rehabilitation Agency: Department of Labor and Industry**
909 Green Street
Harrisburg, PA 17102
717-787-6176
800-622-2842
FAX: 717-787-3210
TTY:717-787-6176
e-mail: cboone@state.pa.us

Rhode Island

8534 **Groden Center**
86 Mt. Hope Avenue
Providence, RI 02906
401-274-6310

Michael Smith, Administration

8535 **Newport County Chapter of Retarded Citizens**
PO Box 4390
Middletown, RI 02842
401-846-0340
FAX: 401-847-9459

John Mahler, Executive Director

8536 **Rhode Island Employment Services and Job Training**
101 Friendship Street
Providence, RI 02903
401-222-3732
FAX: 401-462-8798

8537 **Vocational Resources**
100 Houghton Street
Providence, RI 02904
401-861-2080
FAX: 401-454-0889

Paul Pickes, Director

8538 **Vocational and Rehabilitation Agency**
40 Fountain Street
Providence, RI 02903
401-421-7005
FAX: 401-222-3574
TTY:401-421-7016
e-mail: rcarroll@ors.state.ri.us
www.ri.net

Their goal is to help individuals with physical and mental disabilities prepare for and obtain appropriate employment.

8539 **Vocational and Rehabilitation Agency: Department of Human Services**
Office of Rehabilitation Services
40 Fountain Street
Providence, RI 02903
401-222-2300
FAX: 401-222-1328
TTY:401-222-3010
e-mail: garyw@ors.state.ri.us
www.ors.state.ri.us

Their goal is to help individuals with physical and mental disabilities prepare for and obtain appropriate employment.

South Carolina

8540 **South Carolina Employment Services and Job Training Services**
PO Box 995
700 Taylor Street
Columbia, SC 29202
803-737-9935
FAX: 803-737-0202

8541 **South Carolina Governor's Committee on Employment of the Handicapped**
1330 Boston Avenue
Columbia, SC 29171
803-935-5263
FAX: 803-896-6373

8542 **South Carolina Vocational Rehabilitation Department**
PO Box 15
W Columbia, SC 29171
803-896-6504
FAX: 803-896-6525
TTY:803-896-6635
e-mail: scvrpi@infoave.net
www.scvrd.net

P Charles LaRose Jr, Commissioner

The SCVRD's mission is to enable eligible South Carolinians with disabilities to prepare for, achieve and maintain competitive employment.

8543 **Vocational and Rehabilitation Agency: Vocational Rehabilitation Department**
1410 Boston Avenue
PO Box 15
W Columbia, SC 29171
803-896-6504
800-832-7526
FAX: 803-896-6510
e-mail: kmandeville@scvrd.state.sc.us
www.scvrd.net

Kerry Mandeville, Director, Case Services

8544 **Vocational and Rehabilitation Agency**
1410 Boston Avenue
W Columbia, SC 29170
803-896-6500
800-832-7526
FAX: 803-896-6510
e-mail: lbryant@scvrd.state.sc.us
www.scvrd.net

8545 **Vocational and Rehabilitation Agency: Commission for the Blind**
1430 Confederate Avenue
PO Box 79
Columbia, SC 29202
803-898-8822
800-922-2222
FAX: 803-898-8852

South Dakota

8546 **South Dakota Governor's Advisory Committee on Employment of the Disabled**
700 Governors Drive
Pierre, SD 57501
605-773-3423
FAX: 605-773-4236

8547 **South Dakota Workforce Investment Act Training Programs**
700 Governors Drive
Pierre, SD 57501
605-773-5017
FAX: 605-773-4211
www.sdjobs.org

8548 **Vocational and Rehabilitation Agency**
Department of Human Services
3800 E Highway 34, Hillview Plaza
Pierre, SD 57501
605-773-3195
800-865-9684
FAX: 605-773-5483
TTY:605-773-3195
e-mail: eric.weiss@state.sd.us
www.state.sd.us

8549 **Vocational and Rehabilitation Agency: Divi sion of Services to the Blind/Visually Impaired**
3800 E Highway 34
Hillview Plaza
Pierre, SD 57501
605-773-4644
800-265-9684
FAX: 605-773-5483
TTY:605-773-4644
e-mail: gaye.mattke@state.sd.us
www.state.sd.us

Tennessee

8550 **Tennessee Department of Labor: Job Training Program Liaison**
501 Union Street
Nashville, TN 37219
615-741-6642

8551 **Tennessee Fair Employment Practice Agency**
Human Rights Commission
226 Capitol Boulevard
Suite 602
Nashville, TN 37219
615-741-5825

8552 **Vocational and Rehabilitation Agency**
400 Deaderick Street
Suite 1500
Nashville, TN 37248
615-313-4714
FAX: 615-741-4165
e-mail: carl.w.brown@state.tn.us
www.state.tn.us/humanserv/rehabilitation.html

Carl Brown, Assistant Commissioner

Texas

8553 **Center for Computer Assistance to the Disabled (C-CAD)**
Infomart, Suite 2019
1950 Stemmons Freeway
Dallas, TX 75207
214-800-2223
FAX: 214-800-2224
e-mail: martha@c-cad.org
www.c-cad.org

Martha Surrat, Administrative Assistant
Susan Black, Director of Development

Through assessments, training and workshops, C-CAD provides individuals with all types of disabilities computer access skills to further their education or gain employment.

8554 **Handbook of Career Planning for Students with Special Needs**
Pro-Ed Publications
8700 Shoal Creek Boulevard
Austin, TX 78757
512-451-3246
800-897-3202
FAX: 512-451-8542
e-mail: info@proedinc.com
www.proedinc.com

The practitioner's guide will show you how to help special needs adolescents and young adults overcome barriers to employment by identifying goals and problems, assessing interests and aptitudes, involving client families and developing communication skills. *$42.00*

358 pages

8555 **Texas Employment Services and Job Training Program Liaison**

Texas Workforce Commission
101 E 15th Street
Austin, TX 78778
512-467-7774
800-735-2988
TTY:700-735-2989
www.tec.state.tx.us

8556 **Vocational and Rehabilitation Agency**

State Commission for the Blind
4800 N Lamar Boulevard
Austin, TX 78756
512-377-0500
800-252-5204
FAX: 512-424-4730
TTY:800252520415
e-mail: bill.eastman@tcb.state.tx.us
www.tcb.state.tx.us

8557 **Vocational and Rehabilitation Agency: State Rehabilitation Commission**

4900 N Lamar
Austin, TX 78751
512-424-4000
800-628-5115
FAX: 512-424-4730
TTY:800-628-5115
e-mail: max.arrell@rehab.state.tx.us
www.rehab.state.tx.us

Utah

8558 **Utah Employment Services**

720 S 200 E
Salt Lake City, UT 84111
801-536-7401
FAX: 801-536-7011

8559 **Utah Governor's Committee on Employment of the Handicapped**

PO Box 45500
Salt Lake City, UT]4145
801-538-4222
FAX: 801-538-4446

8560 **Utah Veterans Centers**

750 N 200 W
Suite 105
Provo, UT 84601
801-377-1117
800-246-1197
FAX: 801-377-0227

Ray Ross LCSW, Team Leader

Readjustment counseling services to veterans.

8561 **Utah Vocational Rehabilitation Agency**

Utah State Office of Rehabilitation
250 E 5th S
PO Box 144200
Salt Lake City, UT 84111
801-538-7530
800-473-7530
FAX: 801-538-7522
e-mail: duchida@utah.gov

Blaine Petersen, Executive Director
Don Uchida, Director

Vocational Rehabilitation Services for individuals with disabilities.

8562 **Vocational and Rehabilitation Agency: Division of Services for the Blind/Visually Imp.**

250 N 1950 W
Suite B
Salt Lake City, UT 84116
801-323-4343
800-284-1823
FAX: 801-323-4396
e-mail: wgibson@utah.gov
www.usor.utah.gov

Vermont

8563 **State of Vermont Department of Aging and Disabilities**

103 S Main Street
Waterbury, VT 05671
802-241-2210
888-405-5005
FAX: 802-241-2128
e-mail: fredj@dad.state.vt.us
www.dad.state.vt.us/dbvi

Fred Jones, Director

8564 **Vermont Employment Services and Job Training**

PO Box 488
Montpelier, VT 05601

8565 **Vermont Governor's Committee on Employment of People with Disabilities**

103 S Main Street
Waterbury, VT 05671
802-241-2186
800-361-1239
FAX: 802-241-3359

8566 **Vocational and Rehabilitation Agency**

Vocational Rehabilitation Division
103 S Main Street
Waterbury, VT 05671
802-241-2186
800-361-1239
FAX: 802-241-3359
TTY:802-241-2186
e-mail: diane@dad.state.vt.us
www.dad.state.vt.us

Diane Dalmasse, Director

Virginia

8567 **Alexandria Community Y Head Start**

418 S Washington Street
Alexandria, VA 22314
703-329-2050
FAX: 703-998-5707

Yvonne Walker

Offers social services, on-the-job-training for parents, play therapy, physical therapy, speech therapy and any other specialized services.

8568 **Didlake**

8621 Breeden Avenue
Manassas, VA 20110
703-631-9184
FAX: 703-369-7141

Rexford Parr Jr, President/CEO
John S Craig, Director Rehabilitation Services

Offers situational assessments, work training, employment and job placement services to people with disabilities.

8569 **Learning Services: Shenandoah**

9524 Fairview Avenue
Manassas, VA 20110
703-335-9771
FAX: 703-335-1064

Peter Patrick, Administrator

Postacute rehabilitation program.

8570 **NISH**

2235 Cedar Lane
Vienna, VA 22182
703-560-6800
FAX: 703-560-9345
www.nish.org

E Robert Chamberlin, President/CEO
Mary Jame Williamson

A nonprofit agency desigated by the Committee for Purchase from People Who Are Blind or Severely Disabled to provide technical assistance to rehabilitation programs interested in obtaining federal contracts under Public Law 92-28, the Javits-Wagner-O'Day Act. NISH's primary objective is to assist community rehabilitation programs in providing jobs for people with severe disabilities.

8571 **Richmond Research Training Center**

1314 W Main Street
PO Box 842011
Richmond, VA 23284
804-828-1222

Dr. Paul Wehman, Director

Research and training center report on the supported employment of persons with developmental and other disabilities.

8572 **ServiceSource**

6295 Edsall Road
Suite 175
Alexandria, VA 22312
703-461-6000
800-244-0817
FAX: 703-461-3906
www.ourpeoplework.org

Janet Samuelson

Provides training, job placement and employment services in private sector and government contract employment.

8573 **Sheltered Occupational Center of Virginia**

750 23rd Street S
Arlington, VA 22202
FAX: 703-521-3443

Charles Richman

Employs disabled adults in Northern Virginia.

8574 **Vocational and Rehabilitation Agency**

8004 Franklin Farms Drive
PO Box K300
Richmond, VA 23288
804-662-7000
800-552-5019
FAX: 804-662-9140
TTY:800-464-9950
e-mail: drs@drs.state.va.us

8575 **Vocational and Rehabilitation Agency: Department for the Blind/Visually Impaired**

397 Azalea Avenue
Richmond, VA 23227
804-371-3140
FAX: 804-371-3351
www.vdbvi.org

Washington

8576 **Career Connections**

421 N Mullan Road
Spokane, WA 99206
509-928-0423
FAX: 509-928-0441
e-mail: carconn@mindspring.com
www.peoplelinking.com

Bill Stout, Marketing

8577 **Department of Services for the Blind National Business & Disability Council**

521 E Legion Way
MS:FD-11
Olympia, WA 98504
360-586-1224

8578 **Department of Social & Health Services National Business & Disability Council**

Dddd612 Woodland Square, Loop, SE
PO Box 45340
Lacey, WA 98504
425-902-8400

8579 **Emil Fries School of Piano Tuning and Technology**

2510 E Evergreen Boulevard
Vancouver, WA 98661
360-693-1511
FAX: 360-693-6891
e-mail: pianohospital@pianotuningschool.org
www.pianotuningschool.org

Dr Judy Dresser, President
Donald Mitchell, Director Instruction
Sharon Mitchell, Registar

Teaches piano tuning and repair to blind, visually impaired and sighted men and women, leading to employment and/or self-employment in the piano service industry. Instruction also given in music appreciation and small business operation. Licensed by Washington State and accredited by the Accrediting Commission of Career Schools and Colleges of Technology (ACCSCT). 20-month course.

8580 **SL Stuart and Associates**

25 W Nora Avenue
Spokane, WA 99205
509-328-2740
e-mail: raywhite@sistart.com

Ray White, Contact

8581 **Vocational and Rehabilitation Agency: Division of Vocational Rehabilitation**

Department of Social and Health
PO Box 45340
Olympia, WA 98504
360-438-8000
800-637-5627
FAX: 360-438-8007
TTY:360-438-8000
e-mail: obrien@dshs.wa.gov
www1.dshs.wa.gov/dvr

West Virginia

8582 **Vocational and Rehabilitation Agency**

State Capitol Complex
PO Box 50890
Charleston, WV 25305
304-766-4600
800-642-8207
FAX: 304-766-4905
TTY:304-766-4965
e-mail: johnri@mail.drs.state.wv.us
www.wvdrs.org

8583 **West Virginia Employment Services and Job Training Programs Liaison**

112 California Avenue
Charleston, WV 25305 **304-558-0342**

8584 **West Virginia of Vocational Rehabilitation**

PO Box 1004
Institute, WV 25112 **304-342-9952**

Earl Wolfe, Director

Offers services for the totally blind, legally blind, visually impaired, mentally retarded blind and more with health, counseling, educational, recreational, rehabilitation, computer training and professional training services.

Wisconsin

8585 **Vocational and Rehabilitation Agency**

2917 International Lane
PO Box 7852
Madison, WI 53707 **608-243-5600**
800-442-3477
FAX: 608-243-5680
TTY:6082435601
e-mail: normaju@mail.state.wi.us
www.dwd.state.wi.us

John Conway, Program Specialist

Offers services for the totally blind, legally blind, visually impaired, mentally retarded blind and more with health, counseling, educational, recreational, rehabilitation, computer training and professional training services.

8586 **Wisconsin Employment Services and Job Training Programs Liaison**

Department of Industry, Labor & Human Relations
201 E Washington Avenue
Madison, WI 53702 **608-257-4971**

8587 **Wisconsin Vocational Rehabilitation Agency**

PO Box 7852
2917 International Lane, 3rd Floor
Madison, WI 53707 **608-243-5600**
TTY:608-243-5601
e-mail: normaju@mail.state.wi.us

Judy R Norman-Nunnery, Administrator

Wyoming

8588 **Division of Vocational Rehabilitation of Wyoming**

Wyoming Department of Education
2300 Capitol Avenue
Cheyenne, WY 82002 **307-777-7675**
FAX: 307-777-6234

Robert Dingwall, Administrator

Offers services for the totally blind, legally blind, visually impaired, mentally retarded blind and more with health, counseling, educational, recreational, rehabilitation, computer training and professional training services.

8589 **Vocational Rehabilitation, Division of Department of Workforce Services**

1160 Herschler Building
Suite 1E
Cheyenne, WY 82002 **307-777-7386**
FAX: 307-777-5939
TTY:307-777-7386
e-mail: jmcint@state.wy.us
wydoe.state.wy.us

Jim McIntosh, Administrator

8590 **Wyoming Employment Services and Job Training Programs**

PO Box 2760
Casper, WY 82602 **307-235-3253**
FAX: 307-235-3278

8591 **Wyoming Governor's Committee on Employment of the Handicapped**

Herschler
Room 1102
Cheyenne, WY 82002 **307-777-7230**
FAX: 307-777-5690

Alabama

8592 Lakeshore Rehabilitation Hospital
3800 Ridgeway Drive
Birmingham, AL 35209
205-868-2000
FAX: 205-868-2007

8593 Mobile Infirmary Medical Center: Rotary Rehabilitation Division
5 Mobile Infirmary Drive
Mobile, AL 36617
251-435-3414
FAX: 251-435-3403
www.mimc.com

8594 Montgomery Rehabilitation Hospital
4465 Narrow Lane
Montgomery, AL 36116
334-262-5945
FAX: 334-288-3789

8595 North Alabama Rehabilitation Hospital
107 Governors Drive SW
Huntsville, AL 35801
256-539-2800
FAX: 256-535-2402

8596 UAB Spain Rehabilitation Center
1717 6th Avenue S
Birmingham, AL 35233
205-934-3360
800-UAB-8816
FAX: 205-934-5584

Sonia A Arledge, Marketing Director

Spain offers a comprehensive approach to healing for persons challenged by stroke, spinal cord injury, arthritis, head injury, chronic pain or other disabilities resulting from illness or accident. In addition to a model facility, dedicated physicians and staff, and efficient programs tailored to meet the diverse needs of the physically challenged Spain has a wealth of resources found at the UAB Hospital, the number three health care facility in the United States.

Arkansas

8597 Central Arkansas Rehab Hospital
2201 Wildwood Avenue
Sherwood, AR 72120
501-834-6636
FAX: 501-834-2227

Randy Harris, Admissions

8598 HealthSouth Rehabilitation Hospital
1401 S J Street
Fort Smith, AR 72901
479-785-3300
FAX: 479-785-5203

Raymond Lenz, Administrator

8599 HealthSouth Rehabilitation Hospital of Jonesboro
1201 Fleming Avenue
Jonesboro, AR 72401
870-932-0440
FAX: 870-933-5157

Brenda Antwine, Administrator

Comprehensive physical rehabilitation hospital. Services include inpatient and outpatient services in Jonesboro, Newport, Paragould, Blytheville, and Pocahontas. Programs include stroke, amputee, brain injury, multiple trauma, joint replacement, spinal injury, arthritis, aquatic, pediatric, sports medicine, incontinence and balance.

8600 Northwest Arkansas Rehabilitation Hospital
153 E Monte Painter Drive
Fayetteville, AR 72703
479-444-2207
FAX: 479-444-2390

8601 Rebsamen Rehabilitation Center
1400 Braden Street
Jacksonville, AR 72076
501-982-9515
FAX: 501-985-7384

8602 St. Michael Hospital: RehabCare Unit
6th & Hazel Street
Texarkana, AR 75502
903-792-7380
FAX: 903-614-4060

Arizona

8603 Barrow Neurological Institute Rehab Center
350 W Thomas Road
Phoenix, AZ 85013
602-406-3000
FAX: 602-406-4104

Irwin Altman

8604 Health South Rehab Institute of Tucson
2650 N Wyatt Drive
Tucson, AZ 85712
520-325-1300
800-333-8628
FAX: 520-327-4045

Lora Williams, Admissions

8605 HealthSouth Hospital
9630 E Shea Boulevard
Scottsdale, AZ 85260
480-860-0671
FAX: 480-551-5376
www.healthsouth.com

Kathleen Cahill, Admissions

8606 HealthSouth Rehabilitation Center
1151 S La Canada # 100
Green Valley, AZ 85614
520-625-4625
FAX: 520-648-5272

Shaunna Schelin, Administrator
Greta Bame OTR/L, Director Marketing
Carol Altschuler, Front Office Group Coordinator

Outpatient rehabilitation services, focus on orthopedic, sports and hand rehabilitation. Heavy industrial rehab focus. Accept all major insurances except Cigna and Pacfica.

8607 HealthSouth Rehabilitation Center of Tucson
75 N Wilmot Road
Tucson, AZ 85711
520-790-0900
800-476-2036
FAX: 520-745-0974

Shaunna Schelin, Administrator
Greta Bame OTR/L, Director Marketing
Carol Altschuler, Front Office Group Coordinator

Outpatient rehabilitation services, focus on orthopedic, sports and hand rehabilitation. Heavy industrial rehab focus. Accept all major insurances except Cigna and Pacfica.

8608 **HealthSouth Rehabilitation Centers of Tuscon**
7400 N Oracle
Suite 142
Tucson, AZ 85704
520-742-4822
FAX: 520-742-6711

Shaunna Schelin, Administrator
Greta Bame OTR/L, Director Marketing
Carol Altschuler, Front Office Group Coordinator

Outpatient rehabilitation services, focus on orthopedic, sports and hand rehabilitation. Heavy industrial rehab focus. Accept all major insurances except Cigna and Pacfica.

8609 **HealthSouth Sports Medicine Center**
7900 E Florentine
Prescott Valley, AZ 86314
928-772-6227
FAX: 928-772-1276
e-mail: chamine@wiley@healthsouth.com
www.healthsouth.com

Chamine Wiley, Administrator

8610 **St. Joseph Hospital and Medical Center**
350 W Thomas
Phoenix, AZ 85013
602-406-7007
FAX: 602-406-4190

Rehabilitation programs offered by the clinic assists clients with rehabilitation health needs in the comfort of their own home. The home care rehabilitation team of professionals focuses on correcting deficiencies in self-care, mobility skills and communication. Services offered include physical therapy, occupational therapy, speech pathology, rehabilitative nursing and restorative nursing assistants.

California

8611 **Bakersfield Regional Rehabilitation Hospital**
5001 Commerce Drive
Bakersfield, CA 93309
615-323-5500
800-288-9829
FAX: 661-323-5521

Susan Golino, Admissions

8612 **Brotman Medical Center: RehabCare Unit**
3828 Delmas Terrace
Culver City, CA 90232
310-836-7000
FAX: 310-202-4105

Ellen Graham, Program Manager

8613 **Casa Colinas Centers for Rehabilitation**
255 E Bonita Avenue
Pomona, CA 91767
909-596-7733
FAX: 909-593-0153
e-mail: rehab@casacolina.org
www.casacolina.org

Stephanie Bradhurst, Director of Marketing
Fred Aronow, Director of Public Relations

8614 **Cedars-Sinai Medical Center and Inpatient Rehabilitation Center**
8700 Beverly Boulevard
Los Angeles, CA 90048
310-657-3360
FAX: 310-659-0235
e-mail: jurt.vaillancourt@cshs.com
www.csmc.edu

Kurt Vaillancourt MA, Intake Coordinator

A comprehensive team approach with the primary goal of helping patients achieve optimal physical functioning in their daily activities. The Center also strives to educate both the patient and the patient's family and to help them adjust emotionally and socially. The Center offers various inpatient and outpatient programs including brain injury, spinal cord injury, stroke, orthopedic and a chronic pain management program.

8615 **Community Hospital of Los Gatos Rehabilitation Services**
355 Dardanelli Lane
Los Gatos, CA 95032
408-866-4020
FAX: 408-866-4077
e-mail: CHLG.ask@renethealth.com
www.communityhospitalLG.com

Modestine Fain, Director, Rehab Services

Rehabilitation Services provide individualized treatment programs for inpatient/outpatient care. The team is supervised by a Physiatrist and may include Nurses, Physical Therapists, Occupational Therapists, Speech/Language Therapists, Psychologists, Case Managers, Dietitians, Respiratory Therapists, Recreation Therapists and/or Prosthetists/Orthotists.

8616 **Daniel Freeman Hospitals: Center for Diagnostic and Rehab Medicine**
333 N Prairie Avenue
Inglewood, CA 90301
310-674-7050
FAX: 310-419-8365

Provides a full spectrum of rehabilitation services from sub-acute, skilled nursing, acute rehabilitation, post-acute day program for brain injury, comprehensive outpatient, home health and home/community services. Also offer pediatric rehabilitation and accept ventilator patients. The facility is CARF and JCAHO accredited and have specialized teams for each program such as brain injury, spinal cord injury, stroke/neuro and pain management. Specialized support groups are also offered.

8617 **Garfield Medical Center**
525 N Garfield Avenue
Monterey Park, CA 91754
626-573-2222
FAX: 626-307-2077

Shelly Hansen, Referrals

8618 **Grossmont Hospital Rehabilition Center**
PO Box 158
La Mesa, CA 91944
619-644-4100
FAX: 619-644-4159

Clair Jonesn, Contact

8619 **Holy Cross Comprehensive Rehabilitation Center**
15031 Rinaldi Street N
Mission Hills, CA 91345
818-898-1628
FAX: 818-898-4472

Craig Johnson, Case Manager

8620 **Kentfield Rehabilitation Hospital**
1125 Sir Francis Drake Boulevard
Kentfield, CA 94904
415-485-3541
FAX: 415-485-3613

Susan Jensen, Liaison

8621 **Laurel Grove Hospital: Rehab Care Unit**
19933 Lake Chabot Road
Castro Valley, CA 94546
510-727-2755
FAX: 510-727-2778

Judith Mather, Program Manager

8622 Lodi Memorial Hospital West
800 S Lower Sacramento Road
Lodi, CA 95242
209-333-3100
FAX: 209-368-3745

Gary Sadler, Rehab Services

8623 Long Beach Memorial Medical Center Memorial Rehabilitation Hospital
2801 Atlantic Avenue
Long Beach, CA 90806
562-933-9000

Trish Baeseman, Administrator

The hospital offers rehabilitation after catastrophic injury of disabling disease to give patients the opportunity for maximum recovery. The Hospital offers many of the area's finest rehabilitation specialists and most advanced technology, making it one of Southern California's most respected rehabilitation centers.

8624 Meadowbrook Neurologic Center
340 Northlake Drive
San Jose, CA 95117
408-249-0344
800-826-9152

Mary Ligetti, Marketing

8625 Mercy American River Hospital
4747 Engle Road
Carmichael, CA 95608
916-484-2222
FAX: 916-482-4203

Christine Shipman, Rehab Director

8626 North Coast Rehabilitation Center
151 Sotoyome Street
Santa Rosa, CA 95405
707-433-9600
FAX: 707-525-8413

Joyce Cavagnaro, Admissions

8627 North Valley Rehabilitation Hospital
340 W E Avenue
Chico, CA 95926
530-345-9592
FAX: 530-894-4139

Karen Geissinger, Admissions

8628 Northridge Hospital Medical Center
18300 Roscoe Boulevard
Northridge, CA 91328
818-885-8500
FAX: 818-885-5435

Debra Flaherty, Director Rehab Services

8629 PEERS Program
8912 W Olympic Boulevard
Beverly Hills, CA 90211
310-553-9322
FAX: 310-858-8008

Dr. Paul Berns, Medical Director

Offers a new approach for wheelchair users. PEERS uses a combination of modern physical therapy, the DOUGLAS Reciprocating Gait System and when necessary, functional electrical stimulation to assist selected individuals to walk with recently patented specially made lightweight braces.

8630 Pacifica Nursing and Rehab Center
385 Esplanade
Pacifica, CA 94044
650-993-5576
FAX: 650-359-9388

Bill Connell, Administrator
Lana Ronin, Director Admissions

68 beds offering skilled nursing and complete rehabilitation services, PT, OT, Speech and respiratory therapy, social services, nutritional services, and restorative nursing care.

8631 Providence Holy Cross Medical Center
15031 Rinaldi Street
Mission Hills, CA 91345
818-898-4561
FAX: 818-898-4472

Betsy Jansen, Case Manager

8632 Queen of Angels/Hollywood Presbyterian Medical Center
1300 Vermont Avenue
Los Angeles, CA 90027
213-413-3000
FAX: 323-660-0446
e-mail: maurine.cate@tenethealth.com
www.qahpmc.com

Lu Hallam, Program Manager

8633 Queen of the Valley Hospital
1000 N Trancas Street
Napa, CA 94558
707-252-4411
www.thequeen.org/

Jane Muir, Director

8634 Rancho Los Amigos National Rehabilitation Center
7601 Imperial Highway
Downey, CA 90242
562-401-6554
888-RAN-CHO
FAX: 562-401-7604
www.rancho.org

Consuelo C Diaz, CEO
Mary Miodovski RN, Clinical Director Admissions
Anne Potter, Director Business Development

Specialty programs: APR, AMP, CIR, COR, DYS, HI, MT, NPT, OT, ORT, PED, PT, RN, SS, SLP, ST, TR, VR. Credentials include: JCAHO, CARF, SCI/BI/CARF approved. Prices vary, please call for information.

8635 San Diego Rehabilitation Institute
6645 Alvarado Road
San Diego, CA 92120
619-286-7374
FAX: 619-229-4590
www.alvaradohospital.com

Provides acute and subacute level physical rehab programs specializing in brain injuries, spinal cord injuries and pulmonary/ventilator management. Outpatient programs include brain injury day treatment, pain management, visual rehabilitation and work reconditioning.

8636 San Joaquin Valley Rehabilitation Hospital
7173 N Sharon Avenue
Fresno, CA 93720
559-436-3600
FAX: 559-436-3688

James A Page, Director Marketing

Complete comprehensive rehabilitation services from acute rehab, outpatient and community fitness services.

8637 Santa Clara Valley Medical Center
751 S Bascom Avenue
San Jose, CA 95128
408-885-5000

8638 Scripps Memorial Hospital
354 Santa Fe Drive
Encinitas, CA 92024
760-753-6501
FAX: 760-633-7348
www.scrippshealth.org

8639 **Scripps Memorial Hospital at La Jolla**

9888 Genessee Avenue
La Jolla, CA 92037
858-457-4123
800-727-4777
FAX: 858-626-6122
www.scrippshealth.org

8640 **Sierra Vista Regional Medical Center: Reha bilitation Center**

1010 Murray Street
San Luis Obispo, CA 93405
805-546-7872
FAX: 805-546-7871

Emily Lipscomb PT MBA, Director
Jeanette Petrus PT, Community Liaison

Acute inpatient rehabilitation center provides a seven day comprehensive inpatient treatment program for individuals suffering a disabling injury or illness and outpatient rehabilitation center providing an interdisciplinary treatment approach to rehab patients and the community.

8641 **South Coast Medical Center**

31872 Coast Highway
Laguna Beach, CA 92651
949-499-1311
FAX: 949-499-8644
e-mail: info@southcoastmedcenter.com
www.southcoastmedcenter.com

Maggie Baumann, Marketing Director

A 208 bed acute care hospital. Services include maternity, surgical, subacute care, psychiatric program, eating disorder treatment, chemical dependency treatment, radiology, ICU/CCU and comprehensive rehabilitation services.

8642 **St. Joseph Rehabilitation Center**

2200 Harrison Avenue
Eureka, CA 95501
707-445-5111
FAX: 707-441-4429

Sam Fallon, Admissions Liaison Nurse

Comprehensive inpatient and outpatient rehabilitation services.

8643 **St. Jude Brain Injury Network**

251 E Imperial Highway #440
Fullerton, CA 92835
714-449-4848
866-785-8332
FAX: 714-447-0987
e-mail: jgable@sif.stjoe.org

Jana Gable, Program Coordinator
David Bogdan, Service Coordinator
Lina Marroquin, Servicer Coordinator

Provides comprehensive planning, program referral, assists with funding possibilities, and interagency coordination of services. Areas of emphasis include day treatment, vocational and housing options, and the requirements are adults who have suffered a brain injury from an external force.

8644 **St. Jude Medical Center**

101 E Valencia Mesa Drive
Fullerton, CA 92835
714-871-3280
www.stjudemc.com

A 331 bed full-service regional medical center that serves as a major referral hospital attracting rehabilitation patients throughout southern California for over twenty years.

8645 **St. Mary Medical Center**

1050 Linden Avenue
Long Beach, CA 90813
562-491-9000
FAX: 562-436-6378
www.smmc.com

A 556-bed hospital owned by the Sisters of Charity of the Incarnate World Healthcare Systems, one of the nation's largest Catholic healthcare networks. Services include a trauma unit, a comprehensive Cancer Care Center, complete older adult services, a Low Vision Center, a Rehabilitation Institute, an outpatient Surgi/Center and the only kidney transplant program in Long Beach. St. Mary's is a teaching hospital affiliated with the UCLA School of Medicine.

8646 **St. Mary's Hospital and Medical Center Acute Rehab**

450 Stanyan Street
San Francisco, CA 94117
415-750-5715
FAX: 415-750-4843

8647 **Sunnyside Nursing Center**

22617 S Vermont Avenue
Torrance, CA 90502
310-320-4130
FAX: 310-320-8602

John MacArthur

8648 **Tustin Rehabilitation Hospital**

14851 Yorba Street
Tustin, CA 92780
714-832-9200
FAX: 714-508-4550

Linda McCaskill, CEO

8649 **UCLA Medical Center: Department of Anesthesiology, Acute Pain Services**

200 Medical Plaza
Suite 660
Los Angeles, CA 90095
310-794-1841
FAX: 310-794-1511

Teresa Zaroda, Clinical Director

8650 **White Memorial Medical Center Rehabilitation**

1720 Cesar Chavez Avenue
Los Angeles, CA 90033
323-260-5841
800-995-4389
FAX: 323-260-5786
www.whitememorial.com

Ann Smith, Admission Coordinator

Strokes/neurological disorders, brain injury, musculoskeletal injuries, pulmonary disorders, developmental disorders (arthritis, cardiac rehabilitation), cleft palate, fractures, amputations, joint replacement, burns, swallowing disorders, pain and more.

Colorado

8651 **Children's Hospital Rehabilitation Center**

1056 E 19th Avenue
Denver, CO 80218
FAX: 303-861-6066

Dennis Matthews, Medical Director

8652 **Craig Hospital**
3425 S Clarkson
Englewood, CO 80110 303-789-8000
FAX: 303-789-8219
e-mail: khosack@craighospital.org
www.craighospital.org

Offers the following rehabilitation services: Traumatic Brain Injury Rehab, Spinal Cord Injury Rehab

8653 **Mapleton Center**
Boulder Community Hospital
311 Mapleton Avenue
Boulder, CO 80304 303-440-2273
FAX: 303-441-0484
www.bch.org

Comprehensive inpatient and outpatient rehabilitation services for all age groups. Treatment provided by interdisciplinary teams and staff physicians. CARF accredited in brain injury rehabilitation, pediatric rehabilitation, pain management, work hardening and inpatient rehabilitation.

8654 **Mediplex Rehab: Denver**
8451 Pearl Street
Thornton, CO 80229 303-288-3000
FAX: 303-286-1253

8655 **Rehabilitation Hospital of Colorado Springs**
325 Parkside Drive
Colorado Springs, CO 80910 719-630-2313
FAX: 719-636-3772

8656 **Spalding Rehabilitation Hospital**
900 Potomac Street
Aurora, CO 80011 303-367-1166
FAX: 303-360-8208
e-mail: melissa.francis@healthonecares.com
www.spaldingrehab.com

Melissa Francis, Director Marketing/Volunteers

Rebuilding Lives, Renewing Hope is the mission at Spalding Rehabilitation Hospital. We offer acute inpatient and outpatient rehabilitation services at 3 convenient locations in the Denver metro area. Spalding specializes in treating the neurologically injured patient, including stroke and traumatic brain injury.

Connecticut

8657 **Mariner Health Care: Connecticut**
125 Eugene Oneill Drive
New London, CT 06320 860-701-2000

District of Columbia

8658 **National Rehabilitation Hospital**
102 Irving Street NW
Washington, DC 20010 202-877-1000
TTY:202-877-1450

Edward A Eckanhoff, President/CEO
Robert S Hartmann, VP Communications

A private facility dedicated solely to medical rehabilitation. The hospital offers intensive inpatient programs and full-service outpatient programs.

Florida

8659 **Brooks Rehabilitation**
3599 University Boulevard S
Jacksonville, FL 32216 904-858-7600
800-487-7342
FAX: 904-858-7610
e-mail: rehab@brookshealth.org
www.brookshealth.org

Douglas M Baer, President/CEO
Joanna Buzar, Public Relations

A 127 bed rehabilitation hospital focused on treatment of brain and spinal cord injuries, orthopedic and neurological impairment. Treating adults and pediatrics in our hospital and outpatient network.

8660 **Florida Hospital Rehabilitation Center**
601 E Rollins Street
Orlando, FL 32803 407-893-8055
FAX: 407-893-9459

Diane Lowder, Admissions Director

8661 **HealthSouth Regional Rehab Center/Florida**
20601 Old Cutler Road
Miami, FL 33189 305-251-3800
FAX: 305-251-0498

8662 **HealthSouth Rehab Hospital: Largo**
901 Clearwater Largo Road N
Largo, FL 33770 727-586-2999
FAX: 727-588-3404

Sherri Beasley, Director Marketing Operations

Inpatient acute rehabilitation 70 beds.

8663 **HealthSouth Sports Medicine and Rehabilitation Center**
2141 ALT A1A S
300
Jupiter, FL 33477 561-625-3666
FAX: 561-840-8637

Curtis Becker PT, Administrator

Outpatient orthopedic and sports medicine/physical therapy.

8664 **HealthSouth Sunrise Rehabilitation Hospital**
4399 N Nob Hill Road
Fort Lauderdale, FL 33351 954-746-1501
800-648-9111
FAX: 954-746-1300

Fran Warm Hundley RN, CEO
Dave Rafter, PR Representative

A 108-bed, JCAHO-accredited, comprehensive medical rehabilitation hospital treating patients from throughout South Florida, the Caribbean and Latin America. HEALTHSOUTH Sunrise Rehabilitation Hospital is known for its CARF-accredited specialty programs, including brain injury, spinal cord, pain management, traumatic burns, and pediatrics. Services available on inpatient and outpatient basis.

8665 **HealthSouth Treasure Coast Rehabilitation Hospital**
1600 37th Street
Vero Beach, FL 32960 772-778-2100
FAX: 772-567-7041

Meg McNally, Director Business Development
Barbara Harvey, Case Management Coordinator

HSTCRH is a 90-bed inpatient comprehensive rehabilitation hospital serving Indian River, St. Lucie, Martin, and Okeechobee counties. Outpatient services are available at the hospital including physical, occupational, speech and recreational therapies as well as psychology services.

8666 **Infusion Therapies**

7901 SW 36th Street
Suite 206
Davie, FL 33328

800-342-3777
FAX: 954-452-4262

Specializes in fully managed enteral and parenteral therapies. Offers pharmaceuticals, supplies, pumps, equipment and delivery. Infusion cares for pediatrics to geriatrics, patients at home, in extended care facilities, clinics, physician offices, adult congregate living facilities are on site. Provides IV hydration, chemotherapy, gastric/tube feedings, lab/blood work and medical equipment and supplies.

8667 **Mediplex Rehab: Bradenton**

5627 9th Street E
Bradenton, FL 34203 **941-753-8941**
FAX: 941-756-7563

Kris Hendrix, Admissions Director

Inpatient and outpatient rehabilitation services specializing in subacute, brain injury, neurological and work reconditioning. CARF and JCAHO accredited.

8668 **Miami Rehabilitation Institute**

3280 Ponce De Leon Boulevard
Coral Gables, FL 33134 **305-444-0909**
FAX: 305-444-5760

8669 **Perry Health Facility**

207 Forest Drive
Perry, FL 32347 **850-584-6334**
FAX: 850-838-2370

Jo Ann Gnewuch, Facility Administrator
Michael Brust, Director Rehabilitation

Full rehabilitation team available, Physiatrist, DOR, Psychiatrist, Psychologist, RD, Geriatric Nursing, PT/OT/ST/RT, Orthotiet/Prosthetist. Provider for PPO's & HMO's as well as medicare, private insurance and medicare/medicaid.

8670 **Pinecrest Rehabilitation Hospital and Outpatient Centers**

5360 Linton Boulevard
Delray Beach, FL 33484 **561-495-9266**
FAX: 561-496-4972
e-mail: anna.cohen@tenethealth.com
www.pinecrestrehab.com

Pinecrest Rehabilitation Hospital is a 90 bed, accredited hospital and is comprised of a Specialty Unit, a Neuro Trauma Unit and Joint Replacement Unit. Additional services at Pincrest include six outpatient rehab centers throughout Palm Beach County. The Outpatient Centers each focus on various specialties such as orthopedic and neurological rehab, pain management, cardiac and pulmonary rehab, occupational medicine, Hearing Institute, dizziness and balance and wellness.

8671 **Rehabilitation Institute of Sarasota**

3251 Proctor Road
Sarasota, FL 34231

941-923-4625
FAX: 941-922-6228

8672 **Sea Pines Rehabilitation Hospital**

101 E Florida Avenue
Melbourne, FL 32901

FAX: 321-727-7440

8673 **Shriners Hospitals for Children**

Shriners International Headquarters
2900 N Rocky Point Drive
Tampa, FL 33607 **813-281-0300**
800-237-5055
FAX: 813-281-8496
www.shrinershq.org

Michael C Andrews, PR Director
Michelle Fox, Projects Manager
Sonja Monsen, Corporate Website Manager

Provide specialized acute and reconstructive burn care, orthopaedic care and spinal cord injury rehabilitation to children under 18 at absolutely no cost to the child or family. No insurance monies or government funds are sought or received. Call for application or visit our website.

8674 **Shriners Hospitals for Children: Tampa**

12502 N Pine Drive
Tampa, FL 33612 **813-972-2250**
FAX: 813-975-7125
www.shrinershq.org

Alice Lanford, Administrator
Alicia Argiz-Lyons, Director Public Relations

Pediatric orthopedic.

8675 **South Miami Hospital**

6200 SW 73rd Street
Miami, FL 33143 **305-661-4611**
FAX: 305-662-5302
www.baptisthealth.net

D Wayne Brackin, CEO

8676 **St. Anthony's Hospital**

1200 Seventh Avenue N
St. Petersburg, FL **727-825-1100**

www.stanthonys.com

Ian Payne, Director

Offers the following rehabilitation services: Sub-Acute rehabilitation, Occupational Therapy, Speech/Language Pathology services, Physical Therapy.

8677 **Tampa General Rehabilitation Center**

PO Box 1289
Tampa, FL 33601 **813-251-7000**
FAX: 813-253-4283

Michael Daniels, Director
Norma Fowler, Admission Nurse
Sandra Taylor, Admission Nurse

Offers a full range of inpatient and outpatient programs all aimed at helping patients achieve their full potentials. JCAHO and CARF accredited and V.R. designated center. A wide range of inpatient and outpatient programs are available such as Brain and Spinal Cord Injury Programs, Comprehensive Medical Rehabilitation, Pain Management, Cardiac Rehab, Pediatric Therapy Service, Sleep Disorders, Epilepsy, and Wheelchair Seating.Hosts the Florida Alliance for Assistive Services and Technolgy.

8678 **University of Miami: Jackson Memorial Rehabilitation Center**

1611 NW 12th Avenue
Miami, FL 33136 **305-325-5588**
FAX: 305-585-6092

8679 West Gables Rehabilitation Hospital and Healthcare Center

2525 SW 75th Avenue
Miami, FL 33155 **305-262-6800**
FAX: 305-264-9031

Offers case management services, patient services, a neurological rehabilitation program, cancer rehabilitation, spinal cord injury rehabilitation, orthopedic program, functional restoration and pain management programs, as well as outpatient programs.

8680 Winter Park Memorial Hospital

200 N Lakemount Avenue
Winter Park, FL 32792 **407-646-7000**
FAX: 407-646-7639
e-mail: healthcare@winterparkhospital.com
www.winterparkhospital.com

Terry Barter, Director Rehabilitation

Offers Acute Rehabilitation.

Georgia

8681 Candler General Hospital: Rehabilitation Unit

5353 Reynolds Street
Savannah, GA 31405 **912-354-9211**
FAX: 912-692-2039

Virginia Donaldson, Admissions Director

8682 Children's Healthcare of Atlanta at Egleston

1405 Clifton Road NE
Atlanta, GA 30322 **404-325-6646**
FAX: 404-315-2158

Tricia Easley OTR/L, Satellite Manager

Rehabilitation Center at Egleston accepts children from birth to age 18 with acute or chronic problems. The length of rehab stay varies for each child according to the determined program of care. The center offers inpatient, outpatient & day rehab programs for comprehensive evaluation & treatment. The program emphasizes the development of the child's abilities & concentrates on helping the family & child compensate for any long-term disabilities. Short term stays require one or two weeks.

8683 Cobb Hospital and Medical Center: Rehab Ca re Center

3950 Austell Road
Austell, GA 30106 **770-732-4000**

8684 Emory Healthcare Center for Rehabilitation Medicine

1441 Clifton Road NE
Atlanta, GA 30322 **404-712-7593**
FAX: 404-712-4746
e-mail: sheryl_hope@emoryhealthcare.org
www.emoryhealthcare.org

Sheryl Hope, Manager/Admissions & Referrals
Sara Swanson, Intake Nurse Coordinator
Karen Divito, Manager Outpatient Services

Dedicated to restoring wholeness to a patient after experiencing a stroke, brain injury, spinal cord injury or other disabling injury or illness. Offers an entire interdisciplinary team who work with patients to help them regain or compensate for lost abilities and to adapt to the many changes in their lives. Services provide a continuum of care by offering a wide variety of inpatient/outpatient programs.

8685 HEALTHSOUTH Central Georgia Rehabilitation Hospital

3351 Northside Drive
Macon, GA 31210 **478-471-3500**
FAX: 478-474-6601

Vernona L Moseley, Director Market Operation

HealthSouth Central Georgia rehabilitation hospital is a 55 bed comprehensive medical rehabilitation hospital meeting the medical patients and famloity members in Central Georgia.

8686 Shepherd Center

Shepherd Center
2020 Peachtree Street NW
Atlanta, GA 30309 **404-352-2020**
FAX: 404-350-7773

Gary R Ulicny PhD, President/CEO
James Shepherd, Chairman

A private hospital specializing in treatment of people with spinal cord and acquired brain injury, multiple sclerosis and other neuromuscular diseases, and urological diseases. Houses the largest model spinal cord injury program in the country and the Southeastern Multiple Sclerosis Center, designated by the National Multiple Sclerosis Society. Serving the Southeast since 1975, the 100-bed specialty hospital offers a continuum of services from intensive care through rehabilitation.

8687 Specialty Hospital

Floyd Medical Center Fourth Floor
PO Box 233
Rome, GA 30161 **706-802-2000**
FAX: 706-802-2123

Jon Dixon, CEO

Offers acute rehabilitation.

Hawaii

8688 Shriners Hospital for Crippled Children: Honolulu Unit

1310 Punahou Street
Honolulu, HI 96826
FAX: 808-951-3708

Idaho

8689 Eastern Idaho Regional Medical Center Rehabilitation Program

3100 Channing Way
Idaho Falls, ID 83404 **208-529-6132**
800-575-8426
FAX: 208-529-7075

CARF certified rehabilitation program in Eastern Idaho, providing acute medical rehabilitation services to patients recovering from strokes, spinal cord injury, head trauma, amputation, fractures, arthritis, multiple trauma, neurological disorders, burns, congenital deformity, generalized deconditioning, etc. The rehabilitation team consists of three psychiatrists, physical therapists, occupational therapists, speech pathologists, etc.

8690 Pocatello Regional Medical Center

777 Hospital Way
Pocatello, ID 83201 **208-236-6920**
FAX: 208-239-3719

Illinois

8691 **Builders of Skills**
9021 N Clifton Avenue
Niles, IL 60714 **847-296-6783**

Residential setting for hearing-impaired, developmentally disabled adults who are assisted with daily living skills.

8692 **Center for Learning**
National-Louis University
2840 Sheridan Road
Evanston, IL 60201

Psychoeducational evaluations for children, adolescents, and adults.

8693 **Clearbrook**
1835 W Central Road
Arlington Heights, IL 60005 **847-870-7711**
FAX: 847-870-7741
e-mail: tmartin@clearbrook.org
www.clearbrook.org

Carl M La Mell, President
Tracy Martin, Admissions Director

Offers educational, employment and residential services to the developmentally disabled children and adults.

8694 **Illinois Center for Rehabilitation and Education (ICRE-Wood)**
1151 S Wood Street
Chicago, IL 60612 **312-996-1508**
FAX: 312-633-3575

Residential rehabilitation center for adults who are blind or visually impaired.

8695 **Institute of Physical Medicine and Rehabilitation**
6501 N Sheridan Road
Peoria, IL 61614 **309-692-8110**
800-957-4767
FAX: 309-692-8673
www.ipmr.org

Richard Erickson, President

Comprehensive CARF accredited programs in outpatient medical rehabilitation services. Eight outpatient locations, specialty programs include adult day services, driving evaluations, balance and visual rehabilitation board certified physiatrists.

8696 **LaRabida Children's Hospital and Research Center**
E 65th and Lake Michigan
Chicago, IL 60649
FAX: 773-363-9554

Counseling, educational services, medical and nursing services for children through age 18.

8697 **Marianjoy Rehabilitation Hospital and Clinics**
26 W 171 Roosevelt Road
Wheaton, IL 60189 **630-462-4000**
FAX: 630-462-4440
www.marianjoy.org

Kathleen Yosko, President and CEO

8698 **Regional ADA Technical Assitance Agency**
1640 W Roosevelt Road
Chicago, IL 60608 **312-413-1407**
800-949-4232
e-mail: gldbtac@uic.edu
www.adagreatlakes.org

Robin Jones, Project Director

8699 **Rehabilitation Institute of Chicago**
345 E Superior Street
Chicago, IL 60611 **312-908-6000**
800-354-REHA
FAX: 847-981-6854
TTY:312-908-8523

Each year more than 14,000 children and adults benefit from the full range of inpatient, outpatient, day treatment and subacute services offered by the Rehabilitation Institute of Chicago (RIC) at its 18 sites of care. Specialized treatment programs include: amputee, arthritis, brain injury, burn, general rehab, pain management and more. RIC is an academic affiliate of Northwestern University Medical School and houses the nation's largest residency program in physical medicine.

8700 **Rush Copley Medical Center-Rehab Neuro Physical Unit**
2000 Oden Avenue
Aurora, IL 60504 **630-978-6230**
FAX: 630-978-6846
www.rushcopley.com

Patrick Barnes, Director
Pamela Lewis Scott, Manager Physical Rehabilitation

8701 **Shriners Hospitals for Children: Chicago**
2211 N Oak Park Avenue
Chicago, IL 60707 **773-622-5400**
FAX: 773-385-5453
e-mail: vlwalter@earthlink.net
www.shrinerschicago.org

A James Spang, Administrator
Beth Mikalauskas, Admissions Coordinator
Vickie Walter, Director Public Relations

A leading Midwest children's hospital providing high quality orthopedic treatments, plastic and reconstructive surgery, and spinal cord injury care with innovative education and research, the hospital is one of 22 operated by the Shrine fraternity, the only health care system in the US funded totally through philanthropy. Any child under 18 is eligable for treatment, as long as there is a reasonable possibility that there will benefit the child.

8702 **Wood River Township Hospital: RehabCare Unit**
Edwardsville Road
Wood River, IL 62095 **618-254-3134**
FAX: 618-251-4307

Jo Anne Baker, Clinical Coordinator

Indiana

8703 **ATTAIN**
32 E Washington Street
Suite 1400
Indianapolis, IN 46204 **317-486-8808**
FAX: 317-486-8809
e-mail: attain@attaininc.org
www.attaininc.org

Gary R Hand, Executive Director

8704 **Clark Memorial Hospital: RehabCare Unit**

1220 Missouri Avenue
Jeffersonville, IN 47130
812-282-6631
FAX: 812-283-2656

Jan Goldhammer, Program Manager

8705 **Developmental Disabilities Planning Council**

143 W Market Street
Suite 404
Indianapolis, IN 46204
317-232-7770
e-mail: gpcpd@gpcpd.org
www.state.in.us/gpcpd

Suelle Jackson-Boner, Director

8706 **Down Syndrome Association of North East Indiana**

PO Box 80141
Fort Wayne, IN 46898
260-497-9927
877-713-7264
www.indianadsf.org

8707 **Easter Seals Wayne/Union Counties**

5632 US Highway 40 E
PO Box 86
Centerville, IN 47330
765-855-2482
e-mail: easterseals@juno.com

Pat Bowers, Executive Director

8708 **IN Speechllanguage-Hearing Association**

233 McCrea Street
Suite 200
Indianapolis, IN 46225
317-955-1063
e-mail: isha@in-motion.org
www.isha.org

Michael Flahive, President

8709 **IN-SOURCE**

809 Nosth Michigan Street
South Bend, IN 46601
574-234-7101
800-332-4433
e-mail: insource@insource.org
www.insource.org

Richard Burden, Executive Director

8710 **Indiana Congress of Parent and Teachers**

2525 N Shadeland Avenue
D-4
Indianapolis, IN 46219
317-357-5881
e-mail: www.indianapta.org
in_office@pta.org

Mary Williams, President

8711 **Indiana Parent Information Association**

4755 Kingsway Drive
Suite 105-A
Indianapolis, IN 46205
317-257-8683
e-mail: FamilyNetw@aol.com
www.ai.org/ipin

Donna Gore Olsen, Executive Director

8712 **Indiana Resource Center for Autism**

Indiana Institute on Disability and Community
2853 E 10th Street
Bloomington, IN 47408
812-855-6508
FAX: 812-855-9630
e-mail: prattc@indiana.edu
www.iidc.indiana.edu/irca

The Indiana Resource Center for Autism staff conduct outreach training and consultations, engage in research and develop and disseminate information focused on building the capicity of local communities, organizations, agencies and families to support children and adults across the autism spectrum in typical work, school, home and community settings. Please check our website for our complete list of publications.

8713 **Kokomo Rehabilitation Hospital**

829 N Dixon Road
Kokomo, IN 46901
FAX: 765-868-8108

Brenda Harry, Admissions Director

8714 **Learning Disabilities Association of IN**

PO Box 20584
Indianapolis, IN 46220
800-284-2519
e-mail: dlytle@netusal.net

Dawn Lytle, IN State President

8715 **Memorial Regional Rehabilitation Center**

615 N Michigan Street
South Bend, IN 46601
574-284-7903
FAX: 574-284-3195

Julie Fanner, Unit Director

30-bed CARF accredited inpatient rehabilitation, outpatient orthopedic clinic and work performance program, head injury clinic. Outpatient neuro rehab and TBI Day treatment program, rehab technology center and a driver education and training program are provided.

8716 **Mental Health Association in Indiana**

55 Monumental Circle
Suite 455
Indianapolis, IN 46204
317-638-3501
800-555-6424
e-mail: mhai@indy.net
www.mentalhealthassociation.com

Stephen McCaffrey, President

8717 **Methodist Hospital Rehabilitation Institute**

8701 Broadway
Merrillville, IN 46410
219-738-5500
FAX: 219-738-6636

8718 **NAMI Indiana**

PO Box 22697
Indianapolis, IN 46222
317-925-9399
800-677-6442
e-mail: nami-in@nami.org
www.namiindiana.org

8719 **Office of State Coordinator of Vocational Education for Students with Disability**

10 N Senate Avenue
Room 212
Indianapolis, IN 46207
317-232-1829
e-mail: tfields@dwd.state.in.us
www.state.in.us/dwd/techd

8720 Parkview Regional Rehabilitation Center
2200 Randallia Drive
Fort Wayne, IN 46805 260-484-6636

Elizabeth Williamson, Admissions Coordinator

8721 Programs for Children with Disabilities: Ages 3 Through 5
Division of Special Education
State House, Room 229
Indianapolis, IN 46204 317-232-0567
e-mail: cochra@speed.doe.state.in.us
www.newassessment.org

Sheron Cochran, Preschool Coordinator

8722 Programs for Children with Special Health Care Needs
2 N Meridian Street
Section 7-B
Indianapolis, IN 46204 317-233-5578
e-mail: wgettelf@isdh.state.in.us

Wendy Gettelfinger, Director

8723 Programs for Infants and Toddlers with Disabilities: Ages Birth Through 2
402 W Washington Street
Room W-386
Indianapolis, IN 46204 317-233-9292
e-mail: mgreer@fssa.state.in.us

8724 Protection and Advocacy Agency of Indiana
4701 N Keystone Avenue
Suite 222
Indianapolis, IN 46205 317-722-5555
800-838-1131
e-mail: info@ipas.state.in.us
www.state.in.us

Thomas Gallagher, Executive Director

8725 Riley Child Development Center
702 Barnhill Drive
Room 5837
Indianapolis, IN 46202 317-274-8167
e-mail: jdrau@child-dev.com

8726 Saint Vincent Children's Specialty Hospital
1707 W 86th Street
PO Box 40407
Indianapolis, IN 46240 317-415-5500
FAX: 317-415-5595

Michelle Goff, Clinical Liaison
Diane Reeder, Case Manager

A free-standing pediatric facility providing children with the opportunity to grow physically and emotionally. SVCSH offers specialty programs in burn treatment, Cerebral Palsy, feeding disorders, juvenile rheumatoid arthritis, neuromuscular disorders, orthopedic conditions, spinal cord injuries, traumatic brain injuries, and children who require pulmonary rehab. Patients are involved with a professional interdisciplinary team, nurses, respiratory therapists, social workers and others.

8727 Spina Bifida Association of Northern IN
PO Box 1935
South Bend, IN 46634 574-234-6260

Carla Beres, Director

8728 St. Anthony Memorial Hospital: Rehab Unit
301 W Homer Street
Michigan City, IN 46360 219-877-1734
FAX: 219-877-1838

Doran Lounsbury, Program Manager

8729 State Blind and Visually Impaired Services Agency
402 W Washington Street
Room W-453, PO Box 7083
Indianapolis, IN 46207 317-232-1143
800-962-8408
e-mail: lquarles@fssa.state.in.us
www.state.in.us/fssa/servicedisabl/blind/inde

Linda Quarles, Interim Deputy Director

8730 State Developmental Disability Agency
PO Box 7083
Indianapolis, IN 46207 317-323-7842

Steven C Cook, Director

8731 State Division of Vocational Rehabilitation
402 W Washington Street, Room W453
PO Box 7083
Indianapolis, IN 46207 317-232-1319
800-545-7763
e-mail: martin@fssa.state.in.us
www.state.in.us/fssa

Rita Martin, Deputy Director

8732 State Mental Health Agency
402 W Washington Street
Room W353
Indianapolis, IN 46204 317-232-7845
e-mail: jcorson@fssa.state.in.us
www.IN.gov/fssa

8733 State Mental Health Representative for Children
402 W Washington Street
Room W353
Indianapolis, IN 46204 317-232-7934
e-mail: JPhillips3@fssa.state.in.us

Jim Phillips, Chief

8734 VSA Arts of Indiana
Harrison Center for the Arts
1505 N Delaware Street
Suite 100
Indianapolis, IN 46202 317-974-4123
FAX: 317-974-4124
e-mail: gholtman@vsai.org
www.vsai.org

Gayle Holtman, Director

8735 Wabash Valley Spina Bifida Support Group
PO Box 21
Farmersburg, IN 47850 812-696-2288
e-mail: sbawareness@hoymail.com
www.homestead.com/planetzachary/main.html

Kim Zink, Coordinator

Iowa

8736 Younker Rehabilitation Center of Iowa Methodist Medical Center
1200 Pleasant Street
Des Moines, IA 50309 **515-241-6201**
FAX: 515-241-5872

Fran Wendling, Admissions Coord.

Kansas

8737 Kansas Rehabilitation Hospital
1504 SW 8th Avenue
Topeka, KS 66606 **785-235-6600**
FAX: 785-232-8556

Julie DeJean, Administrator

8738 Mid-America Rehabilitation Hospital HealthSouth
5701 W 110th Street
Overland Park, KS 66211 **913-491-2400**
FAX: 913-491-1097
e-mail: tiffany.wood@healthsouth.com
www.healthsouth.com

Tiffany Wood, Director of Marketing
Laurie English, CEO
Melissa Higgins, Director of Clinical Services

80 bed Acute Rehab hospital offering full continuum from in-patient day treatment to outpatient services fo individuals with rehab needs due to CVA, TBI, SCI, other traumas, joint replacement, etc.

Kentucky

8739 Cardinal Hill Rehabilitation Hospital
2050 Versailles Road
Lexington, KY 40504 **859-254-5701**
800-888-5377
FAX: 859-255-9303
e-mail: sws@cardinalhill.org
www.cardinalhill.org

Sandy Shill CRRN, Manager Referral Relations
Beth A Monarch, COO

CARF-accredited rehab center provides comprehensive inpatient and outpatient services in two locations to people with physical and cognitive disabilities. We provide diagnosis-specific programs to 100 inpatients, outpatient clinics, outpatient therapies, pain management and therapeutic pool services. The Pediatric Center serves children from birth to age 18 years of age.

8740 HealthSouth Rehabilitation of Louisville
1227 Goss Avenue
Louisville, KY 40217 **502-636-1200**
FAX: 502-636-0351
www.healthsouth.com

Michele McCoy, Marketing Representative

8741 Humana Hospital: Lake Cumberland Rehab Uni t
305 Langdon Street
Somerset, KY 42503 **606-679-5488**
FAX: 606-679-5739

Chris Lovelace, Program Manager

8742 Lakeview Rehabilitation Hospital
134 Heartland Drive
Elizabethtown, KY 42701 **270-769-3100**
FAX: 270-769-6870

Diane Stephens, Assistant Director Marketing

40-beds, comprehensive physical rehabilitation.

8743 Shriners Hospitals for Children, Lexington
1900 Richmond Road
Lexington, KY 40502 **859-266-2101**
800-444-8314
FAX: 859-268-5636
www.shrinershq.org

Joan Snowden, Director Family/Cmmty Service

A 50-bed, pediatric orthopedic hospital providing FREE, expert orthopedic medical care to children and adolescents in Kentucky, Tennessee, West Virginia, Ohio, and Indiana.

8744 Shriners Hospitals, Lexington Unit, for Crippled Children
1900 Richmond Road
Lexington, KY 40502 **859-266-2101**
FAX: 859-268-5636

Glenda Ross, Administrator

Louisiana

8745 HealthSouth North Louisiana Rehabilitation
1401 Ezelle Street
Ruston, LA 71270 **318-251-3126**
800-548-9157
FAX: 318-251-5491

8746 Our Lady of Lourdes Rehabilitation Center
611 Saint Landry Street
Lafayette, LA 70506 **337-684-5732**
FAX: 318-289-2681

8747 Rehabilitation Center of Lake Charles Memorial Hospital
1701 Oak Park Boulevard
Lake Charles, LA 70601 **337-494-3253**
FAX: 337-494-2656

Rehabilitation center offering intensive physical, occupational, speech, neuropsychology, recreational therapies along with rehabilitation nursing.

8748 Shriners Hospital, Shreveport Unit, for Crippled Children
3100 Samford Avenue
Shreveport, LA 71103 **318-222-5704**
FAX: 318-424-7610

8749 South Louisiana Rehabilitation Hospital
614 Jackson Street
Thibodaux, LA 70301 **985-448-3088**
e-mail: soberup@powerhouseprograms.com
www.powerhouseprograms.com

Rehabilitation center for substance abuse.

8750 St. Frances Cabrini Hospital: Rehab Unit
3330 Masonic Drive
Alexandria, LA 71301 **318-487-1122**
FAX: 318-448-6822

Judith Rozier, Program Manager

8751 **St. Patrick Hospital: Rehab Unit**
524 Ryan Street
Lake Charles, LA 70601
337-491-7730
FAX: 337-491-7157

8752 **Thibodaux Hospital: Regional Rehabilitatio n Center**
602 N Acadia Road
Thibodaux, LA 70301
985-447-5500

Maine

8753 **Head Injury Treatment Program at Brewer**
74 S Road
Brewer, ME 04412

Mary Goyoi, Program Rep

8754 **New England Rehabilitation Hospital of Portland**
335 Brighton Avenue
Portland, ME 04102
207-775-4000
FAX: 207-879-8168

Amy Weinschenk, Referrals

Maryland

8755 **Mt. Washington Pediatric Hospital**
1708 W Rogers Avenue
Baltimore, MD 21209
419-578-8600
FAX: 410-542-8717

Winne Sherman RN, Admissions Center Manager
Violet Ebbesen RN, Admissions Nurse

8756 **Sinai Rehabilitation Center**
2401 W Belvedere Avenues
Baltimore, MD 21215
410-601-5631
FAX: 410-601-8284

Bonnie Hartley, Senior Field Service Nurse

Provides comprehensive inpatient and outpatient medical rehabilitation services to individuals disabled by head injury, stroke, musculoskeletal/orthopedic disorders, neurologic conditions and other medical diagnoses that impact on their functional capacity. Recognizing that many individuals have special needs, SRC has developed the following specialty programs: driver evaluation and training, electrodiagnostics, oncology, prosthetic/orthotic services, acute and post-acute brain injury services.

Massachusetts

8757 **Braintree Hospital**
250 Pond Street
Braintree, MA 02184
781-848-7740
800-99R-EHAB
FAX: 781-849-9949

Elizabeth Glenn RN BSN CRRN, Patient Access

Since Braintree Hospital's founding in 1975, we have gained recognition as a world class health care provider. Today the Braintree Rehabilitation Network serves as the flagship hospital of Horizon Health Care, the largest independent provider of comprehensive medical rehabilitation in the world. The network consists of a growing number of rehabilitation facilities which provide both inpatient and outpatient services Programs include: amputee, general rehab, neuro rehab and stroke.

8758 **Greenery Extended Care Center**
59 Acton Street
Worcester, MA 01604
508-791-3147
FAX: 508-757-0423

Tom Johnsrud, Admissions

8759 **Greenery Rehab Center Massachusetts**
99 Chestnut Hill Avenue
Boston, MA 02135
617-787-3390
FAX: 617-787-9169

William Garvin, Medical Director

8760 **Mediplex Rehabilitation Hospital**
4499 Acushnet Avenue
New Bedford, MA 02745
508-588-8294
FAX: 508-998-8131

8761 **New England Home for the Deaf**
154 Walter Street
Danvers, MA 01923
978-774-0445
FAX: 781-337-6742

Eddy Laird, Executive Director

Offers services for the deaf, totally blind, legally blind, visually impaired, mentally retarded blind and more with health, counseling, educational, recreational, rehabilitation, computer training and professional training services.

8762 **New England Rehabilitation Hospital: Massachusetts**
2 Rehabilitation Way
Woburn, MA 01801
781-935-5050
FAX: 781-932-8152
www.healthsouth.com

Dianne Landy, Marketing Coordinator

8763 **Shriners Burns Hospital: Boston**
51 Blossom Street
Boston, MA 02114
617-722-3000
FAX: 617-523-1684
e-mail: rburgess@shrinenet.org
www.shrinershq.org

Robert F Bories Jr FACHE, Administrator
Richard W Burgess, Public Relations Director

Provides treatment for children to their 18th birthday with acute, fresh burns, plastic reconstructive surgery for patients with healed burns, severe scarring and facial deformity. Some non-burn conditions such as Scalded Skin Syndrome, Cleft Lip, Cleft Palate and purpura fulminians are also treated. Call the Hospital for information. All medical treatment is without cost to the patient, parents, or any third party.

8764 **Shriners Hospital Springfield Unit for Crippled Children**
516 Carew Street
Springfield, MA 01104
413-787-2000
FAX: 413-735-1226

Michigan

8765 Community Rehabilitation Center
Community Hospital
400 Medical Park Drive
Watervliet, MI 49098 **269-463-5754**
800-463-1164
FAX: 269-463-6729

Sandra L Dugal, Community Relations Coordinator
Linda Beushausen, Program Administrator

Comprehensive medical rehabilitation program in a community hospital setting, providing inpatient and outpatient services to individuals who have become physically challenged by stroke, spinal cord injuries, traumatic brain injuries, major multiple trauma, orthopedic conditions, neurologic disorders, amputation, arthritis conditions and other diagnoses.

8766 Covenant Healthcare Rehabilitation Program
515 N Michigan Avenue
Saginaw, MI 48602 **989-583-2817**
FAX: 989-583-2843

8767 Farmington Health Care Center
34225 Grand River Avenue
Farmington, MI 48335 **248-477-7373**
FAX: 248-477-2888

8768 Flint Osteopathic Hospital: RehabCare Unit
3921 Beecher Road
Flint, MI 48532 **810-762-4682**

Susan Malone, Program Manager

8769 Integrated Health Services of Michigan at Clarkston
4800 Clintonville Road
Clarkston, MI 48346 **248-674-0903**
FAX: 248-674-3359

Carol Doll, Admissions Director
Maggy Canny, Administrator
Rose Berg, Admission

8770 Mecosta County General Hospital Rehabilitation Center
Mecosta County General Hospital
405 Winter Avenue
Big Rapids, MI 49307 **231-592-4444**
FAX: 231-592-4456
e-mail: eriegle@mcghhospital.com
www.mcghhospital.com

Eugene A Riegle, Program Director

Comprehensive medical rehabilitation program in a hospital setting, providing inpatient and outpatient services to individuals who have become physically challenged by stroke, spinal cord injuries, brain injuries, traumatic multiple traumas, arthritis conditions and other diagnoses.

8771 Rehabilitation Institute of Michigan
261 Mack Boulevard
Detroit, MI 48201 **313-745-1203**
FAX: 313-745-1175
e-mail: cangelel@dmc.org
www.RIMrehab.org

Terry Reiley, President
Cheryl Angelelli, Marketing & Public Relations

Rehabilitation Institute of Michigan is a national leader in the delivery of physical medicine and rehabilitation and one of the country's largest freestanding rehabilitation hospitals. A comprehensive spectrum of both inpatient and outpatient services and programs are available for spinal cord injuries, brain injuries, stroke, cerebral palsy, musculoskeletal disorders, low back problems, amputations, sports injuries, work-related injuries and other medical conditions requiring physical rehab.

8772 St. John Hospital: North Shore
26755 Ballard Street
Harrison Township, MI 48045 **586-465-5501**

Susan Looney Smith, Intake Coordinator

8773 Three Rivers Rehabilitation Pavilion
Three Rivers Area Hospital
1111 W Broadway Street
Three Rivers, MI 49093 **269-279-5224**
FAX: 269-279-7375

Christine M Strom RN CRRN, Program Director
Sandra L Cooper, Community Relations

Comprehensive medical rehabilitation program in a community hospital setting, providing inpatient and outpatient services to individuals who have become physically challenged by stroke, spinal cord injuries, traumatic brain injuries, major multiple trauma, orthopedic conditions, neurologic disorders, amputation, arthritis conditions and other diagnoses.

Minnesota

8774 North Memorial Medical Center: Rehabilitat ion Services
3300 Oakdale Avenue N
Minneapolis, MN 55422 **763-520-5090**
FAX: 763-520-1772
www.northmemorial.com

Pete Pytlak, Director
Susan Keeney RN, Inpatient Unit Nurse Manager
Deb Christian, Evaluator

Inpatient unit primarily serves adults and young adults that have a physical disability as a result of TBI, SCI, CVA, multiple trauma, spinal cord dysfunction or tumors and amputation. The interdisciplinary team approach includes the patient and family, as well as representatives from all rehab related disciplines. The program is CARF and JCAHO accredited, consisting of 18 beds.

8775 Sister Kenny Institute
800 E 28th Street
Minneapolis, MN 55407 **612-863-4495**
FAX: 612-863-8942

Helen Kettner, Nurse- Liaison

Missouri

8776 Columbia Regional Hospital: RehabCare Unit
404 Keene Street
Columbia, MO 65201 **573-875-9520**
FAX: 573-875-4417

George Gumbert, Program Manager

8777 **Jewish Hospital of St. Louis: Department of Rehabilitation**

216 N Kings Highway
Saint Louis, MO 63108
314-454-7390
FAX: 314-454-5277

Mary Mitchell, Admitting Clerk

8778 **PremierCare Neurohabilitation Program of Bethesda General Hospital**

3655 Vista Avenue
Saint Louis, MO 63110
314-772-9200
FAX: 314-772-1819

Tim Imhoff, Program Director

8779 **Rusk Rehabilitation Center**

315 Business Loop 70 W
Columbia, MO 65203
573-817-2703
FAX: 573-817-4690

Tracy Rimki, Marketing Coordinator
Patrick Lee, Hospital Administrator

A 60-bed comprehensive rehabilitation hospital. This CARF-accredited facility utilizes a multidisciplinary approach to provide inpatient and outpatient services with specialized programming in head injury, spinal cord injury and chronic pain.

8780 **St. Mary's Regional Rehabilitation Center**

201 W R D Mize Road
Blue Springs, MO 64014
FAX: 816-655-5525

Susan Bottmker RN, Assessment Coordinator

A 17-bed inpatient physical rehabilitation unit offering PT, OT, ST, recreational therapy, psychiatry and all other ancillary services of a full-service hospital. Specialize in orthopedic and neurologic disabilities.

8781 **Three Rivers Health Care**

2620 N Westwood Boulevard
Poplar Bluff, MO 63902
573-785-1657

Montana

8782 **St. Vincent Hospital and Health Center**

1233 N 30th Street
Billings, MT 59101
406-657-8778
FAX: 406-657-8817

John Brewer, Admission

Nebraska

8783 **Madonna Rehabilitation Hospital**

5401 S Street
Lincoln, NE 68506
402-489-7102
800-676-5448
FAX: 402-483-9494
e-mail: information@madonna.org
www.madonna.org

Kent Eichelberger, Admissions Manager
Carol Jess, Marketing/Public Relations Mgr

Nebraska's premier rehabilitation facility for children and adults, Madonna offers many services and programs for both inpatients and outpatients. Programs include: orthopedic, burn, traumatic brain injury, spinal cord injury, adolescent and child rehabilitation and subacute rehabilitation.

Nevada

8784 **University Medical Center**

1800 W Charleston Boulevard
Las Vegas, NV 89102
FAX: 702-383-2536

Debbie Gulo, Rehab Evaluator

New Hampshire

8785 **Head Injury Treatment Program at Dover**

307 Plaza Drive
Dover, NH 03820
603-742-2676
FAX: 603-749-5375

Sue Mills, Program Rep

8786 **Lakeview NeuroRehabilitation Center**

101 Highwatch Road
Effingham Falls, NH 03814
603-539-7451
800-4RE-HAB1
FAX: 603-539-8888
www.lakeviewsystem.com

Susan Bartlett MSW CRC, Director Admissions
Tina Trudel PhD, VP Clinical Services
Edward C Morton Jr, Executive Director

Residential treatment center serving individuals with neurologic/behavioral disorders. Lakeview serves both children and adults in functionally based program environment. Transistional programs in various group homes also available to clients as they progress in their treatment.

8787 **Northeast Rehabilitation Hospital**

70 Butler Street
Salem, NH 03079
603-893-2900
FAX: 603-893-1628

Ellyn Dempsey, Intake Coordinator

8788 **St. Joseph New England Rehabilitation Center**

172 Kinsley Street
Nashua, NH 03060
603-595-3032
FAX: 603-595-3192

Mary Beth Harney, Program Director

A 24-bed acute rehabilitation unit offering general and specialized programs. Located within St. Joseph acute care hospital and affiliated with Advantage Health Corporation.

New Jersey

8789 **Betty Bacharach Rehabilitation Hospital**

Jim Leeds Road
Pomona, NJ 08240
609-652-9057
FAX: 609-748-3586

Virginia Wells, Admissions

8790 **Children's Specialized Hospital**

150 New Providence Road
Mountainside, NJ 07092 **908-233-3720**
FAX: 908-233-4176

Jeannie Brooke RN, Pre-Admission Coordinator

New Jersey's only comprehensive pediatric rehabilitation hospital, treats children and adolescents from birth through 21 years of age. Programs include spinal dysfunction, brain injury, respiratory, burn, Day Hospital, early intervention, preschool, and cognitive rehabilitation.

8791 **Garden State Rehabilitation Hospital**

14 Hospital Drive
Toms River, NJ 08755 **732-244-3100**
FAX: 732-244-2542

Dave Coluzzie, Intake Coordinator

8792 **JFK Johnson Rehab Institute**

65 James Street
Edison, NJ 08820 **732-321-7056**
FAX: 732-321-0994

Patricia Dulin, Client Services

8793 **Kessler Institute for Rehabilitation, Welkind Facility**

201 Pleasant Hill Road
Chester, NJ 07930 **973-584-7500**
800-KES-SLER
FAX: 973-252-6343
e-mail: jkment@kessler-rehab.com
www.kessler-rehab.com

Joyce Kment, Admissions Director
Carol Waggner, Exec Secretary to Administration

Set in the rolling hills of Morris County, this 72 bed facility provides specialized services to brain injury patients, including our unique Cognitive Redmediation Program, as well as a full range of stroke, amputee and orthopedic services. Kessler's team of dedicated rehabilitation professionals, including physicians, nurses and therapists, work with each patient to build physical strength, optimize movement, maximize independence, increase cognitive skills and address any other issues.

8794 **Mediplex Rehab: Camden**

2 Cooper Plaza
Camden, NJ 08103 **856-342-7600**
FAX: 856-342-7979

Beth Crawford, Admissions

New Mexico

8795 **HealthSouth Rehabilitation Center: New Mexico**

7000 Jefferson Street NE
Albuquerque, NM 87109 **505-342-1992**
FAX: 505-344-2851

8796 **St. Joseph Rehabilitation Hospital and Outpatient Center**

505 Elm Street NE
Albuquerque, NM 87102 **505-727-4700**
FAX: 505-727-4793
www.sjhs.org

Sherri Milone, Administrator

A member of the four hospital, St. Joseph healthcare system, this facility provides inpatient and outpatient care for those requiring physical medicine and rehabilitation. Specialty programs include brain injury, stroke, spinal cord, orthopedics, occupational and physical therapies, clinical psychology, speech/language pathology, hand clinic and functional capacity evaluations. The only facility in New Mexico accredited in four areas by the commission on accreditation of rehab facilities.

New York

8797 **Burke Rehabilitation Hospital**

785 Mamaroneck Avenue
White Plains, NY 10605 **914-597-2500**
888-99B-URKE
FAX: 914-597-2787
e-mail: burke@burke.org
www.burke.org

Ann Herring, Marketing

A 150 bed rehabilitation hospital providing both in and out patient physical rehabilitation to people with stroke, spinal cord injury, head injury, pulmonary, cardiac, amputee, orthopedic arthritis and other related diagnoses.

8798 **Rusk Institute of Rehabilitation Medicine**

400 E 34th Street
New York, NY 10016 **212-263-6034**
FAX: 212-263-8510
www.rusknyu.org

North Carolina

8799 **Horizon Rehabilitation Center**

3100 Erwin Road
Durham, NC 27705 **919-383-1546**
800-541-7750
FAX: 919-382-0156

Maureen O'Neal, Administrator

A 125-bed rehabilitation, subacute and long term care facility. HRC is JCAHO and CARF accredited with a physician-directed rehabilitation program, internal case management and a therapy department composed of physical, occupational, speech, recreational and respiratory therapists - pulmonary rehabilitation/ventilator unit.

8800 **Integrated Health Services of Durham- N**

3100 Erwin Road
Durham, NC 27705 **919-383-1546**
FAX: 919-383-0862

Lenon McDaver, Marketing Director/ Admissions

8801 **Learning Services Corporation**

707 Morehead Avenue
Durham, NC 27707 **919-419-9955**
800-765-5327
FAX: 603-425-2176

Randall W Evans PhD, President/CEO

A licensed postacute rehabilitation program for adults who have an acquired brain injury. Individuals who are enrolled in the program participate in active, intensive rehabilitation carried out by a team of neuropsychology, speech/language therapy, physical therapy, occupational therapy, vocational services, family services and life skills training. Services include residential rehabilitation, home based treatment, day treatment, subacute rehabilitation and supported living.

Ohio

8802 Arbors at Columbus

44 S Souder Avenue
Columbus, OH 43222
614-228-5900
FAX: 614-228-3989

Postacute rehabilitation program.

8803 Franciscan Rehabilitation Center

601 S Edwin C Moses Boulevard
Dayton, OH 45402
937-229-6081
800-272-8042
FAX: 937-229-6074

Linda Didas RN CRRN CCM, Case Manager

Acute, inpatient rehabilitation, 77 beds. Twenty-plus years serving the Dayton community. Vocational and assistive technology services are available. Extensive outpatient services include: hand therapy, back school, drivers' training. Accredited by JCAHO and CARF. Liaison with community support groups: SCI, BI, stroke, amputee, ALS, chronic pain. On-site clinics: SCI, MDA, amputee and wheelchair/seating.

8804 Great Lakes Regional Rehabilitation Center

3700 Kolbe Road
Lorain, OH 44053
440-960-3950
FAX: 440-960-4636

Roberta Yehman, Admissions Director

8805 HCR Health Care Services

1 Seagate
Toledo, OH 43604
419-321-5470
800-736-4427
FAX: 419-252-5543

Specialty transitional care and intensive rehabilitation services. Specialized services are focused on patients with catastrophic conditions or whose length of stay at an acute care or rehabilitation hospital can be dramatically reduced by transferring to a subacute level of care.

8806 Heather Hill Rehabilitation Hospital

Heather Hill
12340 Bass Lake Road
Chardon, OH 44024
440-285-9151
800-423-2972

Individualized treatment programs for adults and adolescents can participate in and benefit from three-plus hours a day of active therapy.

8808 Parma Community General Hospital Acute Rehabilitation Center

7007 Powers Boulevard
Parma, OH 44129
440-743-3000
FAX: 440-743-4036
www.parmahospital.org

Dale Winsberg, Administrative Director

The mission of this CARF accredited unit is to provide the most comprehensive, cost-effective, acute rehabilitation program possible in order for every patient and family to adjust to his/her disability and to achieve the maximum potential of independent functioning when returning to community living.

8809 Rehabilitation Hospital at Heather Hill

12340 Bass Lake Road
Chardon, OH 44024
440-285-4040
FAX: 440-285-0946
www.heatherhill.org

Sheila LaRosa, Admissions Director

250-bed, non-profit, multi-level care facility serving the frail elderly and physiclaly disabled.

8810 Rehabilitation Institute of Ohio at Miami Valley Hospital

1 Wyoming Street
Dayton, OH 45409
937-208-2063
FAX: 937-208-4534

Sharyl Kuhnen RN, Rehab Coordinator

Provides inpatient rehab (39 beds), acute inpatient and outpatient physical therapy, occupational therapy and speech pathology services, comprehensive outpatient rehabilitation program, work hardening, head injury return to work, pain center, disabled driving programs, hand therapy and ADA services.

8811 Shriners Burn Institute: Cincinnati Unit

3229 Burnet Avenue
Cincinnati, OH 45229
513-872-6000
FAX: 513-872-6999

Ronald Hitzler, Administrator

8812 St. Francis Health Care Centre

401 N Broadway Street
Green Springs, OH 44836
419-639-2626
800-248-2552
FAX: 419-639-6222
e-mail: jholmer@sfhcc.org
www.sfhcc.org

Greg Raubenolt, Director Marketing
Jane Holmer, Admissions Coordinator
Joy Kinnear CRRN, Dir Admissions/Care Coordinator

8813 St. Rita's Medical Center Rehabilitation Services

730 W Market Street
Lima, OH 45801
FAX: 419-226-9705

Kelly Recker, Administrative of Physical Med

8814 University of Cincinnati Hospital

234 Goodman Street
Cincinnati, OH 45219
513-584-1000
FAX: 513-584-7712

Brook Vargason, Administrator

8815 Upper Valley Medical/Rehab Services

3130 N Dixie Highway
Troy, OH 45373
937-440-4000
FAX: 937-440-7337
www.uvmc.com

Pam Cornett, Director Rehab Services

Oklahoma

8816 HealthSouth Rehab Center: Oklahoma

700 NW 7th Street
Oklahoma City, OK 73102
405-236-3131
FAX: 405-553-1153
www.healthsouth.com

Susan Nelson, Director Business Development

Inpatient Rehab Facility including all therapy services serving people who have been injured and had an illness resulting in a decreased level of independence.

8817 **Hilcrest Medical Center: Kaiser Rehab Cent er**

1125 S Trenton Avenue
Tulsa, OK 74120
918-579-7100
FAX: 918-584-6304

8818 **Jane Phillips Episcopal Memorial Medical Center: RehabCare Unit**

3500 E Frank Phillips Boulevard
Bartlesville, OK 74006
918-335-6655
FAX: 918-331-1360

8819 **Jim Thorpe Rehabilitation Center at Southwest Medical Center**

RehabCare Unit
4401 S Western Avenue
Oklahoma City, OK 73109
405-636-7700
800-677-1238
FAX: 405-636-7501

Gary Zook, Unit Director
Denise Uvino, Marketing Director

Provides inpatient rehabilitation for people with head injuries, spinal cord injuries, orthopedic conditions, pain management, neurological diseases, strokes and a variety of diagnoses that stop individuals from being able to take care of themselves independently. Services available include medical direction, physical therapy, social work, occupational therapy, speech therapy, recreational therapy, and aftercare follow-up.

8820 **Mercy Memorial Health Center-Rehab Center**

1011 14th Avenue NW
Ardmore, OK 73401
580-223-5400
800-572-1182
FAX: 580-220-6681
www.mercyok.net

8821 **St. Anthony Hospital: Rehabilitation Unit**

1000 N Lee Street
Oklahoma City, OK 73102
405-272-7386
FAX: 405-231-8759

8822 **St. Mary's Hospitals: RehabCare Unit**

305 S 5th Street
Enid, OK 73701
FAX: 405-270-7563

Oregon

8823 **Shriners Hospitals for Children: Portland**

3101 SW Sam Jackson Park Road
Portland, OR 97201
FAX: 503-241-5090
www.shrinershq.org

Barbara Flaherty, New Patient Coordinator
Sonia Bouchard, Rehabilation Services Manager
Kerry Grindeland, Care Coordination Manager

Pediatric orthopedic and plastic surgery; inpatient and outpatient services. No charge for any services provided at the Hospital. Diagnosis, rehabilitation, surgery, sports and recreation for ages 0-18 for people with physical disabilities involving bones, muscles or joints or in need of plastic surgery for burn scars or cleft lip/palate.

Pennsylvania

8824 **Allied Services John Heinz Institute of Rehabilitation Medicine**

150 Mundy Street
Wilkes Barre, PA 18702
570-826-3800
FAX: 570-826-3898
www.allied-services.org

Thomas E Pugh, VP/CEO
Gregory Basting MD, VP of Medical Affairs
Karen Kearney, Exec Director Inpatient Services

A 94-bed hospital offering comprehensive inpatient and outpatient rehabilitation services. The Institute specializes in rehabilitation programs in the areas of head trauma, injured worker recovery and outpatient.

8825 **Allied Services Rehabilitation Hospital**

475 Morgan Highway
Scranton, PA 18508
570-348-1300
FAX: 570-348-1281
e-mail: alliedcom@aol.com

Donna Esken, Admissions

8826 **Brighten Place**

131 N Main Street
Chalfont, PA 18914
215-997-7746
FAX: 215-997-0403
e-mail: brightenplace@enter.net
members.aol.com/vmoc3

Suzann Ditzel, Program Director

A residential brain injury program with the mission to encourage growth and foster independence on an individual level for each resident. We are CARF accredited and provide additional services which include a day program and respite care.

8827 **Chestnut Hill Rehabilitation Hospital**

8601 Stenton Avenue
Wyndmoor, PA 19038
215-233-9700
FAX: 215-233-6879

Leslie Gilman, Administrator

8828 **Doylestown Hospital Rehabilitation Center**

595 W State Street
Doylestown, PA 18901
215-345-6412
FAX: 215-345-2007
e-mail: dseife@dh.org
www.dh.org

Donna Seif RN, Outpatient Rehab Case Manager
Gloria Peterson, Inpatient Rehab Services

8829 **Health Care Solutions**

701 Chester Pike
Sharon Hill, PA 19079
610-583-3500
800-451-1671
FAX: 610-583-3550

Donna Sewlin, Regional Sales Manager

Develops unique containment programs, offers equipment set-up, patient instruction, patient assessment and equipment usage. Offers clinical services that include oxygen systems, ventilators, aerosol therapy, suction equipment, T.E.N.S. programs, compression pumps, custom orthotics, enteral feeding.

8830 HealthSouth
143 E 2nd Street
Erie, PA 16507
814-878-1200
FAX: 814-878-1448
www.healthsouth.com

Kathy Lamb, Admissions

8831 HealthSouth Harmarville Rehabilitation Hospital
Guys Run Road
PO Box 11460
Pittsburgh, PA 15238
412-828-1300
FAX: 412-828-7705
www.healthsouth.com

A 202-bed facility providing inpatient and outpatient physical medicine and rehabilitation to adults and adolescents in Pennsylvania, West Virginia, Ohio and Maryland.

8832 HealthSouth Nittany Valley Rehabilitation Hospital
550 W College Avenue
Pleasant Gap, PA 16823
814-359-3421
800-842-6026
FAX: 814-359-5898
www.healthsouth.com

Jodi Drummond MS PT, Program Dir. Neurology/Oncology
Robert Drummond MPT, Program Director Orthopedics

Comprehensive inpatient and outpatient facilities. Treatment for symptoms relating to: stroke, head injury, pulmonary disease, orthopedic conditions, neurological disorders, cardiac illnesses and spinal cord injuries. Healthsouth Nittany Valley Rehabilitation Hospital is a part of Healthsouth's national network of more than 2,000 facilities in 50 states.

8833 HealthSouth Rehabilitation Hospital of Altoona
2005 Valley View Boulevard
Altoona, PA 16602
814-944-3535
FAX: 814-944-6160

Scott Fuler, Administrator/CEO

8834 Healthsouth Rehabilitation Hospital of Greater Pittsburgh
2380 McGinley Road
Monroeville, PA 15146
412-856-2400
FAX: 412-856-2437

8835 Healthsouth Rehabilitation Hospital of Mechanicsburg
175 Lancaster Boulevard
Mechanicsburg, PA 17055
717-691-3700
FAX: 717-697-6524

Roberta Weaver, Director Admissions

8836 Healthsouth Rehabilitation Hospital of York
1850 Normandie Drive
York, PA 17404
717-767-6941
FAX: 717-764-1341

Cheryl Fleming, CEO
Susan Hartman, Business Development
Brent Burger, Controller

A 120-bed rehabilitation hospital dedicated to providing advanced, comprehensive services to patients who have suffered head injury, spinal cord injury, stroke, burns, amputation, chronic pain and other neurological and musculoskeletal disorders. HRH of York provides outpatient services in seven locations. Healthsouth is located in York, Pennsylvania, approximately 50 miles north of Baltimore and 25 miles south of Harrisburg.

8837 Lake Erie Institute of Rehabilitation
137 W 2nd Street
Erie, PA 16507
814-878-2233
FAX: 814-878-1448

Jeff Ondrey, Program Director

8838 Magee Rehabilitation Hospital
6 Franklin Plaza
Philadelphia, PA 19102
215-587-3000
800-96M-AGEE
FAX: 215-568-3736
www.mageerehab.org

Hank Skoczen, Admissions

8839 Moss Rehabilitation Hospital
1200 W Tabor Road
Philadelphia, PA 19141
215-456-9465
FAX: 215-456-9646

Mary Stears, Intake Coordinator

The Philadelphia region's major resource for medical rehabilitation since 1959. This 152 bed facility offers comprehensive care to people with broad ranges of conditions, diagnostic laboratories and a multidisciplinary team of rehabilitation professionals.

8840 Shriners Hospital for Children
1645 W 8th Street
Erie, PA 16505
814-875-8700
FAX: 814-875-8778

8841 Shriners Hospitals for Children, Philadelphia
3551 N Broad Street
Philadelphia, PA 19140
215-430-4000
800-281-4051
www.shrinershq.org/shc/philadelphia

Sharon Rajnic, Administrator

The Shriners Hospital in Philadelphia is a 59-bed pediatric orthopaedic hospital providing a complete range of specialized medical and rehabilitation services at no charge to children with orthopaedic problems or spinal injuries. The hospital is one of 22 Shriners Hospitals for Children throughout North america. In addition to treating children with routine and complex orthopaedic problems, the Philadelphia Hospital provides a comprehensive and individualized rehabilitation program.

8842 Shriners Hospitals for Children, Erie
1645 W 8th Street
Erie, PA 16505
814-875-8700
FAX: 814-875-8756
www.shrinershq.org/shc/erie/index.html

Richard W Brzuz, Administrator
James O Sander MD, Chief of Staff
Bridget Hines, Applications/Admissions Coord.

The Shriners Hospitals for Children, Erie, is a 30-bed pediatric orthopaedic hospital providing comprehensive orthopaedic care to children at no charge. The hospital is one of 22 Shriners Hospitals throughout North America. The Erie Hospital accepts and treats children with routine and complex orthopaedic and neuromuscular problems, utilizing the latest treatments and technology available in pediatric orthopaedics, resulting in early ambulation and reduced length of stay.

8843 Shriners Hospitals, Philadelphia Unit, for Crippled Children
3551 N Broad Street
Philadelphia, PA 19140
215-430-4000
FAX: 215-430-4126
www.shrinershq.org/hospitals/index.html

South Carolina

8844 Colleton Regional Hospital: RehabCare Unit

501 Robertson Boulevard
Walterboro, SC 29488

Johnnie Benson, Program Manager

8845 HealthSouth Rehab Hospital: South Carolina

2935 Colonial Drive
Columbia, SC 29203
803-254-7777
FAX: 803-414-1414

8846 Rebound Head Injury Recovery Services of the Carolinas

800 W Meeting Street
Lancaster, SC 29720
803-286-1418
FAX: 803-286-1824

8847 Shriners Hospitals for Children, Greenville

950 W Faris Road
Greenville, SC 29605
864-271-3444
866-459-0013
FAX: 864-271-4471
www.shrinershp.org

Aenne Doughty, Assistant to the Administration

Tennessee

8848 Health South Cane Creek Rehabilitation Center

180 Mount Pelia Road
Martin, TN 38237
731-587-4231
FAX: 731-587-6716

Dayle Unger RN NHN, Administrator
Martha Stephenson RN, Rehab Liaison
Ray Ann Dudley LPN, Rehab Liaison

8849 HealthSouth Chattanooga Rehabilitation Hospital

2412 McCallie Avenue
Chattanooga, TN 37404
423-698-0221
800-763-5189
FAX: 423-697-9124

Donna L Bourdon, Administrator/CEO
Scooter Brunson, Marketing Coordinator

Offers orthopaedic rehabilitation, stroke rehabilitation, amputee rehabilitation, brain injury program, pain management, ventilator weaning, carpal tunnel screening, low intensity program, oncology program, aquatic therapy, day treatment, burn program and outpatient services.

8850 HealthSouth Rehabilitation Cntr/Tennessee

6100 Primacy Parkway
Suite 115
Memphis, TN 38119
901-682-3730
FAX: 901-685-1968

8851 Healthsouth Rehabilitation at Sumner

555 Hartsville Pike
Gallatin, TN 37066
615-230-3900
FAX: 615-230-3903

Andrea Sanders, Program Director
Doug Danforth, Director Nurses

Inpatient general rehabilitation programs for orthopedic injury, joint replacements, head injury, arthritis, general weakness and cardio/pulmonary diseases.

8852 James H And Cecile C Quillen Rehabilitation Hospital

2511 Wesley Street
Johnson City, TN 37601
423-283-0700
800-235-1994
FAX: 423-283-0153

Dennis Falck, CEO
Jim Perkins, Marketing Director

A 60-bed, freestanding comprehensive medical rehabilitation hospital. Full range of outpatient and day treatment, 14-bed traumatic brain injury unit, in ground therapeutic pool, transitional living apartment, outdoor ambulation course. All inpatient and outpatient programs utilize an interdisciplinary team approach designed to improve a patient's physical and cognitive functioning.

8853 Nashville Rehabilitation Hospital

610 Gallatin Road
Nashville, TN 37206
615-226-4330
800-227-3108
FAX: 615-650-2562

Anne Jacobs RN, Director CM/UR
Sherry Lawlwer LCSW, Social Services

A free-standing physical rehabilitation facility offering services to patients on an inpatient and outpatient basis. Programs include CVA, orthopedic, neuromuscular, traumatic brain injury, spinal cord injury, general rehabilitation and Bridges - geriatric psychiatric unit. Intra-disciplinary team approach is utilized to assist patients in obtaining their maximum fuctional level.

8854 Patricia Neal Rehab Center : Ft. Sanders R egional Medical Center

1901 W Clinch Avenue
Knoxville, TN 37916
865-541-1167
FAX: 865-541-3977

8855 Rebound Comprehensive Rehabilitation Center at Cane Creek

180 Mt Pelia Road
Martin, TN 38237
FAX: 731-587-6716

8856 Rehabilitation Center Baptist Hospital

137 Blount Avenue
Knoxville, TN 37920
865-632-5360
www.baptist.org

8857 Rehabilitation Center at McFarland Hospital

University Medical Center
500 Park Avenue
Lebanon, TN 37087
615-449-0500
FAX: 615-444-7901

Johnny Harrison MS, Director

8858 St. Mary's Medical Center: RehabCare Center

Oak Hill Avenue
Knoxville, TN 37917
865-545-8000
FAX: 865-545-8133

Texas

8859 Bayshore Medical Center: Rehab

4000 Spencer Highway
Pasadena, TX 77504
713-944-6666
FAX: 713-359-1121

Bill Brady, Program Manager

8860 Brown Schools Rehabilitation Center: A Brain Injury Hospital

1106 W Dittmar Road
Austin, TX 78745
512-444-4835
800-252-5151
FAX: 512-462-6636
e-mail: bcollier@brownschools.com
www.brownschools.com/rehabcenter

Admissions Department, Contact

Internationally recognized provider in brain injury/neurobehavioral treatment for children, adolescents, and adults with complex medical, physical and/or behavioral issues. Medical rehabilitation, neurobehavioral, and transitional living programs combine traditional therapies with education, vocational, substance abuse, and outpatient services.

8861 Cecil R Bomhr Rehabilitation Center of Nacogdoches Memorial Hospital

1204 N Mound Street
Nacogdoches, TX 75961
936-568-8547
FAX: 936-569-4616

Bette M Guzman, Director Rehabilitation Serv.

The only JCAHO and CARF, ASHA/PSB certified acute inpatient physical rehab center in East Texas.

8862 Clear Lake Rehabilitation Hospital

655 E Medical Center Boulevard
Webster, TX 77598
281-286-8783
FAX: 281-286-3569

Nancy Dungan

8863 Dallas Rehabilitation Institute

9713 Harry Hines Boulevard
Dallas, TX 75220
FAX: 214-904-6119

Judi McCann, Intake Coordinator

A 126-bed facility offering comprehensive and outpatient programs for brain injury, spinal cord injury, chronic pain, amputation, orthopedic and work-related injuries. Houses a full-service ICU and two surgical suites, a 14,000 square foot physical therapy gym, hydrotherapy pool and an on-site orthotics and prosthetics lab. The Institute is also accredited by CARF, JCAHO and Texas Rehabilitation Commission; certified by Medicare and is an affiliate of the University of Texas Medical School.

8864 Del Oro Institute for Rehabilitation

8081 Greenbriar Street
Houston, TX 77054
800-388-1HCA

Cece Matthews, Admissions

Del Oro offers an interdisciplinary team approach to care, meeting the needs of rehabilitation patients with a wide spectrum of services, including immediate access to surgery, intensive care or other medical treatment which may be required in an emergency.

8865 Ft. Worth Rehabilitation Hospital

6701 Oakmont Boulevard
Fort Worth, TX 76132
817-370-4727
FAX: 817-370-4977

Gala Lewis, Admissions

8866 Gonzales Warm Springs Rehabilitation Hospital

PO Box 58
Gonzales, TX 78629
830-672-6592
FAX: 830-672-8102

8867 Good Shepherd Medical Center: RehabCare Unit

621 N 5th Street
Longview, TX 75601
903-236-3937
FAX: 541-667-3443

Retta Crim, Program Manager

8868 HealthSouth Rehabilitation Center of Humble Texas

18903 S Memorial Drive
Humble, TX 77338
936-760-3443
FAX: 281-446-8022

8869 HealthSouth Rehabilitation Hospital of Bea umont

3340 Plaza 10 Boulevard
Beaumont, TX 77707
409-835-0835
FAX: 409-835-0649
www.healthsouth.com

8871 Hillcrest Baptist Medical Center: Rehab Care Unit

3000 Herring Avenue
Waco, TX 76708
254-202-4262
FAX: 254-202-8975

8872 IHS Hospital at Dallas

7955 Harry Hines
Dallas, TX 75235
800-366-4736
FAX: 214-637-6512

Richard G Allison, Admissions

8873 Institute for Rehabilitation & Research

1333 Moursund Street
Houston, TX 77030
713-799-7011
FAX: 713-797-5289

Karen Hart, VP Education

A national center for information, training, research, and technical assistance in independent living. The goal is to extend the body of knowledge in independent living and to improve the utilization of results of research programs and demonstration projects in this field. It has developed a variety of strategies for collecting, synthesizing, and disseminating information related to the field of independent living.

8874 Mabee Rehabilitation Center

1301 Pennsylvania Avenue
Fort Worth, TX 76104
817-882-2022
FAX: 813-882-2753

8875 Memorial Hospital Nacogdoches: RehabCare Unit

1204 Mound Street
Nacogdoches, TX 75961
936-275-3446
FAX: 936-569-4616

8876 Memorial Hospital and Medical Center

821 Jessee Drive
Drawer H
Midland, TX 79701
432-586-5864

8877 Methodist Hospital Rehabilitation Institute

3615 19th Street
Lubbock, TX 79410
806-793-4251
FAX: 806-793-4037

8878 Navarro Regional Hospital: RehabCare Unit

3201 W Highway 22
Corsicana, TX 75110
903-654-6800
FAX: 903-872-4627

8879 **Neurobehavioral Institute of Houston**
4100 Wellman Road
Conroe, TX 77384
936-788-7742
FAX: 281-367-5610

8880 **Plano Rehabilitation Hospital**
2800 W 15th Street
Plano, TX 75075
972-612-9118
FAX: 972-423-4293

8881 **Pocatello Rehabilitation Center**
777 Hospital Way
Pocatello, ID 83201
208-239-3600
FAX: 208-239-3795
www.ihc.com

R Eric Goodwin, Director Rehab

Provides the full spectrum of medical rehabilitation services including acute inpatient rehab, subacute rehab, home health and comprehensive outpatient services. Accredited by CARF and JCAHO.

8882 **Rebound: San Antonio**
12412 Judson Road
San Antonio, TX 78233
210-650-4949

8883 **Rehabilitation Hospital of Austin**
1215 Red River Street
Austin, TX 78701
512-479-8900
FAX: 512-474-2720

8884 **Rehabilitation Hospital of North Texas**
3200 Matlock Road
Arlington, TX 76015
817-419-0866
FAX: 817-468-3055

8885 **Rehabilitation Hospital of South Texas**
6226 Saratoga Boulevard
Corpus Christi, TX 78414
FAX: 361-994-8998

8886 **Rehabilitation Institute of San Antonio Healthsouth**
9119 Cinnamon Hill
San Antonio, TX 78240
210-691-0737
FAX: 210-558-1297
www.healthsouth.com

Diane B Lampe, CEO
Larry Spriggs, Chief Financial Officer

8887 **Rio Vista Rehabilitation Hospital**
1740 Curie Drive
El Paso, TX 79902
915-544-3399
800-999-8392
FAX: 915-544-4838

8888 **San Antonio Warm Springs Rehabilitation Hospital**
5101 Medical Drive
San Antonio, TX 78229
210-616-0100
FAX: 210-592-5452
www.warmsprings.org

8889 **Shannon Medical Center: RehabCare Unit**
120 E Harris Avenue
San Angelo, TX 76903
915-653-6741
FAX: 915-653-8261

8890 **Shriners Burn Institute: Galveston Unit**
815 Market Street
Galveston, TX 77550
FAX: 409-770-6749

8891 **Shriners Hospitals for Children, Houston**
6977 Main Street
Houston, TX 77030
713-797-1616
800-853-1240
FAX: 713-793-3770
e-mail: shriners@argolink.net

Steven Reiter, Administrator

Shriners Hospitals provides at no charge quality pediatric orthopedic serivces to children ages newborn to 18 years old. These services include both outpatient and inpatient needs. Specialties include cerebrel palsy, spina bifida, scoliosis, hand, hip and feet problems. An application is required and may be completed by phone.

8892 **South Arlington Medical Center: RehabCare Unit**
3301 Matlock Road
Arlington, TX 76015
817-472-4900
FAX: 817-472-4963

8893 **St. David's Rehabilitation Center**
919 E 32nd Street
Austin, TX 78705
512-867-5100
FAX: 512-370-4439

8894 **Valley Regional Medical Center: RehabCare Unit**
100 Alton Glore Boulevard
Brownsville, TX 78520
956-350-7790
FAX: 956-350-7796

Utah

8895 **LDS Hospital Rehabilitation Center**
Eighth Avenue & C Street
Salt Lake City, UT 84143
801-408-5450
888-301-3880
FAX: 801-408-5610

Jeanette Kucharski CRRN, Rehab Liaison

Located within a Trauma I Center, this facility provides comprehensive inpatient and outpatient rehabilitation to people with physical disabilities. CARF/JCAHO accredited. Low cost family housing is available and Medicaid/Medicare is accepted.

8896 **Primary Children's Medical Center**
100 N Medical Drive
Salt Lake City, UT 84113
801-588-2000
FAX: 801-588-2318

8897 **Rehabilitation Services**
University of Utah Hospitals and Clinics
50 N Medical Drive
Salt Lake City, UT 84132
801-581-2267
FAX: 801-585-3778

Sunny Vance-Lauritzen, Director
Trish Jensen, Program Coordinator

Provides quality, comprehensive, rehabilitation services to persons with complex rehabilitation needs, including spinal cord injuries, head trauma, stroke, and other disabling conditions. Rehabilitation Services has been serving physicians, their patients, and the community since 1965. Rehabilitation Services has been an established leader in comprehensive inpatient, outpatient and home/community rehabilitation programs. Accredited by CARF and JCAHO.

8898 **Shriners Hospitals for Children: Intermountain**

Fairfax Avenue @ Virginia Street
Salt Lake City, UT 84103 **801-536-3500**
800-841-0204
FAX: 801-536-3852

James Roach, Chief of Staff
Linda Raccuia, Applications Coordinator

One of nineteen hospitals in North America specializing in pediatric orthopedics (plus four hospitals providing pediatric burn treatment). This hospital serves the Intermountain region. All services provided in the hospital are at no cost to family, insurance company, nor state/federal agency regardless of ability to pay.

8899 **Stewart Rehabilitation Center: McKay Dee Hospital**

4335 S Harrison Boulevard
Suite D
Ogden, UT 84403 **801-387-2080**
FAX: 801-387-7720

Bob Martin, Nurse Coordinator

8900 **Western Rehabilitation Institute**

8074 S 1300 E
Sandy, UT 84094 **801-565-6500**
FAX: 801-565-6576

Vauna Allison, Admissions

Vermont

8901 **Vermont Achievement Center**

88 Park Street
Rutland, VT 05701 **802-775-1360**
FAX: 802-773-9656

Virginia

8902 **Inova Mount Vernon Hospital Rehabilitation Program**

Inova Rehabilitation Center
2501 Parkers Lane
Alexandria, VA 22306 **703-664-7592**
FAX: 703-664-7128
www.inova.com

Toni Jones, Rehab Admissions
Mary Beth Ireland, Inpatient Program Director
Ann Vennell, Outpatient Program Director

Inova Rehabilitation Center at Inova Mount Vernon Hospital provides comprehensive inpatient and outpatient programs for patients with brain injuries, stroke and spinal cord, neurological and orthopedic injuries.

8903 **Kluge Children's Rehabilitation Center**

2270 Ivy Road
Charlottesville, VA 22903 **434-924-5161**
FAX: 434-924-5559

8904 **Portsmouth General Hospital: RehabCare Unit**

850 Crawford Parkway
Portsmouth, VA 23704 **757-465-7772**

Anne Fisher, Program Manager

Washington

8905 **Good Samaritan Healthcare Physical Medicine and Rehabilitation**

407 14th Avenue SE
PO Box 190
Puyallup, WA 98371 **253-841-5849**
FAX: 253-770-5188
www.goodsamhealth.org

Diena Wasson RNC CCM, Rehab Trauma Coordinator

8906 **Northwest Hospital Center for Medical Rehabilitation**

1550 N 115th Street
Seattle, WA 98133 **360-706-7600**
FAX: 206-368-1399

8907 **Providence Medical Center**

500 17th Avenue
Seattle, WA 98122 **206-320-2098**
FAX: 206-320-3387

8908 **Providence Rehabilitation Services**

Providence Rehabilitation Services
Pacific and Nassau
Everett, WA 98206 **425-316-5020**

Elaine Thayer PT, Clinical Director

Continuum of care available: Acute Care, Inpatient Rehabilitation Unit, Transitional Care, Outpatient therapies, and In-home services.

8909 **Shriners Hospitals for Children: Spokane**

PO Box 2472
Spokane, WA 99210 **509-455-7844**
FAX: 509-623-0474
www.shrinershq.org

Chuck Young, Administrator
Cheri Hollenback, Director Nursing
Ron L Ferguson MD, Chief of Staff

Provides pediatric orthopedic services plus burn scar revision to children birth to 18. All services at no charge to the family.

West Virginia

8910 **MountainView Regional Rehabilitation Hospital**

1160 Van Voorhis Road
Morgantown, WV 26505 **304-292-8006**
800-388-2451
FAX: 304-598-1103

Carla Stadelman, Asst. Administrator

An 80-bed freestanding rehabilitation hospital serving central WV, southwestern PA, western MD and northwestern VA. Offers specialized programs to serve the patient population. Brain injury, spinal cord injury, stroke, neuromuscular, pulmonary disorders, pediatrics, ventilator dependence, orthopedics, amputee, case management and pain management.

8911 **Western Hills Rehabilitation Hospital**

3 Western Hills Drive
Parkersburg, WV 26102 **304-420-1300**
FAX: 304-420-1374

Wisconsin

8912 Extendicare
111 W Michigan Street
Milwaukee, WI 53203
414-908-8418
800-395-5000
FAX: 414-908-8123

8913 Midwest Neurological Rehabilitation Center
1701 Sharp Road
Waterford, WI 53185
800-697-5380
FAX: 262-534-8505

A comprehensive, integrated neurological rehabilitation center located only 25 minutes from Milwaukee. The Center provides seven comprehensive programs: acute hospital rehabilitation, pediatric acute rehabilitation, pediatric postacute rehabilitation, rehabilitation and skilled nursing, community-based rehabilitation and vocational rehabilitation.

8914 St. Catherine's Hospital
3556 7th Avenue
Kenosha, WI 53140
FAX: 262-653-5795

Rick Schultz, Program Manager

8915 St. Joseph Hospital
611 Saint Joseph Avenue
Marshfield, WI 54449
FAX: 715-389-3900

Cindy Bokath, Head Nurse

Wyoming

8916 Spalding Rehabilitation Hospital at Memorial Hospital of Laramie
300 E 23rd Street
Cheyenne, WY 82001
307-633-7770

Alabama

8917 Alabama Department of Rehabilitation Services

2129 E S Boulevard
Montgomery, AL 36116 **334-281-8780**
800-441-7607
FAX: 334-281-1973
www.rehab.state.al.us

Steve Shivers, Commissioner

State agency which provides services and assistance to Alabama's children and adults with disabilities.

8918 Alabama Goodwill Industries

2350 Green Springs Highway S
Birmingham, AL 35205 **205-323-6331**
FAX: 205-324-9059

Don Smith, Director

Work adjustment and remunerative work programs.

8919 Alabama Veterans Facility

809 Green Spring Highway
Homewood, AL 35209 **205-916-2700**

Veterans medical clinic offering disabled veterans medical treatments.

8920 American Rehab Center Neuro Care Unit Mobile Infirmary

5 Mobile Infirmary Circle
Mobile, AL 36607 **251-431-5559**
FAX: 251-431-5222

Robert Berg, President

Postacute rehabilitation program.

8921 Arc of Jefferson County

215 21st Avenue S
Birmingham, AL 35205 **205-323-6383**
FAX: 205-323-0085

William F Hoeble II PhD, Executive Director

The Arc of Jefferson County serves children and adults with mental retardation and/or other developmental disabilities. Services are provided through the following programs: the HOPE (Helping Others through Parent Education) Early Intervention Program; Adult Day Services; Residential Services; and Arc-Way Industries, a sheltered and supported employment program.

8922 Association for Retarded Citizens of Jefferson County (The Arc)

215 21st Avenue S
Birmingham, AL 35205 **205-323-6383**
FAX: 205-323-0085

William F Hoehle II PhD, Executive Director

The ARC has four primary components. The HOPE Program provides early intervention therapy services to developmentally delayed infants and toddlers up to the age of three years. The ARC also provides services to adults ages 21 and over with mental retardation. Adult services provides education, pre-vocational screening, and socialization skills training. Employment services provides vocational training, a sheltered workshop, off-site job skills training, job coach services and more. Residential s

8923 Briarcliff Nursing Home & Rehab Facility

850 9th Street NW
Alabaster, AL 35007 **205-663-3859**
FAX: 205-663-9791

Donna Jones, Director Nursing

Postacute rehabilitation program.

8924 Butler Adult Training Center

680 Hardscramble Road
Greenville, AL 36037 **334-382-2353**
FAX: 334-382-9518

Jessica Wyrosdick, Director

Clients 21 years of age and older who are mentally retarded. School age clients are also served at the center and must also be mentally retarded. Clients receive training in Independent Living Skills, Self-Care, Language Skills, Learning, Self Direction and Economic Self-Sufficiency. The clients also participate in Special Olympics activities.

8925 Cheaha Mental Health

PO Box 1248
Sylacauga, AL 35150 **256-245-1340**
FAX: 256-245-1343
http://accmhb.org/members/cheaha/cheaha.html

Larry Morris, Executive Director

Offers mental health rehabilitation, respite care, residential facilities and more for the mentally disabled. Serves Talladega, Coosa, Clay and Randolph counties.

8926 Children's Rehabilitation Service

2121 E S Boulevard
Montgomery, AL 36116
FAX: 334-281-1388

8927 Chilton-Shelby Mental Health Center/ The Mitchell Center

PO Drawer 689
Calera, AL 35040
205-663-1252
FAX: 205-685-0900
www.chiltonshelby.org/

Melodie Crawford, Executive Director

Offers mental health rehabilitation services and more for the recovery of mentally disabled adults. Serves Chilton and Shelby counties.

8928 EL Darden Rehabilitation Center

1001 E Broad Street
Gadsden, AL 35999
FAX: 256-547-5761

Tom Strother

Work hardening and disciplinary programs.

8929 Easter Seals Central Alabama

2125 E S Boulevard
Montgomery, AL 36116
334-288-0240
FAX: 334-288-7171
e-mail: easterseals@worldnet.att.net

J Larry Johnson, Administrator
Dr. Susan McKim, Director Rehab

A private, nonprofit organization offering services audiology, physical, occupational, lymphedemia and speech therapy, psychological counseling, vocational evaluation and assessment, person, social and work adjustment training, GED preparation, computer service training, job placement and follow-up, and special learning disabilities service and supported employment service.

8930 Easter Seals West Alabama

1110 6th Avenue E
Tuscaloosa, AL 35401
205-759-1211
800-726-1216
FAX: 205-349-1162
e-mail: eswa@dbtech.net

Loie Sears Robinson, Administrator

Leading organization in helping children and adults with disabilities to live with equality, dignity and independence. Rehabilitation services are provided in two divisions: outpatient rehabilitation division (physical therapy, occupational therapy, speech therapy, hearing evaluation, sell and service hearind aids) and vocational division (vocational evaulation and vocational development). Services are rendered regardless of age, race, sex, color, creed, national origin, veteran's status.

8931 Geer Adult Training Center

PO Box 419
Carrollton, AL 35447
205-367-8032
FAX: 205-367-8032

Yvonne Williams, Program Coordinator

8932 Goodwill Easter Seals of the Gulf Coast

2448 Gordon Smith Drive
Mobile, AL 36617
251-471-1581
800-411-0068
FAX: 251-476-4303
e-mail: stephanie@gesgc.org
www.goodwill-easterseals.org

Stephanie Constantine, VP Marketing

Vocational, medical, pre-school education, day care, recreation and other support services.

8933 Indian Rivers

1915 6th Street
 # 2190
Tuscaloosa, AL 35401
205-345-1600
FAX: 205-391-0106

Laurie Prentice-Dunn, Director

Services are available to adults who have serious mental illness resulting in personal, family or work-related problems. Counseling may take place in either individual or group settings, identification, evaluation and treatment services are available to persons who experience problems related to alcohol and drug abuse and counseling services are available for children and adolescents who have a severe emotional disturbance causing discipline problems at home and school.

8934 Lighthouse

PO Box 218
Brent, AL 35034
205-926-4681
FAX: 205-926-6016

Gwen Langley, Program Coordinator

8935 Low Vision Clinic/UAB School of Optometry

1716 University Boulevard
Birmingham, AL 35294
205-934-2625
FAX: 205-934-0911

Dr. RW Nowakowski, Chief of Staff
Dr. M Swanson, Chief Low Vision Patient Care
Brenda Watkins, Optometric Technician

Multidisciplinary clinic in a major medical center which provides a comprehensive vision evaluation and prescription of low vision aids for those who are visually impaired. Fees are charged for all examination procedures, special diagnostic tests and materials with most insurance plans accepted. Cost depends on services rendered.

8936 MARC Enterprises

759 Congress Street
Mobile, AL 36603
251-470-0821
FAX: 251-470-0824

Andrew Acklin, Division Director

Serving the mentally retarded of Mobile County both locally and through its state and national affiliations. Their united efforts through this voluntary association assure the availability of services and provide the opportunity for achievement.

8937 North Central Alabama Mental Retardation Authority

1621 Wolverine Drive SE
 # 597
Decatur, AL 35601
256-355-7315
FAX: 256-355-7317

Earl E Brightwell, Director

NCA, MRA, Inc. functions as an entrance to the service delivery system for the Alabama Department of Mental Health and Mental Retardation and is responsible for planning, development, implementation of programs, sanction, monitoring, referral, and case management for persons with mental retardation/developmental disabilities in Morgan, Lawrence and Limestone Counties.

8938 Northwest Alabama: Rehabilitation Center Easter Seal

1450 Avalon Avenue
Muscle Shoals, AL 35661
FAX: 256-381-1110

Robert H Nelson, Administrator
Sheila Phillips, Administrative Assistant

8939 **Southeastern Blind Rehabilitation Center**

Department of Veterans Affairs Medical Center
700 19th Street S
Birmingham, AL 35233 **205-933-8101**
FAX: 205-933-4484

Mark Voorhies, Director
George Sands, Assistant Director

The Center is a 32-bed inpatient blind rehabilitation program which serves the southeastern region. The majority of client services are for basic adjustment and management to sight loss. Basic services include: low vision, orientation and mobility, manual skills, ADL and communications. Training on electronic mobility aids and adapted computers is also available on a restricted basis. The program maintains graduate education affiliations and an active applied research program.

8940 **Tennessee Valley Rehabilitation**

PO Box 1926
Decatur, AL 35602 **256-350-2041**
FAX: 256-350-2806

Charles Harvell

Work hardening and disciplinary programs.

8941 **Vaughn-Blumberg Services**

2715 Flynn Road
PO Box 8646
Dothan, AL 36304 **334-793-3102**
FAX: 334-793-7740

Ed Dorsey, Executive Director

8942 **West Central Alabama Easter Seals Rehabilitation Center**

2906 Citizens Parkway
PO Box 750
Selma, AL 36702 **334-872-8421**
800-801-4776
FAX: 334-872-3907
e-mail: wcarcdw@tomnet.com
www.al.easter-seals.org/selma

Larry F Lewis, Administrator
David White, Program Coordinator

Vocational evaluation, job development, employment development, job coaching, counseling, medical services, audiology, pre-school development programs.

Alaska

8943 **Alaska Center for the Blind and Visually Impaired**

3903 Taft Drive
Anchorage, AK 99517 **907-248-7770**
800-770-7517
FAX: 907-248-7517
e-mail: info@alaskabvi.org
www.alaskabvi.org

Jim King, Executive Director

Services to help the adult residential or community-based student become independent and self-sufficient by offering independent travel, Braille reading and writing, use of assiative technology such as talking computers, manual skills and personal, as well as home management. There is a special program for those 55 years of age and older who are experiencing a vision loss and another program for rural Alaska Native youth who are visually impaired.

8944 **Alaska Veterans Facility**

4201 Tudor Centre Drive
Suite 115
Anchorage, AK 99508 **907-277-3224**

Veterans medical clinic offering disabled veterans medical treatments.

Arizona

8945 **Arizona Center for the Blind and Visually Impaired**

3100 E Roosevelt Street
Phoenix, AZ 85008 **602-273-7411**
FAX: 602-273-7410
e-mail: sgibbs@acbvi.org
www.acbvi.org

James LeMay, Executive Director
Sharon Gibbs, Information/Referral Specialist
Diana Miladin, Communication/Development Coord.

A private, nonprofit organization that provides comprehensive rehabilitation services and more for the blind and visually handicapped. The staff includes 20 instructional and adminstrative professionals.

8946 **Arizona Industries for the Blind**

3013 W Lincoln Street
Phoenix, AZ 85009 **602-269-5131**
FAX: 602-269-9462

DH Peterson, General Manager

Offers rehabilitation services, vocational/pre-vocational evaluation and training, work adjustment, job development and employment and training opportunties for individuals who are blind.

8947 **Beacon Foundation for the Mentally Retarded**

25 E Drachman Street
Tucson, AZ 85705 **520-624-3454**
FAX: 520-623-3494

Paul Wagler, Chief Executive Director

Committed to effectively assisting adults with disabilities to maximize their personal, social, vocational and educational skills in order to attain a successful and meaningful independence within the Tucson community.

8948 **Carondelet Brain Injury Programs and Services (Bridges Now)**

350 N Wilmot Road
Tucson, AZ 85711 **520-873-3994**
FAX: 520-873-3743
e-mail: sascher@carondelet.org

Sarah Ascher, Rehab Coordinator

Comprehensive outpatient rehabilitation program. PT, OT, ST, Psychology and Rehab Counseling Services.

8949 **Casa Grande Rehabilitation Programs**

208 W Main Street
Casa Grande, AZ 85222 **602-254-0754**
FAX: 520-426-9471

James Musick, Executive Director

8950 **Community Rehabilitation Services: Tucson**

1789 W Jefferson
2nd Floor NW
Phoenix, AZ 85007 **602-542-3332**
TTY:602-542-6049

Skip Bingham, Administration

Postacute rehabilitation program.

8951 Desert Life Health Care Center
1919 W Medical Street
Tucson, AZ 85704
FAX: 520-544-0930

Postacute rehabilitation program.

8952 Freestone Rehabilitation Center
10617 E Oasis Drive
Apache Junction, AZ 85220
480-986-1531
FAX: 480-986-1538

Randy Gray, Executive Director

8953 Institute for Human Development
PO Box 5630
Flagstaff, AZ 86011
928-523-7319
FAX: 928-523-9127

Richard Carroll, Director

8954 John C Lincoln Hospital North Mountain
250 E Dunlap Avenue
Phoenix, AZ 85020
602-943-2381
FAX: 602-944-8062
www.jcl.com

Dan Coleman, President

8955 La Frontera Center
502 W 29th Street
Tucson, AZ 85713
520-884-9920

Dr. Floyd Martinez

Provides remunerative work.

8956 Manor Care Nursing and Rehab Center: Tucson
3705 N Swan Road
Tucson, AZ 85718
FAX: 520-529-0038

Mark Bedinger, Administrator
Sheila Powell, Director Admissions & Marketing

Postacute rehabilitation program.

8957 Nova Care
1010 E McDowell Road
Suite 102
Phoenix, AZ 85006
602-256-7232
FAX: 602-256-7292

Work hardening and disciplinary programs.

8958 Perry Rehabilitation Center
3146 E Windsor Avenue
Phoenix, AZ 85008
602-958-0400
FAX: 602-957-7610
e-mail: perrycenteratuswest.com

Robin Ratcliff, Director

Provides services for people with disabilities, cognitive disabilities including residential services, day treatment, job training and job placement.

8959 Phoenix Veterans Center
141 E Palm Lane
Suite 100
Phoenix, AZ 85004
602-379-4769
FAX: 602-379-4130

Veterans medical clinic offering disabled veterans medical treatments.

8960 Progress Valley: Phoenix
4430 N 23rd Avenue
Phoenix, AZ 85015
602-274-5424
FAX: 602-274-5473
e-mail: jlarson@progressvalley.org

Julie Larsson, Associate Director
Joe Brugh, Senior Counselor

Residential aftercare for alcoholism and chemical dependency. Certified chemical dependency counselors provide individual treatment.

8961 Samaritan Rehabilitation Institute
1111 E McDowell Road
Phoenix, AZ 85006
602-239-2635
FAX: 602-239-5868

Ronald Herrick, Associate Administrator

8962 Scottsdale Memorial Hospital Rehabilitation Services
7400 E Osborn Road
Scottsdale, AZ 85251
480-314-2100
FAX: 480-675-4478

Peter Frick, President

8963 Toyei Industries
HC-58 Box 55
Ganado, AZ 86505
928-736-2418
FAX: 928-736-2495

Russell Morgan, Interim Executive Director
Anita Hildreth, Social Services Manager
Walt Jones, HCBS/PR Coordinator

Serves the needs of developmentally disabled and the severely mentally impaired adult citizens of the Navajo Nation and other Indian Nations. Staff of 60+ serves the needs of all the Navajo adults. Services include day treatment programs, home community-based services and residential and group home services.

8964 Tucson Association for the Blind and Visually Imparied
3767 E Grant Road
Tucson, AZ 85716
520-795-1331
FAX: 520-795-1336
e-mail: gluini@tabvi.org

Gene Luini, Executive Director

Offers health services, counseling, social work, home and personal management, computer training, low vision aids and more for the visually handicapped 18 years or older.

8965 Valley of the Sun Rehabilitation Hospital
13460 N 67th Avenue
Glendale, AZ 85304
602-214-2256
FAX: 623-878-5254

Ken Manders, CEO

8966 Yuma Center for the Visually Impaired
2770 S Avenue B
Yuma, AZ 85364
928-726-1310
FAX: 928-783-3261

Calvin Roberts, Director

A private nonprofit agency offering services for totally blind and legally blind children and adults in the Arizona area.

Arkansas

8967 Arkansas Lighthouse for the Blind
PO Box 192666
Little Rock, AR 72219
501-562-2222
FAX: 501-568-5275
e-mail: ALB49799@aol.com

Sue Walker, Executive VP

Offers educational industrial evaluation and training to the legally blind and multihandicapped. Funded by workshop sales and contributions, the staff includes ten full time employees

8968 Beverly Enterprises Network
1200 S Waldron Road
Fort Smith, AR 72903
479-452-0469
800-666-9996
FAX: 479-452-5131

Offers a progressive approach to subacute care. The goal of this organization is to assist injured and disabled individuals regain the level of independence to which they have been accustomed. Provides support and training programs, patient and family services and specialty programs for patients.

8969 Easter Seals: Arkansas
3920 Woodland Heights Road
Little Rock, AR 72212
501-227-3600
877-533-3600
FAX: 501-227-3658
e-mail: mail@ar.easter-seals.org
www.ar.easter-seals.org

Sharon Moone-Jochums, President/CEO
Linda Rogers, VP Programs
Stephanie Smith, VP Finance/Administration

8970 HEALTHSOUTH Rehabilitation Hospital Fort Smith
1401 S J Street
Fort Smith, AR 72901
479-785-3300
FAX: 479-785-8599
www.healthsouth.com

Holli Baker, Director Business Development

A free-standing 80-bed comprehensive physical medicine and rehabilitation hospital offering inpatient and outpatient services. Provides specialized medical and therapy services, designed to assist physically challenged persons to reach their highest level of independent function.

8971 Lions World Services for the Blind
2811 Fair Park Boulevard
Little Rock, AR 72204
501-664-7100
800-248-0754
FAX: 501-664-2743
e-mail: training@lwsb.org
www.lwsb.org

Ramona Sangalli, Executive Director

Offers services in the areas of health, education, recreation, rehabilitation, counseling, social work, employment, computer training and more for all legally blind residents of the U.S. The staff includes 56 full time employees.

8972 Little Rock Vet Center #0713
201 W Broadway Street
Suite A
North Little Rock, AR 72114
501-324-6395
FAX: 501-324-6928

Veterans medical clinic offering disabled veterans medical treatments.

8973 New Medico Rehabilitation Center at Timber Ridge Ranch
PO Box 208
Benton, AR 72018
501-594-5211
FAX: 501-594-5211

California

8974 ARC-VC Magic Muffin Cafe
1661 Pacific Avenue
Oxnard, CA 93033
805-483-0341
FAX: 805-483-2594

Shirley Dove

Provides remunerative work.

8975 ARC: VC Ventura
2647 N Ventura Avenue
Ventura, CA 93001
805-652-0541
FAX: 805-652-0542

Tom Wright, Executive Associate

8976 Accentcare
135 Technology Drive
Suite 150
Irvine, CA 92618
800-834-3059
e-mail: info@accentcare.com
www.accentcare.com

Postacute rehabilitation program: home care aides follow through with rehabilitation instructions given by physical, occupational and speech therapists. Other home care services are available, serving special needs for Alzheimer's, blind, brain injury, MS, ostomies, parkinsonism, spinal injury and stroke.

8977 American Rehab Centers Neuro Care Unit
2776 Pacific Avenue
Long Beach, CA 90806
562-426-4561
FAX: 562-427-0149

Postacute rehabilitation program.

8978 Arrow Center
3035 G Street
San Diego, CA 92102
619-233-8855
FAX: 619-233-4932

Dorothy Cummings

Work hardening and disciplinary programs.

8979 Association for Retarded Citizens: Alameda County
575 Independent Road
Oakland, CA 94621
510-639-4680
FAX: 510-639-4684

Offers the Right Track program in which selected workers are grouped together on a contract basis to maximize work productivity. Provides a full benefit package, as well as a permanent supervisor. A worker is matched to a job of at least 20 hours per week and then trained by the staff of The Right Track.

8980 **Azure Acres Chemical Dependency Recovery Center**

2264 Green Hill Road
Sebastopol, CA 95472 **707-823-3385**
FAX: 707-823-8972

Uwe Gunnersen, President

Offers rehabilitation services and residential care for the person with an alcohol or drug abuse related problems.

8981 **Back in the Saddle**

9775 Mockingbird Avenue
Apple Valley, CA 92308 **760-240-3217**
FAX: 760-240-3274

Richard Smith PhD, Co-Director
Erika Reed, Co-Director

A long term community residential facility for head injured adults. House parents live on-site; and oversee a variety of programs which are individually designed and might include classes in community college, placement in a workshop or on a workstation, volunteer positions and home skills assignments. Recreational outing range from horseback riding to weekend camping. Apartment programs available as set-up. Price: $2800-$3000 per month.

8982 **Ballard Rehabilitation Hospital**

1760 W 16th Street
San Bernardino, CA 92411 **909-473-1200**
FAX: 909-473-1276

Robert Herrick, CEO
Mary Hunt, COO
Patty Meinhardt, Director Marketing/Admissions

Ballard Rehab Hospital is a free standing specialty hospital and provides the complete continuum of acute, subacute and outpatient rehabilitation, dedicated to providing rehab seminars to adults and children. The following inpatient and outpatient programs are available: CNA (Stroke) Rehab; Spinal Cord Injury Rehab; Brain Injury Rehab; Pain Management Rehab; Injured Worker Programs; and Post Amputation Rehab.

8983 **Bayview Nursing and Rehabilitation**

516 Willow Street
Alameda, CA 94501 **510-521-5600**
FAX: 510-865-6441

Postacute rehabilitation program.

8984 **Belden Center**

606 Humboldt Street
Santa Rosa, CA 95404 **707-579-2735**
FAX: 707-579-4145

Wes Killian, Program Director

Postacute rehabilitation program.

8985 **Brotman Medical Center: RehabCare Unit**

3828 Delmas Terrace
Culver City, CA 90232 **310-836-7000**
800-677-1238
FAX: 310-202-4105

Ellen Graham, Program Manager
Kevin McAninch, Director Provider

Culver City is centrally located within the city of Los Angeles. These are two programs offering inpatient rehabilitation. The acute rehab program is designed for patients who need physical rehabilitation due to injury or medical disability. This program requires patients to participate in 3 hours therapy per day. The sub-acute program is designed especially for patients who need rehab but cannot tolerate the intensity of the acute rehab program.

8986 **Build Rehabilitation Industries**

1323 Truman Street
San Fernando, CA 91340 **818-898-0020**
FAX: 818-898-1949

Matthew Lynch, President/CEO
Michele A Utley, VP

Comprehensive C.A.R.F. Accredited vocational rehabilitation services for adults with disabilities or other barriers to employment. Programs include: Sheltered Workshops, Work Evaluation, Work Hardening and Adjustment, Supported Employment, Job Placement, Independent Living Skills, Behavior Management, Adult Development Center, On-the-Job Training, and One-Stop Workforce Development Career Center.

8987 **California Elwyn**

18325 Mount Baldy Circle
Fountain Valley, CA 92708 **714-557-6313**
FAX: 714-963-2961
e-mail: hmichaels@ogelwyn.org
www.elwyn.org

Henry Michales, Program Manager
Joan McKinney, Executive Director

Provides opportunities for people challenged by physical and mental disabilities who are 18 or older. California Elwyn develops an Individual Rehabilitation Plan for all consumers. Contract work, shrinkwrap, janitorial are just some of the types of jobs done. Supported Employment Services are available and over 100 consumers currently are employed. Funded by the State Department of Rehabilitation and Vocational Rehabilitation.

8988 **California Eye Institute**

1360 E Turdan Avenue
Fresno, CA 93720 **559-225-2737**
FAX: 559-499-5090

Virgil Snow

A private, nonprofit agency offering services such as health, educational, recreational, rehabilitation and employment counseling to the totally blind, legally blind and visually impaired. The staff includes two full time workers.

8989 **California Veterans Center**

859 S Harbor Boulevard
Anaheim, CA 92805 **714-776-0161**

Veterans medical clinic offering disabled veterans medical treatments.

8990 **Camp Recovery Centers**

Camp
3192 Glen Canyon Road
Scotts Valley, CA 95066 **831-438-1868**
800-924-2879
FAX: 831-438-5833
www.camprecovery.com

Melissa Preshaw, Marketing Manager

A free-standing social model recovery center for chemical dependency located on 25 wooded acres in the Santa Cruz Mountains. The services include: medical detoxification, complete medical evaluation, psychiatric evaluation and counseling, psychological testing, individual counseling and more. Helps the recovery from chemical dependency in a easier, warm and caring environment.

8991 Campobello Chemical Dependency Recovery Center

3250 Guernville Road
Santa Rosa, CA 95401 **707-579-4066**
800-805-1833
FAX: 707-579-1603
e-mail: campocdrc@aol.com

Kathy Willis NCAC CEAP, Executive Director
James Cody CADC II, Program Director

8992 Casa Colina Centers for Rehabilitation

255 E Bonita Avenue
PO Box 6001
Pomona, CA 91769 **909-596-7733**
800-926-5462
FAX: 909-596-7306
e-mail: rehab@casacolina.org
www.casacolina.org

Fred Arrow, Public Relations

Casa Colina, has pioneered effective programs to create opportunity for health, productivity and self-esteem for persons with disability since 1936. Through medical rehabilitation, transitional living, return to work, residential, community, and prevention and wellness programs. Casa Colina serves more than 6,000 persons annually. Casa Colina, a non-profit organization, offers a unique spectrum of opportunities, achievement and results to patients and their families.

8993 Casa Colina Paova Village

PO Box 6001
Pomona, CA 91769 **909-596-7733**
800-926-5462
FAX: 909-593-0153
e-mail: rehab@casacolina.org
www.casacolina.org

Michelle Stoddard, Director Residential Services
Fred Arotuan, Director Public Relations

Long term residential services for adults with developmental disability. Residences include Malmquist House, Woodbend House, and Hillsdale House, all located in Claremont, California.

8994 Casa Colina Residential Services: Rancho Pino Verde

11981 Midway
Lucerne Valley, CA 92356 **760-248-6245**
FAX: 760-248-2245
e-mail: rehab@casacolina.org
www.casacolina.org

Long term residential services in rural environment for adults with brain injury.

8995 Casa Colina Transitional Living Center

255 E Bonita Avenue
Pomonana, CA 91767 **909-593-7611**
FAX: 909-593-7541
www.casacolina.org

Postacute rehabilitation program.

8996 Casa Colina Transitional Living Center: Pomona

2850 N Garey Avenue
 # 6001
Pomona, CA 91767 **909-596-7733**
800-926-5462
FAX: 909-596-7306
e-mail: ccrehabe@lightside.com
www.casacolina.org

Fred Aronow, Director Public Relations

Post acute short term residential program for persons with brain injury. In a home-like setting, therapy promotes successful re-entry to home and community living.

8997 Cedars of Marin

Bolinas Avenue & Upper Road
PO Box 947
Ross, CA 94957 **415-454-5310**
FAX: 415-454-0573

Brenda McIvor, Executive Director
Alexa Witter, Executive Assistant

Provides residential and day programs for adults with developmental disabilities.

8998 Center for Neuro Skills

2658 Mount Vernon Avenue
Bakersfield, CA 93306 **805-323-4199**
800-843-2943
FAX: 661-872-5150
e-mail: cns@neuroskills.com
www.neuroskills.com/~cns

John Schultz, VP
Steve Katomski, Admissions

A comprehensive, post-acute, community based head-injury rehabilitation program serving over 100 clients per year. Since 1980, CNS has effectively treated the entire spectrum of head-injured clients, including those with severe behavioral disorders, cognitive/perceptual impairments, speech/language problems, physical disabilities and post-concussion syndrome.

8999 Center for the Partially Sighted

12301 Wilshire
Suite 600
Los Angeles, CA 90025 **310-458-3501**
800-481-EYES
FAX: 310-458-8179
e-mail: info@low-vision.org
www.low-vision.org

LaDonna Ringering PhD, Executive Director
Pat Jordan, Public Information Manager
Phyllis Amarai PhD, Clinical Director

Services for partially sighted and legally blind people include low vision evaluations, the design and prescription of low vision devices and adaptive technology, as well as counseling and rehabilitation training (independent living skills and orientation/mobility training). Special programs include children's program, diabetes and vision loss program, HIV and vision loss program. Store carries low vision aids. Catalog available.

9000 Central Coast Neurobehavioral Center OPTIONS

PO Box 877
800 Quintana # 2-C
Morro Bay, CA 93442 **805-772-6066**
FAX: 805-772-6067
www.optionsccnbc.org

Mike Mamot, CEO
Ole Von Frausing-Borch, COO

Serves adults with developmental disabilities, traumatic head injuries, or other neurological impairments. OPTIONS operates two transitional living centers, eight licensed residential facilities, two licensed community integration day programs and a licensed short term stabilization center. Services offered include: supported and independent living services, group and individual vocational services, neuropsychological assessment, occupational therapy, cognitive therapy, speech therapy and more.

9001 Cerebral Palsy: North County Center

205 W Mission
Suite 6
Escondido, CA 92025 **760-743-1050**
FAX: 760-746-0172

Gill Hennessey, Director

Provides remunerative work.

9002 Children's Hospital Central California Reh abilitation Center

9300 Valley Children's Place
Madera, CA 93638
559-353-8030
FAX: 559-353-8650
www.valleychildrens.org

Robin Gomez RN MA CRRN, Manager

We provide rehabilitation services for those birth through 21 years in both inpatient and outpatient settings.

9003 Children's Hospital Los Angeles Rehabilitation Program

4650 W Sunset Boulevard
 # 6
Los Angeles, CA 90027
323-669-2231
FAX: 323-665-4118

Maureen McMorrow, Medical Director

A comprehensive program specializing in the treatment of patients with brain injury.

9004 Children's Therapy Center

770 Paseo Camarillo
Suite 120
Camarillo, CA 93010
805-383-1501
FAX: 805-383-1504
e-mail: ctcinc@paragon,net
www.ctcinc@paragon.net

Jo Murphy Hyland, Administrative Director

Provides individual occupational therapy, speech/language therapy, family/child consulting, education services and physical therapy consultation for children. Evaluations and treatment are on an individual basis and special emphasis is placed on a multidisciplinary approach with information sharing, and often team treatment.

9005 Clausen House

88 Vernon Street
Oakland, CA 94610
510-839-0050
FAX: 510-444-5790
e-mail: info@clausenhouse.org
www.clausenhouse.org

Nan Butterworth, Executive Director
Megan Hornbecker, Development Associate

A private nonprofit organization which emphasizes greater independence for developmentally disabled adults. Programs encompass residential services, adult education, day program training, recreational opportunities, supported employment services, independent living, supported living training and assistance.

9006 Coastline Enterprises

700 Northcrest Drive
Suite D4
Crescent City, CA 95531
707-464-8338
FAX: 707-465-1029

Nancy L Boage, Director

Services people with special needs, and their families.

9007 Community Access Program: Hilltop

2800 Hilltop Mall Road
Suite 1250
Richmond, CA 94806
510-222-8266
FAX: 510-222-8290
e-mail: carolmcap@aol.com
www.ContraCostaARC.com

Carol Anne McCrary, Director
Naomi Santos, Program Coordinator

A private nonprofit membership-based organization dedicated to enhancing the quality of life of individuals with mental retardation and other developmental disabilities.

9008 Community Hospital and Rehabilitation Center of Los Gatos-Saratoga

355 Dardanelli Lane
Los Gatos, CA 95032
408-866-4020
FAX: 408-866-4077
e-mail: CHLG.ask@renethealth.com
www.communityhospitalLG.com

Modestine Fain, Director, Rehab Services

Offers rehabilitation services, inpatient and outpatient care, physical therapy, occupational therapy and more for the physically challenged adult.

9009 Coronado Hospital

250 Prospect Place
Coronado, CA 92118
619-435-6250
FAX: 619-522-3782

Postacute rehabilitation program.

9010 Critical Air Medicine

Montgomery Field
4141 Kearny Villa Road
San Diego, CA 92123
858-514-6060
800-247-8326
FAX: 619-571-0835

Offers emergency medical care by air medical transport carriers. These carriers are fully equipped with medical equipment and supplies for cardiovascular emergencies, respiratory supplies, orthopedic supplies and medications.

9011 Crutcher's Serenity House

50 Hillcrest Drive
PO Box D
Deer Park, CA 94576
877-274-4968
FAX: 707-963-2309
www.crutcherssh.com

Robert Crutcher, CEO/Owner
Lu Crutcher, Executive Director

A privately owned and operated facility that introduces to residents a new lifestyle free of all chemicals, and a new awareness of their total being. The length of the program is four weeks and is within five minutes of an acute care hospital. The Center is licensed for 19 beds, male and female located in a home-like setting with an emphasis on maintaining a family atmosphere.

9012 Daniel Freeman Rehabilitation Centers

333 N Prairie Avenue
Inglewood, CA 90301
310-674-7050
FAX: 310-419-8232

Louis Ceppi, Associate Administrator

Comprehensive rehabilitation services which address needs and issues of the physically diabled and their families. We offer accute input rehabilitation, outpatient and short term skilled nursing rehabilitaion. Specialty areas include: brain injury, stroke, spinal chord injury, chronic pain, arthritis.

9013 Delano Regional Medical Center

1401 Garces Highway
Delano, CA 93215
661-725-4800
FAX: 661-721-5211

Postacute rehabilitation program.

9014 Devereux Santa Barbara
PO Box 6784
Santa Barbara, CA 93160
805-968-2525
FAX: 805-968-3247
e-mail: amcniff@devereux.org
www.devereux.org

Anne McNiff, Director Agency Relations
Anna Martinez, Admissions Coordinator
Janis Johnson, Public Relations Coordinator

Serves ages 8-88, who have developmental disabilities, emotional disturbances, neurological impairments, brain injuries, schizophrenia, autism, and dual diagnosis. The Center has a licensed capacity of 188 served in a continuum of services including residential, vocational, educational and more.

9015 Division of Physical Medicine and Rehabilitation
San Joaquin General Hospital
500 W Hospital Road
French Camp, CA 95231
209-468-6280
FAX: 209-468-6281
www.sjphysicalmedicine.com

Carolyn Genschmer, Rehabilitation Coordinator

Offers rehabilitation services, inpatient and outpatient care, speech therapy, physical therapy, occupational therapy and more for the physically challenged individual.

9016 Dr. Karen H Chao Developmental Optometry Karen H. Chao. O.D.
121 S Del Mar Avenue
Suite A
San Gabriel, CA 91776
626-287-0401
FAX: 626-287-1457
e-mail: drkhchao@yahoo.com
www.BeacoNet.com/Dr.Chao

James Young, Practice Manager

Developmental optometrist specializing in the testing and treatment of vision problems and the enhancement of visual performance. Performs visual perceptual testing and training for children and adults. Undetected vision problems interfere with the ability to achieve and are highly correlated with learning difficulties and developmental problems. Provides the opportunity to overcome vision and visual-perceptual dysfunctions.

9017 Early Childhood Services
216 N Gold Canyon
Ridgecrest, CA 93555
760-375-8494
FAX: 760-375-1288
e-mail: cbridges@iwvisp.com

Cristine Bridges, Director

9018 East County Training Center
1855/1865 John Towers Avenue
El Cajon, CA 92020
619-590-9324
FAX: 619-449-7853

Val Swan

Work adjustment and remunerative work programs.

9019 East Los Angeles Doctors Hospital
4060 Whittier Boulevard
Los Angeles, CA 90023
323-881-1112
FAX: 323-980-9824

Postacute rehabilitation program.

9020 Easter Seals Bay Area
2757 Telegraph Avenue
Oakland, CA 94612
510-835-2131
FAX: 510-444-2470
www.esba.org

Mike Pelfini, Executive VP/CEO
Johnny Jones, VP

9021 Easter Seals Superior California
Sacramento Center & Regional Offices
3205 Hurley Way
Sacramento, CA 95864
916-485-6711
FAX: 916-485-2653
e-mail: info@easterseals-superiorca.org
www.easterseals-superiorca.org

Gary Kasai, President/CEO
Terry Colborn, VP Programs/Government Affairs
Jessica Cone, VP Marketing/Development

Provides outpatient rehabilitation services including day training programs for adults with disabilities and traumatic brain injuries, warm water therapy, non-public agency services to children including pediatric OT and PT services, work training/employment services, medical equipment loans, early intervention services for infants and toddlers. Serving the counties of Alpine, Calaveras, El Dorado, Sacramento, San Joaquin, Sutter, Tuolumne, Yolo, Yuba, Amador, Stanislaus, Nevada and Placer, CA.

9022 El Mirador Rehabilitation Center at Desert Hospital
1180 N Indian Canyon Drive
Suite W214
Palm Springs, CA 92262
760-416-4550
FAX: 760-416-4555

Offers occupational, physical and speech therapy.

9023 Exceed: A Division of Valley Resource Cent er
2050 Trumble Road
PO Box 1776
Perris, CA 92572
909-657-0609
FAX: 909-657-2277
e-mail: vrctwohip@aol.com
www.exceed-aws.com

Kathy Coake, Program Director
Mary Morse, Marketing Director

9024 Eye Medical Clinic of Fresno
1122 S Street
Fresno, CA 93721
559-486-5000
FAX: 559-439-7854

Virgil Snow

A private, nonprofit agency offering services such as health, educational, recreational, rehabilitation, employment and counseling to the totally blind, legally blind and visually impaired. The staff includes hundreds of full time workers.

9025 Fontana Rehabilitation Workshop
Industrial Support Systems
130 N Lilac Avenue
Rialto, CA 92376
909-820-0230

Carole Holt, Executive Director

9026 Foothill Vocational Opportunities
789 N Fair Oaks Avenue
Pasadena, CA 91103
626-449-0218
FAX: 626-449-4802

James Hall, Executive Director

9027 Fred Finch Youth Center
3800 Coolidge Avenue
Oakland, CA 94602 **510-482-2244**
FAX: 510-488-1860
e-mail: adamchase@fredfinch.org
www.fredfinch.org

John Steinfirst MSW, Executive Director
Adame Chase, Admissions Director

A structured, psychiatric (JCAH accredited) residential treatment center for emotionally disturbed girls and boys between the ages of 12 and 18. Our treatment incorporates an on-site, non-public, special education school, an extensive activities and recreational program, a strong professional psychotherapy component (providing individual, group, and family therapy) and a parent support group. We provide 24-hour awake staff.

9028 Friendship Center for the Blind And Visually Impaired
4411 N Cedar
Suite 103
Fresno, CA 93726 **559-222-4447**

Phillip Kimble, Director
Vicki Zehrung, Rehab Social Worker III
Roben Asher, Specialist

A private, nonprofit organization that offers educational, health, recreational and professional training services to the totally blind, legally blind or severely visually impaired. Staff numbers one full- time and four part- time employees.

9029 Gateway Center of Monterey County
850 Congress Avenue
Pacific Grove, CA 93950 **831-372-8002**
FAX: 831-372-2411
www.redshift.com/~gcinc

John Wecker, CEO

Provides residential and day programs for developmentally disabled adults.

9030 Gateway Industries: Castroville
1663 Catalina Street
Sand City, CA 93955 **831-393-1575**

Mike Sweeney, Executive Director

9031 Gilroy Workshop
8855 Murray Avenue
Gilroy, CA 95020 **408-842-0334**
FAX: 408-842-6770

Cathy Andrade

Work adjustment and remunerative work programs.

9032 Glendale Memorial Hospital and Health Center Rehabilitation Unit
1420 S Central Avenue
Glendale, CA 91204 **818-551-0045**
FAX: 818-409-7688

William Parente, President

Offers rehabilitation services, occupational therapy, physical therapy, residential services and more for the disabled.

9033 Goleta Valley Cottage Hospital
351 S Patterson Avenue
Santa Barbara, CA 93111 **805-967-3411**
800-782-2288
FAX: 805-681-6437

Postacute rehabilitation program.

9034 Goose Hill
PO Box 1101
Santa Ynez, CA 93460

Else Wolff, Owner/Operator

A small facility licensed for three developmentally disabled children. Provides residential services for the children currently residing there. The Center is located in a small Danish community of Solvang 45 miles north of Santa Barbara.

9035 Greenery Rehabilitation Center: Pacifica
385 Esplanade
Pacifica, CA 94044
800-356-5959
FAX: 650-359-9388

68 beds offering active/acute rehabilitation, brain injury day treatment, complex care and short-term evaluation.

9036 Hacienda La Puente Adult Education
14101 E Nelson Avenue
La Puente, CA 91746 **626-934-2910**
FAX: 626-934-2900
www.hlpusd.k12.ca.us

Steve Klein, Director
Rachelle Wilson, Counselor
Jerry Fenning, Counselor

9037 Hi-Desert Continuing Care Center
6722 White Feather Road
Joshua Tree, CA 92252 **760-366-2281**
800-782-2288

Postacute rehabilitation program.

9038 Hillhaven Extended Care
1115 Capitola Road
Santa Cruz, CA 95062
FAX: 831-462-9812

Postacute rehabilitation program.

9039 Hillhaven San Francisco at Nobhill
1359 Pine Street
San Francisco, CA 94109 **415-673-8405**
FAX: 415-563-2174

Postacute rehabilitation program.

9040 Home of the Guiding Hands
1100 N Magnolia Avenue
Suite O
El Cajon, CA 92020 **530-579-2501**
FAX: 619-448-7208

Eleanor Lassiter

Work hardening and disciplinary programs.

9041 Hospital of the Good Samaritan Acute Rehabilitation Unit
616 Witmer Street
Los Angeles, CA 90017 **213-977-2358**
FAX: 213-482-2770

Andrew B Leeks, President & CEO
David N Shaw MD, Medical Director Acute Rehab

Physicians, researchers and staff are united by a common mission: to foster growth into one of the most comprehensive medical centers in the West. Services offered include: cardiology and cardiovascular services, neurosciences, movement disorders and Parkinsons disorder, wound care center and transfusion- medicine and surgery center.

9042 **Industrial Therapy Center**

St. John's Regional Medical Center
295 Hueneme Road
Port Hueneme, CA 93041
805-986-3069
FAX: 805-986-3535

Mark Witman PT, Manager

A non-profit health care facility offering multi-disciplinary programs for pain management and work hardening, as well as physical and occupational therapy.

9043 **Janus of Santa Cruz**

200 7th Avenue
Suite 150
Santa Cruz, CA 95062
831-462-1060
FAX: 831-462-4970
www.janussc.org

Jan Tice, Executive Director

9044 **John Muir Medical Center Rehabilitation Services, Therapy Center**

1601 Ygnacio Valley Road
Walnut Creek, CA 94598
925-947-5300
FAX: 925-947-3262

Sandra Reese, VP

9045 **Kelso Activity Center**

404 S Hughes Avenue
Fresno, CA 93706
559-237-5101
FAX: 559-237-5326

Tami Grinstead
Heather Harrison

Serves DTAC and ADP consumers.

9046 **King's View Work Experience Center**

100 Airpark Road
Atwater, CA 95301
FAX: 209-357-0398

Samuel Kalember, Executive Director

9047 **King-Drew Medical Center**

12021 S Wilmington Avenue
Los Angeles, CA 90059
310-668-4321
FAX: 310-632-6965

A private, nonprofit agency offering services such as health, educational, recreational, rehabilitation, employment and counseling to the totally blind, legally blind and visually impaired. The staff includes many full time workers.

9048 **LaPalma Intercommunity Hospital**

7901 Walker Street
La Palma, CA 90623
714-670-7400
FAX: 714-670-6004

Steven Dickson, President

9049 **Lawrence L Frank Center Workshop**

201 S Kinneloa Avenue
Pasadena, CA 91107
626-449-5661

Provides remunerative work.

9050 **Lawrence L Frank Rehabilitation Workshop**

3812 S Grand Avenue
Los Angeles, CA 90037
213-748-7309
FAX: 213-748-7248

Marilyn Graves, Executive Director

9051 **Learning Services of Northern California**

10855 De Bruin Way
Gilroy, CA 95020
408-848-4379

Ann Kent, Marketing Manager

Graduates several hundred individuals each year from its community-integrated rehabilitation programs. These people accomplish renewed productivity in meeting the challenge of their disabling injury, and are more likely to avoid economic and human costs of unnecessary dependency.

9052 **Learning Services: Gilroy**

10855 De Bruin Way
Gilroy, CA 95020
408-848-4379
FAX: 408-848-6509

Mike Howard PhD, Program Director

Flexible sub and post acute rehabilitation for persons with acquired brain injury. Services include subacute long term care and rehab, residential post acute rehab, day treatment, outpatient and home-based rehab.

9053 **Learning Services: South Valley Ranch**

10855 De Bruin Way
Gilroy, CA 95020
408-848-4379
FAX: 408-848-6509

9054 **Learning Services: Supported Living Programs**

10855 De Bruin Way
Gilroy, CA 95020
408-848-4379
800-466-4379
FAX: 408-848-6509

Carol Hughes, Admissions Director
Steven P Johnson PhD, Program Director

Long term living programs provided in normalized community settings. Programs include campus-based living for person in need of high levels of support and/or 24 hour nursing; supervised apartment living and assisted apartment living programs for persons with acquired brain injuries.

9055 **Leon S Peters Rehabilitation Center**

Fresno & R Street
PO Box 1232
Fresno, CA 93715
559-459-3957
800-628-9099
FAX: 559-498-0261

Jeff DiMarco RN, Manager
Jenny Lau RTC CTRS, Community Liaision Rehab Serv.

9056 **Lion's Blind Center**

Lions Blind Center
101 N Bascom Avenue
San Jose, CA 95128
408-295-4016
FAX: 408-295-1308
e-mail: LBCSCV@AOL.Com

Ed Thomas, Executive Director

The Santa Clara Valley BlindCenter, Inc. DBA The Lions Blind Center is a social/recreational training facility for any blind or sight impaired person in Santa Clara County over the age of 12. It provides an hospitable atmosphere that utilizes interactive socialization methods and classes to assist the blind and sight-impaired cope with their disability. Staff includes 2 sighted individuals in management positions.

9057 **Lion's Blind Center of Diablo Valley**

175 Alvarado Avenue
Pittsburg, CA 94565

Phil Sitzman, Director

A private, nonprofit agency offering services such as health, educational, recreational, rehabilitation, employment and counseling to the totally blind, legally blind and visually impaired. The staff includes two full time workers.

9058 Lion's Blind Center of Oakland

3834 Opal Street
Oakland, CA 94609 **510-450-1580**
FAX: 510-654-3603

Peggy Nichols, Executive Director

A private nonprofit organization offering services for the totally blind, legally blind, deaf-blind and multihandicapped blind. Services include: professional training, rehabilitation, educational, counseling, social work, self help and more. The staff includes 17 full time and two part time workers.

9059 Lions Center for the Blind of Oakland

3834 Opal Street
Oakland, CA 94609 **510-450-1580**
FAX: 510-654-3603

Peggy Nichols, Executive Director

Job placement service orientation and mobility services for cane users. Computer training for the blind or visually impaired. Work activity program for the developmentally disabled and the visually impaired. Life enrichment program.

9060 Living Skills Center for the Visually Impaired

2430 Road 20
Apartment B112
San Pablo, CA 94806 **510-234-4984**
FAX: 510-234-4986
e-mail: skillscr@flash.net
www.ci.san-pablo.ca.us/community/skills_cente

Patricia Williams, Director

A private, nonprofit agency offering services such as independent living skills training, recreational, employment and accessible technology training to the totally blind, legally blind and visually impaired. The staff includes six full time teachers.

9061 Loma Linda University Orthopedic and Rehabilitation Institute

11234 Anderson Street
Loma Linda, CA 92354 **909-558-4213**
FAX: 909-558-4133
www.llu.edu/lluhc/rehabilitation.index.htm

Todd Nelson, Senior Intake Officer

Offers a full range of clinical programs for both inpatients and outpatient. The specific diagnosis leading to patient admission includes stroke, spinal cord injury, traumatic or anoxic brain damage, amputation, post neurosurgery, chronic neurological disease, Guillain-Barre syndrome, arthritis, multiple trauma or other complex orthopedic problems. The facilities and professional services are comprehensive and ensure that the best care is provided to pediatric and adult patients.

9062 Manor Care Nursing: Citrus Heights

7807 Uplands Way
Citrus Heights, CA 95610 **916-967-2929**
FAX: 916-965-8439

Postacute rehabilitation program.

9063 Manor Care Nursing: Fountain Valley

11680 Warner Avenue
Fountain Valley, CA 92708 **714-241-9800**
FAX: 714-966-1654

Postacute rehabilitation program.

9064 Manor Care Nursing: Hemet

1717 W Stetson Avenue
Hemet, CA 92545 **909-925-9171**
FAX: 909-925-8186

Postacute rehabilitation program.

9065 Manor Care Nursing: Palm Desert

74350 Country Club Drive
Palm Desert, CA 92260 **760-341-0261**
FAX: 760-779-1564

Postacute rehabilitation program.

9066 Manor Care Nursing: Sunnyvale

1150 Tilton Drive
Sunnyvale, CA 94087 **408-735-7200**
FAX: 408-736-8619

Postacute rehabilitation program.

9067 Manor Care Nursing: Walnut Creek

1226 Rossmoor Parkway
Walnut Creek, CA 94595 **925-975-5000**
FAX: 925-947-2149

Postacute rehabilitation program.

9068 Maynord's Chemical Dependency Recovery Centers

19325 Cherokee Road
PO Box 1657
Tuolumne, CA 95379 **408-279-0136**
800-228-8208
FAX: 209-928-1152
www.maynords.com

Shana Wren, CEO
Walter Reed MFT, Clinical Director
Daniel Meador MD, Medical Director

Maynord's Recovery Centers has always been dedicated to the recovery of good people whose lives are being destroyed by alcohol and drugs. Since 1978, Maynord's residential program has helped thousands of people put their lives back together after addiction has taken its toll. Today, Maynord's offers a treatment system over much of the San Joaquin Valley and the San Francisco Bay Area.

9069 Maynord's Ranch for Men

19325 Cherokee Road
PO Box 1657
Tuolumne, CA 95379 **408-279-0136**
800-228-8208
FAX: 209-928-1152
www.maynords.com

Shana Wren, CEO
Walter Reed MFT, Clinical Director
Daniel Meador MD, Medical Director

Provides treatment for chemical dependency problems to men. The treatment addresses their recovery through a comprehensive plan created for their individual needs. Also offers a program for women called the Meadows.

9070 Meadowbrook Los Angeles: Community Re-Entry Services

4600 Woodley Avenue
Encino, CA 91436 **818-994-4634**

Postacute rehabilitation program.

9071 Meadows

16185 Tuolumne Road
Sonora, CA 95370

Don Blount, Director

Provides treatment designed for women that is directed at every important facet of their lives - mentally, physically and spiritually. Clients receive a variety of treatment approaches to facilitate their recovery and a comprehensive treatment plan is created for their individual needs. Issues relating to the cause of addictions are addressed in lectures, one-on-one counseling sessions, group therapy and re entry groups. Also offers a male treatment programs called Maynord's Ranch.

9072 **Medical Center of La Mirada**
14900 Imperial Highway
La Mirada, CA 90638 **562-944-1900**

John Edwards, Executive Director

9073 **Memorial Hospital of Gardenia**
1145 W Redondo Beach Boulevard
Gardena, CA 90247 **310-532-4200**
800-782-2288

Postacute rehabilitation program.

9074 **Mercy Outpatient Rehab Center**
406-1/2 Sunrise Avenue
Suite 300
Roseville, CA 95661 **916-536-2425**
FAX: 916-780-5770
e-mail: leaton@chw.edu

Lynda Eaton PT, Client Services Liaison

Postacute rehabilitation program for traumatic brain injury survivors.

9075 **Napa County Mental Health**
2344 Old Sonoma Road
Napa, CA 94559 **707-253-4728**
FAX: 707-253-4155

Work hardening and disciplinary programs.

9076 **Napa Valley Support Systems**
650 Imperial Way
Suite 202
Napa, CA 94559 **707-253-7466**
FAX: 707-253-0115

Isabel Harris

Work hardening and disciplinary programs.

9077 **North Valley Services #2**
1350 Vista Way
Red Bluff, CA 95080 **530-529-2100**

Robert Thomas, Assistant Director

9078 **Northridge Hospital Medical Center: Center for Rehabilitation Medicine**
18300 Roscoe Boulevard
Northridge, CA 91328 **818-885-5330**
FAX: 818-701-7367
northridgehospital.com

Debra Flaherty, Director Rehabilitation Services

9079 **Old Adobe Developmental Services**
235 Casa Grande Road
Petaluma, CA 94954 **707-763-0646**
FAX: 707-763-7708
e-mail: nickbobo@aol.com

Dennis Orner, Executive Director

Provides remunerative work.

9080 **PRIDE Industries**
10030 Foothills Boulevard
Roseville, CA 95747 **916-788-2100**
800-550-6005
FAX: 916-788-2560
e-mail: info@prideindustries.com
www.prideindustries.com

Michael Ziegler, President
Rosemary Elston, Director of Rehabilitation
Roxanne Snyder, Employment Services Manager

To provide opportunities through employment, training, evaluation and placement maximizing community access, independence and quality of life for people with barriers to employment.

9081 **Pain Center**
9888 Genesee Avenue
La Jolla, CA 92037 **858-626-6952**
FAX: 858-626-7213

Corinna Nyquist, Outreach Coordinator

Offers both inpatient and outpatient programs including: physical activity management, individual pain management, group therapy, medication adjustment, pain control classes, occupational therapy, biofeedback training, family counseling, vocational and leisure counseling and recreational therapy.

9082 **Parents and Friends**
350 Cypress Street
PO Box 656
Fort Bragg, CA 95437 **707-964-4692**
800-222-0343
FAX: 707-964-2701
e-mail: friends1@mcn.org
www.mendochairs.com

Linda Rosengarten, Executive Director
Teri Scott, Controller
Russ Pals, Vocational Director

Parents and Friends provides opportunities for persons with developmental challenges and similar needs to participate fully in our community.

9083 **Peninsula Center for the Blind & Visually Impaired**
2470 El Camino Real
Suite 107
Palo Alto, CA 94306 **650-858-0202**
800-660-2009
FAX: 650-858-0214
e-mail: pbrandin@pcbvi.org
www.pcbvi.org

Pam Brandin, Executive Director

Private nonprofit agency that serves the visually impaired in the San Mateo, Santa Clara and San Benito counties. Offers rehabilitation services, counseling, social work, self help and education. The staff includes 12 full time employees and five part time.

9084 **Peninsula ReCare**
1764 Marco Polo Way
Burlingame, CA 94010 **650-259-8500**
FAX: 650-697-5010

Kirk F Cunningham, President/CEO

Vocational, health and recreational services for individuals with disabilities.

9085 People Services
4195 Lakeshore Boulevard
Lakeport, CA 95453 707-263-3810
FAX: 707-263-0552
e-mail: peopleservices@mindspring.com
www.peopleservices.org

F Ilene Dumont, Executive Director
Martin Diesman, Director Community Services

Providing an array of services for adults with developmental disabilities and other people with disabilities. Services include supported employment, work services, supported living, personal, social and community training, transportation, specialized individual services and much more.

9086 Petaluma Recycling Center
315 2nd Street
Petaluma, CA 94952 707-763-4761
FAX: 707-763-4921

David Donati, Executive Director

9087 Pomerado Rehabilitation Outpatient Service
15708 Pomerado Road
Suite N102
Poway, CA 92064 858-613-4636
FAX: 858-613-4248

Sheila Brown, Director Rehab Services

A modern outpatient rehabilitation facility featuring state-of-the-art therapies, techniques and equipment in the areas of physical therapy, occupational therapy and speech/language pathology.

9088 Pride Industries: Grass Valley
12451 Loma Rica Drive
Grass Valley, CA 95945 530-477-1832
FAX: 530-477-8038

Kimberly Jonesad, Site Manager
Lisa Bowers, Counselor
Craig Hays, Adult Day Program Coordinator

Work adjustment and remunerative work programs. We offer an adult day program as well.

9089 Rancho Adult Day Care Center
Rancho Los Amigos Medical Center
7600 Consuelo Street
Downey, CA 90242 562-940-7981

Provides personal care, social services and a therapeutic program to older adults in order to improve their quality of life. Offers a Clinical Gerontology Service, an Alzheimer's Disease Diagnostic and Treatment Center and a Geriatric Assessment and Rehabilitation Unit.

9090 Redlands Psychological and Psychiatric Group
Maxine McGowan Smith
440 Cajon Street
Redlands, CA 92373 909-793-4475

Marjorie Smith, Director

9091 Redwoods United
45 Ericson Court
Arcata, CA 95521 707-822-2352
FAX: 707-822-7075

Rochelle Parkinson, Executive Director

9092 Regional Center for Rehabilitation
2288 Auburn Boulevard
Sacramento, CA 95821 916-421-4167
FAX: 916-925-1586

Postacute rehabilitation program.

9093 Regional Infant Center
3010 W Harvard Street
Santa Ana, CA 92704

Joan Hess, Public Health Nurse

9094 Rehabilitation Center at Corona Community Hospital
800 S Main Street
Corona, CA 91720 909-737-4343

Michael Schultz, President

Offers inpatient and outpatient rehabilitation services. The Center consists of an acute rehab unit, a subacute rehab unit containing modules for long-term ventilator care, respiratory rehab, coma intervention and orthopedics. In addition to inpatient therapies, the Center's outpatient programs include sports and industrial medicine.

9095 Rehabilitation Institute Glendale Adventist Medical Center
1509 Wilson Terrace
Glendale, CA 91206 818-409-8071
FAX: 818-546-5609
www.glendaleadventist.com

Patricia Prouty OTR, Program Development Specialist

Complete inpatient and outpatient programs for orthopedic and neurological disabilities.

9096 Rehabilitation Institute of Santa Barbara
427 Camino Del Remedio
Santa Barbara, CA 93110 805-683-3788
FAX: 805-683-0381

Rusty Pollock, President/CEO
Rosemary Resch, Admission Manager

A regional rehabilitation system with an acute care hospital at the center, the Institute provides specialized inpatient and outpatient programs for brain injury, spinal cord injury, stroke, work-related injury, chronic pain, orthopedic problems and more. Offers a 46-bed acute-care rehabilitation hospital, a free-standing outpatient center, the brain injury continuum, chronic pain program.

9097 Rehabilitation Institute of Southern California
1800 E La Veta Avenue
Orange, CA 92866 714-633-7400
FAX: 714-633-4586
e-mail: rhayes@rio.rehab
www.rio-rehab.com

Raylene Hays, Director Programs

Outpatient rehabilitation serving physically and disabled children and adults. Child development programs, adult day care for disabled seniors, child care for disabled and non-disabled children, outpatient therapy, aquatics, adult day healthcare, independent living, vocational services, social services, and housing.

9098 Rehabilitation Unit, Northridge Hospital Medical Center

18300 Roscoe Boulevard
Northridge, CA 91328 **818-885-5330**
FAX: 818-701-7367

Debra Flaherty, Director Rehabilitation Services

9099 Rex Industries

9575 Aero Drive
San Diego, CA 92123 **760-471-0250**
FAX: 858-715-3788

Gary Luce, Operations Manager

Offers many different programs including: North County Parent/Infant Program which is an educational program for children, birth to three years who are showing delays in development or who are at risk for developmental delays. The Adult Development Center is a program for adults, eighteen and over, with a developmental disability in the severe to profound range. The program focuses on self-help, communication, daily living and pre-vocational skills. Other programs are available.

9100 Rohnert Park Services (Behavioral)

6800 Hunter Drive
Suite B
Rohnert Park, CA 94928 **707-585-6700**
FAX: 707-664-8057

Patricia Vreeland, Program Director
Judith Clover, Assistant Program Director

The program services are designed to assist individuals who demonstrate basic work skills, to develop social skills and work habits necessary to succeed in supported or competitive employment. Most often individual program services involve working with the client to replace those behavioral excesses that have been a barrier to vocational placement.

9101 Rubicon Programs

2500 Bissell Avenue
Richmond, CA 94804 **510-235-1516**
FAX: 510-235-2025
www.rubiconpgms.org

Jane Fischberg, Deputy Director

Provides remunerative work, placement and training.

9102 San Bernardino Valley Lighthouse for the Blind

762 N Sierra Way
San Bernardino, CA 92410 **909-884-3121**
FAX: 909-884-2964

Robert McBay, Executive Director
Sandra Wood, Administrative Assistant

Provides training in independent living skills - cooking, mobility and orientation, sewing, Braille and typing. Also, we have classes in macrame, ceramics and basket weaving. Weekly support group and Bible study.

9103 San Diego Center

3821-C Calle Fortunada
San Diego, CA 92123 **619-263-7600**
FAX: 619-571-0919

Nancy Oro

Provides remunerative work.

9104 San Gabriel Valley Training Center and Workshop for the Handicapped

400 S Covina Boulevard
La Puente, CA 91746 **626-285-6407**
FAX: 626-330-5966

Randall Hyatt, Executive Director

9105 Shriners Hospitals for Children: Los Angeles

3160 Geneva Street
Los Angeles, CA 90020 **213-388-3151**
888-486-KIDS
FAX: 213-387-7528
e-mail: edever@shrinenet.org
www.shrinershq.org

Elizabeth Dever, Director Public Relations
Faviola Ramirez, Applications Coordinator
G Frank LaBonte, Hospital Administrator

Treats children under the age of 18 with burn scars and orthopedic conditions. All medical care is provided completely free of charge for patients and their families. Conditions commonly treated include scoliosis, club feet, leg length discrepancies, arthrogryposis, orthopedic problems related to cerebral palsy and spina bifida. Treats amputation or limb deficiency. Also treated are deformities due to burns, scar revision and reconstructive surgery.

9106 Shriners Hospitals, San Francisco Unit, for Crippled Children

2425 Stockton Boulevard
Sacramento, CA 95817 **916-451-7025**
FAX: 415-661-3615

9107 Society for the Blind

2750 24th Street
Sacramento, CA 95818 **916-452-8271**
FAX: 916-452-2622
www.societyfortheblind.org

Bryan Bashin, Executive Director

A private, local nonprofit organization providing blind and visually impaired people with the training supplies and support they need to live independent, productive and fulfilled lives with limited vision. Services include the Low Vision Clinic, Braille classes, computer training, support groups, living skills instruction, mobility training and the Products for Independence Store.

9108 Solutions at Santa Barbara: Transitional Living Center

1135 N Patterson Avenue
Santa Barbara, CA 93111 **805-683-1995**
FAX: 805-683-4793
e-mail: 5011135@aol.com

Susan Hannigan OTR CCM, Director
Susan Farber MA, Case Manager

Postacute rehabilitation program. Short-term transitional living program for individuals with traumatic brain injury, stroke, aneurysm and other neurological disorders.

9109 South Bay Rehabilitation Center at Paradise Valley Hospital

2400 E 4th Street
National City, CA 91950 **619-470-4239**
FAX: 619-470-4126

Fred Harder, President

9110 Southeast Industries

9501 Washburn Road
Downey, CA 90242 **562-803-4606**
FAX: 562-803-4080

Howard Buswell

Work hardening and disciplinary programs.

9111 St. John's Pleasant Valley Hospital Neuro Care Unit
2309 Antonio Avenue
Camarillo, CA 93010 **805-389-5846**
FAX: 805-389-5968

Rosa Vasquez, Director

Subacute rehabilitation program; ventilator dependent.

9112 Starlight Center
1280 Nolan Avenue
Chula Vista, CA 91911 **619-427-7524**
FAX: 619-427-4657

Laura Orcutt

Provides remunerative work.

9113 Sub-Acute Saratoga Hospital
18611 Sousa Lane
Saratoga, CA 95070 **408-378-1382**
FAX: 408-866-8144

Postacute rehabilitation program.

9114 Synergos Neurological Center: Hayward
27200 Calaroga Avenue
Hayward, CA 94545 **510-264-4000**

Postacute rehabilitation program.

9115 Synergos Neurological Center: Mission Hills
15031 Rinaldi Street
Mission Hills, CA 91345 **818-898-4412**

Postacute rehabilitation program.

9116 Tehama County Opportunity Center
13315 Baker Road
Red Bluff, CA 96080 **530-527-0407**
FAX: 530-527-7091

Delbert Brownfield, Executive Director

9117 Temple Community Hospital
235 N Hoover Street
Los Angeles, CA 90004 **213-382-7252**
FAX: 213-389-4559

Postacute rehabilitation program.

9118 Ukiah Valley Association for Habilitation
564 S Dora Street
Suite D
Ukiah, CA 95482 **707-468-8824**
FAX: 707-468-9149
e-mail: roy@uvah.org
www.uvah.org

Roy Smith, Executive Director
Elaine Thaler, Mayacama Industries Director
George Mayers, Rural Adult Program Director

Work adjustment and remunerative work programs.

9119 Valley Center
546 Brunken Avenue
Salinas, CA 93901 **831-754-5509**
FAX: 831-758-0250

Ruth Grigsby, Executive Director

9120 Valley Rehabilitation Industries
2701 E Hammer Lane
Stockton, CA 95210 **209-948-2065**
FAX: 209-463-1511
e-mail: arcsj@gotnet.net

Ronald Tognoli, Executive Director
Sandra Monroe, Director

Vocational training, supported employment and job placement for persons with mental retardation and other developmental disabilities. Valley Rehabilitation Industries is a program of the Association for Retarded Citizens-San Joaquin.

9121 Variety Club Blind Babies Foundation
1200 Gough Street
San Francisco, CA 94109 **415-771-9035**
FAX: 415-771-9026

Dr. Phillip Hatlen, Executive Director

A private, nonprofit agency offering services in the areas of health, counseling, social work, self help and education to blind and visually impaired infants. The educated staff includes 8 full time and 3 part time employees.

9122 Villa Esperanza Services
2116 E Villa Street
Pasadena, CA 91107 **626-449-2919**
FAX: 626-449-3141
www.villaesperanzaservices.org

Dottie Cebula Nelson, CEO

Serving disabled infants to seniors in a school, adult day program, adult work program and residences and adult day health care program and care management program.

9123 Village Square Nursing Center
1586 W San Marcos Boulevard
San Marcos, CA 92069 **760-471-2986**
FAX: 760-471-5176

Postacute rehabilitation program.

9124 Western Neuro Care Center
165 N Myrtle Avenue
Tustin, CA 92780 **714-832-9200**
FAX: 714-508-4550

John Fenton, Chief Exec. Officer

9125 Winways
7732 Santiago Canyon Road
Orange, CA 92869 **714-771-5276**
FAX: 714-771-1452
e-mail: helpdesk@winwaysrehab.com
www.winwaysrehab.com

Nancy R Silver MACCM, Director Admissions

Postacute rehabilitation program.

Colorado

9126 Capron Rehabilitation
Penrose/St. Francis Healthcare System
2215 N Cascade Avenue
Colorado Springs, CO 80907
FAX: 719-776-2534

Gary A Morse, Director

Southern Colorado's most complete inpatient and outpatient rehabilitation center.

9127 Cerebral Palsy of Colorado
2200 S Jasmine Street
Denver, CO 80222
303-691-9339
FAX: 303-691-0846
e-mail: info@cpco.org
www.cpco.org

Judith I Ham, Executive Director

Provides services for children birth-5 years, employment services for adults, information and referral, donation pickup and cell phone/ink cartridge recycling services.

9128 Cherry Hills Health Care Center
3575 S Washington Street
Englewood, CO 80110
303-789-2265
FAX: 303-781-8808

Jody Porupski, Administrator

Postacute rehabilitation program.

9129 Community Hospital Back and Conditioning Clinic
1060 Orchard Avenue
Grand Junction, CO 81501
970-243-3400
800-621-0926
FAX: 970-856-6510

Amy Hibberd, Executive Director

9130 Developmental Preschool
1333 Elm Avenue
Canon City, CO 81212
719-275-0550

Paulette Bolton, Deputy Director

9131 Laradon Hall Society for Exceptional Children and Adults
5100 Lincoln Street
Denver, CO 80216
303-296-2400
FAX: 303-296-0737

Timothy C Hall, Executive Director

Laradon provides educational, vocational and residential services to children and adults with developmental disabilities and other special needs. Laradon was founded in 1948. It is among the largest and most comprehensive service providers in Colorado.

9132 Learning Services: Bear Creek
7201 W Hampden Avenue
Lakewood, CO 80227
303-989-6660
FAX: 303-989-2830

Supported living program for persons with acquired brain injury.

9133 Manor Care Nursing and Rehabilitation Center: Boulder
2800 Palo Parkway
Boulder, CO 80301
303-440-9100
FAX: 303-440-9251

Sherry Howell PhD CCC-SLP, Rehab. Director

Postacute rehabilitation program. Inpatient and Outpatient programs.

9134 Manor Care Nursing: Denver
290 S Monaco Parkway
Denver, CO 80224
303-355-2525
FAX: 303-355-6960

Nancy Schwalm, Administrator
Rose Reinhardt, Admissions Director

Postacute rehabilitation program.

9136 Martin Luther Homes: Colorado Springs
3707 Parkmoor Village Drive
101
Colorado Spgs, CO 80917
FAX: 719-531-0582

Coleen Abeyta, Administrator
Fred Naumann III, Communications

Providing a wide array of services to assist individuals and families in achieving positive life goals. Services to persons with disabilities and other special needs include community living options, training and employment options, spiritual growth and development options, training and counseling support.

9137 Mediplex of Colorado
8451 Pearl Street
Thornton, CO 80229
303-288-3000
FAX: 303-286-1253

Peggy DiTommaso, Marketing Director

Our programs and services help each patient along the road to recovery toward our ultimate aim; the greatest possible restoration of the individual's self-esteem, ability to set goals, and self-sufficiency. Also offer specialized acute inpatient rehabilitative services, including special programs in Trauma Rehabilitation.

9138 Platte River Industries
490 Bryant Street
Denver, CO 80204
303-825-0041
FAX: 303-825-0564

Robert Smith, Executive Director

9139 Pueblo Diversified Industries
2828 Granada Boulevard
Pueblo, CO 81005
FAX: 719-564-3407

Karen Lillie, President
Will Dell, Director Operations

9140 SHALOM Denver
2498 W Second Avenue
Denver, CO 80223
303-623-0251
FAX: 303-620-9584
e-mail: akover@jewishfamilyservice.org
www.shalomdenver.com

Arnold Kover, Director

Work hardening and disciplinary programs.

9141 Schaefer Rehabilitation Center
500 26th Street
Greeley, CO 80631
FAX: 970-353-2779

Richard Kuhn

Work hardening and disciplinary programs.

9142 Spalding Rehab Hospital West Unit
150 Spring Street
Morrison, CO 80465
303-697-4334
FAX: 303-697-0570

Postacute rehabilitation program.

Connecticut

9143 ACES/ACCESS Inclusion Program
60 United Drive
North Haven, CT 06473 **203-234-1344**
FAX: 203-234-1369

Provides a person centered planning approach for integrated employment, volunteer community based opportunities for adults who have developmental disabilities.

9144 APT Residential Services
1 Third Street
PO Box 1587
Newtown, CT 06470 **203-781-4790**
FAX: 203-270-3729

Sharon Sokolowski, Executive Director

9145 Apria Healthcare
40 Sebethe Drive
Cromwell, CT 06416 **860-613-4900**
800-277-4288
e-mail: contact_us@apria.com
www.apria.com

Provides a broad range of high quality and cost effective specialty infusion therapies and related services to patients in their homes throughout the Northeastern United States. Offer home infusion antibiotic therapy, quality pharmacy services, skilled nursing services and related support services.

9146 Central Connecticut Association for Retarded Citizens
1 Hartford Square
New Britain, CT 06052 **860-224-6993**

James McCann, Executive Director

9147 Connecticut Subacute Corporation
955 S Main Street
Middletown, CT 06457 **860-347-6300**
800-257-6300
FAX: 860-347-2446

Evan K Lyle, Managed Care Director
Cheri Kauset, Corporate Rep.

Specializes in subacute medical and rehabilitation programming. The strength of our system is in its' ability to service a broad range of clinical and psychosocial needs which enable each individual to attain his/her optimal potential. Programming includes neurological and orthopedic rehabilitation, post-surgical and wound care management, intravenous therapy, pulmonary rehabilitation including ventilator services, and long term care.

9148 Datahr Rehabilitation Institute
135 Old State Road
Brookfield, CT 06804 **203-775-2418**
888-8DA-TAHR
FAX: 203-740-7129
www.datahr.org

Thomas Fanning, President

Providers of comprehensive rehabilitation services with a history of nearly 5 decades of service. This institute is recognized as a leading resource in meeting the needs of those disabled by illness, injury or developmental disorders in Connecticut and New York. A team of rehabilitation and health care professionals offering career development, residential services, supported employment, volunteer services, occupational therapy, day activities and more.

9149 Eastern Blind Rehabilitation Center
950 W Spring Street
W Haven, CT 06516 **203-937-4850**
FAX: 203-937-3806
www.visn1.va.gov/vact

Penny Schuckers, Director Chief Eastern Blind
Pamela Redmond, Public Affairs

Provides residential rehabilitation services to eligible legally blind veterans in the Northeast and Middle Atlantic portions of the country. Referral applications by Veterans Administration Medical Centers and Outpatient Clinics in the geographical area served by the Blind Rehabilitation Center.

9150 FAVRAH
Avon Park N
Building 23
Avon, CT 06001
FAX: 860-676-0275

Provides remunerative work.

9151 Farmington Valley ARC
225 Commerce Drive
Canton, CT 06019 **860-677-2971**
FAX: 860-693-8662
e-mail: favarh@favarh.org
www.favarh.org

Nancy Thompson, Director Of Clinical Services
Ginger Alexander, Assistant To The Exec. Director

Serving over 300 mentally retarded adults through a comprehensive program of residential and support services. These include three group homes, three apartments, competitive and supported employment options, a day program for mentally retarded seniors, community experience day services for severe and profoundly disabled adults, recreation and leisure services, advocacy, transportation, case management, in-home respite and other support services.

9152 Gaylord Hospital
PO Box 400
Wallingford, CT 06492 **203-284-2800**
800-64R-EHAB
FAX: 203-284-2894
e-mail: pjohnson@gaylord.org
www.gaylord.org

Paul Johnson, President

Works to restore ability and build courage. Offers rehabilitation care with one goal in mind: to help patients return to their homes, communities and jobs.

9153 Hockenum Greenhouse
Route 44A And Bone Mill Road
Mansfield, CT 06251 **860-429-6697**

Sarah Beardsley, Program Director

9154 Kuhn Employment Oppurtunities
165 Pratt Street
Meriden, CT 06480 **203-235-2583**
FAX: 203-235-0827

Robert L Stephens, Executive Director

9155 Lake Grove at Durham
Christopher Ezzo
459R Wallingford Road
Durham, CT 06422 **203-265-0413**
FAX: 860-349-1382

9156 **Litchfield County Association for Retarded Citizens**
84-R Main Street
Torrington, CT 06790 **860-567-9401**
FAX: 860-489-2492

Lawrence Cassella, Executive Director

A private, nonprofit organization whose mission is to improve the quality of life for individuals with mental retardation or associated disabilities and their families through its vocational, residential and community services departments. The vocational component of LARC, provides adults with vocational opportunities with supports in mobile work crews, enclaves, and individual placements.

9157 **Meriden-Wallingford Society for the Handic**
226 Cook Avenue
Meriden, CT 06451 **203-272-8911**
FAX: 203-639-0946
e-mail: mwshinc@snet.net

Pamela Smithus, Executive Director
Diane Morra, Director Program Services
Pauline Bouffard, Director Employment Services

Provides remunerative work, supported employment and job placement.

9158 **Rehabilitation Associates**
60 Katona Drive
Fairfield, CT 06824 **203-384-8681**
FAX: 203-384-0722
www.rehabassociatesinc.com

Carol Landsman, Director
Myra Watnick, Director

A comprehensive outpatient rehabilitation facility offering physical therapy, occupational therapy, speech-language pathology, clinical social work services and nutritional services to all age groups. Facility locations in Fairfield, Stratford, Milford, Shelton and Westport. All facilities are CARF accredited.

9159 **Rehabilitation Center of Fairfield County**
226 Mill Hill Avenue
Bridgeport, CT 06610 **203-378-0092**
FAX: 203-336-5465

Sally Gammon, President

Medical services are provided by physicians who are specialists in physical medicine and rehabilitation. The physical therapy department provides a variety of services and utilizes sophisticated modalities to restore and reinforce physical abilities.

9160 **Reliance House**
40 Broadway
Norwich, CT 06360 **860-887-6536**
FAX: 860-885-1970

David Burnett, Executive Director

A residential vocational and recreational support network. An active and productive clubhouse where people with mental illness can gain skills, strength and self-esteem.

9161 **Section of Physical Medicine and Rehabilitation**
Norwalk Hospital 24 Stevens Street
Norwalk, CT 06856
FAX: 203-852-2027

Dr. Claudio Petrillo, Director

9162 **South Church Activity Program**
99 Main Street
New Britain, CT 06051 **860-224-9480**
FAX: 860-827-8681

Margaret Stowell, Supervisor

Delaware

9163 **Alfred I DuPont Hospital for Children**
Division of Rehabilitation
1600 Rockland Road
Wilmington, DE 19803 **302-651-5600**
FAX: 302-651-5612
www.nemours.org

Thomas Ferry, Administrator

Offers rehabilitative services for the physically challenged individual.

9164 **Community Systems**
3204 Drummond Plaza
Newark, DE 19711 **302-322-5066**
FAX: 302-456-5733

George Baer, Executive Director

9165 **Delaware Association for the Blind**
800 W Street
Wilmington, DE 19801 **302-655-2111**
888-777-3925
FAX: 302-655-1442
www.dabdel.org

Linda Lauria, Executive Director

A private, nonprofit organization that offers adjustment to blindness counseling, recreation activities, summer camps and financial assistance for the legally blind. The staff includes five full time, nine part time and twelve seasonal. Operates a store selling items for the blind.

9166 **Delaware Elwyn**
321 E 11th Street
Wilmington, DE 19801 **302-657-5601**
FAX: 302-654-5815

Lewis C Monges, Executive Director

9167 **Delaware Veterans Center**
1601 Kirkwood Highway
Wilmington, DE 19805 **302-764-0848**
FAX: 302-633-5250

Veterans medical clinic offering disabled veterans medical treatments.

9168 **Easter Seal Rehabilitation Center: New Castle County**
61 Corporate Circle
New Castle Common
New Castle, DE 19720 **302-324-4488**
FAX: 302-324-4481

Bill Adami, Executive Director

9169 **Edgemoor Day Program**
500 Duncan Road
Office A
Wilmington, DE 19809 **302-762-1391**
FAX: 302-762-2416

Betty Brown, Executive Director

9170 **First State Senior Center**
291A N Rehoboth Boulevard
Milford, DE 19963
302-422-1510
FAX: 302-422-1354

Marcella Wilson, Supervisor

9171 **Georgetown Day Program**
5 Academy Street
Georgetown, DE 19947
302-856-5366
FAX: 302-856-5360

Joyce Oliver, Supervisor

9172 **Salvation Army Developmental Service**
701 N Broad Street
Philadelphia, PA 19123
215-787-2804

Michael Paoli, Executive Director

9173 **Woodside Day Program**
941 Walnut Shade Road
Dover, DE 19901
302-739-4494
FAX: 302-697-4490

Connie Grace, Supervisor

District of Columbia

9174 **Barbara Chambers Children's Center**
1470 Irving Street NW
Washington, DC 20010
202-387-6755
FAX: 202-319-9066

Francisca Torres
Offers special education, play and speech therapy services to children 2-5 years of age with developmental delays.

9175 **District of Columbia General Hospital Physical Medicine & Rehab Services**
19th and Mass Avenue
Room 1358
Washington, DC 20003
202-529-6211
FAX: 202-675-7819

Dr. Maribel Bieberach, Chairperson PM&R
Dr. Raman Kapur, Staff Physiatrist
Offers comprehensive physical medicine and rehabilitation services including in and outpatient consultations and electrodiagnostic testing; in and outpatient physical and occupational therapy; inpatient recreational therapy, and a multidisciplinary prosthetic clinic which meets once a month.

9176 **George Washington University Medical Center**
2150 Pennsylvania Avenue NW
Washington, DC 20037
202-994-0825
FAX: 202-994-4005
Offers an Ambulatory Physical Therapy/Sports Medicine Center, a Medical Center Prosthetics/Orthotics Clinic and a Speech and Hearing Center to persons in the District of Columbia, Virginia and Maryland.

9177 **Hospital for Sick Children**
1731 Bunker Hill Road NE
Washington, DC 20017
202-832-4400
800-226-4444
FAX: 202-635-5780
hfscsite.org

Nancy Burch, Manager, Communications

9178 **Howard University Child Development Center**
1911 5th Street NW
Washington, DC 20089
202-865-4620

Offers children with developmental problems diagnosis, treatment, evaluation and follow along visits.

9179 **Psychiatric Institute of Washington**
4228 Wisconsin Avenue NW
Washington, DC 20016
202-885-5600
FAX: 202-966-7374

Psychiatric intensive care, crisis intervention, adult day treatment, drug treatment and other services to children and adults who have psychiatric and chemical dependency problems.

9180 **Spina Bifida Program of DC Children's Hospital**
Department of Physical Medicine and Rehabilitation
111 Michigan Avenue NW
Washington, DC 20010
202-884-3092
FAX: 202-884-3422
e-mail: sreid@onme.org
www.cnmc.org

Eileen Donovan MD, Medical Director Spina Bifida
Lisa Barber, Senior Administrative Assistant
Offers neurosurgery, orthopedics,physical medicine, social work, urology and nursing.

Florida

9181 **Back Technology of Miami**
545 San Esteban Avenue
Miami, FL 33146

Jerry Fogel
Provides remunerative work.

9182 **Bayfront Rehabilitation Center**
Bayfront Medical Center
701 6th Street S
St Petersburg, FL 33701
727-893-6702
FAX: 727-893-6779
www.bayfront.org

JoAnn W Gardner MA RPT, Director of Rehab Services
Bayfront Medical Center has an Inpatient Rehabilitation Hospital and two outpatient rehabilitation clinics that each provide progressive, comprehensive, individualized treatment. Specialized care in Physiatry (physical medicine), rehab nursing, occupational therapy, speech language pathology, recreational therapy, patient/family services and psychology is tailored to each patient from admission to community and/or school reintegration.

9183 **Bon Secours Hospital**
1050 NE 125th Street
North Miami, FL 33161
305-893-0068

Julie Rog, Executive VP
Offers rehabilitation services, occupational therapy, physical therapy, inpatient and outpatient care and more for the physically challenged.

9184 Brain Injury Rehabilitation Center Sand Lake Hospital

9400 Turkey Lake Road
Orlando, FL 32819 **407-351-8500**
FAX: 407-351-8584

Tina Whatley, BIRC Admissions

Dedicated to restoring brain injured patients with rehabilitation potential to their highest level of functioning. This is accomplished through an interdisciplinary team demonstrating personal responsibility to the patient, their family and each other.

9185 Center for Pain Control and Rehabilitation

2780 Cleveland Avenue
Suite 607
Fort Myers, FL 33901 **239-337-4332**

Dr. Harris Bonnette, Medical Director

9186 Comprehensive Rehabilitation Center at Lee Memorial Hospital

2776 Cleveland Avenue
Fort Myers, FL 33901 **239-334-5200**

Palma Fuson, Director

Offers rehabilitation services, occupational therapy, physical therapy, respite services and more for the physically challenged individual.

9187 Comprehensive Rehabilitation Center of Naples Community Hospital

350 7th Street N
Naples, FL 34102 **239-436-5324**
FAX: 239-436-5250

William Crone, President
Heather Baker, Administrative Director
Ken Schields, Marketing Coordinator

Offers rehabilitation services, inpatient and outpatient care at 5 locations in the county and more for the benefit of the disabled.

9188 Conklin Center for the Blind

405 White Street
Daytona Beach, FL 32114 **386-258-3441**
FAX: 386-258-1155
e-mail: robert@conklincenter.org
www.conklincenter.org

Robert Kelly, Executive Director

Offers services for the totally blind, legally blind, visually impaired, mentally retarded blind and more with health, counseling, educational, recreational, rehabilitation, through computer training and professional training services. Serves people who are blind and who are challenged by one or more additional disabling conditions. Functional skills training and employment services, including supported employment.

9189 Davis Center for Rehabilitation Baptist Hospital of Miami

8900 N Kendall Drive
Miami, FL 33176 **305-596-6520**
FAX: 305-270-3640

Elizabeth Matalon, Administrative Director

A full-service, nonprofit community hospital providing a full range of inpatient and outpatient rehabilitation services. The overall commitment to excellence has extended to this specialized field. Access to medical expertise and services ensures that the best in medical resources are available should an unforeseen medical problem arise.

9190 Division of Blind Services

2551 W Executive Center Circle
Lafayette Building, Suite 200
Tallahassee, FL 32399 **850-488-1330**
800-342-1828
FAX: 850-487-1804
e-mail: randy_touchton@fdles.state.fl.us

Randy Touchton, Director

Serves the totally blind, legally blind, visually impaired, deaf-blind, learning disabled, mentally retarded and other multiply handicapped by offering health, counseling, educational, recreational and computer training services.

9191 Easter Seal Society of Dade County

1475 NW 14th Avenue
Miami, FL 33125 **305-325-0470**

Joan L Bornstein PhD, Acting President
Lillianne Camargo MSW, Admissions Social Worker

9192 Easter Seals Broward County

6951 W Sunrise Boulevard
Plantation, FL 33313 **954-792-8772**
FAX: 954-791-8275
e-mail: info@esbc-fl.easter-seals.org
www.esbc-fl.easter-seals.org

Becky Dausman, President/CEO
Leni Ulrich, Program Director
Kate Pelletier, Vocational Services Director

A nonprofit health agency dedicated to helping individuals of all ages with temporary and long-term physical disabilities become as self-reliant as possible. Coordinates and guides each client through the therapy process. All treatment is done by licensed and supervised therapists.

9193 Easter Seals Southwest Flordia

350 Braden Avenue
Sarasota, FL 34243 **941-355-7637**
800-807-7899
FAX: 941-351-4997
e-mail: info@easterseal.org
www.swfl.easter-seals.org

Mary Hitchcock, President/CEO
Mark Dobosz, VP Development and Programs
Amy Spears, Director Health/Childern Svcs.

9194 Easter Seals: Volusia and Flagler Counties , FL

1219 Dunn Avenue
Daytona Beach, FL 32114 **386-255-4568**
877-255-4568
FAX: 386-258-7677
e-mail: info@eseals-vf.org
www.easterseals-volusiaflagler.org

Lynn Sinnott, President
Penny Young, Comunication Director

Provides early intervention services: inclusive pre-school, aquatherapy and sensory processing therapy, OT, PT, ST and parenting programs, audiology services, equipment loan program, assistive technology information and referral. Residential summer camp and respite.

9195 FIRE

1286 Cedar Center Drive
Tallahassee, FL 32301 **850-942-3658**
FAX: 850-942-4518
e-mail: ibskip@earthlink.net

Skip Koch, Executive Director

Provides independent living and vocational rehabilitation services to Florida residents who are legally blind. Services include instruction in orientation and mobility, accessible technology, daily living skills and employability skills. Information, referral and counseling services are also offered. All services are provided without charge.

9196 Florida CORF

Columbia Medical Center: Peninsula
264 South Atlantic Avenue
Ormond Beach, FL 32176 **386-672-4161**

www.memorial-health.com

John Feore, Executive VP

Offers Medicare authorized therapy programs for seniors, disabled and others who need rehabilitation. CORF can provide coordinated and extended services in the home after a hospital stay, or when physical status changes. Patients who are treated at CORF, include amputations, arthritis, chronic/acute pain, depression/anxiety, nerve injury, sports injury, stroke and swallowing problems.

9197 Florida Community College at Jacksonville/ Services for Students with Disabilities

101 W State Street
Jacksonville, FL 32202 **904-632-5007**
FAX: 904-633-8110

Cecilia Sumner, Director

9198 Florida Institute for Neurologic Rehabilitation, Inc

1962 Vandolah Road
PO Box 1348
Wauchula, FL 33873 **863-773-2857**
800-697-5390
FAX: 863-773-0867
e-mail: info@finr.net
www.finr.net

Stephen C Freeley, Director of Marketing

A residential rehabilitation facility providing a therapeutic environment in which children, adolescents and adults who have survived head-injury can develop the independence and skills necessary to re-enter the community.

9199 Florida Veterans Centers

713 NE 3rd Avenue
Fort Lauderdale, FL 33304 **954-356-7926**
FAX: 954-356-7609

Veterans medical clinic offering disabled veterans medical treatments.

9200 Goodwill Industries-Suncoast

10596 Gandy Boulevard N
St Petersburg, FL 33702 **727-523-1512**
888-279-1988
FAX: 727-563-9300
www.goodwill-suncoast.org

Deborah A Passerini, VP for Operations
Jean-Marie Moore, HS Operations Director

A nonprofit community-based organization whose purpose is to improve the quality of life for people who are handicapped, disabled and/or disadvantaged or aged. This mission is accomplished through providing independent living skills, affordable housing, training and placement in useful employment. Annually, the organization serves more than 1,400 handicapped, disabled or disadvantaged people in various components within the Human Services Department. Staff consists of 120+ full time employees.

9201 Halifax Hospital Medical Center Eye Clinic Professional Center

306 N Clyde Morris Boulevard
Daytona Beach, FL 32114 **386-322-4700**
FAX: 386-274-5889

James Clower

Offers services for the totally blind, legally blind, visually impaired, mentally retarded blind and more with health, counseling, educational, recreational, rehabilitation, computer training and professional training services.

9202 HealthQuest Subacute and Rehabilitation Programs

Regenta Park
7130 Southside Boulevard
Jacksonville, FL 32256
FAX: 904-641-7896

HealthQuest offers four centers within the state of Florida offering exceptional staff, comfortable surroundings and individually designed, closely monitored programs dedicated to enabling patients to achieve their goals. Each location offers a progressive and cost effective alternative to in-hospital subacute and rehabilitative care. Centers are offered in Jacksonville, Winter Park, Sarasota and Sunrise.

9203 HealthSouth Regional Rehabilitation Center

20601 Old Cutler Road
Miami, FL 33189 **305-251-3800**
FAX: 305-251-5978

Les Alt, Administrator

A comprehensive source of medical rehabilitation services for Pinellas County, Florida area residents, their families and their physicians. Offers the people of Florida all the clinical, technical and professional resources of the nation's leading provider of comprehensive rehabilitation care.

9204 HealthSouth Rehabilitation Hospital of Tallahassee

1675 Riggins Road
Tallahassee, FL 32308 **850-656-4800**
FAX: 850-656-4809

Lynn Streetman, Administrator
Paige Mitchell, Director Business Development
Donna Crawford, Director Clinical Services

North Florida's sole acute rehabilitation hospital between Jacksonville \, Panama City, and Gainesville. With 250 employees providing a full continuum of care form its 70 bed facility, the hospital is accredited by JCAHO, CARF and state designated and certified by Vocational Rehabilitation for traumatic brain injury, as well as a wide variety of other diagnoses. With the addition of our outpatients, the facility has served the greater community by touching the lives of over 50,000 patients.

9205 HealthSouth Rehabilitation Hospital of Sarasota

3251 Proctor Road
Sarasota, FL 34231 **941-921-8600**
800-873-4222
FAX: 941-925-7526

Laurie Boggus, Administrator

9206 HealthSouth Sports Medicine & Rehabilitation Center/Worksite Program

1710 Lisenby Avenue
Panama City, FL 32405 **850-784-4878**
FAX: 850-769-7566

Jim McGonley MPT/ATC, Director Clinical Services

Outpatient sports medicine and rehabilitation center providing physical therapy, occupational therapy, industrial rehab, work hardening/work simulation, worksite and ergonomic analysis, FCE's, work assessment and pre-employment goals of returning the clients back to work, and returning to all recreational, sports and functional activities safely.

9207 Holy Cross Hospital

4725 N Federal Highway
Fort Lauderdale, FL 33308 **954-771-8000**
FAX: 954-351-5994

Barbara Dale, Director

9208 Lee Memorial Hospital

PO Box 2218
Fort Myers, FL 33902 **239-332-1111**

Mary Kalina, Marketing Director

Offers a complete inpatient program of intensive rehabilitation designed to restore a patient to a more independent level of functioning. The comprehensive care includes medical rehabilitation and training for spinal cord injury, brain injury, stroke and neurological disorders.

9209 Lighthouse for the Blind of Palm Beach

7810 S Dixie Highway
W Palm Beach, FL 33405 **561-586-5600**
FAX: 561-586-5630

William S Thompson, President & CEO
Sandra L Lamb, VP Administration/HR
Dawn M Clemons, VP Development/Services

A private, non-profit rehabilitation and education agency in its 55th year of service. Offers programs to assist persons who areblind or visually impaired, an on-site Industrial Center, a technology training center, an Aids and appliances Store, special equipment grant programs, outreach services for children and adults, Early Intervention and Preschool Services, and a variety of support groups. These programs provide services and education for blind children and their parents.

9210 Lighthouse for the Visually Impaired and Blind

8610 Galen Wilson Boulevard
Port Richey, FL 34668 **727-815-0303**
FAX: 727-815-0203
e-mail: dgriffin@lighthouse-pasco.org
www.lighthouse-pasco.org

Don Griffin PhD, Executive Director
Nancy TerKeurst, Director Clinical Services

The Lighthouse offers services for visually impaired or blind adults and children ages 0-5 years old. Counseling, educational services, recreational services, rehabilitation, computer training and support groups.

9211 MacDonald Training Center

5420 W Cypress Street
Tampa, FL 33607
FAX: 813-872-6010
TTY:813-873-7631
www.mcginc.com/Training/default.htm

Jim Freyvogel, President
Mara Brad, Director Communication Services
Scott Gaedtke, Director Day Services

A private, non-profit, community-based human services organization serving adults with disabilities (since 1953). Persons are provided the opportunity to achieve their highest potential through the Center's various programs that include day training, employment, community living and various support services.

9212 Medical Rehabilitation Center of Jacksonville

836 Prudential Drive
Jacksonville, FL 32216 **904-202-1611**
FAX: 904-202-3147

Mark Kosier, Executive Director

9213 Medicenter of Tampa

4411 N Habana Avenue
Tampa, FL 33614 **813-872-2271**

Robert Westhoff, Administrator

Postacute rehabilitation program.

9214 Memorial Hospital Rehabilitation Center

3599 University Boulevard S
Jacksonville, FL 32216 **904-858-7600**
FAX: 904-858-7610

Dr Charles Schauer, President

An entire care facility featuring five day inpatient evaluation, pre-operative evaluation programs, five week pain management program, referral criteria and treatment goals, therapy services, psychological services and more to the physically challenged.

9215 Miami Heart Institute Adams Building

4701 N Meridian Avenue
Suite 601
Miami Beach, FL 33140 **305-674-5956**
www.msmc.com

David Lehrman, M.D.

Dr. Lehrman now works with Dr. Sher and Dr. Lozman in orthopaedic surgery

9216 Miami Lighthouse for the Blind

601 SW 8th Avenue
Miami, FL 33130 **305-856-2288**
FAX: 305-285-6967
e-mail: info@miamilighthouse.ncom
www.miamilighthouse.com

Roxann Mayros, Chief Executive Officer
Dr Elly du Pre, Adult Services Chair
Carol Brady-Simmons, Children Services Chair

Offers services for the legally blind and severely visually impaired (including those who are developmentally delayed) of all ages in the areas of counseling and educational, recreational, rehabilitation, computer and vocational training services.

9217 Mount Sinai Medical Center Rehabilitation Unit

4300 Alton Road
Miami Beach, FL 33140 **305-674-2590**
FAX: 305-674-2606
e-mail: Dharma-m@msmc.com
www.msmc.com

Dharma Mirabent, Director

9218 Neuropsychiatric Pain Rehabilitation Clinic

5330 George Street
New Port Richey, FL 34652 **727-849-2005**
FAX: 727-849-2087

Charlene Evina, Administrative Assistant
Vickie Penick, Administrator

A multidisciplinary outpatient program for the evaluation and treatment of chronic pain. Consultation services for hospitalized patients are also provided upon request.

9219 **North Broward Rehab Unit**
North Broward Medical Center
201 E Sample Road
Pompano Beach, FL 33064 **954-786-6405**
FAX: 954-786-6476

Wendy Burkholder, Regional Manager

CARF accredited, 30-bed inpatient rehabilitation unit treating adults with brain injuries, spinal cord injuries, stroke, orthopedic and neurologic injuries.

9220 **Northwest Medical Center**
5901 Colonial Drive
Margate, FL 33063 **954-974-0400**
FAX: 954-984-1463

9221 **Pain Institute of Tampa**
4178 N Armenia Avenue
Tampa, FL 33607 **813-875-5913**
FAX: 813-872-6215

Dave Braughton

Pain management.

9222 **Pain Treatment Center, Baptist Hospital of Miami**
8900 N Kendall Drive
Miami, FL 33176 **305-596-6525**
FAX: 305-273-2406

Brian Keeley, President

9223 **Pine Castle**
4911 Spring Park Road
Jacksonville, FL 32207 **904-733-2650**
FAX: 904-733-2681
e-mail: pcastle@ilnk.com
www.edcationcentral.org/fdlsr/Special%20Place

Jonathan May, Executive Director

Provides remunerative work, training, community employment and community living options for adults with developmental disabilities.

9224 **Polk County Association for Handicapped Citizens**
1038 Sunshine Drive E
Lakeland, FL 33801 **863-665-3846**
FAX: 863-665-2330

Shirley Balogh

Work adjustment and remunerative work programs.

9225 **Quest**
210 W 4th Street
Orlando, FL 32811 **407-880-3731**
FAX: 407-880-3964
www.questinc.org

Donna Smith, Executive Director
Michele Cardinal, Associate Exec Director/Programs
Cheryl Lyng, Associate Exec Dir/Production

A multi-faceted vocational rehabilitation facility. Programs offered are vocational evaluation and assessment, work adjustment, placement, supported employment, community employment, developmental training, long-term sheltered care and residential services.

9226 **Rehab of Melbourne**
Sea Pines Rehabilitation Hospital
101 E Florida Avenue
Melbourne, FL 32901
FAX: 321-952-6532

Mark Tellier, Administrator

9227 **Rehabilitation Center for Children and Adults**
300 Royal Palm Way
Palm Beach, FL 33480 **561-655-7266**
FAX: 561-655-3269
e-mail: info@rcca.org
www.rcca.org

Pamela Henderson, Executive Director

A private, nonprofit organization whose purpose is to improve physical function, independence and communication of people with physical disabilities. Any child or adult with a physical or speech disability is eligible for services.

9228 **Renaissance Center**
PO Box 17067
Jacksonville, FL 32245 **904-743-1883**
FAX: 904-743-5109

Dr Robert Sommers, President

9229 **Sarasota Memorial Hospital/Comprehensive Rehabilitation Unit**
1700 S Timiami Trail
Sarasota, FL 34239 **941-952-2535**

Phillip Beauchamp, President

9230 **South Dade Nursing Home**
2525 SW 75th Avenue
Miami, FL 33155 **305-262-6800**

Frank Jimenez, Executive Director

9231 **Strive Physical Therapy Centers**
2620 SE Maricamp Road
Ocala, FL 34471 **352-351-8883**
FAX: 352-351-4219
e-mail: cwabbersen@striverehab.com
www.striverehab.com

Chuck Wabbersen PT, ATC, Clinical Director

9232 **Sunbridge Care and Rehabilitation**
5627 9th Street E
Bradenton, FL 34203 **941-753-8941**
FAX: 941-739-4409

Anita Faulmann, Administrator

A comprehensive medical rehabilitation facility that is committed to helping individuals with disabilities improve their quality of life. This is a 120-bed facility offering a full range of acute and sub-acute inpatient programs as well as community-based outpatient programs.

9233 **Tampa Bay Academy**
12012 Boyette Road
Riverview, FL 33569 **813-677-6999**
FAX: 813-671-3145

Malcolm Harriman

A psychiatric residential treatment center and partial hospitalization program for ages 7 to 17.

9234 **Tampa General Rehabilitation Center**
PO Box 1289
Tampa, FL 33601 **813-251-7000**
FAX: 813-253-4283

Cindy Leistner, Development Director

Offers a full range of programs all aimed at helping patients achieve their full potentials. It is one of three centers in the state that provides Driver Training and Evaluation Programs for persons with disabilities, and also an Assisted Reproduction Program for neurologically impaired males. A Community Re-entry Day Treatment Program is available for individuals who have recovered from a brain injury. A wide variety of inpatient and outpatient programs are available.

9235 Tampa Lighthouse for the Blind

1106 W Platt Street
Tampa, FL 33606 **813-251-2407**
FAX: 813-254-4305

CE Olstrom, Executive Director

Offers services for the totally blind, legally blind, visually impaired, mentally retarded blind and more with health, counseling, educational, recreational, rehabilitation, computer training and professional training services.

9236 University of Miami Comprehensive Pain and Rehabilitation Center

600 Alton Road
Miami Beach, FL 33139 **305-532-7246**
FAX: 309-534-3974

Renee Stelle-Rosomoff, Programs Director

9237 UpReach Pavilion

8900 NW 39th Avenue
Gainesville, FL 32606

Cindy Toth, Administrator

9238 Upper Pinellas Association for Retarded Citizens

1501 N Belcher Road
Clearwater, FL 33765 **727-799-3330**
FAX: 727-799-4632
e-mail: uparc@aol.com
www.members.aol.com/uparc/index.htm

Thomas J Buckley EdD, Executive Director

Offers services to more than 500 persons with mental retardation and other developmental disabilities. Services include two early intervention pre-schools, physical, speech and occupational therapies, homebound education and family support for children, birth to five years and transitional, vocational, habilitation, employment and placement services for adolescents and adults. UPARC operates 31 group homes, a 22 unit apartment complex, and Supported Living options to provide for residential need

9239 Visually Impaired Persons of Southwest Florida

35 W Mariana Avenue
North Fort Myers, FL 33903 **239-997-7797**
FAX: 239-997-8462
e-mail: sherryd@vipcenter.org
www.vipcenter.org

Sherry Danko, Executive Director
Kat Newland, Social Worker

Provides training in independent living skills, orientation and mobility, counseling, computer and other communication skills, family support groups, peer counseling, socialization and a low vision clinic. Second location in Collier County.

9240 West Florida Hospital: The Rehabilitation Institute

8391 N Davis Highway
Pensacola, FL 32514 **850-494-6000**
FAX: 850-494-4881
www.westfloridahospital.com

Dennis A Taylor, President/CEO
Carol Saxton, Sr VP Paient Care Services

A 58-bed comprehensive rehabilitation facility offering inpatient and outpatient services. JCAHO and CARF accredited and a State designed head and spinal cord injury center. CARF accredited programs include: comprehensive inpatient rehab, spinal cord injury, brain injury and work hardening.

9241 Willough at Naples

9001 Tamiami Trail E
Naples, FL 34113 **239-775-4500**
800-722-0100
FAX: 239-775-0534

A licensed psychiatric hospital in Southwest Florida which provides quality management and treatment for eating disorders and chemical dependency in adults.

Georgia

9242 Annandale at Suwanee

3500 Annandale Lane
Suwanee, GA 30024 **770-945-8381**
FAX: 770-945-8693
e-mail: administration@annandale.org
www.annandale.org

Patricia M Brown, Executive Director

Private nonprofit residential facility for adults with developmental disabilities. Located on 124 acres just north of Atlanta. Annandale provides full program and 24 hour residential services.

9243 Atlanta Institute of Medicine and Rehabilitation

2915 Piedmont Road
Suite A
Atlanta, GA 30305 **404-365-0160**
FAX: 404-365-0751

9244 Bobby Dodd Institute (BDI)

2120 Marietta Boulevard NW
Atlanta, GA 30318 **678-365-0071**
FAX: 678-365-0098
e-mail: wmcmillan@bdi-atl.org
www.bobbydodd.org

Wayne McMillan, President & CEO
David Turner, Director Of Finance
Barbara Massey, Vice President, Ops & Marketign

BDI annually serves approximately 400 clients in Atlanta, GA. BDI works primarily with people with developmental disabilities such as autism, down syndrome or mental retardation, but includes clients with physical or acquired disabilities. Client age varies from teenagers to adults.

9245 Cave Spring Rehabilitation Center

Georgia Avenue
Cave Spring, GA 30124 **706-777-3382**

Loring Kirk, Executive Director

9246 Center for Assistive Technology and Environmental Access

490 10th Street
Atlanta, GA 30332 **404-894-4960**
FAX: 404-894-9320
www.catea.org

Barbara Christopher, Administrative Coordinator
Elizabeth Bryant, Project Director II

The Center for Assistive Technology and Environmental Access (CATEA) promotes maximum function, activity and access of persons with disabilities through the use of technology. The foci of the Center includes the development, evaluation and utilization of Assistive Technology and the design and development of Accessible Environments.

9247 **Center for the Visually Impaired**

739 W Peachtree Street NW
Atlanta, GA 30308
404-875-9011
FAX: 404-607-0062
www.cviatlanta.org

Susan B Green, Executive Director
Karen Cheatham, Development Director

Offers services to people of all ages who are blind or visually impaired with training in orientation and mobility, computer technology, activities of daily living, communication skills and employment readiness. Aso offers two children's programs, a community-based rehabilitation program for senior citizens, and a low vision clinic.

9248 **Devereux Georgia Treatment Network**

1291 Stanley Road NW
PO Box 1688
Kennesaw, GA 30156
770-427-0147
800-342-3357
FAX: 770-427-4030
e-mail: jzdencan@devereux.org
www.devereuxgeorgia.org

John Zdencanovic, Director Agency Relations

Serves ages 11 to 17, males and females with a capacity for up to 135. Serves moderate to severe emotional, behavioral and/or learning disabilities. A specialized psychiatric hospital/intensive residential treatment program for low average to superior intelligence.

9249 **Easter Seals East Georgia**

1500 Wrightsboro Road
PO Box 2441
Augusta, GA 30903
706-667-9695
FAX: 706-667-8831
e-mail: sthomas@esega.org
www.ga-ea.easter-seals.org

Sheila H Thomas, President/CEO

9250 **Georgia Industries for the Blind**

PO Box 218
Bainbridge, GA 31718
229-248-2666
FAX: 229-248-2669

Jim Hughes, Executive Director

Offers services for the totally blind, legally blind, visually impaired, mentally retarded blind and more with health, counseling, educational, recreational, rehabilitation, computer training and professional training services.

9251 **Head Injury Treatment Program at Marietta**

26 Tower Road
Marietta, GA 30060
770-422-8913
800-526-5782

Karen Erlinger, Program Director

Postacute rehabilitation program.

9252 **Hillhaven Rehabilitation**

26 Tower Road
Marietta, GA 30060
770-422-8913
800-526-5782
FAX: 770-425-2085

Leslie Ann Marie Parrish, Case Manager

Routine skilled and subacute medical and rehabilitation care including physical therapy, occupational therapy, speech pathology and therapeutic recreation. Programs include stroke and head injury rehab; orthopedic rehab; complex IV therapy; woundcare; cancer; total parental nutrition and dialysis.

9253 **In-Home Medical Care**

CareMaster Medical Services
1428 US 41 Bi-Pass S
PO Box 278
Griffin, GA 30224
800-542-8889
FAX: 770-412-0014
e-mail: caremaster@accesunited.com
www.caremastermedical.com

Nancy Frederick, VP

Offers the devoted attention of a professional nurse, the use of I.V. therapies, pain management and provision of medical equipment and supplies right where the patient wants to be.

9254 **Learning Services: Peachtree**

337 W Pike Street
Suite B
Lawrenceville, GA 30045
770-962-4828
FAX: 770-995-1253
www.learningservices.com

Greg Lang, Admissions

Postacute rehabilitation program.

9255 **Pain Control & Rehabilitation Institute of Georgia**

2784 N Decatur Road
Suite 120
Decatur, GA 30033
404-897-1400
FAX: 404-297-1427

Dr. Shulim Spektor, CEO
Anna Britman, Office Manager

Provides pain management for chronic and acute pain resulted from injuries, diseases of muscles and nerve, Reflex Sympathetic Dystrophy, perform disabilities and impairment ratings.

9256 **Savannah Association for the Blind**

214 Drayton Street
Savannah, GA 31401
912-236-4473
FAX: 912-234-4156

W Chandler Simmons, Executive Director

Offers services for the totally blind, legally blind, visually impaired, mentally retarded blind and more with health, counseling, educational, recreational, rehabilitation, computer training and professional training services.

9257 **Shepherd Center for Treatment of Spinal Injuries**

2020 Peachtree Road NW
Atlanta, GA 30309
404-352-2020
FAX: 404-350-7479

James Collins, Administrator

Dedicated exclusively to the care of patients with spinal cord injuries and other paralyzing spinal disorders. It serves predominately residents of Georgia and neighboring states as one of the only 14 hospitals designated by the U.S. Department of Education as a Model Spinal Cord Injury System Program.

9258 **Transitional Hospitals Corporation**
7000 Central Parkway NE
Suite 1000
Atlanta, GA 30328 **404-378-8353**
800-683-6868
FAX: 770-913-0015

A national network of intensive care hospitals providing care for patients who suffer from a chronic illness and/or catastrophic accident. The mission is founded on providing quality health care to patients who require highly skilled nursing care and access to technologically advanced therapies.

9259 **Walton Rehabilitation Hospital**
1355 Independence Drive
Augusta, GA 30901 **706-823-8511**
866-492-5866
FAX: 706-724-5752
e-mail: postmaster@wrh.org
www.wrh.org

Dennis Skelley, President
Frank Lewis, Chief Operating Officer
Mike Harrell, CFO

A 58-bed comprehensive physical rehabilitation hospital offering inpatient and outpatient services. Services offered include: stroke recovery, orthopedic injury, pediatrics, head injury, pain management for chronic pain syndrome, TMJ/Craniofacial pain and chronic headache disorders, spinal cord injury, driving instruction, work re-entry, independent living, assistive technology and ADA consulting.

Hawaii

9260 **Rehabilitation Hospital of the Pacific**
226 N Kuakini Street
Honolulu, HI 96817 **808-531-3511**
FAX: 808-544-3335
www.rehabhospital.org

Stuart Wo, President/CEO
Pauline Osborne, VP/CFO
Dr Thomas Au, VP Clinical Affairs/Medical Dir

Idaho

9261 **Ashton Memorial Nursing Home and Chemical Dependency Center**
801 Main
Ashton, ID 83420 **208-652-7461**
FAX: 208-652-7252

Sheila King, Executive Director

9262 **Easter Seal Society**
1465 Vinnell Way
Boise, ID 83709 **208-378-9924**
800-374-1910
FAX: 208-378-9965

Donna Grummer, VP

9263 **Idaho Elks Rehabilitation Hospital**
PO Box 1100
Boise, ID 83701 **208-343-2583**
FAX: 208-489-4005

A nonprofit hospital serving Idaho and the Pacific Northwest. All inpatient and outpatient programs and services are supervised by the hospital's full-time medical directors whose specialty is psychiatry, the profession of physical rehabilitative medicine. Services include: occupational therapy, rehabilitative nursing, social skills, head injury program, physical therapy, speech pathology, audiology and cardiac rehabilitation.

9264 **Portneuf Medical Center Rehabilitation**
651 Memorial Drive
Pocatello, ID 83201 **208-239-1836**

Robbie Oyler, Director/Manager

Illinois

9265 **Alexian Brothers Medical Center**
800 Biesterfield Road
Elk Grove Village, IL 60007 **847-437-5500**

A threefold mission: Works toward maximizing physical function, enhance independent social skills and optimize communication skills consistent with an individual's ability. The Center helps those disabled by accident or illness achieve a new personal best.

9266 **Back in the Saddle Hippotherapy Program**
Corcoran Physical Therapy
PO Box 597901
Chicago, IL 60659 **773-286-2266**
847-604-4145
FAX: 847-673-8895
e-mail: info@hippotherapychicago.com
www.hippotherapychicago.com

Julie Naughton, Program Coordinator
Maureen Corcoran, Physical Therapist

A direct medical treatment used by licensed physical therapists who have a strong treatment background in posture and movement, neuromotor function and sensory processing. The benefits of Hippotherapy are available to individuals with just about any disability. Two locations: Glen Grove, IL and Morton Grove, IL. Accepts all insurance.

9267 **Barbara Olson Center of Hope**
3206 N Central Avenue
Rockford, IL 61101 **815-964-9275**
FAX: 815-964-9607
www.b-olsoncenterofhope.org

Carm Kilker, Executive Director
Jackie Neil Boss, Director Administrative Serv.
Susan Nagy, Accountant

We provide vocational employment, educational and social opportunities for adults with developmental disabilities.

9268 **Baxter Healthcare Corporation**
1 Baxter Parkway
Deerfield, IL 60015 **847-948-2000**
FAX: 847-948-3948
www.baxter.com

Ed Dobryzkowski, Executive Director

9269 **Beacon Therapeutic Diagnostic and Treatment Center**

10650 S Longwood Drive
Chicago, IL 60643 **773-881-1005**
FAX: 773-881-1164

Offers community day treatment, education, diagnostic services, family counseling, learning disabled, speech and hearing and psychiatric services.

9270 **Blind Service Association**

22 W Monroe Street
11th Floor
Chicago, IL 60603 **312-236-0808**
FAX: 312-236-8679

Debbie Grossman, Executive Director

Offers services for the totally blind, legally blind and visually impaired with reading and recording low vision network, social services, referrals and support groups.

9271 **Brandecker Rehabilitation Center**

9455 S Hoyne Avenue
Chicago, IL 60620 **773-239-2191**
FAX: 773-239-6229

Mary Howell PhD, Executive Director

We offer early intervention services for infants and toddlers with developmental delays and disabilities. Our outpatient Medical Rehabilitation Program offers direct therapy services for children from age birth-16.

9272 **Caremark Healthcare Services**

2211 Sanders Road
Northbrook, IL 60062 **847-559-4700**
800-423-1411

An 80-service-center network providing services anywhere in the U.S. Offers 24 hour access to nursing and pharmacy services, case management resource centers, HIV/AIDS services, women's health services, transplant care services, nutrition support services, infectious disease management and other therapies and programs.

9273 **Center for Comprehensive Services**

306 W Mill Street
Carbondale, IL 62901 **618-529-3060**
800-582-4227
FAX: 618-457-5372
e-mail: sandy.boston@thementornetwork.com
www.thementornetwork.com

Sandra Boston, National Director of Admissions

Post-acute rehabilitation services for adults and adolescents with acquired brain injuries. Residential, day-treatment and out-patient services tailored to individual needs.

9274 **Center for Rehabilitation at Rush Presbyterian: Johnston R Bowman Health Center**

710 S Paulina Street
Chicago, IL 60612 **312-942-3600**
FAX: 312-942-3601
e-mail: teri_sommerfeld@rush.edu
www.rush.edu

Teri Sommerfeld, Administrator

Postacute rehabilitation program.

9275 **Center for Spine, Sports & Occupational Rehabilitation**

1030 N Clark Street
Suite 500
Chicago, IL 60610 **312-238-7767**
FAX: 312-238-7709
www.rehabchicago.org

Offers evaluation and treatment of patients with acute and subacute musculoskeletal and sports injuries.

9276 **Children's Home and Aid Society of Illinois**

125 S Wacker Drive
Suite 14
Chicago, IL 60606 **312-424-0200**
www.chasisystems.org

Private state-wide. Multi-service, racially integrated staff and client populations. Provides educational, placement and community services for children-at-risk and their families. Advocacy, consultation and follow-up services provided according to our philosophy of continuum of care. No one, child or adult, is denied service because of disabilities, if the program services meet their needs. Higher quality in-service training for staff as well as parenting figures.

9277 **Christ Hospital and Medical Center**

4440 W 95th Street
Oak Lawn, IL 60453 **708-346-3144**
FAX: 708-346-2072

Ronald Struxness, Executive Director

9278 **Clinton County Rehabilitation Center d/b/a CCRC Community Link**

1665 N Fourth Street
PO Box 157
Breese, IL 62230 **618-526-2252**
FAX: 618-526-2021
e-mail: John@commlink.org
www.commlink.org

John Sedivy, Executive Director

9279 **Continucare, A Service of the Rehab Institute of Chicago**

West Suburban Hospital Medical Center
Erie at Austin
Oak Park, IL 60302 **708-383-6200**
800-354-7342
FAX: 312-908-1369

Offers inpatient subacute rehabilitation program.

9280 **Delta Center**

1400 Commercial Avenue
Cairo, IL 62914 **618-734-3626**
FAX: 618-734-1999

Frederica Garnett, Executive Director

9281 **Division of Rehabilitation-Education Services, University of Illinois**

1207 S Oak Street
Champaign, IL 61820 **217-333-4600**
FAX: 217-333-0248

Brad Hedrick, Director

Offers services for the totally blind, legally blind, visually impaired, mentally retarded blind and more with health, counseling, educational, recreational, rehabilitation, computer training and professional training services.

9282 **Easter Seal Rehabilitation Center**

1230 N Highland Avenue
Aurora, IL 60506
FAX: 630-896-6257

Beverly Brownel, Program Services
Richard N Merz, Executive Director

Provides comprehensive outpatient rehabilitation services for physical, developmental and speech/language disabilities. Serves all ages. Also operates short-term residential camp for children with disabilities. Charges bases on third party coverage and family ability to pay. Private, non-profit organization.

9283 **Easter Seals**

212 Barney Drive
Joliet, IL 60435 **815-725-2194**
FAX: 815-725-5150

Debra Condotti, President

Services for children and adults with disabilities and their families. Pediatric outpatient medical rehabilitation, inclusive childcare, fostercare, residential homes, clinics.

9284 **Easter Seals DuPage Dold Center for Children**

830 S Addison Avenue
Villa Park, IL 60181 **630-620-4433**
FAX: 630-620-1148

James A Johnson, Executive Director
Linda Matheson, Program Services

Maximizes independence for infants, children and adults with disabilities by providing physical, occupational and speech therapy, audiology, social work, early intervention, assistive technology, toy lending, equipment loan and special needs day care.

9285 **El Valor Corporation**

Early Intervention Program
1951 W 19th Street
Chicago, IL 60608 **312-997-2021**
FAX: 312-432-9849

Catalina Ariza, Director

Mission is to challenge people with disabilities. It is a center for people with disabilities and their families and serves Chicago and surrounding areas, providing services in English and Spanish to individuals whose lives would be drastically impoverished without them.

9286 **Elgin Rehabilitation Center**

1485 Davis Road
Elgin, IL 60123 **847-888-5540**

Robert Borchert, VP

9287 **Family Counseling Center**

Washington & Market Street
Golconda, IL 62938 **618-683-2461**
FAX: 618-683-2066
e-mail: fccgolconda@shawneelink.com

Larry Mizell, Executive Director
Beci Gates, Behavioral Health Division Dir.
Donna Perez, Housing Coordinator

Provides counseling, developmental training, evaluations, assisted living services, referrals, psychosocial rehabilitation, and a variety of work services.

9288 **Family Matters**

ARC Community Support Systems
2502 S Veterans Drive
Effingham, IL 62401 **217-347-5118**
866-436-7842
FAX: 217-347-5119
e-mail: deinhorn@arc-css.org
www.fmptic.org

Debbie Einhorn, Director Family Support

Parent Training and Information Center and family support programs for families of children who have disabilities from the ages of birth through 21. Services include: Parent support and training, school advocacy, home visits, information and referral, parent-to-parent networking, special education rights workshops and other training sessions on special education topics for parents and school personnel throughout Illinois except in the Chicago area.

9289 **Five Star Industries**

PO Box 60
Du Quoin, IL 62832 **618-542-5421**
FAX: 618-542-5556

Thomas Hamlin, Executive Director

Incorporated as a private, non-profit corporation under the laws of the State of Illinois, is an equal opportunity employer and provides equal opportunity in compliance with the Civil Rights Act of 1964 and all other appropriate laws, rules and regulations referring to civil rights.

9290 **Gilchrist-Marchman Rehabilitation Center**

2345 W N Avenue
Chicago, IL 60647
FAX: 773-276-5653

Therese O'Shea, Executive Director

9291 **HSI Austin Center For Development**

1819 S Kedzie
Chicago, IL 60623 **773-854-1676**
FAX: 773-854-8300

Provides an educational program designed to enhance academic, behavioral and social performance of children 4-14 years of age experiencing emotional disorders that result in exclusion from the public school setting.

9292 **Hardin County Center**

580 Westport Road
Elizabethtown, KY 42701 **207-765-6196**

9293 **Henry County Clinic**

117 S E Street
Cambridge, IL 61238 **309-937-5391**
FAX: 309-937-2023

Individual, group, marital and family therapy, psychological testing and evaluation services offered.

9294 **Hyde Park-Woodlawn**

950 E 61st Street
Chicago, IL 60637 **773-702-0660**
FAX: 773-493-2397

William Cinwell, Executive Director

9295 **IHS at Brentwood Rehabilitation**

5400 W 87th Street
Burbank, IL 60459 **708-423-1200**
800-430-0098
FAX: 708-423-1266
ihs.com

Roxane Sanderson, Provider Relations Sr Director

Postacute rehabilitation program and ventilator weaning.

9296 **ILC Enterprises**

6415 Stanley Avenue
Berwyn, IL 60402 **630-789-0511**
FAX: 708-788-0831

Cindy Holbrook, Program Director

A nonprofit tax exempt private social service agency serving suburban Chicago offering day treatment and vocational counseling to individuals who encountered a pattern of job loss due to emotional problems.

9297 **Illinois Center for Autism**

548 S Ruby Lane
Fairview Heights, IL 62208 **618-398-7500**
FAX: 618-397-9869

A community-based mental health/educational treatment center dedicated to serving autistic clients.

9298 **Illinois Masonic Medical Center**

836 W Wellington Avenue
Chicago, IL 60657 **773-975-1600**

Consultation, education, family counseling, parent training in behavior modification techniques offered to developmentally disabled adults.

9299 **Infant Program**

409 W New Indian Trail
Aurora, IL 60506 **630-879-9119**

E Duane Thompson, Executive Director

9300 **Jayne Shover Easter Seal Rehabilitation Center**

799 S McLean Boulevard
Elgin, IL 60123 **847-742-3264**
FAX: 847-742-9436
e-mail: jeastersea@aol.com
www.il-js.easter-seals.org

Peggy Muetterties, President

A free-standing, comprehensive outpatient rehabilitation center serving children and adults with physical and developmental disabilities.

9301 **Julius and Betty Levinson Center**

332 Harrison Street
Oak Park, IL 60304 **708-383-8887**
FAX: 708-383-9025
e-mail: soneill@ucp.net.org

Houses one of its three adult developmental training programs for substantially physically disabled men and women.

9302 **Lake County Health Department**

3012 Grand Avenue
Waukegan, IL 60085 **847-377-8180**
FAX: 847-336-1517
www.co.lake.il.us

Includes counseling, crisis intervention, emergency management, psychotherapy and chemotherapy management for individuals and families.

9303 **Little Friends**

140 N Wright Street
Naperville, IL 60540 **630-355-6533**
FAX: 630-355-3176
www.littlefriendsinc.com

Jack Ryan, President/CEO

Nonprofit early intervention and special education programs with focus on children with autism or other developmental, emotional or behavioral disabilities. Vocational and residential services for adults with developmental disabilities.

9304 **MAP Training Center**

7th and McKinley Street
Karnak, IL 62956 **618-634-9401**
FAX: 618-634-9090

Larry Earnhart, Executive Director

Training, employment, residential and support services, targeted for adults with developmental disabilities.

9305 **Macon Resources**

PO Box 2760
Decatur, IL 62524 **217-875-1910**
FAX: 217-875-8899
TTY:217-875-8898
e-mail: kscrogin@maconresources.org

Kay Scrogin, Executive Director
Shirley Paceley, Associate Director
Tommy Nelson, Deputy Director Clinical Svcs.

The purpose is to provide a comprehensive array of habilitative/rehabilitative training programs and support services to assist individuals and/or family units of an individual with a developmental disability, mental illness, or other handicapping condition to live, attend school or day program, and/or work in the least restrictive, most normalized environment possible.

9306 **Marianjoy Rehablink**

26 W 171 Roosevelt Road
Wheaton, IL 60187 **630-462-4000**
FAX: 630-462-4440
www.marianjoy.org

Kathleen C Yosko, President/CEO

Marinjoy Rehabilitation Hospital is a 120-bed hospital in Wheaton, Illinois that is dedicated to the delivery of rehabilitative medicine. Founded in 1972 by the Wheaton Franciscan Sisters, the hospital is a division of Marianjoy provides comprehensive inpatient and outpatient rehabilitation services, including programs that assist patients with re-entry, such as driver rehabilitation and return-to-work programs.

9307 **Mary Bryant Home for the Blind**

2960 Stanton Avenue
Springfield, IL 62703 **217-529-1611**
FAX: 217-529-6975
e-mail: MBHA@springnet1.com

Jerry Curry, Administrator

Residential living facility for the blind or visually impaired.

9308 **Northern Illinois Medical Center**

4201 W Medical Center Drive
McHenry, IL 60050 **815-363-1220**
800-734-7342
FAX: 815-759-8062

Kathryn Murauskas, Inpatient Rehabilitation Unit
Nora Connors, Director Rehabilitation Network
Lisa Forino, Marketing Coordinator

Providing rehabilitation services in Lake and McHenry Counties, the Rehabilitation Unit is a complete living environment for up to 15 patients after a debilitating illness of trauma. Various locations offering a multitude of services: PT, OT, speech, HT, RT aquatics, work hardening, FCE's, vocational counseling, rehab nursing, physiatry, neuropsychology, case management. Comprehensive Inpatient Rehabilitation Unit, and many more services.

9309 **Northern Illinois Special Recreation Association**
820 E Terra Cotta Avenue
Suite 125
Crystal Lake, IL 60014
815-459-0737
FAX: 815-459-0388
e-mail: nisra@mc.net
www.NISRA.org

Leisure and recreation services to those who are unable to participate successfully in park district and city recreation programs.

9310 **Oak Forest Hospital of Cook County**
15900 Cicero Avenue
Oak Forest, IL 60452
708-687-7200
FAX: 708-687-7979

Cyntjia T Henderson, Interim Hospital Director
Joe Turner, Public Information

A 654 bed health care center devoted to the diagnosis, rehabilitation and long-term care of adults suffering from chronic illnesses, diseases and physical impairments.

9311 **Peoria Area Blind People's Center**
2905 W Garden Street
Peoria, IL 61605
309-637-3693
FAX: 309-673-3699

Mabel VanDeusen, Executive Director

Offers services for the totally blind, legally blind, visually impaired, mentally retarded blind and more with health, counseling, educational, recreational, rehabilitation, computer training and professional training services.

9312 **Peoria Association for Retarded Citizens**
PO Box 3418
Peoria, IL 61612
309-691-3800
FAX: 309-689-3613
www.peoriaarc.org

Ron Wisecarver, President/CEO
Roy Ricketts, VP/COO
Anne Follis, Executive Director

Serves all ages that are diagnosed with mental retardation and other developmental and physical disabilities. Programs include early intervention, family support, respite care, vocational training, supported employment, adult day programs and residential services. Serves 1,000 clients with 400 staff members.

9313 **Phoenix I**
3075 Grand Avenue
Galesburg, IL 61401
309-343-6126
FAX: 309-344-1754
e-mail: kccdd@galesburg.net

Ned Hippensteel, Executive Director

9314 **Pioneer Center of McHenry County**
4001 W Dayton Street
McHenry, IL 60050
815-344-1230
FAX: 815-344-3815

Jeff A Epstein PhD, Executive Director
Lorraine Kopczynski, Associate Director

Early intervention, sheltered employment, developmental training, employment services, residential services, mental health services and respite care.

9315 **Prosthetics and Orthotics Center in Blue Island**
2310 York Street
Blue Island, IL 60406
708-597-2611
800-354-7342
FAX: 800-908-1932
www.rehabchicago.org/about/blue_island.php

Provides orthotic and prosthetic fittings and follow-up services to adults and children in the south suburbs of Chicago.

9316 **RB King Counseling Center**
2300 N Edward Street
Decatur, IL 62526
217-877-8121
FAX: 217-875-0966

Offers outpatient, individual, group, divorce and meditation, family and re-adjustment counseling.

9317 **REHAB Products and Services**
3715 N Vermilion Street
Danville, IL 61832
217-446-1146
FAX: 217-446-1191

Larry McConkey, President/CEO

9318 **RIC Northshore**
345 E Superior Street
Chicago, IL 60611
800-354-7342
e-mail: webmaster@rehabchicago.org
www.rehabchicago.org

Provides rehabilitation for sports-related injuries, musculoskeletal conditions, neurological conditions, stroke, arthritis, amputation, burns, and general deconditioning.

9319 **RIC Prosthetics and Orthotics Center**
2310 York Street
Blue Island, IL 60406
708-597-2611
FAX: 708-597-5373
e-mail: webmaster@rehabchicago.org
www.rehabchicago.org

Offers almost all the prosthetics and orthotics services provided at RIC's main hospital in downtown Chicago, including consultations, fittings and training.

9320 **RIC Windermere House**
5548 S Hyde Park Boulevard
Chicago, IL 60637
312-908-9554
800-354-7342
FAX: 773-256-5060
www.rehabchicago.org

Evaluation, therapeutic services and patient education are offered in the areas of arthritis, multiple sclerosis, musculoskeletal conditions, orthopedics, stroke, spinal cord injury, brain injury and sports medicine.

9321 **RIC and Swedish Covenant Hospital Rehabilitation Services**
5145 N California Avenue
Chicago, IL 60625
773-989-3990
FAX: 773-256-5060
www.rehabchicago.org

Provides acute rehabilitation services, subacute care and outpatient services for many types of disabling injuries and conditions, including amputation, arthritis, brain injury, general deconditioning, multiple sclerosis, musculoskeletal injuries, stroke, and joint replacements.

9322 **Ray Graham Association for People with Disabilities**
2801 Finley Road
Suite 3C
Downers Grove, IL 60515 **630-620-2222**
FAX: 630-628-2350
www.ray-graham.org

William Murphy, President
John Voit, VP

Provides developmental services at 15 sites to infants, children and adults with disabilities. Services range from 1 hr/wk respite to full-time residential.

9323 **Reach Rehabilitation Program: Americana Healthcare**
9401 S Kostner Avenue
Oak Lawn, IL 60453

Postacute rehabilitation program.

9324 **Rehabilitation Achievement Center**
5150 Capitol Drive
Wheeling, IL 60090 **847-215-9977**
FAX: 847-215-9376

Richard Green, Program Director
Mary Helen Ekstam, Director Clinical Relations

A post-acute head injury program designed specifically to help survivors and their families meet the challenge of community re-entry after discharge from acute care settings. RAC uses an integrated team approach to develop and implement a realistic program to suit each person's individual needs.

9325 **Rehabilitation Institute of Chicago: Alexian Brothers Medical Center**
800 Biesterfield Road
Elk Grove Village, IL 60007 **847-981-3694**
800-354-7342
FAX: 312-908-9561

A 32-bed rehabilitation unit under the medical direction and supervision of the Rehabilitation Institute of Chicago.

9326 **Riverside Medical Center**
Mental Health Unit
350 N Wall
Kankakee, IL 60901
FAX: 815-935-7485

Offers recreation, parenting therapy, emergency services, psychological testing and inpatient treatment programs.

9327 **Robert Young Mental Health Center Division of Trinity Regional Haelth System**
2701 17th Street
Rock Island, IL 61201 **309-779-2031**
FAX: 309-779-2027

Services include comprehensive inpatient rehabilitation, chronic pain management programs, outpatient medical rehabilitation, work hardening programs, vocational evaluation, alcohol and other drug dependency rehabilitation programs, Burn Center, and mental health services for inpatient, partial hospitalization, residential treatment, case management, emergency/crisis intervention and outpatient therapy. Licensed for 443 beds, it is the largest health care institution in the Iowa/Illinois area.

9328 **Sampson-Katz Center**
2020 W Devon Avenue
Chicago, IL 60659
FAX: 773-764-3131

Jim Balark, Executive Director

9329 **Shelby County Community Services**
1810 W S 3rd Street
Shelbyville, IL 62565 **217-774-3911**
FAX: 217-774-5120

Richard Gloede, Executive Director

9330 **St Elizabeth Hospital Physical Rehabilitation Unit In-Patient/CARFT Certified**
211 S 3rd Street
Belleville, IL 62220 **618-234-2120**
FAX: 618-234-8741

Lucy Beaver, Rehab Services Director
Patricia Parsaghian, Rehab Nurse Manager
Tom Dibadj, Rehab Therapy Manager

Comprehensive inpatient and outpatient physical rehab services that include the services of a psychiatrist, rehab nursing, OT, PT, Speech, RT, social service, neuro psychologist and other resource and support personnel that support the rehab program.

9331 **Streator Unlimited**
305 N Sterling Street
Streator, IL 61364 **815-675-5574**
FAX: 815-673-1714

Jeffrey Dean, Executive Director
Beth Lawless, Director Rehabilitation

Vocational and personal skills training, residential services, client and family support, CARF accredited.

9332 **TCRC Sight Center**
111 W Washington Street
Suite 410
E Peoria, IL 61611 **309-698-4001**
FAX: 309-698-9227

Linda Haas RN, VP Visual/Medical Services

Offers services for persons who are totally blind, legally blind, partially sighted or visually impaired along with other disabilities. Have support group, rehabilitation classes, orientation and mobility services, counseling services, low vision clinic, Braille transcription services, technology services and specialized aids and appliances for sale.

9333 **Tazewell County Resource Center**
RR 1 Box 12
Tremont, IL 61568 **309-477-2272**
FAX: 309-925-4241

Gus Van Den Brink, Executive Director

A private, nonprofit agency providing programs for the special needs of infants, adults, children and their families residing in Tazewell County. Services offered include: birth-three infant/parent program, adult day care services, family support, residential, vocational services, sheltered work and activity services programs.

9334 **Thresholds AMISS**
12145 Western Avenue
Blue Island, IL 60406 **708-597-8073**
FAX: 708-597-8053

Natalie Marsh, Program Director
Malissa Landis, Assistant Program Director
Camille Rucks, Team Leader

Services offered include psychosocial, vocational and residential programs for ages 18 or older with a primary diagnosis of mental illness. Facility is wheelchair accessible.

9335 **Thresholds Bridge Deaf North**
4814 N California Avenue
Chicago, IL 60625
773-989-8991
FAX: 773-989-1075
TTY:773-989-1875
www.thresholds.org

Herminio Cardona Jr, Program Director

A private, nonprofit psychosocial rehabilitation center that serves the hearing impaired mental health consumers at the highest risk of hospitalization, those with serious and persistent mental illness. The program provides residential and assertive treatment case management services focused on rehabilitation.

9336 **Tri-County Rehabilitation Center**
1650 S Kanner Highway
Stuart, FL 34994
772-221-4050
FAX: 772-286-4364

Suzanne Hutcheson, President/CEO

9337 **Trumbull Park**
10530 S Oglesby Avenue
Chicago, IL 60617
773-375-7022
FAX: 773-375-5528

Gregory Terry, Director
Diana Moore, Site Supervisor

Offers consultation, education, general counseling, recreation, self-help and social services for children and adults.

9338 **University of Illinois Medical Center**
1855 W Taylor Street
Chicago, IL 60612
312-355-0746
FAX: 312-996-7770

Timothy McMahon, Chief

Offers services for the totally blind, legally blind, visually impaired, mentally retarded blind and more with health, counseling, educational, recreational, rehabilitation, computer training and professional training services.

9339 **VanMatre Rehabilitation Center**
2400 N Rockton Avenue
Rockford, IL 61103
815-971-3737
800-752-9907
FAX: 815-969-5797

Vicki McDonnough, Administrative Services

A CARF-accredited comprehensive rehabilitation center based within the Rockford Memorial Hospital providing inpatient and outpatient services for physically and cognitively challenged persons with debilitating illness and injuries.

9340 **Warren Achievement Center**
1220 E 2nd Avenue
Monmouth, IL 61462
309-734-3131
FAX: 309-734-7114
e-mail: jmae@maplecity.com

J McVey, President

For developmentally disabled children and adults. Parent-infant education programs are for parents of infants with disabilities or developmental delays; Children's Group Homes which serve children on a fulltime basis and can serve additional children on a respite basis; Vocational training and residential programs assist the handicapped adult and developmental training for adults; adult residential community living; manufacturing, capabilities in workshop includes packaging, and assembly.

Indiana

9341 **Ball Memorial Hospital**
2401 W University Avenue
Muncie, IN 47303
765-285-8431
FAX: 765-747-3313

Robert Brodhead, President

Offers rehabilitation services, occupational therapy, physical therapy and more for the physically challenged child or adult.

9342 **Community Hospitals, Indianapolis**
1500 N Ritter Avenue
Indianapolis, IN 46219
317-633-8210
FAX: 317-351-7723

Barbara Gebhardt, Executive Director

9343 **Crossroads Industrial Services**
4740 Kingsway Drive
Indianapolis, IN 46205
317-254-0228
FAX: 317-897-9763

Jack Costello, Executive Director

9344 **Department of Veterans Affairs Vet Center #418**
311 N Weinbach Avenue
Evansville, IN 47711
812-473-5993
FAX: 812-473-4028
e-mail: vcen418@evansvilla.net

Jack Weber LCSW MPA, Team Leader

Provides readjustment counseling to combat veterans of all eras. Onsite assistance for employment problems and Department of Veteran Affairs, Vocational Rehabilitation and Sexual Trauma Counsel.

9345 **Frasier Rehabilitation Center Division of Clark Memorial Hospital**
2201 Greentree N
Clarksville, IN 47129
812-282-4257
FAX: 812-288-1161

Designed to help patients in their adjustment to a physically limiting condition, both psychologically and physically, by helping to maximize each patient's abilities so he or she can function as independently as possible. The program treats patients whose functional impairment may range from temporary to permanent, from partial to total disability.

9346 **HealthSouth Tri-State Rehabilitation Hospital**
4100 Covert Avenue
Evansville, IN 47714
800-677-3422
FAX: 812-476-4270
www.healthsouth.com

Barb Butler, CEO
Myra Wetzel, Marketing Coordinator
Dick Ondrey, Clinical Services Director

An 80-bed JCAHO accredited freestanding hospital specializing in comprehensive medical rehabilitation for Brain Injury, Spinal Cord Injury, Orthopedic, Pulmonary, Cardiac, Oncology and disabilities and general disabilities.

9347 **Healthwin Specialized Care**
20531 Darden Road
South Bend, IN 46637
574-272-0100
FAX: 574-277-3233

Patrock Pingel, Administrator

Postacute rehabilitation program.

9348 **Memorial Regional Rehabilitation Center**

221 W Wayne Street
South Bend, IN 46601 **574-232-4861**
FAX: 574-282-4692

Margaret Sak OTR, Manager, ILC

CARF accredited outpatient medical rehabilitation and post acute brain injury program. Serves neurologically impaired adults and young adults.

9349 **Saint Joseph Regional Medical Center- South Bend**

801 E LaSalle
South Bend, IN 46616 **574-237-7314**
e-mail: sgersp@sjrmc.com

Phyllis Syers MSN CRRN, Director, Inpatient Rehab

Continuum of rehabilitation services offered. Included are: acute rehabilitation, a 26 bed CARF accredited comprehensive inpatient unit, a CARF certified inpatient brain injury program, a CARF outpatient day treatment brain injury program, comprehensive outpatient services, with available case management, and Driver's Training Program, a 30 bed state of the art subacute rehab unit, CARF accredited Industrial Rehabilitation Programs and CARF accredited Pain and Complimentary Medicine Program.

Iowa

9350 **Adults Incorporated**

3420 University Avenue
Waterloo, IA 50701 **319-236-0901**
888-879-1365
FAX: 319-236-3701
e-mail: ainc@cedarnet.org
www.cedarnet.org/ainc

Mark Witmer, Executive Director
Denise Hinders, Director Rehabilitation
Donna Davis, Director Development/Public Rel.

Provides adult day services, employment services and supported community living so people with disabilities can live and work in the community. Populations served include, but are not limited to: senior adults with age-related disabilities, youth with disabilities (age 15+), adults with disabilities, including those with mental and physical disabilities. CARF accredited. Serves northeast, north and central Iowa. Head Injury Program serves the whole state.

9351 **Crossroads of Western Iowa**

One Crossroads Place
Missouri Valley, IA 51555 **712-642-4114**
FAX: 712-642-4115
e-mail: crwi@inebraska.com
www.crwi.com

David Lovell, CEO

CWI provides services in Missouri Valley, Onawa and Council Bluffs, Iowa. An array of services for people with mental illness, mental retardation and brain injury are provided in each location.

9352 **Easter Seals Iowa**

PO Box 4002
Des Moines, IA 50333 **515-289-1933**
FAX: 515-289-1281
e-mail: essia@netins.net
ia.easter-seals.org

Martha H Wittkowski, President/CEO

Easter Seals is a leading nonprofit provider of services to Iowans with disabilities. Services include vocational and employment training, camping recreation and respite services, craft training and sales, home and farm adaptations, transportation, scholarships and a club for stroke survivors and their families.

9353 **Genesis Regional Rehabilitation Center**

2720 W Locust
Suite 2B
Davenport, IA 52804 **563-421-3495**
FAX: 563-421-3499

Janet King, Executive Director

Serves persons of all ages experiencing a disability, whether acquired at birth or following a serious interdisciplinary service. Rehabilitation programs include acute rehabilitation; adult rehabilitation, pediatric rehabilitation, outpatient orthopaedics. LIFT, a community based, nontraditional approach to the treatment of adolescents and adults with brain injuries is also offered at Genesis. It is designed to facilitate re-entry into the community or return to appropriate employment.

9354 **Homelink**

Van G Miller & Associates
PO Box 2817
Waterloo, IA 50704 **319-235-7100**
800-482-1993
FAX: 319-235-7822

A national network of home medical equipment, respiratory therapy, rehabilitation and infusion therapy service providers with over 2,500 locations serving all fifty states.

9355 **Iowa Central Industries**

127 Avenue M
Fort Dodge, IA 50501 **515-576-2126**
FAX: 515-576-2251

Quentin Weidner, Director

Services include evaluation and training in pre-vocational and vocational skills, personal behavior management, cognitive skills, communication skills, self-care skills and social skills. Services arranged include: independent living training, medical services, psychological services, therapeutic services and social services.

9356 **Iowa Veterans Centers**

2600 Harding Road
Des Moines, IA 50310 **515-285-6701**
FAX: 515-284-4901

Veterans medical clinic offering disabled veterans medical treatments.

9357 **Life Skills Laundry Division**

1510 Industrial Road SW
Le Mars, IA 51031 **712-546-4786**
FAX: 712-546-4985

Cindi Kruse, Executive Director

9358 **MIW**

909 S 14th Avenue
Marshalltown, IA 50158
FAX: 641-752-1614
e-mail: jstegmamann@miwi.org

Janet Stegmann, Services Manager

Vocational services for adults with disabilities. Includes organizational employment services, supported employment, job placement.

9359 **Mercy Pain Center**
400 University Avenue
Des Moines, IA 50314
FAX: 515-248-8867

Dianne Alber EdD, Administrative Director

An outpatient program dedicated to helping people with chronic pain live more productive, satisfying lives. The program is not designed for conditions that are surgically curable, but rather approaches the problem using a comprehensive, holistic treatment.

9360 **Mercy Physical Rehabilitation Unit**
Mercy Drive
Dubuque, IA 52001
FAX: 563-589-8162

Joan Hentges, Director

Provides services which open the door to improved communication, offering the opportunity to enrich the quality of life. Mercy offers many other branches of services including, rehabilitation services for children, pulmonary rehabilitation program, services for the head-injured patient, back to school, and the disabled driver program.

9361 **Nishna Productions**
902 Day Street
PO Box 70
Shenandoah, IA 51601
712-246-1242
FAX: 712-246-1243

Sherri Clark, Executive Director

Shelter, workshop and job training for the disabled.

9362 **Options of Linn County**
1019 7th Street SE
Cedar Rapids, IA 52401
319-892-5800
FAX: 319-892-5849
www.linncounty.org/dhrm/options

Vivian Davis, Director
Reggie Ancelet, Associate Director
Jim Nagel, Associate Director

Provides employment services to adults with disabilities. Options serves over 300 people annually in community based and facility based services.

9363 **RISE**
107 Gunder Road
Elkader, IA 52043
563-245-1868
FAX: 563-245-2859

Edward Josten, Executive Director

9364 **Ragtime Industries**
116 N 2nd Street
Albia, IA 52531
641-932-7813
FAX: 641-932-7814

Diana Shehan, Executive Director

A work-oriented rehabilitation organization which provides training for mentally and physically disabled adults in Monroe County. A variety of programs which help to develop each person's individual potential are offered so that the person may live as normal a life as possible.

9365 **Sunshine Services**
PO Box 225
Spencer, IA 51301
712-262-7805
FAX: 712-262-8369

Dan Penkert, Executive Director

9366 **Tenco Industries**
710 Gateway Drive
 # 1287
Ottumwa, IA 52501
641-682-8114
FAX: 641-684-4223
e-mail: luehlingtech@lisco.com
www.tenco.org

Lorraine Uehling-Techel, Executive Director

To advocate and provide opportunities for people with disabilities, or conditions that limit their abilities, to develop and maintain the skills necessary for personal dignity and independence in all areas of life. Provide a wide array of services to individuals with disabilities. By looking at each person as individuals, we are able to work with them to maximize their skills. Residentials services, including HCBS and CSALA are also provided in all communities.

Kansas

9367 **Arrowhead West**
1100 E Wyatt Earp Boulevard
PO Box 1417
Dodge City, KS 67801
620-227-8803
FAX: 620-227-8812
www.arrowheadwest.org

Lori Pendergast, President
Janet Heit, Admission Coordinator
Julie Nelson, Public Relations Coordinator

Services and programs offered include: developmental and therapy services for children birth to age 3. Adult center-based work services and community integrated employment options; adult life skills and retirement programs; adult residential services including supervised living, supported living and independent living services. Staff includes over 200 employees. Services are provided over a 14 county area with service centers in Dodge City, Kinsley, Pratt, Medicine Lodge and Wichita.

9368 **Bethany Rehabilitation Center**
51 N 12th Street
Kansas City, KS 66102
913-281-8400
FAX: 913-281-7696

Wayne Kutz, VP

Offers rehabilitation services, inpatient and outpatient care, respite programs, psychiatric evaluations and more.

9369 **Big Lakes Developmental Center**
1416 Hayes Drive
Manhattan, KS 66502
785-776-9201
FAX: 785-776-9830
e-mail: biglakes@biglakes.org
www.biglakes.org

James Shaver, President/CEO

Work services, community employment and residential services. Serving adults with developmental disabilities. Family support services also available.

9370 **Developmental Services of Northwest Kansas**
2703 Hall Street, Suite 10
PO Box 1016
Hays, KS 67601
785-625-5678
FAX: 785-625-8204
e-mail: jim_blume@notes1.dsnwk.org
www.dsnwk.org

James W Blume, President
Ruth Lang, Administrative Assistant

A private nonprofit organization serving both children and adults with disabilities. Offers services to children ages birth to three years, youth and adults through a network of community-based and outreach programs and inter-agency agreements with other service providers in the eighteen counties of Northwest Kansas.

9371 ENVISION

2301 S Water
Wichita, KS 67213
316-267-2244
FAX: 316-267-4312
e-mail: envision@envisionus.com
www.envisionus.com

David Austin, Manager of Public Relations

Provides jobs, job training and vision rehabilitation services to people who are blind or low vision.

9372 Heartspring

8700 E 29th Street N
Wichita, KS 67226
316-634-8700
800-835-1043
FAX: 316-634-0555
www.heartspring.org

Charles Wolford, Admissions Director
Jennifer Wolthaa, PR Director
Charlene Kuzma LMSW CLP, Life Care Planner

Private, not-for-profit residential school for children from across the country ages five to twenty-one with multiple disabilities. Heartspring students are diagnosed with mental retardation and one or more of the following: autism, cerebral palsy, maladaptive behaviors, seizures, or other disabilities. Services are provided by an interdisciplinary team of specialists. Assessments and therapies are provided in the areas of speech/language, physical, occupational and hearing development.

9373 Indian Creek Nursing Center

6515 W 103rd Street
Overland Park, KS 66212
913-648-5093
FAX: 913-642-3982

Linnea Brandt, Administrator

Postacute rehabilitation program.

9374 Johnson County Developmental Supports

10501 Lackman Road
Lenexa, KS 66219
913-492-6161
FAX: 913-492-5171

Mark Elmore, Executive Director
Shelly Toft, Executive Assistant

9375 Ketch Industries

201 Ida Street
Wichita, KS 67211

Kaye Herman, Executive Director

9376 Lakemary Center

100 Lakemary Drive
Paola, KS 66071
913-557-4000
FAX: 913-294-4361

William R Craig PhD, President

A private, not-for-profit day and residential training facility which provides for the assessment, education, training, therapy and social development of children and adults, moderate and severe mental retardation. The Center is based 28 miles southwest of Kansas City in Paola, Kansas.

9377 Northview Developmental Services

700 E 14th Street
Newton, KS 67114
316-283-5170
FAX: 316-283-5196
e-mail: nds@northviewdsi.com

Stan Zienkewicz, President

Kentucky

9378 Cardinal Hill Outpatient Center

2050 Versailles Road
Lexington, KY 40504
859-254-5701
800-428-7755
FAX: 859-224-2081

Karen J Miller, Manager Referral Relations
Elizabeth A Monarch, VP Patient Services

Provides occupational health services, therapy services and urgent medical treatment of injured workers.

9379 Frazier Rehab Institute

220 Abraham Flexner Way
Louisville, KY 40202
502-582-7400
FAX: 502-582-7477
www.jewishhospital.org

Joanne Berryman, Senior VP
Barth Weinberg, VP Inpatient Rehab
Jean Russell, VP Rehab Operations

Frazier Rehab Institute is a regional healthcare system dedicated entirely to rehabilitation. Through an expansive network of inpatient and outpatient facilites in Kentucky and southern Indiana, Frazier offers a wide array of services based on one common goal - helping people with disabilities reach their full potential.

9380 HealthSouth Northern Kentucky Rehabilitation Hospital

201 Medical Village Drive
Edgewood, KY 41017
859-341-2044
800-860-6004
FAX: 859-341-2813

Marty Lautner, CEO/Administrator
Mary Pfeffer, Director of Clinical Services
Lynn Bean, Director of Nursing

Offers all types of rehabilitation services such as occupational therapy, physical therapy, speech therapy, inpatient and outpatient care and more for the disabled.

9381 King's Daughter's Medical Center's Rehab Unit/Work Hardening Program

2201 Lexington Avenue
Ashland, KY 41101
800-633-6388
FAX: 606-327-7542
www.komc.com

Harry Bell, Medical Director
Sue Strehle, Service Line Manager

Offers a 27-bed, inpatient rehabilitation services unit treating physical disabilities related to accident or illness. The program provides an interdisciplinary inpatient program designed to restore the individual to the highest level of independence. It is the goal of the staff to provide rehabilitative services that will enable the disabled or injured person to return home and re-enter the community at the maximum level of efficiency.

9382 **LifeSkills Industries**
2420 Russellville Road
Bowling Green, KY 42101 **270-842-8813**
FAX: 270-782-0058

Joe Miller, Executive Director

9383 **Low Vision Services of Kentucky**
120 N Eagle Creek Drive
Suite 501
Lexington, KY 40509
800-627-2020
FAX: 859-263-3757

William Wood MD, Clinical Director
Jeanne Van Arsdall, Low Vision Specialist
Helen T Wade, Administrator
Offers devices and services for the totally blind, legally blind, visually impaired educational, recreational and rehabilitation.

9384 **Muchlenberg County Opportunity Center**
Opportunity Way
Greenville, KY 42345 **502-338-5970**
FAX: 502-338-0301

Michael Morgan, Executive Director

9385 **New Vision Enterprises**
1900 Brownsboro Road
Louisville, KY 40206 **502-893-0211**
800-405-9135
FAX: 502-893-3885

Robert Jarboe, CEO
Offers employment training and services for the blind and legally blind.

9386 **Northfield Manor Healthcare Facility**
6000 Hunting Road
Louisville, KY 40222
FAX: 502-426-1401

Mark Malone, Administrator
Postacute rehabilitation program.

9387 **Park DuValle Community Health Center**
1817 S 34th Street
Louisville, KY 40211 **502-774-4401**
FAX: 502-775-6195

Richard Jones, Executive Director
Offers services for the totally blind, legally blind, visually impaired, mentally retarded blind and more with health, counseling, educational, recreational, rehabilitation, computer training and professional training services.

Louisiana

9388 **Alliance House**
2902 Florida Boulevard
Baton Rouge, LA 70802 **225-343-5393**
FAX: 225-346-0857

A non-residential facility serving male and female chronically mentally ill. Services include: social service, vocational evaluation, pre-vocational training and job placement.

9389 **Assumption Activity Center**
4201 Highway 1
Napoleonville, LA 70390 **985-369-2907**
FAX: 985-369-2657

Teal Stroud, Project Manager
A community work center providing prevocational training and extended employment for adults with disabilities. Services include: social services, work activities, specialized training and supported employment.

9390 **Caddo-Bossier Association for Retarded Citizens**
4103 Lakeshore Drive
Shreveport, LA 71109 **318-425-8888**
FAX: 318-221-4262

A community operated workshop for male and female mentally retarded individuals. It provides work evaluation and transitional and extended employment.

9391 **Deaf Action Center of GNO**
1000 Howard Avenue
Suite 1200
New Orleans, LA 70113 **504-523-3755**

Kathy Treubig, Administrator
Shari Bernius, Interpreter Coordinator
This community service and resource center serves deaf, deaf-blind, hard of hearing and speech-impaired persons in the greater New Orleans area regardless of age, religion, race or secondary disability. DAC provides interpreting services, equipment distribution, sign language classes, case management and advocacy.

9392 **Donaldsville Association for Retarded Citizens**
1030 Clay Street
Donaldsonville, LA 70346

A private, nonprofit sheltered work program working with the mentally retarded and developmentally disabled adults.

9393 **East Jefferson General Hospital Rehab Center**
3601 Houma Boulevard
Metairie, LA 70006 **504-885-4677**
FAX: 504-456-7381

Yolanda Cameron, Program Manager
Postacute rehabilitation program.

9394 **Family Service Society**
2515 Canal Street
Suite 201
New Orleans, LA 70119
FAX: 504-822-0831

Robert Quintana, Executive Director
Offers services for the totally blind, legally blind, visually impaired, mentally retarded blind and more with health, counseling, educational, recreational, rehabilitation, computer training and professional training services.

9395 **Foundation Industries**
9995 Highway 64
Zachary, LA 70791 **225-654-6283**
FAX: 225-654-3988

A private, nonprofit sheltered workshop providing extended employment and work activities for the mentally retarded and developmentally disabled clients.

9396 **Handi-Works Productions**

2700 Lee Street
Alexandria, LA 71301 **318-442-3377**
FAX: 318-473-0858

This is a nonprofit workshop for male and female clients who have vocational handicapping conditions. All types of handicapped persons are served in this non-residential workshop.

9397 **Iberville Association for Retarded Citizens**

PO Box 201
Plaquemine, LA 70765 **225-687-4062**
FAX: 225-687-3272
e-mail: arci@eatel.net

A private sheltered work program operating out of one facility and providing transitional, extended employment and work activities for mentally and developmentally ill adults.

9398 **Lighthouse for the Blind in New Orleans**

123 State Street
New Orleans, LA 70118 **504-899-4501**
FAX: 504-895-4162

RG Harmer, Executive Director

Offers services for the totally blind, legally blind, visually impaired, mentally retarded blind and more with health, counseling, educational, recreational, rehabilitation, computer training and professional training services.

9399 **Louisiana Center for the Blind**

101 S Trenton Street
Ruston, LA 71270 **318-251-2891**
800-234-4166
FAX: 318-251-0109
e-mail: allenp@lcb-ruston.com
www.lcb-ruston.com

Pam Allen, Director

A new kind of orientation and training center for blind persons. The center is privately operated and provides quality instruction in the skills of blindness. Offers employment assistance, computer literacy training, summer training and employment project, special seminars, outreach and referral services.

9400 **Louisiana State University Eye Center**

2020 Gravier Street
New Orleans, LA 70112 **504-412-1200**
FAX: 504-412-1315

9401 **New Orleans Speech and Hearing Center**

1639 Toledano Street
New Orleans, LA 70115 **504-524-9631**
FAX: 504-891-6048

Lesley Jernigan, Executive Director
Patty Connolly, Coordinator Clinical Services

This non-residential facility serves male and female clients for purposes of evaluating speech and hearing problems and providing speech therapy, hearing aids and other assistive technology for speech and hearing.

9402 **Port City Enterprises**

PO Box 113
Port Allen, LA 70767 **225-344-1142**
FAX: 225-344-1192

Christine Dunlevy, Executive Director

Offers supported employment, sheltered work and supervised programs for the mentally retarded, ages 22 and over.

9403 **Rehabilitation Center at Thibodeaux Regional**

RehabCare
602 N Acadia Road
Thibodaux, LA 70301 **985-493-4435**
FAX: 985-493-4436

Jan Torres, Program Manager
Rose Pipes, Clinical Coordinator

Designed to help patients in their adjustment to a physically limiting condition, both physically and psychologically, by helping to maximize each patients abilities so he or she can function as independently as possible.

9404 **Rehabilitation Hospital of Baton Rouge**

8595 United Plaza Boulevard
Baton Rouge, LA 70809 **225-927-0567**
800-264-0567
FAX: 225-926-2357

Jill Root, Admissions Director
Amy Searles, Community Relations

Dedicated to one field of medicine - physical rehabilitation medicine - and are committed to one goal, helping patients achieve the highest level of functioning possible after a debilitating injury or illness.

9405 **Rehabilitation Living Centers**

3434 Canal Street
New Orleans, LA 70119 **225-482-3075**
FAX: 504-483-2135

Dr. Robert Voogt, Owner

Postacute rehabilitation program.

9406 **St. Patrick RehabCare Unit**

RehabCare
524 S Ryan Street
Lake Charles, LA 70601 **337-491-7789**
FAX: 337-491-7194

Annette Harlow, Program Manager
Ruth Thornton, Admissions

Provides inpatient rehabilitation services in acute-care and sub-acute facilities. Treatment is provided for neurological and degenerative disorders.

9407 **Touro Rehabilitation Center**

1401 Foucher Street
New Orleans, LA 70115 **504-897-8560**
FAX: 504-897-8393
e-mail: haunj@touro.com
www.touro.com

Dr Gary Glynn, Medical Director
Suzy Laborde, Director of Inpatient Service
Keith Randazzo, Neuro Rehab Coordinator

Located in New Orleans' Garden District, Touro Rehabilitation is a comprehensive rehabilitation facility dedicated to the restoration of function and independence for individuals with disabilities. The scope of rehabilitation services is broad, with 4 CARF accreditations for Brain Injury, Spinal Cord Injury, Chronic Pain and General Rehabilitation. TRC opened in 1984 and offers 69 rehab beds. TRC is part of Touro Infirmary which has a proud 150 year history as a nonprofit teaching hospital.

9408 **Training, Resource & Assistive-Technology**

University of New Orleans
Lakefront Campus
New Orleans, LA 70148 **504-280-5700**
FAX: 504-280-5707
www.uno.edu/~trac

Kenneth Zangla, Program Director

This facility provides a curriculum utilizing innovative technology for people with disabilities, emphasizing microcomputer training, assessments, self-employment, disability awareness, education and international exchange.

9409 **University of New Orleans Training and Resource Center for the Blind**

Metro Campus Lakefront Campus
New Orleans, LA 70148 **504-280-6603**
FAX: 225-286-7294

This center offers a range of computer courses for the blind and visually impaired; maintains a resource lab with adaptive technology; conducts vocational evaluations for persons with disabilities; and provides information on the ADA.

Maine

9410 **Charlotte White Center**

572 Route 15
PO Box 380
Dover Foxcroft, ME 04426 **207-564-2499**
888-440-4158
FAX: 207-564-2404

Richard Brown, Executive Director
Anthony Zambrono, Director Operations

9411 **Iris Network for the Blind**

189 Park Avenue
Portland, ME 04102 **207-774-6273**
FAX: 207-774-0679
e-mail: sobremski@theiris.org
www.theiris.org

Steven Obremski, President/CEO

Offers services to persons who are blind, visually impaired or multi-disabled blind with rehabilitation, counseling, educational, recreational, computer training and professional training services.

9412 **Limerick Adult Day Program**

Foss Road
Limerick, ME 04048

Carol Snyder, Executive Director

9413 **Roger Randall Center**

50 Green Street
Houlton, ME 04730 **207-532-9196**
FAX: 207-532-9494

Dawn Ledger, Director Day Programs

The Roger Randall Cneter is one of five Day Habilitation Programs adminsitered by Community Living Association, a private, non-profit agency. These programs may provide a supportive environment that allows the individual to achieve their maximum growth potential. Individualized services address but are not limtied to the following areas: fine/gross motor skills, communication, community awareness and involvement, appropriate social skills, and independent living skills.

9414 **Sebasticook Farms**

PO Box 65
Saint Albans, ME 04971 **207-938-4615**
FAX: 207-938-5670

Tom Davis, Executive Director

Provides residential, educational and vocational services to adults who are developmentally disabled in order to maximize independent living and to provide assistance in obtaining an earned income.

9415 **Social Learning Center**

984 Sabattus Street
Lewiston, ME 04240 **207-783-4672**
FAX: 207-783-4673

Deborah Beam, Unit Manager

Maryland

9416 **Blind Industries and Services of Maryland**

2901 Strickland Street
Baltimore, MD 21223 **410-233-4567**
888-322-4567
FAX: 410-233-0544
www.bism.com

Rosemary Lerdahl, Rehab Director

Offers a comprehensive residential rehabilitation training program for people who are blind. Areas of instruction: braille, cane travel, independent living, computer, adjustment and blindness seminars.

9417 **Center for Neuro-Rehabilitation**

222 Severn Avenue
2340238 N Cary Street
Annapolis, MD 21223 **410-263-1704**
410-462-4711
e-mail: cnrnhq@erols.com

Jeanne Fryer
Laurent Pierre-Philippe

Provide community-based inpatient and outpatient acute rehabilitation, vocational services and long-term care. Specializing in treating complex neurological conditions including spinal cord injuries, multiple sclerosis, strokes, and other brain injuries resulting from trauma, anoxia, tumors, genetic malformations and other related conditions. Locations in Annapolis, Bethesda, Frederick, Towson, MD and Fairfax, Va. CNR is licensed, a Medicare provider and CARF accredited.

9418 **Child Find/Early Childhood Disabilities Unit Montgomery County Public Schools**

10731 Saint Margaret's Way
Suite A4
Kensington, MD 20895 **301-929-2224**
FAX: 301-929-2223

Julie Bader, Supervisor

Offers free developmental screening for children ages 2 years 9 months through 4 years, evaluation and placement services.

9419 **Greenery Extended Care Center: Baltimore**

1300 S Ellwood Avenue
Baltimore, MD 21224 **410-342-6644**
FAX: 301-327-3949

150 beds offering complex care treatment, extended rehabilitation and neurological restorative care.

9420 **James Lawrence Kerman Hospital**

2200 N Forest Park Avenue
Baltimore, MD 21207 **410-285-6566**
FAX: 410-448-6854

Dennis Grote, Executive Director

9421 **Levindale Hebrew Geriatric Center**
2434 W Belevedere Avenue
Baltimore, MD 21215 **410-601-2400**
FAX: 410-367-9066
www.lifebridgehealth.org

Ronald Rothstein, President and COO

9422 **Meridan Medical Center For Subacute Care**
770 York Road
Towson, MD 21204 **410-821-5500**
FAX: 410-337-7233

Patients receive around-the-clock professional nursing care; physical and occupational, speech and respiratory therapists also assist patients. Each patient's individualized plan of care is reviewed and updated as patient needs change. Careful discharge planning prepares patients and their families for success at home by teaching them how to avoid complications that might lead to rehospitalization.

9423 **Rehabilitation Opportunities**
5100 Philadelphia Way
Suite A
Lanham Seabrook, MD 20706 **301-731-4242**
FAX: 301-322-5891

Rory Brett, Executive Director

Organization offering day programs, evaluation, work adjustments and sheltered workshops for persons who are mentally retarded or developmentally disabled.

9424 **Richard E Hoover Rehabilitation for Low Vision and Blindness**
6569 N Chales Street
Physicians Pavilion W, Suite 305
Baltimore, MD 21204 **443-849-2658**
800-597-9142
FAX: 443-849-2631
http://www.gbmc.org/medicine/hoover

Nicole Love MD, Director Hoover Services

Offers services for the visually impaired and blind with low vision exams. Rehabilitation teaching and orientation and mobility in the home or workplace. Also offers a bimonthly newsletter for $12/yr for Hoover patients and monthly share group.

9425 **Rosewood Center**
200 Rosewood Lane
Owings Mills
Baltimore County, MD 21117 **410-951-5301**
FAX: 410-581-6157

Michael G Edukat, Facility Director
James Anzalone, Deputy Director

Offers a full range of habilitation services.

9426 **TLC: Treatment and Learning Centers**
9975 Medical Center Drive
Rockville, MD 20850 **301-424-5200**
FAX: 301-424-8063
www.ttlc.org

Patricia A Ritter PhD, Assistant Executive Director

Provides audiological evaluations, testing and hearing aids, physical and occupational therapy and evaluation; speech-language evaluation and therapy, psycho-educational testing and tutoring services for learning disabled students, head injury services and infant and early childhood services including child care, summer therapeutic camp and a special education preschool-8th grade.

9427 **Workforce and Technology Center**
2301 Argonne Drive
Baltimore, MD 21218 **410-554-9439**
FAX: 410-554-9112
e-mail: sschaffer@dors.state.md.us
www.dors.state.md.us

Susan Schaffer, Program Director
Kathi Long, Public Information and Planning

Is one of nine state operated comprehensive rehabilitation facilities in the country providing a wide range of services to individuals with disabilities. The Maryland Division of Rehabilitation Services operates the Workforce and Technology Program. Available services include medical functional evaluation, career training, mobility training, placement assistance, career assessment, rehab. technology assessments, driver's education and independent living skills training.

Massachusetts

9428 **Baroco Corporation**
PO Box 574
Williamsburg, MA 01096 **413-584-9978**
FAX: 413-585-9010
www.baroco.com

Provides training and therapeutic support for its recipients with developmental disabilities in order to aid them in securing and maintaining placement in a less-restrictive setting.

9429 **Berkshire Meadows**
249 N Plain Road
Housatonic, MA 01236 **413-528-2523**
FAX: 413-528-0293
e-mail: gcharpentier@jri.org
www.berkshiremeadows.org

Gail Charpenter, Executive Director

Private, non profit school for children, adolescents, young adults who are severely, developmentally disabled. approved special education learning center, work site program and foster care. Physical therapy, speech and language development, behavioral programming, occupational therapy, aquatic therapy, round-the-clock nursing. Also included is our state of the art equipment. *$8200.00*

9430 **Blueberry Hill Healthcare**
75 Brimbal Avenue
Beverly, MA 01915 **781-598-2107**
FAX: 978-922-4643

Phil Sher, Administrator

Postacute rehabilitation program.

9431 **Boston University Hospital Vision Rehabilitation Services**
720 Harrison Avenue
Boston, MA 02118 **617-638-8340**
FAX: 617-638-8321

Offers services for the totally blind, legally blind, visually impaired, mentally retarded blind and more with health, counseling, educational, recreational, rehabilitation, computer training and professional training services.

9432 **Burbank Rehabilitation Center**
275 Nichols Road
Fitchburg, MA 01420 **978-343-5660**
FAX: 978-343-5342

Diane O'Brien, Program Director

The largest community hospital and regional referral center in the area. Offers the most extensive high quality, cost-effective healthcare services in the region. The hospital provides outstanding hospital-based services such as case management of high risk elderly and the region's only comprehensive geriatric evaluation service. Also offers patients access to a complete continuum of healthcare, skilled nursing homes, and adult day care. This range of services affords patients prompt care.

9433 CPB/WGBH National Center for Access Media

WGBH Educational Foundation
125 Western Avenue
Boston, MA 02134 **617-300-3400**
FAX: 617-300-1035
TTY:617-492-9258
e-mail: ncam@wgbh.org
www.wgbh.org/ncam

Larry Goldberg, Director

A division within the WGBH Educational Foundation that works to make media accessible to under-served populations, such as disabled persons, minority language users, and people with low literacy skills. NCAM researches and develops new technologies that create access to public mass media (TV, radio, movies, newspapers, etc.), investigates how existing access technologies may benefit other populations, and conducts community outreach to educate people about media access issues.

9434 Carroll Center for the Blind

770 Centre Street
Newton, MA 02158 **617-969-6200**
800-852-3131
FAX: 617-969-6204
e-mail: rrosenbaum@carroll.org
www.carroll.org

Rachel Rosenbaum, Executive Director/President
Arthur O'Neill, Public Relations Director

Offers services for the totally blind, legally blind, visually impaired, mentally retarded blind and more with health, counseling, educational, in dependent living, tronell skills, computer traing, recreational, rehabilitation, computer training and professional training services.

9435 Center for Psychiatric Rehabilitation

Boston University
940 Commonwealth Avenue W
Boston, MA 02215 **617-353-3549**
FAX: 617-353-7700
www.bu.edu/cpr

William A Anthony PhD, Executive Director
Renee Sheppard, Publications Manager
Kathy Furlong-Norman, Director, Resource Information

The mission of the Center is to increase knowledge, to train treatment personnel, to develop effective rehabilitation programs and to assist in organizing both personnel and programs into efficient and coordinated service delivery systems for people with mental illness.

9436 Clark House of Fox Hill Village

30 Longwood Drive
Westwood, MA 02090 **781-326-5652**
FAX: 781-326-4034

Jim Brusstar, Administrator

Postacute rehabilitation program.

9437 College Internship Program at the Berkshire Center

18 Park Street
PO Box 160
Lee, MA 01238 **413-243-2576**
FAX: 413-243-3351
e-mail: gshaw@berkshirecenter.org
www.berkshirecenter.org

Gary Shaw, Admissions Director
Margaret Katz, Admissions Counselor

A highly individualized postsecondary program for learning disabled young adults 18-30. Provides job placement services and follow-ups; college support; money management and social skills. Residential students share an apartment and have their own room. They learn independent living skills and leisure skills. Clinically, each student has individual and group therapy. Psychiatric consultation is available as well as medication supervision if necessary.

9438 Eagle Pond

One Love Lane
PO Box 208
South Dennis, MA 02660 **508-385-6034**
FAX: 508-385-7064
eaglepond.com

James Des Rosiers, Administrator
Ellen Reil, Marketing Director

Postacute rehabilitation program. Alzheimer's disorder and related dementia long-term care.

9439 FOR Community Services

75 Litwin Lane
Chicopee, MA 01020 **413-592-6142**
FAX: 413-598-0478

Gina M Golash, Executive Director

9440 Fairlawn Rehabilitation Hospital

189 May Street
Worcester, MA 01602 **508-791-6351**
FAX: 508-753-2087

Ellen Ferrante, President

Offers comprehensive rehabilitation on both an inpatient and outpatient basis. Specialty programs include: head injury, spinal cord injury, young/senior stroke, oncology, geriatrics and orthopedics.

9441 Greenery Extended Care Center: Worcester

59 Acton Street
Worcester, MA 01604 **508-791-3147**
800-633-0887
FAX: 508-753-6267

173 beds offering complex care, extended rehabilitation and neurobehavioral intervention.

9442 Greenery Rehabilitation Center: Boston

PO Box 1330
Middleboro, MA 02346 **617-787-3390**
FAX: 617-787-9169

201 beds offering programs of active/acute rehabilitation, cognitive rehabilitation, respiratory care and short-term evaluations.

9443 Harrington House

160 Main Street
Walpole, MA 02081 **508-660-3080**
FAX: 508-660-1634

William McGinley, Administrator

Postacute rehabilitation program, sub-acute medical services and respiratory therapy program. Subacute accreditation by JCAHO.

9444 Holiday Inn Boxborough Woods
242 Adams Plaza
Boxborough, MA 01719 978-263-8701
FAX: 978-263-0518
e-mail: box_sales@fine-hotels.com
www.hotels-gauranteed.com/Massachusetts/Boxbo

Kathleen Kelly, Director Sales

Located on 35 acres of wooded countryside just off I-495 at exit #28. Minutes from the Mass Turnpike, Route 2, 290 and 9. Conference center located on main level with 30,000 square feet of meeting space. Guest rooms feature two-line telephones, voice mail and dataports, irons and ironing boards, hair dryers and coffemakers. $129-$159.

$129 - $159

9445 Kolburne School
Southfield Road
New Marlborough, MA 01230 413-229-8787
FAX: 413-229-7708

Peter Weinstein, Executive Director

A family owned residential treatment center offering psychiatric services, clinical services, special education programs, vocational programs and occupational therapy.

9446 Lifeworks Employment Services
588 Pleasant Street
Norwood, MA 02062 781-769-1212
FAX: 781-551-0045

Ruth Antonucci, Director

9447 Mariner Health Care: Massachusetts
4 5th Street
Peabody, MA 01960 508-229-0185
800-348-7676

Postacute rehabilitation program.

9448 Massachusetts Eye and Ear Infirmary & Vision Rehabilitation Center
243 Charles Street
Boston, MA 02114 617-573-4177
FAX: 617-573-4178
www.meei.harvard.edu

Joel Kraut MD FACS, Medical Director
Pat McCabe MPH, Director
Paulette Demors-Turco, Associate Director

Visual rehabilitation encompasses a low vision rehabilitation evaluation, occupational therapy evaluation (with home visit if necessary), and social service evaluation.

9449 New England Center for Children
33 Turnpike Road
Southborough, MA 01772 508-481-1015
FAX: 508-485-3421
e-mail: cwelch@necc.org
www.necc.org

Catherine Welch, Director Admissions

A comprehensive year-round program for students with autism and PDD who require a highly specialized educational and behavior management program. Students are from all over the country and receive intensive, positive, behavioral counseling and social skills training free of aversive treatment and excessive medication.

9450 New England Medical Center
Vision Rehabilitation Service
750 Washington Street
Boston, MA 02111
800-231-3316
FAX: 617-636-4867
e-mail: eli@vision.eri.harvard.edu

Eli Peli OD, Director Vision Rehabilitation
Maria Mercuri OD, Optometrist

Offers services for the legally blind, visually impaired, mentally retarded blind and more with health, counseling, educational, recreational, rehabilitation, computer training and professional training services.

9451 New Medico Rehabilitation and Skilled Nursing Center at Lewis Bay
89 Lewis Bay Road
Hyannis, MA 02601 508-775-7601
FAX: 508-790-4239

Edmund Steinle, Executive Director

9452 Protestant Guild
411 Waverly Oaks Road
Waltham, MA 02452 781-899-0222
FAX: 781-893-1171

Edmund Hagerty, Executive Director

Offers services for the diagnostically disabled adolescents with health, counseling, educational, recreational, rehabilitation, computer training and professional training services.

9453 Rehabilitation Hospital of Western New England
14 Chestnut Plaza
Ludlow, MA 01056 413-547-9063
FAX: 413-547-6530

Bonnie Breit, Outpatient Services

Postacute rehabilitation program.

9454 Shaughnessy-Kaplan Rehabilitation Hospital
Dove Avenue
Salem, MA 01970 978-745-9000
FAX: 978-741-1967
www.shaughnessy-kaplan.org

Anthony Sciola, President CEO

Rehabilitation for disabled and skilled nursing facility.

9455 Son-Rise Program
2080 S Undermountain Road
Sheffield, MA 01257 413-229-2100
800-714-2779
FAX: 413-229-3202
e-mail: sonrise@option.org
www.son-rise.org

Glenna Klein, Publicist

Provides innovative training programs for parents and professionals and caring for children challenged by Autism, Autism Spectrum Disorders, PDD and other developmental difficulties. The Son-Rise Program teached a specific yet comprehensive system of treatment and education designed to help families and caregivers enable their children to dramatically improve in all areas of learning, development and communication.

9456 Southern Worcester County Rehabilitation Center
44 Morris Street
Webster, MA 01570 508-943-0700
FAX: 508-949-6129
e-mail: swcrc@swcrc.inc.org

J Thomas Amick, Executive Director

Provides day habilitation services, residential services, evaluation and personal adjustment training, sheltered employment, supported employment services, supported work services for individuals with mental health problems. Serves the physically disabled, developmentally disabled, mental health and mental retardation. Vocational services and job placement programs are available as well.

9457 **Vinfen Corporation**
950 Cambridge Street
Cambridge, MA 02141
617-441-1800
877-284-6336
FAX: 617-441-1858

Gary W Lamson, President/CEO

A private, nonprofit company, Vinfen Corporation is the largest human services provider in Massachusetts. Vinfen offers clinical, educational, residential and support services to individuals of all ages with mental illness and or mental retardation, who also may have another disability (e.g. substance abuse, homelessness, AIDS). The company also trains professionals in the mental health field and helps consumers to learn to live in community-based settings at the highest levels.

9458 **Visiting Nurse Association of North Shore**
5 Federal Street
Danvers, MA 01923
978-777-6100
800-457-8999
FAX: 978-777-6517

Susan Comparone, President

Home health services including nurses, physical, occupational and speech therapy, home health aides and more. Special programs include nutrition counseling, IV care, pediatric therapy, HIV/AIDS services and wound management. Provides services 7 days a week, 365 days a year and we accept Medicare, Medicaid and most HMO's and health insurers.

9459 **Weldon Center for Rehabilitation**
233 Carew Street
Springfield, MA 01104
413-748-6800
FAX: 413-748-6806

Dr. James Lomastro, VP

9460 **Westridge Healthcare Center**
121 Northboro Road
Marlborough, MA 01752
FAX: 508-481-5585

Ivan Howard, Administrator

Postacute rehabilitation program.

9461 **Youville Hospital & Rehab Center**
1575 Cambridge Street
Cambridge, MA 02138
FAX: 617-547-5501

T Richard Quigley, President

Meets the long and short term health care and rehabilitation needs of patients who are physically disabled and chronically ill. Strives to develop and maintain health as a human right on physical, social, vocational and spiritual levels. The ultimate goal of the hospital is to treat and assist each individual patient in reaching his or her optimal level of living. Services include: stroke, brain injury, spinal cord trauma, orthopedic disabilities and more.

Michigan

9462 **Botsford General Hospital Inpatient Hospitalization Unit**
28050 Grand River Avenue
Farmington Hills, MI 48336
248-471-8000
FAX: 313-471-8773

Gina Massengill, ACSW

A 20 bed inpatient physical rehabilitation unit, servicing individuals who have experienced a stroke, amputation, orthopedic fracture, or other neurological impairment.

9463 **Chelsea Community Hospital Rehabilitation Unit**
775 S Main Street
Chelsea, MI 48118
734-475-4102
FAX: 734-475-4102
www.cch.org

Sally Flack, Coordinator IP Services
Diane Fenske, Coordinator of Services

A private, non-profit, acute care facility that combines the best of small town values with national standards of healthcare excellance. The hospital has a 19-bed acute care inpatient rehabilitation unit with comprehensive outpatient programs, including a coordinated brain injury program.

9464 **Clare Branch**
790 Industrial Drive
Clare, MI 48617
989-386-7707
FAX: 989-386-2199

Sherrie Johnson, Executive Director

9465 **Eight CAP**
904 Oak Drive Turk
Greenville, MI 48838
616-754-9315
FAX: 616-754-9310

Ralph Loeschner, Executive Director

9466 **Greenery Healthcare Center: Clarkston**
4800 Clintonville Road
Clarkston, MI 48346
248-674-0903
800-837-1913
FAX: 313-674-3431

120 beds offering active/acute rehabilitation, complex care, day treatment, extended rehabilitation, neurobehavioral intervention and short-term evaluation.

9467 **Haggerty Center for Neurorehabilitation**
42005 W 12 Mile Road
Novi, MI 48377
248-305-7575
FAX: 248-347-4578

Helene Rimer, Intake Coordinator

Postacute rehabilitation program.

9468 **Lakeland Center**
26900 Franklin Road
Southfield, MI 48034
248-350-8070
FAX: 248-350-8078
www.thelakelandcenter.net

Adrienne Shepperd, Marketing Associate
Moira Donnelly-Kempf, Marketing Associate

Subacute rehabilitation program directed toward those with severe neurologic diagnoses, ie: TBI, cerebral aneurysm, anoxic encephalopathy, CVA and cerebral hemorrhage and spinal cord injury. Subacute rehabilitation is provided for those who recover slowly and require individualized treatment plans.

9469 Mary Free Bed Hospital and Rehabilitation Center
235 Wealthy Street SE
Grand Rapids, MI 49503
616-242-0474
800-528-8989
FAX: 616-493-9666
e-mail: mderrer@mfbrc.com
www.mfbrc.com

Meg Derrer, Marketing Director/Webmaster

9470 Men-O-Mee Activity Center
W5522 First Street
Hermansville, MI 49847
FAX: 906-498-7606

Thomas Warren, Executive Director

9471 Michigan Commission for the Blind Training Center
1541 Oakland Drive
Kalamazoo, MI 49008
269-337-3848
FAX: 269-337-3872
www.mcb1.gov

Melody Lindsey, Director

Residential facility that provides instruction to legally blind adults in Braille, computers, handwriting, keyboarding, cane travel, adaptive kitchen skills, daily living, industrial arts and also crafts. Clients may also learn to use a variety of adaptive devices such as raised dot timers and watches, hand tools, talking calculators, tape recorders, reading machines and computers. Special training is also offered in vending stand operation, college preparation and job seeking skills.

9472 Mid-Michigan Industries
2426 Parkway Drive
Mt Pleasant, MI 48858
989-773-6918
888-773-7664
FAX: 989-773-1317
e-mail: mail@mmionline.com
www.mmionline.com

M Judith Garland, President
Andrea Christopher, Director Admissions

Providing training program for persons with barriers to employment. Services include vocational evaluation, job placement, supported employment, work services, prevocational training and case management

9473 New Medico Community Re-Entry Service
216 Saint Marys Lake Road
Battle Creek, MI 49017
FAX: 269-962-2241

James Rekshan, Executive Director

9474 Rehabilitation Services
Hope Network
1490 E Beltline Avenue SE
Grand Rapids, MI 49506
616-940-0040
FAX: 616-940-8151

Tom Stranz MA, Director Rehab
Elizabeth Lock, Admissions Manager

A department of Hope Network, one of the largest, private, nonprofit organizations of its kind in Michigan. The purpose is to assist people with brain injuries and/or physical disabilities in achieving an optimal level of self-determination, dignity, and independence as they develop and attain goals to overcome environmental barriers and mobilize adaptive skills.

9475 Sanilac County Community Mental Health
217 E Sanilac
Suite 1
Sandusky, MI 48471
810-648-0330
888-225-4447
FAX: 810-648-0319

Dr. Roger Dean, Executive Director

9476 Special Tree Rehabilitation System
1640 Axtell Road
Troy, MI 48084
248-649-0101
800-649-5011
FAX: 248-649-5445

Michael Malley, Communications

Postacute rehabilitation program.

9477 State Technical Institute and Rehabilitation Center
Alber Drive
Plainwell, MI 49080
269-664-9257
FAX: 269-664-5850

Leonard Lee, Executive Director

9478 Thumb Industries
1263 Sand Beach Road
Bad Axe, MI 48413
989-269-9229
FAX: 989-269-9229

Teresa Rabideau, Executive Director

Provides job training and employment for disabled persons.

9479 Upshaw Institute for the Blind
16625 Grand River Avenue
Detroit, MI 48227
313-272-3900
FAX: 313-272-6893
www.upshawinst.org

Gail L McEntee, Interim Executive Director

Offers services for seniors 60 and over who are legally blind. Also provides eye health information, counseling, education and rehabilitation services.

9480 Visually Impaired Center
1422 W Court Street
Flint, MI 48503
810-235-2544
FAX: 810-235-2597
e-mail: info@vicflint.org
www.vicflint.org

Sharon Reigle, Executive Director
Criss Kellogg, Social Worker

Committed to developing resources and collaborative programs as well as providing services that enable independent life for people with vision loss. Services include: Information and referals, assessments of needs, peer support groups, training by a Rehabilitation teacher of the blind and visually impaired, independent living skills, computer skills, training by an Orientation and Mobility Specialist, safe traveling skills, Diabetes management/education.

a pages

9481 Welcome Homes Retirement Community for the Visually Impaired
1953 Monroe Avenue NW
Grand Rapids, MI 49505
616-363-9088
888-939-9292
FAX: 616-363-3099
e-mail: info@welcomehomes.org
www.welcomehomes.org

Kathy Higgins, Executive Director/CEO

Offers services for the totally blind, legally blind, visually impaired, mentally retarded blind and more with health, counseling, educational, recreational, rehabilitation, computer training and professional training services.

9482 William H Honor Rehabilitation Center Henry Ford Wyanclotte Hospital
2333 Biddle Street
Wyandotte, MI 48192 **734-284-2400**
FAX: 734-246-6926

Denise Dailing, Admin. Leader/Rehabiliation Svcs

Minnesota

9483 Brown-Nichollet Industries
21st N Street & Broadway
New Ulm, MN 56073
FAX: 507-345-4507

Arne Berg, Executive Director

9484 Industries
500 Walnut Street S
Mora, MN 55051 **320-679-2354**
FAX: 320-679-2355

Nonprofit organization that does vocational assessment and training for people with disabilities.

9485 Shriners Hospitals for Children: Twin Cities
2025 E River Parkway
Minneapolis, MN 55414 **612-596-6100**
888-293-2832
FAX: 612-339-5954
www.shrinershq.org

Erin Jurkovich, Public Relations Specialist

Shriners Hospital for Children-Twin Cities offers quality orthopedic medical care at no cost. Shriners Hospitals provide inpatient and outpatient services, surgery, casts, braces, artificial limbs, X-rays and physical and occupational therapy to any child under 18 who may benefit from treatment. To obtain an application, call toll free at (888)293-2832.

9486 Vision Loss Resources
1936 Lyndale Avenue S
Minneapolis, MN 55403 **612-871-2222**
FAX: 612-872-0189
www.visionlossresources.com

Steven Fischer, Executive Director

Offers services for the totally blind, legally blind, visually impaired, and more with health, counseling, educational, recreational, rehabilitation, computer training and professional training services.

Mississippi

9487 Addie McBryde Rehabilitation Center for the Blind
2550 Peachtree Street
PO Box 5314
Jackson, MS 39296 **601-364-2700**
FAX: 601-364-2677
e-mail: cponder@mdrs.state.ms.us

Carrie Ponder, Director
Karen Wallace, Assistant Director
Rosie Gibson, Assistant Director

Offers services for the totally blind, legally blind, visually impaired, mentally retarded blind and more with health, counseling, educational, recreational, rehabilitation, computer training services and orientation and mobility.

9488 Mississippi Methodist Rehabilitation Center
1350 E Woodrow Wilson Avenue
Jackson, MS 39216 **601-364-3481**
800-981-2611
FAX: 601-364-3465

Rebuild lives that have been broken by disabilities and impairments from serious illness or severe injury. The challenge is to help patients regain abilities, restore function and movement, and renew emotionally. It features personal rehabilitation treatment plans administered by specialized teams of health care professionals through a variety of outpatient programs, treatments and other services.

Missouri

9489 Alpine North Nursing and Rehabilitation Center
4700 NW Cliff View Drive
Kansas City, MO 64150
FAX: 816-746-1301

Sharon Garcia, Clinical Director

Postacute rehabilitation program.

9490 Christian Hospital Northeast
11133 Dunn Road
Saint Louis, MO 63136 **314-653-5000**
FAX: 314-653-4174

Nancy Bartmess, Executive Director

9491 Integrated Health Services of St. Louis at Gravois
10954 Kennerly Road
Saint Louis, MO 63128 **314-843-4242**
FAX: 314-843-5370

Cathy Deffendall, Administrator
Fran Jackson, Marketing Director

Subacute, skilled and intermediate care; ventilator/tracheostomy management program; wound management program and complex rehabilitation program.

9492 Joplin House Healthcare
2502 S Moffet Avenue
Joplin, MO 64804
FAX: 417-623-0880

Jan Zacny, Administrator

Postacute rehabilitation program.

9493 Metropolitan Employment & Rehabilitation Service
1727 Locust Street
Saint Louis, MO 63103 **314-241-3464**
FAX: 314-241-9348
www.mers.org

Dr. Lewis C Chartock, President
Zip Rzeppa, VP Public Affairs

Vocational rehabilitation, primarily with the disabled, skills training and placement services.

9494 Missouri Easter Seal Society: Southeast Region

5025 Northrup Avenue
St. Louis, MO 63110 **314-664-6014**
FAX: 314-664-4838
www.mo.easter-seals.org

The mission of the Easter Seal Society is to work with individuals, their families and the community to enhance the independence and quality of life for persons with disabilities.

9495 Poplar Bluff RehabCare Program

Lucy Lee Hospital
PO Box 88
Poplar Bluff, MO 63902 **573-686-7320**
FAX: 573-686-7307

Jim Martin, Program Manager
Chris Murray, Care Coordinator
Darlene Hill, Care Admissions Coordinator

Provides physical medicine and rehabilitation to individuals with a physically limiting condition. The program is designed to help individuals function as independently as possible by maximizing their strength and abilities.

9496 Service Club for the Blind

3719 Watson Road
Saint Louis, MO 63109 **314-647-3306**
FAX: 314-647-3306

Fred Keller, President
Joann Hall, Office Assistant
Kathleen Demsky, Office Assistant

Offers services for the totally blind, legally blind, visually impaired, mentally retarded blind and more with health, counseling, educational, recreational, rehabilitation, computer training and professional training services.

9497 Shriners Hospitals for Children St. Louis

2001 S Lindbergh Boulevard
Saint Louis, MO 63131 **314-432-3600**
800-850-2960
FAX: 314-432-2930
www.shrinershq.org/SHC/STLOUIS

Carolyn P Golden, Administrator
Tammy M Dugan, Director Community Relations

Medical care is provided free of charge for children 18 and under with orthopaedic conditions.

9498 St. Louis Society for the Blind and Visually Impaired

8770 Manchester Road
Saint Louis, MO 63144 **314-968-9000**
FAX: 314-968-9003
e-mail: info@slsbvi.org
www.slsbvi.org

David C Ekin, Executive Director
Brenda Dunn, Client Services Coordinator

Offers vision rehabilitation services for the totally blind, legally blind, visually impaired, including counseling, educational, recreational, rehabilitation, computer training and professional training services. Low vision aids and appliance available through low vision clinic by appointment.

9499 TNC Community Truman Neurological Center

15600 Woods Chapel Road
Kansas City, MO 64139 **816-373-5060**
FAX: 816-373-5787
e-mail: debbietnc@aol.com

Scott Litten, Executive Director

A licensed habilitation center established for the purpose of assisting persons with developmental disabilities and/or mental retardation. The minimum age is 18. Residential care is provided in four group homes in the community licensed by the DMH and CARF accredited.

9500 Visual Independence Program

Eye Foundation of Kansas City
2300 Holmes Street
Kansas City, MO 64108 **816-881-6157**
FAX: 816-881-6246

Camille Matta MD, Medical Director
Brendan Smith OTR, Program Director

Program offers in home rehabilitation services to older adults with visual impairments including training in use of magnifying devices for reading and other activities of daily living. Specialized rehabilitation program for persons with visual impairment secondary to stroke or head trauma.

Montana

9501 Benefis Healthcare

1101 26th Street S
Great Falls, MT 59405 **406-761-1200**
FAX: 406-455-2110

Lloyd Smith, President/CEO

9502 Disability Services Division

111 Sanders Street
PO Box 4210
Helena, MT 59604 **406-444-2995**
FAX: 406-444-0230
www.dphhs.state.mt.us/dsd

Joe A Mathews, Administrator
Karen Cech, Administrative Assistant
Janice Frisch, Chief Management Operations

Responsible for coordinating, developing and implementing comprehensive programs to assist Montanans with disabilities with activities of daily living, community base services and coordinated programs of habilitation, rehabilitation and independent living.

9503 Montana Department of Developmental Disabilities Program

111 Sanders Street
PO Box 4210
Helena, MT 59604 **406-444-2590**
FAX: 406-444-0230
www.dphhs.state.mt.us/dsd

Information on developmental disabilities and automated systems.

Nebraska

9504 Career Achievement Center

PO Box 83589
Lincoln, NE 68501 **402-476-5097**
FAX: 402-483-1127

Susie Feistner, Executive Director

9505 Las Vegas Convalescent Center

2832 S Maryland Parkway
Las Vegas, NV 89109 **702-796-3855**
FAX: 702-735-6218

Postacute rehabilitation program.

9506 **Sierra Pain Institute**
265 Golden Lane
Reno, NV 89502 **775-323-7092**
FAX: 775-323-5259

The program consists of a medically supervised outpatient program managed by an interdisciplinary team with input from specialties of Pain Medicine, Physical Therapy and Occupational Science. The format insures that each patient receives the full range of behavioral techniques in a well-integrated, individually tailored therapeutic regimen.

New Hampshire

9507 **Adroscoggin Valley Mental Health Center**
Page Hill Road
Berlin, NH 03570
FAX: 603-752-5194

Arthur Froburg, Executive Director

9508 **Crotched Mountain Adult Brain Injury Center**
Crotched Mountain Rehabilitation Center
1 Verney Drive
Greenfield, NH 03047 **603-547-3311**
FAX: 603-547-3232
e-mail: admissions@cmf.org
www.info@cmf.org

Brant A Elkind MS CBIS-CE, Brain Injury Center Director
Rita Phinney, Admissions Director
John Young, Registrar

Adult Brain Injury Unit provides sub-acute rehabilitative services and individualized care to survivors of acquired (including traumatic) brain injury. Ambulatory and non-ambulatory adults are served. Ages range from 18-59, the staff to client ratio is 4:1 and services are provided by experienced interdisciplinary clinical and therapeutic teams. Crotched Mountain is a licensed Special Hospital providing 24 hour medical coverage and skilled nursing. Clients reside in semi-private rooms w/supervis

9509 **Department of Physical Medicine and Rehabilitation**
Exeter Hospital
10 Buzell Avenue
Exeter, NH 03833 **603-778-7311**
FAX: 603-778-6671

Robert Haskins, Administrator

Offers patient treatment, committed to enhancing the lives of individuals with short and long term physically disabling conditions.

9510 **Farnum Rehabilitation Center**
580 Court Street
Keene, NH 03431 **603-357-3018**
FAX: 603-355-2078

Susan Loughrey, Program Director

Offers rehabilitation services, occupational therapy, physical therapy and more for the physically challenged individual.

9511 **Hackett Hill Nursing Center and Integrated Care**
191 Hackett Hill Road
Manchester, NH 03102 **603-668-8161**
FAX: 603-622-2584

Claudia Gallo, Case Manager

Postacute rehabilitation program.

9512 **New Hampshire Rehabilitation and Sports Medicine**
Catholic Medical Center
769 S Main Street
Suite 201
Manchester, NH 03102 **603-663-5863**
800-437-9666
FAX: 603-668-5348

Heidi George, Director

A specialized facility for comprehensive rehabilitation for individuals who have been injured or have a disability.

9513 **New Medico, Highwatch Rehabilitation Center**
Highwatch Road
Effingham Falls, NH 03814
FAX: 603-539-8888

Dr. William Burke, Executive Director

9514 **Northern New Hampshire Mental Health and Developmental Services**
87 Washington Street
Conway, NH 03818 **603-430-2101**
FAX: 603-447-8893

Stanley Marsden, Director

Provides mental health and developmental services to northern New Hampshire, including early intervention, elderly services, residential program, outpatient services, employee assistance programs, inpatient services, etc.

New Jersey

9515 **All Garden State Physical Therapy**
750 Broadway
Paterson, NJ 07514 **973-345-1312**
FAX: 973-742-0669

Evelyn Perez, General Manager

Postacute rehabilitation program.

9516 **Bancroft NeuroHealth**
PO Box 20
Haddonfield, NJ 08033 **856-429-5637**
FAX: 856-429-1613
e-mail: inquiry@bancroft.org
www.bancroft.org

Dr. George Niemann, President/CEO
Jim Powers, VP Marketing/Public Affairs
Michelle Stewart, Director of Communciations

Private, not-for-profit organization serving people with disabilities since 1883. Based in Haddonfield, New Jersey, help more than 1000 children and adults with autism, developmental disabilities, brain injuries, and other neurological impairments. Operates more than 140 sites throughout the U.S. and abroad.

9517 **Cerebral Palsy of Monmouth & Ocean Counties**
Schroth School & Technical Education Center
1701 Kneeley Boulevard
Asbury Park, NJ 07712 **732-493-5900**
FAX: 732-493-5980

K David Holmes, Executive Director
Patti Carbone, Executive Director

Provides an array of services and programs specifically for children and adults with developmental and physical disabilities. Services include approved Department of Education school programs; adult education and training; vocational training, personal care assistance services, in-home and Saturday respite; child care programs, housing opportunities, and more.

9518 Daughters of Miriam Center for the Aged
155 Hazel Street
Clifton, NJ 07011 **973-772-3700**
FAX: 973-772-7117

Harvey Adelsburg, Executive Director

9519 Devereux Center in New Jersey
230 Pottersville Road
 # 520
Chester, NJ 07930
FAX: 908-879-6370

Kristy Hartman, Admissions Director
Lynn Jones, Executive Director
Carol Poirier, Admissions Assistant

Serves emotionally disturbed females, ages 5-21, who have affective disorders, bi-polar disorders, adjustment reactions, behavioral disorders, specific developmental disorders, identity disorders, attention deficit disorders, schizoid disorders, anxiety disorders, enuresis, runaway behavior, substance abuse, in remission and personality disturbances. The center offers 95-100 full-time staff including, teachers, administrators, counselors, therapists, recreation staff and support services.

9520 Integrated Health Services of New Jersey at Somerset Valley
1621 Route 22 W
Bound Brook, NJ 08805 **732-469-2000**
FAX: 732-469-8917
www.ihs-inc.com

Carolyn Allen, Executive Director
Janine Vyzas, Social Work/Admissions Director

Postacute rehabilitation program.

9521 Lourdes Regional Rehabilitation Center
1600 Haddon Avenue
Camden, NJ 08103 **856-757-3840**
FAX: 856-968-2522

Tammy Feuer, Admin., Rehab & Post Acute Serv.

9522 Mt. Carmel Guild
494 Broad Street
Newark, NJ 07105 **973-639-9534**

Edda Stewart, Coordinator

Offers services for the totally blind, legally blind, visually impaired, mentally retarded blind and more with health, counseling, educational, recreational, rehabilitation, computer training and professional training services.

9523 Pediatric Rehabilitation Department, JFK Medical Center
2050 Oak Tree Road
Edison, NJ 08820 **732-548-7610**
FAX: 732-548-7751

Dr. Patricia Munday, Director Pediatric Rehab

Comprehensive interdisciplinary, family focused outpatient pediatric rehabilitation services including evaluation and individual and group treatment programs for children birth-21.

9524 REACH Rehabilitation Program: Leader Nursing and Rehabilitation Center
550 Jessup Road
Paulsboro, NJ 08066 **856-848-9551**

Karen Fattore, Case Manager

Postacute rehabilitation program.

9525 REACH Rehabilitation and Catastrophic Long-Term Care
1180 Route 22
Mountainside, NJ 07092 **908-654-0020**

Linda Sweeney, Program Director

Postacute rehabilitation program.

9526 Rehabilitation Specialists
33 Sicomac Road
North Haledon, NJ 07508 **973-636-9366**
800-441-7488
FAX: 973-427-1463

Doug Cerminaro, Admissions Coordinator

Rehabilitation Specialists, founded in 1983, is a quality, cost effective community re-entry center treating individuals with acquired brain injury. A non clinical environment based in the community is utilized that offers professional services enabling participants to learn skills they need to return to a productive life. Both our Day and Residential programming emphases focus on Functional Life Skills, Work Skills and Learning Skills. Each participant's program is tailored to meet their needs.

9527 Summit Ridge Center
20 Summit Street
W Orange, NJ 27052 **973-736-2000**
FAX: 973-731-4582
www.ghv.com

Charlene Harn, Admissions & Marketing Director

Offers rehabilitation services, occupational therapy, physical therapy and more for the physically challenged.

New Mexico

9528 Lifecourse Rehabilitation Services
525 S Schwartz Avenue
Farmington, NM 87401 **505-325-6645**
FAX: 505-327-6562

Bobi Logsdon RN CRRN, Case Manager

Uses a team of professionals to provide a comprehensive rehabilitation program. Accomplishing the best possible physical and cognitive improvement is the aim of the following treatment members: nurses, physical therapists, physicians, speech and occupational therapists, therapeutic recreation specialist. Providing inpatient and out patient services.

9529 Southwest Communication Resource
PO Box 788
Bernalillo, NM 87004 **505-867-3396**
FAX: 505-867-3398
e-mail: info@swcr.org
www.swcr.org

Norman Segel, Executive Director

Services for infants, children and adults with developmental disabilities in Sandoval County New Mexico.

New York

9530 Bronx Continuing Treatment Day Program
1527 Southern Boulevard
Bronx, NY 10460
718-893-1414
FAX: 718-893-0707

Ellen Stoller, Executive Director

9531 Brooklyn Bureau of Community Service
285 Schermerhorn Street
Brooklyn, NY 11217
718-885-5600
FAX: 718-855-1517

Leslie Klein, Director Adult Rehabilitation
Maryclare Scerbo, Director Volunteer Services

Offers independent living skills, counseling, work readiness, vocational trianing, job placement and job follow-up services to individuals with disabilities (to include individuals with psychiatric, physical, and developmental disabilities). Special programs to move disabled welfare recipients from welfare to work. Publishes a bi-annual newsletter.

9532 Buffalo Hearing and Speech Center
50 E N Street
Buffalo, NY 14203
716-885-8318
FAX: 716-885-4229
www.buffalohearingandspeech.org

Janet Maher, President

Assists individuals with speech, language and/or hearing impairments to achieve maximum communication potential.

9533 Cora Hoffman Center
2324 Forest Avenue
Staten Island, NY 10303
718-447-8205
FAX: 718-815-2182

Kevin Kenney, Executive Director

9534 Elmhurst Hospital Center
7901 Broadway
Elmhurst, NY 11373
718-334-2600
FAX: 718-334-2623

Offers rehabilitation services, occupational therapy, physical therapy and more for the physically challenged individual.

9535 F-E-G-S
315 Hudson Street
New York, NY 10013
212-366-8400
FAX: 212-366-8441
e-mail: execoffice@fegs.org
www.fegs.org

Jill Colon-Regus, Day Habilitation Services
Loel Tayler, Continuing Day Treatment Prgms
Rena Moore, Intensive Psychiatric Rehab Prgm

9536 Flushing Hospital
4500 Parsons Boulevard
Flushing, NY 11355
718-670-3134
FAX: 718-670-3082

David Karan MD, Director Clinic

Offers services for the totally blind, legally blind, visually impaired, mentally retarded blind and more with health, counseling, educational, recreational, rehabilitation, computer training and professional training services.

9537 Gateway New Palz
137 N Chestnut Street
New Paltz, NY 12561
845-255-6700
FAX: 845-255-6706

Mark Hildebrandt, Executive Director

9538 Henkind Eye Institute Division of Montefiore Hospital
3400 Bainbridge Avenue
Bronx, NY 10467
718-920-6244
FAX: 718-920-6244

Lanny M Binstock

Offers services for the totally blind, legally blind, visually impaired, mentally retarded blind and more with health, counseling, educational, recreational, rehabilitation, computer training and professional training services. Low vision services offered.

9539 Industries for the Blind of New York State
230 Washington Avenue
Albany, NY 12210
518-456-8671
FAX: 518-456-3587

Steven M Ennis, President

Offers services for the totally blind, legally blind, visually impaired, mentally retarded blind and more with health, counseling, educational, recreational, rehabilitation, computer training and professional training services.

9540 Inpatient Pain Rehabilitation Program
301 E 17th Street
New York, NY 10003
212-598-6606
FAX: 212-598-6468
e-mail: isaac.pinter@med.nyu.edu
www.hjd.edu/hjd/hjd-home.jsp

Isaac Pinter PhD, Administrative Director

The Inpatient Rehabilitation Program, established in 1983 specializes in the treatment of chronic pain. Our inpatient program is one of the oldest and well established pain programs in the country. It is the only interdisciplinary inpatient pain program in the tri-state area and one of only 20 pain programs in the entire US to have CARF accreditation. Upon completion of an extensive evaluation, patients are admitted for an 18-day inpatient stay.

9541 Koicheff Health Care Center
2324 Forest Avenue
Staten Island, NY 10303
718-447-0200
FAX: 718-981-1431

P Jeanne DeLaRosa, Clinic Director

9542 Marcus Pain Institute
30 E 40th Street
New York, NY 10016
212-532-7999
FAX: 212-532-5957
e-mail: njm@nmpi.com
www.nmpi.com

Norman Marcus MD, Medical Director

We focus on muscles as the cause of most common pains, i.e. back, neck, shoulders, and headaches. We make specific muscle diagnoses and have specific treatments that in many cases will eliminate the need for surgery or relieve the pain. Patients diagnosed with herniated disc, spinal stenosis, rotator cuff tear, impingement syndrome, sciatica, fibromyalgia and headache will generally find relief.

9543 **Pain Alleviation Center**
125 S Service Road
Jericho, NY 11753 **718-258-9222**
FAX: 516-997-7281

Dr. Richard Linchitz, Medical Director
One of the first pain clinics to gain national accreditation from the Commission on Accreditation of Rehabilitation Facilities. This is due largely to a patient-centered program based on the latest research.

9544 **Pathfinder Village**
3 Chenango Road
Edmeston, NY 13335 **607-965-8377**
FAX: 607-965-8655
e-mail: info@pathfindervillage.org
www.pathfindervillage.org

Edward Shafer, CEO
Pathfinder Village is a warm, friendly community in the rolling hills of Central New York. Here children and adults with Down Syndrome gain independence, build lasting friendships, become partners in the world and take in all that life has to offer.

9545 **Pilot Industries: Ellenville**
48 Canal Street
Ellenville, NY 12428 **845-647-7711**
FAX: 845-647-7711

Peter Pierri, Executive Director

9546 **Presbyterian Hospital in the City of New York**
622 W 168th Street
New York, NY 10032 **212-874-6633**
FAX: 212-305-1017

Michael Bradley, Executive Director

9547 **Skills Unlimited**
405 Locust Avenue
Oakdale, NY 11769 **516-567-3320**
FAX: 516-567-3285

Richard Kassnove, Executive Director

9548 **United Cerebral Palsy of Western New York**
7 Community Drive
Buffalo, NY 14225 **716-894-0130**
FAX: 716-894-8257

Virginia C Purcell, Executive Director
Provides comprehensive services, to individuals with disabilities from infancy through adulthood. Also serves people with all types of developmental disabilities as well as providing clinical services to persons with other types of disabilities such as: spinal cord injury, multiple sclerosis, head trauma and others. The center employs over 750 people.

North Carolina

9549 **Center for Vision Rehabilitation**
Academy Eye Associations
3115 Academy Road
Durham, NC 27707 **919-493-7456**
800-942-1499
FAX: 919-493-1718
e-mail: hgeyesomindspring.com
www.academyeye.com

Henry A Greene OD, President
Vision rehabilitation and low-vision care for the visually impaired, post-stroke, head trauma and for neuro-oncology vision complications.

9550 **Diversified Opportunities**
610 N Pender Street
Wilson, NC 27893 **252-291-0378**
FAX: 252-291-1402

Mike Petty, Executive Director

9551 **Hillhaven Convalescent Center**
616 Wade Avenue
Raleigh, NC 27605
FAX: 919-828-3294

Dennis Redmond, Administrator
Postacute rehabilitation program.

9552 **Industries of the Blind**
920 W Lee Street
Greensboro, NC 27403 **336-274-1591**
FAX: 336-274-9207

Anette Klinard, Personnel/Safety Administrator
Offers services for the totally blind, legally blind, visually impaired, mentally retarded blind and more with health, counseling, educational, recreational, rehabilitation, computer training and professional training services.

9553 **John C Whitaker Regional Rehabilitation**
3333 Silas Creek Parkway
Winston Salem, NC 27103 **336-718-5780**
FAX: 336-718-9272
www.forsythmedicalcenter.org/services

Mary Jo Weavil, Director

9554 **Johnston County Industries**
912 Bright Leaf Boulevard
Smithfield, NC 27577 **919-934-0677**

Vicki Shore, Executive Director

9555 **Learning Services: Carolina**
707 Morehead Avenue
Durham, NC 27707 **919-419-9955**
FAX: 919-687-0530

Gary Ulciny, Admission
Postacute rehabilitation program.

9556 **LifeSpan**
940 Beaumont Avenue
High Point, NC 27260 **336-883-0111**
FAX: 336-883-0031
www.lifespanservices.org

Patti Huggins, Program Director
Provide vocational and enrichment program for adults with developmental disabilities.

9557 **Lions Club Industries for the Blind**
1810 E Main Street
Durham, NC 27703
FAX: 919-598-1179

William Hudson, Executive Director
Offers services for the totally blind, legally blind, visually impaired, mentally retarded blind and more with health, counseling, educational, recreational, rehabilitation, computer training and professional training services.

9558 **Lions Services**

4600 N Tryon Street
A
Charlotte, NC 28213
704-921-1527
FAX: 704-921-1577

Charles Lamb, Adminstrator

Offers services for the totally blind, legally blind, visually impaired, mentally retarded blind and more with health, counseling, educational, recreational, rehabilitation, computer training and professional training services.

9559 **McLeod Center West**

Old Highway 70
Black Mountain, NC 28711
FAX: 828-669-4164

Steve Lee, Executive Director

9560 **Regional Rehabilitation Center Pitt County Memorial Hospital**

2100 Stantonsburg Road
Greenville, NC 27834
252-816-4715
FAX: 252-816-7552
e-mail: mdixon@pcmh.com

Martha M Dixon, VP General Services

9561 **Rehab Home Care**

2660 Yonkers Road
Raleigh, NC 27604
800-447-8692
FAX: 919-831-2211

Alan Silver, CEO
Janis Hansen, Chief Operating Officer

A Medicare/Medicaid certified, state-licensed home health agency with emphasis on rehabilitation.

9562 **Thoms Rehabilitation Hospital**

Thoms Rehabilitation Hospital
68 Sweeten Creek Road
Asheville, NC 28803
828-274-6179
FAX: 828-274-9452

Kathi Petersen, Dir. of Planning & Communication
Edgardo Diez MD, Medical Director Brain Injury
Kathy Price, Director Admissions

Freestanding physical rehabilitation hospital, founded 1938 - 100 beds, including 90 acute and 10 transitional - JCAHO accredited.

9563 **Winston-Salem Industries for the Blind**

7730 N Point Drive
Winston Salem, NC 27106
336-759-0551
FAX: 336-759-0990

Daniel Boucher, President

Offers services for the totally blind, legally blind, visually impaired, mentally retarded blind and more with health, counseling, educational, recreational, rehabilitation, computer training and professional training services.

Ohio

9564 **Bellefaire Jewish Children's Bureau**

22001 Fairmount Boulevard
Shaker Heights, OH 44118
216-932-2800
800-879-2522
FAX: 216-932-8520
e-mail: yulishj@bellefairejcb.org
www.bellefairejcb.org

Jill Yulish, Intake Coordinator

Residential treatment for ages 12 to 17 1/2 at time of admission offering individualized psychotherapy, special education, and group living for severaly emotionally disturbed children and adolescents. Also offers a variety of other programs including specialized and therapuetic foster care, partial hospitilization, outpatient counseling, home-based intensive counseling and adoption services.

9565 **Christ Hospital Rehabilitation Unit**

2139 Auburn Avenue
Cincinnati, OH 45219
513-585-2205
FAX: 513-585-3300

Richard Seim, Senior VP

9566 **Cleveland Society for the Blind**

Cleveland Sight Center
1909 E 101st Street
PO Box 1988
Cleveland, OH 44106
216-791-8118
FAX: 216-791-1101
e-mail: jdsidley@clevelandsightcenter.org
www.clevelandsightcenter.org

John David Sidley, Manager Public Education
Michael E Grady, Executive Director

Social, rehabilitation, education and support services for blind and visually impaired children and adults, early intervention program for children birth to age 6, low vision clinic, aid and appliance shop, Braille and taping transcription, training for rehabilitation, orientation, mobility and computer access, employment services and job placement, recreation program, resident camping, talking books, radio reading services, food service training and snack bar employment. Free screening.

9567 **Columbus Speech and Hearing Center**

510 E N Broadway
Columbus, OH 43214
614-263-5151
FAX: 614-263-5365
www.columbusspeech.org

Dawn Gleason, Acting President/CEO
Joanne Shannon, Director Vocational Services

Serves persons who have speech-language and hearing challenges. Provides vocational rehabilitation services for individuals who are deaf, hard-of-hearing or deaf-blind.

9568 **CommuniCare of Clifton Nursing and Rehabilitation Center**

625 Probasco Street
Cincinnati, OH 45220
513-281-2464
FAX: 513-281-2559

Lisa Renaker, Director Nursing

A long term care facility which specializes in rehabilitation. Offers a full range of rehabilitative services including physical therapy, occupational therapy and speech therapy.

9569 Doctors Hospital
5100 W Broad Street
Columbus, OH 43228 **614-297-5639**
FAX: 614-870-9639

Janet Hymiak, Executive Director

9570 Dodd Hall at the Ohio State University Hospitals
480 W 9th Street
Columbus, OH 43215 **614-293-3300**

Sue Arnold, Admissions Coordinator
Dr. William Pease, Medical Director

Dodd Hall is a full service medical rehabilitation hospital offering comprehensive inpatient and outpatient rehabilitation.

9571 Easter Seal Society of Mahoning
299 Edwards Street
Youngstown, OH 44502 **330-743-1168**
FAX: 330-743-1616
www.mtc.easter-seals.org

Kenan J Sklenar, President/CEO

Outpatient medical rehabilitation - physical therapy, speech therapy, occupational therapy, warm-water therapy and adult day services.

9572 Four Oaks School
623 Dayton Xenia Road
Xenia, OH 45385 **937-222-7474**

Judith Pierce, School Administrator

Starts children on the road to discovery by providing a learning environment rich in opportunities and encouragement. The program was designed to give children with delays or disabilities, or those at-risk the extra help needed to develop fully. Any child under the age of six who exhibits developmental delays, handicapping conditions, or is considered at risk may qualify to participate.

9573 Genesis Healthcare System
Rehabilitation Center
800 Forest Avenue
Zanesville, OH 43701 **740-454-5000**
800-322-4762
FAX: 740-455-7527
e-mail: llynn@genesishcs.org
www.genesishcs.org

Keela Barker, Outpatient Manager
Lisa Lynn, Inpatient Manager
Karen Eyberger, Rehab Development Manager

A CARF and JACHO accredited 19-bed rehabilitation facility located within Genesis Healthcare System, a 732 bed, non-profit hospital system, located in Zanesville, Ohio. Freestanding outpatient services, including work hardening, pain management, vocational services, audiology, lymphedema, vestibular rehab, off-the-road driving evals, womens health and sports enhancement.

9574 George A Martin Center
3603 Washington Avenue
Cincinnati, OH 45229 **513-961-0144**

William Poole, Administrator

Offers services for the totally blind, legally blind, visually impaired, mentally retarded blind and more with health, counseling, educational, recreational, rehabilitation, computer training and professional training services.

9575 Grady Memorial Hospital
561 W Central Avenue
Delaware, OH 43015 **740-369-8711**
FAX: 740-363-3175

Everett Weber, Executive Director

9576 Hamilton Center
3400 Symmes Road
Hamilton, OH 45015 **513-867-5970**
FAX: 513-874-2977

Donald Musnuff, Executive Director

9577 Holzer Clinic
90 Jackson Pike
Gallipolis, OH 45631 **740-446-5411**
e-mail: webmaster@holzerclinic.com
www.holzerclinic.com

J. Craig Strafford, President

Serves medical needs of patients in an 8 county area, including counties in Ohio and West Virginia.

9578 Holzer Medical Center RehabCare
100 Jackson Pike
Gallipolis, OH 45631 **740-446-5000**
FAX: 740-446-5904

Carol Wellman, Program Manager
Kaye Rutherford, Nurse Manager

Offers an individualized quality comprehensive rehabilitation program for people with disabilities by an interdisciplinary team including physical therapy, occupational, speech, nursing and social services to restore the patient to the highest degree of rehab outcomes attainable.

9579 Human Resource Consultants
1946 N 13th Street
Toledo, OH 43624

9580 IKRON Institute for Rehabilitative and Psychological Services
2347 Vine Street
Cincinnati, OH 45219 **513-621-1117**
FAX: 513-621-2350

Randy E Strunk, Executive Director
Chris Etter, Fiscal Officer
Ann Webb, Program Director

An accredited mental health facility and a certified rehabilitation center. Through a variety of creative treatment and rehabilitation services, IKRON assists adults with mental health and/or substance abuse problems to attain greater independence, to lead lives of sobriety, to obtain competitive work and live more satisfying lives. IKRON places a strong emphasis on respect and support for persons with problems of adjustment. Special contracts to persons desiring job placement.

9581 Integrated Health Services at Waterford Commons
955 Garden Lake Parkway
Toledo, OH 43614 **419-382-2200**
FAX: 419-381-0188

Mary E McConnell, Provider Relations

A subacute and rehabilitation program specializing in ventilator weaning and management, I.V. therapeutics and pain management, wound management and subacute rehabilitation.

9582 **Lake County Society for Rehabilitation**
9521 Lake Shore Boulevard
Mentor, OH 44060 **440-255-8835**
FAX: 330-652-6632

Ahby Mansour, Executive Director

9583 **Lester H Higgins Adult Center**
2950 Whipple Avenue NW
Canton, OH 44708 **330-484-4814**

Dr. Joseph James, Superintendent

9584 **Live Oaks Career Development Campus**
5956 Buckwheat Road
Milford, OH 45150 **513-575-1900**
FAX: 513-771-6575

Dr. Harold Carr, Superintendent

9585 **Metro Health: St. Luke's Medical Center Pain Management Program**
11311 Shalar Boulevard
Cleveland, OH 44104 **216-778-7800**
FAX: 216-368-7140

CARF accredited comprehensive multidisciplinary pain management program.

9586 **MetroHealth Medical Center**
3395 Scranton Road
Cleveland, OH 44109 **216-459-5192**
FAX: 216-778-8376

Henry Manning, Executive Director

9587 **Middletown Regional Hospital: Inpatient Rehabilitation Unit**
105 McKnight Drive
Middletown, OH 45044 **513-423-9265**
FAX: 513-420-5718

Bob Gauder, Program Manager

9588 **Newark Healthcare Center**
75 McMillen Drive
 # 85
Newark, OH 43055
FAX: 740-344-8615

Joanne Whiteman, Administrator
Subacute rehabilitation program.

9589 **Parma Community General Hospital Acute Rehabilitation Center**
7007 Powers Boulevard
Parma, OH 44129 **440-743-3000**
FAX: 440-743-4036
www.parmahospital.org

Dale Winsberg, Administrative Director
The mission of this CARF accredited unit is to provide the most comprehensive, cost-effective, acute rehabilitation program possible in order for every patient and family to adjust to his/her disability and to achieve the maximum potential of independent functioning when returning to community living.

9590 **Peter A Towne Physical Therapy Center**
447 Nilles Road
Suite 10
Fairfield, OH 45014 **513-829-6100**
FAX: 513-829-7726

Debbie Wilkerson, Office Manager
Outpatient, private practice physical and occupational therapy. Three other offices in Hamilton, Monroe and West Chester.

9591 **Philomatheon Society of the Blind**
2810 Tuscarawas Street W
Canton, OH 44708 **330-453-9157**

Gerald Deffecker, President
Offers services for the totally blind, legally blind, visually impaired, mentally retarded blind and more with health, counseling, educational, recreational, rehabilitation, computer training and professional training services.

9592 **Providence Hospital Work**
2270 Banning Road
Cincinnati, OH 45239 **513-853-5261**
FAX: 513-853-5910

Christopher West, Executive Director

9593 **SCI: Six County**
2927 Bell Street
Zanesville, OH 43701 **740-452-9953**
FAX: 740-455-4134

David O Wesner PhD, Program Research

9594 **Southeast Ohio Sight Center**
358 Lincoln Avenue
Unit A
Lancaster, OH 43130 **740-687-4785**
800-969-3490
FAX: 740-689-9753
e-mail: frvrc@thevisioncenter.org
www.uwayfairfieldco.org/center.html

John Sterba, Director
Offers services for the blind and visually impaired to include functional low vision evaluations, community rehabilitation trading, counseling, educational, recreational, rehabilitation and vocational services.

9595 **St. Francis Rehabilitation Hospital**
401 N Broadway Street
Green Springs, OH 44836 **419-639-6218**
FAX: 419-639-6222

Martha Stevens, Marketing Coord.
Program offers specialized treatment for patients who have suffered a head injury, spinal cord injury, or stroke, or who have an orthopedic injury. The Head Injury Program provides a continuum of care from coma stimulation through transitional living. Their physicians, nurses, counselors and therapists are dedicated to helping our patients develop the motivation, strength and skills needed to overcome or adapt to their disability.

9596 **TAC I**
110 W Leffel Lane
Springfield, OH 45506
FAX: 937-325-4623

William Hoke, Executive Director

9597 **TAC II**
110 W Leffel Lane
Springfield, OH 45506
FAX: 937-325-4623

William Kent Hoke, Executive Director

Oklahoma

9598 **Dean A McGee Eye Institute**
608 Stanton L Young Boulevard
Oklahoma City, OK 73104 **405-271-1092**

Dr. Amelia Miranda, Director

Offers services for the totally blind, legally blind, visually impaired, mentally retarded blind and more with health, counseling, educational, recreational, rehabilitation, computer training and professional training services.

9599 **Jane Phillips Rehab Services**
RehabCare
3500 E Frank Phillips Boulevard
Bartlesville, OK 74006 **918-335-6655**
FAX: 918-333-7801

Scott Smith, Program Manager
Kathy Potts, Social Worker

Comprehensive inpatient rehabilitation services are provided to patients with orthopedic, neurologic, and other medical conditions of recent onset or regression, who have experienced a loss of function in activities of daily living, mobility, cognition and communication.

9600 **McAlester Regional Health Center RehabCare Unit**
1 Clark Bass Boulevard
McAlester, OK 74501 **918-421-8063**
FAX: 918-426-1016

A 19-bed inpatient physical rehabilitation unit serving the Southeast Oklahoma area. Offers physical therapy, occupational therapy, social work, speech and psychological services in an interdisciplinary framework.

9601 **Oklahoma League for the Blind**
PO Box 24020
Oklahoma City, OK 73124 **405-232-4644**
FAX: 405-236-5438
www.olb.org

Lauren White, Executive Director
Mike Bruce, Controller

Offers services for the blind and visually impaired, counseling, educational, recreational, rehabilitation, computer training and professional training services.

9602 **Valley View Regional Hospital RehabCare Unit**
430 N Monte Vista Street
Ada, OK 74820 **580-332-2323**
FAX: 580-421-1395

Rita Baumgartner, Program Manager

Comprehensive physical medicine and rehabilitation services designed to help patients in their adjustment to a physically limiting condition.

Oregon

9603 **Emanuel Rehabilitation Center**
3025 N Vancouver
Portland, OR 97227 **503-335-2000**
FAX: 503-413-1501

Gary Guidetta, Executive Director

9604 **Garten Services**
3334 Industrial Way NE
Salem, OR 97303 **503-581-4472**
FAX: 503-581-4497
e-mail: garten@garten.org

Emil Graziani, Executive Director

9605 **Oakcrest Care Center**
2933 Center Street NE
Salem, OR 97301
FAX: 503-588-5251

Postacute rehabilitation program.

9606 **Oakhill-Senior Program**
1190 Oakhill Avenue SE
Salem, OR 97302 **503-364-9086**
FAX: 503-365-2879

Jan Dillon, Senior Services Manager

Garten Senior Services provides an adult day service program to seniors with and without developmental disabilities. The program will provide community opportunities, college classes and a wide variety of leisure activities in group and individual settings.

9607 **Pacific Spine and Pain Center**
1801 Highway 99 N
Ashland, OR 97520 **541-482-5515**
FAX: 541-482-2433

Linda Dunn, Executive Director

9608 **Vision Northwest**
621 SW Alder
Portland, OR 97205 **503-221-0705**
FAX: 503-243-2537

Evelyn Maizels, Executive Director

Offers services for the totally blind, legally blind, visually impaired, mentally retarded blind and more with health, counseling, educational, recreational, rehabilitation, computer training and professional training services.

9609 **Willamette Valley Rehabilitation Center**
4390 S Santiam Highway
Lebanon, OR 97355 **541-258-8121**
FAX: 541-451-1762

Pennsylvania

9610 **Alcohol and Drug Abuse Services**
2 Main Street
Bradford, PA 16701 **814-362-6517**
FAX: 814-362-3202

Carma Horner, Supervisor

Offers rehabilitation services to individuals with an alcohol or drug related problem.

9611 Alpine Nursing and Rehabilitation Center of Hershey

820 Rhue Haus Lane
Hershey, PA 17033
FAX: 717-533-8698

Abe Locker, Executive Director

Postacute rehabilitation program.

9612 Alpine Ridge and Brandywood

Devereux Foundation
600 Boot Road
Downingtown, PA 19335 **610-942-5915**
800-345-1292
FAX: 610-873-4961

Offers a continuum of services for residents requiring services ranging from minimal care and supervision to total physical and medical care.

9613 Amity Lodge

Devereux Foundation
600 Boot Road
Downingtown, PA 19335 **610-520-3000**
800-345-1292
FAX: 610-524-3000

Offers residents a continuum of services ranging from minimal care and supervision to total physical and medical care.

9614 Beechwood Rehabilitation Services A Community Integrated Brain Injury Program

469 E Maple Avenue
Langhorne, PA 19047 **215-750-4299**
800-782-3299
FAX: 215-750-4327
e-mail: dcerra-tyl@wood.org
www.beechwoodrehab.com

Deborah Cerra-Tyl, Director Program Development

Services include residential, day treatment and community based support services. Beechwood has programs in both Pennsylvania and New Jersey. Individuals with an acquired brain injury are served.

9615 Bryn Mawr Rehabilitation Hospital

414 Paoli Pike
PO Box 3007
Malvern, PA 19355 **610-251-5400**
888-734-2241
FAX: 610-647-3648
www.brynmawrrehab.org

Patricia M Ryan, President

9616 Clara Burke Nursing Home

251 Stenton Avenue
Plymouth Meeting, PA 19462 **610-828-2272**
FAX: 610-828-2519

Terri Herd, Admissions

Postacute rehabilitation program.

9617 Concord Training Center

105 Loudon Road
Suite 3103
Concord, NH 03301 **603-230-9994**
FAX: 603-230-9696

Scott Selkowitz, Executive Director

9618 Daman Villa

Devereux Foundation
889 Boot Road
Downingtown, PA 19335 **610-942-5915**
800-345-1292
FAX: 215-873-4961

Offers residents a continuum of services ranging from minimal care and supervision to total physical and medical care.

9619 Devereux

444 Devereux Drive
Villanova, PA 19085
800-345-1292
FAX: 610-542-3100
e-mail: knash@devereux.org
www.devereux.org

Kimberleigh Nash, Dir. of Corporate Communications
Michele Petti, Director Client Services

Nationwide network of residential, day, and community-based services for children and adults who have special emotional and/or developmental needs.

9620 Devereux Foundation Health Services Center

600 Boot Road
Downingtown, PA 19335 **610-942-5915**
800-345-1292
FAX: 610-971-4600
www.devereux.org

Provides a continuum of residential services for adults with developmental disabilities. active treatment is offered in a safe and therapeutic environment which allows on-going assessment and individual growth that will enhance the quality of life for each of its residents. Candidates could have needs that range from minimal care and supervision to those requiring medical and behavioral assistance with an intensive support system. $145-$161.00 per day.

9621 Devereux's Kanner Center

390 E Boot Road
W Chester, PA 19380 **610-431-8126**
FAX: 610-430-0567
www.devereux.org

Steve Silverman, Admissions Director
Kelly McCool, Admissions Coordinator

A private nonprofit nationwide network of treatment services for individuals of all ages with emotional and/or developmental disabilities. Located in twelve states and the District of Columbia, Devereux's continuum includes inpatient and partial hospitalization, residential treatment, community based programs and outpatient services. Provides a continuum of care to children, adolescents and young adults who have developmental disabilities, mental retardation, autism and emotional disturbances.

9622 Fox Subacute Center

2644 Bristol Road
Warrington, PA 18976 **215-491-1191**
FAX: 215-343-8023

Gerry Nevilln, Admissions

Postacute rehabilitation program.

9623 Greater Pittsburgh Guild for the Blind

311 Station Street
Bridgeville, PA 15017 **724-224-8700**
FAX: 412-257-8573

Leroy Bectwy, Director

Offers services for the totally blind, legally blind, visually impaired, mentally retarded blind and more with health, counseling, educational, recreational, rehabilitation, computer training and professional training services.

9624 **IHS of Greater Pittsburgh**
890 Weatherwood Lane
Greensburg, PA 15601 **724-837-8076**
FAX: 724-837-7456

Sue Wojciechowski, Case Manager
Laurie Tamay, Director Admissions

Subacate care, ventilator and pulmonary managment, comprehensive rehabilitation.

9625 **Pediatric Center at Plymouth Meeting Integrated Health Services**
491 Allendale Road
King of Prussia, PA 19406 **610-265-9290**
800-220-7337
FAX: 610-265-2772

Subacute programs such as intensive respiratory care, stressing ventilator dependent children, pre and post transplant care, total parenteral nutrition, IV therapy, intensive/behavioral oral feeding programs. Provides extensive discharge planning including teaching or review for all the above programs with an emphasis on development and accessing community resources.

9626 **Pennsylvania Pain Rehabilitation Center**
252 W Swamp Road
Bailiwick #2, PO Box 1802
Doylestown, PA 18901 **215-348-5104**
FAX: 215-348-5106

Dr. Reza Azar, Executive Director

9627 **Robert L Miller Rehab Center**
Good Samaritan Hospital
PO Box 1281
Lebanon, PA 17042 **717-270-7500**
FAX: 717-270-7840

Joanne Ebert, Rehab Coordinator
Stuart Hartman, Medical Director

Comprehensive inpatient rehab unit for adults regarding general physical rehabilitation. Specific programs include orthopedic, neurological, stroke, amputee, etc.

9628 **Therapy Services Department of Orthopedic and Rehabilitation Center**
Hershey Medical Center at Penn State University
PO Box 850
Hershey, PA 17033 **717-531-8070**
FAX: 717-531-4558

9629 **Willis Eye Hospital**
Nonth & Walnut Street
Philadelphia, PA 19107
FAX: 215-238-0804

John Jeffers

Offers services for the totally blind, legally blind, visually impaired, mentally retarded blind and more with health, counseling, educational, recreational, rehabilitation, computer training and professional training services.

Rhode Island

9630 **In-Sight**
43 Jefferson Boulevard
Warwick, RI 02888 **401-941-3322**
FAX: 401-941-3356

Judith Smith, Executive Director

Offers services for the totally blind, legally blind, visually impaired, mentally retarded blind and more with health, counseling, educational, recreational, rehabilitation, computer training and professional training services.

9631 **Vanderbilt Rehabilitation Center**
Friendship Street
Newport, RI 02840 **401-783-9718**
FAX: 401-845-1087

Robert Healey, Executive Director

South Carolina

9632 **Association for the Blind**
1071 Morrison Drive
Charleston, SC 29403 **843-723-6915**
FAX: 843-577-4312

Bettye Dorn, Director Programs & Planning

Offers services for people who are blind, or are visually impaired with health, counseling, educational, recreational, rehabilitation, computer training and professional training services.

9633 **Hitchcock Rehabilitation Center**
690 Medical Park Drive
Aiken, SC 29801 **803-648-8344**
800-207-6924
FAX: 803-649-4639
e-mail: dhillman@hitchcockrehab.com
www.hitchcockrehab.com

Pat Samuel, Executive Director
Dan Hillman, Case Manager
Carrie Morgan, Finance Director

Comprehensive outpatient rehabilitation for adults, children, geriatrics, pediatric therapy, special needs preschool, sports medicine, home health and hospice.

9634 **Mentor of South Carolina**
3200 Devine Street
Columbia, SC 29205 **803-799-9025**
FAX: 803-931-8959

Lynny Morton-Epps, State Director

Mentor provides a full network of individually tailored services for people with development disabilities and their families. Individuals may be served in their homes, shared living home, or in a host home.

Tennessee

9635 **Humana Hospital: Morristown RehabCare**
726 McFarland Street
Morristown, TN 37814 **423-586-2930**
FAX: 423-581-6988

Nickie Tabor, Program Director
Chuck Olson, Clinical Director

Designed to help patients in their adjustment to a physically limiting condition by helping to maximize each patient's abilities so he or she can function as independently as possible.

9636 **Opportunity East Rehabilitation Services for the Blind**

758 W Morris Boulevard
Morristown, TN 37814 **423-586-3998**
FAX: 423-586-2004
e-mail: vic@volblind.org
www.opportunityeast.tripod.com

Fred Overbay, Executive Director
Vic Mende, Director Rehabilitation Services
Dorothy Moyers, Client Services Coordinator

Offers services for the totally blind, legally blind, visually impaired, mentally retarded blind and more with health, counseling, educational, recreational, rehabilitation, computer training and professional training services.

9637 **Patrick Rehab Wellness**

Lincoln County Health System
1001 Huntsville Highway
Fayetteville, TN 37334 **931-433-0273**
FAX: 931-438-0378

Laura Clark, Director Rehab
Gloria Meadows, Administrator

Provides rehabilitation services of physical, occupational, and speech therapy. Also, wellness memberships are available to the public.

9638 **PharmaThera**

Corporate Offices, Suite 107
1785 Nonconnah Boulevard
Memphis, TN 38132 **901-754-5485**
800-767-6714
FAX: 901-348-8270

Offers 10 locations serving patients throughout the southern United States, each with an in-house, expertly trained staff. All locations use the latest technologies and techniques in infusion care to provide a broad range of individualized home infusion therapies.

9639 **Siskin Rehabilitation Hospital**

3 Siskin Plaza
Chattanooga, TN 37403 **423-634-1700**

Debby Barker, VP of Development

9640 **St. Mary's RehabCare Center**

Oak Hill Avenue
Knoxville, TN 37917
FAX: 865-545-8133

Debbie Keeton, Director

Provides comprehensive rehabilitation services for patients experiencing CVA, head trauma, orthopedic conditions, spinal cord injury or neurological impairment.

Texas

9641 **Baylor Institute for Rehabilitation**

3505 Gaston Avenue
Dallas, TX 75246 **214-826-7030**
888-7BA-YLOR
FAX: 214-841-2679

Alice Douden, Admissions Manager

A 92-bed specialty hospital offering comprehensive rehabilitation services for persons with spinal cord injury, traumatic brain injury, stroke, amputation, and other orthopedic and neurological disorders.

9642 **Brown-Karhan Health Care**

PO Box 419
Dripping Springs, TX 78620 **512-894-0801**
FAX: 512-858-4627
e-mail: info@brown-karhan.com
www.brown-karhan.com

Dr. Jim Misko, Clinical Director/VP

Postacute rehabilitation program, long-term neuropsychiatric program, apartment living and full compliment of therapies, including cognitive rehabilitation. $225-$800/day.

9643 **Center for Neuro Skills**

3501 N Macarthur Boulevard
Suite 200
Irving, TX 75062 **972-597-7715**
FAX: 972-255-3162

Rocky Brogdon, Admissions

Postacute rehabilitation program.

9644 **Center for Neuro Skills: Texas**

3501 N Macarthur Boulevard
Suite 200
Irving, TX 75062 **972-597-7715**
FAX: 972-255-3162
e-mail: cns@neuroskills.com
www.neuroskills.com/~cns

David Krych, Executive Director
Peter O'Neill, Admissions
Rocky Brogdon, Admissions

A comprehensive, post-acute, community based head-injury rehabilitation program serving over 100 clients per year. Since 1985, CNS has effectively treated the entire spectrum of head-injured clients, including those with severe behavioral disorders, cognitive/perceptual impairments, speech/language problems, physical disabilities and post-concussion syndrome.

9645 **Comprehensive Rehabilitation**

Hillcrest Baptist Medical Center
3000 Herring Avenue
Waco, TX 76708 **254-202-5100**
FAX: 254-202-5674

Carl Lutz MSW, Program Director
Ann Gammel, Nurse Manager

Designed to assist patients in adjustment to a physically limiting condition, utilizing interdisciplinary strategies to maximize each patient's ability and capability.

9646 **Dallas Services for Visually Impaired Children**

4242 Office Parkway
Dallas, TX 75204 **214-828-9900**
FAX: 214-828-9901

Robert Berger, Executive Director

Offers services for the totally blind, legally blind, visually impaired, mentally retarded blind and more with health, counseling, educational, recreational, rehabilitation, computer training and professional training services.

9647 **Devereux Texas Treatment Network Adult Community**

120 David Wade Drive
PO Box 2666
Victoria, TX 77902 **361-575-8271**
800-383-5000
FAX: 361-575-6520

Ric Tinney, Adult Services Administrator
Shirley Heron, Program Manager

Provides a permanent home for individuals with chronic psychiatric and/or developmental disabilities who require long term or lifelong care, support or a transitional home for individuals who progress to a less structured setting. Located on a beautiful 400+ acre campus in sunny south Texas, the primary focus is to offer, in keeping with the philosophies of least restrictive alternatives and normalization, active treatment which will facilitate growth.

9648 El Paso Lighthouse for the Blind

200 Washington Street
El Paso, TX 79905 **915-542-1969**
FAX: 915-532-6338
e-mail: tomdyles@whc.net

Tom Doyle, Executive Director

Enables people of all ages to embody blindness and vision impairment through training, rehabilitation, employment opportunity, advocacy and research. Provides access to opportunities and quality of life so that the blind and visually impaired can reach their fullest potential for self-sufficiency and independence.

9649 Harris Methodist Fort Worth/Mabee Rehabilitation Center

1301 Pennsylvania Avenue
Fort Worth, TX 76104 **817-882-2364**
FAX: 817-882-2753

Michelle Wilson, Speciality Program Manager
Peggyo Ehrlich, Rehab Manager

A hospital based inpatient rehab program and outpatient day programs in chronic pain management, work hardening and brain injury transitional services.

9650 Heights Hospital Rehab Unit

1917 Ashland Street
Houston, TX 77008 **713-861-6161**
FAX: 713-802-8537

Leticia Bravo, Program Manager
Kim Willis, Admissions

This program is designed to assist patients with physical disabilities achieve their maximum functional abilities.

9651 Houston Rehabilitation Institute

17506 Red Oak Drive
Houston, TX 77090 **713-223-5971**
FAX: 281-580-6714

Jerome Lengel, Executive Officer

Offers an individualized approach to the process of rehabilitation for severely injured or disabled individuals. The process begins with a pre-admissions assessment of each referred patient. The Center combines state-of-the-art technology and equipment with multi-disciplinary therapy and education in a cheerful, secure environment.

9652 IHS Hospital at Dallas

7955 Harry Hines
Dallas, TX 75235
800-366-4736
FAX: 214-637-6512

Richard G Allison, Admissions

66 beds offering active/acute rehabilitation, brain injury day treatment, cognitive rehabilitation, complex care, extended rehabilitation, pediatric brain injury rehabilitation and short-term evaluation.

9653 Institute for Rehabilitation & Research

1333 Moursund Street
Houston, TX 77030 **713-799-7011**
FAX: 713-797-5289

Karen Hart, VP Education

A national center for information, training, research, and technical assistance in independent living. The goal is to extend the body of knowledge in independent living and to improve the utilization of results of research programs and demonstration projects in this field. It has developed a variety of strategies for collecting, synthesizing, and disseminating information related to the field of independent living.

9654 Integrated Health Services of Amarillo

5601 Plum Creek Drive
Amarillo, TX 79124 **806-351-1000**
FAX: 806-355-9650

Jackie Forbis, Case Manager
Neal Duncan, Executive Director
Paula Washington, Administrator

Postacute rehabilitation program including ventilator weening, complex wound program and interdisciplinary team case management.

9655 Lighthouse of Houston

3602 W Dallas Street
Houston, TX 77019 **713-527-9561**
FAX: 713-284-8451
e-mail: gduterroil@houstonlighthouse.org
www.thelighthouseofhouston.org

Gibson M DuTerroil, President
Shelagh Moran, VP and COO
Jennifer Blando, Director Education

Serves the blind, visually impaired, deaf-blind and multihandicapped blind. Provides workshops, vocational training and placement, low vision clinic, orientation and mobility, housing, Braille, volunteer services, senior center, visual aid sales, counseling and support, diabetic education and day health activity services and day summer camp, Summer Transition for Youth.

9656 Mainland Center Hospital RehabCare Unit

Highway 1764
Texas City, TX 77592 **281-534-3522**
FAX: 409-938-5501

David Roberts, Program Manager

The RehabCare program is designed and staffed to assist functionally impaired patients improve to their maximum potential. The opportunities for improvement and adjustments are provided in a pleasant, supportive inpatient environment by therapists from the occupational, physical, recreational and speech therapy disciplines.

9657 North Texas Rehabilitation Center

1005 Midwestern Parkway
Wichita Falls, TX 76302 **940-322-0771**
FAX: 940-766-4943

Lesa Enlow, Director Programs

Provides outpatient rehabilitation services to maximize independence or promote development to children and adults with disabilities. Programs include: physical, occupational, speech therapy, closed head injury, infant/child development, support groups, aquatics and wellness program and a child achievement program.

9658 South Texas Lighthouse for the Blind

PO Box 9697
Corpus Christi, TX 78469 **361-883-6553**
FAX: 361-883-1041

Barbara Russell, Executive Director

Offers services for the totally blind, legally blind, visually impaired, mentally retarded blind and more with health, counseling, educational, recreational, rehabilitation, computer training and professional training services.

9659 **Transitional Learning Center at Galveston**

1528 Postoffice Street
Galveston, TX 77550
409-762-6661
800-TLC-GROW
FAX: 409-763-3930

Lee Kinard, Managed Care & Account Manager
Jim McCurdy, Director Business Development

The Transitional Learning Center at Galveston has specialized in post-acute brain injury since 1982. TLC is a leader who offers comprehensive therapies in a residential setting, 24-hour monitoring, outcome focused pathways, superior staff credentials - including physician and nursing staff on-site to address medical issues, innovative clinical research integrated into treatment plans, discharge lifecare planning, and long-term living at Tideway Lodge.

9660 **Treemont**

5550 Harvest Hill Road
Dallas, TX 75230
972-404-0833
FAX: 972-715-5550

Donna Snyder, Administrator

Postacute rehabilitation program.

9661 **West Texas Lighthouse for the Blind**

2001 Austin Street
San Angelo, TX 76903
325-653-4231
FAX: 325-657-9367
e-mail: wtlb@wee.net
www.lighthousefortheblind.org

Robert Porter, Executive Director
Ron Beard, Operations Manager
Margene Hale, Office Manager

Offers services for the totally blind, legally blind, visually impaired, mentally retarded blind and more with health, counseling, educational, recreational, rehabilitation, computer training and professional training services.

Utah

9662 **Quincy Rehabilitation Institute of Holy Cross Hospital**

1050 E S Temple
Salt Lake City, UT 84102
801-350-8140
FAX: 801-350-4483

Postacute rehabilitation program.

9663 **Wasatch Villa**

2200 E 3300 S
Salt Lake City, UT 84109
801-328-2020
FAX: 801-486-0105

Postacute rehabilitation program.

Vermont

9664 **Rutland Mental Health Services**

78 S Main Street
Rutland, VT 05701
FAX: 802-747-7699

Mark G Monson, President/CEO

A private, non-profit comprehensive community mental health center. It provides services to individuals and families for mental health and substance abuse related problems and also to persons who are mentally retarded.

Virginia

9665 **Bay Pine-Virginia Beach**

1148 First Colonial Road
Virginia Beach, VA 23454
757-481-3321
FAX: 757-481-4413

Willie Alston Jr, Administrator

Postacute rehabilitation program.

9666 **Carilion Rehabilitation: New River Valley**

2900 Tyler Road
PO Box 5
Radford, VA 24141
540-731-2992
FAX: 540-731-2011
e-mail: jsmith@carilion.com

Jennie Smith, Clinical Team Leader
Rhonda Fanning, Department Secretary/Referrals
Robin Sutphin, Rehabilitation Assistant

CARF-accredited pain management program, work hardening program and comprehensive outpatient therapy clinic, massage therapy, outpatient programs and more. Program emphasis is on interdisiplinary behavioral rehab based pain management and functional restoration in conjunction with medical treatment. Work hardening is a transdisciplinary work simulation program taylored to the individual. Comprehensive outpatient program is multi-disciplinary with emphasis on manual treatment.

9667 **Faith Mission Home**

3540 Mission Home Lane
Free Union, VA 22940
434-985-2294
FAX: 434-985-7633

Merle Miller, Administrator
Reuben Yoder, Director

A Christian residential center that serves 60 mentally retarded children, including individuals with Down Syndrome, Cerebral palsy and other similar conditions. Children may be admitted from the time they are ambulatory until they reach 15 years of age. He or she may stay as long as it is in the child's best interests. The training program stresses the following areas: self-care, social, academic, vocational, crafts, speech and physical development.

9668 **Pines Residential Treatment Center**

825 Crawford Parkway
Portsmouth, VA 23704
757-391-6602
FAX: 757-393-1029

Dr. Leonard Lexier MD, Medical Director
Judy Kemp, Admissions Director

A 310-bed residential treatment center in Portsmouth Virginia, providing a therapeutic environment for severely emotionally disturbed children and youth. Five unique programs meet behavioral, educational and emotional needs of males and females, five to twenty-two years of age. Multi-disciplinary teams devise individual service plans to enhance strengths and reverse self-defeating behavior. A highly effective positive reinforcement program with a proven track record.

9669 **Reach Rehabilitation Program: Manor Care**
550 S Carlin Springs Road
Arlington, VA 22204
703-379-7200
FAX: 703-820-2535

Barb Feege, Program Director
Ruth Gurinsky RN, Referral/Marketing

Postacute rehabilitation program.

9670 **Resurrection Children's Center**
2280 N Beauregard Street
Alexandria, VA 22311
703-578-1314

Charlie Armstrong, Administrative Director
Kim Messinger, Program Director

Offers children ages 2-5 with varying disabilities academic education, parent education, opportunities including classes, workshops, support groups and individual counseling.

9671 **Roanoke Memorial Hospital**
PO Box 13367
Roanoke, VA 24033
540-981-8215
FAX: 540-981-8233

Kathy Robertson, Director

9672 **Southside Virginia Training Center**
PO Box 4110
Petersburg, VA 23803
804-520-2275
FAX: 804-524-7228

Richard Buckley

Offers residential, vocational, occupational, physical, and speech therapies.

9673 **Woodrow Wilson Rehabilitation Center**
Box W-528
PO Box 1500
Fishersville, VA 22939
540-332-7000
800-345-9972
FAX: 540-332-7132
e-mail: coleman1@wwrc.state.va.us
www.wwrc.net

Barbie Ostrander, Admissions Director
Wendell L Coleman, Public Information Director

Comprehensive residential rehabilitation center offering complete medical and vocational rehabilitation services including: vocation evaluation, vocational training, transition from school to work, occupational therapy, physical therapy, speech, language and audiology, assistive technology, rehabilitation engineering, counseling/case management, behavioral health services, nursing and physician services, etc.

Washington

9674 **Arden Nursing Home**
16357 Aurora Avenue N
Seattle, WA 98133
FAX: 206-546-5480

Postacute rehabilitation program.

9675 **Bellingham Care Center**
1200 Birchwood Avenue
Bellingham, WA 98225
360-734-9295
FAX: 360-671-4368

Postacute rehabilitation program.

9676 **Division of Vocational Rehabilitation Department of Social and Health Services**
PO Box 45340
Olympia, WA 98504
360-438-8000
800-637-5627
FAX: 360-438-8007
e-mail: krulik@dshs.wa.gov
www1.dshs.wa.gov/dvr

Mike O'Brien, Director

Information on computers, supported employment, marketing rehabilitation facilities and transition.

9677 **First Hill Care Center**
1334 Terry Avenue
Seattle, WA 98101
206-624-1484
FAX: 206-624-3090

Postacute rehabilitation program.

9678 **Harborview Medical Center, Low Vision Aid Clinic**
325 9th Avenue
Seattle, WA 98104
206-521-1600

Thomas Gillette, Director

Offers services for the totally blind, legally blind, visually impaired, mentally retarded blind and more with health, counseling, educational, recreational, rehabilitation, computer training and professional training services.

9679 **Integrated Health Services of Seattle**
820 NW 95th Street
Seattle, WA 98117
206-782-0100
FAX: 206-781-1448

Jerry Harvey, Administrator
Marlette Basada, Director Nursing
Flavia Lagrange, Director Admissions

Postacute rehabilitation program. IHS provides 24 hour subacute and long-term care. We can handle vent/trach/hemo andritoneal dialysis and provide a full scope of rehabilitation services.

9680 **Intergrated Health Services**
820 NW 95th Street
Seattle, WA 98117
206-782-0100
FAX: 206-781-1448

Postacute rehabilitation program longterm acute care. Gero Psych.

9681 **Lakeside Recovery Centers**
535 E Dock Street
Tacoma, WA 98402
253-573-0250
FAX: 253-272-0171

Hugh Long, Administrator

9682 **Lakewood Health Care Center**
11411 Bridgeport Way SW
Tacoma, WA 98499
253-581-9002
FAX: 253-581-7016

Janice Olson, Admissions Coordinator
Patty Wood, Administrator
Linda Doll, Social Services

Postacute rehabilitation program.

9683 **Manor Care Nursing: Tacoma**
5601 S Orchard Street
Tacoma, WA 98409
FAX: 253-474-8172

Postacute rehabilitation program.

9684 **ManorCare Health Services**
3701 188th Street SW
Lynnwood, WA 98037
425-775-9222
FAX: 425-744-1602

Renee Beste, Admissions Director

Postacute rehabilitation program.

9685 **ManorCare Health Services: Spokane**
6025 N Assembly Street
Spokane, WA 99205
FAX: 509-326-4790

Susan Cooper, Admissions Director

Postacute rehabilitation program.

9686 **Northwest Continuum Care Center**
128 Beacon Hill Drive
Longview, WA 98632
360-423-4060
FAX: 360-636-0958

Postacute rehabilitation program.

9687 **Park Manor Convalescent Center**
1710 Plaza Way
Walla Walla, WA 99362
509-529-4218
FAX: 509-522-1729

Postacute rehabilitation program.

9688 **Queen Anne Health Care**
Queen Anne Health Care
2717 Dexter Avenue N
Seattle, WA 98109
206-284-3936
FAX: 206-283-3936

Postacute rehabilitation program.

9689 **Rainier Vista Care Center**
920 12th Avenue SE
Puyallup, WA 98372
253-875-9999
FAX: 253-848-3937

Postacute rehabilitation program.

9690 **Rehabilitation Enterprises of Washington**
2626 12th Center SW
Suite 6
Olympia, WA 98502
360-943-7654
FAX: 360-943-7680
e-mail: phaney@cco.net

Penny Jo Hanley, Business Manager

REW is the professional trade association representing community rehabilitation programs before government and other publics. These organizations provide a wide array of employment and training services for people with disabilities. The goal is to assist member organizations to provide the highest quality rehabilitative and employment services to their customers.

9691 **Seattle Medical and Rehabilitation Center**
Evergreen Healthcare
555 16th Avenue
Seattle, WA 98122
206-362-6998
800-877-3422
FAX: 206-324-4345

Donna Stromski, Executive Director
Christine Lafrenz, Director Nursing
Matt Murray, Director Admissions

103 beds offering subacute rehabilitation, complex care, subacute treatment and short-term evaluation. Pulmonary unit offering long and short term care for ventilator dependent patients.

9692 **Slingerland Institute for Literacy**
Educators Publishing Service
411 108th Avenue
Suite 2060
Bellevue, WA 98004
425-453-1190
FAX: 425-635-7762
e-mail: SlingInst@aol.com
www.slingerland.org

Madeline P Beery, Executive Director
Annette Calvagno, Program Support
Sue Heinz, Dean

A nonprofit public corporation founded in 1977 to carry on the work of Beth H. Slingerland in providing classroom teachers with the techniques, knowledge and understanding necessary for identifying and teaching children with Specific Language Disability. The main objective is to educate teachers in successful methods of identifying, diagnosing and instructing children and adults with SLD and to promote literacy through reading, writing and oral expression.

9693 **Synergos NeuroMedical Rehab Unit: Seattle**
Highline Community Hospital
12844 Military Road S
Tukwila, WA 98168
206-248-4552
FAX: 206-248-4663

Matt Crockett, Director Rehab Services
Debbie Link RN, Intake Coordinator

Sub-acute rehabilitation program specializing in brain injuries.

9694 **Timberland Opportunities Association**
T00 W Curtis Street
Aberdeen, WA 98520
360-533-5823
FAX: 360-533-5848

Jim Eddy, Executive Director

Provides training and employment for disabled people.

9695 **Vancouver Health and Rehabilitation Center**
400 E 33rd Street
Vancouver, WA 98663
360-696-2561
FAX: 360-750-0665

Postacute rehabilitation program.

West Virginia

9696 **West Virginia Rehabilitation Center**
Barron Drive
Institute, WV 25112
304-766-4696
800-642-8207
FAX: 304-766-4989
www.wvdrs.org

Michael Meadows, Assistant Director Client
Bill Tanzey, Manager Center Services
Tracy Carr, Mgr State and Federal Relations

The West Virginia Rehabilitation Center has been called West Virginia's best kept secret. Set on a 33-acre campus near Charleston, WV, the Center complex houses a school with 9 training areas, dormitories, a full-service rehabilitation hospital, a recreation program, a state-of-the-art assistive technology program and extension services statewide.

Wisconsin

9697 **Christian League for the Handicapped**
PO Box 948
Walworth, WI 53184 **262-275-6131**
FAX: 262-275-3355

Steven Jensen, Executive Director
Tim Schnake, Director Resident Services

Multifaceted ministry including independent living apartments, assisted living housing, employment, camping, retreats, employment counseling, and more. 103 people with physical disabilities live and work on 160 acre campus. The League generally serves those over 18.

9698 **Colonial Manor of Wausau: Extended Rehab Services**
1010 E Wausau Avenue
Wausau, WI 54403 **715-842-2028**
FAX: 715-848-0510

Jean Burgener, Administrator

Postacute rehabilitation program.

9699 **Waushers Industries**
210 E Townline Road
Wautoma, WI 54982
FAX: 920-787-4698

Richard King, Executive Director

9700 **Woodstock/Kenosha Health Center**
3415 Sheridan Road
Kenosha, WI 53140
FAX: 262-657-5756

Mary Petersen, Administrator

Postacute rehabilitation program.

Alabama

9701 **Rehabilitation & Healthcare Center Of Birm ingham**
2728 10th Avenue S
Birmingham, AL 35205 **205-933-7010**
FAX: 205-933-8052

Alaska

9702 **Fairbanks Memorial Hospital/Denali Center**
1650 Cowles Street
Fairbanks, AK 99701 **907-452-8181**
FAX: 907-458-5324

Linda Smith, Assistant Administrator

Offers the following rehabilitation services: Physical Therapy, Occupational Therapy, Speech Therapy, Sub-Acute Rehab.

Arizona

9703 **Desert Life Rehabilitation & Care Center**
1919 W Medical Street
Tuscon, AZ 85704 **520-297-8311**
FAX: 520-544-0930

Renee Tank, District Rehab Services Dir

Offers the following rehabilitation services: Physical Therapy, Occupational Therapy, Speech Therapy, Sub-Acute Rehab.

9704 **Hacienda Rehabilitation and Care Center**
660 Coronado Drive
Sierra Vista, AZ 86351 **520-459-4900**
FAX: 520-458-4082

Maria Ritter, Administrator

Offers the following rehabilitation services: In-patient, Out-patient, Sub-Acute.

9705 **Kachina Point Health Care and Rehabilitati on Center**
505 Jacks Canyon Road
Sedona, AZ 86351 **928-284-1000**
FAX: 928-284-0626

Christine Walker, Administrator

Offers the following rehabilitation services: Occupational Therapy, Speech Therapy, Physical Therapy, Sub-Acute Rehab.

9706 **Mayo Clinic Scottsdale**
13400 E Shea Boulevard
Scottsdale, AZ 85259 **480-301-8000**
FAX: 480-301-4391

9707 **Sonoran Rehabilitation and Care Center**
4202 N 20th Avenue
Phoenix, AZ 85015 **602-264-3824**
FAX: 602-279-6234

Tim Badgley, Administrator

Offers the following rehabilitation services: Respiratory Therapy, Physical Therapy, Speech Therapy, Occupational Therapy, Restorative Therapy, Sub-Acute Rehabilitation, Wound Care.

9708 **Valley Health Care and Rehabilitation Cent er**
5545 E Lee Street
Tuscon, AZ 85712 **520-296-2306**
FAX: 520-296-4072

Wayne Wisniewski, Administrator

Offers the following rehabilitation services: Physical Therapy, Occupational Therapy, Speech Therapy, Sub-Acute Rehab.

California

9709 **Alamitos-Belmont Rehab Hospital**
3901 E Fourth Street
Long Beach, CA 90814 **562-434-8421**
FAX: 562-433-6732

Darien Dahl, Administrator

Offers the following rehabilitation services: Speech Therapy, Occupational Therapy, Physical Therapy, Sub-Acute Rehab.

9710 **Bay View Nursing and Rehabilitation Center**
516 Willow Street
Alameda, CA 94501 **510-521-5600**
FAX: 510-865-6441

9711 **Canyonwood Nursing and Rehab Center**
2120 Benton Drive
Redding, CA 96003 **530-243-6317**
FAX: 530-243-4646

9712 **Foothill Nursing and Rehab Center**
401 W Ada Avenue
Glendora, CA 91741 **626-335-9810**
FAX: 626-914-4679

Dan Husband, Administrator

Offers the following rehabilitation services: Physical Therapy, Occupational Therapy, Speech Therapy, In and Out Patient Rehab.

9713 **Long Beach Memorial Medical Center Memorial Rehabilitation Hospital**
2801 Atlantic Avenue
Long Beach, CA 90806 **562-933-9000**

Trish Baeseman, Administrator

The hospital offers rehabilitation after catastrophic injury of disabling disease to give patients the opportunity for maximum recovery. The Hospital offers many of the area's finest rehabilitation specialists and most advanced technology, making it one of Southern California's most respected rehabilitation centers.

9714 **Mercy Medical Center Mt. Shasta**
914 Pine Street
PO Box 239
Mt. Shasta, CA 96067 **530-926-6111**
FAX: 530-926-0517
mtshasta.mercy.org

9715 Northridge Hospital Medical Center
18300 Roscoe Boulevard
Northridge, CA 91328
818-885-8500
FAX: 818-349-1546
www.northridgehospital.org

Offers the following rehabilitation services: Physical Therapy, Occupational Therapy, Speech Therapy, Sub-Acute Rehab.

9716 Riverside Community Hospital
4445 Magnolia Avenue
Riverside, CA 92501
909-788-3000
FAX: 909-788-3616
www.riversidecommunityhospital.org

9717 Saint Jude Medical Center
101 E Valencia Mesa Drive
Fullerton, CA 92835
714-871-3280
FAX: 714-992-3912

Winkie Sonnefield, Director Rehab/Therapy Services

Offers the following rehabilitation services: Out-patient Rehab, Sub-Acute Rehab, Occupational Therapy, Physical Therapy, Speech and Audiology Therapy, Pain Management Program.

9718 South Coast Medical Center
31872 Coast Highway
Laguna Beach, CA 92651
949-499-1311
FAX: 949-499-8644
e-mail: info@southcoastmedcenter.com
www.southcoastmedcenter.com

Maggie Baumann, Marketing Director

Offers the following services: physical therapy, occupational therapy, speech therapy, cardica rehabilitation, incontinence program, sub-acute rehabilitation.

9719 Valley Garden Health Care and Rehabilitati on Center
1517 E Knickerbocker Drive
Stockton, CA 95210
209-957-4539
FAX: 209-957-5831

Colorado

9720 Boulder Community Hospital Mapleton Center
311 Mapleton Avenue
PO Box 9130
Boulder, CO 80301
303-443-0230
www.bch.org

Offers comprehensive rehabilitation services for individuals of all ages on both an inpatient and outpatient basis. Specialty programs include brain injury, chronic pain management, and pediatric rehabilitation.

9721 Fairacres Manor
1700 18th Avenue
Greeley, CO 80631
970-353-3370
FAX: 970-353-9347

Kathy Mekelburg, Administrator

Offers the following rehabilitation services: Physical Therapy, Occupational Therapy, Speech Therapy, Restorative Therapy, Skilled Nursing, and Sub-Acute Rehabilitation.

9722 Rowan Community
4601 E Asbury Circle
Denver, CO 80222
303-757-1228
FAX: 303-759-3390
www.pinonmgt.com

Sixty bed skilled nursing facility in southwest Denver, serving younger residents with multiple sclerosis traumatic brain injury, chronic mental illness, 24 hour care need behavior.

Connecticut

9723 Hamilton Rehabilitation and Healthcare Cen ter
50 Palmer Street
Norwich, CT 06360
860-889-8358
FAX: 860-889-0395

Jim Christofori, Administrator

Offers the following rehabilitation services: Sub-Acute, Occupational Therapy, Speech Therapy, Physical Therapy.

9724 Hospital For Special Care
2150 Corbin Avenue
New Britain, CT 06053
860-223-2761
FAX: 860-832-6236
e-mail: info@hfsc.org

9725 Masonic Healthcare Center
22 Masonic Avenue
Wallingford, CT 06492
203-679-5900
800-982-3919
FAX: 203-679-6427

9726 Stamford Hospital
30 Shelburne Road
Stamford, CT 06902
203-325-7000
FAX: 203-325-7905

9727 Windsor Rehabilitation and Healthcare Cent er
581 Poquonock Avenue
Windsor, CT 06095
860-688-7211
FAX: 860-688-6715

Laurie Tillestie, Director
Melissa Romano, Admissions

Offers the following rehabilitation services: Physical Therapy, Occupational Therapy, Speech Therapy, Sub-Acute Rehabilitation

Delaware

9728 Arbors at New Castle Subacute and Rehab Ce nter
32 Buena Vista Drive
New Castle, DE 19720
302-328-2580
FAX: 302-328-2036

Dan Deitzel, Administrator

Offers the following rehabilitation services: Sub-Acute Rehab, Occupational Therapy, Physical Therapy, Speech Therapy.

Florida

9729 Boca Raton Rehabilitation Center
755 Meadows Road
Boca Raton, FL 33486
561-391-5200
FAX: 561-391-0685

Mark Rayner, Administrator
Offers the following rehabilitation services: Occupational Therapy, Speech Therapy, Physical Therapy, Sub-Acute Rehabilitation

9730 Evergreen Woods Health and Rehabilitation Center
7045 Evergreen Woods Trail
Spring Hill, FL 34608
352-596-8371
FAX: 352-596-8032

Richard Brady, Administrator
Offers the following rehabilitation services: Sub-Acute rehabilitation, Occupational therapy, Speech pathology therapy, Physical therapy.

9731 Healthcare and Rehabilitation Center of Sanford
950 Mellonville Avenue
Sanford, FL 32771
407-322-8566
FAX: 407-322-0121

Mark Niemeyek, Administrator
Rexine Fernandez, Director of Admissions
Offers the following rehabilitation services: Sub-Acute rehab, Stroke rehab, Cardiac rehab, Orthopedic rehab, Occupational therapy, Speech therapy, Physical therapy.

9732 Highland Pines Rehabilitation Center
1111 S Highland Avenue
Clearwater, FL 33756
727-446-0581
FAX: 727-442-9425

Dennis Miller, Administrator
Offers the following rehabilitation services: Sub-Acute rehabilitation, Occupational Therapy, Speech Therapy, Physical Therapy.

9733 Jupiter Medical Center-Pavilion
1210 S Old Dixie Highway
Jupiter, FL 33458
561-744-4444
FAX: 561-743-5042

Jay Mikosch, Administrator
Offers the following rehabilitation services: Sub-Acute Rehabilitation, Occupational Therapy, Speech Therapy, Physical Therapy.

9734 Kindred Rehab
401 E Sample Road
Pompano Beach, FL 33064
954-941-4100
FAX: 954-941-4233

Scott Lipman, Administrator
Offers the following rehabilitation services: Sub-Acute rehabilitation, Physical Therapy, Occupational Therapy, Speech Therapy, Respiratory Therapy.

9735 Oaks at Avon Nursing and Rehabilitation Ce nter
1010 US 27 N
Avon Park, FL 33825
863-453-5200
FAX: 863-453-5308

Robert Seymour, Administrator
Offers the following rehabilitation services: Sub-Acute rehabilitation, Occupational Therapy, Speech Therapy, Physical Therapy.

9736 Pompano Rehabilitation and Nursing Center
51 W Sample Road
Pompano Beach, FL 33064
954-942-5530
FAX: 954-942-0941

Offers the following rehabilitation services: Sub-Acute Rehabilitation, Physical Therapy, Occupational Therapy, Speech Therapy

9737 Rehabilitation Center of the Palm Beaches
301 Northpoint Parkway
W Palm Beach, FL 33407
561-712-1717
FAX: 561-712-1118

Anna Fortune, Administrator
Offers the following rehabilitation services: Sub-Acute Rehabilitation, Physical Therapy, Occupational Therapy, Speech Therapy

9738 Rehabilitation and Healthcare Center Of Ca pe Coral
2629 Del Prado Boulevard
Cape Coral, FL 33904
239-574-4434
FAX: 239-574-6968

9739 Rehabilitation and Healthcare Center of Ta mpa
4411 N Habana Avenue
Tampa, FL 33614
813-872-2771
FAX: 813-871-2831

Kate Hawk, Administrator
Offers the following rehabilitation services: Sub-Acute Rehabilitation, Physical Therapy, Occupational Therapy, Speech Therapy, Respiratory Therapy.

9740 Shands Rehab Hospital
8900 NW 39th Avenue
Gainesville, FL 32606
352-338-0091
FAX: 352-265-5430
http://shands.org/find/service/rehab/

Marina Cecchini, Director
Linda Brown, Director Marketing
Offers the following rehabilitation services: Sub-acute rehabilitation, traumatic brain injury, spinal cord injury, stroke, degenerative neurological conditions, amputations, burns, organ transplantation.

9741 St. Anthony's Hospital
1200 Seventh Avenue N
St. Petersburg, FL
727-825-1100
www.stanthonys.com

Ian Payne, Director
Offers the following rehabilitation services: Sub-Acute rehabilitation, Occupational Therapy, Speech/Language Pathology services, Physical Therapy.

9742 Winkler Court
3250 Winkler Avenue Extension
Fort Myers, FL 33916
239-939-4993
FAX: 239-939-1743

Rachel Rudd, Administrator
Offers the following rehabilitation services: Sub-Acute Rehabilitation, Physical Therapy, Speech Therapy, Occupational Therapy.

9743 **Winter Park Memorial Hospital**
200 N Lakemount Avenue
Winter Park, FL 32792
407-646-7000
FAX: 407-646-7639
e-mail: healthcare@winterparkhospital.com
www.winterparkhospital.com

Terry Barter, Director Rehabilitation

Offers the following rehabilitation services: Sub-Acute Rehabilitation, Occupational Therapy, Speech Pathology, Physical Therapy.

Georgia

9744 **Athena Rehab of Clayton**
2055 Rex Road
Lake City, GA 30260
404-361-1028
FAX: 404-363-6366

Carol Beavers, Administrator

Offers the following rehabilitation services: Sub-Acute rehabilitation, Occupational therapy, Speech therapy, Physical therapy, Restorative care.

9745 **Lafayette Nursing and Rehabilitation Cente r**
110 Brandywine Boulevard
Fayetteville, GA 30214
770-461-2928
FAX: 770-461-8507

Offers the following rehabilitation services: Sub-Acute rehabilitation, Physical Therapy, Occupational Therapy, Speech Therapy.

9746 **Savannah Rehabilitation and Nursing Center**
815 E 63rd Street
Savannah, GA 31405
912-352-8615
FAX: 912-355-4642

Melanie McCain, Administrator

Offers the following rehabilitation services: Sub-Acute rehabilitation, Physical Therapy, Occupational Therapy, Speech Therapy

9747 **Specialty Hospital**
Floyd Medical Center Fourth Floor
PO Box 233
Rome, GA 30161
706-802-2000
FAX: 706-802-2123

Jon Dixon, CEO

Offers the following rehabilitation services: Sub-Acute rehabilitation, Physical Therapy, Occupational Therapy, Speech Therapy.

9748 **Walton Rehabilitation Hospital**
1355 Independence Drive
Augusta, GA 30901
706-823-8511
866-492-5866
FAX: 706-724-5752
e-mail: postmaster@wrh.org
www.wrh.org

Dennis Skelley, President
Frank Lewis, Chief Operating Officer
Mike Harrell, CFO

Has Centers of Excellence in Stroke Brain Injury, Complex Orthopedics, Spinal Cord Injury and Pain Management. 58-bed nonprofit facility.

9749 **Warner Robins Rehabilitation and Nursing C enter**
1601 Elberta Road
Warner Robins, GA 91093
478-922-2241
FAX: 478-328-1984

Bill Sampson, Administrator

Offers the following rehabilitation services: Sub-Acute rehabilitation, Physical Therapy, Occupational Therapy, Speech Therapy.

Hawaii

9750 **Aloha Nursing and Rehab Center**
45-545 Kamehameha Highway
Kaneohe, HI 96744
808-247-2220
FAX: 808-235-3676

Idaho

9751 **Eastern Idaho Regional Medical Center**
3100 Channing Way
Idaho Falls, ID 83404
208-529-6111
FAX: 208-529-7021

9752 **Emmett Rehabilitation and Healthcare**
714 N Butte
Emmett, ID 83617
208-365-4425
FAX: 208-365-6989

Joan Buck, Administrator

Offers the following rehabilitation services: Sub-acute rehab, physical therapy, occupational therapy, speech therapy.

9753 **Hillcrest Rehabilitation and Care Center**
1001 S Hilton Street
Boise, ID 83705
208-345-4464
FAX: 208-345-2998

Phil Herink, Administrator

Offers the following rehabilitation services: Sub-acute rehabilitation, occupational therapy, speech therapy, physical therapy.

9754 **Lewiston Rehabilitation and Care Center**
3315 8th Street
Lewiston, ID 83501
208-743-9543
FAX: 208-743-3945

Offers the following rehabilitation services: Sub-acute rehabilitation, physical therapy, occupational therapy, speech therapy.

9755 **Mountain Valley Care and Rehabilitation Ce nter**
601 W Cameron Avenue
PO Box 689
Kellogg, ID 83837
208-784-1283
FAX: 208-784-0151

Illinois

9756 Chevy Chase Nursing and Rehabilitation Cen ter
3400 S Indiana Avenue
Chicago, IL 60616 **312-842-5000**
FAX: 312-842-3790

Barbara Casey, Administrator
Offers the following rehabilitation services: Sub-acute rehabilitation, physical therapy, occupational therapy, speech therapy.

9757 Glenview Terrace Nursing Center
1511 Greenwood Road
Glenview, IL 60025 **847-729-9090**
FAX: 847-729-9135

9758 Halsted Terrace Nursing Center
10935 S Halsted Street
Chicago, IL 60628 **773-928-2000**
FAX: 773-928-9154

Joleynn Johnson, Administrator
Offers the following rehabilitation services: Sub-acute rehabilitation, physical therapy, occupational therapy, speech therapy, cardiac rehabilitation.

9759 Harmony Nursing and Rehabilitation Center
3919 W Foster Avenue
Chicago, IL 60625 **773-588-9500**
FAX: 773-588-9533

9760 Imperial
1366 Fullerton Avenue
Chicago, IL 60614 **773-248-9300**
FAX: 773-935-0036

David Hartman, Administrator
Offers the following rehabilitation services: Sub-acute rehabilitation, physical therapy, occupational therapy, speech therapy.

9761 Jackson Square Nursing and Rehabilitation Center
5130 W Jackson Boulevard
Chicago, IL 60644 **773-921-8000**
FAX: 773-928-3980

Wayne Hanik, Administrator
Offers the following rehabilitation services: Sub-acute rehabilitation, physical therapy, occupational therapy, speech therapy.

9762 Renaissance at 87th Street
2940 W 87th Street
Chicago, IL 60652 **773-434-8787**
FAX: 773-434-8717

Tom Smith, Administrator
Offers the following rehabilitation services: Sub-acute rehabilitation, occupational therapy, physical therapy, speech therapy.

9763 Renaissance at Hillside
4600 N Frontage Road
Hillside, IL 06162 **708-544-9933**
FAX: 708-544-9966

Colleen Kamin, Administrator
Offers the following rehabilitation services: Sub-acute rehabilitation, physical therapy, occupational therapy, speech therapy.

9764 Renaissance at Midway
4437 S Cicero Avenue
Chicago, IL 60632 **773-884-0484**
FAX: 773-884-0485

Robin Harris, VP of Marketing
Debra Kroner, Director of Admissions

9765 Renaissance at South Shore
2425 E 71st Street
Chicago, IL 60649 **773-721-5000**
FAX: 773-721-6850

David Schecter, Administrator
Offers the following rehabilitation services: Sub-acute rehabilitation, physical therapy, occupational therapy, speech therapy.

9766 Schwab Rehabilitation Hospital
1401 S California Boulevard
Chicago, IL 60608 **773-522-2010**
www.sinai.org/rehabilitation/

Suzan Rayner MD, Medical Director
Treats medically stable patients who require nursing and medical care that cannot be supplied at home, in an outpatient facility or in a nursing home. Treats stroke patients, amputees, individuals with brain injuries, burns, diabets and spinal cord injuries.

Indiana

9767 Angel River Health and Rehabilitation
5233 Rosebud Lane
Newburgh, IN 47630 **812-473-4761**
FAX: 812-473-5190

Kay Tongleton, Administrator
Offers the following rehabilitation services: Sub-acute rehabilitation, speech therapy, occupational therapy, physical therapy.

9768 Chalet Village Health and Rehabilitation C enter
1065 Parkway Street
Berne, IN 46711 **260-589-2127**
FAX: 260-589-3521

Steven Schaaf, Administrator
Offers the following rehabilitation services: Sub-acute rehabilitation, physical therapy, occupational therapy, speech therapy, respiratory therapy.

9769 Columbus Health and Rehabilitation Center
2100 Midway Street
Columbus, IN 47201 **812-372-8447**
FAX: 812-375-5117

9770 Harrison Health and Rehabilitation Centre
150 Beechmont Drive
Corydon, IN 47112 **812-738-0550**
FAX: 812-738-6273

Inez Voyles, Administrator
Offers the following rehabilitation services: Sub-Acute rehabilitation, speech therapy, physical therapy, occupational therapy.

9771 **Indian Creek Health and Rehabilitation Center**
240 Beechmont Drive
Corydon, IN 47112 **812-738-8127**
877-380-7211
FAX: 812-738-2917
e-mail: sherry.leclair@kindredhealthcare.com
www.indiancreekhealthcare.com

Marianne Keller ACSW, Administrator
Sherry LeClair, Admissions Director

140 bed facility offering the following rehabilitation services: Sub-Acute rehabilitation, Physical therapy, Occupational Therapy, Speech Therapy, pain management, Wound rehabilitation. Short and long term skilled nursing care certified for Medicare, Medicaid, Private Pay and Private Insurance. Hospice and respite care rated #1 in clinical care in southern Indiana district for 2002.

9772 **Meadowvale Health and Rehabilitation Cente r**
1529 W Lancaster Street
Bluffton, IN 46714 **260-824-4320**
FAX: 260-824-4689

Vicki Shepherd, Administrator

Offers the following rehabilitation services: Sub-acute rehabilitation, physical therapy, occupational therapy, speech therapy.

9773 **Muncie Health Care and Rehabilitation**
4301 N Walnut Street
Muncie, IN 47305 **765-282-0053**
FAX: 765-282-3290

Douglas Roberts, Administrator

Offers the following rehabilitation services: Sub-Acute rehabilitation, physical therapy, occupational therapy, speech therapy.

9774 **Rehabilitation Hospital of Indiana**
4141 Shore Drive
Indianapolis, IN 46254 **317-329-2000**
FAX: 317-329-2104
www.rhin.com

Denny Armington, Chief Executive Officer
Joe Kubala, Chief Financial Officer
Nancy Stover, Director of Operations

Offers the following rehabilitation services: Sub-acute rehabilitation, brain injury, spinal cord injury programs.

9775 **Sellersburg Health and Rehabilitation Cent re**
7823 Old State Road 60
Sellersburg, IN 47172 **812-246-4272**
FAX: 812-246-8160

9776 **Westpark Rehabilitation Center**
25 S Boehne Camp Road
Evansville, IN 47712 **812-423-7468**
FAX: 812-423-7568

Raymond Bell, Administrator

Offers the following rehabilitation services: Sub-acute rehabilitation, occupational therapy, physical therapy, speech therapy, respiratory therapy.

9777 **Westview Nursing and Rehabilitation Center**
1510 Clinic Drive
Bedford, IN 47421 **812-279-4494**
FAX: 812-275-8313

Sandi Harpe

Offers the following rehabilitation services: Sub-acute rehabilitation, physical therapy, occupational therapy, speech therapy.

9778 **Windsor Estates Health and Rehab Center**
429 W Lincoln Road
Kokomo, IN 46902 **765-453-5600**
FAX: 765-455-0110

Iowa

9779 **Madison County Rehab Services**
300 Hutchings
Second Floor
Winterset, IA 50273 **515-462-2373**
FAX: 515-462-5108

Marcia Jones, Utilization Review Nurse

Offers the following rehabilitation services: Sub-acute rehabilitation, occupational therapy, physical therapy, speech therapy, home health rehab, wellness programs.

9780 **Mercy Subacute Care**
300 Laurel Street
Des Moines, IA 50314 **515-247-4400**
FAX: 515-643-8871

Bonnie McCoy, Administrator
Pam Nelson, Intake Coordinator

Offers the following rehabilitation services: Sub-acute rehabilitation, physical therapy, speech therapy, occupational therapy.

Kentucky

9781 **Danville Centre for Health and Rehabilitat ion**
642 N 3rd Street
Danville, KY 40422 **859-236-3972**
FAX: 859-236-0033

Lisa White, Administrator

Offers the following rehabilitation services: Sub-acute rehabilitation, physical therapy, occupational therapy, speech therapy.

9782 **Lexington Center for Health and Rehabilita tion**
353 Waller Avenue
Lexington, KY 40504 **859-252-3558**
FAX: 859-233-0192

Susan Middleton, Administrator

Offers the following rehabilitation services: Sub-acute rehabilitation, speech therapy, occupational therapy, physical therapy.

9783 **Paducah Centre For Health and Rehabilitati on**
501 N 3rd Street
Paducah, KY 42002 **270-444-9661**
FAX: 270-443-9407

9784 **Pathways Brain Injury Program**
4200 Brown's Lane
Louisville, KY 40220 **502-459-8900**
FAX: 502-459-5026

Pam Pearson, Program Director

Offers the following rehabilitation services: Sub-acute rehabilitation, speech therapy, occupational therapy, physical therapy, recreational therapy.

9785 **Winchester Centre For Health and Rehabilit ation**

200 Glenway Road
Winchester, KY 40391 859-744-1800
FAX: 859-744-0285

Robert Hollon, Administrator

Offers the following rehabilitation services: Sub-acute rehabilitation, speech therapy, physical therapy, occupational therapy.

Louisiana

9786 **Guest House of Slidell Sub-Acute and Rehab Center**

4051 S Robert Boulevard
Slidell, LA 70458 985-643-5630
800-303-9872
FAX: 985-649-6065
e-mail: jburch@ghslidell.com

Jeff Burch, Administrator

116 bed healthcare center offering the following subacute services within the skilled nursing setting: physical, occupational, and speech therapies, infusion therapy, respiratory care, wound care, neurological rehabilitation, cardiac reconditioning, pain management, post surgical recovery, orthopedic rehabilitation.

9787 **Irving Place Rehabilitation and Nursing Ce nter**

1736 Irving Place
Shreveport, LA 71101 318-221-1983
FAX: 318-222-2095

Maine

9788 **Augusta Rehabilitation Center**

187 Eastern Avenue
Augusta, ME 04330 207-622-3121
FAX: 207-623-7666

9789 **Brentwood Rehabilitation and Nursing Cente r**

122 Portland Street
Yarmouth, ME 04096 207-846-9021
FAX: 207-846-1479

9790 **Den-Mar Rehabilitation and Nursing Center**

44 S Street
Rockport, MA 01966 978-546-6311

9791 **Eastside Rehabilitation and Living Center**

516 Mount Hope Avenue
Bangor, ME 04401 207-947-6131
FAX: 207-942-0884

9792 **Kennebunk Nursing and Rehabilitation Cente r**

158 Ross Road
Kennebunk, ME 04043 207-985-7141
FAX: 207-985-1946

9793 **Norway Rehabilitation and Living Center**

29 Marion Avenue
Norway, ME 04268 207-743-7075
FAX: 207-743-9269

9794 **Shore Village Rehabilitation and Nursing C enter**

201 Camden Street
Rockland, ME 04841 207-596-6423
FAX: 207-596-7751

Maryland

9795 **Greater Baltimore Medical Center**

6701 N Charles Street
Baltimore, MD 21204 443-849-2000
FAX: 443-849-3024

Massachusetts

9796 **Bolton Manor Nursing Home**

400 Bolton Street
Marlborough, MA 01752 508-481-6123
FAX: 508-481-6130

9797 **Brigham Manor Nursing and Rehabilitation C enter**

77 High Street
Newburyport, MA 01950 978-462-4221
FAX: 978-463-3297

9798 **Country Gardens Skilled Nursing and Rehabilitation Center**

2045 Grand Army Highway
Swansea, MA 02777 508-379-9700
FAX: 508-379-0723
www.countrygardensnursing.com

, Social Worker

9799 **Country Manor Rehabilitation and Nursing C enter**

180 Low Street
Newburyport, MA 01950 978-465-5361
FAX: 978-463-9366

9800 **Franklin Skilled Nursing and Rehabilitation Center**

130 Chestnut Street
Franklin, MA 02038 508-528-4600
FAX: 508-528-7976

9801 **Great Barrington Rehabilitation and Nursing Center**

148 Maple Avenue
Great Barrington, MA 01230 413-528-3320
FAX: 413-528-2302

9802 **Ledgewood Rehabilitation and Skilled Nursi ng Center**

87 Herrick Street
Beverly, MA 01915 978-921-1392
FAX: 978-927-8627

9803 **Leo P La Chance Center for Rehabilitation and Nursing**

59 Eastwood Circle
Gardner, MA 01440 978-632-8776
FAX: 978-632-5048

9804 **Oakwood Rehabilitation and Nursing Center**

11 Pontiac Avenue
Webster, MA 01570 508-943-3889
FAX: 508-949-6125

9805 **Walden Rehabilitation and Nursing Center**

785 Main Street
Concord, MA 01742 978-369-6889
FAX: 978-369-8392

Michigan

9806 **Boulder Park Terrace**
14676 W Upright Street
Charlevoix, MI 49720
231-547-1005
FAX: 231-547-1039

Minnesota

9807 **Park Health And Rehabilitation Center**
4415 W 36 1/2 Street
St. Louis Park, MN 55416
952-927-9717
FAX: 952-927-7687

Missouri

9808 **Barnes-Jewish Hospital Washington University Medical Center**
One Barnes-Jewish Hospital Plaza
St Louis, MO 63110
314-747-3000
FAX: 314-286-0305

Montana

9809 **Parkview Acres Care and Rehabilitation Cen ter**
200 Oregon Street
Dillon, MT 59725
406-683-5105
FAX: 406-683-6388

Nebraska

9810 **Homestead Healthcare and Rehabilitation Ce nter**
4735 S 54th Street
Lincoln, NE 68516
402-488-0977
FAX: 402-488-4507

9811 **Madonna Rehabilitation Hospital**
5401 South Street
Lincoln, NE 68506
402-489-7102
FAX: 402-486-8285
www.madonna.org

Marsha Lommel, President/CEO

Patients who need only one or two types of therapy for a specific condition are served in the subacute program. Patients who have a diagnosis suggesting a positive course of recovery are typical for the subacute level of care.

9812 **Mary Lanning Memorial Hospital**
715 N St. Joseph Avenue
Hastings, NE 68901
402-463-4521
FAX: 402-461-5321
e-mail: tanderson@mlmh.org
www.mlmh.org

Nevada

9813 **Las Vegas Healthcare and Rehabilitation Ce nter**
2832 Maryland Parkway
Las Vegas, NV 89109
702-735-5848
FAX: 702-735-6218

New Hampshire

9814 **Dover Rehabilitation and Living Center**
307 Plaza Drive
Dover, NH 03820
603-742-2676
FAX: 603-749-5375

9815 **Northeast Rehab Clinic**
70 Butler Street
Salem, NH 03079
603-893-2900
FAX: 603-893-1628
www.northeastrehab.com

Subacute rehabilitation at NRH was designed for people who have experienced an acutely disabling orthopedic, medical, or neurologic condition but who either do not require or are unable to participate in a full acute inpatient program. Impairment groups pertinent to this level of care include brain injury, spinal cord injury (traumatic/non-traumatic), stroke, orthopedic injury, amputation, and neurologic disorder.

New Jersey

9816 **Atlantic Coast Rehabilitation & Healthcare Center**
485 River Avenue
Lakewood, NJ 08701
732-364-7100
FAX: 732-364-2442
e-mail: info@atlanticcoastrehab.com
www.atlanticcoastrehab.com

Offers the following rehabilitation services: Sub-acute rehab, physical therapy, occupational therapy, speech therapy.

9817 **Crestwood Nursing and Rehabilitation Cente r**
101 Whippany Road
Whippany, NJ 07981
973-887-0311
FAX: 973-887-8355

9818 **Lakeview Subacute Care Center**
130 Terhune Drive
Wayne, NJ 07470
973-616-5802
FAX: 973-839-2729
state.nj.us/cgi-bin/health/ltc/reportcard.pl

Susan R Ahlers, Case Manager

Offers physical therapy, occupational therapy, speech therapy, recreational therapy, respiratory therapy, aqua therapy. 68-bed subacute unit.

9819 **Merwick Rehabilitation and Sub-Acute Care**
79 Bayard Lane
Princeton, NJ 08540
609-497-3000
FAX: 609-497-3024
www.mcp.org

Kathy Ales, Medical Director

76-bed skilled nursing and residential center as well as a separate 17-bed comprehensive rehabilitation center. Offers rehabilitation, physiatry, occupational therapy, respite care, speech/hearing therapy, sub-acute care.

9820 **Seacrest Village Nursing Center**
1001 Center Street
Little Egg Harbor, NJ 08087 609-296-9292
FAX: 609-296-0508
e-mail: info@seacrestvillagenj.com

9821 **St. Lawrence Rehabilitation Center**
2384 Lawrencville Road
Lawrenceville, NJ 08648 609-896-9500
FAX: 609-895-0242

9822 **Summit Ridge Center Genesis Eldercare**
20 Summit Street
W Orange, NJ 07052 973-736-2000
800-699-1520
FAX: 973-731-4582
www.ghv.com

Charlene Harn, Admissions/Marketing Director

Skilled nursing facility with a total of 152 beds. 40 bed sub-acute unit and 24 bed secure dementia unit. Able to care for a wide variety of rehab and medical cases from orthopedics to TPN and tracheostomies.

New York

9823 **Beth Abraham Health Services**
612 Allerton Avenue
Bronx, NY 10467 718-881-3000
888-238-4223
FAX: 718-519-4010
e-mail: info@bethabe.org
www.bethabe.org

Offers the following rehabilitation services: Sub-Acute rehabilitation, brain injury rehabilitation, pain management, post-operative recovery. Home visits and a network of community-based programs help patients and their families with a successful transition home.

9824 **Central Island Healthcare**
825 Old Country Road
Plainview, NY 11803 516-433-0600
FAX: 516-868-7251
www.centralislandhealthcare.net

9825 **Clove Lakes Health Care and Rehabilitation Center**
25 Fanning Street
Staten Island, NY 10314 718-289-7900
FAX: 718-761-8701

9826 **Dr. William O Benenson Rehabilitation Pavi lion**
36-17 Parsons Boulevard
Flushing, NY 11354 718-961-4300
FAX: 718-939-5032

9827 **Flushing Manor Nursing and Rehab**
35-15 Parsons Boulevard
Flushing, NY 11354 718-961-3500
FAX: 718-461-1784
e-mail: jenella.nh@flushingmanors.com
www.flushingmanors.com

Jerry Enella, Administrator

Skilled nursing facility and subacute rehabilitation.

9828 **Glengariff Health Care Center**
Dosoris Lane
Glen Cove, NY 11542 516-676-1100
FAX: 516-759-0267
www.glenhaven.org

Jean Campo, Director of Admissions

Licensed skilled nursing and subacute medical and rehabilitation facility.

9829 **Haym Salomon Home for Nursing and Rehab**
2340 Cropsey Avenue
Brooklyn, NY 11214 718-373-1700
FAX: 718-449-9028

9830 **Kings Harbor Multicare Center**
2000 E Gun Hill Road
Bronx, NY 10469 718-320-0400
FAX: 718-320-0557
e-mail: info@kingsharbor.com
www.kingsharbor.com

9831 **Northwoods of Cortland**
28 Kellog Road
Cortland, NY 13045 607-753-9631
FAX: 607-756-2968

9832 **Port Jefferson Health Care Facility**
Dark Hollow Road
Port Jefferson, NY 11777 631-473-5400
FAX: 631-474-5362
www.glenhaven.org

Anne Kohlmann, Director of Admissions
Kathy Peets, VP Corporate & External Affairs

Subacute medical and rehabilitative care and long term residential skilled nursing care.

9833 **Rehab Institute at Florence Nightingale He alth Center**
1760 Third Avenue
New York, NY 1009 212-410-8760
800-786-8968
FAX: 212-410-8792
e-mail: info@rehabinstitute.org

9834 **Schnurmacher Center for Rehabilitation and Nursing**
12 Tibbits Avenue
White Plains, NY 10606 914-287-7200
FAX: 914-428-1216
e-mail: knodiff@bethabe.org
www.bethabe.org

Karen Nodiff, Director Admissions
Diane McKillop, Director Nursing
Karen Kaplan Blick, Director Social Services

9835 **South Shore Healthcare**
275 W Merrick Road
Freeport, NY 11520 516-868-6097
FAX: 516-868-7251
www.southshorehealthcare.net

9836 **St. Camillus Health and Rehabilitation Cen ter**
813 Fay Road
Syracuse, NY 315-488-2951
FAX: 315-488-3255
www.st-camillus.org

North Carolina

9837 **Chapel Hill Rehabilitation and Healthcare Center**
1602 E Franklin Street
Chapel Hill, NC 27514
919-967-1418
FAX: 919-918-3811

9838 **Cypress Pointe Rehabilitation and Healthca re Center**
2006 S 16th Street
Wilmington, NC 28401
910-763-6271
FAX: 910-351-9803

9839 **Pettigrew Rehabilitation and Healthcare Ce nter**
1551 W Pettigrew Street
Durham, NC 27705
919-286-0751
FAX: 919-286-7065

9840 **Raleigh Rehabilitation and Healthcare Cent er**
616 Wade Avenue
Raleigh, NC 27605
919-828-6251
FAX: 919-828-3294

9841 **Rehabilitation and Healthcare Center of Al manace**
779 Woody Drive
Graham, NC 27253
336-228-8394
FAX: 336-228-8170

9842 **Rehabilitation and Healthcare Center of Mo nroe**
1212 Sunset Drive
Monroe, NC 28112
704-283-8548
FAX: 704-283-4664

9843 **Winston-Salem Rehabilitation and Healthcar e Center**
1900 W 1st Street
Winston Salem, NC 27104
336-724-2821
FAX: 336-725-8314

Ohio

9844 **Arbors East Subacute and Rehabilitation Ce nter**
5500 E Broad Street
Columbus, OH 43213
614-575-9003
FAX: 614-575-9101

9845 **Arbors at Canton Subacute And Rehabilitati on Center**
2714 13th Street NW
Canton, OH 44708
330-456-2842
FAX: 330-456-5343

9846 **Arbors at Dayton**
320 Albany Street
Dayton, OH 45408
937-496-6200
FAX: 937-496-1990

9847 **Arbors at Marietta**
400 Seventh Street
Marietta, OH 45750
740-373-3597
FAX: 740-373-3597

9848 **Arbors at Milford**
5900 Meadowcreek Drive
Milford, OH 45150
513-248-1655
FAX: 513-248-0466

9849 **Arbors at Sylvania**
7120 Port Sylvania Drive
Toledo, OH 43617
419-841-2200
FAX: 419-841-2822

9850 **Arbors at Toledo Subacute and Rehab Centre**
2920 Cherry Street
Toledo, OH 43608
419-242-7458
FAX: 419-242-6514

9851 **Bridgepark Center for Rehabilitation and N ursing Services**
145 Olive Street
Akron, OH 44310
330-762-0901
FAX: 330-762-0905

9852 **Broadview Multi-Care Center**
5520 Broadview Road
Parma, OH 44134
216-749-4010
FAX: 440-748-6860

9853 **Caprice Care Center**
9184 Market Street
North Lima, OH 44452
330-965-9200
FAX: 330-726-6097

9854 **Cleveland Clinic**
9500 Euclid Avenue
Cleveland, OH 44195
216-444-2200
800-223-2273
FAX: 216-444-7021

9855 **Columbus Rehabilitation And Subacute Insti tute**
44 S Souder Avenue
Columbus, OH 43222
614-228-5900
FAX: 614-228-3989

9856 **LakeMed Nursing and Rehabilitation Center**
70 Normandy Drive
Painesville, OH 44077
440-357-1311
FAX: 440-352-9977

9857 **Oregon Nursing And Rehabilitation Center**
904 Isaac Streets Drive
Oregon, OH 43616
419-691-2483
FAX: 419-697-5401

9858 **Sunset View Castle Nursing Homes**
434 N Washington Street
Millersburg, OH 44654
330-674-0015
FAX: 330-763-2215
e-mail: info@castlenursinghomes.com

Oregon

9859 **Care Center East Health & Specialty Care C enter**
11325 Ne Weidler Street
Portland, OR 97220
503-253-1181
FAX: 503-253-1871

9860 **Medford Rehabilitation and Healthcare Cent er**
625 Stevens Street
Medford, OR 97504
541-779-3551
FAX: 541-779-3658

Pennsylvania

9861 **Dresher Hill Health and Rehabilitation Cen ter**
1390 Camp Hill Road
Dresher, PA 19034 215-643-0600
FAX: 215-641-0628

9862 **Good Shepherd Home Long Term Care Facility**
601 St. John Street
Allentown, PA 18103 610-776-3199
FAX: 610-776-3143

9863 **Statesman Health and Rehabilitation Center**
2629 Trenton Road
Levittown, PA 19056 215-943-7777
FAX: 215-943-1240

9864 **UPMC Braddock**
Holland Avenue
Braddock, PA 15104 412-636-5000
FAX: 412-636-5398
braddock.upmc.com

Christine Phillips, Director

Offers the following rehabilitation services: Sub-acute rehabilitation, speech therapy, occupational therapy.

9865 **UPMC McKeesport**
1500 Fifth Avenue
McKeesport, PA 15132 412-664-2000
FAX: 412-664-2318
mckeesport.upmc.com

Offers 56 beds for patients who need skilled nursing care. Offers ongoing rehabilitation and educational programs to patients with cardiac, neurologic, and orthopaedic diagnosis.

9866 **UPMC Passavant**
9100 Babcock Boulevard
Pittsburg, PA 15237 412-367-6541

e-mail: tomazichcw@ph.upmc.edu
www.upmc.edu/Passavant/

Cynthia Tomazich, Dir Inpatient Physical Therapy

Patients who have had an acute illness, injury, or exacerbation of a disease and no longer need the intensity of services in the acute care setting, but still require some complex medical care or supervision and rehabilitation services, may be appropriate to be transferred into the Subacute Unit.

Rhode Island

9867 **Health Havens Nursing and Rehabilitation C enter**
100 Wampanoag Trail
E Providence, RI 02915 401-438-4275
FAX: 401-438-8093

9868 **Oak Hill Nursing and Rehabilitation Center**
544 Pleasant Street
Pawtucket, RI 02860 401-725-8888
FAX: 401-727-6731
e-mail: scott_sanborn@kindredhealthcare.com
www.oakhillnursingandrehabilitationcenter.com

Scott Sanborn, Administrator
Heidi Capela, Director of Nursing
Amybeth Almeida, Director of Admissions

Subacute unit with Program Specific Medical Director. Complex pain and wound management. Long term beds and dedicated Alzheimers Unit.

9869 **Southern New England Rehab Center**
21 Peace Street
Providence, RI 02907 401-456-4500
FAX: 401-456-4019

South Carolina

9870 **Tuomey Healthcare System**
129 N Washington Street
Sumter, SC 29150 803-778-9000
FAX: 803-778-9551

Tennessee

9871 **Camden Healthcare and Rehabilitation Cente r**
197 Hospital Drive
Camden, TN 38320 731-584-3500
FAX: 731-584-2753

9872 **Centennial Medical Center Tri Star Health System**
2300 Patterson Street
Nashville, TN 37203 615-342-1000
FAX: 615-342-1045

9873 **Cordova Rehabilitation and Nursing Center**
955 Germantown Road
Cordova, TN 38018 901-754-1393
FAX: 901-754-3332

9874 **Erlanger Medical Center Baronness Campus**
975 E Third Street
Chattanooga, TN 37403 423-778-7000
FAX: 423-778-7615

9875 **Horizon Medical Center**
111 Highway 70 E
Dickson, TN 37055 615-446-0446
FAX: 615-441-9695
www.horizonmedctr.com

9876 **Huntington Health and Rehabilitation Cente r**
635 High Street
Huntington, TN 38344 731-986-8943
FAX: 731-986-3188

9877 **Madison Healthcare and Rehabilitation Cent er**
431 Larkin Springs Road
Madison, TN 37115 615-865-8520
FAX: 615-868-4455

9878 **Mariner Health of Nashville**
3939 Hillsboro Circle
Nashville, TN 37215 615-297-2100
FAX: 615-463-1990

9879 **Pine Meadows Healthcare and Rehabilitation Center**
700 Nuckolls Road
Bolivar, TN 38008 731-658-4707
FAX: 731-658-4769

9880 **Primacy Healthcare and Rehabilitation Cent er**
6025 Primacy Parkway
Memphis, TN 38119
901-767-1040
FAX: 901-685-7362

9881 **Ripley Healthcare and Rehabilitation Cente r**
118 Halliburton Road
Ripley, TN 38063
731-635-5180
FAX: 731-635-0663

9882 **Shelby Pines Rehabilitation and Healthcare Center**
3909 Covington Pike
Memphis, TN 38135
901-377-1011
FAX: 901-377-0032

9883 **Siskin Hospital Subacute Rehabilitation Program**
1 Siskin Plaza
Chattanooga, TN 37403
423-634-1631
FAX: 423-634-4538
www.siskinrehab.org

Texas

9884 **North Hills Hospital**
4401 Booth Calloway Road
North Richland Hills, TX 76180
817-255-1000
FAX: 817-255-1967
www.northhillshospital.com

9885 **Valley Regional Medical Center**
100 A E Alton Gloor Boulevard
Brownsville, TX 78526
956-350-7000
FAX: 956-350-7999
www.valleyregionalmedicalcenter.com

Utah

9886 **Crosslands Rehabilitation and Healthcare C enter**
575 E 11000 S
Sandy, UT 84070
801-571-7600
FAX: 801-571-4875

9887 **Federal Heights Rehabilitation and Nursing Center**
41 S Ninth Street
Salt Lake City, UT 84102
801-532-3539
FAX: 801-553-0314

9888 **St. George Care and Rehabilitation Center**
1032 E 100th S
Saint George, UT 84770
435-628-0488
FAX: 435-628-7362

9889 **St. Mark's Hospital**
1200 E 3900 S
Salt Lake City, UT 84124
801-268-7111
FAX: 801-270-3353
www.stmarkshospital.com

9890 **Wasatch Valley Rehabilitation**
2200 E 3300 S
Salt Lake City, UT 84109
801-486-2096
FAX: 801-484-3443

Virginia

9891 **Nansemond Pointe Rehabilitation and Health care Center**
200 Constance Road
Suffolk, VA 43434
757-539-8744
FAX: 757-539-6128

9892 **Rehabilitation and Research Center Virginia Commonwealth University**
PO Box 980661
Richmond, VA 23298
804-828-2156
FAX: 804-828-5074
e-mail: beagle@hsc.vcu.edu
www.rrc.pmr.vcu.edu

9893 **Warren Memorial Hospital**
1000 Shenandoah Avenue
Front Royal, VA 22630
540-636-0300
FAX: 540-636-0475

9894 **Winchester Rehabilitation Center**
333 W Cork Street
Winchester, VA 22601
540-536-5114
800-382-0772
FAX: 540-536-1122
www.valleyhealthlink.com

Dena Kent, Administrator

Offers the following rehabilitation services: Sub-Acute inpatient rehabilitation, Speech therapy, Physical therapy, Occupational therapy, Disability evaluations. 30-bed inpatient center.

Washington

9895 **Aldercrest Health and Rehabilitation Center**
21400 72nd Avenue W
Edmonds, WA 98026
425-775-1961
FAX: 425-771-0116

9896 **Arden Rehabilitation and Healthcare Center**
16357 Aurora Avenue N
Seattle, WA 98133
206-542-3103
FAX: 206-542-4562

9897 **Bellingham Health Care and Rehabilitation Services**
1200 Birchwood Avenue
Bellingham, WA 98225
360-734-9295
FAX: 360-671-1583

9898 **Bremerton Convalescent and Rehabilitation Center**
2701 Clare Avenue
Bremerton, WA 98310
360-377-3951
FAX: 360-377-9756

9899 **Edmonds Rehabilitation and Healthcare Cent er**
21008 76th Avenue W
Edmonds, WA 98026
425-778-0107
FAX: 425-776-9532

9900 **Heritage Health and Rehabilitation Center**
3605 Y Street
Vancouver, WA 98663
360-693-5839
FAX: 360-693-5515

9901 **North Auburn Rehabilitation And Health Cen ter**
2830 I Street Ne
Auburn, WA 98002 253-833-1260
FAX: 253-833-3743

9902 **Northwoods Lodge**
2321 Schold Place NW
Silverdale, WA 98383 360-698-3930
FAX: 360-613-9520

9903 **Pacific Specialty and Rehabilitation Cente r**
1015 N Garrison Road
Vancouver, WA 98664 360-694-7501
FAX: 360-694-8148

9904 **Puget Sound Healthcare Center**
4001 Capitol Mall Drive SW
Olympia, WA 98502 360-754-9792
FAX: 360-754-2455

9905 **Vencor of Vancouver Healthcare and Rehabil itation Center**
400 E 33rd Street
Vancouver, WA 98663 360-696-2561
FAX: 360-750-0665

West Virginia

9906 **War Memorial Hospital**
1124 Fairfax Street
Berkeley Springs, WV 24511 301-258-1234
FAX: 304-258-2048
www.warmemorialhospital.com

Linda Carl, Nurse Manager

Offers physical therapy, occupational therapy, speech therapy, social services, and patient/family education for individuals who have experienced a recent physical disability due to disease, dysfunction, or general debilitation. Helps patients to maximize their abilities through activities of daily living, mobility, self-medication, and self-care and restore their ability to return to their previous lifestyle.

Wisconsin

9907 **Brain Injury Rehabilitation Center at Mequ on Care Center**
10911 N Port Washington Road
Mequon, WI 53092 262-241-2080
FAX: 262-241-2090

9908 **Cedar Spring Health and Rehabilitation Cen ter**
N27 W5707 Lincoln Boulevard
Cedarburg, WI 53012 262-376-7676
FAX: 262-376-7808

9909 **Clearview-Brain Injury Center**
199 Home Road
Juneau, WI 53039 920-386-3400
877-386-3400
FAX: 920-386-3800
www.dodgecountywi.com

9910 **Colonial Manor Medical and Rehabilitation Center**
1010 E Wausau Avenue
Wausau, WI 54403 715-842-2028
FAX: 715-845-5810

9911 **Eastview Medical and Rehabilitation Center**
729 Park Street
Antigo, WI 54409 715-623-2356
FAX: 715-623-6345

9912 **Family Heritage Medical and Rehabilitation Center**
130 Strawberry Lane
Wisconsin Rapids, WI 54494 715-424-1600
FAX: 715-424-4817

9913 **Hospitality Nursing and Rehabilitation Cen ter**
8633 32nd Avenue
Kenosha, WI 53142 262-694-8300
FAX: 262-694-3622

9914 **Kennedy Park Medical and Rehabilitation Ce nter**
6001 Alderson Street
Schofield, WI 54476 715-359-4257
FAX: 715-355-4867

9915 **Lakeside Nursing and Rehabilitation Center**
7490 156 Street
Chippewa Falls, WI 54729 715-723-9341
FAX: 715-723-3376

9916 **Middleton Village Nursing and Rehabilitati on Center**
6201 Elmwood Avenue
Middleton, WI 53562 608-831-8300
FAX: 608-831-9408

9917 **Mount Carmel Health and Rehabilitation Cen ter**
5700 W Layton Avenue
Milwaukee, WI 53220 414-281-7200
FAX: 414-281-7183

9918 **Mount Carmel Medical and Rehabilitation Center**
677 E State Street
Burlington, WI 53105 262-763-9531
FAX: 262-763-7579

9919 **North Ridge Medical and Rehabilitation Cen ter**
1445 N 7th Street
Manitowoc, WI 54220 920-682-0314
FAX: 920-682-0553

9920 **Oshkosh Medical and Rehabilitation Center**
1580 Bowen Street
Oshkosh, WI 84901 920-233-4011
FAX: 920-233-5177

9921 **San Luis Medical and Rehabilitation Center**
2305 San Luis Place
Green Bay, WI 54304 920-494-5231
FAX: 920-494-1958

Wyoming

9922 **Mountain Towers Healthcare and Rehabilitat ion Center**
3128 Boxelder Drive
Cheyenne, WY 82001 307-634-7901
FAX: 307-634-7910

9923 **South Central Wyoming Healthcare and Rehab ilitation**
542 16th Street
Rawlins, WY 82301 307-324-2759
FAX: 307-324-7579

9924 **Wind River Healthcare and Rehabilitation C enter**
1002 Forest Drive
Riverton, WY 82501 **307-856-9471**
FAX: 307-856-1757

AIDS

Aging

Alternative Therapies

Amputation

Amythrophic Lateral Sclerosis

Art Therapies

Arthritis

Asthma

Attention Deficit Disorder

Autism

Behavioral Disorders

Birth Defects

Brain Injuries

Cancer

Cerebral Palsy

Chronic Disabilities

Cleft Palate

Cognitive Disorders

Cystic Fibrosis

Dementia

Dental Issues

Depression

Developmental Disabilities

Diabetes

Down Syndrome

Dyslexia

Education & Counseling

Emergency Alert

Environmental Disoders

Epilepsy

Head & Neck Injuries

Hearing Impairments

Hemophilia

Human Interaction Disabilities

Immune Deficiencies

Incontinence

Language Disorders

Learning Disabilities

Lung Disorders

Mental Health Disorders

Mental Retardation

Multiple Disabilities

Multiple Sclerosis

Muscular Dystrophy

Neurological Impairments

Orthopedical Disabilities

Pain Management

Parkinson Disease

Pediatric Disorders

Phenylketonuria

Physical Disabilities

Polio

Prader-Willi Syndrome

Rare Disabilities

Respiratory Disorders

Severe Disabilites

Sexual Abuse & Related Conditions

Sjogren's Syndrome

Speech Disorders

Spina Bifida

Spinal Cord Disorders

Stroke

Tinnitus

Tourette Syndrome

Visual Impairments

A

B

C

D

E

F

G

H

I

J

K

L

M

N

O

P

Q

R

S

T

U

V

W

X

Y

Z

Alabama

Alaska

Arizona

Arkansas

California

Colorado

Connecticut

Delaware

District of Columbia

Florida

Georgia

Hawaii

Idaho

Illinois

Indiana

Iowa

Kansas

Kentucky

Louisiana

Maine

Maryland

Massachusetts

Michigan

Minnesota

Mississippi

Missouri

Montana

Nebraska

Nevada

New Hampshire

The Directory of Venture Capital Firms, 2003

This brand new Sixth Edition has been extensively updated and broadly expanded to offer direct access to over 2,800 Domestic and International Venture Capital Firms, including address, phone & fax numbers, e-mail addresses and web sites for both primary and branch locations. Entries include details on the firm's Mission Statement, Industry Group Preferences, Geographic Preferences, Average and Minimum Investments and Investment Criteria. You'll also find details that are available nowhere else, including the Firm's Portfolio Companies and extensive information on each of the firm's Managing Partners, such as Education, Professional Background and Directorships held, along with the Partner's E-mail Address. *The Directory of Venture Capital Firms* offers five important indexes: Geographic Index, Executive Name Index, Portfolio Company Index, Industry Preference Index and College & University Index. With its comprehensive coverage and detailed, extensive information on each company, *The Directory of Venture Capital Firms* is an important addition to any finance collection.

"The sheer number of listings, the descriptive information provided and the outstanding indexing make this directory a better value than its principal competitor, Pratt's Guide to Venture Capital Sources. Recommended for business collections in large public, academic and business libraries." –Choice

1,300 pages; Softcover ISBN 1-930956-77-0, $450.00 ◆ Online Database (includes a free copy of the directory) $889.00

Thomas Food and Beverage Market Place, 2002/03

Thomas Food and Beverage Market Place is bigger and better than ever with thousands of new companies, thousands of updates to existing companies and two revised and enhanced product category indexes. This comprehensive directory profiles over 18,000 Food & Beverage Manufacturers, 12,000 Equipment & Supply Companies, 2,200 Transportation & Warehouse Companies, 2,000 Brokers & Wholesalers, 8,000 Importers & Exporters, 900 Industry Resources and hundreds of Mail Order Catalogs. Listings include detailed Contact Information, Sales Volumes, Key Contacts, Brand & Product Information, Packaging Details and much more. *Thomas Food and Beverage Market Place* is available as a three-volume printed set, a subscription-based Online Database via the Internet, on CD-ROM, as well as mailing lists and a licensable database.

"An essential purchase for those in the food industry but will also be useful in public libraries where needed. Much of the information will be difficult and time consuming to locate without this handy three-volume ready-reference source." –ARBA

8,500 pages, 3 Volume Set; Softcover ISBN 1-930956-95-9, $495.00 ◆ CD-ROM ISBN 1-930956-33-9, $695.00 ◆ CD-ROM & 3 Volume Set Combo ISBN 1-930956-34-7, $895.00 ◆ Online Database $695.00 ◆ Online Database & 3 Volume Set Combo, $895.00

The Grey House Safety & Security Directory, 2003

The Grey House Safety & Security Directory is the most comprehensive reference tool and buyer's guide for the safety and security industry. Published continuously since 1943 as Best's Safety & Security Directory, Grey House acquired the title in 2002. Arranged by safety topic, each chapter begins with OSHA regulations for the topic, followed by Training Articles written by top professionals in the field and Self-Inspection Checklists. Next, each topic contains Buyer's Guide sections that feature related products and services. Topics include Administration, Insurance, Loss Control & Consulting, Protective Equipment & Apparel, Noise & Vibration, Facilities Monitoring & Maintenance, Employee Health Maintenance & Ergonomics, Retail Food Services, Machine Guards, Process Guidelines & Tool Handling, Ordinary Materials Handling, Hazardous Materials Handling, Workplace Preparation & Maintenance, Electrical Lighting & Safety, Fire & Rescue and Security. The Buyer's Guide sections are carefully indexed within each topic area to ensure that you can find the supplies needed to meet OSHA's regulations. Six important indexes make finding information and product manufacturers quick and easy: Geographical Index of Manufacturers and Distributors, Company Profile Index, Brand Name Index, Product Index, Index of Web Sites and Index of Advertisers. This comprehensive, up-to-date reference will provide every tool necessary to make sure a business is in compliance with OSHA regulations and locate the products and services needed to meet those regulations.

1,500 pages, 2 Volume Set; Softcover ISBN1-930956-71-1, $225.00

International Business and Trade Directories, 2003/04

Completely updated, the Third Edition of *International Business and Trade Directories* now contains more than 10,000 entries, over 2,000 more than the last edition, making this directory the most comprehensive resource of the worlds business and trade directories. Entries include content descriptions, price, publisher's name and address, web site and e-mail addresses, phone and fax numbers and editorial staff. Organized by industry group, and then by region, this resource puts over 10,000 industry-specific business and trade directories at the reader's fingertips. Three indexes are included for quick access to information: Geographic Index, Publisher Index and Title Index. Public, college and corporate libraries, as well as individuals and corporations seeking critical market information will want to add this directory to their marketing collection.

1,800 pages; Softcover ISBN 1-930956-63-0, $225.00 ◆ Online Database (includes a free copy of the directory) $450.00

To preview any of our Directories Risk-Free for 30 days, call (800) 562-2139 or fax to (518) 789-0556